Cover illustration

The picture on the cover shows the Robert Wood Johnson Medical School Fetal Surgery team in action, performing fetoscopic laser ablation for twin-to-twin transfusion syndrome at the Regional Perinatal Center, Robert Wood Johnson University Hospital.

Operative Obstetrics

Third Edition

Joseph J Apuzzio MD

Department of Obstetrics, Gynecology and Women's Health
UMDNJ–New Jersey Medical School
Newark, NJ, USA

Anthony M Vintzileos MD

Department of Obstetrics, Gynecology and Reproductive Sciences
UMDNJ–Robert Wood Johnson Medical School
New Brunswick, NJ, USA

Leslie Iffy MD

Department of Obstetrics, Gynecology and Women's Health
UMDNJ–New Jersey Medical School
Newark, NJ, USA

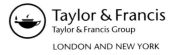

Taylor & Francis
Taylor & Francis Group

LONDON AND NEW YORK

©2006 Taylor & Francis, an imprint of the Taylor & Francis Group

First published in the United Kingdom in 2006
by Taylor & Francis, an imprint of the Taylor & Francis Group, 2 Park Square, Milton Park, Abingdon, Oxon OX14 4RN

Tel.: +44 (0)20 7017 6000
Fax.: +44 (0)20 7017 6699
E-mail: *info.medicine@tandf.co.uk*
Website: *www.tandf.co.uk/medicine*

All rights reserved. No part of this publication may be
reproduced, stored in a retrieval system, or transmitted,
in any form or by any means, electronic, mechanical,
photocopying, recording, or otherwise, without the
prior permission of the publisher or in accordance with
the provisions of the Copyright, Designs and Patents
Act 1988 or under the terms of any licence permitting
limited copying issued by the Copyright Licensing
Agency, 90 Tottenham Court Road, London W1P 0LP.

Although every effort has been made to ensure that all owners of
copyright material have been acknowledged in this publication,
we would be glad to acknowledge in subsequent reprints or
editions any omissions brought to our attention.

The Author has asserted his right under the Copyright, Designs and Patents
Act 1988 to be identified as the Author of this Work.

Although every effort has been made to ensure that drug doses and
other information are presented accurately in this publication, the
ultimate responsibility rests with the prescribing physician.
Neither the publishers nor the authors can be held responsible for errors or
for any consequences arising from the use of information contained
herein. For detailed prescribing information or instructions on the
use of any product or procedure discussed herein, please consult the
prescribing information or instructional material issued by the manufacturer.

A CIP record for this book is available from the British Library.

Library of Congress Cataloging-in-Publication Data
Data available on application

ISBN 1–84184–284–4
ISBN 978–1–84214–284–4

Distributed in North and South America by
Taylor & Francis
2000 NW Corporate Blvd
Boca Raton, FL 33431, USA
Within Continental USA
Tel: 800 272 7737; Fax: 800 374 3401
Outside Continental USA
Tel: 561 994 0555; Fax: 561 361 6018
E-mail: *orders@crcpress.com*

Distributed in the rest of the world by
Thomson Publishing Services
Cheriton House
North Way
Andover, Hampshire SP10 5BE, UK
Tel.: +44 (0)1264 332424
E-mail: salesorder.tandf@thomsonpublishingservices.co.uk

Composition by J&L Composition, Filey, North Yorkshire
Printed and bound in Spain by Grafos SA

WQ
400
O608
2006

Contents

63185241

Contributors

Abdulla Al-Khan, MD
Assistant Profesor
UMDNJ-New Jersey Medical School
Department of Obstetrics, Gynecology and Women's Health
Newark, NJ, USA

Jesus R Alvarez, MD
Fellow, Division of Maternal-Fetal Medicine
Department of Obstetrics and Gynecology
UMDNJ-New Jersey Medical School
Newark, NJ, USA

Joseph J Apuzzio, MD
Professor & Director Division Maternal Fetal Medicine
Department of Obstetrics, Gynecology and Women's Health
UMDNJ-New Jersey Medical School
Newark, NJ, USA

Michael S Baggish, MD
Chairman
Department of Obstetrics and Gynecology
Good Samaritan Hospital
Cincinnati, OH, USA

Asha G Bale, MD
Chief Division of Minimally Invasive Surgery and Bariatric Surgery
Assistant Professor of Surgery
Department of Surgery
UMDNJ-New Jersey Medical School
Newark, NJ, USA

Robert H Ball, MD
Associate Professor
Department of Obstetrics, Gynecology, and Reproductive Sciences
Fetal Treatment Center
University of California, San Francisco
San Francisco, CA, USA

György Bártfai, MD
Professor, Department of Obstetrics & Gynecology,
Szent-Györgyi Albert University
School of Medicine,
Szeged, Hungary

Jason Baxter, MD
Division of Maternal-Fetal Medicine
Department of Obstetrics and Gynecology
Jefferson Medical College of Thomas Jefferson University
Philadelphia, PA, USA

Michele Berghella, MD
Department of Obstetrics and Gynecology
Universitá degli studi 'L'Aquila'
L'Aquila, Italy

Vincenzo Berghella, MD
Associate Professor
Director, Division of Maternal-Fetal Medicine
Department of Obstetrics and Gynecology
Jefferson Medical College of Thomas Jefferson University
Philadelphia, PA, USA

Isaac Blickstein, MD
Department of Obstetrics and Gynecology
Kaplan Medical Center
Rehovot, Israel

Watson A Bowes Jr., MD
Emeritus Professor
Department of Obstetrics and Gynecology
University of North Carolina at Chapel Hill
Chapel Hill, NC, USA

David A Britt, PhD
Institute for Genetics
New York, NY, USA

Anthony Caggiano, MD
Clinical Associate Professor of Obstetrics & Gynecology
UMDNJ-New Jersey Medical School
Newark, NJ, USA

Howard JA Carp, MB BS FRCOG
Professor of Obstetrics and Gynecology
Sheba Medical Center
Tel Hashomer, Israel

Curtis L Cetrulo, MD
Professor of Obstetrics and Gynecology
Tufts University School of Medicine
Boston, MA, USA

Frank A Chervenak, MD
Professor
Director, Division of Maternal-Fetal Medicine
Department of Obstetrics and Gynecology
Weill Medical College of Cornell University,
Professor and Chair
New York, NY, USA

Doina Ciorica, MD RDMS
Institute for Genetics
New York, NY, USA

Timothy M Crombleholme, MD
Director of the Fetal Care Center of Cincinnati
Richard G & Geralyn Azizkham Chair in Pediatric Surgery
Division of Pediatric General, Thoracic and Fetal Surgery
Cincinnati Children's Hospital Medical Center
Professor of Surgery, Molecular and Developmental Biology,
and Obstetrics and Gynecology
University of Cincinnati College of Medicine
Cincinnati, OH, USA

David N Dhanraj, MD
Assistant Director
Residency Training, Department of Obstetrics and Gynecology
Good Samaritan Hospital
Cincinnati, Ohio, USA

Elaine K Diegmann, CNM ND
Professor of Midwifery
UMDNJ-School of Health Related Professions
Newark, NJ, USA

Edwin A Deitch, MD
Professor and Chair Department of Surgery
UMDNJ-New Jersey Medical School
Newark, NJ, USA

Mark I Evans, MD
Director, Institute for Genetics
New York, NY, USA

†John C Fletcher PhD

Vijaya Ganesh, MD
Associate Professor of Clinical Obstetrics and Gynecology
UMDNJ-New Jersey Medical School
Newark, NJ, USA

Javier Garcia, MD
Resident
Department of Obstetrics, Gynecology and Women's Health
UMDNJ-New Jersey Medical School
Newark, NJ, USA

Raymond F Gasser, PhD
Professor
Department of Cell Biology & Anatomy
Louisiana State University Health Sciences Centre
New Orleans, LA, USA

Márta Gávai, MD
Senior Lecturer
I. Department of Obstetrics and Gynecology
Semmelweis University
Budapest, Hungary

Darlene G Gibbon, MD
Assistant Professor
Department of Obstetrics and Gynecology
Division of Gynecologic Oncology
UMDNJ-Robert Wood Johnson Medical School
and Cancer Institute of New Jersey
New Brunswick, NJ, USA

Shamshad H Gilani, PhD
Professor
Department of Anatomy
UMDNJ-MSB G685
Newark, NJ, USA

Shimon Ginath, MD
Instructor
Department of Obstetrics & Gynecology, Edith Wolfson
Medical Center, Holon
Sackler Faculty of Medicine, Tel Aviv University
Tel Aviv, Israel

Lisa N Gittens-Williams, MD
Associate Professor
Department of Obstetrics and Gynecology,
UMDNJ-New Jersey Medical School
Newark, NJ, USA

Abraham Golan, MD FRCOG
Professor
Department of Obstetrics & Gynecology, Edith Wolfson
Medical Center, Holon, Sackler Faculty of Medicine
Tel Aviv University
Tel Aviv, Israel

Jeffrey Hammond, MD MPH
Section Chief, Trauma/Surgical Critical Care
Professor of Surgery
UMDNJ-Robert Wood Johnson Medical School
New Brunswick, NJ, USA

Gerard Hansen, MD MPH
Associate Professor,
Department of Obstetrics & Gynecology
UMDNJ-New Jersey Medical School
Newark, NJ, USA

Joanie Hare-Morris, MD
Houston Perinatal Associates
Houston, TX, USA

Ursula F Harkness, MD MPH
Fellow, Maternal Fetal Medicine
University of Cincinnati, College of Medicine
Cincinnati, OH, USA

Christopher R Harman, MD
Professor and Vice Chairman
University of Maryland School of Medicine
Department of Obstetrics, Gynecology and
Reproductive Sciences
Baltimore, MD, USA

Michael R Harrison, MD
Professor of Surgery, Pediatrics,
Obstetrics, Gynecology, and Reproductive Sciences
Director, Fetal Treatment Center
Chief, Division of Pediatric Surgery
University of California
San Francisco, CA, USA

Armando E Hernandez-Rey, MD, Fellow
Department of Obstetrics, Gynecology, & Women's Health
Division of Reproductive Endocrinology & Infertility
UMDNJ-New Jersey Medical School
Newark, NJ, USA

Jonathan J Hwang, MD
Assistant Professor
Director, Robotics/Laproscopic and Minimally
Invasive Urology
UMDNJ-Robert Wood Johnson Medical School
Department of Surgery
Division of Urology
New Brunswick, NJ, USA

Leslie Iffy, MD
Professor of Obstetrics and Gynecology
Department of Obstetrics, Gynecology & Women's Health
UMDNJ-New Jersey Medical School
Newark, NJ, USA

Akos Jakobovits, MD PhD
Senior Consultant, Division of Perinatology
Department of Obstetrics and Gynecology
Cegled General Hospital
Cegled, Hungary

Mark P Johnson, MD
Associate Professor
Obstetrics & Gynecology, Surgery and Pediatrics
University of Pennsylvania School of Medicine
Director of Obstetrical Services
The Center for Fetal Diagnosis and Treatment
Children's Hospital of Philadelphia
Philadelphia, PA, USA

Louis G Keith, MD PHD
Department of Obstetrics and Gynecology,
The Feinberg School of Medicine
Northwestern University, and the Center for Study of
Multiple Birth
Chicago, IL, USA

Stuart S Kesler, MD
Chief Resident
UMDNJ-Robert Wood Johnson Medical School
Department of Surgery
Division of Urology
New Brunswick, NJ, USA

Sundeep J Keswani
The Center for Fetal Diagnosis and Treatment
Children's Hospital of Philadelphia
Philadelphia, PA, USA

Steve H Kim, MD
Assistant Professor of Surgery Division Surgical Oncology
Department of Surgery
UMDNJ-New Jersey Medical School
Newark, New Jersey
Newark, NJ, USA

Wendy Kinzler, MD
Assistant Professor
UMDNJ-Robert Wood Johnson Medical School
Department of Obstetrics, Gynecology and Reproductive
Sciences
Division of Maternal Fetal Medicine
New Brunswick, NJ, USA

Brian Kirshon, MD
Houston Perinatal Associates
Houston, TX, USA

Pierre F Lespinasse, MD
Clinical Instructor
Department of Obstetrics, Gynecology and Women's Health
UMDNJ-New Jersey Medical School
Newark, NJ, USA

Gábor Németh, MD
Associate Professor
Department of Obstetrics & Gynecology
Szent-Györgyi Albert University
School of Medicine
Szeged, Hungary

Rhonda Nichols, MD
Chairperson
Department of Obstetrics & Gynecology
Jersey City Medical Center
Jersey City, NJ, USA

Wilberto Nieves-Niera, MD
Assistant Professor
Department of Obstetrics and Gynecology
Division of Gynecologic Oncology
UMDNJ-Robert Wood Johnson Medical School
and Cancer Institute of New Jersey
New Brunswick, NJ, USA

Yinka Oyelese, MD
Fellow
Division of Maternal-Fetal Medicine
Department of Obstetrics, Gynecology and Reproductive
Sciences
UMDNJ-Robert Wood Johnson Medical School
New Brunswick, NJ, USA

Zoltán Papp, MD PhD DSc, FACOG (Hon)
Professor and Chairman
I. Department of Obstetrics and Gynecology
Semmelweis University
Budapest, Hungary

Sriram C Perni, MD
Division of Maternal-Fetal Medicine
Department of Obstetrics and Gynecology
Weill Medical College of Cornell University
New York, NY, USA

Joseph Ramieri, MD
Department of Obstetrics & Gynecology
Morristown General Hospital
Morristown, NJ, USA

E Albert Reece, MD PhD MBA
Professor of OB/GYN, Internal Medicine and Biochemistry
Vice Chancellor and Dean, College of Medicine
University of Arkansas College of Medicine
Little Rock, AR, USA

Lorna Rodriguez-Rodriguez, MD PhD
Associate Professor
Department of Obstetrics and Gynecology
Division of Gynecologic Oncology
UMDNJ-Robert Wood Johnson Medical School
and Cancer Institute of New Jersey
New Brunswick, NJ, USA

Joseph J Rovinsky, MD
Professor of Obstetrics & Gynecology
Albert Einstein Medical College
New York, NY, USA

Charbel G Salamon, MD
Senior Resident
Department of Obstetrics, Gynecology and Women's Health
UMDNJ-New Jersey Medical School
Newark, NJ, USA

Jahir C Sama, MD
Associate Professor of Obstetrics and Gynecology,
UMDNJ-New Jersey Medical School
Newark, NJ, USA

Marlene Schwebel, JD CNS RNC
Instructor, Department of Obstetrics, Gynecology
and Reproductive Sciences
UMDNJ-Robert Wood Johnson Medical School
New Brunswick, NJ, USA

Neel Shah, MD
UMDNJ-Robert Wood Johnson Medical School
Department of Surgery
Division of Urology
New Brunswick, NJ, USA

Josef Shalev, MD
Professor of Obstetrics and Gynecology
Rabin Medical Center, Campus Beilinson
Petach Tiqua, Israel

Neil S Silverman, MD
Geffon School of Medicine
UCLA
Los Angeles, CA, USA

Morton A Stenchever, MD
Professor and Chairman Emeritus
Department of Obstetrics and Gynecology
University of Washington School of Medicine
Seattle, WA, USA

Patrice ML Trauffer, MD
Associate Professor
Department of Obstetrics and Gynecology
Drexel University College of Medicine
Philadelphia, PA, USA

Anthony M Vintzileos, MD
Professor and Chair
Department of Obstetrics, Gynecology and Reproductive
Sciences
UMDNJ-Robert Wood Johnson Medical School
New Brunswick, NJ, USA

Allison Wagreich, MD
Instructor
Department of Obstetrics and Gynecology
Division of Gynecologic Oncology
UMDNJ-Robert Wood Johnson Medical School
and Cancer Institute of New Jersey
New Brunswick, NJ, USA

Ronald J Wapner, MD
Associate Professor of Obstetrics and Gynecology
Director of Maternal-Fetal Medicine
NY Presbyterian Hospital
New York, NY, USA

Peter T Watson, MD
Director, Northwest Perinatal Center
Assistant Professor
Department of Obstetrics and Gynecology
Oregon Health Sciences University
Portland, OR, USA

Jonathan Weinberg, MD
Department of Anesthesiology
New York Methodist Hospital
Brooklyn, NY, USA

Richard M Weinberg, MD CPE
Medical Director, Quality Improvement and Patient Safety
Officer
University Hospital
Newark, NJ, USA

Carl P Weiner, MD
Professor, Department of Obstetrics, Gynecology and
Reproductive Sciences
Professor, Department of Physiology
University of Maryland School of Medicine
Baltimore, MD, USA

Gerson Weiss, MD
Professor and Chairman
Department of Obstetrics, Gynecology, & Women's Health
Division of Reproductive Endocrinology & Infertility
UMDNJ-New Jersey Medical School
Newark, NJ, USA

R Douglas Wilson, MS MSc FRCSC
The Center for Fetal Diagnosis and Treatment
Children's Hospital of Philadelphia
Philadelphia, PA, USA

Joel Mann Yarmush, MD MPA
Program Director
Department of Anesthesiology
New York Methodist Hospital
New York, NY, USA

Lami Yeo, MD
Associate Professor of Obstetrics and Gynecology
Director of Perinatal Ultrasound
Director of Fetal Cardiovascular Unit
Department of Obstetrics, Gynecology, and Reproductive
Sciences
Division of Maternal-Fetal Medicine
UMDNJ-Robert Wood Johnson Medical School
Robert Wood Johnson University Hospital
New Brunswick, NJ, USA

Preface

This third edition of *Operative Obstetrics* has been updated significantly in order to define the current state of the art of operative obstetric and perinatal techniques. The authors of the chapters are renowned experts in the topic about which they have written and each has done an extremely meticulous job in updating their chapter from the previous edition. As a result the reader is provided with current information written by those who are best able to describe the fine details of the procedures.

A new chapter on patient safety has been added to the book. This is a matter of particular importance today as the medical community tries to devise ways to make the medical environment safer for their patients.

In the preface of the previous edition of this book it was written that the exact role of new operative or technical approaches is sometimes difficult to define. This statement still holds true. Therefore the reader is advised to keep abreast of the comtemporary medical literature as it further defines the role of operative and perinatal techniques.

The authors expect that this book will be useful for obstetricians, residents, perinatologists and others who care for pregnant women. To help them with their difficult endeavor has been the primary goal of our efforts. However, the production of this edition would not have been possible without the devoted support and cooperation of the contributors and the publishers. For their invaluable help with the development of this textbook, we express our profound gratitude.

Joeseph J Apuzzio
Anthony M Vintzileos
Leslie Iffy

Dedications and Acknowledgements

Joseph J Apuzzio
This book is dedicated to my family – my parents Ann and Ralph, who gave me the ideals that I have; my brothers Lou and Ralph, who made my path in life enormously easier as I followed them; my wife Marili, who is the most courageous person that I know; and my daughter Leila and son Kevin – all of whom have inspired me and whose love and support have carried me through life.

Anthony M Vintzileos
To my sister Elisavet, to my 'brother' Spyros and to my wife Cathy, with all my love and gratitude.

Leslie Iffy
To the memory of my mother.

Acknowledgements from the Editors
The editors wish to express their gratitude for the support and cooperation provided by Taylor & Francis Medical Books and, in particular, by Mr Nick Dunton, Head of Medical Publishing, Dr Kelly Cornish, Development Editor and Abigail Griffin, Senior Production Editor. We are also greatly indebted to Ms Margaret Lesniak and Mrs Carol Musso for their valuable administrative and secretarial support, and to Mr Christopher Apuzzio and Mr Julian Gaspar for the development of some of the art work.

Obituaries
Since the publication of the last edition of Operative Obstetrics, Dr David Charles, Co-Editor and Drs Moshe Lancet, David Serr and Leo Stern, Associate Editors of the first edition have died. Their contributions to the development of this textbook are gratefully remembered by the Editors.

1 Anatomy of the anterior abdominal wall, uterus, and pelvic organs

Raymond F Gasser

A 3-D model of the female abdomen and pelvis has been built from the cross-sectional image data set of the US National Library of Medicine, Visible Human Female.[1] The female pelvis has been three-dimensionally reconstructed and more than 300 structures are delineated. In addition, the anatomy of the female pelvis has been reviewed with emphasis on avoiding anatomic complications of laparoscopic pelvic surgery[2] and on structures important in pelvic organ support and urinary continence.[3,4]

Anterior abdominal wall

Boundaries and surface landmarks

The anterior abdominal wall is bound above by the xiphisternal junction in the midline and the arching margin of the lower costal cartilages (costal margin) laterally. Below, it is bound by the symphysis pubis in the midline and laterally by the pubic crest, inguinal (Poupart's) ligament, and iliac crest (Figure 1.1). There are no bony structures laterally, the wall being limited by a vertical line from the middle of the axillary depression (midaxillary line) that crosses the tenth rib to the iliac crest. Additional bony landmarks are the xiphoid process in the midline above, the pubic tubercle located below at the lateral end of the pubic crest, and the anterior superior iliac spine at the anterior end of the iliac crest. The inguinal ligament courses from the pubic tubercle to the anterior superior iliac spine, separating the abdominal wall from the thigh. The pubic bone and symphysis pubis separate the wall from the genitalia.

In addition to the above bony landmarks, several soft tissue landmarks are apparent, their degree of visibility largely dependent upon the amount of fat in the subcutaneous tissue. Most obvious is the umbilicus, which lies in the midline about two-thirds of the distance between the suprasternal (jugular) notch and the symphysis pubis[5] at approximately the level of

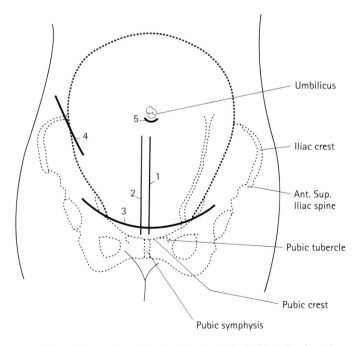

Figure 1.1 Surface landmarks and the sites of popular incisions for obstetric surgery: (1) vertical median incision; (2) vertical paramedian incision; (3) transverse incision; (4) oblique incision; (5) umbilical incision.

the lumbar (L3–4) intervertebral disk. The aponeuroses of the lateral abdominal muscles unite in the midline with their equivalent on the other side, forming the linea alba, which runs from the xiphoid process to the symphysis pubis. The linea alba is usually the strongest point in the aponeurotic part of the wall. In lean, muscular subjects, it is represented on the surface as a vertical midline depression. On each side the lateral margin of the rectus muscle is evident in similar subjects, appearing as a slightly curved, vertical depression called the linea semilunaris.

The surface markings and contour of the anterior abdominal wall vary considerably with age, nutritional and muscular status, parity, and period of gestation. The normal landmarks mentioned above usually are present during pregnancy, and, in some instances, the umbilicus and linea alba may be more intensified because of the distention of the wall by the expanding uterus. Abdominal contents sometimes protrude through a weak umbilicus, resulting in an umbilical hernia. The distention during pregnancy also may widen the linea alba, thereby separating the rectus muscles and creating diastasis recti of varying degrees. In severe cases the uterus is covered only by skin, a thin layer of fascia, and peritoneum. A brown black pigment frequently is deposited in the midline skin, forming the linea nigra.

Skin and subcutaneous tissue

Usually the skin of the abdomen is smooth, very elastic, and firmly attached to the deeper tissue in the midline. The cleavage lines of the skin (Langer's lines) mainly run transversely.[6] Transverse incisions through the skin course mainly parallel to the lines of tension, whereas vertical incisions cut perpendicular to them. The cutaneous lips of vertical incisions, therefore, tend to retract. In the latter months of pregnancy about one-half of all pregnant women develop reddish, slightly depressed streaks (striae gravidarum) in the abdominal skin. In addition to reddish striae, the abdominal skin of multiparous women frequently exhibits glistening, silvery, vertical lines that represent cicatrices of previous striae.

The subcutaneous tissue (superficial fascia) of the anterior abdominal wall, like other areas of the body, is composed mainly of fat and connective tissue and contains cutaneous blood vessels, lymphatics, and nerves (Figure 1.2). The quantity of fat in this region varies remarkably from one individual to another. In fatty subjects, the outer portion of the superficial fascia in the lower abdominal wall appears more fatty in texture than the deeper portions, where sheets (lamellae) of overlapping fibrous connective tissue tend to concentrate.[7] The fibrous sheets do not always form on the deep surface of the fat. Often they are enclosed in fat themselves and, on occasion, may comprise more than one layer.[8,9] In thin individuals, it may be impossible to demonstrate distinct fatty and fibrous portions. The subcutaneous tissue is continuous inferiorly into the labia majora and perineum. Often a vertical, thickened, fibrous band is present in the midline in the lower abdominal wall which is

adherent to the linea alba. It represents the fundiform ligament, which usually is described only in the male. On each side of the midline the subcutaneous layer is loosely separated from the deep fascia over the lower part of the external abdominal aponeurosis. This fascial cleft is quite definite and is continuous below with a similar cleft in the perineum.

The superficial (subcutaneous) arteries arise from various sources and freely anastomose with each other in the subcutaneous layer. Most of the skin below the umbilicus is supplied by three small branches that ascend from the femoral artery passing superficial to the inguinal ligament: the superficial epigastric courses obliquely toward the umbilicus, the superficial circumflex iliac passes laterally just above the iliac crest, and the superficial external pudendal runs medially, superficial to the round ligament of the uterus to the perineum and lowermost part of the wall (Figure 1.2). The superficial (subcutaneous) veins accompany the arteries but are more numerous and form extensive anastomoses. Below the umbilicus they course mainly downward, also crossing superficial to the inguinal ligament to empty into the great saphenous vein in the upper thigh. The subcutaneous veins in the lower abdominal wall anastomose with those draining the upper wall. When the deeper, main venous drainage of the lower limb is obstructed, these anastomoses enlarge, forming a large venous channel, the thoracoepigastric vein that connects the great saphenous vein with the axillary vein. The superficial (subcutaneous) lymph vessels generally follow the course of the veins. Below the umbilicus they course downward to the superficial inguinal nodes located just below the inguinal ligament. The cutaneous nerves arise from the lower six thoracic nerves and the first lumbar nerve (T7–12 and L1). The seventh thoracic nerve supplies the skin over the xiphoid process, the tenth thoracic nerve courses to the umbilicus, and the eleventh and twelfth thoracic nerves and the iliohypogastric nerve (L1) innervate the skin of the infraumbilical portion of the wall. The nerves to the skin on each side of the midline are arranged in two vertical rows, a small, anterior, cutaneous series that pierce the anterior rectus sheath a short distance from the midline, and a larger, lateral, cutaneous series that enter the subcutaneous layer near the midaxillary line. The anterior branches of the lateral cutaneous series supply a large segment of the anterior wall.

Muscles and rectus sheath

The anterior abdominal wall contains five pairs of muscles that support and protect the abdominal viscera in front and laterally (Figure 1.2). The muscles are mainly attached above and laterally to the sternum and lower ribs, and below to the pelvic bone. Three of the muscles are located laterally and superimpose as sheets one on the other. From superficial to deep, they are the external oblique, the internal oblique, and the transversus muscles. The rectus and pyramidalis muscles make up the medial group lying adjacent to the linea alba and enclosed in varying degrees by the rectus sheath. The rectus sheath is formed by the fusion of the sheet-like tendons (aponeuroses) of

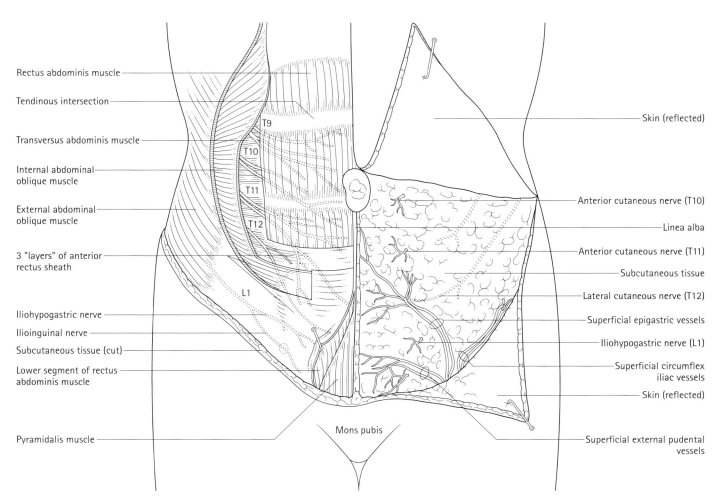

Figure 1.2 Front view of the layers and components of the infraumbilical part of the anterior abdominal wall. The more superficial subcutaneous layer is exposed on the left side of the body; the deeper muscular layer and the anterior rectus sheath are shown on the right side.

the three lateral muscles as they course to the midline. The linea alba might be considered the common area of decussation of the aponeuroses of the three lateral muscles rather than their insertion.[10]

The external oblique muscle originates from the outer surface of the lower eight ribs, its fibers coursing downward and forward. The more posterior fibers insert directly on the outer lip of the iliac crest. The remaining muscle fibers give rise to a broad aponeurosis that passes in front of the rectus muscle to attach to the linea alba. Above, the aponeurosis attaches to the sternum; below, it attaches to the anterior superior iliac spine, pubic tubercle, and symphysis pubis. The lower border of the aponeurosis is thickened and folded back on itself to form the inguinal (Poupart's) ligament between the anterior superior iliac spine and the pubic tubercle. The inguinal ligament is bound down to the deep fascia of the thigh (fascia lata). A small oval opening in the external oblique aponeurosis, the superficial inguinal ring, is located about 2.5 cm above and lateral to the pubic tubercle. Its inferior margin lies close to the inguinal ligament. The round ligament of the uterus passes

through the ring into the labium majus, where it attaches to the subcutaneous tissue.

Immediately deep to the external oblique is the internal oblique muscle. Its fibers arise from the lateral half of the inguinal ligament, iliac crest, and lumbodorsal fascia. The posterior fibers run upward and forward to insert into the lower ribs and their cartilages. The anterior fibers course medially and give rise to an aponeurosis. Most of the fibers of the external and internal oblique muscles run at right angles to each other, an arrangement that contributes strength to the wall. The internal oblique aponeurosis divides at the lateral border of the rectus into anterior and posterior lamellae. The anterior lamella joins the aponeurosis of the external oblique to form the anterior rectus sheath in front of the rectus and pyramidalis muscles. In the upper three-fourths of the wall, the posterior lamella joins the aponeurosis of the transversus muscle to form the posterior rectus sheath, passing deep to the rectus muscle to attach in the midline to the linea alba (Figure 1.3). Approximately midway between the umbilicus and the symphysis pubis, the entire aponeurosis of the internal oblique

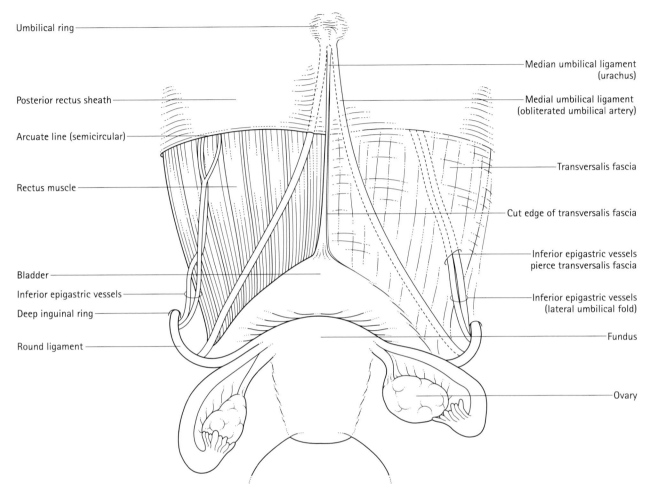

Figure 1.3 Posterior view of the infraumbilical part of the anterior abdominal wall. The parietal peritoneum and extraperitoneal (preperitoneal) tissue are removed from the right side, exposing the layer of transversalis fascia. On the left side, the transversalis fascia is removed, revealing the deep surface of the rectus muscle, below the arcuate line, and the posterior rectus sheath, above the line.

muscle unites with the aponeurosis of the external oblique and transversus muscles, and together they pass in front of the lowest part of the rectus muscle in the anterior rectus sheath. The posterior rectus sheath, therefore, is lacking below this point, its lower border referred to as the arcuate line (semilunar line of Douglas).

The deepest of the lateral muscles is the transversus muscle. Like the internal oblique, its fibers originate from the inguinal ligament, iliac crest, and lumbodorsal fascia, but it has an additional origin from the inner aspect of the lower six costal cartilages. Its fibers are directed mainly transversely, coursing medially to give rise to an aponeurosis at the lateral border of the rectus muscle. Its aponeurosis helps form the posterior rectus sheath in the upper three-fourths of the wall and the anterior rectus sheath in the lower one-fourth (see above). The lowermost fibers of the transversus muscles join similar fibers of the internal oblique muscle, and together they arch inferiorly and medially over the inguinal canal as the falx inguinalis. More medially, the combined fibers give rise to the conjoined

tendon that inserts below on the pecten of the pubis. The conjoined tendon blends medially with the lowermost part of the anterior rectus sheath and lies just deep to the superficial inguinal ring.

The rectus muscle arises from the xiphoid process and the anterior surface of the fifth, sixth, and seventh costal cartilages. Passing inferiorly as a thick, flat, strap-like muscle, it inserts on the front of the pubic bone and symphysis pubis. It is broad and thin above, narrow and thick below. The rectus muscle is enclosed by the rectus sheath except posteriorly in its lower one-fourth. Above the umbilicus the muscle is attached to the anterior rectus sheath at approximately three levels by transverse bands called tendinous intersections or inscriptions (Figure 1.2).

The pyramidalis muscle lies deep to the lowest part of the anterior rectus sheath in front of the rectus muscle (Figure 1.2). It arises from the pubic crest and courses superiorly and medially to insert into the lower part of the linea alba. This muscle is absent approximately 10–20% of the time; it is more frequently missing in whites than African-Americans and is usually missing bilaterally.[11,12]

The anterior wall muscles are innervated mainly by the lower six thoracic nerves (T6–12) (Figure 1.2). The iliohypogastric and ilioinguinal branches of the first lumbar nerve (L1) are primarily cutaneous nerves. The lower five intercostal nerves and the subcostal nerve enter the anterior wall after giving off lateral cutaneous branches. They spiral forward and inferiorly between the internal oblique and transversus muscles, sending motor branches to them and the external oblique muscle. The nerves then enter the lateral aspect of the rectus sheath, innervate the rectus muscle, and terminate by piercing the anterior rectus sheath as anterior cutaneous nerves. The lateral border of the rectus muscle, therefore, cannot be easily freed and retracted medially without injuring its nerve supply. It can be retracted safely laterally, however. The infraumbilical portion of the rectus muscle usually is innervated by the tenth, eleventh, and twelfth thoracic nerves. The pyramidalis muscle receives its motor innervation from the subcostal nerve (T12). The iliohypogastric and ilioinguinal nerves often arise in common with the first lumbar nerve and enter the anterior wall in series with the lower thoracic nerves. They divide close to the iliac crest but do not enter the rectus sheath. The ilioinguinal nerve may send a branch to the lower part of the internal oblique muscle, and then passes through the inguinal canal to emerge through the superficial ring to supply cutaneous branches to the labium majus.

The deep arteries to the anterior wall include branches of the lower five intercostal arteries and the subcostal artery that accompany their respective nerves. They sometimes enter the rectus sheath, where they anastomose with the superior and inferior (deep) epigastric arteries. The smaller superior epigastric artery is the inferior continuation of the internal thoracic (mammary) artery. It passes downward behind the seventh costal cartilage, enters the rectus sheath, and becomes buried in the deep portion of the rectus muscle. The larger inferior epigastric artery arises from the external iliac artery behind the middle of the inguinal ligament. It courses medial to the deep inguinal ring and then runs diagonally upward and medially between the transversalis fascia and peritoneum (Figure 1.3). Close to the lateral border of the rectus muscle, the inferior epigastric artery pierces the transversalis fascia and enters the rectus sheath by passing in front of the arcuate line. It ascends on the deep surface of the rectus muscle, gradually becoming buried in it. In only about one-half the cases studied did the superior and inferior epigastric arteries anastomose to form a vertically coursing channel within the rectus sheath.[13] The course of the inferior epigastric vessels can be more difficult to identify in overweight patients at laparoscopy.[14] The lower lateral part of the anterior wall is supplied by branches of the deep circumflex iliac artery. This vessel also arises from the external iliac artery and ascends between the internal oblique and transversus muscles.

The veins draining the deeper portions of the anterior wall correspond to the arteries. Below the umbilicus they course downward to the external iliac vein, but above this level they pass upward to the internal thoracic vein and laterally to the intercostal veins.

Transversalis fascia, extraperitoneal tissue, and peritoneum

The fascia deep to the transversus muscle is better developed than it is between the abdominal wall muscles, and it is referred to as the transversalis fascia. This relatively strong fascial layer is a part of the endoabdominal fascia that lines the entire abdominal cavity. It is continuous with that of the other side in the midline deep to the linea alba and lies adjacent to the deep surface of the rectus muscle in the lower one-fourth of the anterior wall, where the posterior rectus sheath is absent (Figure 1.3). Above the arcuate line, it lies adjacent to the deep surface of the posterior rectus sheath. Superiorly, it becomes the fascia on the underside of the diaphragm. Inferiorly, it attaches to the pubis, but more laterally in the pelvis it helps form the femoral sheath and is continuous with the iliopsoas fascia. Posteriorly, the transversalis fascia blends with the fascia on the anterior surface of the quadratus lumborum muscle. The transversalis fascia is separated from the peritoneum by loose extraperitoneal (preperitoneal) tissue that contains a variable quantity of fat and, in the lower portion of the anterior wall, remnants of fetal structures. The peritoneum forms the deepest layer of the anterior wall and is the serous membrane lining the peritoneal cavity. In the lower part of the anterior wall, it extends laterally on the deep side of the inguinal canal and reflects superiorly to line part of the iliac fossa on each side. Inferiorly, the parietal layer of peritoneum becomes visceral by continuing onto the superior surface of the bladder into the vesicouterine pouch to the anterior aspect of the uterus. In the infraumbilical part of the anterior wall, there may be little or no fat in the extraperitoneal layer, or there may be a considerable quantity. The ligamentous remnants of fetal structures course superiorly within this layer to the deep side of the umbilicus (Figure 1.3). In or near the midline is the single median (middle) umbilical ligament that represents the remains of a tubular structure called the urachus. The urachus connected the fetal bladder to the body wall at the umbilicus. The proximal part of the ligament retains its tubular structure and attaches to the apex of the bladder. Its distal segment is a fibrous cord that usually divides into three strands as it approaches the umbilicus.[15] This ligament is often hypertrophied during pregnancy and is sectioned during mobilization of the bladder. Located farther laterally on either side is the medial (formerly called lateral) umbilical ligament, a remnant of the distal part of the umbilical artery. It sometimes is referred to as the obliterated umbilical or hypogastric artery. During fetal life the umbilical artery arose as a large, rounded trunk from the uppermost part of the internal iliac artery. It actually represented the main stem of the parent artery that continued along the lateral pelvic wall, up the deep side of the anterior abdominal wall to the umbilicus, and then through the umbilical cord to the placenta. The definitive branches of the internal iliac artery during fetal life were relatively small. Thin sheets of connective tissue that stretch between the medial umbilical ligaments have been observed in the extraperitoneal tissue but are of little clinical importance. Of more importance is the fact that the extraperitoneal tissue in the lower anterior abdominal wall continues below to the prevesical or retropubic space (cave of Retzius), allowing for easy separation of the bladder. The peritoneum in the lower anterior wall in the gravid female is mobilized in an extraperitoneal cesarean section by the development of this space from the suprapubic approach (Figure 1.4).

Incisions

The main incisions used in obstetric surgery are in the infraumbilical portion of the abdominal wall and are as follows (Figure 1.1):

A. vertical
   1. median (1)
   2. paramedian (2)
B. transverse (3)
C. oblique (4)
D. umbilical (5).

The ideal incision is one that affords maximum exposure with minimal damage to the tissue, especially nerves and blood vessels. Sites that predispose to the formation of postoperative hernias should be avoided whenever possible. Many factors influence the surgeon's choice.

Perhaps the most commonly used is the median vertical incision. It has the advantage of good exposure and comparative avascularity, cuts through no muscle fibers or nerves, and can be repaired to produce a strong abdominal wall. The linea alba is incised, using the pyramidalis muscles as a guide to the midline (Figure 1.2). The medial margins of the rectus muscles are exposed and retracted laterally. The rectus muscles lie in close proximity, unless diastasis has occurred. The deeper median umbilical ligament usually is pushed to one side (Figure 1.3).

The paramedian vertical incision is made through similar layers as in the median incision, except that the anterior rectus sheath is cut rather than the linea alba. The rectus muscle may be retracted medially or laterally; medial retractions tend to jeopardize its nerve supply. In muscle-splitting incisions, the rectus muscle is dissected vertically along the length of the wound. When the posterior rectus sheath is divided, the inferior epigastric vessels are retracted laterally (Figure 1.3). Below the arcuate line (semicircular line of Douglas), since the

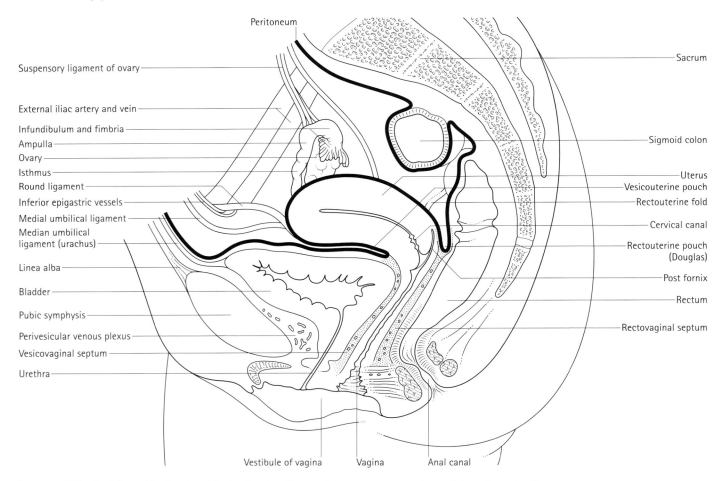

Figure 1.4 Midsagittal view of the female pelvis, showing the relations of the viscera to each other and the peritoneal cavity.

posterior rectus sheath is absent, the transversalis fascia is encountered immediately.

The transverse incision is made in a curved manner above the symphysis pubis just below the hair line.[16] The anterior rectus sheath is cut transversely on both sides. The median sagittal septum (linea alba) that separates the rectus muscles is freed above and below the cut. The rectus muscles are retracted laterally, and the peritoneal cavity is entered by a vertical incision through the transversalis fascia, extraperitoneal tissue, and peritoneum. When additional exposure is required, the rectus muscles are cut transversely (Maylard or Mackenrodt technique), or their insertion on the symphysis pubis is detached.[17] When the need for even greater exposure is anticipated, the skin incisions may extend from one anterosuperior iliac spine to the other (Mackenrodt's approach). As the rectus muscles are cut transversely in this approach, the inferior epigastric vessels are ligated and cut. The transversalis fascia, extraperitoneal tissue, and peritoneum also are cut transversely.

The oblique incision (McArthur or McBurney incision) is a muscle-splitting incision in the lower lateral part of the anterior wall, providing good postoperative support because of the grid type of closure. The three flat abdominal muscles (external oblique, internal oblique, and transversus) are divided in the direction of their fleshy and tendinous fibers. The aponeurosis of the external oblique muscle is encountered first and is separated inferiorly and medially in the direction of its fibers. The internal oblique and transversus muscles are then encountered and separated in the direction of their fibers. Last, the incision is made through the underlying transversalis fascia, extraperitoneal tissue, and peritoneum. In the pregnant patient, consideration must be given to the possible upward and lateral displacement of the underlying viscera by the gravid uterus. The more advanced the pregnancy, the higher must be the incision in the abdominal wall for exposure of the appendix and uterine adnexa.

The umbilical incision is a short semilunar incision made at the lower edge of the umbilicus. The incision is made through stretched skin and the underlying subcutaneous layer. Transversely cutting the underlying transversalis fascia and peritoneum is now preferred to the initial vertical incision.

Uterus

Parts and relations of the nongravid uterus

The nongravid uterus is a hollow, flat, pear-shaped, muscular organ located in or near the midline of the pelvis between the bladder and small intestine, in front, and the rectum and sigmoid colon, behind (Figure 1.4). It is best divided into three major parts: an upper triangular portion, the body; a lower, tubular portion, the cervix; and an intervening, short, constricted segment, the isthmus (Figure 1.5). The dome-shaped portion of the body, above the entrance of the uterine tubes, is the fundus. The cervix is continuous inferiorly with the vagina, the wall of which attaches to the cervix along an oblique line dividing it into supravaginal and vaginal segments. The nongravid uterus usually has an anteverted and anteflexed position with the convex fundus directed anteriorly. The anterior surface of the body is flat and rests on the superior surface of the bladder. Its posterior surface is convex and lies close to the rectum and sigmoid colon. The cervix is directed downward and backward, resting against the posterior wall of the vagina. Its external os lies at about the level of the ischial spine and the upper border of the symphysis pubis. The ureter lies immediately lateral to the cervix, making it very susceptible to injury at this level (Figures 1.6, 1.7, and 1.8). The fundus and body are covered by peritoneum that is reflected anteriorly at the level of the isthmus to the upper surface of the bladder, forming the

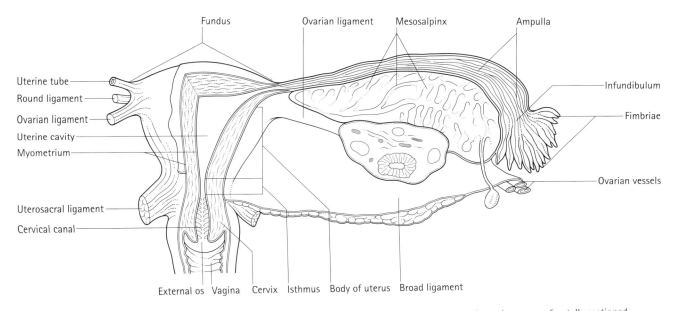

Figure 1.5 Posterior view of the mature, nongravid uterus and adnexa. Part of the uterus and the right uterine tube and ovary are frontally sectioned.

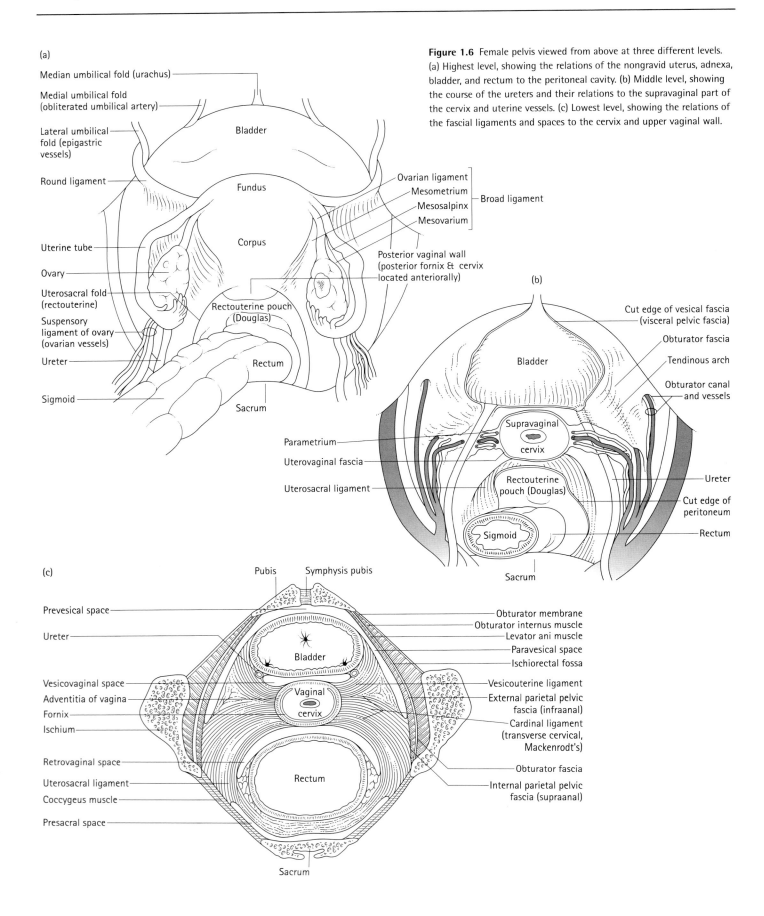

(a)

Median umbilical fold (urachus)

Medial umbilical fold (obliterated umbilical artery)

Lateral umbilical fold (epigastric vessels)

Round ligament

Bladder

Fundus

Corpus

Ovarian ligament
Mesometrium
Mesosalpinx
Mesovarium
— Broad ligament

Uterine tube

Ovary

Uterosacral fold (rectouterine)

Suspensory ligament of ovary (ovarian vessels)

Ureter

Sigmoid

Posterior vaginal wall (posterior fornix & cervix located anteriorly)

Rectouterine pouch (Douglas)

Rectum

Sacrum

Figure 1.6 Female pelvis viewed from above at three different levels. (a) Highest level, showing the relations of the nongravid uterus, adnexa, bladder, and rectum to the peritoneal cavity. (b) Middle level, showing the course of the ureters and their relations to the supravaginal part of the cervix and uterine vessels. (c) Lowest level, showing the relations of the fascial ligaments and spaces to the cervix and upper vaginal wall.

(b)

Cut edge of vesical fascia (visceral pelvic fascia)
Obturator fascia
Tendinous arch
Obturator canal and vessels

Bladder

Supravaginal cervix

Parametrium

Uterovaginal fascia

Uterosacral ligament

Rectouterine pouch (Douglas)

Sigmoid

Ureter

Cut edge of peritoneum

Rectum

Sacrum

(c)

Pubis   Symphysis pubis

Prevesical space

Ureter

Bladder

Vesicovaginal space
Adventitia of vagina
Fornix
Ischium

Vaginal cervix

Retrovaginal space
Uterosacral ligament
Coccygeus muscle

Presacral space

Rectum

Sacrum

Obturator membrane
Obturator internus muscle
Levator ani muscle
Paravesical space
Ischiorectal fossa

Vesicouterine ligament
External parietal pelvic fascia (infraanal)
Cardinal ligament (transverse cervical, Mackenrodt's)
Obturator fascia
Internal parietal pelvic fascia (supraanal)

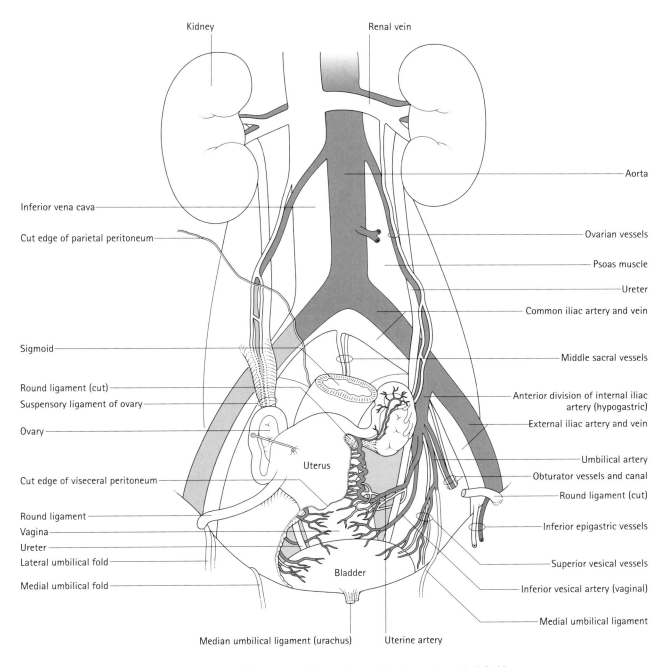

Figure 1.7 Anterior view of the origin, course, and relations of the ureter and the ovarian and uterine vessels on the left side.

vesicouterine pouch (Figure 1.4). Posteriorly, the peritoneum extends farther inferiorly, covering the isthmus, supravaginal cervix, and posterior fornix of the vagina before reflecting to the rectum to form the rectouterine pouch of Douglas.

Size and positional changes of the gravid uterus

First trimester

The dimensions of the nongravid uterus vary considerably. The body averages approximately 5 cm in length, 5 cm at its widest part, and 3–4 cm in thickness (anteroposteriorly). The isthmus and cervix together measure about 2.5 cm in length and 3 cm in diameter. The uterus that has accommodated a previous pregnancy is usually slightly larger than one that has not. For the first few weeks of pregnancy, the original pear shape is maintained. By the end of the second month of gestation, the uterus triples in size and changes from the typical flat pear shape to a rounded form, a shape it retains throughout the second trimester. Because of the rapid increase in size and weight during the second month, the uterus may assume exaggerated positions of anteflexion, retrocession, and retroversion.[15] By the end

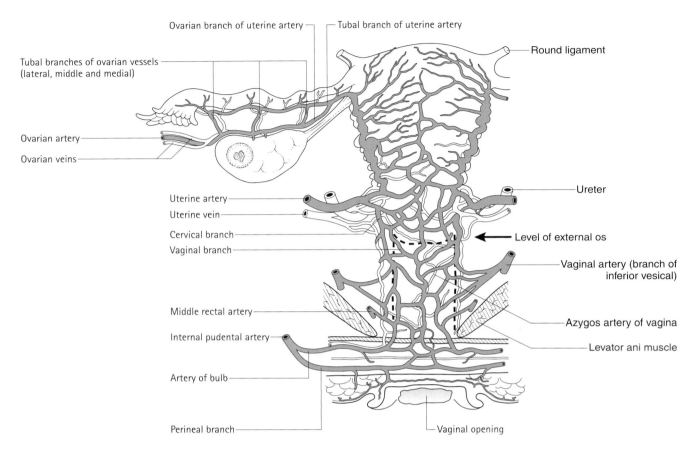

Figure 1.8 Posterior view of the course, relations, and anastomoses of the ovarian and uterine vessels.

of the first trimester, the fundus usually can be palpated above the symphysis (Figure 1.9).

Second and third trimesters

During the second trimester, the uterus expands superiorly out of the pelvic cavity, through the superior pelvic aperture, and into the abdominal cavity (Figure 1.9). It contacts the anterior abdominal wall and displaces the intestines laterally and superiorly. Midway through pregnancy (fifth month), the fundus is at the level of the umbilicus. By 8½ months, the fundus reaches the level of the xiphoid process, but during the last month it recedes slightly when the presenting part of the fetus descends into the pelvis (lightening). At the beginning of the third trimester, the uterus assumes an ovoid shape, the vertical axis increasing more rapidly than either the transverse or antero-posterior axis.[18] The pregnant uterus is quite mobile and tends to rotate to the right with the left side moving anteriorly toward the midline. Rotation to the right is considered to result from the pressure of the sigmoid colon in the left side of the pelvic cavity. Occasionally, rotation of the uterus to the left occurs when there is a pelvic or lower abdominal mass on the right side. In the erect standing position, the abdominal wall supports the uterus. In the supine position, the uterus lies backward, resting upon the aorta and inferior vena cava.

The myometrium during pregnancy

The wall of the uterus is composed of a thin outer covering of peritoneum (serosa), a thick, intermediate layer of variable proportions of muscle and connective tissue (myometrium), and an inner mucosal layer (endometrium). The body of the uterus contains the most muscle, with the content of muscle fibers diminishing below as the cervix is approached. The cervix is composed mainly of connective tissue and only about 10% muscle fiber.[19] The arrangement of the muscular fibers within the myometrium of the body is complex as a result of its development from the fused portion of the paramesonephric (müllerian) ducts (Figure 1.10), but generally they can be divided into three layers. The external longitudinal layer of the uterine tube blends with the outer layer of vertical fibers of the uterus.[20] Muscle fibers in the outer part of the inner circular layer of the tube spiral around each tube and continue into the uterus, spiraling in a clockwise direction from the right and a counterclockwise direction from the left. This interlacing network of muscle fibers is in the middle layer that forms the main part of the uterine wall. Bundles of smooth muscle contained in the supportive ligaments interlace and blend with the middle layer. The inner layer of muscle consists of circularly arranged, sphincter-like fibers at the isthmus and, at the orifices of the

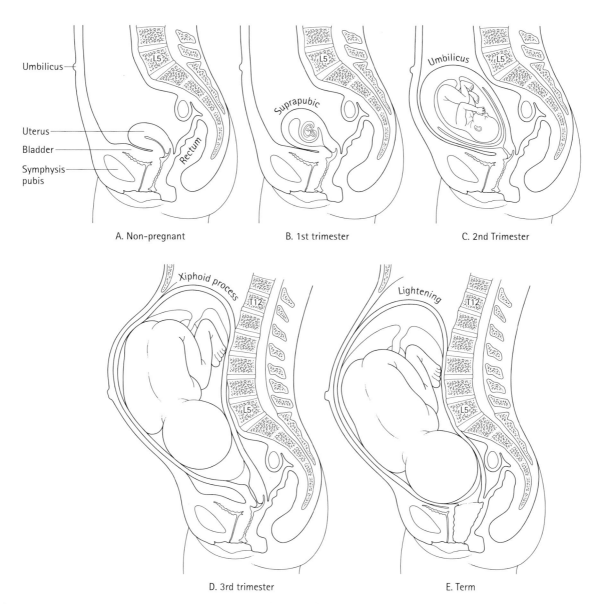

A. Non-pregnant

B. 1st trimester

C. 2nd Trimester

D. 3rd trimester

E. Term

Figure 1.9 Relations of the body of the uterus and superior extent of the fundus at different periods of gestation.

tubes, it is continuous with the inner portion of the inner circular layer of the tube. Two muscle bundles, the fasciculi cervicoangulares, are present at the lateral aspect of the uterus, bridging the cervix and fundus. The bundles may serve as a system for conduction or coordination of muscle contraction.[21] During pregnancy, the muscle fascicles in the lower portion of the uterus overlap one another like shingles on a roof.

Uterine enlargement during pregnancy involves stretching and marked hypertrophy of the muscle layer. At term the body of the uterus weighs over 1000 g compared to approximately 70 g in the nongravid state. Since mitotic activity is rarely observed in the myometrium, the smooth muscle cells are considered to undergo hypertrophy rather than hyperplasia. The new muscle cells which do form likely originate from growth of the media of the myometrial arteries and veins.[22] Hypertrophy

of the myometrium begins during the first few weeks and overall increases five- to tenfold, mainly during the third month. Increases in fibrous and elastic tissue accompany the hypertrophy. During the second and third trimesters, the increased uterine size is caused mainly by the pressure exerted by the expanding conceptus. In early pregnancy the myometrium of the body is 2–3 cm thick but thins to 1–2 cm in late pregnancy. Thinning of the uterine wall may be exaggerated in multigravid women, during multiple pregnancy, and in hydramnios.

The musculature in the wall of the isthmus must dilate during labor rather than contract and, after the second month, makes up the major portion of the lower uterine segment. It is poorly defined during the early weeks of pregnancy when the area feels softer than either the body or cervix. The isthmus hypertrophies like the body during the first trimester, and its

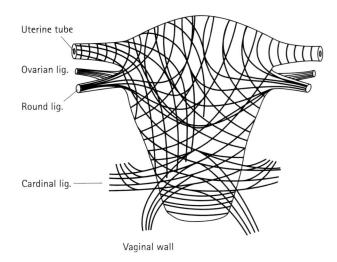

Figure 1.10 Course and arrangement of smooth muscle fibers in the myometrium and their continuities with those in the uterine tube, vaginal wall, and lateral ligaments.

canal triples in length to approximately 3 cm (Figure 1.11). During the second trimester, the isthmus becomes incorporated into the body of the uterus, and the isthmic canal becomes part of the uterine cavity.[23–25] Since the wall of the isthmus and the wall of the body are approximately the same thickness during this time, their junction region no longer is visible externally. This condition persists until the middle of the last trimester, when a transverse linear depression appears in the junction region. The musculature above the depression is thicker than that below. The transverse depression forms just below the vesico-uterine pouch and is thought to correspond to the level of the anatomic internal os. It is sometimes referred to as the physiologic contraction ring, which rises to a higher level during labor. After delivery the ring appears as a marked constriction between the body and the cervix.

The cervix of the gravid uterus

The size of the cervix in relation to the body of the uterus varies with age and parity. The cervix is twice the size of the body in a young child, about equal in nulliparous women, and about one-third the size of the body in a multiparous woman. It is composed mainly of collagen-rich connective tissue, and only approximately 10% is muscle.

The cervix undergoes profound changes during pregnancy and labor. Two of the earliest signs of pregnancy are cervical softening and cyanosis caused by increased vascularity and edema. Soon after conception, the cervical glands secrete a very thick mucus into the cervical canal, forming a plug that closes off the canal during the gestation period. In the nonpregnant state, the glands usually comprise only a small fraction of the cervical mass. They undergo such remarkable proliferation during pregnancy that by term they make up approximately one-half its mass. There is no appreciable change in the muscle content of the cervix during pregnancy. The cervix dilates during labor as a result of collagen dissociation. The incompetent cervix dilates painlessly during the second or early third trimester, resulting in rupture of the membranes, followed by the delivery, usually, of a previable fetus.[26] Previous cervical trauma from such procedures as dilation, curettage, and cauterization appears to be a major causative factor. The ratio of muscle to collagen has been reported to change, resulting in more abundant muscle fibers. Cervical weakness is reinforced surgically by the placement of a purse-string suture around the vaginal cervix after the first trimester but before significant dilation occurs.

Changes in the uterine cavity during pregnancy

The uterine cavity in the nongravid state is little more than a slit, when viewed laterally, with close anterior and posterior walls (Figure 1.4). From the front, the cavity has the shape of an inverted triangle with a base superiorly, where it is continuous on each side with the lumen of the uterine tube, and an apex inferiorly, where it is continuous with the canal through the isthmus and cervix (Figure 1.5). The cervical canal is slightly expanded in its middle and opens into the vagina through the external os. It is continuous superiorly with the constricted canal of the isthmus, which may be 6–10 mm long (Figure 1.11). The point where the lower end of the isthmic canal widens into the cervical canal is known as the histologic internal os, as it is the point where an abrupt microscopic change occurs in the mucosa. Its upper end widens into the uterine cavity at the anatomic internal os. The uterine cavity in the gravid condition enlarges as the myometrium hypertrophies. Initially, its rate of enlargement is greater than the growth rate of the conceptus. Later, during the early part of the second trimester, the uterine cavity becomes completely filled by the rapidly expanding conceptus. Uterine enlargement is not symmetric, but is sometimes most marked in the fundus and other times in the body below the tubes. This probably is influenced greatly by the location of the implantation site.

Uterine tube

A long, narrow, trumpet-shaped uterine (fallopian) tube extends laterally from each side of the uterine body, arching over the upper pole of the ovary and then downward on the posterior part of its medial surface (Figures 1.4, 1.5, and 1.6). Its canal runs from the superior angle of the uterine cavity to the ovary and gradually increases in diameter as it courses laterally. When straightened, the tube in the nongravid state measures approximately 10 cm long. It can be divided into four parts. The intramural portion passes through the uterine wall and has the smallest lumen diameter (1 mm or less). The portion that extends laterally from the uterus is the narrow isthmus. It continues laterally into a broad, sometimes tortuous, portion called

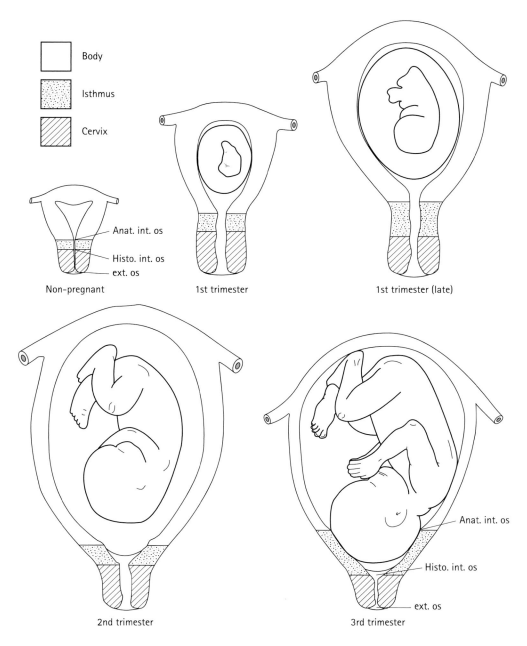

Body

Isthmus

Cervix

Anat. int. os
Histo. int. os
ext. os

Non-pregnant

1st trimester

1st trimester (late)

2nd trimester

3rd trimester

Anat. int. os

Histo. int. os

ext. os

Figure 1.11 Location and extent of the three parts of the uterine wall at different periods of gestation.

the ampulla. The ampulla terminates near the ovary as the funnel-shaped infundibulum. Finger-like fimbriae extend from the periphery of the infundibulum surrounding the abdominal ostium. One or more fimbriae are in contact with the ovary (ovarian fimbria). The wall of the uterine tube is made up of three layers: an outer serosa, an intermediate smooth muscle layer (myosalpinx), and an inner mucosal lining (endosalpinx). The endosalpinx is arranged into longitudinal folds that become highly branched in the ampullary segment. The uterine tube occupies the upper border of the broad ligament and stretches with it as tension is exerted on them by the rising,

gravid uterus. It becomes hyperemic but undergoes little hypertrophy during pregnancy.

Ovary

Medial to the curved segment of the uterine tube on each side lies the solid, almond-shaped ovary (Figures 1.4, 1.5, and 1.6). Each ovary measures approximately 4 cm long, 2 cm wide, and 1 cm thick and usually has a grayish-pink color and a puckered, uneven surface. Its long axis is nearly vertical, with the upper pole located close to the uterine tube and the lower pole nearer the uterus. One surface faces medially, and the other laterally. Its posterior border is free, but its anterior border is attached to the broad ligament by a short, two-layered fold of peritoneum, the mesovarium, through which vessels and nerves pass to the hilum of the ovary. The ovary in the nulliparous woman usually lies in the upper part of the pelvic cavity in a slight depression on the lateral pelvic wall between the diverging external and internal iliac vessels (ovarian fossa). However, in the multiparous woman, it may lie anywhere against the lateral pelvic wall and sometimes in the rectouterine pouch.[27] During the first pregnancy, the ovary becomes displaced and probably never returns to its original position. In nulliparous women, the upper pole of the ovary lies near the external iliac vein, and attached to it is a vascular fold of peritoneum, the suspensory ligament of the ovary (infundibulopelvic), containing the ovarian vessels and nerves. The lower pole is attached to the lateral angle of the uterus behind the uterine tube by a round cord, the ligament of the ovary, that is made up mainly of fibrous tissue but also contains some smooth muscle fibers.

During the first month of pregnancy, the ovary enlarges, and the corpus luteum reaches its maximal size of 2–2.5 cm in diameter. After the second month, the ovary becomes smaller, and its surface often is covered by patches of the reddish-appearing decidual reactions in the underlying stroma. Regressive changes appear in the corpus luteum within 2–3 weeks after implantation. Parts of the corpus luteum persist until the middle of pregnancy, but eventually it involutes and becomes the corpus albicans.

As pregnancy progresses, the adnexal structures move superiorly. An adnexal mass may present in the upper abdominal quadrant during the last trimester.

Ligaments of the uterus

The broad ligament is the mesentery of the uterus, uterine tube, and ovary. It is formed by extensions laterally of the peritoneum on the anterior and posterior surfaces of the uterus to the lateral pelvic wall (Figures 1.5 and 1.6a). Enclosed between the two peritoneal layers are important structures related to the uterus, tubes, and ovaries. A reflection from the posterior surface of the broad ligament forms the mesovarium portion. That part above the mesovarium containing the tube in its free border is the mesosalpinx, while the part below this level is the mesometrium. The suspensory ligament of the ovary and its contained vessels and nerves continue into the lateral aspect of the broad ligament. The ligament of the ovary lies within the broad ligament as it courses to the lateral border of the uterus. The base of the broad ligament encloses the uterine vessels and nerves and part of the uterus (Figure 1.6b). As the gravid uterus enlarges and rises, it exerts tension on the broad ligament and the structures within it.

The connective tissue and smooth muscle within the broad ligament are referred to as the parametrium. The parametrium

is scant medially near the uterus and superiorly near the tube where the two layers of the ligament are close. Laterally and inferiorly, the ligament thickens, and the parametrial tissue is more abundant. The connective tissue in the base of the ligament is continuous with the connective tissue of the pelvic floor. Its densest portion is referred to as the cardinal ligament (transverse cervical or Mackenrodt's) that blends medially with the supravaginal portion of the cervix and upper vaginal wall and laterally with the fascia on the lateral pelvic wall (Figure 1.6c). Continuous with the posterior aspects of the cardinal ligament is another fascial condensation known as the uterosacral ligament. It extends posterolaterally from the supravaginal portion of the cervix, encircles the rectum, and becomes continuous with the fascia over the second and third sacral vertebrae. It is covered by peritoneum forming the uterosacral fold, which is the lateral boundary of the rectouterine pouch (Figure 1.6). While the cardinal and uterosacral ligaments have long been regarded as important supports of the uterus, they are considered primarily perivascular sheaths or simple condensations of intrapelvic fibrous tissue rather than distinct anatomic ligaments.[28] The uterosacral fold does not contain thick fibrous tissue. In nulliparous women, pregnancy is associated with increased pelvic organ prolapse.[29]

The round ligament of the uterus is attached to the lateral uterine border in front of the attachment of the ovarian ligament. It passes laterally through the broad ligament to reach the pelvic wall. There it ascends over the external iliac vessels, enters the deep inguinal ring, and passes through the inguinal canal to anchor in the tissue of the labium majus. The round ligament of the uterus is composed of smooth muscle fibers and connective tissue, and it has a diameter of 3–5 mm. As the gravid uterus rises, the round ligament of the uterus increases substantially in both length and diameter (Figures 1.3, 1.4, and 1.6a).

Uterine blood vessels, lymphatics, and nerves

Arteries

Knowledge of the origin, course, and branching pattern of the vessels that supply the uterus is important in controlling bleeding during surgery. The uterine artery is the main blood supply to the uterus, although the ovarian artery assists through its large anastomoses with the uterine artery (Figures 1.7 and 1.8). The uterine artery arises in a variable manner from the anterior division of the internal iliac (hypogastric) artery.[30] Nearly half of the time, it arises independently from the internal iliac artery, but very often it may originate from the umbilical artery.[31] Origins from the internal pudendal, inferior vesical, vaginal, and a stem in common with two other anterior division vessels have been observed, as well as doubling of the artery. From its origin, the uterine artery courses along the lateral pelvic wall downward, forward, and medially, passing in front of and above the ureter, to which it may send a branch. It turns sharply medially in the base of the broad ligament running toward the cervix. The surrounding connective tissue binds it to the accompanying veins, the ureter, and the cardinal ligament (Figure 1.6b and c). As the uterine artery approaches the cervix, it supplies the cervix with several tortuous, penetrating branches that allow for rapid cervical expansion. It then divides into a large, very tortuous ascending branch and one or more smaller descending branches to the upper vaginal wall and adjacent portions of the bladder (Figure 1.8). The ascending or main branch courses superiorly along the side of the uterus supplying arcuate branches to the body of the uterus. The arcuate arteries circle the uterus just beneath the serosa and, at intervals, give off radial branches that penetrate directly inward, passing between interlacing muscle fibers of the myometrium. When the muscle fibers contract after delivery, their interlacing arrangement constricts the radial branches, thus acting as ligatures. The arcuate arteries rapidly diminish in size as they pass toward the midline. This arrangement explains why midline sections of the uterus bleed relatively less than lateral ones.

As the ascending branch of the uterine artery approaches the uterine tube, it turns laterally in the upper part of the broad ligament, where it divides into tubal and ovarian branches (Figure 1.8). The tubal branch courses laterally in the mesosalpinx close to the uterine tube, which it supplies through a series of branches. The ovarian branch passes into the mesovarium, where it forms a broad anastomosis with the ovarian artery proper from the abdominal aorta. The anastomotic channel supplies the ovary and gives a series of tubal branches through the mesosalpinx that anastomose with the tubal branch of the uterine artery.

Both the uterine and ovarian arteries undergo marked enlargement during pregnancy, the latter vessel bringing blood to the uterus through its broad anastomosis with the ovarian branch of the uterine artery. The tortuous arrangement of the ascending branch of the uterine artery allows the vessel to elongate and accommodate to the growth of the uterus during pregnancy. The unspiraled descending branches are felt easily along the lateral side of the cervix at vaginal examination as a result of their increased size during pregnancy. A vast ipsilateral and contralateral arterial anastomotic network forms throughout the uterus.[32] There is an increase in the size and degree of arborizations of the arcuate arteries in and around the implantation site.

Veins

The uterine venous plexus drains inferiorly, and the vaginal venous plexus drains superiorly into a plexiform arrangement of uterine veins that surround the uterine artery lateral to the cervix (Figures 1.7 and 1.8). Near the lateral pelvic wall, the uterine veins unite to form usually two trunks that drain into the internal iliac vein. The major portion of venous blood from the uterus is drained by way of the uterine veins. The

remainder drains through the ovarian or pampiniform plexus. On the right, the ovarian plexus drains superiorly through the suspensory ligament of the ovary, crosses the right ureter obliquely, and then empties into the inferior vena cava. On the left, the ovarian plexus drains into the left renal vein and usually does not cross the ureter on that side. The ovarian veins on both sides dilate to enormous size during pregnancy and are possible routes for thrombus formation. They can be injured by external trauma and occasionally rupture spontaneously. The diameter of the ovarian vascular pedicle nearly triples during pregnancy.[33] The veins surrounding the uterus (plexus of Santorini), including those beneath the bladder, within the broad ligament, and around the cervix and upper vagina, become greatly enlarged during pregnancy.

Dissection during cesarean section must remain near the midline to avoid excessive bleeding from these dilated venous plexuses. Those veins in the broad ligament appear medusa-like and may be 1 cm or more in diameter. The ovarian and uterine veins are devoid of valves, so that constant venous pressure within the uterus is probably maintained by their expansion and contraction. Hypervascularity of the uterine wall during pregnancy may occur 20% of the time, probably representing dilation of myometrial veins.[34] Hypervascularity of the anterior uterine wall may cause excessive bleeding during invasive procedures.

Lymphatics

Lymph channels are especially numerous in the walls of the female genital tract.[35] Intramural plexuses drain both the endometrium and myometrium into a subserous plexus from which efferent vessels arise. Studies on the rhesus monkey show the intramural plexuses much enlarged during pregnancy.[36] Efferent vessels from the lower uterus empty mainly into sacral nodes and nodes along the external, internal, and common iliac vessels. Some empty into lower lumbar nodes around the aorta, and a few empty into superficial inguinal nodes. Most of the lymphatics from the upper uterus pass laterally in the broad ligament, where they join those from the uterine tube and ovary. Together, they leave the pelvis by coursing superiorly through the suspensory ligament of the ovary, accompanying the ovarian vessels on the posterior body wall to empty into nodes along the lower part of the abdominal aorta.

Nerves

Nerves to the uterus and vagina are derived from the pelvic plexus (Frankenhauser's ganglion) and consist of afferent and sympathetic fibers but few, if any, parasympathetic fibers. The uterovaginal portion of the plexus passes medially toward the cervix around the uterine vessels in the upper part of the cardinal ligament. Most of the nerves accompany the branches of the uterine artery, with the cervix supposedly receiving more fibers than the body of the uterus. During pregnancy, the nerve supply to the uterus hypertrophies and is accompanied by an increase in size of the pelvic plexus. The function of the motor supply to the uterus is not well understood and is not essential to normal activity at parturition. Catecholamines exert a greater inhibiting effect on the pregnant than the nonpregnant uterus,[37] and norepinephrine can both excite and inhibit the musculature of both the uterus and uterine tube.[38]

Preganglionic sympathetic fibers to the uterus course from the aortic plexus through the hypogastric plexus just below the sacral promontory to the pelvic plexus, where they synapse in ganglia contained within the plexus. Afferent pain fibers from the body apparently travel also through the hypogastric plexus and lumbar sympathetic trunk to enter the spinal cord through the T11 and T12 nerves. Pain in cancer of the uterus has been relieved by blocks of the first three lumbar sympathetic ganglia,[39] and hypogastric resection makes biopsy of the fundus painless.[40] Sensory pain fibers from the cervix and upper vagina pass through the pelvic nerves to enter the spinal cord through the sacral (S2, S3, and S4) nerves.

Pelvic portion of ureter

The course and relations of the pelvic ureter can be clearly demonstrated by endovaginal magnetic resonance imaging.[41] Both ureters can usually be identified with laparoscopy even in overweight patients.[14] As the ureter enters the pelvis, it crosses the common or external iliac artery, coursing medial to the ovarian vessels (Figure 1.7). The base of the pelvic mesocolon lies between the left ureter and the midline. In the pelvis the ureter on both sides passes medial to the internal iliac artery, its branches, and the obturator nerve (Figures 1.6b and 1.7). It courses in a curved manner just posterior to the ovary on the upper part of the pelvic wall where it lies just beneath the peritoneum (Figure 1.6a). If the uterus is elevated anteriorly by traction, the course of the ureter frequently can be seen clearly through the transparent peritoneum and posterior leaf of the broad ligament to below the cervical level without involving dissection.[42] The ureter is in close proximity to the suspensory ligament of the ovary through which the ovarian vessels course (Figures 1.5 and 1.6). It adheres to the undersurface of the peritoneum and may be accidentally drawn into the jaws of artery forceps if traction is placed on the peritoneum when the suspensory ligament is clamped.[43] Dissection of the bladder off the anterior surface of the supravaginal cervix displaces the ureter downward and laterally. As the uterosacral fold is approached, the ureter loses its peritoneal relation by passing deeply into the connective tissue of the uterosacral and cardinal ligaments at the base of the broad ligaments of the uterus. Here it passes obliquely medially, behind and beneath the uterine artery (Figures 1.7 and 1.8). The ureter and uterine artery are closely related for 1–2.5 cm of their length[44] and are enclosed in a common connective tissue sheath.[27] At this point the ureter lies approximately 1.5–2 cm lateral to the cervix, varying 1–4 cm.[45] This segment of the ureter is most susceptible to injury during surgery, its ligation apparently being the most

common accident,[46] but ligation of the uterine vessels also may produce injury.[47] Identification of the cord-like medial umbilical ligament (obliterated hypogastric or umbilical artery) and following it to its lateral origin help locate the distal ureter.[48]

After the ureter leaves the base of the broad ligament, it inclines medially and downward in front of the upper vaginal wall to terminate in the bladder. This segment is eminently palpable.[42] At the posterior wall of the bladder, the ureters are approximately 5 cm apart. Their slit-like openings inside the bladder are only 2.5 cm apart approximately because of their very oblique downward and medial course through the thick wall of the empty bladder. The oblique course of the ureter through the bladder wall is important in preventing reflux. It is unclear whether or not reflux, which may occur with chronic bladder distention, causes the hydroureter that often accompanies pregnancy. The connective tissue sheath that encloses the lower one-third of the ureter and uterine vessels hypertrophies during pregnancy. This, together with the accompanying massive enlargement of the uterine vessels, would favor urinary stasis and dilation of the upper portion of the ureter. After the pregnant uterus rises completely out of the pelvis (fourth month), it may compress the ureter at the pelvic brim, also producing hydroureter.[49] Ureteral dilation above the pelvic brim is usually more marked on the right side.[50] The right ovarian vein, which becomes greatly dilated during pregnancy, obliquely crosses the right ureter, possibly contributing to dilation on the right side.[51] The pressure of the enlarged uterus frequently causes lateral displacement and elongation of both the abdominal and pelvic portions of the ureter.

The chief arterial supply to the pelvic portion of the ureter arises close to the pelvic brim from the common, external, or internal iliac arteries rather than descending with it from higher levels.[52,53] Since this branch reaches it from the lateral side, the pelvic ureter should be exposed from its medial side. The lower end of the ureter close to the bladder regularly receives a branch from the uterine and inferior vesical arteries. As many as 10–15% of ureters may have inadequate anastomoses in their pelvic portions.[54] Interruption of one of the supplying vessels in such cases may damage the ureter.

Nerves to the pelvic portion of the ureter are limited to a few branches from the hypogastric nerve and the pelvic plexus. Although ureteric peristalsis is not dependent upon a nerve supply, the lower part of the ureter receives both sympathetic and sacral, parasympathetic fibers.

Bladder and urethra

Bladder

The bladder is a hollow, muscular organ lined with a mucous membrane and covered superiorly with peritoneum (Figures 1.4 and 1.6). The shape and relations of the bladder vary, depending upon its state of distention. The place when empty, the bladder has a pyramidal shape with an apex directed forward and slightly upward, a base (fundus) directed backward and slightly downward, and a superior and two lateral surfaces. The place where the two lateral surfaces meet the base is the neck, which lies on the superior layer of the urogenital diaphragm and is continuous with the urethra. The apex is continued superiorly as the median umbilical ligament, which runs to the umbilicus in the extraperitoneal tissue between the peritoneum and transversalis fascia. Below the vesicouterine pouch, the base of the bladder is related to the cervix and the anterior vaginal wall, from which it is separated by a concentration of connective tissue called the vesicovaginal septum. This region contains a large venous plexus (vesical, pudendal, or Santorini's) that drains the posterior surface of the bladder, the cervix, and upper vagina. An awareness of these veins is important during low cervical cesarean section and total hysterectomy. Toward the end of pregnancy, the base of the bladder is moved superiorly out of the pelvis by the enlarging uterus to a position in the lower abdomen. The pressure of the presenting part may impair the drainage of blood and lymph from the base of the bladder, causing the area to swell and become traumatized. During parturition, the anterior vaginal wall is enlarged and is the site of possible vesicovaginal fistulas.

The superior surface of the bladder is covered by peritoneum and, when empty, is flat or concave and in contact with the body of the nongravid uterus which lies directly upon it (Figure 1.4). When the bladder fills, the superior surface becomes convex and comes into close relation with coils of small intestine. As the pregnant uterus expands, it compresses the superior surface from above. The lateral surfaces are separated from the symphysis pubis and pubic bones by a loose connective tissue space called the prevesical or retropubic space (of Retzius) that allows for easy separation of the bladder from the pubis. The space may contain a large amount of fat and extend around the sides of the bladder, upward through extraperitoneal tissue to the umbilicus. An extraperitoneal cesarean section is performed through the upper part of this space with mobilization of the peritoneum over the bladder.[55] More laterally, the lateral surface of the bladder lies close to the levator ani and obturator internus muscle (Figure 1.6c); between these muscles and the bladder passes the obliterated umbilical artery that courses forward and upward on the anterior abdominal wall as the medial umbilical ligament.

Adjacent to the bladder wall and surrounding it is a loose layer of visceral pelvic fascia allowing for great distention. Between the bladder and the cervix, there are sometimes thickened bands of parietal pelvic fascia (called the vesicouterine or pubocervical ligament) that course obliquely anteriorly to the symphysis pubis as the pubovesical ligament. The bladder is supported by this fascia and the underlying pelvic floor.

The mucous membrane lining the interior of the bladder is loosely attached to the muscular coat and appears folded when the bladder is empty. Only in a smooth triangular area at the base of the bladder (called the trigone) is the lining smooth. Here the mucous and muscular layers are bound firmly. The lateral angles of the trigone are formed by the orifices of the ureters. Underlying muscle fibers between the ureteral orifices raise the mucosa into an interureteric ridge. After the fourth month of pregnancy, the bladder becomes hyperemic, the trigone elevates, and the interureteric ridge thickens. The trigone region progressively deepens and widens until the end of pregnancy.

Urethra

The female urethra is a short tube approximately 3–4 cm long that extends from the bladder neck to the external urethral orifice (meatus) in the vestibule of the vagina (Figure 1.4). The upper end begins at the level of the middle of the symphysis pubis, where it is surrounded by dense fascia and the vesical plexus of veins. It extends downward and forward in a gentle curve to terminate posterior to the lower border of the symphysis pubis. Intact pubourethral ligamentous and muscular attachments aid in stabilizing the urethra to its normal anatomic position and help maintain continence.[56] Posteriorly, the urethra is applied closely to the anterior vaginal wall, from which its upper half is separated by dense connective tissue and blood vessels. Its lower half is actually embedded in the anterior wall of the vagina. While superiorly the bladder and vagina are separated from each other by a cleavage plane, called the vesicovaginal septum, this plane does not extend inferiorly to separate the urethra and vagina.[57] The urethra pierces the urogenital diaphragm where it is surrounded by the sphincter urethrae muscle. Its mucosa is arranged into longitudinal folds that contribute to the ease with which the female urethra can be dilated.

The arteries to the bladder vary in origin, number, and branching pattern. One to four superior vesical arteries usually arise from the proximal, patent segment of the umbilical artery and supply the apex and superior and lateral surfaces of the bladder.[58] In about 10% of the cases, a superior vesical artery arises from the uterine artery. Anastomoses occur with the inferior epigastric artery in the extraperitoneal tissue, but none were found in the bladder wall. The usually single inferior vesical artery has a variable origin directly or indirectly from the internal iliac artery to supply the base and neck of the bladder and the upper part of the urethra and vagina (Figure 1.8). The vesical plexus of veins around the neck of the bladder drains most of the bladder wall, receives the deep dorsal vein of the clitoris, and communicates with the vaginal plexus. It drains laterally by three channels into the internal iliac vein.[59] Lymphatics from the bladder drain laterally into the external and internal nodes.

The nerves to the bladder are derived from the superior hypogastric plexus, the sacral sympathetic trunk, and the pelvic splanchnic nerves, all of which join together in the pelvic plexus. The vesical plexus of nerves is an anteroinferior continuation of the pelvic plexus that turns medially toward the bladder. Numerous cholinergic (parasympathetic) nerves supply the bladder neck and the proximal urethra,[60] although there are few adrenergic (sympathetic) nerves in these areas except in the trigone area, where they are abundant.[61] The connective tissue lateral to the bladder containing the arteries, veins, and nerves to the bladder and the terminal part of the ureter is known as the lateral (true) ligament of the bladder. The connective tissue blends inferiorly and laterally with the fascia on the upper surface of the levator ani muscle. It sometimes thickens to form the vesicouterine ligament, which laterally binds the shallow vesicouterine pouch (Figure 1.6c). No muscular connections are found between the levator ani muscle and the pelvic organs.[62] A layer of fascia is always interspersed between them.

Sigmoid colon, rectum, and anal canal

Sigmoid colon

The sigmoid (pelvic) colon is the continuation of the descending colon, beginning in the left iliac fossa near the pelvic brim and ending in front of the third sacral vertebra by becoming the rectum. The course of the sigmoid colon is S-shaped, entering the true pelvis by passing over the medial border of the left psoas major muscle, crossing the midline in front of the sacrum, and then swinging back to the left and inferiorly to become the rectum in the posterior pelvic wall. The uterus, uterine tubes, and ovaries are anterior to this segment of the colon (Figure 1.4). Structures crossing the left pelvic brim are posterior to the sigmoid colon, including the left ovarian vessels, left ureter, and left common iliac vessels (Figure 1.7). In the midline the sacral promontory and first three sacral vertebrae are posterior. The sigmoid colon is covered completely with peritoneum and is suspended by the sigmoid mesocolon. After pelvic surgery, the sigmoid colon sometimes is used to cover the operative site and thereby prevent adhesions to the small intestine.

Rectum

At the level of the third sacral vertebra, the sigmoid colon loses its mesentery and becomes the rectum. The rectum is approximately 10 cm long and extends downward and forward in the back of the true pelvis, following the curve of the sacrum and coccyx (Figure 1.4). Below the coccyx, it turns sharply backward to become the anal canal. The highest one-third of the rectum is covered with peritoneum on its front and sides. Only the front of the middle one-third is covered with peritoneum where it is reflected upward in the floor of the rectouterine pouch onto the posterior fornix of the vagina and supravaginal cervix. The lowest one-third of the rectum has no peritoneal covering and is sometimes dilated, forming the ampulla. Posterior to the rectum are located the lower sacrum, coccyx, and anococcygeal raphe. Related laterally are, from above downward, the sigmoid colon in the pararectal fossa, the sacral

plexus, and the piriformis, coccygeus, and levator ani muscles. Anteriorly, the upper part of the rectum usually is separated from the cervix and posterior fornix of the vagina by coils of intestine that fill the rectouterine pouch. The posterior vaginal wall is directly anterior to the lower part of the rectum, from which it is separated by a thin layer of fascia named the rectovaginal septum. Although its existence has been controversial, the rectovaginal septum can be separated from the rectum by a cleavage space but is associated more closely with the vaginal fascia.[63]

Anal canal

The anal canal is the terminal segment of the large intestine, beginning at the lower flexure of the rectum as the intestinal tract passes through the pelvic diaphragm between the pubococcygeus portions of the levator ani muscles (Figure 1.4). The canal is 3–4 cm long, extending downward and backward to end at the anus. It is separated from the ischiorectal fossa by the levator ani muscle and is surrounded by an upper, involuntary internal anal sphincter and a lower, voluntary external anal sphincter. Anorectal varicosities or hemorrhoids are very frequent during pregnancy and arise from the venous plexus just deep to the surface lining of the anal canal. The upper part of the plexus drains into the hepatic portal system by the superior rectal (hemorrhoidal) vein. There are no valves in this system of veins, and the plexus therefore is affected particularly by the pressure from the growing uterus.

References

1. Bajka M, Manestar M, Hug J, et al. Detailed anatomy of the abdomen and pelvis of the visible human female. Clin Anat 2004; 17: 252–60.
2. Scott-Conner CE, Hedican S. Laparoscopic anatomy of the pelvis. Semin Laparosc Surg 1999; 6: 43–50.
3. Kluteke CG, Siegel CL. Functional female pelvic anatomy. Urol Clin North Am 1995; 22: 487–98.
4. Strohbehn K. Normal pelvic floor anatomy. Obstet Gynecol Clin North Am 1998; 25: 683–705.
5. Johnson MM. A study in surface anatomy with special reference to the position of the umbilicus. Anat Rec 1911; 5: 461–71.
6. Cox HT. The cleavage lines of the skin. Br J Surg 1941; 29: 234–40.
7. Tobin CE, Benjamin JA. Anatomic and clinical re-evaluation of Camper's, Scarpa's and Colles' fascia. Surg Gynecol Obstet 1949; 88: 545–59.
8. Forster DS. A note on Scarpa's fascia. J Anat 1937; 72: 130–1.
9. Howell AB. Anatomy of the inguinal region. Surgery 1939; 6: 653–62.
10. Rizk NN. A new description of the anterior abdominal wall in man and mammals. J Anat 1980; 131: 373–85.
11. Chouke KS. The constitution of the sheath of the rectus abdominis muscle. Anat Rec 1935; 61: 341–9.

12. Beaton LE, Anson BJ. The pyramidalis muscle: its occurrence and size in American whites and negroes. Am J Phys Anthropol 1939; 25: 261–9.

13. Milloy FJ, Anson BJ, McAfee DK. The rectus abdominis muscle and the epigastric arteries. Surg Gynecol Obstet 1960; 110: 293–302.

14. Nezhat CH, Nezhat F, Brill AI et al. Normal variations of abdominal and pelvic anatomy evaluated at laparoscopy. Obstet Gynecol 1999; 94: 238–42.

15. Begg RC. The urachus: its anatomy, histology and development. J Anat 1930; 64: 170–83.

16. Pfannenstiel J. Über die Vorteile des suprasymphysaren Fascien – Querschnitts für die gynakologischen Koliotomien, zugleich ein Beitrag zu der Indikationsstellung der Operationswege. Samml Klin Vortr (Neue Folge) Gynaekol 1900; 97: 1735–56.

17. Cherney LS. A modified transverse incision for low abdominal operations. Surg Gynecol Obstet 1941; 72: 92–5.

18. Gillespie EC. Principles of uterine growth in pregnancy. Am J Obstet Gynecol 1950; 59: 949–59.

19. Schwalm H, Dubrauszky V. The structure of the musculature of the human uterus – muscles and connected tissue. Am J Obstet Gynecol 1966; 94: 391–404.

20. Kipfer K. Das Muskelsystem des menschlichen Eileiters. Schweiz Med Wochenschr 1948; 78: 65–7.

21. Toth A. Studies on the muscular structure of the human uterus. Obstet Gynecol 1977; 49: 190–6.

22. Schwarz OH, Hawker WD. Hyperpasia and hypertrophy of the uterine vessels during various stages of pregnancy. Am J Obstet Gynecol 1950; 60: 967–76.

23. Danforth DN. The fibrous nature of the human cervix and its relation to the isthmic segment in gravid and nongravid uteri. Am J Obstet Gynecol 1947; 53: 541–60.

24. Danforth DN, Ivy AC. The lower uterine segment – its derivation and physiologic behavior. Am J Obstet Gynecol 1949; 57: 831–41.

25. Danforth DN, Chapman JCF. The incorporation of the isthmus uteri. Am J Obstet Gynecol 1950; 59: 979–88.

26. Lockwood CJ, Senyei AE, Dische MR et al. Fetal fibronectin in cervical and vaginal secretions as a predictor of preterm delivery. N Engl J Med 1991; 325: 669–74.

27. Waldeyer W. Topographical sketch of the lateral wall of the pelvic cavity, with special reference to the ovarian groove. J Anat Physiol 1897; 32: 1–10.

28. Tamakawa M, Murakami G, Takashima K et al. Fascial structures and autonomic nerves in the female pelvis: a study using microscopic slices and their corresponding histology. Anat Sci Int 2003; 78: 228–42.

29. O'Boyle AL, Woodman PJ, O'Boyle JD et al. Pelvic organ support in nulliparous pregnant and nonpregnant women: a case control study. Am J Obstet Gynecol 2002; 187: 99–102.

30. Ashley FL, Anson BJ. The hypogastric artery in American whites and negroes. Am J Phys Anthropol 1941; 28: 381–95.

31. Roberts WH, Krishingner GL. Comparative study of human internal iliac artery based on Adachi classification. Anat Rec 1967; 158: 191–6.

32. Itskovitz J, Lindenbaum ES, Brandes JM. Arterial anastomosis in the pregnant human uterus. Obstet Gynecol 1980; 55: 67–71.

33. Hodgkinson CP. Physiology of the ovarian veins during pregnancy. Obstet Gynecol 1953; l: 26–37.

34. Hadlock FP, Deter RL, Carpenter R et al. Hypervascularity of the uterine wall during pregnancy: incidence, sonographic appearance and obstetrical implications. J Clin Ultrasound 1980; 8: 399–403.

35. Nesselrod JP. An anatomic restudy of the pelvic lymphatics. Ann Surg 1936; 104: 905–16.

36. Wislocki GB, Dempsey EW. Remarks on the lymphatics of the reproductive tract of the female rhesus monkey (Macaca mulatta). Anat Rec 1939; 75: 341–63.

37. Nakanishi H, McLean J, Wood C et al. The role of sympathetic nerves in control of the nonpregnant and pregnant human uterus. J Reprod Med 1969; 2: 20–33.

38. Nakanishi H, Wansbrough H, Wood C. Postganglionic sympathetic nerve innervating human fallopian tube. Am J Physiol 1967; 213: 613–19.

39. Pereira A de S. A basis for sympathectomy for cancer of the cervix uteri. Arch Surg 1946; 52: 260–85.

40. Meigs JV. Excision of the superior hypogastric plexus (presacral nerve) for primary dysmenorrhea. Surg Gynecol Obstet 1939; 68: 723–32.

41. Tan IL, Stoker J, Zwamborn AW et al. Female pelvic floor: endovaginal MR imaging of normal anatomy. Radiology 1998; 206: 777–83.

42. Skinner D. The pelvic ureter. J R Soc Med 1978; 71: 541.

43. Brundenell M. The pelvic ureter. J R Soc Med 1977; 70: 188–90.

44. Hollinshead WH. Anatomy for Surgeons. Vol. 2, The Thorax, Abdomen, Pelvis (2nd edition). Harper and Row: New York, 1971.

45. Burch JC, Lavely HT. Avoidance of ureteral injury by routine palpation during total hysterectomy. Am J Surg 1950; 79: 819.

46. Niceley EP. Injuries of the ureters following pelvic surgery. J Urol 1950; 64: 283–9.

47. Remington JH. Prevention of ureteral injury in surgery of the pelvic colon. Dis Colon Rectum 1959; 2: 340–9.

48. Fischman JL, Weiner I, Wexler N. Relationship of distal ureter to obliterated hypogastric artery. Urology 1976; 8: 387–8.

49. Rubi RA, Sala NL. Ureteral function in pregnant women. III. Effect of different positions and of fetal delivery upon ureteral tonus. Am J Obstet Gynecol 1968; 101: 230–7.

50. Schulman A, Herlinger H. Urinary tract dilatation in pregnancy. Br J Radiol 1975; 48: 638–45.

51. Bellina JH, Dougherty CM, Mickal A. Pyeloureteral dilation and pregnancy. Am J Obstet Gynecol 1970; 108: 356–63.

52. Meigs N. The Wertheim operation for carcinoma of the cervix. Am J Obstet Gynecol 1945; 49: 542–53.

53. Michaels JP. Study of ureteral blood supply and its bearing on necrosis of the ureter following the Wertheim operation. Surg Gynecol Obstet 1948; 86: 36–44.

54. Daniel O, Shackman R. The blood supply of the human ureter in relation to ureterocolic anastomosis. Br J Urol 1952; 24: 334–43.

55. Ricci JV. Simplification of the Physick–Frank–Sellheim principle of extraperitoneal cesarean section. Am J Surg 1940; 47: 33–40.

56. Cruikshank SH, Kovac SR. The functional anatomy of the urethra: role of the pubourethral ligaments. Am J Obstet Gynecol 1997; 176: 1200–3.

57. Ricci JV, Thom CH, Kron WL. Cleavage planes in reconstructive vaginal plastic surgery. Am J Surg 1948; 76: 354–63.

58. Shehata R. The arterial supply of the urinary bladder. Acta Anat 1976; 96: 128–34.

59. Shehata R. Venous drainage of the urinary bladder. Acta Anat 1979; 105: 61–4.

60. Gosling JA, Dixon JS, Lendon RG. The autonomic innervation of the human male and female bladder neck and proximal urethra. J Urol 1977; 118: 302–5.

61. Ek A, Alm P, Andersson KE et al. Adrenergic and cholinergic nerves of the human urethra and urinary bladder. A histochemical study. Acta Physiol Scand 1977; 99: 345–52.

62. Frohlich B, Hotzinger H, Fritsch H. Tomographical anatomy of the pelvis, pelvic floor, and related structures. Clin Anat 1997; 10: 223–30.

63. Milley PS, Nichols DH. A correlative investigation of the human rectovaginal septum. Anat Rec 1969; 163: 443–51.

2 Topographic anatomy of the perineum, vulva, vagina, and surrounding structures

Shamshad H Gilani

Vulva

The region of the external genital organs, known as the vulva (or pudendum), lies in front of and below the pubis (Figure 2.1). It is the term applied to the mons pubis and labia majora, and the structures that lie between the labia (i.e., labia minora, vestibule of the vagina, clitoris, bulbs of the vestibule, and greater vestibular glands).

Mons pubis

The mons pubis is a rounded, median elevation lying anterior and inferior to the pubic bone. It consists mostly of a pad of fat. After puberty, the overlying skin is covered by coarse hair.

Labia majora

The labia majora are two large folds of skin that run downward and backward from the mons pubis. These elongated folds enclose between them the median pudendal cleft and are largely filled with subcutaneous fat. After puberty, their outer aspects are overlaid by pigmented skin that contains sweat and sebaceous glands and are covered by coarse hair. Their interval aspects are hairless and smooth. Anteriorly, the labia majora meet in the midline at the anterior labial commissure. They are not united posteriorly, but the forward projection of the tendinous center of the perineum into the pudendal cleft gives the appearance of a posterior labial commissure. Each labium majus contains the termination of the round ligament of the uterus.

Labia minora

The labia minora are fleshy, smaller lips located between the labia majora at either side of the opening of the vagina. The two lips are without hairs and are in contact with each other. Posteriorly, the labia minora may be united by a small fold of the skin called the frenulum of the labia. Anteriorly, each labium minus divides into a lateral and a medial part. The lateral part joins the corresponding one from the opposite side to form the prepuce of the clitoris. The medial parts unite below the clitoris to form the frenulum of the clitoris.

Vestibule of the vagina

The vestibule of the vagina is the space between the labia minora. It contains the orifices of the urethra, vagina, and ducts of the greater vestibular glands. The external urethral orifice (meatus) is located about 2 cm or more behind the glans clitoris and immediately in front of the vaginal orifice. It is usually a median slit with slightly everted margins. The vaginal orifice is considerably larger than the urethral one and is also a median cleft. Its appearance and size depend upon the condition of the hymen, which is a thin fold of mucous membrane that partially or sometimes wholly occludes the vaginal orifice. It varies much in shape and extent.

Clitoris

The clitoris lies between the anterior ends of the labia minora. The parts of the labia minora lying anterior to the clitoris form

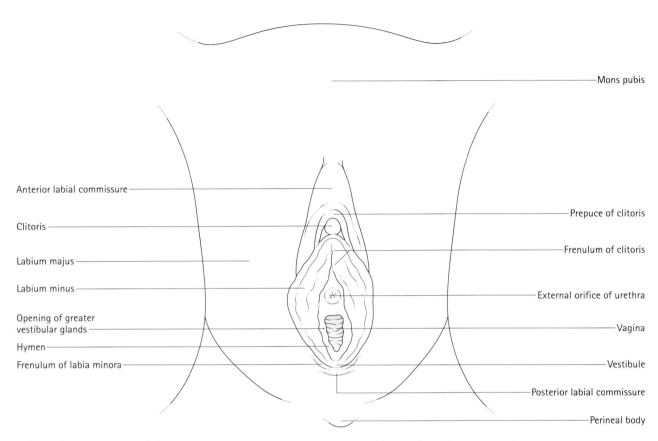

Figure 2.1 Vulva showing mons pubis, labia majora, labia minora, vestibule, glans clitoris, and the opening of the greater vestibular glands.

the prepuce of the clitoris, whereas the parts lying posterior to it form the frenulum. The clitoris consists mainly of erectile tissue and is capable of enlargement like the penis as a result of engorgement with blood. It is composed of two corpora cavernosa which form the body of the clitoris, which is about 2.5 cm long. The corpora cavernosa are enclosed by a fibrous envelope and are separated from each other by an incomplete septum. The body of the clitoris separates posteriorly into two crura, each of which is attached to its respective ischiopubic ramus. The glans of the clitoris is the small elevation on the free end of the body. It also is composed of erectile tissue and, like the glans of the penis, is covered by sensitive epithelium. The suspensory ligament of the clitoris connects the organ to the front of the pubic symphysis.

Bulbs of the vestibule

The bulbs of the vestibule are two elongated masses of erectile tissue, one lying at each side of the vaginal opening under the bulbospongiosus muscle. They are narrow in front where they unite with each other to form a thin strand which is connected to the underside of the glans clitoris. Their posterior ends are broad and in contact with the greater vestibular glands.

Greater vestibular glands

The greater vestibular glands are small ovoid bodies, one located on each side of the vaginal vestibule posterolateral to the vaginal orifice. The duct of each gland opens into the groove between the labium minus and the attached margin of the hymen. During sexual intercourse, the greater vestibular glands are compressed and secrete mucus which lubricates the vagina. There are many smaller, lesser vestibular glands on each side of the vestibule which open between the urethral and vaginal orifices.

Perineum

The perineum is a diamond-shaped area which forms the most inferior part of the trunk (Figure 2.2). It extends from the symphysis pubis, anteriorly, to the sacrum and the tip of the coccyx, posteriorly, with an ischial tuberosity on each lateral side. Its superior limit is the pelvic diaphragm consisting of the levator ani and coccygeus muscles. It is restricted to the region immediately around and between the anal and vaginal orifices. The perineum is divided into two parts, the urogenital region and the anal region. The urogenital region is anterior to an imaginary horizontal line joining the midpoints of the two ischial tuberosities. The anal region is posterior to this line.

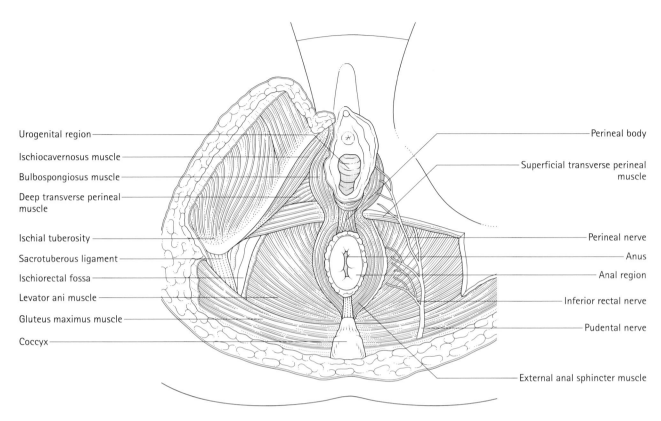

Urogenital region
Ischiocavernosus muscle
Bulbospongiosus muscle
Deep transverse perineal muscle
Ischial tuberosity
Sacrotuberous ligament
Ischiorectal fossa
Levator ani muscle
Gluteus maximus muscle
Coccyx

Perineal body
Superficial transverse perineal muscle
Perineal nerve
Anus
Anal region
Inferior rectal nerve
Pudental nerve
External anal sphincter muscle

Figure 2.2 Female perineum showing urogenital and anal regions.

The perineal body or tendinous center of the perineum is a fibromuscular mass that is located in the median plane between the anal canal and the lower vagina. It contains smooth and skeletal muscle fibers bound with elastic and collagenous tissue. Attached to it are the superficial and deep transverse perineal, the bulbospongiosus, the levator ani, and the external anal sphincter muscles. The superficial and deep perineal fasciae and the superior and inferior fasciae of the urogenital diaphragm blend with it.

Urogenital region

The urogenital region contains the external genital organs and the associated muscles and glands. This region is divided into a superficial and a deep perineal compartment.

Superficial perineal compartment

The superficial compartment lies superficial to the inferior layer of fascia of the urogenital diaphragm and contains on each side the bulbospongiosus muscle with the underlying bulb of the vestibule, the ischiocavernosus muscle with the underlying crus of the clitoris, the superficial transverse perineal muscle, and the greater vestibular gland. All of the muscles in the superficial compartment are supplied by the perineal branch of the pudendal nerve.

Bulbospongiosus muscle
This muscle arises from the tendinous center of the perineum and passes forward around the lower part of the vagina covering the bulb of the vestibule. It is inserted partly into the side of the pubic arch and partly into the dorsum and body of the clitoris. The muscle with its counterpart on the other side constricts the vagina.

Ischiocavernosus muscle
This muscle originates from the inner surface of the ramus of the ischium and inserts on the lower and medial aspects of the crus of the clitoris. It helps to maintain erection of the clitoris by compressing the crus and thus retarding the flow of blood from the clitoris.

Superficial transverse perineal muscle
This muscle arises from the lower part of the inner surface of the ramus of the ischium adjacent to the tuberosity and inserts into the tendinous center of the perineum. It is poorly developed, and its action is insignificant.

Deep perineal compartment

The deep compartment is enclosed between the superior and inferior layers of fascia of the urogenital diaphragm. The inferior layer of fascia also is called the perineal membrane. The deep compartment contains the deep transverse perineal and sphincter urethrae muscles and is traversed by the urethra and vagina (Figure 2.2). Both muscles are innervated by the perineal branch of the pudendal nerve. Their arrangement varies considerably, and often they are poorly developed.

Deep transverse perineal muscle
This muscle arises from the inner surface of the ramus of the ischium. Its anterior fibers insert into the lateral wall of the vagina, and its posterior fibers insert into the tendinous center of the perineum. It helps fix the tendinous center.

Sphincter urethrae muscle
This muscle arises from the inner surface of the inferior ramus of the pubis. Most of its fibers insert into the lateral wall of the vagina, but a few pass in front of the urethra and between the urethra and vagina. Since the urethra and vagina are fused inferiorly, the fibers of the sphincter urethrae muscle do not surround the urethra completely.

The superior fascia of the urogenital diaphragm is indistinct, but the inferior fascia is relatively dense and strong. The deep compartment contains the internal pudendal vessels, the dorsal nerve of the clitoris, and branches of the perineal nerve that supply the two muscles located there.

Anal region

The anal region contains the anus, the external anal sphincter muscle, and the ischiorectal fossa (Figure 2.1). The anal canal passes through the pelvic diaphragm and opens onto the surface of the perineum as the anus. The skin around the anus is pigmented and contains sweat and sebaceous glands.

The external anal sphincter muscle surrounds that part of the anal canal which is located in the anal triangle below the pelvic diaphragm. This muscle forms a broad band on each side of the anal canal and is divided into three parts: subcutaneous, superficial, and deep. The external anal sphincter muscle is under voluntary control and is supplied mainly by the inferior rectal nerve. The anterior portion of the muscle is innervated by the perineal division of the pudendal nerve. An additional innervation may be the perineal branch of the forth sacral nerve. The coccygeal nerve can be found near the posterior part of the external anal sphincter muscle close to where this muscle attaches to the coccyx. It is sensory to the skin over the coccyx.

The ischiorectal fossa is a wedge-shaped space located between the skin of the anal region below and the levator ani muscle above. It is filled with fat which allows the rectum and anal canal to distend during the passage of feces. The ischiorectal fossa is not limited to the anal region but extends anteriorly and posteriorly. Anteriorly, when the fossa reaches the posterior border of the urogenital diaphragm, it extends forward above the diaphragm but below the levator ani muscle. When the surfaces of these two structures meet near the symphysis pubis, the fossa is obliterated. Posteriorly, the fossa extends above the gluteus maximus muscle to the sacrotuberous ligament. Laterally, it is limited by the ischium and the fascia covering the inferior part of the obturator internus muscle. The fossa extends medially to the levator ani and external anal sphincter muscles which separate the fossa from the rectum and anal canal.

In addition to the ischiorectal pad of fat, the ischiorectal fossa contains branches of the internal pudendal vessels and pudendal nerve that run in its lateral wall in a channel through the obturator fascia called the pudendal canal. Posteriorly, these vessels and this nerve give off the inferior rectal (hemorrhoidal) vessels and nerve which cross the fossa to supply the external anal sphincter muscle and the skin and fascia around the anus. Other cutaneous branches, such as the perforating branch of the second and third sacral nerves and the perineal branch of the fourth sacral nerve, also pass through the ischiorectal fossa.

Nerves and vessels of the perineum

The pudendal nerve is the principal nerve to the perineum and divides into three terminal branches. The nerve contains fibers from S2, S3, and S4 spinal cord segments and leaves the pelvis through the greater sciatic (ischiatic) foramen. It passes behind the spine of the ischium and enters the ischiorectal fossa through the lesser sciatic (ischiatic) foramen. The pudendal nerve divides near the ischial spine into three branches: (1) the inferior rectal nerve, which crosses the ischiorectal fossa and innervates the external anal sphincter muscle, the skin around the anus, and the lining of the anal canal below the pectinate line; (2) the perineal nerve, which enters the urogenital region and divides into superficial and deep branches (the superficial perineal branch gives posterior labial branches to the labia majora and lower vagina, whereas the deep perineal branch supplies the levator ani and external anal sphincter muscles, the muscles of the superficial and deep perineal compartments, and the bulb of the vestibule); and (3) the dorsal nerve of the clitoris, which runs forward in the urogenital diaphragm, and then passes through the inferior layer to the dorsum of the clitoris.

The internal pudendal artery is the principal artery to the perineum, where it gives off many branches. It arises from the internal iliac artery and leaves the pelvic cavity by passing out the greater sciatic foramen. It crosses behind the spine of the ischium and enters the pudendal canal in the lateral wall of the ischiorectal fossa through the lesser sciatic foramen. Its inferior rectal branch crosses the ischiorectal fossa to the muscles and skin around the anal canal. The perineal branch enters the superficial perineal compartment to supply the structures there and continues as posterior labial branches to the labium majus and minus. The internal pudendal artery enters the deep perineal compartment, where it gives branches to the bulb of the vestibule, urethra, and greater vestibular gland. It terminates near the pubic symphysis by dividing into the deep and dorsal arteries to the clitoris.

The veins primarily accompany the arteries and drain into the internal iliac vein. An exception is the deep dorsal vein of the clitoris, which passes entirely or mainly into the pelvis through a gap in the perineal membrane to the vesical venous plexus.

The lymph vessels from the perineum course mainly to the superficial inguinal lymph nodes, but some also pass to the deep inguinal nodes. A few lymph vessels from the clitoris follow the deep dorsal vein to join lymphatics from the upper part of the urethra and bladder to empty into the internal iliac nodes.

Vagina

The vagina is the female organ of copulation, extending from the uterus to the vestibule. Its walls are distensible and serve as the lower end of the birth canal. The upper part of the vagina is located in the pelvic cavity and the lower part lies in the perineum. The longitudinal axes of the vagina and uterus are almost at right angles. The vagina extends forward and downward in a plane parallel to that of the pelvic inlet. This plane is about 60° from the horizontal. The vagina forms an angle of about 90° with the uterus.

The anterior and posterior walls of the vagina are in contact with each other below the entrance of the cervix. The anterior wall is about 7 cm in length; the posterior wall is 2.5–3 cm longer. The lateral walls are attached above to the cardinal ligament and below this to the pelvic diaphragm. The vaginal lumen surrounding the cervix forms a recess called the fornix. Since more of the posterior part of the cervix enters the vagina than the anterior part, the posterior fornix is deeper than the anterior fornix. The vaginal recess lateral to the cervix is called the lateral fornix.

The opening of the vagina into the vestibule is partially covered by the hymen. After the hymen ruptures, small fragments remain attached to its margin called hymenal caruncles.

Relationship to surrounding structures

Anteriorly
The upper part of the vagina is related to the base of the urinary bladder, the terminal parts of the ureter, and the urethra, whose lower half is actually embedded in the vaginal wall. The vagina is connected to the pubis by the pubovesical ligament.

Posteriorly
The upper third of the vagina lies close to the rectouterine peritoneal pouch (pouch of Douglas); below this, it is adjacent to the ampulla of the rectum. The lower part is related to the tendinous center of the perineum, which separates it from the anal canal.

Laterally
The ureter and uterine vessels are closely related to this part of the vagina. More inferiorly, the pubococcygeal portion of the levator ani muscle, the greater vestibular gland, the bulb of the vestibule, and the bulbospongiosus muscle are near. The levator ani muscles together act as a sphincter of the vagina by decreasing the size of the lumen about 3 cm above the orifice.

The uppermost part of the vagina is supplied by a branch of the uterine artery. The lowermost part has a blood supply from the internal pudendal artery. The middle portion of the vagina may be supplied by vaginal branches from the internal iliac, inferior vesical, and middle rectal arteries. The vessels anastomose on and in the vaginal wall, forming a longitudinal channel anteriorly and posteriorly known as the azygos artery. All the arteries to the vagina directly or indirectly originate from the internal iliac artery.

The veins from the vagina drain into a vaginal venous plexus, then upward to the uterine plexus, and then to the internal iliac vein. The lymphatics from the upper part of the vagina accompany the uterine artery and drain to the external and internal iliac nodes. From the middle part, the lymph vessels accompany the vaginal artery and drain to the internal iliac nodes. Lymph from the lower part of the vagina adjacent to the hymen drains into the superficial inguinal nodes.

The nerves to the upper vagina are derived from the uterovaginal portion of the hypogastric plexus. Parasympathetic, sympathetic, and afferent fibers pass through this plexus to supply the cervix and superior part of the vagina. The lowermost part of the vagina receives its innervation from the pudendal nerve, which has its origin from the same sacral nerves (S2, S3, and S4) that supply the viscera in the pelvis.

For a more extensive review of the anatomic relationships of the female reproductive organs, see Clemente,[1] Hollinshead,[2] Leeson and Leeson,[3] Moore,[4] and Snell.[5]

References

1. Clemente CD. Gray's Anatomy (30th edition) Lea & Febiger: Philadelphia, 1985.
2. Hollinshead WH. Textbook of Anatomy (5th edition) Lippincott Williams & Wilkins: Baltimore, MD, 1997.
3. Leeson CT, Leeson TS. Human Structure (2nd edition) Elsevier: New York, 1989.
4. Moore KL. Clinically Oriented Anatomy (4th edition) Lippincott Williams & Wilkins: Baltimore, MD, 1999.
5. Snell RS. Clinical Anatomy (7th edition) Lippincott Williams & Wilkins: Baltimore, MD, 2003.

3 Clinical pelvimetry

Elaine K Diegmann and Rhonda Nichols

Power, passenger, and passage; this is the triad that controls the birth process. Unaffected by the ebbs and tides of modern technology, the dimensions of the bony pelvis remain constant. Therefore, it is of utmost importance to understand the role of the pelvis and to commit to memory the types, the dimensions, and prognosis for birth of the basic pelvic types, since the practitioner will be making decisions regarding the route of birth that may have grave consequences for mother and infant. Therefore, this chapter will focus on the bony pelvic structures, the best predictors of birth outcomes. Knowledge of pelvic adequacy is an essential component in the decision to allow a trial of labor and plan for a vaginal birth.

Pelvic anatomy

The pelvis is composed of the two innominate bones (each of which is further divided into the ilium, the ischium, and the pubis), the sacrum and the coccyx (Figure 3.1).

Each innominate bone has several points of obstetric significance. The ilium contains the greater sacrosciatic notch between the inferior iliac spine and the ischial spine. The ischium contains the ischial spine, the landmark for the smallest pelvic diameter, the ischial tuberosity, located at the lowest border of the ischium; and the lesser sacrosciatic notch housed between them. The side walls of the ischium can be slightly convergent in the normal pelvis.

The pubis joins the two innominate bones anteriorly to form the symphysis pubis, the lower border of which serves as the apex of the pubic arch. The inferior pubic rami form the

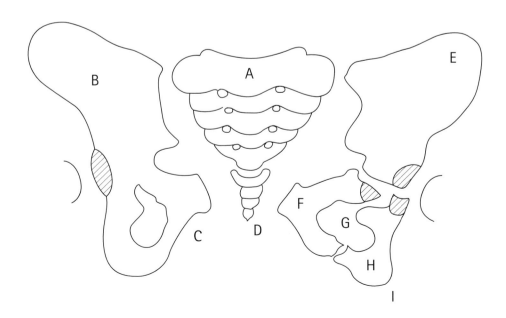

Figure 3.1 Pelvic bones: (A) sacrum; (B) innominate bone; (C) inferior rami; (D) coccyx; (E) ilium; (F) pubis; (G) ischial spine; (H) ischium; (I) ischial tuberosity.

side walls of this significant anatomic structure, the angle of which is a predictor of successful vaginal birth.

The sacrum comprises the posterior pelvic boundary. It has five fused vertebrae, the angle and inclination of which predict birth outcome. The sacral promontory is the anterior surface of the first sacral vertebra. It is a significant obstetric landmark of the pelvis.

The coccyx, composed of four vestigial vertebrae, forming the 'tail bone', articulates with the sacrum.

Four joints articulate with the pelvic bones. Laterally, the sacroiliac joints join the sacrum to the two innominate bones at the iliac portions. Anteriorly, the symphysis connects the pubic portions of the innominate bones. Posteriorly, the sacrococcygeal joint joins the sacrum and the coccyx.

The sacrospinous ligament spans the greater sacrosciatic notch from the junction of the fifth sacral and first coccygeal vertebrae to the ischial spine. The sacrosciatic notch is a landmark in determining the posterior capacity of the pelvis. The sacrotuberous ligament is attached to the level of the third, fourth, and fifth sacral vertebrae posteriorly and to the ischial tuberosities anteriorly. The two ligaments form the side walls of Alcock's canal, through which the pudendal nerve passes.

The obstetric pelvis

The pelvis is divided into the false and the true pelvis. The linea terminalis, also known as the iliopectinal line, is the structural boundary which separates the two. The false pelvis provides support for the abdominal and pelvic organs and has no obstetric significance. The true pelvis is located beneath the false pelvis and is of paramount importance to the birth process. As the fetus enters the pelvis, the pelvic axis curves gradually downward and backward. Once the fetus traverses the midpelvis, the axis is gradually directed downward and forward.

There are four planes of the pelvis through which the passenger (fetus) must pass: the pelvic inlet, the plane of greatest pelvic dimensions, the plane of least pelvic dimensions, and the pelvic outlet.

The pelvic inlet is shaped like a rounded heart. Its boundaries are the sacral promontory, the iliopectinal line, and the upper aspect of the symphysis pubis. The anteroposterior diameter, known as the anatomic (true) conjugate, extends from the top of the symphysis to the sacral promontory and measures 11.5 cm. It has no obstetric relevance, since it is not the smallest diameter of the inlet. The anteroposterior diameter, known as the obstetric conjugate, is the shortest distance between the sacral promontory and the posterosuperior surface of the symphysis pubis. It should measure at least 10 cm and is the shortest anteroposterior diameter of the pelvis through which the presenting part must pass. Since this distance cannot be measured clinically, the diagonal conjugate is used to estimate it. The diagonal conjugate, which can be determined by bimanual examination, is measured from the lower margin of the symphysis to the sacral promontory. It usually measures 12.5 cm or more. By subtracting 1–1.5 cm (depending on the inclination of the symphysis), the obstetric conjugate can be estimated. The normal transverse diameter is 13 cm or more at the inlet. The average oblique diameter is 12.5 cm. Right/left designation of the oblique diameters is determined by the sacral crest.

The midpelvis has two planes. The plane of greatest dimensions runs from the middle of the symphysis through the second and third sacral vertebrae. It is the roomiest plane and, therefore, does not have obstetric significance. On the other hand, the plane of least dimensions is very important obstetrically, since it is the smallest plane of the pelvis, accounting for most cases of arrest of labor. This plane circles at the level of the ischial spines, the apex of the pubic arch, and the fourth and fifth sacral vertebrae (Figure 3.2).

The anteroposterior diameter of the midpelvis extends from the fourth and fifth sacral vertebrae to the lower margin of the symphysis. It usually measures 11.5 cm. The transverse diameter, also known as the bispinous diameter, is the smallest midplane measurement through which the fetus must travel. A less than 10.5 cm measurement of this diameter may have adverse effects on the birth progress. The posterior segment of the midpelvis is predictive of the birth outcome. This diameter extends from the midpoint between the ischial spines to the junction of the fourth and fifth sacral vertebrae. It should measure 4.5 cm or more.

The pelvic outlet is diamond shaped. It has been described as two triangles with the bituberous diameter as the common base.

Anteriorly, the landmarks are the lower margin of the symphysis pubis, the pubic rami, and the tuberosities. Posteriorly, the landmarks are the sacrotuberous ligaments and the sacrococcygeal joint. Again, there are two anteroposterior diameters which must be addressed. The anatomic anteroposterior diameter is measured from the apex of the pubic arch to the tip of the coccyx. This diameter measures only about 9.5 cm but is not considered in the determination of pelvic capacity, since the

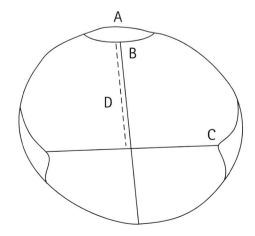

Figure 3.2 Pelvic midplane: (A) sacrum; (B) anteroposterior diameter; (C) bispinous diameter; (D) posterosagittal diameter.

coccyx is mobile and is pushed backward at the time of birth. Of clinical significance is the obstetric anteroposterior diameter. It extends from the lower border of the symphysis to the sacro-coccygeal joint and measures 11.5 cm. The transverse (or bituberous) diameter is the distance between the ischial tuberosities. It measures an average of 11 cm. In the pelvic outlet, both the anterior and posterior sagittal diameters are important. The posterior sagittal diameter extends from the midpoint between the ischial tuberosities to the sacro-coccygeal joint and measures 9 cm. The anterior sagittal diameter extends from the same point to the apex of the pubic arch and measures 6 cm.

Pelvic shapes

There are four basic pelvic shapes classified by Caldwell and Moloy,[1,2] recognized authorities on pelvic architecture. The four types are gynecoid, android, anthropoid, and platypelloid.[3]

The gynecoid pelvis is the typical female type configuration. Its inlet is rounded in shape. The measurements of this pelvic type reflect the optimum dimensions of the pelvic planes. The average inlet measurements include the obstetric conjugate (11 cm), the diagonal conjugate (12.5 cm), and the transverse diameter (13 cm). The midplane measurements include the anteroposterior diameter (12 cm), the transverse diameter (bispinous) (10.5 cm), and the posterosagittal diameter (4.5 cm). The greater sacrosciatic notch is wide and short, the ischial spines are blunt and not encroaching, and the sacrum is concave and inclined backward. The side walls of the pelvis are straight. The postero-sagittal diameter is spacious, encouraging the passage of the fetus through the midpelvis without obstruction. The measurements of the outlet include the anteroposterior diameter (11.5 cm) and the transverse diameter (bituberous) (11 cm). The pubic arch is wide: about 90° at its apex. The inferior rami are short and gently splay outward. The fetal head typically enters this pelvic type in the transverse diameter. Labor usually progresses without complications and culminates in spontaneous vaginal birth (Figure 3.3).

The android pelvis is the male-type configuration. Its inlet is wedge shaped, with the sacral promontory deeply encroaching on the anteroposterior diameter of this plane, reducing the posterosagittal diameter as well. The transverse diameter is usually adequate, but the anterior pelvis is sharply angulated. In the midpelvis the anteroposterior and the transverse diameters are reduced. The spines are usually prominent and encroaching. This further reduces the already small midpelvic diameter. The side walls are convergent. This reduces the capacity of the midplane as well as that of the outlet. The sacrum is flat, narrow, thick, and inclined forward. The greater sacrosciatic notch is narrow and high. This combination reduces the capacity of the posterior midpelvis and diminishes the posterosagittal diameter. Coupled with the angulation of the anterior pelvis, the dimensions of the midpelvis are so reduced that the fetal head may not be able to engage. The measurements of the outlet may also be reduced. The anteroposterior diameter is short, due to the flatness of the sacral curve. The transverse or bituberous diameter is decreased. The pubic arch is narrow, and the inferior rami are long and straight. The angle of the arch is less than 90°. Occipitoposterior and transverse rotations of the vertex are common with this pelvic type. In occipitoposterior positions, especially because the head is often not well flexed until it hits the pelvic floor, engagement is difficult. Thus, the progression of labor may be delayed. If the head negotiates the inlet in the transverse position, deep transverse arrest in the midplane is common. The android pelvis frequently is the source of labor dystocia requiring operative delivery (Figure 3.4).

The anthropoid pelvis is commonly known as the ape-like pelvis. Its inlet is a long oval. All the planes of this pelvis are adequate. The anteroposterior diameter of the inlet usually is long. The transverse diameter tends to be the least adequate. The sagittal diameters are deep. In the midplane, again, the anteroposterior diameter generally is long and the transverse diameter adequate. The posterosagittal measurement is deep. The greater sacrosciatic notch is wide and long, and the sacrum is narrow, long, and inclined backward. The spines are variable, and the side walls usually are straight. The measurements of the outlet are also adequate. The anteroposterior measurement is

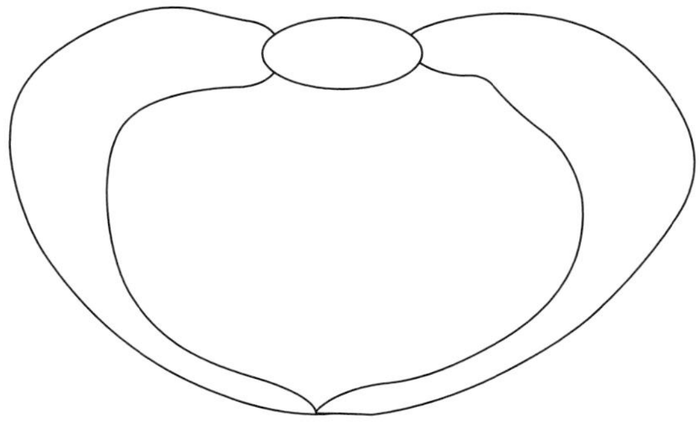

Figure 3.3 Gynecoid pelvis.

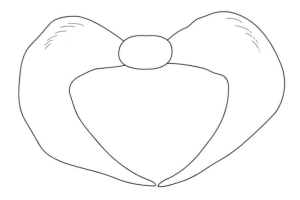

Figure 3.4 Android pelvis.

the longest. The pubic arch may be somewhat narrow, depending upon the length and angulation of the inferior rami. The fetal head often engages in the oblique diameter. Occipitoposterior rotation of the vertex is common. Face presentation is prevalent in this pelvic type. The progress of labor is usually normal, and the prognosis for vaginal birth is good (Figure 3.5).

The platypelloid pelvis is commonly known as the flat pelvis. Its inlet is a horizontal oval. The antero-posterior diameter is short, and the antero- and posterosagittal diameters are shallow. The transverse diameter is wide. The midplane has the same characteristics: a short anteroposterior diameter, a long transverse diameter, and reduced antero- and posterosagittal diameters. The greater sacrosciatic notch is wide and shallow. The sacrum is wide and deeply curved, with sharp angulation. The sacral vertebrae tend to be thick. The side walls are straight or divergent.

The outlet measurements mirror the other planes, the anteroposterior diameter being short, and the pubic arch wide. The inferior pubic rami are also wide, with decreased angulation. The fetal head engages in transverse rotation, but, due to the reduced anteroposterior dimensions, cannot rotate to complete the mechanisms of labor. Thus, deep transverse arrest often occurs. The prognosis for vaginal birth is unfavorable, and cesarean section is a frequent mode of delivery (Figure 3.6). The above quoted pelvic configurations represent the pure prototypes. In any individual gravida, these types may be mixed to various extents.

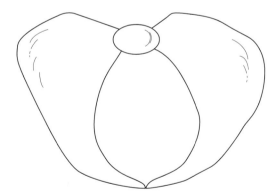

Figure 3.5 Anthropoid pelvis.

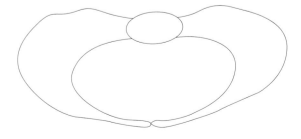

Figure 3.6 Platypelloid pelvis.

Clinical pelvimetry

Due to the potential hazards associated with x-rays, radiologic examinations have little place in obstetric practice today. Computed tomography (CT) scanners can be utilized to calculate pelvic measurements, with negligible amounts of radiation to mother and fetus, but at great expense.[4] However, the obstetrician and the nurse midwife have at their fingertips an effective and readily available tool with few working parts to break down: clinical pelvimetry.[5–7] All the clinician needs is a pair of gloves and awareness of a few measurements.

It is important to measure from the angle of the thumb to the third finger for the determination of the diagonal conjugate. The measurement should be made in centimeters. The width of the fist of the examining hand should also be measured in centimeters. This measurement will assist in determining the bituberous diameter.

There are several sequences for doing a clinical pelvimetry. One's preference is the main prerequisite for choosing a particular sequence. As with all procedures, the clinician should choose one and refine his or her skills. An explanation to the patient both before and during the examination is of paramount importance. The patient should empty her bladder prior to the examination and be instructed not to hold her breath or lift her head during the procedure in order to avoid tension of the vaginal muscles. Table 3.1 illustrates one effective technique. Documentation for clinical pelvimetry should be succinct, as follows:

- pubic arch
- angle of symphysis
- notch
- spines
- side walls
- sacrum
- coccyx
- diagonal conjugate measured by the examining finger
- obstetric conjugate (calculated)
- bituberous diameter measured by the fist.

Knowledge of pelvic measurements and a sequential technique for clinical pelvimetry should facilitate the assessment of pelvic capacity and the formulation of a prognosis for vaginal birth. The size of the examiner's hand and the length of the fingers probably have little effect on the accuracy of clinical pelvimetry. If they do, one's reach can be extended by the placement of a thimble on the middle finger under the glove. Knowledge of pelvic architecture and expertise in recognizing the pelvic landmarks are important. The practitioner who has small hands must be more inventive in hand placement and must learn to position patients to the best advantage. One should remember that, when positioning the hand to begin the examination, the middle and index fingers should be straight, with the thumb extended at greater than 90°. The ring finger and the pinky should be flexed across the palm, with the first and second joints extended. This position decreases the angulation of the hand

Table 3.1 Sequence for performing clinical pelvimetry

Technique	Findings
1. Slide the index and middle fingers into the vagina and evaluate the width of the subpubic arch in FB. Then slide fingers up along the *symphysis* to determine the angle of the pubic bones (separate fingers slightly to 'splint' urethra, thereby eliminating discomfort).	Slide arch: average about 2 FB. Angle of the symphysis: about 90°.
2. Next outline the sacrosciatic notch. Feel the *sacrospinous ligament* by placing the gloved fingers between the ischial spine and the lateral edge of the sacrum	Sacrosciatic notch: note depth; it gives clue to pelvic type. Sacrospinous ligament: short, average, or long.
3. Continue down to the back until reaching the *ischial spine.* Determine its prominence.	Ischial spines: blunt, defined, palpable, prominent, sharp, encroaching. Side wall slope: convergent, straight, divergent.
4. Proceed either to left or right and palpate the side walls to determine their splay. The splay is determined by following a line from the point of origin of the widest transverse diameter of the inlet downward to the inner aspect of the tuberosity. (Placing the thumb or the examining hand on the patient's buttocks over the tuberosity may increase spatial conceptualization.)	
5. Sweep the fingers down the sacrum, noting its curvature. Note angle and mobility of coccyx.	Straight, concave or convex, forward, or backward inclination. Coccyx mobile or rigid.
6. Measure the diagonal conjugate. Keep vaginal hand relaxed by placing your corresponding foot on a stool and rest your arm against your thigh or hip if comfortable. Exert downward pressure on the perineum and keep away from the symphysis to prevent undue discomfort to the patient. With the examining fingers directed upward at an acute angle toward the upper sacrurn and with the longest finger touching the sacral vertebrae, walk up the sacrum until the promontory is reached or fingers lose contact with the sacrum. Raise fingers to the symphysis. Drop elbow and mark off on your hand the point that touches the symphysis. Measure this distance on a ruler or cm scale. This measurement is done last, since it usually causes discomfort and may increase patient's emotional tension.	Exact measurement in cm if reached. Greater than your measurement limit if not reached.
7. The *ischial tuberosities* are measured by following the descending rami down to the tuberosities and placing your fist between them.	Average, 10 cm. Note exact measurement in cm if your fist fits snugly between the tuberosities. Chart greater-than-fist measurement if there is room between your fist and the bones.

FB: Finger breadth.

between the extended middle finger and the flexed first and second fingers, allowing partial admission of these two fingers posteriorly into the vagina to increase the reach of the examining fingers. When positioning the patient, ask her to place her fists under her buttocks. This will decrease the angle between the pelvis and the examining table and thus increase the efficiency of the small examining hand.

Until the 1950s, assessment of the gravida's pelvic capacity by external measurements was a routine procedure. It was discarded almost overnight when an anonymous 'expert' declared that 'the size of the dining room cannot be determined by measuring the outside walls of the house'. Members of the profession overlooked that, whereas a house may contain as many as 20 chambers, the various pelvic bones surround only one. Thus, in keeping with the experience of early twentieth-century obstetricians, external pelvic measurements may provide useful information about a woman's pelvic dimensions. When the technique was discarded, x-ray pelvimetry was a routine procedure and accurate enough to make external pelvimetry unnecessary. Today, since x-ray pelvimetry is not considered appropriate in current practice, only practitioners who have mastered the technique of clinical pelvimetry can perform accurate pelvic assessments. Therefore, the obstetric calipers may deserve to be reintroduced into clinical practice as a practical method for assessing a woman's pelvis with acceptable accuracy (Figure 3.7).

The external pelvic diameters to be measured are indicated in Table 3.2. The tips of the arms of the instrument are to be placed onto the quoted anatomic points. Representing the best palpable pelvic prominence (anterosuperior spines) and the most distant points of the pelvic side walls (iliac crests), the critical anatomic landmarks are easily identifiable. The same is true for the anteroposterior diameter. The predictive value of 'normal', 'borderline', and 'contracted' pelvic measurements approaches that obtainable by internal manual pelvimetry performed by an experienced examiner. This alternative method can be helpful for those accoucheurs who are not comfortable with their manual skills in clinical pelvimetry as well as for those who may utilize it to check their accuracy. It can be invaluable in a clinical situation when a previously unregistered gravida is hospitalized after premature rupture of the membranes, prior to the onset of labor, a situation which renders manual pelvimetry contraindicated.

Table 3.2 External pelvic diameters

Measurable pelvic diameter	Normal pelvis	Borderline pelvis	Contracted pelvis
Distance between the anterosuperior iliac spines	26 cm or more	23–25 cm	Less than 23 cm
Distance between the iliac crests	29 cm or more	26–28 cm	Less than 26 cm
Distance between the middle of the symphysis and the deepest point of Michaelis's rhomboid	20 cm or more	18–19 cm	Less than 18 cm

With considerable approximation, these pelvic measurements permit the identification of various pelvic types as well as pelvic adequacy or inadequacy.

References

1. Caldwell WE, Moloy HC. Anatomical variations in the female pelvis and their effect on labor with a suggested classification. Am J Obstet Gynecol 1933; 26: 479.
2. Steer C. Moloy's Evaluation of the Pelvis in Obstetrics. Plenum Medical Book: New York, 1975, pp. 793–831.
3. Beck A, Rosenthal A. Pelvic variations – contracted pelves. In: Obstetrical Practice, p. 793. Williams & Wilkins: Baltimore, MD, 1958.
4. Lenke RR, Sherman WP. Computed tomographic pelvimetry. J Reprod Med 1996; 31: 958–60.
5. Cunningham FG, Gant NF, Leveno K et al. Williams' Obstetrics (21st edition), p. 51. McGraw-Hill: New York, 2001, pp. 51–61.
6. Suono S, Saarikoski S, Raty E, Vohlonen I. Clinical assessment of the pelvic cavity and outlet. Arch Gynecol 1986; 239: 11–16.
7. Varney H, Kriebs J, Gegor C. Varney's Midwifery (4th Edition), p. 1205. Jones & Bartlett: Boston, MA, 2004.

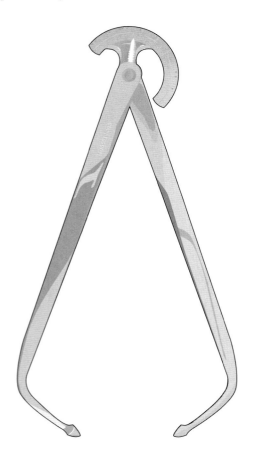

Figure 3.7 Obstetric calipers.

4 First-trimester embryofetoscopy

E Albert Reece and Anthony M Vintzileos

First-trimester embryofetoscopy is a technique that allows visualization and access to the developing embryo/fetus and its environment. The procedure can be performed by the introduction of an endoscope into the extracoelomic space transcervically or transabdominally. The procedure uses high-resolution fiber-optic equipment attached to a camera for direct visualization of the embryo/fetus. The need for first-trimester embryofetoscopy has been created by the recent technological advances of ultrasound for first-trimester prenatal diagnosis. Improved high-resolution of transvaginal ultrasound has made possible the morphologic evaluation of a developing embryo/fetus. However, certain fetal anomalies cannot be diagnosed with certainty by using ultrasound alone. Direct visualization of the fetus may be necessary to confirm some ultrasonically diagnosed fetal anomalies in the first trimester of pregnancy, and also to help in the management in selected families affected by recurrent genetic syndromes with recognizable external fetal abnormalities. An additional reason for introducing first-trimester embryofetoscopy is its potential for early in utero therapy, opening the way of a new era of early pregnancy intervention.

History

Transcervical fetal visualization in three early pregnancies was first reported by Westin in 1954,[1] using the McCarthy panendoscope. The gestational ages were not stated by the author, and measurements of fetal length suggested that these pregnancies were in the second trimester. It is unclear, however, whether fetal size had been overestimated by the varying magnification factor of the fiber-optic scope. Westin described the exploration of 'the space between the uterine wall and the membranes up to the site of the placenta', a description which is suggestive of the unobliterated extracoelomic cavity of the first trimester. In the 1960s, several groups of investigators performed transcervical chorion villus biopsy under endoscopic guidance; however, fetal anatomy and development were not a main focus. In 1974, MacKenzie[2] described his experience with transcervical fetoscopy between 8 and 20 weeks' gestation in 28 patients. He used a 5-mm, flexible-tip bronchofiberscope, which was introduced through an undilated cervix and without anesthesia or sedation. Gallinat et al[3] reported in 1979 on transcervical embryoscopy using a hysteroscope and CO_2 inflation of the uterus. Pregnancies which were intended to be terminated at 12 weeks' gestation were followed weekly from 5 weeks' gestation on, and gross fetal anatomy was described. Roume et al[4] and Dumez[5] from the Port Royal Maternity Hospital in Paris incorporated embryoscopy into their prenatal diagnosis program in 1979, and reported on the utility of this tool in the diagnosis of limb abnormalities. The largest experience in non-continuing pregnancies was reported in 1990 by Cullen et al.[6] They confirmed the utility of embryoscopy in the detection of fetal anomalies other than limb abnormalities. In 1990, Reece et al demonstrated the accessibility of the embryonic blood circulation.[7]

Technique

The technique of first-trimester embryofetoscopy consists of fiber-optic endoscopy, and it can be done as early as 5 weeks' menstrual age transcervically or transabdominally.[6] The first attempts of early embryofetoscopy were performed transcervically with rigid fiber-optic endoscopes 30 cm in length with diameters 2–3.5 mm and angle lengths of 0° or 30°.[6] Under continuous sonographic guidance, the endoscope is passed through the cervix into the extracoelomic cavity with extreme care, so that the amnion is not ruptured. The chorion is identified by its opaque character, and it is bluntly penetrated by the tip of the endoscope. The site of penetration is very carefully chosen in order to avoid the placenta and also areas where the chorion and amnion are juxtaposed (Figure 4.1). Another technique of first-trimester embryofetoscopy uses the transabdominal approach. This approach was developed in recent years and it is also performed under continuous sonographic guidance.[7] Instrumentation consists of an 0.8-mm fiber-optic endoscope and a 27-gauge needle, which are accommodated by a specially designed 16-gauge, double-barrel instrument sheath. Under

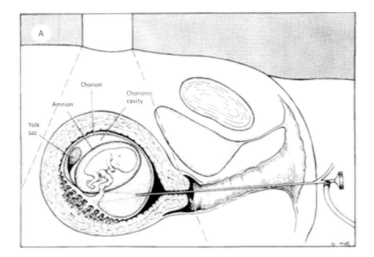

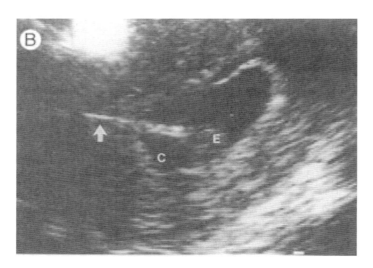

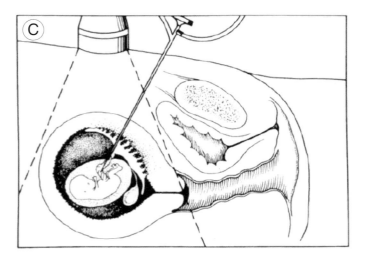

Figure 4.1 (A) Schematic representation of transcervical embryofetoscopy; (B) ultrasound image of transcervical embryofetoscopy; (C) access to the umbilical cord via transabdominal embryofetoscopy.

sonographic guidance, the endoscope and needle are passed transabdominally into the extracelomic or amniotic cavity. The morphology of the fetus, as well as any blood-sampling procedures, is viewed through a video camera and recorded. The procedure is very similar to performing an amniocentesis, and it avoids the potential risk of fetal trauma and introduction of infection that are associated with the transcervical route.

Application

First-trimester embryofetoscopy has several current as well as potential applications. Applications include: a) documentation of normal early human development; b) confirmation of first-trimester ultrasound findings; c) evaluation of embryonic morphology and cytogenetic analysis in early failed pregnancies. Future applications may involve access to the fetal circulation for early fetal therapy.

Documentation of normal early human development

Embryoscopy can be a valuable tool for primary diagnosis of congenital anomalies in the first trimester and for the confirmation of ultrasonographically suspected anomalies. Since this technique can be used as early as 5 menstrual weeks and allows for direct visualization of normal and abnormal development, it is of significant importance to our understanding of human embryology. Much of our knowledge of early human development has been based on the investigation of human abortuses or animal research. However, the stages of embryonic development in animals are not necessarily representative of human development. Embryoscopy visualizes the human embryo *in vivo* unaffected by any pathology of the uterine environment. The embryonic period, during which all major external and internal structures develop, extends from conception to 8 weeks (or 10 menstrual weeks). This is the period of greatest susceptibility to the effects of teratogens. At the end of this early development, the fetus has all external features of the human species.

The head and neck
The endoscopic view of the fetal face at 6 conceptual weeks reveals a prominent forehead, widely spaced eyes, and confluent oral and nasal cavities. At 8 conceptual weeks and beyond, greater facial detail is seen. Some congenital malformations of the head and neck can be visualized in early pregnancy. These include anencephaly, acrania, hydrocephaly, microcephaly, and macrocephaly. However, the most likely diagnosable malformations include anencephaly and acrania. Potentially diagnosable anomalies of the face include micrognathia and cleft lip.

The trunk
Development of the gut occurs at a time when the abdominal cavity is still small; hence, herniation occurs in the body stalk at about 5 weeks' gestation. The gut remains extruded until

about 10 weeks' gestation, when reinsertion occurs, followed by complete closure of the ventral wall. These normal developmental events can be documented by embryoscopy. The ventral hernia is seen as early as 4 conceptual weeks, and by 8 conceptual weeks the hernia is almost completely resolved. It is likely, therefore, that dorsal and ventral wall defects are diagnosable by embryoscopy.

The neural tube

The neural tube is seen with the cephalic end open at about 5 conceptual weeks. By about 7 conceptual weeks, there is complete closure of the neural tube (Figures 4.2 and 4.3).

The limbs

The normal development of the limb buds is manifested first as lateral swellings or paddle-shaped structures in the late fourth week after conception (Figure 4.4). At 7 weeks' gestation, a fully developed hand is seen (Figures 4.5 and 4.6). Foot paddles and well-developed feet are usually visible 2 weeks later than the equivalent in the upper extremities (Figure 4.7). Since the limbs are clearly visualized by embryoscopy, this technique is likely to diagnose limb anomalies such as hemimelia, phocomelia, sirenomelia, missing digits, lobster claw, polydactyly (Figure 4.8), syndactyly, brachydactyly, clubhand, and clubfoot.

Other structures

The yolk sac can be visualized as early as 5 weeks' gestation. Embryoscopically, the early yolk sac has a confluent and prominent vasculature in contrast to the yolk sac at 10 conceptual weeks, which contains smaller, more numerous, but less prominent vessels. The anomalous development and external appearance of the yolk sac have been described under experimental conditions and have been associated with embryonic malformations. It is likely that similar changes of yolk-sac morphology

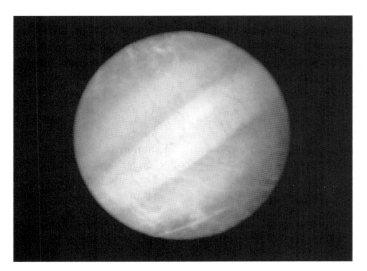

Figure 4.2 The completely closed neural tube is seen at 7 conceptual weeks.

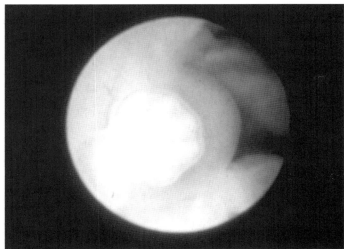

Figure 4.4 Hand paddle at 4 conceptual weeks with subtle demarcations of finger rays.

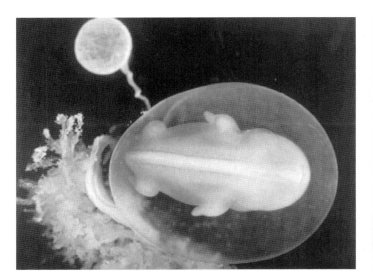

Figure 4.3 Posterior view of neural tube at 7 conceptual weeks.

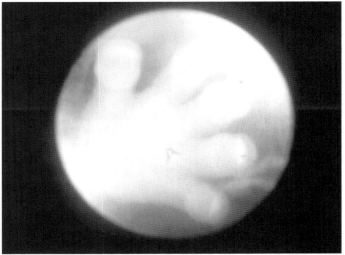

Figure 4.5 Hand at 7 conceptual weeks.

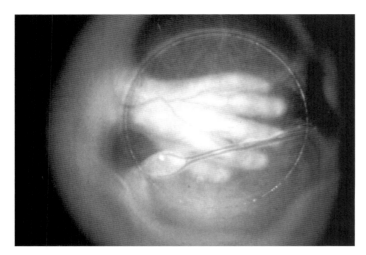

Figure 4.6 At 9 conceptual weeks, a fully developed hand is observed without webbing.

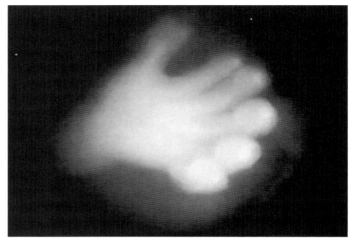

Figure 4.8 Hand at 7 conceptual weeks shows polydactyly.

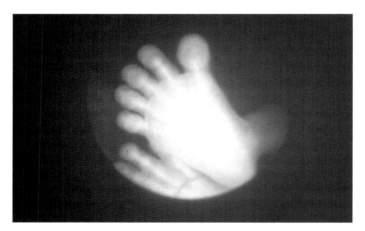

Figure 4.7 Well-developed fetal foot at 9 conceptual weeks with well-developed toes without webbing.

will be detected by embryoscopy and correlated with pathologic states. The genitalia can also be seen to develop from a 'nonspecific' genital ridge to typical male genitalia.

With first-trimester embryofetoscopy, a thorough examination of the embryo/fetus is possible in the overwhelming majority of cases, including visualization of the head, face, dorsal and ventral walls, limbs, umbilical cord, and yolk sac. According to Reece et al, the duration of the procedure is approximately 5 minutes, and fetal visualization is achieved in approximately 90% of the cases.[7,8] The risk of infection, uterine perforation or any other maternal morbidity related to the procedure is very small. The possibility of trauma to the amnion is increased with increasing gestational age and is the least between 7½–11 menstrual weeks' gestation.

Other investigators have reported similar success rates of visualization. Dumez has reported his experience with over 60 continuing pregnancies in using transcervical embryofetoscopy.[5] There were six pregnancy losses in the latter stage of his experience in using transcervical embryofetoscopy, but after intro-

ducing the transabdominal approach in 20 cases, there was no adverse outcome. Quintero et al reported their experience with transabdominal embryofetoscopy using an 18- or 19-gauge, thin-wall needle and a 0.7-mm endoscope in 18 patients undergoing first-trimester or early second-trimester termination of pregnancy.[9] A thorough visualization of fetal anatomy from 7–13 weeks was obtained in 85% of cases. Ville et al reported that the procedure-related risk of transabdominal, first-trimester embryofetoscopy is approximately 12%.[10] Yin et al reported on 12 pregnant women scheduled for legal termination of pregnancy at 6–12 weeks' gestation.[11] A flexible fiber-optic endoscope was used transcervically under ultrasound guidance. Complete visualization of the embryo/fetus was accomplished in 50% of the cases. There were no procedure-related complications. Greco et al reported on their experience with nine cases at 10–14 weeks' gestation, using transabdominal embryofetoscopy.[12] They reported complete visualization of the embryo/fetus in all cases, and they concluded that fetal examination was easier at 10–12 weeks of gestation than 13–14 weeks. Surbek et al performed transabdominal embryofetoscopy in 14 patients scheduled for termination of pregnancy, using a 1-mm, semirigid, fiber-optic telescope with an 18-gauge examination sheath and a single-chip digital camera.[13] A 25-gauge needle was inserted through a 21-gauge side port to access the fetal circulation. The fetal head, face, abdomen, and complete upper and lower limbs were visualized in over 80% of the cases. However, the fetal back and external genitalia were visualized in only 35.7% and 64.3% of the cases, respectively. Injection of 10–20 ml saline improved visibility in 43% of the cases. The investigators attempted successful funipuncture in two of three attempts. Zwinger and Krofta attempted transabdominal embryofetoscopy at 7–8 postconceptional weeks and were successful in all seven cases.[14] Miliou-Paouleskou et al attempted transabdominal embryofetoscopy during the first 12 weeks of pregnancy in 20 women prior to pregnancy termination.[15] A complete methodological survey of the embryo/fetus was possible in all cases. Access to embryonic circulation was attempted, and a small quantity of blood was obtained in 71.4% of the cases. The average length of the procedure was approximately 15 minutes. There were no maternal complications.

Confirmation of first-trimester ultrasound findings

The introduction of high-resolution vaginal sonography has tremendously improved our ability to diagnose fetal anomalies in the first trimester of pregnancy. However, when congenital anomalies are diagnosed at such an early stage of pregnancy and patients choose to terminate the pregnancy, pathologic confirmation and anatomic studies are not possible due to the destructive nature of first-trimester induced abortions. First-trimester embryofetoscopy prior to pregnancy termination can be used to confirm prenatally diagnosed anomalies and ensure accurate patient counseling for subsequent pregnancies. In addition, embryofetoscopy can be used in cases where the ultrasound diagnosis is not certain or an ultrasound diagnosis may not be possible, depending upon the type and nature of the genetic disorder. In several cases, embryofetoscopy was used for early pregnancy prenatal diagnosis. In 1993, Quintero et al diagnosed a case of Meckel–Gruber syndrome at 11 weeks' menstrual age by visualizing postaxial polydactyly and occipital encephalocele.[9] Dommergues et al used embryofetoscopy to diagnose a case of van der Woude's syndrome at 11 weeks' menstrual age, allowing for early pregnancy termination.[16] Reece et al used transabdominal embryofetoscopy to rule out a suspected neural tube defect based on suspicious ultrasound findings.[17] In addition, Robert's syndrome has been ruled out in a mother who had previously given birth to an affected infant.[18] Complete visualization of the embryo was achieved in this case, and no limb or facial abnormalities were seen. Similarly, Hobbins et al ruled out Smith–Lemli–Opitz type 2 syndrome in a patient at risk by using transabdominal embryofetoscopy after transvaginal ultrasound had suggested polydactyly.[19] Embryofetoscopy revealed a normal fetal hand and the patient chose to continue with the pregnancy, resulting in a healthy, normal baby at birth. Recently, Rankine et al were able to confirm the diagnosis of acrania at 12 weeks' gestation by using transcervical endoscopy.[20] In addition, they were able to demonstrate other abnormalities, including a small omphalocele, hexadactylism on both sides, and bilateral clubfoot.

In summary, first-trimester embryofetoscopy has been used by various clinicians and investigators to confirm congenital anomalies in patients who wish to continue their pregnancies, as well as those who have already decided for a pregnancy termination.

Evaluation of embryonic fetal morphology and cytogenetic analysis in early failed pregnancies

One of the applications of embryofetoscopy is to evaluate the morphology of the embryo/fetus in early failed pregnancies. In such cases, the embryofetoscopy is performed transcervically in order to assess fetal morphology and obtain material directly from fetal tissues, so that successful fetal cytogenetic analysis is possible. Yin et al reported on transcervical embryoscopic diagnosis of conjoined twins in a 10-week missed abortion.[21] Philipp and Kalousek reported on the use of transcervical embryofetoscopy in diagnosing localized and systemic defects in the embryonic morphogenesis of missed abortions in a population of 24 women with missed abortions.[22] They used the rigid hysteroscope, which was passed transcervically into the amniotic cavity. An embryo was visualized in 80% of the cases, and half of the embryos showed multiple developmental defects. Philipp et al subsequently reported on 272 patients with missed abortion in whom they used transcervical embryofetoscopy prior to dilation and curettage in order to study the morphology of the embryo/fetus and also to perform cytogenetic analysis of chorionic villi by either standard, G-banding cytogenetic techniques or comparative genomic hybridization in combination with flow-cytometry analysis.[23] Visualization of the embryo or early fetus was successful in 86% of the cases, and a successful karyotype was obtained in 81% of the cases.

Approximately 75% of the cases had an abnormal karyotype, 18% had a morphologic defect with a normal karyotype, and no embryonic or chromosomal abnormality could be found in 7% of the cases. The authors concluded that transcervical embryofetoscopy for the evaluation of missed abortions provides valuable information for genetic counseling in planning for future pregnancies. Philipp et al also reported on the use of transcervical embryofetoscopy in the evaluation of structural defects in four first-trimester, monochorionic twin, intrauterine deaths.[24] One case was diagnosed with trisomy 21, a second with thoracophagus twins, and a third with acardiac twins, while a fourth case was remarkable because of the concordance of limb-reduction defects.

It appears that the use of transcervical embryofetoscopy in accurate evaluation of embryonic morphology and cytogenetic analysis can be a helpful tool for understanding the reasons for early pregnancy failure; most importantly, it may provide extremely useful information for genetic counseling and planning for future pregnancies.

Access to the embryonal/fetal circulation and future applications of first-trimester embryofetoscopy

Cannulation of the vitelline and umbilical blood vessels under direct embryofetoscopic guidance is feasible. Reece et al were the first to attempt fetal blood sampling by using first-trimester, transabdominal needle embryofetoscopy.[7,8] These investigators were able to infuse indigo carmine dye into the circulation of three patients at 8–12 weeks' gestation prior to pregnancy termination. Surbek et al reported on the use of transabdominal, first-trimester embryofetoscopy as a potential approach to early in utero stem-cell transplantation and gene therapy, since they succeeded in funipuncture in two of three attempts in patients prior to pregnancy termination.[13] The best results in achieving access to the embryonal/fetal circulation during the first trimester of pregnancy were reported by Miliou-Paouleskou et al, who attempted first-trimester, transabdominal embryofetoscopy in 20 women.[15] Access to the embryonic circulation was attempted in 14 cases and was performed successfully in 10 (success rate 71.4%). There is no question that such high success rates, if confirmed by other investigators, would provide the vehicle for early intravascular stem-cell transplantation.

The prospects of human gene and cell therapy have become excellent in recent years. First-trimester embryofetoscopy allows accessibility to the circulation of the developing embryo/fetus at a time when it is immunologically naive, and therefore more receptive to grafts. The early *in utero* application of this technology may be advantageous in genetic diseases that produce irreversible damage by the time of birth. At present, the only technique that can be used effectively for gene transfer is bone marrow. In the near future, more should be learned about how to package DNA and make it tissue-specific. If so, the use of embryofetoscopy for intravenous injection of genetic material will hold great promise. Although fetal gene therapy is still experimental, the availability of first-trimester embryofetoscopy brings fetal gene therapy within our reach, and this therapy may be proven in the future to be critical in preventing irreversible perinatal disease manifestations in many inherited conditions. However, it is prudent to investigate this approach extensively, first in animal models in order to improve the technological aspects of the procedure and assess the efficacy of gene expression, as well as possible side effects, before application in humans is considered.

Another future application of first-trimester embryofetoscopy is research on the role of the human yolk sac. A major question awaiting elucidation is the role of the yolk sac in early human development. The yolk sac provides blood cell precursors, gonadocytes, and epithelia of the digestive and respiratory tracts, and has been demonstrated to be structurally altered when exposed to high glucose concentrations in embryo-culture experiments.[25] Therefore, the yolk sac may play an essential role in the pathogenesis of congenital anomalies in the fetuses of diabetic mothers. Direct observation of the yolk sac by embryoscopy, as well as aspiration of its contents for laboratory analysis, could enhance our understanding of human malformations considerably.

Ethical considerations

Patients undergoing embryofetoscopy for either fetal diagnosis or therapy should be selected very carefully. The risks versus benefits should be carefully weighed in each individual case. The ability to treat terminal or debilitating congenital disorders before birth will lead to complex ethical questions with respect to the rights of the mother and fetus. The hospital ethics committee and other noninvolved physicians should be consulted in difficult or controversial cases.

Conclusion

In recent years, prenatal diagnosis has focused on the first trimester of pregnancy due to the improved resolution of transvaginal ultrasound and other first-trimester screening techniques such as nuchal translucency evaluation. We now have the ability to diagnose many fetal anomalies in the first trimester of pregnancy, and the opportunity may be given for early intervention in terms of termination of pregnancy or fetal therapy, depending upon the particulars of each situation and the parents' wishes. Soon the availability of first-trimester embryofetoscopy may allow access to the embryo/fetus for early diagnosis as well as potential therapy. At the present time, in everyday practice, early embryofetoscopy may be considered in the evaluation of embryonic morphology and for fetal tissue retrieval for cytogenetic analysis in patients with early failed pregnancies.

References

1. Westin B. Hysteroscopy in early pregnancy. Lancet 1954; 2: 872–5.
2. MacKenzie IZ. Transcervical fetoscopy. Lancet 1974; 2: 346–7.
3. Gallinat A, Lueken RP, Lindemann HJ. A preliminary report about transcervical embryoscopy. Endoscopy 1978; 10: 47–50.
4. Roume J, Aubry MC, Labbe F et al. Diagnostic prénatal des anomalies des membres et des extrémités. J Genet Hum 1985; 33: 457–61.
5. Dumez Y. Embryofetoscopy and congenital malformations. Proceedings of International Conference on Chorionic Villus Sampling and Early Prenatal Diagnosis, 28–29 May 1990, Athens, Greece.
6. Cullen MT, Reece EA, Whetham J et al. Embryofetoscopy: description and utility of a new technique. Am J Obstet Gynecol 1990; 162: 82–6.
7. Reece EA, Goldstein I, Chatwani et al. Transabdominal needle embryofetoscopy: a new technique paving the way for early fetal therapy. Obstet Gynecol 1994; 84: 634–6.
8. Reece EA. First trimester prenatal diagnosis: embryoscopy and fetoscopy. Semin Perinatol 1999; 23: 424–33.
9. Quintero RA, Abuhamad A, Hobbins JC et al. Transabdominal thin-gauge embryofetoscopy: a technique for early prenatal diagnosis and its use in the diagnosis of a case of Meckel–Gruber syndrome. Am J Obstet Gynecol 1993; 168: 1552–7.
10. Ville Y, Khalil A, Homphray T et al. Diagnostic embryofetoscopy and fetoscopy in the first trimester of pregnancy. Prenat Diagn 1997; 17: 1237–46.
11. Yin CS, Liu JY, Yu MH. Transcervical flexible endoscopy for first trimester embryonic/fetal evaluation. Int J Gynaecol Obstet 1996; 54: 149–53.
12. Greco P, Vimercati A, Bettocchi S et al. Endoscopic examination of the fetus in early pregnancy. J Perinat Med 2000; 28: 34–8.
13. Surbek DV, Tercanli S, Holzgreve W. Transabdominal first trimester embryofetoscopy as a potential approach to early in

utero stem cell transplantation and gene therapy. Ultrasound Obstet Gynecol 2000; 15: 302–7.

14. Zwinger A, Krofta L. Embryo-fetoscopy – present possibilities of endoscopy in obstetrics. Ceska Gynekol 2000; 65: 3–6.

15. Miliou-Paouleskou D, Antsaklis A, Papantoniou N et al. First trimester transabdominal embryo fetoscopy. Early Pregnancy 2001; 5: 36–7.

16. Dommergues M, Lemerrer M, Couly G et al. Prenatal diagnosis of cleft lip at 11 menstrual weeks using embryoscopy in the van der Woude syndrome. Prenat Diag 1995; 15: 378–81.

17. Reece EA, Homko CJ, Wiznitzer A et al. Needle embryofetoscopy and early prenatal diagnosis. Fetal Diagn Ther 1995; 10: 81–2.

18. Reece EA, Homko CJ, Koch S et al. First-trimester needle embryofetoscopy and prenatal diagnosis. Fetal Diagn Ther 1997; 12: 136–9.

19. Hobbins JC, Jones OW, Gottesfeld S et al. Transvaginal ultrasonography and transabdominal embryofetoscopy in the first-trimester diagnosis of Smith–Lemli–Optiz syndrome, type II. Am J Obstet Gynecol 1994; 171: 546–9.

20. Rankine M, Hafner E, Schuchter K et al. Ultrasound and endoscopic image of exencephaly (acrania) in the 12th week of pregnancy. Z Geburtshilfe Neonatol 2000; 204: 236–8.

21. Yin CS, Chen WH, Wei RY et al. Transcervical embryoscopic diagnosis of conjoined twins in a ten-week missed abortion. Prenatal Diagn 1998; 18: 626–8.

22. Philipp T, Kalousek DK. Transcervical embryoscopy in missed abortion. J Assist Reprod Genet 2001; 18: 285–90.

23. Philipp T, Philipp K, Reiner A et al. Embryoscopic and cytogenetic analysis of 233 missed abortion factors involved in the pathogenesis of developmental defects of early failed pregnancies. Human Reprod 2003; 18: 1724–32.

24. Philipp T, Separovic ER, Philipp K et al. Transcervical fetoscopic diagnosis of structural defects in four first-trimester monochorionic twin intrauterine deaths. Prenat Diagn 2003; 23: 964–9.

25. Reece EA, Pinter E, Leranth C et al. Yolk sac failure in embryopathy due to hyperglycemia: horseradish peroxidase uptake in the assessment of yolk sac function. Obstet Gynecol 1989; 74: 755.

5 Chorionic villus sampling

Patrice ML Trauffer, Neil S Silverman, and Ronald J Wapner

Although transabdominal puncture of the uterus has been carried out often for therapeutic and experimental reasons without accidents, mere curiosity does not justify the procedure, and its practical value is probably limited in the human. If the results are confirmed in animals, however, it might become of great significance in veterinary practice.[1]

Innovation and technology have advanced genetic counseling and diagnosis exponentially over the past three decades, past the point of cautions such as the one cited above. Where, previously, parents at risk of abnormal offspring had no more to plan with than statistics and odds, geneticists and obstetricians are able today to provide them with precise answers based upon analysis of cells from the fetus. It is the evolving access to the developing fetal compartment that has moved the science of prenatal diagnosis squarely into the arena of operative obstetrics.

The reports of Barr and Bertram in 1949[2] suggested that sex differences could be distinguished from isolated animal cells. The technique was applied by Fuchs and Riis to human fetal cells extracted from amniotic fluid obtained at the time of rupture of the membrane for induction of labor. Yet, the knowledge of fetal gender was of value only in X-linked diseases, and here the destruction of all male conceptuses was necessary to prevent the birth of an affected child. As a result, the technique of transabdominal amniocentesis had few enthusiasts. Interest in amniocentesis was revived in the mid-1960s, with the use of amniotic fluid to evaluate fetal erythroblastosis. Of at least equal significance was the successful demonstration in 1966 that a complete fetal karyotype, not simply sex chromatin determination, could be obtained from amniotic fluid.[3]

During the ensuing years, second-trimester amniocentesis for prenatal diagnosis, in conjunction with directed genetic counseling, became an accepted practice.[4] The safety and reliability of the method and the accuracy of its results set amniocentesis as the 'reference standard' against which newer methods of fetal diagnosis were measured. The technical limitations of the methods for obtaining and culturing fluid were such that results were not available until well after 16 weeks' gestation. As such, parents wishing to abort an abnormal fetus were required to make a decision well after the pregnancy was apparent to both the mother and other observers. In addition, pregnancy termination in the second trimester was associated with risks much greater than those of first-trimester suction curettage.

It was against this background that the development and refinement of chorionic villus sampling began. Mohr, in 1968, was the first to utilize chorionic tissue obtained via endoscopic biopsy for fetal diagnosis.[5] The biopsy was made transvaginally, with uterine puncture performed after peritoneal entry through one of the vaginal fornices. Modification of the technique via a transcervical approach was developed later. With both techniques, direct visualization of the chorionic membrane, via an adapted, 6-mm endoscope, was required. The optics were then removed from the cannula and continuous suction was applied through the hollow tube to achieve bulging of the chorion into the tip of the device. A tubular knife was then inserted and used to cut off the tissue drawn in by suction. The procedure was attempted with some success on patients prior to pregnancy termination. Accurate karyotyping was accomplished when chorion was obtained, but only half of the samples were found to contain chorionic tissue. In addition, the presence of amniotic membrane in many specimens suggested that the integrity of the amniotic sac had been interrupted.[6,7]

In Sweden, Kullander and Sandahl reported on their experience with transcervical villus biopsy, using a device similar to the one engineered by Hahnemann and Mohr in Denmark.[8] Patients seeking abortion at 8–20 weeks' gestation, who allowed their pregnancies to be observed up to 3 weeks after sampling but before termination, were recruited. Two patients developed intrauterine infection after the procedure and aborted spontaneously. This complication resolved after the institution of prophylactic antibiotics for 3–4 days after the procedure. Overall, only about 35% of the specimens could be cultured successfully. Nulliparous patients were noted to be particularly difficult to sample, with many requiring mechanical dilation. In 1974, Hahnemann reported a series of attempted transcervical biopsies, using a modified endoscope adapted with a trigger device to provide intermittent rather than continuous suction through the cannula.[9] In 30% of the subjects, the pregnancy continued for at least 8 days after the biopsy; but in almost one-half of this group, complications 'inconsistent with continued pregnancy' were observed. Again, nulliparous cervices presented significant obstacles to successful visualization, and many 'blind' biopsies were found to be contaminated with decidua.

The resolution of most major problems in genetic amniocentesis had been achieved around the time of these reports; thus, further investigations concerning first-trimester diagnostic procedures drew little attention. Reports like Kullander's, moreover, did little to dispel the impression that an abdominal procedure would have a lower infectious complication rate than a biopsy through the vagina. In 1975, Chinese investigators described a technique for the aspiration of chorionic villi.[10] Without optical guidance, they inserted a 3-mm diameter blunt metal cannula transcervically until they felt 'a soft resistance'. A smaller internal tube was then inserted and advanced 0.5–1.0 cm past the tip of the outer cannula. Syringe suction was then applied. When performed at 6–14 weeks' gestation, a single aspiration yielded adequate tissue for analysis in 73% of cases. In 93 of 100 sampled cases, the fetal sex was correctly identified by sex chromatin alone, without tissue culture. Of the pregnancies allowed to continue (keeping in mind that the procedure was developed as a family-planning tool), slight bleeding was the only maternal morbidity. Only 4% of the continuing pregnancies were lost to miscarriage. Unfortunately, attempts in the USA to adapt this approach via endocervical saline lavage, followed by aspiration behind the cervical mucus plug, were plagued by contamination of samples by maternal cells, leading to incorrect fetal sex predictions.[11–13] The unreliability of the procedure led one group to conclude that 'first-trimester prenatal diagnosis is not feasible at this time'.[12]

Interest in first-trimester prenatal diagnosis was restored in the early 1980s, largely as the product of two major advances in the field. First, the development of DNA techniques of gene analysis held the promise of a variety of diagnostic capabilities utilizing milligram amounts of tissue. Second, the quality of visualization afforded by real-time ultrasound made tissue retrieval under direct ultrasound guidance feasible. Kazy et al in the USSR reported success with placental biopsies, using a forceps apparatus under ultrasound guidance. After over 100 biopsies in pretermination patients, 26 gravidas with genetically at-risk pregnancies who intended to carry the pregnancy to term were successfully sampled without complications. One-half of the pregnancies were subsequently terminated at the patient's request. The remaining 13 gave birth to normal babies.[14] Around the same time, a team of British biochemists and obstetricians reported the successful diagnosis of hemoglobinopathies by DNA analysis from chorionic villus specimens obtained by aspiration just before pregnancy termination.[15] Ward and his group in London described the chorionic villus sampling method currently in use.[16] A 1.5-mm plastic catheter, threaded over a blunt, malleable metal obturator, was introduced under real-time ultrasound guidance to the lower border of the chorion frondosum. After withdrawal of the obturator, a syringe was attached to the catheter and suction was applied to aspirate villi. The following year the same group demonstrated a 90% sampling success rate when using the catheter apparatus for obtaining villi at 7–14 weeks' gestation.[17]

In contrast, Simoni et al,[18] using either a direct endoscopic approach, blind insertion of a plastic cannula, or blind insertion of the flexible (Ward) catheter, achieved no better than a 76% sampling success, with a 17% rate of bleeding complications. The addition of ultrasound guidance with the Ward catheter raised the success rate to 96%, with only 5% bleeding morbidity. These authors also developed a process for the rapid, direct preparation of karyotypes that took advantage of spontaneous mitoses in the dividing villi.[18] Using this method, the group reported the diagnosis of trisomy 21 within 5 hours of transcervical sampling in an 11-week gestation.[19] Subsequently, in addition to karyotypic evaluation, the use of first-trimester villi was described in the detection of hemophilia, Tay–Sachs disease, sickle-cell disease, Duchenne's muscular dystrophy, and argininosuccinicaciduria.[20–27] Most recently, transabdominal ultrasound-guided needle retrieval of chorionic villi has received increasing favor. This approach, along with both transcervical villus sampling and midtrimester amniocentesis, provides the armamentarium needed for prenatal diagnosis.

The sampling procedure

Embryology and histology

During the 9–12 weeks from the last menstrual period, the amniotic sac does not yet fill the uterine cavity. This relationship offers an ideal opportunity for the passage of a sampling instrument transcervically into the developing placenta. The chorion has begun its differentiation into the chorion frondosum, which will become the placental site, and the smooth chorion laeve, from which the villi have begun to degenerate (Figure 5.1). The chorion frondosum contains the mitotically active villi cells and is, therefore, the area to be biopsied. At this early gestational age, the villi float relatively freely in the intervillous space and are anchored loosely to the underlying decidua; this is why sampling via aspiration at this stage is only minimally traumatic. The individual villi have a distinctive branched appearance with an outer single-cell layer, the syncytiotrophoblast, bordering on the proliferative cytotrophoblast. Fetal capillaries are visible within the mesenchymal core of the villus (Figure 5.2). The mitotically active cytotrophoblastic buds provide the tissue for the rapid direct karyotype preparation, while the mesenchymal core is used as the source of chromosomes in tissue culture.

Transcervical sampling

Before sampling, real-time abdominal or vaginal ultrasound is used to evaluate the pregnancy.[28] Fetal cardiac activity is docu-

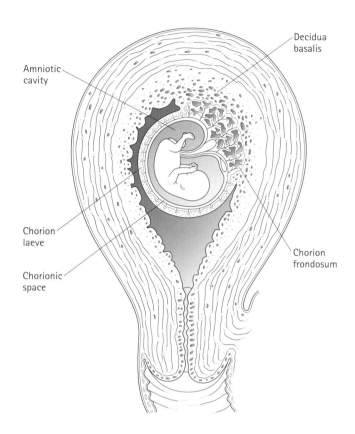

Figure 5.1 Chorionic villus sampling is performed at 9–11 weeks' gestation. At this stage of gestation, the chorion has already differentiated into the frondosum, in which the villi are present, and the chorion laeve, in which the chorionic villi have degenerated. The chorionic space remains, since the amnion and the chorion have not yet fused.

mented, and measurements of the fetal crown–rump length (CRL) and gestational sac size are taken and compared to expected values for the gestational age by menstrual dates. If the fetal measurement is over 1 week smaller than expected by dates, we delay sampling until appropriate growth by CRL is shown, since an early discrepancy, in our experience, may predict an impending miscarriage. Over 10% of our patients have had blighted ova diagnosed on this initial scan. Scheduling the procedure after 9 weeks' gestation appears to eliminate much of the potential early pregnancy loss and may prevent sampling of karyotypically abnormal embryos destined to perish spontaneously.[29] Ultrasound is also used preprocedurally to map out the area of the chorion frondosum, which is recognizable as a homogeneous, hyperechoic area. Visualization of the cord insertion can be used as confirmation, and is especially useful when difficulty in precisely locating the chorion frondosum is encountered. The positions of the uterus and cervix should be noted and may be altered, to assist sampling, by distention or emptying of the maternal bladder, though overfilling, in correcting for uterine anteversion, can prevent uterine mobility, which is a requisite for safe sampling. Uterine contractions are frequently encountered, and can interfere with the passage of the catheter (Figure 5.3). Frequently, waiting 10–20 minutes for dissipation of the contraction will make the procedure much easier and, therefore, safer.

After the condition and position of the uterus are satisfactory, the patient is placed in the lithotomy position; a speculum is inserted; and the vulva, vagina, and cervix are aseptically prepared with a povidone-iodine (Betadine) solution. Some centers use a tenaculum to grasp the anterior lip of the cervix and to aid in positioning the cervical/uterine path to the chorion. We have moved away from doing this routinely, as it is usually the only part of the procedure that produces significant discomfort. It is, however, a useful adjunct for operators beginning to learn the technique, and also in certain cases in which uterine manipulation is required to reach the frondosum. The

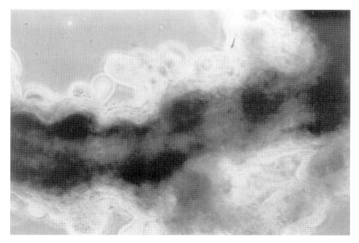

Figure 5.2 A high-power view of the chorionic villus. Cytotrophoblast buds are seen emanating from the villus core. Within the mesenchymal core of the villus, fetal blood vessels are easily identified.

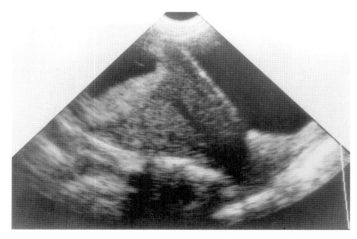

Figure 5.3 A uterine contraction is seen in the lower uterine segment displacing the sac upward. Waiting 15–20 minutes will frequently allow the contraction to dissipate and make sampling easier.

uterine position is then again confirmed by ultrasound. The distal 3–5 cm of the 1.5-mm sampling catheter is bent into a slight curve (Figure 5.4) and passed, avoiding touching the vaginal walls, through the cervix until loss of resistance is detected at the internal os. At this point, the operator waits until the tip of the catheter is seen on ultrasound, and then directs the catheter, under continuous ultrasound guidance, to the sampling site well in the substance of the chorion frondosum. A combination of movement of the speculum by an assistant to change the angle of approach, rotation of the catheter, and, if required, manipulation of the cervix with the tenaculum is used to guide the catheter into place. The catheter must be inserted slowly, without excessive force, along the unresisting tissue plane provided by the freely floating villi. Excessive force against resistance may cause disruption of the underlying vessels or injury to the chorionic membrane. The catheter is inserted parallel to the axis of the chorion frondosum and passed almost to its distal end (Figure 5.5). The flexible obturator is then

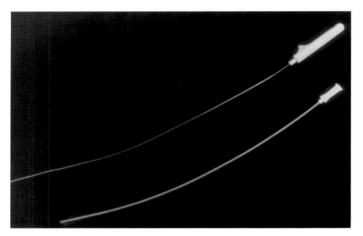

Figure 5.4 The catheter used for transcervical sampling includes a stainless steel inner stylet which is easily malleable. The polyethylene outer sheath is also seen.

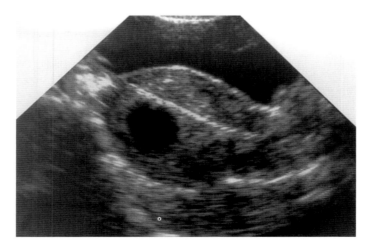

Figure 5.5 The CVS catheter is seen well within the chorion frondosum. The catheter is inserted into the distal end of the frondosum in order to maximize sample size.

removed, the outer plastic catheter is held in place, and a 20-ml syringe containing 5 ml of nutrient medium with added heparin is attached to the catheter. Approximately 15–20 ml of negative pressure is applied through the syringe as the catheter and attached syringe are withdrawn slowly. Villi can be seen within the syringe as white, branched structures. If inadequate material is obtained on the first pass, up to three passes, each with a fresh catheter, may be attempted, though the risk of adverse outcome appears to be proportional to the number of passes required.[30]

Once the technique is mastered, however, one can achieve sufficient tissue retrieval with one or two insertions in about 97% of the cases. After an adequate sample is obtained, the patient is discharged home with no required recovery period, except for mild reduction of activity for the first 24 hours. She is instructed to contact the sampling center if heavy bleeding or fever develop, though mild to moderate spotting is not uncommon up to 1 week after the procedure.

Transabdominal approach

Though accumulated data suggest the safety and reliability of transcervical chorion villus sampling (CVS) for first-trimester prenatal diagnosis, the technique has two major imitations. First, not all patients are appropriate candidates for a transcervical procedure. For example, that approach would be difficult or relatively contraindicated in women with genital herpes, cervical polyps, or a severely retroverted uterus. Second, many practitioners, because of experience gained by performing amniocenteses, are more comfortable with a transabdominal than with a transcervical approach. Two basic techniques for transabdominal CVS have been described. Originally, Smidt-Jensen and Hahnemann recommended a two-needle technique, using a larger outer needle as a trocar, through which a thinner sampling needle was inserted to obtain a suction biopsy.[31] More recently, Brambati's group described a single-needle, 'free-hand' method, using a 20-gauge spinal needle, under direct ultrasound guidance.[32] Although the two-needle technique has the advantage of allowing reinsertion of the sampling needle without requiring a second skin puncture if sufficient tissue is not initially aspirated, the single-needle procedure is quicker, less uncomfortable, and able to retrieve adequate tissue with minimal number of insertions.

We use this second procedure for transabdominal CVS at our center, and it is the one which appears to be gaining wider acceptance. As with the transcervical technique, a careful ultrasound evaluation is performed before the procedure. The biopsy path is selected by ultrasound so that the needle will be inserted parallel to the chorionic plate. In most cases, a relatively empty bladder is preferred so that the uterus is closer to the abdominal wall, minimizing the possibility of an inadvertent visceral injury. Povidone iodine preparation of the skin of the abdominal wall is performed, as in amniocentesis. We do not employ local anesthesia as a rule, though some centers do. At our center, an ultrasound biopsy guide is used to direct insertion of the needle tip into the myometrium just above the chorionic sampling site. Other centers prefer not to use a biopsy guide. Either approach appears to be equally successful, depending upon the operator's preference.[33] Once the needle is in place, the stylet is removed, a syringe is placed into the needle's luer lock, and, by continuous negative pressure from the syringe, the biopsy needle is moved up and down three or four times through the entire length of the chorion before removal. If the sample is inadequate, a new needle is reinserted and the procedure is repeated. As with the transcervical technique, no recovery period is required. Patients experience little if any bleeding after transabdominal CVS, but significantly more transient cramping than with the transcervical approach.

Twin gestations

It has been demonstrated that CVS can be performed successfully and safely in twin gestations.[34,35] There are, however, a number of potential pitfalls that are not present when a singleton is sampled. Whereas dye can be injected into the amniotic sac of one twin to allow confirmation that each fetus has been sampled at the time of amniocentesis, no such marker is available for CVS sampling in twin gestations. Therefore, the operator must be certain that each placental site is separately identified by ultrasound and individually sampled. The ultrasound is important in determining whether monochorionic or dichorionic placentation is present. A thick, well-defined membrane separating the two fetuses is a reliable indicator in the first trimester of dichorionic pregnancy. The absence of a membrane or a thin, wispy membrane is seen with a monochorionic pregnancy. In order to avoid errors, we attempt to sample near each placental cord insertion site whether a monochorionic or dichorionic placentation is demonstrated by ultrasound. In cases in which a membrane is not demonstrated and individual cord insertion sites are not visible, only one sample is retrieved. In our experience of over hundreds of chorionic villus samplings in multiple gestations, utilization of this sampling technique has consistently led to correct information, given the fact that monozygotic gestations have the same karyotype.

Theoretically, mosaicism from postzygotic nondysjunctional events could occur and be missed with this sampling technique. Cases in which the operator is not convinced that both fetuses have been sampled should be followed up with an amniocentesis. With experience, this should occur in less than 1% of cases. Contamination of one tissue sample with villi from the other fetus can lead to misinformation. Clinically, this is usually not a problem when karyotype alone is to be analyzed, since the presence of an abnormal cell line in one fetus will be identified even if some of these villi are contaminating the other sample. However, this can lead to a completely inaccurate result when biochemical enzyme analysis is performed. Contamination is best avoided by choosing sampling routes that do not pass through both frondosums. Combinations of both abdominal and cervical sampling make this possible. For biochemical testing, analysis of individual villi rather than combining all villi in one sample will also diminish the possibility

of an error. Requests for multifetal pregnancy reductions will also occur when multiple gestations are diagnosed. In our experience, 1–2% of pregnancies in advanced maternal age patients will have at least one fetus with a karyotypic abnormality. Fortunately, reduction can be performed safely in early gestation.[36] However, the ability to perform this procedure mandates that an accurate and detailed graph of fetal position be drawn at the time of sampling so that the aneuploid fetus can be identified 1–2 weeks later. In cases in which uterine rotation makes identification of the affected fetus inconclusive, a repeat CVS with a 1–3-hour direct preparation to confirm the karyotype is suggested.

Since twins present unique difficulties, it is suggested that only experienced operators sample these gestations. Multiple gestations of higher order such as triplets and quadruplets have also been successfully sampled, but in these cases the patient must be informed of the potential additive risks of the procedure. At this point it should be emphasized that all patients with either singleton or twin gestations who have had first-trimester CVS should receive ultrasound examination and maternal serum alpha-fetoprotein (AFP) testing at 15–18 weeks' gestation. Should the maternal serum AFP be elevated, the CVS should not be regarded as the cause of this elevation, and these patients should have the appropriate workup to explain the high maternal serum AFP, including targeted ultrasound examination or amniocentesis. Patients who have undergone fetal reduction are not candidates for maternal serum alphafetoprotein screening because of the residual fetal tissue but should receive targeted ultrasound for malformation screening.

Laboratory aspects of CVS

Tissue preparation

The average sample from a transcervical CVS contains 15–30 mg wet weight of villus material for analysis. Transabdominal samples are slightly smaller, on average, but are adequate for routine procedures.[37] When larger samples are required for both karyotyping and biochemical diagnosis, we will usually proceed from the outset with a transcervical aspiration. The tissue, once obtained, is aseptically transferred to a 60-mm Petri dish and inspected under an inverted microscope, where contaminating maternal tissue adherent to the villi is teased away with a fine forceps. Decidual tissue is distinguishable for its structurelessness in contrast to the villi, and has a sheetlike or membranous appearance. To avoid errors, atypical villi are discarded. Cleaned villi are then transferred to a clean dish containing Hanks' balanced salt solution (HBSS), gently washed with a swirling motion, and transferred again to smaller dishes for tissue culture, incubation, or further preparation and analysis for biochemical or DNA diagnoses. Cytogenetic analysis processing of the villi for cytogenetic analysis may be performed by two distinct methods. The 'direct' method described by Simoni et al[38] makes use of the actively mitotic cytotrophoblast cells in the buds of the villi. This method may give a result in as little as 2 hours, but most laboratories use an overnight incubation and report results 3–4 days after the procedure. The second approach is to culture the cells of the villous mesenchymal core in standard monolayer cultures, for about 5–8 days (Tables 5.1 and 5.2). It is recommended that all samples be set up by both direct and culture methods. Though the direct method is rapid and rarely plagued with decidual contamination, tissue culture is superior in identifying and evaluating discrepancies between the cytotrophoblast and the actual fetal state, which is more closely represented by the cells of the mesenchymal core.

Biochemical and DNA analysis

For biochemical studies, extracts of chorionic villi may be prepared by the same methods used to prepare fibroblast or cultured amniotic fluid cell extracts. In many cases, the procedure can be made more rapid and efficient by using villi, since the enzyme is present in sufficient quantities for analysis in the aspirated tissue itself. The analysis for Tay–Sachs disease, for example, can be performed in less than 30 minutes using fresh villi.[39] In performing biochemical analysis, the process of removing maternal decidua from the specimen is especially critical, since small amounts of decidua may contain relatively large quantities of the enzyme being investigated. Once cleaned and rinsed,

Table 5.1 Chorionic villus sampling tissue preparation: direct/rapid preparation of chorionic villi

Procedural steps	Results
Clean villi and remove decidua and place in RPMI 1640 with fetal calf serum	Prevents maternal cell contamination
Add FUDR (17 h) and then thymidine (5 h) and incubate overnight	Synchronizes chromosome division to enhance chromosome metaphase quality and quantity (for same-day results, this step is eliminated)
Add colcemid for 2 h	Arrests cell division
Add hypotonic solution (20 ml Na citrate)	Swells the cell membrane
Wash with and place in methanol/acetic acid solution	Stops the action of the hypotonic solution and fixes the tissue
Add 50% acetic acid	Releases metaphase cells from the villus
Drop on warm slide and spread suspension slowly while drying	Allows cells to settle from fixative and adhere to the slide and spread out
Stain to band	Allows microscope analysis of chromosomes

Table 5.2 Chorionic villus sampling tissue preparation: long-term culture of chorionic villi

Procedural steps	Results
Clean villi and remove decidua	Prevents maternal cell contamination
Place in Chang medium overnight (37°C CO$_2$ incubation)	Restores and enhances cell viability after initial manipulation
Wash villi in HBSS and expose to trypsin (1 h) and collagenase (30 min); villus skeleton aspirated with Pasteur pipette and planted in culture flask with Chang medium, RPMI, glutamine, and antibiotics	First dissociates and removes both the remaining maternal cells (if any) and syncytiocyto-trophoblast which will not grow; dissociates mesenchymal core into single cells for tissue culture growth
Single-cell suspension plated onto cover slips and incubated for 24 h (37°C CO$_2$)	Initiates cell attachment to cover slips
Change media and incubate for 24 h	Begins cell growth and eliminates toxic cell factors
Change media and incubate for 1–3 days	Allows continued cell division and growth of cell colonies
Cell harvest begins	
Colcemid added to cover slip for 1 h	Arrests dividing cells on cover slip in metaphase
Process as usual *in situ* tissue culture with hypotonic and fixative, and then prepare by controlled drying	Produces metaphase with well-spread, high quality morphology
Stain and examine chromosomes with microscope	Bands on chromosomes are stained for analysis

the tissue is transferred to 1.5-ml polypropylene tubes, where it is weighed and suspended in 25 ml of saline for each 5 μg of tissue. Cells are disrupted by freezing and thawing five times, along with maceration of the tissue by a sealed Pasteur pipette between each freeze–thaw cycle. The suspension is centrifuged at 15 000 g for 5 minutes, and the supernatant is extracted for analysis, according to the test's specific protocol. Deoxyribonucleic acid may be prepared similarly from villi by standard methods for restriction enzyme analysis. Approximately 2–5 mg of wet tissue is obtained from each average-sized villus, and about 5 μg of DNA may be obtained per mg of tissue weight. These amounts provide adequate tissue samples for standard assays.

Evaluation of fetal red blood cells

Vessels within the mesenchymal core of the chorionic villi contain small amounts of fetal red blood cells. Microdissection of these vessels, followed by mixed agglutination[40] or counterstaining[41] techniques, has been described in evaluating the presence or absence of fetal red cell antigens. This analysis had been valuable for patients in whom a previous pregnancy has been affected by hemolysis via isoimmunization. With the advent of expanded molecular techniques to diagnose red cell suface antigens, the use of this technique has become noteworthy for historic purposes only.

Safety of CVS

Despite the increasing acceptance of CVS as a first-trimester diagnostic procedure, the desired advantage of earlier diagnosis must be weighed against any increased risks encountered by sampling the developing placental site. Since September 1984, a registry of CVS procedures, results, and pregnancy outcomes has been sponsored by the World Health Organization's Inherited Disease Program and the March of Dimes Birth Defects Foundation. Reports to the registry have been voluntary, without stringent reporting criteria, and usually submitted in groups of 'procedures performed', with pregnancy outcomes and losses lagging months behind. Despite these limitations, the registry, by virtue of its large volume of cases, offered early investigators a rapid assessment of the status and progress of the procedure. As of June 1990, over 60 000 procedures had been reported by over 120 centers via a variety of techniques and approaches. Although the registry continues to collect data and serves as a communication source for investigators, there are now sufficient single-center and collaborative reports to provide a more controlled and standardized database.

Evaluation of the risks of CVS has focused on the issues of fetal loss, particularly in regard to spontaneous abortion (Table 5.3). Procedure-related spontaneous abortion has generally been defined as spontaneous fetal loss or diagnosed intrauterine fetal death prior to 28 completed weeks of gestation. Calculating such procedure-related losses is complicated, however, by the background pregnancy loss rate. Investigators have demonstrated that 2–5% of pregnancies shown by ultrasound to be viable at 7–12 weeks' gestation were either nonviable when rescanned at 18 to 20 weeks prior to amniocentesis[42–45] or were lost spontaneously prior to 28 weeks' gestation. The rate of spontaneous loss increases with maternal age and is highest in women whose age places them at particular risk of chromosomal abnormalities, and thus in need of prenatal diagnosis.[43,45,46] Overall, these spontaneous losses appear to occur predominantly in early pregnancy, with losses after 16 weeks occurring uncommonly.[47]

The largest compilations of data regarding the risks of CVS have come from two collaborative reports. In early 1989, the Canadian Collaborative CVS-Amniocentesis Clinical Trial Group documented an excess loss of only 0.6% for CVS over amniocentesis, a difference which was not statistically significant.[48] No significant differences were noted between the two groups in terms of incidence of preterm birth or low birth weight. Maternal complications were infrequent in each group.

An American collaborative report described a prospective but nonrandomized trial of over 2200 women who had chosen either transcervical CVS or second-trimester amniocentesis for prenatal diagnosis.[30] As in the Canadian study, advanced maternal age was the primary indication for the procedures. When the losses were adjusted for group differences in gestational age and maternal age, an excess pregnancy loss of 0.8% referable to CVS, over amniocentesis, was calculated, which again was not significant.

Multiple single-center reports have confirmed the results of these collaborative trials regarding the safety and accuracy of transcervical CVS.[49–54] After adjustments for background loss, no significant increases in pregnancy losses were related to CVS, though a procedural 'learning curve' was observed. The latter must be taken into account with any new technical development. Data from all studies show that loss rates increase with the number of insertions required to obtain an adequate sample and that the number of insertions is inversely proportional to the expertise of the operator.

Table 5.3 CVS and pregnancy loss

Reference	Total procedures (technique used)	Induced abortions (%)	Spontaneous abortions (%) (Losses to 28 weeks/ continuing pregnancies	Procedural success (%)
Rhoads et al[30]	2248 (TC)*	45 (2.0)	77 (3.5)	97.8
Brambati et al[34]	1159 (TA)†	71 (6.1)	25/716 (3.5) ‡	99.7
Canadian Group[47]	1191 (TC)	26 (2.2)	57 (4.9)	98.5
Ward et al[53]	163 (TC)	43 (26.3)	13 (10.8)	96.8
Green et al[49]	940 (TC)	27 (2.9)	23 (2.5)	99.4
Wade & Young[52]	714 (TC)	29 (4.1)	31 (4.5)	N/A
Jahoda et al[51]	1550 (TC)	101 (6.5)	73 (5.0)	97.8
Clark et al[48]	211 (TC)	8 (3.8)	6 (2.9)	N/A
	8029	350/8176 = (4.3%)	305/7454 = 4.1%	

*TC: transcervical CVS; † TA: transabdominal CVS; ‡ includes only completed pregnancies.

Refinement of the transabdominal technique for CVS has ensured its place in the prenatal diagnostic arena. Where initial reports described simply the feasibility of the method in the first trimester,[31,32,34,55,56] more recent trials have compared the transcervical and transabdominal approaches in a randomized fashion.[37,57] In the USA with over 1000 patients in each arm of the study, procedural success (over 99%) and total pregnancy loss rates (2.4–2.8%, not increased over baseline) were equivalent for both groups.[37] In addition, comparable numbers of patients required only one attempt to retrieve tissue (87%) or had unsuccessful procedures (less than 1%). These results were confirmed by others, who also suggested that, because of pre-existing operator experience with transabdominal invasive procedures, that approach might be the method of first choice for most CVS.[58] Since fetal loss rates tend to stabilize once expertise is gained with the technically more difficult transcervical approach, it would be reasonable to conclude that the integration of both methods into any single center's program offers the most practical approach to first-trimester diagnosis.[59]

Because of the success with transabdominal CVS for diagnosis in the first trimester, investigators have suggested extending its use to rapid karyotyping in the second and third trimesters as well. Pijpers et al reported successful chromosomal analysis beyond 13 weeks' gestation.[60] This confirmed the work by others[61,62] who advocated second-trimester transabdominal CVS for rapid chromosomal evaluation of at-risk fetuses. A recent study demonstrated the efficacy of the procedure performed in the second and third trimesters and showed its special value in oligohydramnios, where amniocentesis was technically unfeasible.[63] Exact determination of the pregnancy loss rates associated with these placental biopsies is difficult, since many procedures are performed for abnormal pregnancies. Documented losses occurred in less than 1% of the reported cases within 2 weeks of the procedures.

Complications of CVS

Infection

There has been concern, from the initial introduction of transcervical CVS, that transvaginal passage of the catheter would introduce vaginal flora into the uterus with subsequent chorioamnionitis. This potential risk was first suggested by Schialli et al,[64] who isolated bacteria from 30% of the catheters used for CVS, and has been confirmed by other studies.[65–68] However, no associations between bacteria cultured from the cervical swab and/or aspirating cannula and adverse pregnancy outcome have been demonstrated.[66] Two life-threatening infections have been reported after transcervical CVS.[69,70] In both, a single catheter was used for repeated insertions. Since these reports, the practice of using a new sterile catheter for each insertion has been adopted. Similarly, for transabdominal procedures, a fresh spinal needle is used for repeat passes.

The incidence of post-CVS chorioamnionitis is low. One study found an incidence of 0.3% prior to 20 weeks' gestation,[71] while another reported only two clinically detected infections in 1000 procedures.[72] These results were confirmed by the large CVS collaborative series.[30,48] In our own series of over 8000 patients, we have observed no case of chorioamnionitis requiring uterine evacuation. We do not prescribe prophylactic antibiotics periprocedurally. Among our pregnancy losses, the suspected incidence of periabortion chorioamnionitis was 0.08%, about the same as seen in series of spontaneous abortions that had not been previously sampled.[43,45]

Bleeding

Vaginal bleeding or spotting is relatively uncommon after transabdominal CVS procedures, but not unusual after transcervical CVS. Most centers report this occurrence in 15–20% of transcervically sampled patients, though heavy bleeding occurs in only a small percentage. Subchorionic hematoma formation immediately after sampling was seen in 4% of sampled pregnancies and was associated with up to 7 days of vaginal bleeding.[72] The hematoma usually disappeared before week 16 of pregnancy and was rarely associated with adverse outcome. The heavy bleeding and resulting hematoma formation result from accidental placement of the transcervical catheter into the vascular decidua basalis underlying the chorion frondosum. In many of these cases, a distinct 'pop' is felt prior to the bleeding, and a gritty feeling indicates penetration into the decidual layer. In extreme cases the development of a hematoma can be seen on ultrasound, and its expansion charted (Figure 5.6). Careful attention to the feel of the catheter, which is gained with experience, can prevent many of these hemorrhagic episodes.

Rh sensitization

An acute and consistent rise in maternal serum AFP levels after CVS has been reported, implying a detectable degree of fetal-maternal bleeding.[73–75] In Rh-negative women, this fact is critical, since Rh-positive cells in volumes as low as 0.1 ml can cause Rh sensitization.[76] The risk of fetal-maternal bleeding has been shown to be independent of CVS method (transcervical or transabdominal), and dependent on the amount of tissue aspirated, though all women with even a single pass by either method had detectable rises in AFP.[75] For these reasons, all Rh-negative, nonsensitized women undergoing CVS receive Rho (D) immunoglobulin subsequent to the procedure. The risk of worsening already-existing Rh immunization in previously sensitized women has been described and presents a relative contraindication to CVS in this population.[77]

Rupture of the membranes

Acute rupture of the membranes, documented either by obvious gross fluid leakage or by a decrease in amniotic fluid volume

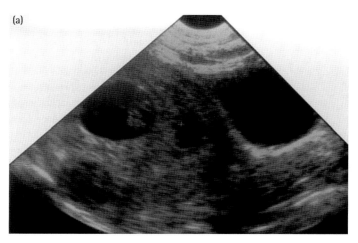
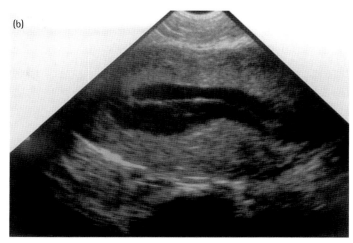

Figure 5.6 (a) Demonstrates a small subchorionic hematoma seen shortly after transcervical chorionic villus sampling. (b) Demonstrate a much larger hematoma found on 16-week follow up scan. Both of these hematomas resolved spontaneously and were not visible at follow-up scanning at 20 weeks.

on ultrasound, is a very rare complication of CVS. In a collaborative review of over 6000 procedures from three centers, acute membrane rupture was not observed. In fact, attempts intentionally to rupture membranes with a transcervical catheter in pregnancies scheduled for termination have confirmed that the chorion can withstand significant pressure without rupturing.

Rupture of the membranes days or weeks after the procedure may occur, however, either from injury to the chorion allowing exposure and damage of the amnion, or as a result of low-grade chorioamnionitis. Various groups have reported a 0.3% incidence of delayed rupture of the membranes after CVS.[71,72] A significant finding confirmed by our own experience is the presence of oligohydramnios in the second trimester in 6 of 1000 sampled patients, in the absence of clinical evidence of fluid leakage.[71] In one of our cases, blue dye injected transabdominally into the amniotic sac was subsequently detected transvaginally, confirming the leak.

Perinatal complications

Absence of increase in the rate of congenital abnormalities after CVS was noted in the large collaborative series and in our own experience of over 6000 deliveries. Prolonged follow-up of 53 children born after placental biopsy found all of them in good health, with normal development and school performance.[78] No series to date has demonstrated late perinatal complications. There has been no reported increase in preterm labor, premature rupture of the membranes, small-for-date infants, or other obstetric complications.[79]

Risk of fetal abnormalities after CVS

It has recently been suggested that CVS may be associated with the occurrence of specific fetal malformations. The first suggestion of this was reported by Firth et al.[80] In a series of 539 CVS-exposed pregnancies, they identified five infants with severe limb abnormalities, all of which came from a cohort of 289 pregnancies sampled at 66 days' gestation or less. Four of these infants had the unusual or rare oromandibular-limb hypogenesis syndrome, and the fifth had a terminal transverse limb reduction defect. Oromandibular-limb hypogenesis syndrome occurs with a birth prevalence of 1 per 175 000 live births,[81] and limb reduction defects occur in 1 per 1690 births.[82] Therefore, the occurrence of these abnormalities in more than 1% of CVS-sampled cases raised strong suspicion of an association. In this initial report, all of the limb abnormalities followed transabdominal sampling performed at 55–66 days' gestation.

Subsequent to this initial report, others added supporting cases to this list. Using the Italian multicenter birth defects registry, Mastroiacovo et al reported in a case-control study an odds ratio of 11.3 (CI 5.6–2.13) for transverse limb abnormalities after first-trimester CVS.[83] When stratified by gestational age at sampling, pregnancies sampled prior to 70 days had a 19.7% increased risk of transverse limb reduction defects, while patients sampled later did not demonstrate a significantly increased risk. Subsequent case-control studies, however, did not find an association between CVS and limb reduction defects.[84]

There have been additional reports of transverse limb defects following very early CVS. Most notably, Brambati et al, an extremely experienced group that found no increased risk of limb defects in patients sampled after 9 weeks, had a 1.6% incidence of severe limb reduction defects in a group of patients sampled at 6 and 7 weeks.[85] This rate decreased to 0.1% for sampling at 8–9 weeks. Hsieh, in a report of the Taiwan CVS experience, reported 29 cases of limb reduction defects following CVS from September 1990 until June 1992; four cases had oromandibular-limb hypogenesis syndrome.[86] There were two remarkable aspects of this report. First, although the gestational age at sampling was not known with certainty in all cases, the majority were performed at less than 63 days after the last menstrual period. Secondly, the cases with limb reduction defects were performed by very inexperienced, community-based operators, whereas no defects were reported from the major centers. This experience suggests that early gestational sampling and excessive placental trauma may be etiologic in the reported clusters of post-CVS limb reduction defects.

The question continues to be debated of whether CVS sampling after 10 weeks has the potential of causing more subtle defects, such as shortening of the distal phalanx or nail hypoplasia.[87] At present, there are few data to substantiate this concern. On the contrary, most experienced centers performing CVS after 10 weeks have not seen an increase in limb defects of any type. A review of the almost 140 000 CVS procedures reported to the WHO registry has demonstrated no increase in the overall incidence of limb reduction defects after CVS nor in any specific type or pattern of defects.[88] The absence of defects in most centers has led to speculation that the few reported clusters are either statistical flukes or related to center-specific practices.

Mechanisms by which CVS could potentially lead to fetal malformations continue to be disputed. Placental thrombosis with subsequent fetal embolization has been raised as a potential etiology, but this is unlikely, since fetal clotting factors appear to be insufficient at this early gestational age. Inadvertent entry into the extraembryonic celoem with resulting amnionic bands has also been raised as a potential mechanism, but this appears unlikely as well, since actual bands have not been observed in the majority of the cases. Additionally, many of the cases of oromandibular-limb hypogenesis syndrome had internal central nervous system anomalies which cannot be accounted for by fetal entanglement or compression.

Uterine vascular disruption appears to be the most plausible mechanism at present.[81] In this hypothesis, CVS causes injury, vasospasm, or compression of the uterine vessels, resulting in underperfusion of the fetal peripheral circulation. After the initial insult, there may be subsequent rupture of the thin-walled vessels of the damaged distal embryonic circulation, leading to further hypoxia, necrosis, and eventually resorption of pre-existing structures. Theoretically, an overly traumatic CVS technique could lead to significant uterine or placental disruption with secondary fetal hypovolemia, vasospasm, and peripheral shutdown, especially in very early gestation. A similar mechanism leading to limb defects has been demonstrated in animal models after uterine vascular clamping, maternal cocaine exposure, or even simple uterine palpation.[89,90]

A variation of this hypothesis implicates fetal hemorrhage, rather than vasospasm, as the cause of fetal hypoperfusion. Since the fetal and maternal circulations are contiguous, a significant fetal bleed will result in a fetal-to-maternal hemorrhage detectable as an increase in the maternal serum AFP level. Smidt-Jensen et al found that spontaneous fetal loss occurs more frequently among women whose serum AFP increased substantially after transabdominal CVS.[91] This suggested that severe fetal hemorrhage may result in fetal death, while lesser degrees of hemorrhage may allow the pregnancy to continue, but result in transient episodes of fetal hypoperfusion.

In a report in *The Lancet*, Quintero et al have added additional information about the possible etiologic mechanisms.[92] Using transabdominal embryoscopic visualization of the first trimester embryo, they demonstrated the occurrence of fetal facial, head, and thoracic ecchymotic lesions after traumatically induced detachment of the placenta with subchorionic hematoma formation. No changes in fetal heart rate were seen. While these lesions consistently appeared after significant physical trauma to the placental site, they could not be produced by the passage of a standard CVS catheter.

Any theory of CVS-induced limb defects must consider the varying stages of fetal sensitivity and should demonstrate a correlation between the severity of the defects and the gestational age at sampling. Firth et al have recently presented evidence that appears to illustrate that sampling prior to 9 weeks' gestation induces severe fetal limb defects, which are not increased after later CVS.[93] However, Froster and Jackson have reviewed the severity of the post-CVS limb defects reported to the World Health Organization (WHO) registry and found no such correlation.[88,94] Table 5.4 summarizes the studies evaluating the association between CVS and fetal limb defects for procedures performed after 63 days of gestation.

At the present time, the possible association of fetal limb abnormalities and CVS appears to have sufficient credibility that patients should be informed of the controversy prior to having the procedure performed. Centers performing CVS should have aggressive follow-up systems in place and should be able to give patients information about the rates of congenital abnormalities in their center. Sampling prior to 10 weeks' gestation should be limited to exceptional cases. CVS beyond 10 weeks, in experienced hands, continues to have a very low (if any) risk of fetal abnormalities and should continue to be routinely offered.

Accuracy of CVS

Maternal cell contamination

Direct preparations of chorionic villus tissue is generally thought to exclude maternal cell contamination (MCC),[18] though the preparations are of a suboptimal quality compared to long-term culture techniques. Comparison of direct and long-term culture processing shows a low rate of MCC in long-term cultures, of 0.1–1.3%.[109–111] Of interest is the fact that, in a different series of placental biopsies performed later in pregnancy, the risk of MCC, even using DNA-probe analysis techniques on direct-prepared specimens, appears to be significantly lower than with first-trimester procedures.[112]

Mosaicism

A consistent finding in the majority of reports on both methods of CVS is the small but notable proportion of patients in whom an initial report of mosaicism is disproved subsequently by analysis of amniotic fluid, fetal blood, or neonatal blood. This

Table 5.4 Studies evaluating the association of CVS and LRDs: procedures performed after 63 days of gestation

No association			Association		
Author	No. of post-CVS Livb	No. of LRD	Author	No. of CVS	No. of LRD
Jahoda et al[95]	3973	3		Burton et al[106]	394	4
Halliday et al[96]	2071	3 U	Mastroiacovo et al[107]	2759	3
Canadian Group[48]	905	0	Bissonnette (A)[104]	507	5
Schloo et al[97]	3120	2			
Monni et al[98]	2752	2			
Blakemore et al[99]	3709	3			
Silver et al[100]	1048	1 U			
Mahoney–USNICHD[101]	4588	8			
Jackson et al[102]	12863	5			
Smidt-Jensen et al[103]	2624	0			
Bissonnette (B)[104]	269	0			
Case control studies	OR	CI		OR	CI
Eurocat[84]	1.8	0.7–5	Italian Multicenter <76 days[108]	19	9–37
US Multi-State[105]			US Multistate[105]		
Overall LRD	1.7	0.4–6	Terminal Digital		
Transverse LRD	4.7	0.8–28	LRD	6.4	1.1–38

CI: Confidence interval. LRD: limb reduction defects. OR: odds ratio. U: uncertain association.

suggests that the identical composition of the fetus and the extraembryonic tissue cannot always be assumed. The earlier quoted multicenter studies confirmed reports from single centers indicating that 0.6–0.8% of CVS samples yielded mosaics, with approximately three-quarters of follow-up analyses demonstrating normal karyotypes.[30,48]

The issue of mosaicism in CVS samples was addressed specifically in a large European collaborative study involving 36 centers and over 11 000 specimens.[113] Overall, mosaicism was reported in 1.3%, with 70% of the mosaics restricted to extraembryonic tissue after follow-up analysis of both continuing and noncontinuing pregnancies. Mosaicism was seen twice as frequently in direct preparations as in long-term cultures. Confirming CVS mosaics with amniocentesis is suggested, therefore, before final patient counseling. A recent report showed that, in similar circumstances, no increase in the rate of fetal loss was seen if a second, confirmatory procedure, such as amniocentesis, was required later in pregnancy to evaluate CVS mosaicism.[114]

Placental mosaicism may affect fetal outcome. In one study, two of nine fetuses with unexplained growth retardation had documented placental mosaicism.[115] Isolated placental mosaics seen at our center were also shown to be associated with perinatal complications.[116] In over 4300 CVS samples, mosaicism isolated to the placenta was seen in 0.6%. The rate of fetal loss in this group was 16.7%. It rose to 24% when mosaicism was confined exclusively to the cytotrophoblast. Many of these losses occurred well into the second and third trimesters. As in cases of suspected maternal cell contamination, with isolated mosaics or other unusual findings (such as satellites or marker chromosomes), amniocentesis and fetal blood sampling are available to aid in clinical interpretation. A mosaic culture with a karyotype which is associated with viable aneuploid neonates requires further testing by amniocentesis or by fetal blood analysis. In general, if the mosaicism is confined to the cytotrophoblast, and the tissue culture is normal, no further follow-up is indicated. However, delineation of the parental origin of the diploid karyotype in the case of a trisomic/disomic mosaic may be necessary. Uniparental disomy, the inheritance of two identical chromosomes from a single parent, has been identified as a mechanism for genetic diseases. Usually, each chromosome pair involves a chromosome contributed from each parent, which balances recessively mutated or imprinted genes. In pregnancies which involve a trisomic cell line, rescue of the pregnancy occurs by loss of one of the chromosomes to produce a euploid cell. If the cell contains a chromosome pair that is of a single parental origin and that chromosome carries a mutated or unbalanced gene, then a genetic syndrome may result. Detection of uniparental disomy requires comparison of parental karyotype with the fetal specimen. In no case should a decision to terminate a pregnancy be based on a CVS mosaic result alone.

Recommendations

Evaluations of cost/benefit ratios, diagnostic accuracy, speed of diagnosis, and bacterial contamination have drawn lines between two camps regarding the preferable cytogenetic method to use if a center is to rely on a single technique, either direct preparation or long-term culture.[109] Unless extremely rapid diagnosis is essential (as before multifetal pregnancy reduction), we await the results of both cytogenetic methods at our center before reporting a fetal karyotype.

Establishing a CVS program

Although CVS has been demonstrated to be safe and efficacious in the hands of experienced operators, gaining this experience has proven difficult for a number of centers. Whereas transabdominal sampling utilizes skills that many operators already have, ultrasound-guided transcervical sampling requires the learning of a new approach. However, the availability of both techniques dramatically improves the ability to retrieve tissue safely and easily. Transcervical sampling is best learned on pretermination patients. In general, 25–50 such procedures should be performed prior to beginning sampling on continuing pregnancies. It is suggested that the operator continue to practice sampling until he or she is able to retrieve sufficient villi from over 95% of patients. If pretermination procedures are unavailable, sampling in patients with blighted ova is useful and has the added advantage of offering the patients karyotype information on the abnormal pregnancy. At the present time, CVS sampling should be performed in centers in which samplers and cytogeneticists are in close proximity to each other, working as a single system. This allows the tissue to be reviewed prior to the discharge of the patient, and permits a comprehensive and complete service for the patient.

Acceptance of CVS

Initial experiences reporting on the technical feasibility of first-trimester sampling of the placenta for the purposes of prenatal diagnosis were followed by large-scale series that confirmed the safety of the procedure.[30,48,117] Still to follow were reports on the acceptability of the method by patients presenting for genetic diagnosis. The ability to move prenatal diagnosis into the first trimester found approval for a number of reasons. Once the safety and accuracy of CVS were documented, the advantage of added privacy inherent in an earlier procedure became evident. One study showed that 70% of women at high genetic risk who had terminated an abnormal pregnancy diagnosed by CVS returned in future pregnancies for similar genetic testing.[52] As transabdominal CVS became available, reports appeared that patients preferred that method for reasons of comfort, speed, and avoidance of embarrassment.[118] Added to this asset is the ease of adapting amniocentesis skills to transabdominal sampling.[119]

Psychologic studies on populations of women undergoing prenatal diagnosis demonstrated that first-trimester procedures lowered maternal anxiety levels earlier and more consistently than traditional midtrimester amniocentesis. Measurable and significant decreases in anxiety scores were seen after normal results were available. Chorionic villus sampling results, logically, produced lower scores earlier than did amniocentesis.[120,121] In addition, women undergoing CVS reported greater attachment to the pregnancy during the second trimester than did women undergoing amniocentesis, assessed in terms of both attachment between mother and fetus and self-comparison to attachment perceived to be felt by other pregnant women.[122] These authors assessed the perceived benefits afforded by CVS as confirming earlier reports demonstrating a patient preference for CVS,[123] though lower than the 100% elicited in the earlier study. The increased acceptance of prenatal diagnosis earlier in pregnancy, coupled with our expanding ability to manipulate genetic material to give up its information antenatally, has made researchers realize that, as earlier procedures become available, they quickly become the preferred procedure.[124] CVS has become the standard against which the safety and accuracy of even newer technologies applied to first-trimester gestations have to be measured.

References

1. Fuchs F, Riis P. Antenatal foetal sex determination. Nature 1956; 177: 330.
2. Barr ML, Bertram EG. A morphological distinction between neurones of the male and female, and the behavior of the nucleolar satellite during accelerated nucleoprotein synthesis. Nature 1949; 163: 676.
3. Steele MW, Breg WR Jr. Chromosome analysis of human amniotic-fluid cells. Lancet 1966; 1(7437): 383–5.
4. Golbus MS, Loughman WD, Epstein CJ et al. Prenatal genetic diagnosis in 3000 amniocenteses. N Engl J Med 1979; 300: 157.
5. Mohr J. Foetal genetic diagnosis: development of techniques for early sampling of foetal cells. Acta Pathol Microbiol Scand 1968; 73: 73.
6. Hahnemann N, Mohr J. Genetic diagnosis in the embryo by means of biopsy from extraembryonic membranes. Bull Eur Soc Hum Genet 1968; 2: 23.
7. Hahnemann N, Mohr J. Antenatal foetal diagnosis in genetic disease. Bull Eur Soc Hum Genet 1969; 3: 47.
8. Kullander S, Sandahl B. Fetal chromosome analysis after transcervical placental biopsies during early pregnancy. Acta Obstet Gynecol Scand 1973; 52: 355.
9. Hahnemann N. Early prenatal diagnosis: a study of biopsy techniques and cell culturing from extraembryonic membranes. Clin Genet 1974; 6: 294.
10. Department of Obstetrics and Gynecology, Tietung Hospital of Anshan Iron and Steel Company. Fetal sex prediction by sex chromatin of chorionic villi cells during early pregnancy. Chin Med J 1975; 1: 117.

11. Goldberg MF, Chen ATL, Ahn YW et al. First-trimester fetal chromosomal diagnosis using endocervical lavage: a negative evaluation. Am J Obstet Gynecol 1980; 138: 436.

12. Rhine SA, Cain JL, Cleary RE et al. Prenatal sex detection with endocervical smears: successful results utilizing Y-body fluorescence. Am J Obstet Gynecol 1975; 122: 155.

13. Rhine SA, Palmer CG, Thompson JF. A simple alternative to amniocentesis for first trimester prenatal diagnosis. Birth Defects 1977; 12(3D): 231.

14. Kazy Z, Rozovsky IS, Bakharev VA. Chorion biopsy in early pregnancy: a method of early prenatal diagnosis for inherited disorders. Prenat Diagn 1982; 2: 39.

15. Williamson R, Eskdale J, Coleman DV et al. Direct gene analysis of chorionic villi: a possible technique for first-trimester antenatal diagnosis of haemoglobinopathies. Lancet 1981; 2: 1125.

16. Old JM, Ward RHT, Karagozlu F et al. First-trimester fetal diagnosis for haemoglobinopathies: three cases. Lancet 1982; 2: 1413.

17. Ward RHT, Modell B, Petrou M et al. Method of sampling chorionic villi in first trimester of pregnancy under guidance of real time ultrasound. BMJ 1983; 286: 1542.

18. Simoni G, Brambati B, Danesino C et al. Efficient direct chromosome analyses and enzyme determinations from chorionic villi samples in the first trimester of pregnancy. Hum Genet 1983; 63: 349.

19. Brambati B, Simoni G. Diagnosis of fetal trisomy 21 in first trimester. Lancet 1983; 1: 586.

20. Chistolini A, Papacchini M, Mazzucconi MG et al. Carrier detection and renatal diagnosis in haemophilia A and B. Haematologica 1990; 75: 424.

21. Goossens M, Dumez Y, Kaplan L. Prenatal diagnosis of sickle-cell anemia in the first-trimester of pregnancy. N Engl J Med 1983; 309: 831.

22. Grebner EE, Wapner RJ, Barr MA, Jackson LG. Prenatal Tay–Sachs diagnosis by chorionic villi sampling. Lancet 1983; 2: 286.

23. Gustavii B. First-trimester chromosomal analysis of chorionic villi obtained by direct vision technique. Lancet 1983; 2: 507.

24. Lilford R, Maxwell D, Coleman D et al. Diagnosis, four hours after chorion biopsy, of female fetus in pregnancy at risk of Duchenne muscular dystrophy. Lancet 1983; 2: 1491.

25. Permagent E, Ginsberg N, Verlinksy Y et al. Prenatal Tay–Sachs diagnosis by chorionic villi sampling. Lancet 1983; 2: 286.

26. Rodeck CH, Nicolaides KH, Morsman JM et al. A single-operator technique for first-trimester chorion biopsy. Lancet 1983; 2: 1340.

27. Vimal CM, Fensom AH, Heaton D et al. Prenatal diagnosis of argininosuccinicaciduria by analysis of cultured chorionic villi. Lancet 1984; 2: 521.

28. Popp LW, Ghirardini G. The role of transvaginal sonography in chorionic villi sampling. J Clin Ultrasound 1990; 18: 315.

29. Dolk H, Bertrend F, Lechat MF. Chorionic villus sampling and limb abnormalities. Lancet 1992; 339; 876.

30. Rhoads GG, Jackson LG, Schlesselman SE et al. The safety and efficacy of chorionic villus sampling for early prenatal diagnosis of cytogenetic abnormalities. N Engl J Med 1989; 320: 609.

31. Smidt-Jensen S, Hahnemann N, Jensen PU et al. Experience with fine needle biopsy in the first trimester – an alternative to amniocentesis. Clin Genet 1984; 26: 272.

32. Brambati B, Oldrini A, Lanzati A. Transabdominal chorionic villus sampling: a freehand ultrasound-guided technique. Am J Obstet Gynecol 1987; 157: 134.

33. Nicolaides KH, Rodeck CH, Soothill PW et al. Why confine chorionic villus (placental) biopsy to the first trimester? Lancet 1986; 1: 543.

34. Brambati B, Lanzani A, Oldrini A. Transabdominal chorionic villus sampling: clinical experience of 1,159 cases. Prenat Diagn 1988; 8: 609.

35. Wapner RJ, Johnson A, Davis GH, et al. The prenatal diagnosis of twin gestations: a prospective comparison between second trimester amniocentesis and first trimester chorionic villus sampling. Am J Obstet Gynecol 1993; 82: 49–56.

36. Wapner RJ, Davis GH, Johnson A et al. Selective reduction of multifetal pregnancies. Lancet 1990; 335: 90.

37. Wapner RJ, Davis GH, Johnson A et al. A prospective comparison between transcervical and transabdominal chorionic villus sampling. Abstract no. 8. Society of Perinatal Obstetricians, 1990 Meeting, Houston.

38. Simoni G, Terzoli G, Rossella F. Direct chromosome preparation and culture using chorionic villi: an evaluation of the two techniques. Am J Med Genet 1990; 35: 181.

39. Grebner EE, Jackson LG. Prenatal diagnosis for Tay–Sachs disease using chorionic villus sampling. Prenat Diagn 1985; 5: 313.

40. Gemke RJBJ, Kanhai HHH, Overbeeke MAM et al. ABO and rhesus phenotyping of fetal erythrocytes in the first trimester of pregnancy. Br J Haematol 1986; 64: 689.

41. Rodesch F, Lambermont M, Donner C et al. Chorionic biopsy in management of severe cell alloimmunization. Am J Obstet Gynecol 1987; 156: 124.

42. Casner KA, Christopher CR, Dysert GA. Spontaneous fetal loss after demonstration of a live fetus in the first trimester. Obstet Gynecol 1987; 70: 827.

43. Gilmore DH, McNay MB. Spontaneous fetal loss rate in early pregnancy. Lancet 1985; 1: 107.

44. Simpson JL, Bombard AT. Chromosomal abnormalities in spontaneous abortion, frequency, pathology, and genetic counseling. In: Edmonds K, Bennet MJ (eds), Spontaneous Abortion, pp. 51–76. Blackwell: London, 1987.

45. Wilson RD, Kendrick V, Wirtman BK et al. Risk of spontaneous abortion in ultrasonographically normal pregnancies. Lancet 1984; 2: 920.

46. Warburton D, Stein Z, Kline J, Susser M. Chromosome abnormalities in spontaneous abortion: data from the New York City study. In: Porter IH, Hook EB (eds), Human Embryonic and Fetal Death, pp. 261–87. Academic Press: New York, 1980.

47. Simpson JL. Incidence and timing of pregnancy losses: relevance to evaluating safety of early prenatal diagnosis. Am J Med Genet 1990; 35: 165.

48. Canadian Collaborative CVS–Amniocentesis Clinical Trial Group: multicentre randomized clinical trial of chorion villus sampling and amniocentesis. Lancet 1989; 1: 1.

49. Clark BA, Bissonnette JM, Olson SB et al. Pregnancy loss in a small chorionic villus sampling series. Am J Obstet Gynecol 1989; 161: 301.

50. Green JE, Dorfman A, Jones SL et al. Chorionic villus sampling: experience with an initial 940 cases. Obstet Gynecol 1988; 71: 208.

51. Gustavii B, Claesson V, Kristoffersson U et al. Risk of miscarriage after chorionic biopsy is probably not higher than after amniocentesis. Lakartidningen 1989; 86: 4221.

52. Jahoda MGJ, Pijpers L, Reuss A et al. Evaluation of transcervical chorionic villus sampling with a completed follow-up of 1,550 consecutive pregnancies. Prenat Diagn 1989; 9: 621.

53. Wade RV, Young SR. Analysis of fetal loss after transcervical chorionic villus sampling: a review of 719 patients. Am J Obstet Gynecol 1989; 161: 513.

54. Ward RHT, Petrou M, Modell BM et al. Chorionic villus sampling in a high-risk population: 4 years' experience. Br J Obstet Gynecol 1988; 95: 1030.

55. Elias S, Simpson JL, Shulman LP et al. Transabdominal chorionic villus sampling for first-trimester prenatal diagnosis. Am J Obstet Gynecol 1989; 160: 879.

56. Smidt-Jensen S, Hahnemann N. Transabdominal chorionic villus sampling for fetal genetic diagnosis. Technical and obstetric evaluation of 100 cases. Prenat Diagn 1988; 8: 7.

57. Brambati B, Terzian E, Tognoni G. Randomized clinical trial of transabdominal versus transcervical chorionic villus sampling methods. Prenat Diagn 1991; 11: 285.

58. Brambati B, Lanzani A, Tului L. Transabdominal and transcervical chorionic villus sampling: efficacy and risk evaluation of 2,411 cases. Am J Hum Genet 1990; 35: 160.

59. Copeland KL, Carpenter RJ, Fenolio KR et al. Integration of the transabdominal technique into an ongoing chorionic villus sampling program. Am J Obstet Gynecol 1989; 161: 1289.

60. Pijpers L, Jahoda MGJ, Reuss A et al. Transabdominal chorionic villus sampling in second and third trimesters of pregnancy to determine fetal karyotype. BMJ 1988; 297: 822.

61. Hogdall CK, Doran TA, Shime J et al. Transabdominal chorionic villus sampling in the second trimester. Am J Obstet Gynecol 1988; 158: 345.

62. Holzgreve W, Miny P, Basaran S et al. Safety of placental biopsy in the second and third trimesters. N Engl J Med 1987; 317: 1159.

63. Holzgreve W, Miny P, Gerlach B et al. Benefits of placental biopsies for rapid karyotyping in the second and third trimesters (late chorionic villus sampling) in high-risk pregnancies. Am J Obstet Gynecol 1990; 162: 1188.

64. Schialli AR, Neugebauer DL, Fabro SE. Microbiology of the endocervix in patients undergoing chorionic villus sampling. In: Fracaro M, Simoni G, Brambati B (eds), First Trimester Fetal Diagnosis, pp. 69–73. Springer-Verlag: Berlin, 1985.

65. Brambati B, Matarrelli M, Varotto F. Septic complications after chorionic villus sampling. Lancet 1987; 1: 1212.

66. Garden AS, Reid G, Benzie RJ. Chorionic villus sampling. Lancet 1995; 1: 1270.

67. McFadyen JR, Taylor-Robinson D, Furr PM et al. Infection and chorionic villus sampling. Lancet 1985; 2: 610.

68. Wass D, Bennett MJ. Infection and chorionic villus sampling. Lancet 1985; 2: 338.

69. Barela A, Kleinman GE, Golditch IM et al. Septic shock with renal failure after chorionic villus sampling. Am J Obstet Gynecol 1986; 154: 1100.

70. Blakemore KH, Mahoney MH, Hobbins JC. Infection and chorionic villus sampling. Lancet 1985; 2: 339.

71. Hogge WA, Schonberg SA, Golbus MS. Chorionic villus sampling: experience of the first 1,000 cases. Am J Obstet Gynecol 1986; 154: 1249.

72. Brambati B, Oldrini A, Ferrazzi E et al. Chorionic villus sampling: an analysis of the obstetric experience of 1,000 cases. Prenat Diagn 1987; 7: 157.

73. Blakemore KJ, Baumgarten A, Schoenfeld-Diamaio M et al. Rise in maternal serum alpha-fetoprotein concentration after chorionic villus sampling and the possibility of isoimmunization. Am J Obstet Gynecol 1986; 155: 988.

74. Brambati B, Guercilena S, Bonacchi I et al. Fetomaternal transfusion after chorionic villus sampling: clinical implications. Hum Reprod 1986; 1: 37.

75. Shulman LP, Meyers CM, Simpson JL et al. Fetomaternal transfusion depends on amount of chorionic villi aspirated but not on method of chorionic villus sampling. Am J Obstet Gynecol 1990; 162: 1185.

76. Zipursky A, Israels LG. The pathogenesis and prevention of Rh immunization. Can Med Assoc J 1967; 97: 1245.

77. Moise KJ, Carpenter RJ, Wapner RJ et al. Increased severity of rhesus alloimmunization after first trimester transcervical chorionic villus biopsy. Fetal Diagn Ther 1990; 5: 76.

78. Angue H, Bingru Z, Hong W. Long-term follow-up results after aspiration of chorionic villi during early pregnancy. In: Fracaro M, Simoni G, Brambati B (eds), First Trimester Fetal Diagnosis, pp. 1–18. Springer-Verlag: New York, 1985.

79. Williams J, Medearis AL, Bear MB et al. Chorionic villus sampling is associated with normal fetal growth. Am J Obstet Gynecol 1987; 157: 708.

80. Firth HV, Boyd PA, Chamberlain P et al. Severe limb abnormalities after chorion villus sampling at 56–66 days' gestation. Lancet 1991; 337: 762.

81. Hoyme F, Jones KL, Van Allen MI et al. Vascular pathogenesis of transverse limb reduction defects. J Pediatr 1982; 101: 839.

82. Foster-Iskenius U, Baird P. Limb reduction defects in over 1,000,000 consecutive live births. Teratology 1989; 39: 127.

83. Mastroiacovo P, Botto LD, Cavalcanti DP. Limb anomalies following chorionic villus sampling: a registry based case control study. Am J Med Genet 1992; 44: 856–63.

84. Dolk H, Bertrend F, Lechat MF. Chorionic villus sampling and limb abnormalities. Lancet 1992; 339; 876.

85. Brambati B, Simoni G, Traui M. Genetic diagnosis by chorionic villus sampling before 8 gestational weeks: efficiency, reliability, and risks on 317 completed pregnancies. Prenat Diagn 1992; 12: 784–99.

86. Hsieh FJ, Shyu MK, Sheu BC et al. Limb defects after chorionic villus sampling. Obstet Gynecol 1995; 85: 84.

87. Burton BK, Schultz CJ, Burd LI. Spectrum of limb disruption defects associated with chorionic villus sampling. Pediatrics 1993; 91: 989–93.

88. Froster UG, Jackson L. Limb defects and chorionic villus sampling: results from an international registry, 1992–1994. Lancet 1996; 347(9000): 489.

89. Brent RL. Relationship between uterine vascular clamping, vascular disruption syndrome and cocaine teratology. Teratology 1990; 41: 757.

90. Webster W, Brown-Woodman T. Cocaine as a cause of congenital malformations of vascular origin: experimental evidence in the rat. Teratology 1990; 41: 689.

91. Smidt-Jensen S, Philip J, Zachary J et al. Implications of maternal serum alpha- fetoprotein elevation caused by transabdominal and transcervical CVS. Prenat Diagn 1994; 14: 35–46.

92. Quintero R, Romero R, Mahoney M et al. Fetal hemorrhagic lesions after chorionic villus sampling. Lancet 992; 339: 193.

93. Firth HV, Boyd PA, Chamberlain PF et al. Analysis of limb reduction defects in babies exposed to chorionic villus sampling. Lancet 1994; 343(8905): 1069.

94. Froster UG, Jackson LG. Safety of chorionic villus sampling: results from an international registry. Am J Hun Genet 1994; 55: A1.

95. Jahoda MGJ, Brandenberg H, Cohen-Overbeek et al. Terminal transverse limb defecta and early chorionic villus sampling: evaluation of 4,300 cases with completed follow-up. Am J Med Genet 1993; 46: 483.

96. Halliday J, Lumley J, Sheffield LJ et al. Limb deficiencies, chorion villus sampling, and advanced maternal age. Am J Med Genet 1993; 47: 1096.

97. Schloo R, Miney P, Holzgreve W et al. Distal limb deficiency following chorionic villus sampling? Am J Med Genet 1992; 42: 404.

98. Monni G, Ibba RM, Lai R et al. Limb-reduction defects and chorion villus sampling. Lancet 1991; 337: 1091.

99. Blakemore K, Filkins K, Luthy DA et al. Cook obstetrics and gynecology catheter multicenter chorionic villus sampling trial: comparison of birth defects with expected rates. Am J Obstet Gynecol 1993; 169: 1022.

100. Silver RK, Macgregor SN, Muhlbach LH et al. Congenital malformations subsequent to chorionic villus sampling: outcome analysis of 1048 consecutive procedures. Prenat Diagn 1994; 14: 421.

101. Mahoney MJ for the USNICHD Collaborative CVS Study Group. Limb abnormalities and chorionic villus sampling. Lancet 1991; 337: 1422.

102. Jackson LG, Wapner RJ, Brambati B. Limb abnormalities and chorionic villus sampling. Lancet 1991; 337: 1423.

103. Smidt-Jensen S, Permin M, Philip J et al. Randomized comparison of amniocentesis and transabdominal and transcervical chorionic villus sampling. Lancet 1992: 340: 1237.

104. Brezinka C, Hagenaars AM, Wladimiroff JW et al. Fetal ductus venous flow velocity waveforms and maternal serum AFP before and after first-trimester transabdominal chorionic villus sampling. Prenat Diagn 1995; 15: 699.

105. Olney RS, Khoury MJ, Alo CJ et al. Increased risk for transverse digital deficiency after chorionic villus sampling: results of the United States Multistate Case-Control Study, 1988–1992.

106. Burton BK, Schulz CH, Burd LI. Limb anomalies associated with chorionic villus sampling. Obstet Gynecol 1992; 79: 726.

107. Mastroiacovo P, Tozzi AE, Agosti S et al. Transverse limb reduction defects after chorion villus sampling: a retrospective cohort study. Prenat Diagn 1993; 13: 1051.

108. Mastroiacovo P, Botto LD. Chorionic villus sampling and transverse limb deficiencies: maternal age is not a confounder. Am J Med Genet 1994; 53: 182.

109. Ledbetter DH, Martin AO, Verlinsky Y et al. Cytogenetic results of chorionic villus sampling: high success rate and diagnostic accuracy in the United States collaborative study. Am J Obstet Gynecol 1990; 162: 495.

110. Roberts E, Duckett DP, Lang GD. Maternal cell contamination in chorionic villus samples assessed by direct preparations and three different culture methods. Prenat Diagn 1988; 8: 635.

111. Wright DJ, Brindley BA, Koppitch FC et al. Interpretation of chorionic villus sampling laboratory results is just as reliable as amniocentesis. Obstet Gynecol 1989; 74: 739.

112. Ganshirt-Ahlert D, Pohlschmidt M, Gal A et al. Transabdominal placental biopsy in the second and third trimesters of pregnancy: what is the risk of maternal contamination in DNA diagnosis? Obstet Gynecol 1990; 75: 320.

113. Vejerslev LO, Mikkelsen M. The European collaborative study on mosaicism in chorionic villus sampling: data from 1986 to 1987. Prenat Diagn 1989; 9: 575.

114. Brandenburg H, Jahoda MGJ, Pijpers L et al. Fetal loss rate after chorionic villus sampling and subsequent amniocentesis. Am J Med Genet 1990; 35: 178.

115. Kalousek D, Dill F. Chromosomal mosaicism confined to the placenta in human conceptions. Science 1983; 221: 665.

116. Johnson A, Wapner RJ, Davis GH, Jackson LG. Mosaicism in chorionic villus sampling: an association with poor perinatal outcome. Obstet Gynec 1990; 175: 573.

117. Goldsmith MF. Trial appears to confirm safety of chorionic villus sampling procedure. JAMA 1988; 259: 3521.

118. Monni G, Olla G, Cao A. Patient's choice between transcervical and transabdominal chorionic villus sampling. Lancet 1988; 1: 1057.

119. Bovicelli L, Rizzo N, Montacuti V, Morandi R. Transabdominal versus transcervical routes for chorionic villus sampling. Lancet 1986; 2: 290.

120. Robinson GE, Garner DM, Olmsted MP et al. Anxiety reduction after chorionic villus sampling and genetic amniocentesis. Am J Obstet Gynecol 1988; 159: 953.

121. Sjogren B, Uddenberg N. Prenatal diagnosis and psychological distress: amniocentesis or chorionic villus biopsy? Prenat Diagn 1989; 9: 477.

122. Spencer JW, Cox DN. A comparison of chorionic villi sampling and amniocentesis: acceptability of procedure and maternal attachment to pregnancy. Obstet Gynecol 1988; 72: 714.

123. McGovern MM, Goldberg JD, Resnick RJ. Acceptability of chorionic villi sampling for prenatal diagnosis. Am J Obstet Gynecol 1986; 155: 25.

124. Evans MI, Drugan A, Koppitch FC et al. Genetic diagnosis in the first trimester: the norm for the 1990s. Am J Obstet Gynecol 1989; 160: 1332.

6 Amniocentesis

Sriram C Perni and Frank A Chervenak

Historical background

Amniocentesis is the most commonly performed invasive diagnostic prenatal test. Initial reports of extracting amniotic fluid from the gravid uterus appeared over a century ago for the treatment of polyhydramnios.[1] Since the emergence of this invasive technology, indications for its use have evolved over time. Amniocentesis was performed in the 1930s to identify the placental location and for the purpose of pregnancy termination by the instillations of dye and hypertonic saline, respectively.[2] Subsequently, in the 1950s, amniocentesis was utilized to monitor the progression of rhesus isoimmunization[3] and for fetal sex determination.[4] It was not until the 1960s that amniocentesis was used for the prenatal diagnosis of fetal abnormalities,[5] including evaluation of metabolic derangements.[6] In the 1970s, amniocentesis was used to assess fetal lung maturity[7] and as an adjunct in the diagnosis of fetal neural tube defects with the amniotic fluid alpha-fetoprotein assay.[8] Currently, the role for amniocentesis in the field of prenatal diagnosis has greatly expanded.

Indications for genetic amniocentesis

Invasive prenatal diagnosis remains the reference standard for diagnosis of pregnancies at increased risk of fetal aneuploidy, genetic disorders, and metabolic derangements. Midtrimester amniocentesis continues to be the most common procedure performed in invasive prenatal diagnosis.[9,10] Amniocentesis is a safe and accurate procedure.

There are a number of indications to counsel patients for prenatal diagnosis by amniocentesis. The results obtained can be used to determine future management options. Unlike ultrasound markers such as nuchal translucency and serum biochemical marker tests, which are screening tests for aneuploidy, amniocentesis is a diagnostic test. Indications for genetic amniocentesis include advanced maternal age at time of delivery, a pregnancy previously affected by aneuploidy, parental carriage of a balanced chromosomal translocation, a phenotyp-

ically normal mother with known sex chromosomal mosaicism, a female carrier of a sex-linked recessive condition, heterozygous parental carriers of a single-gene mutation disorder, evaluation of fetal neural tube defects in conjunction with maternal serum alpha-fetoprotein levels and fetal anatomic survey by ultrasonography, abnormal multiple serum marker biochemical screening, and maternal request.[11] The most common of these indications for amniocentesis is a maternal age greater than or equal to 35 years of age at the time of delivery,[9] although the clinical use of an age cutoff has been questioned.[12] Amniocentesis may be selectively performed by the clinician to identify conditions after collecting amniocytes; chorionic villus sampling (CVS), in contrast, may be indicated if there is a need to examine fibroblasts from the mesodermal core or cytotrophoblasts for different biologic conditions.

Timing of amniocentesis

Genetic amniocentesis

Genetic amniocentesis is usually performed between 15 and 20 weeks of gestation.[10,11,13] At this gestational age, there should be a sufficient amount of amniotic fluid surrounding the fetus to allow for adequate sampling. As fetal size and micturition steadily increase with advancing gestational age, approximately 100 cc of fluid is present at 14 weeks' gestation and greater than 300 cc surrounds the fetus by 17 gestational weeks.[14] In addition, results from the amniocentesis will be available to offer the patient the option of pregnancy termination. Fetal cells exfoliated from the gastrointestinal and urogenital tracts, from the skin, and from the amnion are used for genetic analysis. Since these cells are not actively proliferating, they are cultured. Culture failure rates are low, owing to the fact that there are 1.2×10^4 cells per milliliter of amniotic fluid collected; however, culture failure is more likely if the fetus is abnormal.[15] Cell culture production for genetic analysis is undertaken by setting up multiple flask cultures or by allowing amniocytes to settle individually on a slide and form discrete colonies.[11] However, conclusive results may take weeks. Amniocentesis performed at this gestational age yields greater than 99% diagnostic accuracy.[16,17] The amniotic fluid collected can be used to test for fetal chromosomes, alpha-fetoprotein and acetylcholinesterase levels, and fetal metabolic disorders when indicated.

Due to the significant recent advances in ultrasound visualization and laboratory techniques, efforts have been made to shift prenatal diagnosis into the first trimester of pregnancy to provide parents with an earlier diagnosis. The available diagnostic options available in the first trimester for fetal karyotyping include CVS and early amniocentesis (EA). A few studies have demonstrated the possibility of performing amniocentesis at 11–14 weeks of gestation,[18,19] the so-called EA. The primary concerns that the clinician faces when performing an EA are the reliability in obtaining a specimen and the potential for culture failure. A study evaluating EA in 600 patients demonstrated that a specimen could not be obtained in only 1.6% of patients.[20] Another study, however, demonstrated a higher culture failure rate with EA than in later gestational ages.[21] In our opinion, EA should probably not be performed. CVS may be a safer alternative for earlier diagnosis.

Most new information on the safety and efficacy of EA comes from the Canadian Early and Midtrimester Amniocentesis Trial (CEMAT), a large, prospective, randomized clinical trial, of over 4000 pregnant women, with significant power to detect clinical outcome differences.[17,22,23] In this trial, EA was associated with a higher rate of total fetal loss, an increase in the incidence of talipes equinovarus, and a higher incidence of postprocedural amniotic fluid leakage compared to the midtrimester amniocentesis group. However, culture success (97.7%) and accuracy (99.8%) rates were high for the patients in the EA group; culture of EA fluid required one more day than the midtrimester amniocentesis group.

Studies have also evaluated and compared CVS with EA. These studies have also demonstrated a higher incidence of talipes equinovarus in the EA than the CVS group.[24,25] In addition, higher rates of fetal loss after EA has also been demonstrated compared to CVS,[24,26] and a higher rate of repeat testing was required in the EA group due to culture and sample failure.[26]

There are a few other technical considerations that make EA challenging to the clinician. Membrane tenting may be more likely to occur with EA due to the incomplete fusion of the amnion and chorion. With EA, the presence of physiologic gut herniation or bladder exstrophy between the abdominal wall and uterus makes the procedure difficult and potentially dangerous. We believe EA should not be performed in most situation.

Fetal lung maturity testing

Utilization of amniocentesis for determination of fetal lung maturity is usually performed in the mid-to-late third trimester of pregnancy. It usually is indicated at various late gestational ages depending on the maternal, fetal, and obstetric conditions that are involved. A variety of diagnostic laboratory tests are available to determine the relative concentrations of the surfactant-active phospholipids. Prior to 34 weeks' gestation, lecithin and sphingomyelin are present in similar concentrations in the amniotic fluid. However, after 34 weeks' gestation, the relative concentration of lecithin to sphingomyelin begins to increase. Some clinicians, in contrast, utilize the presence of phosphatidylglycerol in amniotic fluid as the definitive test to ensure fetal pulmonary maturity. A myriad of other tests, including the foam stability, lamellar body counting, surfactant-to-albumin ratio, and infrared spectroscopy tests, may also be performed by various reference laboratories on amniotic fluids obtained by amniocentesis.[13,27–29]

Isoimmunization in pregnancy

Hemolytic disease of the newborn resulting from rhesus alloimmunization was previously a major contributor to perinatal morbidity and mortality. Since the widespread availability of rhesus immunoglobulin (RhoGam), the prevalence of this condition has substantially decreased to 1–6 cases per 1000 live births.[30] Today, alloimmunization is more likely to result from the 'atypical' antibodies (e.g. anti-Kell or non-D Rh-antigens). Amniocentesis with spectrophotometric examination of the amniotic fluid is the most accepted invasive diagnostic test for assessing the severity of erythroblastosis *in utero*.[31] Amniotic fluid bilirubin, derived from fetal pulmonary and tracheal secretions, is quantified by spectrophotometrically measuring its absorbance at the 450-nm wavelength (ΔOD_{450}). Care must be taken to shield the amniotic fluid specimen from light. Fetal status is estimated by plotting the results from the ΔOD_{450} measurement on the Liley curve and assessing which zone (i.e. zone I lowest, zone II middle, zone III uppermost) the measurement falls in. Amniocentesis is repeated as indicated, usually every 3–4 weeks if it is in zone I and every 1–4 weeks if in zone II.

Technique of amniocentesis

Before one performs amniocentesis, the patient should be counseled. In our view, this is best done by a genetic counselor. A careful assessment of the patient's medical history and family pedigree analysis will provide useful information for both the patient and the obstetric caregivers. This time will also allow for a discussion regarding the risks and benefits involved in the amniocentesis procedure itself. At this initial encounter, the patient's laboratory tests (ABO blood type and indirect Coombs' tests status) should be verified to assess the need for RhoGAM after the amniocentesis. An ultrasound evaluation should also be performed prior to the procedure to document the viability, number, limited anatomic survey, gestational age, and position of the fetus(es) and to identify the placental location. Amniocentesis should be performed only by clinicians familiar with its indications and technique.[32]

High rates of infection and failure to obtain amniotic fluid have been reported with amniocentesis performed transvaginally.[1] This technique also potentially causes greater patient discomfort and requires appropriate patient positioning. Thus, transabdominal amniocentesis is the approach of choice for this prenatal diagnostic technique.

Initially, transabdominal amniocentesis was performed without ultrasound guidance.[33] Later, static and real-time ultrasound was utilized during amniocentesis. The possibility of continuous ultrasound guidance during amniocentesis was first reported in the early 1980s.[34] Studies have demonstrated the superiority of continuous ultrasound visualization of the needle during amniocentesis to 'blind' amniocentesis, in which ultrasound is performed prior to the procedure, with subsequent removal of the transducer and immediate sampling. Continuously monitored amniocentesis resulted in a lower number of dry and bloody taps of the first needle insertion, a decrease in the number of patients requiring multiple attempts, and a reduction in the number of spontaneous losses following the procedure.[35,36] Other studies have also corroborated the safety and efficacy of continuous visualization of the needle during amniocentesis.[37]

After the maternal abdomen is prepped in a sterile manner (e.g. Betadine), the transducer should be placed into a sterile plastic bag, sheath, or glove with gel. Sterile gel can then be applied to the abdomen for improved sonographic visualization of the intrauterine environment. Alternatively, the transducer can be held at a 90° angle outside the sterile field.

After the initial ultrasonic evaluation, the obstetrician locates an appropriate site for the needle insertion. An area that does not contain fetal parts (especially the head) or the umbilical cord, has an adequate volume of amniotic fluid, and avoids the lower uterine segment and placental tissue, should be selected, if possible (see Figure 6.1).[10] Utilization of a local anesthetic agent (e.g. 1% lidocaine without epinephrine) prior to needle insertion is at the individual discretion of the physician and patient. Some would argue that this is an unnecessary step because the site of the initial needle insertion may change if the fetus moves; therefore, the anesthetic would have to be applied to another site. In addition, this may actually increase patient discomfort because an extra skin puncture would be required.

A variety of spinal needles can be utilized for amniocentesis. The procedure has been reported to use an 18-, 20-, or 22-gauge spinal needle.[1,10,11] The 18-gauge needle is used the least. In our center, we prefer to use a 22-gauge needle to

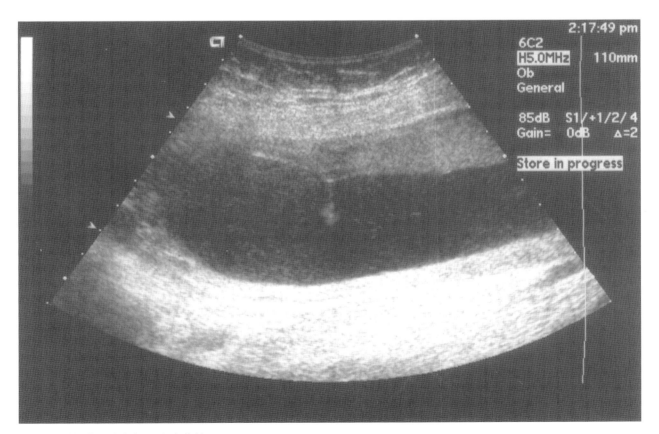

Figure 6.1 Needle and tip in amniotic fluid.

minimize maternal discomfort and maintain uterine quiescence if possible. However, some clinicians prefer a 20-gauge spinal needle to the 22-gauge because of the decreased resistance to amniotic fluid flow, increased resistance to bending, and more echogenic visibility of the tip on real-time ultrasound. Needle guidance can adequately be performed with a linear or curvilinear transducer, and great care must be taken to ensure that the echogenic needle tip is always visualized by the clinician, and does not go outside the beam of the ultrasound. In addition, minimal pressure should be applied to the transducer so as not to distort the spatial relationship between the maternal abdomen and uterine cavity. Some obstetricians also prefer to use a needle guide during the procedure; however, there is a limited range of motion compared to the free-hand technique.

After meticulous asepsis of the maternal abdomen is completed and the puncture site has been selected after ultrasonic evaluation, the spinal needle is introduced into the maternal skin. After dermal and uterine penetration, the amniotic sac is perforated, with a characteristic 'pop' or loss of resistance being perceived by the obstetrician. During this time, careful attention is paid to continuous visualization of the needle tip. Upon confirmation of appropriate entry into the amniotic cavity, the needle stylet should be removed. A 5-ml syringe can be attached and approximately 2–3 ml of amniotic fluid is aspirated and discarded to minimize the potential of maternal cell contamination of the specimen. Maternal cell contamination is much more pronounced in women with anterior placentas than in posterior placentation.[38] This most likely is the result of introduction of maternal cells from placental bleeding into the amniotic fluid cavity. Some investigators have evaluated different techniques of amniocentesis and their impact on maternal cell contamination; one study found no difference between amniocentesis technique and influence on maternal cell contamination.[39] For the initial syringe application, a 5- or 10-ml syringe should be chosen for easier removal of amniotic fluid under less tension. If no fluid is aspirated, the needle should be slowly rotated. This 'dry tap' is not uncommon in early gestation and may result from a tenting of the membranes. In the 1980s, two techniques were introduced to overcome tenting. The first technique involved withdrawing the needle tip back into the myometrium and reinserting it with a forceful thrust.[40] The second involved further needle penetration into the posterior myometrium under ultrasound guidance and then withdrawing the needle into the amniotic fluid pocket in an attempt to displace physically the obstructing membrane.[41] In 1996, a modified stylet technique was introduced to relieve membrane tenting.[42] In this technique, the membrane can be entered by using a stylet that is made longer than the inserted needle by advancing the stylet tip 10 mm beyond the needle tip.

After initial removal of the 2–3 ml of amniotic fluid to be discarded, a second syringe is attached. This syringe is usually a 20- or 30-ml syringe. The amount of amniotic fluid to be aspirated depends on the indication for the procedure. A volume of 15–40 ml of amniotic fluid is usually required for chromosomal and alpha-fetoprotein analysis.[10,11] The amount of amniotic

fluid to be removed depends on the gestational week in which the procedure is being preformed. In general, earlier in gestation, less fluid is removed. If large quantities of amniotic fluid are being removed in cases of polyhydramnios to alleviate maternal symptoms, a gravitational drainage system, multiple syringe aspirations, or a negative-pressure vacuum bottle aspiration system can be used safely to remove amniotic fluid at a rate of 89 ml/minute.[43] If amniotic fluid is required for assessment of fetal lung maturity, a smaller volume of amniotic fluid (10–15 ml) is sufficient.

After obtaining the appropriate volume of amniotic fluid, the stylet should be reinserted, and the needle removed under continuous ultrasound visualization. If no fluid is obtained after more than two attempts, the patient should be offered the opportunity to repeat the procedure after 1 week. Fetal cardiac activity should be observed after the completion of the amniocentesis, whether successful or not. The patient can be discharged after the appropriate postprocedural counseling is completed and the results of the indirect Coombs test are confirmed.

Amniocentesis in a multifetal gestation

Multifetal gestations have increased over the past decade owing to an increase in absolute number and proportion as a result of assisted reproductive technologies and women delaying childbirth. The twin birth rate has increased 50% over the past two decades in the USA and represented over 3% of all births in 2001.[44] The first genetic amniocentesis in a multifetal gestation was performed in the 1970s.[45] Prenatal diagnosis of chromosomal abnormalities in multifetal gestation requires the sampling of two or more gestational sacs. Great care must be taken to ensure that all gestational sacs have been sampled. The clinician can instill 1 ml of a dilute indigo carmine dye solution (1 ml indigo carmine/9 ml normal saline) into the first gestational sac after amniotic fluid has been removed. In this manner, with sampling of the second sac, the amniotic fluid should be clear and colorless. If the fluid is not clear, this may indicate that the same sac was sampled twice. Methylene blue dye is contraindicated for this purpose because of the potential for fetal hemolysis. This technique usually requires two different skin puncture wounds under continuous ultrasound guidance.

Other techniques have been described for amniocentesis in a multifetal gestation. Two techniques were described in the early 1990s. In the first technique described, two separate needles are introduced sequentially into two different gestational sacs with visualization of the dividing membrane without altering the position of the transducer. This technique permits verification of the sampling of two different sacs without introduction of a foreign dye substance.[46] The second technique requires a single-needle insertion, does not require dye, and can potentially be performed quicker than the other techniques. In this technique, an amniotic fluid pocket is identified that contains the dividing membrane. Once fluid is aspirated from the first sac, the needle is guided to penetrate the dividing membrane, and fluid is removed from the second sac.[47] This technique cannot be encouraged at this point until larger studies evaluating the possibility of cross-contamination are adequately addressed. A recent study, however, utilizing quantitative fluorescent polymerase chain reaction assays of amniotic fluid samples obtained by the single-needle technique, allowed detection of all aneuploid fetuses quickly and had great sensitivity in detecting small traces of contaminating cell lines.[48] In our opinion, amniocentesis in a multifetal gestation is best performed by the two separate skin punctures technique.

Complications of amniocentesis

As previously mentioned, amniocentesis is an invasive diagnostic procedure which should be performed only after careful patient counseling for an appropriate indication. Due to the nature of the procedure, there are minimal risks, to both the mother and fetus, that the patient must understand. Amniocentesis is generally safe for both the mother and her fetus. Maternal risks, overall, are much less than fetal risks.

Although a major common concern for a patient undergoing amniocentesis is the risk of spontaneous abortion,[49] maternal factors also need to be addressed prior to performing amniocentesis. Maternal complications occur in approximately 1 in 1000 procedures.[50] The risk of developing chorioamnionitis after the procedure is 0–1%, and subclinical infection may complicate under 0.5% of pregnancies requiring repeated sampling.[10,50,51] If chorioamnionitis is confirmed, expeditious delivery is advised with utilization of the appropriate broad-spectrum, intravenous antibiotic regimen. Significant maternal sequelae can occur, including septic shock and death, if chorioamnionitis is not promptly handled. There are reports of maternal septicemia with Escherichia coli after midtrimester amniocentesis that resulted in septic shock, multiorgan failure, and ultimate demise.[50] The incidence of amniotic fluid leakage after amniocentesis has been reported to occur in 1–2% of patients.[52] This usually does not represent frank rupture of the membranes, but rather a transient condition of extraovular leakage of fluid that should spontaneously resolve in 2–3 days. Other maternal complications, such as premature rupture of the membranes, preterm delivery, fetomaternal transfusion, and placental abruption, are rare. There has been a report that women undergoing amniocentesis more often had an operative vaginal delivery and opted for elective cesarean delivery.[49]

The most common and concerning fetal complication of amniocentesis is spontaneous loss. A spontaneous loss rate of 1.0% has been reported from randomized, controlled, prospective clinical trials.[53,54] However, lower loss rates have been reported.[50] The fetal loss rate has been reported to be higher (2.7%) when amniocentesis is performed in a multifetal gestation.[55] Although it is impossible to predict which pregnancies will end in a fetal loss, certain variables have been identified that could increase the spontaneous loss rate, including older maternal age, uterine myoma, multifetal gestation, and earlier gestational age.[56] A recent review of 4600 amniocentesis procedures by one clinician over a 28-year period demonstrated that the indications for amniocentesis and the technique used have evolved over time; however, the procedure-related fetal loss rate did not improve significantly with increasing operator experience.[57] The reported loss rate in this study (0.95%) is consistent with loss rates described in other large series.

Before continuous ultrasound guidance was used for amniocentesis, fetal injuries, such as gangrene of the fetal limb and porencephalic cysts,[58,59] were reported to be due to direct needle trauma. Other reported neonatal morbidities with amniocentesis include potentially higher rates of pneumonia, respiratory distress syndrome, and ear infections.[1,56]

Conclusion

Amniocentesis is the most common invasive procedure used in prenatal diagnosis. It is a very accurate and safe technique that can be used to diagnose many genetic and metabolic conditions. The procedure should be performed only after careful patient counseling.

References

1. Chervenak JL, Chervenak FA. Amniocentesis. In: Iffy L, Apuzzio JJ, Vintzileos AM (eds), Operative Obstetrics (2nd edition), pp. 64–9. McGraw-Hill: New York, 1992.
2. Menees TO, Miller JD, Holly LE. Amniography. Preliminary report. Am J Roentgenol 1930; 24: 363.
3. Liley AW. The technique and complications of amniocentesis. Aust N Z J Med 1960; 59: 581.
4. Fuchs F, Riis P. Antenatal sex determination. Nature 1956; 117: 330.
5. Jacobsen CB, Barter RH. Intrauterine diagnosis and management of genetic defects. Am J Obstet Gynecol 1967; 99: 795.
6. Nadler HL, Gerbie AB. Role of amniocentesis in the intrauterine detection of genetic disorders. N Engl J Med 1970; 282: 596.
7. Gluck L, Kulovich MV, Barer RC. The interpretation and significance of the lecithin/sphingomyelin ratio in amniotic fluid. Am J Obstet Gynecol 1971; 109: 1432.
8. Brock DJH, Sutcliffe RG. Alphafetoprotein in the antenatal diagnosis of anencephaly and spina bifida. Lancet 1972; ii: 197.
9. Wilson RD. Amniocentesis and chorionic villus sampling. Curr Opin Obstet Gynecol 2000; 12: 81–6.
10. D'Ercole C, Shojai R, Desbriere R et al. Prenatal screening: invasive diagnostic approaches. Childs Nerv Syst 2003; 19: 444–7.
11. Robinson A, Henry GP. Prenatal diagnosis by amniocentesis. Annu Rev Med 1985; 36: 13–26.

12. Druzin ML, Chervenak F, McCullough LB et al. Should all pregnant patients be offered prenatal diagnosis regardless of age? Obstet Gynecol 1993; 81: 615–18.

13. Cunningham FG, Gant NF, Leveno KJ, et al. Williams' Obstetrics (21st edition), pp. 989–92. McGraw-Hill: New York, 2001.

14. Fuchs F. Volumes of amniotic fluid at various stages of pregnancy. Clin Obstet Gynecol 1966; 9: 449–60.

15. Persutte WH, Lenke RR. Failure of amniotic-fluid-cell growth: is it related to fetal aneuploidy? Lancet 1995; 345: 96–7.

16. NICHD National Registry for Amniocentesis Study Group: midtrimester amniocentesis for prenatal diagnosis. JAMA 1976; 236: 1471.

17. The Canadian Early and Mid-Trimester Amniocentesis Trial (CEMAT) Group. Randomized trial to assess safety and fetal outcome of early and midtrimester amniocentesis. Lancet 1998; 351: 242–7.

18. Evans MI, Drugan A, Koppitch FC et al. Genetic diagnosis in the first trimester: the norm for the 1990s. Am J Obstet Gynecol 1989; 160: 1332.

19. Elejalde BR, de Elejalde MM. Early genetic amniocentesis, safety, complications, time to obtain results and contraindications. Am J Hum Genet 1988; 43: A232.

20. Godmillow L, Weiner S, Dunn LK. Early genetic amniocentesis: experience with 600 consecutive procedures and comparison with chorionic villus sampling. Am J Hum Genet 1988; 43: A234.

21. Sundberg K, Jorgensen FS, Tabor A et al. Experience with early genetic amniocentesis. J Perinat Med 1995; 23: 149–58.

22. Winsor EJT, Tompkins DJ, Kalousek D et al. Cytogenetic aspects of the Canadian Early and Mid-Trimester Amniotic Fluid Trial (CEMAT). Prenat Diagn 1999; 19: 620–7.

23. Johnson JM, Wilson RD, Singer J et al. Technical factors in early amniocentesis predict adverse outcome. Results of the Canadian Early (EA) vs Mid-Trimester Amniocentesis (MA) Trial (CEMAT). Prenat Diagn 1999; 19: 732–8.

24. Nicolaides KH, Brizot ML, Patel F et al. Comparison of chorion villus sampling and early amniocentesis for karyotyping in 1,492 singleton pregnancies. Fetal Diagn Ther 1996; 11: 9–15.

25. Sundberg K, Bang J, Smidt-Jensen S et al. Randomised study of risk of fetal loss related to early amniocentesis versus chorionic villus sampling. Lancet 1997; 350: 697–703.

26. Cederholm M, Axelsson O. A prospective comparative study on transabdominal chorionic villus sampling and amniocentesis performed at 10–13 weeks' gestation. Prenat Diagn 1997; 17: 311–17.

27. Anceschi MM, Piazze Garnica JJ, Unfer V et al. A comparison of the shake test, optical density, L/S ratio (planimetric and stechiometric) and PG for the assessment of fetal lung maturity. J Perinatal Med 1996; 24: 355–62.

28. Carlan SJ, Gearity D, O'Brien WF. The effect of maternal blood contamination on the TDx-FLM II assay. Am J Perinatol 1997; 14: 491–4.

29. Liu K, Dembinski TC, Mantsch HH. Rapid determination of fetal lung maturity from infrared spectra of amniotic fluid. Am J Obstet Gynecol 1998; 178: 234–41.

30. Moise KJ. Management of rhesus alloimmunization in pregnancy. Obstet Gynecol 2002; 100: 600–11.

31. American College of Obstetricians and Gynecologists. Management of isoimmunization in pregnancy. Washington, DC, 1996; ACOG Technical Bulletin No. 227.

32. Verp MS, Gerbie AB. Amniocentesis for prenatal diagnosis. Clin Obstet Gynecol 1981; 24: 1007–21.

33. Crandon AJ, Peel KR. Amniocentesis with and without ultrasound guidance. Br J Obstet Gynecol 1979; 86: 1.

34. Jeanty P, Rodesch F, Romero R. How to improve your amniocentesis technique. Am J Obstet Gynecol 1983; 146: 593–6.

35. Romero R, Jeanty P, Reece EA et al. Sonographically monitored amniocentesis to decrease intraoperative complications. Obstet Gynecol 1985; 65: 426–30.

36. De Crespigny LC, Robinson HP. Amniocentesis: a comparison of 'monitored' versus 'blind' needle insertion technique. Aust N Z J Obstet Gynecol 1986; 26: 124–8.

37. Benacerraf BR, Frigoletto FD. Amniocentesis under continuous ultrasound guidance: a series of 232 cases. Obstet Gynecol 1983; 62: 760–3.

38. Nuss S, Brebaum D, Grond-Ginsbach C. Maternal cell contamination in amniotic fluid samples as a consequence of the sampling technique. Hum Genet 1994; 93: 121–4.

39. Steed HL, Tompkins DJ, Wilson DR. Maternal cell contamination of amniotic fluid samples obtained by open needle versus trocar technique of amniocentesis. J Obstet Gynaecol Can 2002; 24: 233–6.

40. Platt LD, DeVore GR, Gimovsky ML. Failed amniocentesis: the role of membrane tenting. Am J Obstet Gynecol 1982; 144: 479.

41. Bowerman RA, Barclay ML. A new technique to overcome failed second-trimester amniocentesis due to membrane tenting. Obstet Gynecol 1987; 70: 806–8.

42. Dombrowski MP, Isada NB, Johnson MP et al. Modified stylet technique for tenting of amniotic membranes. Obstet Gynecol 1996; 87: 455–6.

43. Dolinger MB, Donnenfeld AE. Therapeutic amniocentesis using a vacuum bottle aspiration system. Obstet Gynecol 1998; 91: 143–4.

44. Kalish RB, Vardhana S, Gupta M, Perni SC, Witkin SS. Interleukin-4 and -10 gene polymorphisms and spontaneous preterm birth in multifetal gestations. Am J Obstet Gynecol 2004; 190: 702–6.

45. Toth-Pal E, Papp C, Beke A et al. Genetic amniocentesis in multiple pregnancy. Fetal Diagn Ther 2004; 19: 138–44.

46. Bahado-Singh R, Schmitt R, Hobbins JC. New technique for genetic amniocentesis in twins. Obstet Gynecol 1992; 79: 304–7.

47. Jeanty P, Shah D, Roussis P. Single-needle insertion in twin amniocentesis. J Ultrasound Med 1990; 9: 511–17.

48. Cirigliano V, Canadas P, Plaja A. Rapid prenatal diagnosis of aneuploidies and zygosity in multiple pregnancies by amniocentesis with single insertion of the needle and quantitative fluorescent PCR. Prenat Diagn 2003; 23: 629–33.

49. Cederholm M, Haglund B, Axelsson O. Maternal complications following amniocentesis and chorionic villus sampling for prenatal karyotyping. Br J Obstet Gynaecol 2003; 110: 392–9.

50. Elchalal U, Shachar IB, Peleg D. Maternal mortality following diagnostic 2nd-trimester amniocentesis. Fetal Diagn Ther 2004; 19: 195–8.

51. Terzic MM, Plecas DV, Stimec BV et al. Risk estimation of intraamniotic infection development after serial amniocentesis. Fetal Diagn Ther 1994; 9: 35–7.

52. Crane JP, Rohland BM. Clinical significance of persistent amniotic fluid leakage after genetic amniocentesis. Prenat Diagn 1986; 6: 25.

53. Tabor A, Philip J, Madsen M et al. Randomised controlled trial of genetic amniocentesis in 4606 low-risk women. Lancet 1986; 1: 1287–93.

54. Bettelheim D, Kolinek B, Schaller A et al. Complication rates of invasive intrauterine procedures in a centre for prenatal diagnosis and therapy. Ultraschall Med 2002; 23: 199–22.

55. Yukobowich E, Anteby EY, Cohen SM et al. Risk of fetal loss in twin pregnancies undergoing second trimester amniocentesis. Obstet Gynecol 2001; 98: 231–4.

56. Papp C, Papp Z. Chorionic villus sampling and amniocentesis: what are the risks in current practice? Curr Opin Obstet Gynecol 2003; 15: 159–65.

57. Horger EO, Finch H, Vincent VA. A single physician's experience with four thousand six hundred genetic amniocenteses. Am J Obstet Gynecol 2001; 185: 279–88.

58. Lamb MP. Gangrene of a fetal limb due to amniocentesis. Br J Obstet Gynaecol 1975; 82: 829.

59. Youroukos S, Papadelis F, Matsaniotis N. Porencephalic cysts after amniocentesis. Arch Dis Child 1980; 55: 814.

7 Fetal transfusion

Christopher R Harman

The concept of fetal therapy has been successfully realized in treating fetal anemia by using ultrasound-guided, intrauterine transfusion (IUT). Detecting the fetus at risk, evaluating the extent of disease, and delivery of transfusion blood continue to improve. So have results, with even the worst alloimmune fetal anemia. The advent of fetal blood sampling has further modified treatment regimes and has extended application to other causes. Fetal transfusions were developed to address the staggering perinatal mortality of severe Rh disease. Strict adherence to Rh prophylaxis produced a marked drop in the number of such cases, but IUT remains a critical resource for those most severely affected. This chapter highlights the evolution of IUT, emphasizing fetal evaluation and transfusion techniques.

Mechanisms of fetal anemia

Alloimmunization

Maternal sensitization to foreign paternal-fetal red blood cell (RBC) antigens commonly follows transplacental hemorrhage (TPH). TPH occurs in many pregnancies, including over 50% at delivery and at least 15% antenatally.[1] Volumes are usually inconsequential, but Rh-negative 'high responders' may immunize with as little as 0.01 ml Rh-positive fetal blood.[2] Rh prophylaxis is indicated in routine pregnancies at 28 weeks and after delivery of an Rh-positive fetus, and in virtually all unusual pregnancies where TPH before 28 weeks is a concern (Table 7.1).[3] Infrequently, TPH is so large that sensitization would not be prevented by standard treatment, and additional Rh-immunoglobulin may be required.[4]

While universal prophylaxis has dramatically decreased the incidence of severe Rh disease, maternal D-alloimmunization remains the leading cause of severe fetal anemia requiring intrauterine therapy. Causes of serious anti-D-alloimmunization include failure to provide prophylaxis for obstetric events, failure to administer the routine 28-week dose, inadequate Rh-immunoglobulin for TPH, misidentification of Rh-negative women, absent prenatal care, and patient refusal.[5] Sources outside pregnancy are unusual, because RhD cross-matching for transfusion is routine. However, maternal intravenous drug abuse, with 'boosting' (injection of blood from another narcotic abuser) may produce extremely potent alloimmunization before any pregnancy.[6]

Non-D Rh disease is important, as transfusion blood is not typically matched for other Rh system components (CcEe). Anti-C disease is just as dangerous as classic Rh disease and is monitored and treated by similar protocols.[7,8] Anti-C disease is rarer, with less hydrops, but may require invasive testing and treatment in the third trimester.[9] Anti-E is more common, but milder still, while isolated anti-e virtually never causes fetal disease. Many other RBC antigens may induce maternal sensitization and (in subsequent pregnancies) fetal anemia due to transplacental IgG.[10]

Among responders, RBC antigen immune processing generates plasma cells producing both IgM and IgG. IgM production is usually an initial response, followed by IgG production

---

Table 7.1 Indications for Rh-immunoglobulin (D-negative woman, unsensitized, with all pregnancy events when the fetus/baby is not proven Rh-negative)

Any instance of:
Spontaneous abortion (with or without D & C)
Therapeutic abortion (any method)
Chorionic villus sampling
Genetic amniocentesis
Amniocentesis for lung profile

Treat, additional RhIG depending on Kleihauer test:
Antepartum hemorrhage
Molar pregnancy
Large transplacental hemorrhage
Stillbirth
Obstetric manipulation
Manual removal of placenta

Routine prophylaxis (none of the above has occurred):
28 weeks' gestation, and
40 weeks, if undelivered, or
delivery of Rh-positive baby

after second exposure. IgG is the critical vector of fetal disease. It crosses the placenta by facilitated transport, reaches high concentration in the fetus, binds to paternal/fetal antigens, and induces fetal immune-mediated trapping of these antibody-labeled RBCs. Immune-based microphagocytosis and extravascular hemolysis rapidly eliminate labeled cells. Anemia and corresponding waste products result. Ultimately, severe Rh disease demands extreme erythropoietic effort, with release of many immature forms; hence, the term 'erythroblastosis fetalis'.

Kell alloimmunization has an additional complement-fixing mechanism, inducing hemolysis intravascularly and within fetal bone marrow.[11] The Kell antigen is an active RBC membrane component, and immunization may also inhibit cell division and erythropoietin response.[12] The result is more complete hemolysis, hemolysis of progenitor cells, and unexpectedly profound and sudden fetal anemia. For all alloimmune anemias, since the fetus simply produces more RBC with the same offending antigen, an accelerating process is inevitable.

Immune responsiveness is important. Up to 30% of Rh-negative women and 20–30% of Kell-negative women immunized by mismatched blood transfusion will not produce antibody sufficient to cause fetal disease.[1]

Anemia due to fetal infection

Fetal infection may produce anemia in varying patterns: (1) hydrops with profound anemia, potentially remediable by serial IUT (e.g., *Parvovirus B19*) and (2) hydrops with moderate anemia without improvement despite maintenance of normal hemoglobin levels by IUT (most other infections and even some *Parvovirus*).

Parvovirus generates aplastic anemia by specific mechanism. The P antigen on RBC precursors facilitates integration of virus into the cellular genome, arresting cell division of colony-forming erythroid precursors (CFU-E) and more primitive burst-forming units (BFU-E).[13] Fetal RBC production is halted, almost absolutely.[14] There is no direct viral effect on circulating cells, although the RBC half-life may be shortened by associated hepatitis and myocarditis.[15] As erythropoiesis stops, natural attrition of 1–2% per day results in progressive anemia. Immunity, acquired from the mother transplacentally, reverses this viral suppression. Of course, reactivation of BFU-E and CFU-E takes some time, and recovery may be further complicated by liver failure with hypoproteinemia, and/or cardiac failure with nonanemic hydrops. In some fetuses, serious anemia lasts only a few days, and the disease is self-limited. In other fetuses, absent RBC production is so profound and sustained that recovery starting with release of very immature forms (another example of erythroblastosis) is too little, and hydropic stillbirth results. Lifesaving serial transfusions may be necessary in up to 50% of such fetuses.[16]

Other infections generate fetal anemia by chronic debilitation, induced hemolysis by hepatosplenomegaly, and sequestration in the enlarged placenta. In some cases of congenital syphilis, listeriosis, and coxsackie infection, fetal anemia may be severe enough to warrant transfusion, but, in general, anemia is a rather modest manifestation of hydrops, not a cause.

Hydrops fetalis

As anemia worsens, physical manifestations become apparent, paralleling different patterns of response. In the fetus compensating effectively for low-grade hemolysis, with increased reticulocytosis and bilirubin resulting in a very slow rate of anemia, physical changes may be restricted. Slight increase in liver diameter (due to extramedullary erythropoiesis), modest cardiovascular changes (slight cardiac chamber dilation, increased peak systolic velocities in cerebral and systemic circulations, increased cardiac output, increased heart rate – 'hyperdynamic' fetal circulation), and increased amniotic fluid volume (increased cardiac output leads to increased fetal glomerular filtration rate) may occur.[17]

More severe anemia results in localized endovascular hypoxemia, with vasodilation in major vascular beds. Fewer RBCs result in decreased blood viscosity, further potentiating increased velocity, which is the basis for Doppler prediction of anemia. Fetal liver and, after 26–28 weeks, fetal kidney are potent sources of oxygen-dependent erythropoietin release. Erythropoietin acts not only on intramedullary BFU-E but also on dormant lines within liver, spleen, and other organs. Once erythropoietin rises, extramedullary RBC production displaces normal hepatic function. Hypersplenism, low production in bone marrow congested with hematopoiesis, and oxygen-sensitive life span, may produce associated thrombocytopenia. Devotion of hepatic architecture to erythropoietic cells results in metabolic defects, including hypoproteinemia, disordered fixed-acid buffering, and mechanical obstruction of venous cardiac return. Lymphatic blockade by the enlarged liver, decreased oncotic pressure due to hypoproteinemia, increased peritoneal vascular permeability from hypoxemia, and increased venous pressure all combine to produce ascites as hydrops begins. Worsening hypoproteinemia, venous congestion, and hypoxemic tissue fluid mishandling result in progressive anasarca, serous accumulations in pleural spaces and pericardium, and scalp and subcutaneous edema. The placenta also becomes increasingly edematous.[18] This full-blown picture is hydrops fetalis (Figure 7.1). Further decline features loss of heart rate variability and biophysical variables, as anemia becomes lethal. Once blamed for the onset of hydrops, fetal heart failure is now understood to be terminal, caused by hypoxemic myocardial malfunction. Classification of ultrasound hydropic manifestations (Table 7.2) serves as a system for description of fetal compromise.[19] There are direct hematologic correlates (Figure 7.2). Disease severity described by this classification also reflects prognosis.

These physical manifestations reflect pathophysiology, within limits. For instance, small pericardial effusions are common in mild to moderate anemia. Large pericardial effusions in end-stage hydrops are components of anasarca, not cardiac mal-

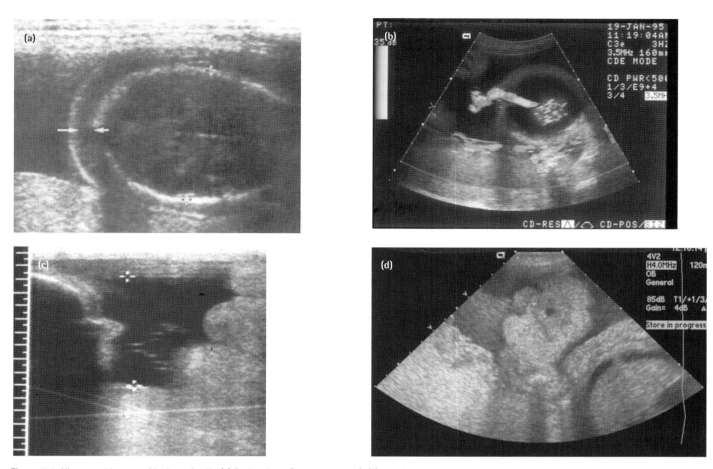

Figure 7.1 Ultrasound images of hydrops fetalis. (a) Scalp edema (between arrows), (b) massive ascites with umbilical cord stretched from the edematous abdominal wall to its insertion at the base of the fetal liver, (c) polyhydramnios (between calipers), edematous placenta with multiple folds (right of image), (d) grossly edematous fetal face (upper left of image), hepatomegaly, and rim of ascites (lower right of image).

function, while pericardial effusions seen with *Parvovirus* may follow anemia and/or viral myocarditis. Often, onset of hydrops is apparent only on serial observations by experienced operators in terminal fetal disease. Especially in midtrimester, ambient fetal P_{O_2} is very high, so hydropic changes may be modest and, due to mechanical effects, the hypoxemic abnormalities readily inducible in third-trimester anemic fetuses do not usually occur prior to 22 weeks' gestation unless the fetus is preterminal.

Table 7.2 Ultrasound classification of fetal alloimmune disease

Class	Elevated MCA Doppler	Placentomegaly	Ascites	Effusion	Anasarca	Abnormal BPS <4/10
			Ultrasound appearance			
0	−	−	−	−	−	−
I	+	+	−	−	−	−
II	+	+	+	−	−	−
III	+	+	+	+	+	−
IV	+	+	+	+	+	+

− = absent; + = present; MCA = middle cerebral artery; BPS = biophysical profile score.

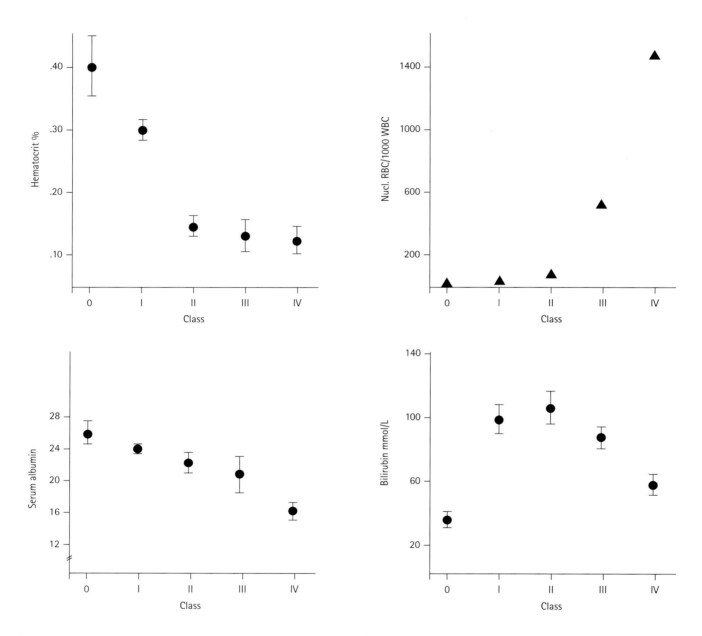

Figure 7.2 The relationship between disease severity by ultrasound classification (Table 7.2) and fetal hematologic parameters measured at the time of cordocentesis. In all parameters, there is a significant reflection of disease severity and prognosis.

Thus, physical changes in anemic fetuses are important correlates of disease, but are too complex to use as sole determinants of therapy.

The presence of fetal hydrops on ultrasound mandates immediate blood sampling. With known etiology (e.g., alloimmunization, *Parvovirus*), starting transfusing before the opening hemoglobin value is known may be appropriate. However, in many cases of nonimmune hydrops, comprehensive fetal sampling is important before transfusion with adult donor cells permanently obscures diagnosis. High-level ultrasound examination and careful planning of sample requirements are imperative before the procedure is started.

Subjective 'prehydropic' changes may have relevance to preprocedure monitoring in patients at very early gestational ages. For instance, abdominal circumference may accelerate before hydrops appears (Figure 7.3). Amniotic fluid volume and placental thickness, subjective appearance of fetal organs outlined by fluid, and minor reductions in fetal heart rate (FHR) variability determined by computerized interpretation are all features which may predict hydrops. However, the use of fetal middle cerebral artery (MCA) Doppler velocimetry has increased our ability today to predict fetal anemia accurately.

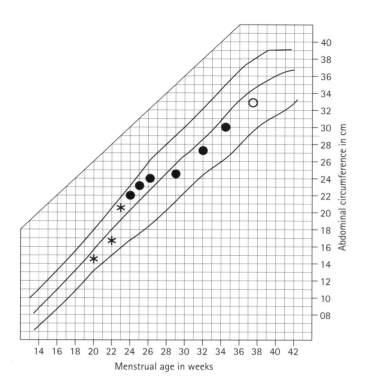

Figure 7.3 The relationship between abdominal circumference (AC) measured by ultrasound, and disease progression. Asterisks show AC in a severely affected fetus without ascites, before treatment. Rapid increase in AC is a result of gross hepatosplenomegaly. With treatment by IVT, liver size and, therefore, AC, are reduced to previously established percentiles. Open circle represents AC at delivery.

Table 7.3 Indications for invasive fetal testing

Test to determine whether treatment is necessary

Antibody specificity
Frequent: D, c, E, C^w, K
Uncommon: C, e, Kp^a, Kp^b, Fy^a, Cellano, s

Antibody strength
D: Albumin titer ≥1.6
                       Absolute anti-D level ≥2 µg/ml
                       (10 IU/ml)
Kell: Indirect Coombs' test titer ≥1 : 4–8
All others: Indirect Coombs' test ≥1 : 16

Antibody pattern (serial testing)
Late-appearing IgM–IgG conversion
Recent 2-dilution rise from any level

Test to determine when treatment should begin

History
Previous affected infant, heterozygous father
Homozygous father, previous infant no/mild effect
Homozygous father, albumin titer ≥1.64
Homozygous father, previous infant ≥
    moderate disease

Fetal blood type positive
Previous affected infant, new antibody rise
Fetal blood typing done, albumin titer ≥64

Evidence of significant fetal hemolysis
Ultrasound examination
Amniotic fluid spectrophotometry
Cordocentesis results

Noninvasive monitoring of fetal anemia

History

In alloimmune disease, the timing of invasive testing depends on the onset and severity of previous disease, as subsequent antigen-positive fetuses are often more severely affected (Table 7.3). Recurrence is not invariable and not always as severe, so historical factors are always weighed against more relevant evidence from the index pregnancy.

Maternal antibody titers

The concept of 'critical titer' is important. For each regional laboratory and for each antibody, there is a threshold concentration below which fetal disease is unlikely (Table 7.3).[20,21] Local standards may range from 1:16 to 1:128 depending on the test and control antigen-positive cells used.[22] Typical titers at our institution (anti-D 1:16, anti-C 1:32, anti-K 1:4–8; direct antiglobulin test) may not apply to the reader's experience.[23,24] Serial titrations, done by the same laboratory using identical cell lines, performed monthly or sooner with important obstetric events, provide the most accurate assessment, but this remains controversial.[25] Reaching the critical titer, or a rise of two dilutions, mandates enhanced surveillance.

Physical examination

Ultrasound provides interesting data on disease progression, but may incompletely represent the onset of anemia. Many fetuses with hemoglobin under the 10th percentile have normal ultrasound. Among fetuses referred for emergency IUT, 15% had procedures deferred because 'the fetus looks normal', only to develop overt hydrops within 10–14 days.[5] Suspicious findings may prompt invasive testing *earlier* than planned, but a normal scan should not postpone invasive testing scheduled for objective prognostic factors.[17]

Doppler velocimetry

Several vascular beds reflect regionalized effects of anemia,[17] but MCA Doppler velocimetry is now the standard for noninvasive prediction.[26] Mari et al, correlating anemia with MCA peak systolic velocity in untreated fetuses,[27] in fetuses with anemia following transfusion,[28] and in fetuses with anemia other than alloimmune causes,[29] provide a solid experiential basis for application in prospective management of fetuses at risk (100% for detection of moderate to severe anemia, 95% CI 86–100%).[30] In fetuses with mild anemia, MCA Doppler velocimetry has a significant false-positive rate (up to 30% in unselected patients undergoing fetal blood sampling for nonanemic reasons) and a more concerning false-reassuring rate of 5–10%. In the latter case, normal MCA peak systolic velocity delayed invasive testing. When a significant rise finally occurred, fetal hemoglobin levels were below 5.0 g/dl.[31]

Some investigators have not duplicated Mari et al's high level of accuracy in predicting anemia. However, in all studies, the detection of fetal anemia improves as disease becomes more severe. Several factors may interact in this relationship. In mild anemia, blood viscosity may singly influence MCA changes (thinner blood is easier to push, volume cardiac output increases, and peak systolic velocity rises) With worsening anemia, additional mechanisms, including vasodilation due to endovascular hypoxemia, optimized ejection fraction due to mild cardiac dilation, increased sympathetic tone, and advancing gestational age, may interact, enhancing the accuracy of MCA peak systolic velocity.

The MCA is readily accessible, the Doppler angle is usually optimal, and adding color Doppler imaging helps in differentiating from other intracranial arterial waveforms. Gestational age variation appears predictable and thresholds for invasive testing seem applicable to all forms of fetal anemia. IUT produces Doppler changes concurrent with measured hematocrit (Figure 7.4). Incorporated in a routine of fetal physical and functional assessment, MCA Doppler velocimetry has become the standard for noninvasive fetal testing.

Invasive monitoring of fetal anemia

Invasive procedures require caution because of their potential aggravation of existing disease. Transplacental amniocentesis causing TPH may provoke maternal antibody production.[32] Cordocentesis for fetal blood typing with subcritical sensitization may convert a benign situation into one needing repetitive early IUT.[33] The goal of testing must be clear. If the father is a known homozygote, there is no reason to perform an invasive procedure for blood typing alone. In known alloimmunized pregnancies, when hydrops is present, cordocentesis for fetal blood sampling without transfusion is equally pointless.

Fetal blood typing

Noninvasive techniques are fallible and invasive techniques have potential complications, so knowing whether the fetus is at risk is extremely important. If the father is heterozygous, 50% of the fetuses will be antigen-negative, and completely unaffected. Fetal blood typing for Kell and Rh system antigens requires simple amniocentesis only.[34,35] Standard DNA tech-

nology, as early as 14–16 weeks, can mandate ongoing surveillance (positive fetuses) or make it irrelevant (negative fetuses). When the father is known to be heterozygous, in D-alloimmunization (where father's zygosity cannot be proven, but only estimated by CcDEe phenotype), and when paternal blood type is unavailable, we advocate amniocentesis, which is associated with minimal risk of aggravating sensitization. The same methodology allows typing of fetal platelets for critical antigens in neonatal alloimmune thrombocytopenia (NAIT).[36] Currently, alloimmune disease from other sources requires fetal blood typing from RBCs obtained at cordocentesis.

Amniocentesis for ΔOD450

The endpoint of hemolytic degradation is bilirubin. As hemolysis increases, much is transported across the placenta, fetal serum bilirubin levels are modestly elevated, and amniotic fluid bilirubin also rises. Amniotic fluid bilirubin normally changes over gestation, requiring specific norms (Figure 7.5).[5] Amniocentesis done under continuous ultrasound guidance, through a placenta-free window, under sterile procedure, can provide reassurance in most cases, so that more invasive methods are not necessary. Serial values are more reliable than a single value, especially early in gestation when norms may vary widely. Amniocentesis is performed together with detailed fetal physical examination, and is deferred in favor of immediate fetal transfusion if hydrops is suspected/present. In the presence of a completely anterior placenta, we do not advocate transplacental amniocentesis, even with a 25- or 27-gauge needle. In such cases, cordocentesis for fetal blood sampling is preferred.

Amniocentesis was established by the landmark work of Liley in 1961.[37] It is generally easy to perform, it is within the technical range of many obstetricians, and it does not require specialized laboratory services. With proper interpretation, and within stringent limits, it remains useful, but there are significant pitfalls. These include contamination from blood and meconium, difficult interpretation before 22 weeks, a false-alarm rate of about 10%, and a life-threatening false-reassuring rate of 3–5%. It is not recommended as the sole predictor of Kell disease, and a single value should be interpreted cautiously, especially when the antibody titer is rising. IUT is indicated when serial ΔOD450 values are rising to the 80% zone 2 or higher, or in the presence of a single value in zone 3.

Fetal blood sampling

Cordocentesis for fetal blood sampling without IVT is not considered for hydropic fetuses with known etiology. In nonhydrops, blood sampling is performed separately with IVT readily available. With suspicious history, ultrasound findings, rising ΔOD450 or antibody titers, or difficulty in obtaining rare donor blood types, a combined procedure (cordo-IVT) is prepared, but infusion of blood is withheld until the hemoglobin value is known at bedside. Here, the portable hemoglobin machine is

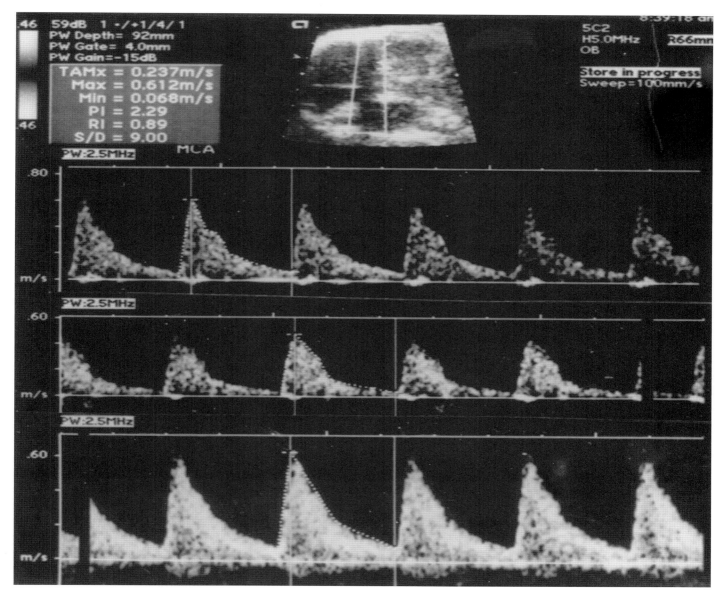

Figure 7.4 Serial Doppler waveforms from the middle cerebral artery of a fetus severely affected by Rh disease. Top panel: MCA peak velocity is 61.2 cm/s, more than two standard deviations above the mean; fetal hemoglobin = 5.7g/dL. Middle panel: post-IVT, MCA peak systolic velocity is 38.5 cm/s; fetal hemoglobin = 13.4. Bottom panel: 3 weeks later, pre-IVT MCA peak systolic velocity is 72.9 cm/s, as predicted by the post-IVT hemoglobin; the pretransfusion level is 6.0.

invaluable, saving donor blood, but at the same time avoiding a repeat procedure, if transfusion is necessary.

Cordocentesis procedure

For simple cordocentesis, maternal sedation, prophylactic antibiotics, hospital admission, and antenatal steroids are not used. Meticulous identification of an umbilical vein target often takes as long as the procedure itself. The ideal image shown in Figure 7.6 is not always available. Alternative targets include umbilical vein within the fetal abdomen, free cord loop which can be pinned against adjacent uterine or placental surfaces,

umbilical cord at its fetal abdominal skin insertion, and fetal cardiac puncture, in order of preference. Mother or fetus can be manipulated to improve target imaging. Only when a safe approach is identified, not traversing surface placental vessels or maternal vascular compartment, should cordocentesis proceed. Other prerequisites are shown in Table 7.4.

Cordocentesis is performed under continuous ultrasound visualization, with a 22-gauge spinal needle of appropriate length.[38] Once the needle is positioned on the vessel, it is inserted with a vigorous 'pop', and the tip should be readily seen within the lumen of the vessel (Figure 7.7). An initial sample is aspirated for immediate hemoglobin measurement, and further

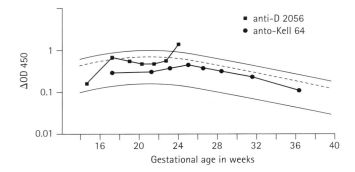

Figure 7.5 Gestational age application of ΔOD450 shows a curvilinear relationship. Depicted are two patients with significant alloimmunization. Upper profile in an Rh-alloimmunized woman shows a sudden rise in ΔOD450 at 24 weeks, associated with ultrasound evidence of accelerating hydrops (class II). This fetus survived intact with four IVT. ΔOD450 measurements in Kell disease may not accurately reflect disease severity; therefore, in this case (shown by circles), amniocenteses were performed frequently from 18 to 36 weeks. Serial results did not cross 80% zone II line, fetal blood sampling was not utilized, no IVT were done, and a healthy baby was delivered at 37 weeks, requiring only exchange transfusions for elevated bilirubin. (This case was managed in 1984, prior to use of cordocentesis – undoubtedly Kell management would not be based on amniocentesis results now.)

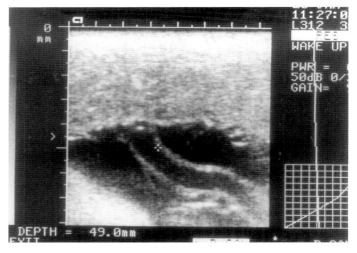

Figure 7.6 Sonogram of the insertion site of the umbilical cord on the surface of an anterior placenta. The umbilical vein, the prime target for IVT, is well visualized.

samples are slowly withdrawn while the reading is taken. Blood typing, the direct Coombs' test, hematologic values in duplicate, and biochemistry normally require 3.0 ml. Once samples are secured, a small 'puff' of sterile saline identifies the vessel sampled, to validate results.

The following critical values may indicate proceeding directly to fetal transfusion.

Table 7.4 Prerequsites for performing invasive fetal testing/ therapy

Detailed indication
Informed consent
Experienced team
High-resolution ultrasound
Accessible target
Bedside testing
Detailed blood typing laboratory
Transfusion blood available
Fetal monitoring capability*
Emergency obstetric services*
Tertiary-level neonatal intensive care*
Maternal/family support systems

*Usually applicable only when gestation is >25–26 weeks.

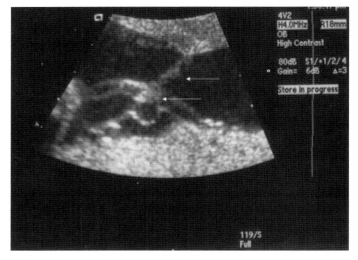

Figure 7.7 With a posterior placenta, the needle traverses the amniotic fluid, with the shaft indicated by the upper arrow. The needle tip is within the umbilical vein, the larger of the two vessels seen overlapping (lower arrow).

Hemoglobin concentration

This rises throughout gestation; therefore, an age-correlated curve is used (Figure 7.8). Transfusing at the 5th percentile avoids unnecessary transfusion of fetuses not requiring it (some have simplified this to a threshold of 9.0 g/dl for all gestations).

Serum bilirubin[39]

In hemolytic disease, clearance from the fetal compartment is rapid, but not complete. Total bilirubin over 80 mmol/l, indicates potential hemolytic crisis, and normal hemoglobin is interpreted cautiously – it may fall rapidly. Bilirubin 60–80 mmol/l indicates accelerated hemolysis. In this intermediate group, an elevated reticulocyte count may indicate adequate erythropoietic response.[40] For bilirubin under 40 mmol/l, hemolysis is most likely mild, and timing of repeat cordocentesis is based on hemoglobin concentration and other disease inputs.

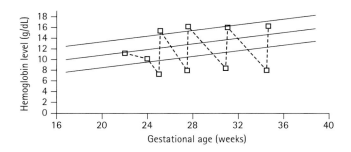

Figure 7.8 Normal hemoglobin concentration rises throughout gestation, depicted by lines indicating the 95th, 50th, and 5th percentiles. The case was that of a sensitized Rh-negative woman in her third pregnancy, undergoing invasive testing, starting 3 weeks earlier than the severe anemia that had occurred in the second pregnancy. Serial cordocentesis, begun at 21.5 weeks, showed declining hemoglobin levels, reaching threshold for transfusion at 24+ weeks. Four transfusions, shown by rapid rise in hemoglobin concentration, allowed continuation of pregnancy until induction and vaginal delivery at 37+ weeks, with delayed cord clamping and newborn hemoglobin level of 11.8 g/dl.

RBC precursors

Some authors have evaluated nucleated red blood cell counts (NRBC)[41] (in our experience, NRBC vary with technical difficulties and may remain elevated for days following difficult cordocentesis), reticulocyte count[40] (in our experience, only levels under 2% predict anemia), and mean corpuscular volume (MCV), which rises as earlier/younger RBCs are elaborated. In the latter instance, microphagocytosis of older RBC produces smaller damaged forms, tending to lower MCV.[5]

Blood gases/pH

Most fetuses show minor changes in P_{O_2} through mild to moderate anemia. Tissue hypoxemia responsible for local perfusion changes is not usually detectable in blood-gas analysis.[42] Increased concentration of carboxyhemoglobin may indicate intravascular oxygen depletion, but is very difficult to measure it clinically.

Preparing for IUT: amniocentesis versus cordocentesis

Amniocentesis is easier than cordocentesis but provides relatively modest information of imperfect accuracy. However, cordocentesis provides greatly superior data. Amniocentesis may be chosen primarily to avoid aggravation of mild to moderate maternal disease. As well as making existing conditions worse, cordocentesis may alloimmunize against other RBC antigens (e.g., Kell or Duffy in an Rh-negative woman), causing fetal disease, and at the least, complicating the cross-matching process. In the final analysis, however, if any doubt exists, cordocentesis provides the definitive data.[43]

Invasive treatment of fetal anemia

Goals of transfusion

The goals of transfusion are as follows:

(1) restore hemoglobin concentration and, therefore, oxygen-carrying capability
(2) suppress production of antigenic RBCs
(3) elevate hemoglobin concentration enough to allow significant interval between procedures, while minimizing the risk of high-volume infusion.

Preparation

Patients are counseled according to the likelihood of intact survival (Table 7.5). Maternal cooperation is critical; in selected patients, premedication with narcotic analgesic and mild sedation is used. However, much has become simplified in our experience with over 1000 IUTs. Nowadays, in the ultrasound era, maternal sedation, prophylactic antibiotics, and tocolytics are rarely used. Once viability is attained, mothers are NPO from midnight, and have an intravenous started. Hospital admission is rarely required.

Transfusion blood

Fresh RBC, group O, Rh-negative, HIV/CMV-negative, buffy coat poor, and fully cross-matched with mother, are irradiated immediately prior to the procedure. Centrifugation for approximately 10 minutes at 4000 RPM achieves donor hematocrit 80–85%. With class IV hydrops, platelet concentrate is also obtained for suspension of the packed RBCs. We usually order 30–40 ml more than the target volume to account for tubing, residue, and sampling losses.

Intravascular transfusion (IVT)

The history of fetal transfusion includes hysterotomy and open cannulation of fetal vessels, repetitive transfusion via indwelling catheters, fetal exchange transfusions, IVT, and combined (intravascular and intraperitoneal) transfusions.[44, 45] All had detailed justifications, and most had some success. It has become clear, however, that the shortest, simplest procedure, giving high-volume, highly concentrated RBCs in 20-ml

Table 7.5 Likelihood of intact survival with fetal intravascular transfusions (IVTs)

	Nonhydropic	Hydrops
First IVT <24 weeks	95%	70%
First IVT >24 weeks	99%	88%

aliquots, sampling halfway and at completion of the target volume, maximizes therapeutic effect and minimizes complications. Uterine tone and maternal complications, such as emesis, supine hypotension, and anxiety, are time-dependent. Quickly reaching a high concentration of donor (adult) blood meets therapeutic targets. There appears no measurable advantage to extra blood intraperitoneally, or fetal exchange transfusion because these do increase the time, technical difficulties, and complications.

Maternal preparation

Standard Betadine prep, maternal tilt, and 1% Xylocaine infiltration, directly above the targeted vessel, are used.

Needle insertion

A 22-gauge spinal needle is used, 20-gauge after 28 weeks. If needle removal is required, it is changed to preserve maximum sharpness. We do not use 'echo tip' needles for this same reason. We have not found a rigid needle guide necessary for stability. The needle is directed under continuous ultrasound to the umbilical vein, the picture format is zoomed, and gentle bouncing indents the vein wall. Vessel entry is a 'pop'. Pressing forward does not enter the vessel cleanly; a 3-mm staccato advance achieves the necessary motion. Without follow-through, drag on the needle penetrating the vessel wall will usually stop it in the ideal position. The stylet is removed, and blood wells into the hub. Only light aspiration pressure is required – aspirating too hard may pull the vessel wall up against the needle. The vein is preferred – larger lumen, turbulence along the cord (vs on placental surface), no risk of vascu-

lar spasm – but we have performed over 50 full-volume intra-arterial IVT without complication. The stylet should not be reinserted above the target, as this may obscure the approach. After preliminary sampling, proper cannulation is confirmed by injecting 0.4–0.6 ml sterile saline. This produces intravascular turbulence, confirming free placement (Figure 7.9). The first sample is used for bedside hemoglobin level. After correct vessel placement is ensured, it is common to inject 0.4–0.6 mg pancuronium for fetal paralysis.[46] We use this approach in most transamniotic procedures and in about one-third of transplacental procedures in order to avoid needle displacement by fetal movement. Vecuronium (causes frequent fetal arrhythmia) and atracurium (has shorter onset and duration) have not worked as well. Postprocedure monitoring is more complicated when the fetus is paralyzed, as an initial period of pseudosinusoidal heart rate follows pancuronium, and movement may not resume for several hours.[5]

Transfusion volume

Pressurizing the donor blood bag facilitates filling the 20-ml syringe connected via stopcock. The amount of used blood volumes aims to raise fetal hemoglobin concentration to approximately 10.0 g/l.[5] However, for hydropic fetuses with pre-IVT hemoglobin under 4.0 g/l, or previously transfused fetuses with pre-IVT hemoglobin over 10.0 g/l, such blood volumes may not be tolerated. Sampling halfway verifies that the total volume will reach the desired target. If the needle is dislodged, it is reinserted, and target volume attained, unless one of the following occurs: there is significant change in FHR (monitored by audi-

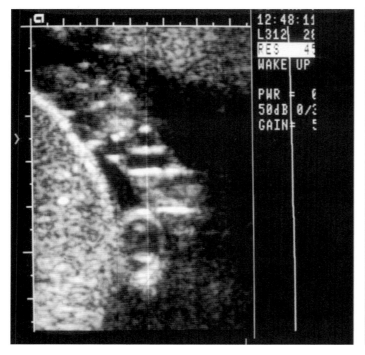 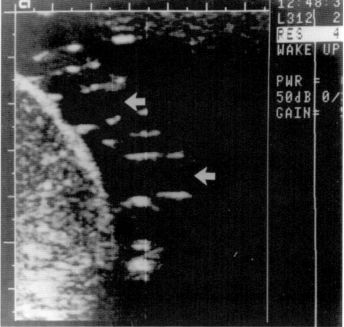

Figure 7.9 The umbilical vein is infused with concentrated donor red blood cells, producing turbulence during infusion (left), which stops immediately when the infusion stops (right) well shown by ultrasound.

ble PW-Doppler), there is severe maternal supine hypotension, over 75% target volume is reached, or visualization declines. *Blood should be injected if intravascular turbulence is absent.*

Needle removal

When the total volume is administered, the intravenous tubing is disconnected and the posttransfusion sample is obtained (Figure 7.10). This is not always simple. After large transfusions, dense blood coats the inner lumen and aspiration may be difficult; uterine tone may increase and preclude needle manipulation; visualization may decline; and all these may prevent

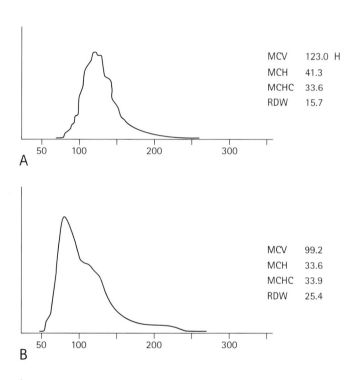

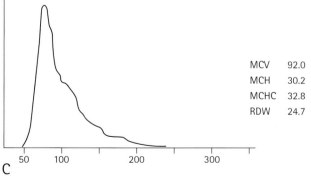

Figure 7.10 Serial red blood cell histograms taken during an IVT. Top panel: pretransfusion shows high MCV (123.0) typical of an anemic fetus. Middle panel: bimodal curve demonstrates substantial addition of adult (donor) red blood cells, lowering average MCV to 99.2. Lower panel: post-transfusion final MCV of 92 reflects the addition of donor hemoglobin, raising the initial pre-IVT hemoglobin value of 4.8 g/dl to a post-IVT value of 11.4 g/dl.

post-IVT sampling. Calculation (*versus* measurement) of posttransfusion hemoglobin is approximate, but correlates with midpoint sampling and posttransfusion MCA Doppler.[47] We do not reinsert the needle just for a posttransfusion value. Back-bleeding after needle removal is common, but may be reduced if vessel penetration is via cord substance, and if the needle is removed very gradually. In severe hydrops, combination of elevated intravascular pressure and thrombocytopenia may result in excessive bleeding.[48] Arterial back-bleeding averages about 25% longer than venous.[49] In either case, it is watched until cessation. The threshold for cardiovascular collapse due to blood loss is 300 seconds (5 minutes) and this may indicate an immediate repeat procedure. Since tiny volumes of blood leaking from vessel punctures are detectable by ultrasound, it is common to overestimate blood loss. Periodic checks of FHR, cardiac filling, cord artery, and MCA Doppler waveforms provide ample reassurance of circulating volume stability.

Complications

Most complications occur during the IVT (Table 7.6). Cord tamponade may be lethal, so IVT over 24 weeks are done on the delivery suite, with emergency cesarean section available. Deaths of hydropic fetuses not improving with serial IVTs have occurred despite retransfusion within 12 hours of first IVT. In 10 cases (1.1%), post-IVT monitoring was abnormal enough to prompt emergency cordocentesis, but the most common finding was normal post-IVT hemoglobin, and normal pH and blood gases.

Table 7.6 Complications of fetal intravascular transfusions

Fetuses treated	202	
Transfusions	903	
Overall survival	172	(85%)
Survivors class I	114/117	(97%)
Survivors classes II–III	48/56	(86%)
Survivors class IV	24/32	(75%)
Failed procedures	40	(4.2%)*
Compressive cord hematoma	10	1.1%
Bradycardia, unknown cause	35	3.9%
Severe bradycardia	5	0.6%
Exsanguinating bleed	17	1.9%
Rupture of membranes	5	0.6%
Supine hypotension	30	3.3%
<50% target volume	21	2.3%

*28 of these had successful cordocentesis, noncritical hemoglobin level, procedure deferred for 24 hours for various reasons.

Intraperitoneal transfusion (IPT)

Transfusion blood is absorbed from the peritoneal cavity via subdiaphragmatic and intrathoracic lymphatics. Absorption is directly related to volume, duration after transfusion, and presence of fetal diaphragmatic and body movements.[50] Poor response of hydropic fetuses to IPT relates to dilution of transfused blood by ascites and, importantly, absence of fetal breathing movement accompanying low biophysical profile scores.[51] Only under 17 weeks, when fetal blood vessels are too small to cannulate, is IPT used in hydrops. IPT (without fetal blood sampling) is less precise than IVT. Transplacental IPT is hazardous, featuring fetal mortality of up to 5% per procedure.[52]

Preparation

In addition to the prerequisites indicated for all transfusions, mandatory IPT criteria include:

a. non-hydropic fetus
b. ideal fetal position
c. team experience in IPT
d. posterior placenta.

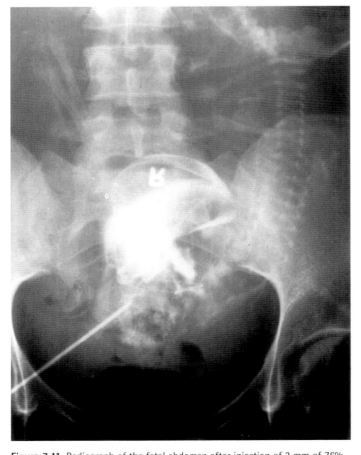

Figure 7.11 Radiograph of the fetal abdomen after injection of 3 mm of 76% Renografin via intraperitoneal catheter. The fetus, in a breech position, shows radiopaque dye along the dome of the diaphragm. Lower in the fetal abdomen, dye dispersed between loops of fetal bowel causes discrete scalloping, confirming that the catheter tip is free within the peritoneal cavity.

Further, IPT application is generally limited to times when fetal vascular access is not available, for example, very early in gestation when vessels are too small, or very late in gestation when fetal size, spine anterior, blocks vascular access.

Technique

Classical IPT uses a 16-gauge Tuohy needle with curved lumen, inserted into the peritoneal cavity, allowing threading of a no. 18 epidural catheter.[54] Placement of the catheter free within the abdomen is confirmed by infusion of radiopaque dye (Figure 7.11). A simpler procedure is to visualize by ultrasound the turbulence produced by pushing saline to prove free placement (Figure 7.12). However, many fetal complications may result from inadvertent injection of highly packed donor blood (prepared as for IVT) into a confined space.[55] Considerable force is required to push this thick blood through the catheter in 10-ml aliquots.[56] FHR is monitored throughout, showing characteristic tachycardia, probably indicating pain as the peritoneum distends. Bradycardia, failure of transfused blood to produce a fluid interface on ultrasound, and maternal complications are the most common reasons for terminating IPT before target volume. Post-IPT monitoring is extended, as traumatic fetal bleeding may take time to produce detectable effects. Timing of repeat IPT is similar to IVT, averaging 3–4 weeks, but serial IPTs are seldom used.

IPT versus IVT

Theoretically, it might be easier to place a needle within the fetal peritoneal cavity than into a vessel. Also, more blood can be delivered intraperitoneally, according to the following formula:[52]

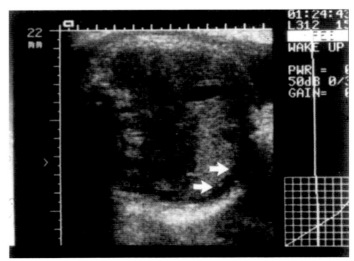

Figure 7.12 Intraperitoneal transfusion, with ultrasound verification of proper placement. With ideal fetal position (spine at 11 o'clock position), a 20-gauge spinal needle was used to enter the peritoneal cavity, and placement free in the abdomen was confirmed with agitated saline. Arrows show intraperitoneal fluid rim forming (infused blood), at the 50-ml point in the transfusion.

$$\text{IPT volume in ml} = (\text{weeks gestation} - 20) \times 10$$

The major drawback of IPT, in addition to limited ability to treat fetal hydrops, is fetal trauma. This is worse at premature gestation and with anterior placenta. Death from laceration of a major vessel, cardiac penetration, and neurologic injury have been reported. While these are decreased with continuous ultrasound guidance, data from a matched control trial display dramatic differences in safety and efficacy, all favoring IVT (Table 7.7).[53]

Table 7.7 Intraperitoneal fetal transfusion (IPT) – 1980–6*

Fetuses treated	75	
Total procedures	202	
Overall survival	57	(76%)
Survivors/class I[†]	41/46	(89%)
Survivors/classes II–III	16/21	(76%)
Survivors/class IV	0/8	(0%)
Procedures total	216	
Successful	202	
Attempts/IPT	2.4	
Failed procedures	14	
Deaths		
Trauma	18	
Fetal	4	
Neonatal	3	
Moribund hydropic disease	8	
Newborn complications‡	3	

* Does not include eight fetuses who had single IPT in the course of management with intravenous fetal transfusion (IVT).
† Class assigned at first IPT.
‡ Hyaline membrane disease due to prematurity (two cases), and iatrogenic complications of exchange transfusion (one case).

Table 7.8 Choice of management (IVT vs IPT) (matched control trial – 1990)[53]

Factor	IPT	IVT	p
Number of procedures	2.4	3.9	0.03
Attempts/transfusions	1.8	1.2	0.02
Procedural complications	38%	10%	0.004
Traumatic death	18%	3%	0.001
Delivery (GA)	31	34	0.011
Exchange transfusions	1.8	0.8	0.007
ICN days	8.2	6.1	0.044
Nonhydrops alive	83%	98%	NS
Hydrops alive	48%	86%	0.01
Class IV alive	0/6	4/6	

IVT = fetal intravascular transfusion; IPT = (fetal) intraperitoneal transfusion; GA = mean gestational age; ICN = intensive care nursery..

Intracardiac transfusion (ICT)

In severe early disease treated with IVT, fetal exsanguination occasionally occurs due to vessel trauma and/or thrombocytopenia. In such critical situations, the opportunity for resuscitation may pass in seconds. Vascular collapse makes repeating venous puncture impossible and fetal death is probable. ICT in such circumstances may be lifesaving. Even more rarely, ICT may be the only means of transfusing very early hydrops.[56]

Our experience includes 16 ICTs in 15 fetuses. Ten of these fetuses were exsanguinating. Twelve fetuses survived the acute event after successful intracardiac resuscitation (Figure 7.13). Intracardiac blood sampling and transfusion were semielective in two Rh-positive fetuses whose mothers had hydropic demise at 16-weeks in prior pregnancy.[5] Without life-threatening hypovolemia, ICT is relatively straightforward. The rigidity of a 20-gauge needle may allow improved maneuverability. While the right ventricle seems most appropriate, it is usually not easy to be that selective. IVT principals are utilized, with blood return and 'puffs' of saline confirming placement and RBC infusion under continuous ultrasound visualization. Turbulence should be visible in umbilical arteries exiting the fetus. The initial response to severe hypovolemia is profound bradycardia. After the first few milliliters of intracardiac infusion, FHR rises to normal, and then to tachycardia. Cold blood straight from the blood bank produces cardiac slowing and ventricular dysfunction. Therefore, one should warm several capped, 5-ml syringes of donor blood under running water. The catheter should not be removed from the needle hub for repeated sampling. We simply give 50% of anticipated IVT volume, sample once, and remove the needle. In fetuses recovering from this procedure, it

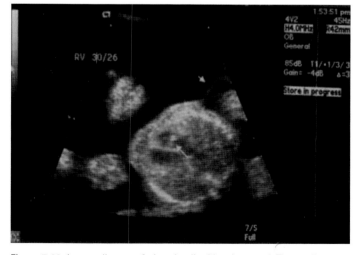

Figure 7.13 Intracardiac transfusion visualized by ultrasound. The needle enters the chest in the right anterior axillary line (upper arrow), and the tip sits in the right ventricle (lower arrow). Just below the needle tip, echogenicity is apparent, due to infusion of densely packed donor blood. Hydropic fetus at 17.1 weeks, with pretransfusion hemoglobin of 3.0 g/dl. An initial attempt via the intrahepatic umbilical vein resulted in significant intraperitoneal hemorrhage and fetal bradycardia. The ICT was lifesaving. At last follow-up, this child was 8 years old, and developmentally normal.

is perhaps surprising that only one had a significant pericardial effusion. All class III or class IV hydropic fetuses have the potential for thrombocytopenia, vessel wall edema, and exsanguination at IVT. It is useful before starting IVT for such severe illness, to perform a complete anatomic survey of the fetal heart.[17]

Disorder-specific issues

Transplacental hemorrhage

Chronic anemia due to blood loss follows fetomaternal hemorrhage (FMH) either spontaneously or post-trauma. IUT to replace blood loss has been successful in FMH, but chronic hemorrhage often continues. Because donor cells are adult, Kleihauer–Betke testing cannot assess post-IVT fetal bleeding. MCA Doppler and serial cordocenteses should be used for this situation.[57] In many cases, delivery is a better option once viability has been reached.

TTTS

In twin-to-twin transfusion syndrome (TTTS), IVT has been suggested for the donor twin after laser ablation of placental anastomoses.[58] This practice assumes the TTTS donor is anemic due to fetofetal blood loss. However, donors have contracted intravascular volume that will eventually re-expand if placental function is adequate and, except in the minority, still have enough hemoglobin for oxygenation. IVT in TTTS is currently undergoing active research.

Parvovirus

Parvovirus hydrops with profound anemia is quite treatable with IVT. An average of 2.2 transfusions is enough to raise the hemoglobin and sustain it until fetal erythropoiesis resumes. Results will vary, as *Parvovirus* may cause permanent deficits in cardiac function, hepatic function, cerebral function, and growth. Cautious counseling about the potential for permanent injury in other systems should accompany transfusion therapy in *Parvovirus*.[59]

Anemia beyond 32 weeks

In most centers, 32 weeks marks a watershed between mortality and morbidity of the neonate. Should one deliver the anemic fetus for transfusions in the neonatal intensive care unit (NICU) rather than 'risking' IVT? For experienced teams, IVT up to 36 weeks has measurable advantages. The *neonate* challenged with rapid, high-volume transfusion suffers cardiac failure and pulmonary edema. Due to the distensibility of fetoplacental vasculature, the *fetus* simply makes volume corrections into the maternal space and amniotic cavity. For the nonhydropic fetus, arrhythmia, NICU accidents, operator experience with exchange transfusion, and infectious issues all may mean that a simple IUT is safer than multiple neonatal exchange transfusions.[5, 60]

Lethal fetal anemias

Inherited hemoglobinopathies and RBC membrane disorders may cause severe fetal anemia and/or anemic hydrops. Serial fetal transfusions are timed similarly to those in Rh disease, suppressing production of abnormal RBCs, and allowing recovery from RBC breakdown products, while maintaining homeostasis. Hemosiderosis is a significant problem with potentially lethal complications in childhood. Advances in transfusion medicine, iron chelation, and bone marrow and liver transplantation in infancy have salvaged small numbers.[61, 62] This demonstrates the potential for early and sustained fetal transfusion, but the unaltered high rate of complication in these children has limited widespread acceptance.

Class III/IV hydrops

In such compromised fetuses, rapid transfusion to usual target volumes leads to cardiovascular collapse, due to the already high intravascular pressures, poor placental respiratory function caused by edema, and direct cardiac failure.[63] One gives 50–60% target volume for gestational age, and 3–5 days later, the same volume is repeated. Response to the first two transfusions is highly predictive of outcome (Figure 7.14). In class IV disease, with abnormal biophysical profile, maternal oxygen is started preprocedure, and maintained until heart rate and activity are normal. Rarely, thrombocytopenia is so severe that fetal platelet transfusion is required. Usually, a short, single-puncture procedure restoring hemoglobin concentration to 6.0–8.0 g/dl produces rapid return to normal neurologic function and normal vascular integrity, although physical changes of hydrops may take weeks to regress. Unexpected elevation in post-IVT intravenous pressure may be treated with fetal intravenous digoxin.[64]

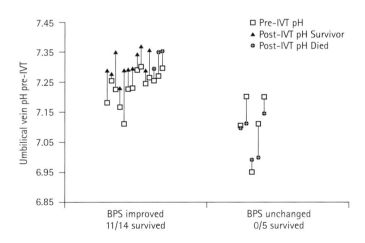

Figure 7.14 Initial response to fetal transfusion indicates prognosis in moribund class IV hydrops. On the left, 14 fetuses showed improvement in biophysical profile score (BPS) between first and second transfusions. Eleven of 14 survived. On the right, five fetuses, equally sick, showed no improvement in pH, and no return of fetal activity, and all died during or after the second transfusion. The return of normal behavior after the transfusion, even when the physical findings are severe, is reassuring.

Neonatal alloimmune thrombocytopenia (NAIT)

This is a significant source of transfusion patients, meriting attention. Maternal sensitization against platelet antigens (primarily PLA1 and Bak[a]), causes alloimmune destruction of fetal platelets via transplacental antiplatelet IgG. High-dose maternal IgG therapy may treat up to 70% of these fetuses at risk of intracranial hemorrhage antenatally. However, the problem with NAIT in its most severe form is that not all cases respond to IV IgG, and the worst may have platelet counts so low that intracranial hemorrhage is probable.[65] Thus, after a significant course of therapy (starting at 14 weeks, and extending for 6–8 weeks, until placental and fetal receptors are saturated with IgG), fetal blood sampling for platelet count may be appropriate to confirm therapeutic effect. However, there is controversy about this approach because bleeding after cordocentesis depends not only on thrombocytopenia, but also on the fact that the offending antigen is present in fetal endothelial cells.[66] Both vascular integrity and platelet count and function are impaired, and both remain impaired in the 30% treatment failures. Exsanguination from uncomplicated cordocentesis in PLA1 disease caused our only fetal losses in hundreds of procedures. Because of this danger, every blood-sampling procedure for NAIT includes a fetal platelet transfusion. The platelets are fresh, moderately concentrated, at 10 ml/kg of anticipated fetal weight. The transfusion technique is similar, with a 25- or 22-gauge needle in the intrahepatic umbilical vein. If cord needling is utilized, it is in midcord where Wharton's jelly may assist in closing the puncture. Adjunctive, high-dose dexamethasone and early delivery further maximize therapeutic results. In our experience of 22 severely thrombocytopenic fetuses, of the 19 survivors, only two required serial fetal platelet transfusion.[67]

Post-transfusion monitoring

In class IV hydrops, FHR monitoring is continuous with maternal oxygenation until the biophysical profile score is normal. In less severe disease, oxygen is not used, and the mother is discharged when FHR reactivity and fetal movement have returned and there are no uterine contractions. Weekly MCA Doppler and biophysical profile scoring are performed until the following transfusion.[68] The following transfusion is planned for pre-IVT donor hemoglobin of 80–90 g/dl subtracting 0.3 g/dl per day from post-IVT donor level (e.g., if closing level is 16.6 g/dl, 10% residual fetal, repeat IVT in 20–24 days). This interval lengthens as gestational age advances and is modified by MCA results.[69, 70]

Outcome studies

The results of our transfusion program are shown in Tables 7.8 and 7.9.[5,17] We have seen substantial improvement in IVT technique and outcome statistics since its first inception, with renewed focus on preventing prematurity and related morbidity.

Table 7.9 Progress with fetal intravascular transfusions.

1986–9		1994–2004
67	Fetuses	73
287	IVT	212
41%	Hydrops	49%
30%	Class IV*	56%
37%	First IVT <24 weeks	42%
75	Interval (days)[M]	89
34.4	Weeks at delivery[M]	37.3
5	ICN days[M]	1
40%	'Ideal'	79%

Ideal outcome: term delivery, no 'crash', C/S, normal Apgars, normal pH, Hb >10 g/dl, no respirator, home with mother

*% of all hydrops.
M = mean.

Long-term follow-up is key, whenever fetal therapy is considered. For many intrauterine interventions, infancy and childhood are marked with multiple complications and a very challenging course. However, in general, this is not the case for survivors of fetal transfusion, regardless of severity of disease. In class IV hydrops, with poor fetal behavior, outcomes include 10% incidence of cerebral palsy.[71] Other than this discrete group, long-term results are excellent, with very low incidence of permanent handicap.[5, 72, 73]

Over the short-term, most fetuses with serial IVT have delayed erythropoietic response.[74] In the transfused fetus, erythropoietin levels have been suppressed for weeks or months prior to delivery. Donor cells have a reduced half-life in the newborn. With this combination of delayed response and rapid attrition, it is very common for IVT survivors to have two or more neonatal 'top-up' transfusions, typically at 6 and 10 weeks. In many cases, this is the only hematologic manifestation of disease. The fully transfused neonate has normal bilirubin, ample iron to make new RBC, and an excellent birth hemoglobin level if cord clamping is delayed, and often needs no transfusion during its short NICU stay. For many fetal transfusion teams, these neonatal benefits clearly justify the application of transfusion therapy until late in gestation.

Summary

Access to the fetal circulation has made precise monitoring and pretransfusion evaluation routine. More recently, data obtained by cordocentesis have validated noninvasive Doppler techniques using MCA Doppler velocimetry, reliably identifying fetuses at risk of anemia, while reliably excluding fetuses not yet anemic. Fetal IVT techniques have been simplified, and now account for almost all IUT procedures. This has resulted in a high level of success, even in the presence of fetal hydrops. The success of these techniques has led to the application of IVT in many other areas with promising results. Against a background of continued vigilance to prevent alloimmunization by proper transfusion and prophylaxis techniques, IUT stands as a model of successful fetal therapy.

References

1. Harman CR, Manning FA. Alloimmune disease. In: Pauerstein CJ (ed), Clinical Obstetrics, pp. 441–69. Wiley: New York, 1987.

2. Bowman JM. Blood group immunization in obstetric practice. Curr Probl Obstet Gynecol 1983; 7: 1–61.

3. Bowman JM. The prevention of Rh immunization. Transfusion Med Rev 1988; 2: 129–50.

4. Bowman JM. Suppression of Rh isoimmunization. Obstet Gynecol 1978; 52: 385–93.

5. Harman CR. Invasive techniques in the management of alloimmune anemia. In: Harman, CR (ed), Invasive Fetal Testing and Treatment, pp. 107–91. Blackwell Scientific: Boston, MA, 1995.

6. Bowman JM, Harman CR, Manning FA et al. Intravenous drug abuse causes Rh immunization. Vox Sang 1991; 61: 96–8.

7. Bowell PJ, Brown SE, Dike AE et al. The significance of anti-c alloimmunization in pregnancy. Br J Obstet Gynaecol 1986; 93: 1044–8.

8. Hackney DN, Knudtson EJ, Rossi KQ et al. Management of pregnancies complicated by anti-c isoimmunization. Obstet Gynecol 2004; 103: 24–30.

9. Bowman JM, Pollock JM, Manning FA et al. Severe anti-C hemolytic disease of the newborn. Am J Obstet Gynecol 1992; 166: 1239–43.

10. Bowman JM. Maternal blood group immunization. In: Creasy RK, Resnick R (eds.), Maternal-Fetal Medicine: Principles and Practice, pp. 613–49 (2nd edition) Saunders: Philadelphia, 1989.

11. Bowman JM, Pollock JM, Manning FA et al. Maternal Kell blood group alloimmunization. Obstet Gynecol 1992; 79: 239–44.

12. Vaughan JI, Manning M, Warwick RM et al. Inhibition of erythroid progenitor cells by anti-Kell antibodies in fetal alloimmune anemia. N Engl J Med 1998; 338: 798–803.

13. Norbeck O, Tolfvenstam T, Shields LE et al. K. *Parvovirus B19* capsid protein VP2 inhibits hematopoiesis in vitro and in vivo: implications for therapeutic use. Exp Hematol 2004; 32: 1082–7.

14. Corcoran A, Doyle S. Advances in the biology, diagnosis and host–pathogen interactions of *Parvovirus B19*. J Med Microbiol 2004; 53(Pt 6): 459–75.

15. Vogel H, Kornman M, Ledet SC et al. Congenital *Parvovirus* infection. Pediatr Pathol Lab Med 1997; 17: 903–12.

16. Crane J. *Parvovirus B-19* infection in pregnancy. J Obstet Gynaecol Can 2002; 24: 727–43.

17. Harman CR. Ultrasound in the management of the alloimmunized pregnancy. In: Fleischer AC, Manning FA, Jeanty P, Romero R (eds), Sonography in Obstetrics and Gynecology [Principles and Practice], pp. 683–709 (6th edition) McGraw-Hill: New York, 2001.

18. Harman CR. Specialized applications of obstetric ultrasound: management of the alloimmunized pregnancy. Semin Perinat 1985; 9: 184–97.

19. Harman CR. Fetal monitoring in the alloimmunized pregnancy. Clin Perinatol 1989; 16: 691–733.

20. Moise KJ Jr. Management of rhesus alloimmunization in pregnancy. Obstet Gynecol 2002; 100: 600–11.

21. Moise KJ Jr, Perkins JT, Sosler SD et al. The predictive value of maternal serum testing for detection of fetal anemia in red blood cell alloimmunization. Am J Obstet Gynecol 1995; 172: 1003–9.

22. Hadley AG, Kumpel BM, Leader KA et al. Correlation of serological, quantitative and cell-mediated functional assays of maternal alloantibodies with the severity of haemolytic disease of the newborn. Br J Haemat 1991; 77: 221–8.

23. Nicolaides KH, Rodeck CH. Maternal serum anti-D antibody concentration and assessment of rhesus isoimmunization. BMJ 1992; 304: 1155–6.

24. van Dijk BA, Dooren MC, Overbeeke AM. Red cell alloantibodies in pregnancy: there is no 'critical titer'. Transfusion Med 1995; 4: 199–202.

25. Clark DA. Red-cell antibodies in pregnancy: evidence overturned. Lancet 1996; 347: 485–6.

26. Mari G, Detti L, Oz U et al. Accurate prediction of fetal hemoglobin by Doppler ultrasonography. Obstet Gynecol 2002; 99: 589–93.

27. Mari G, Adrignolo A, Abuhamad AZ et al. Diagnosis of fetal anemia with Doppler ultrasound in the pregnancy complicated by maternal blood group immunization. Ultrasound Obstet Gynecol 1995; 5: 400–5.

28. Mari G, Rahman F, Olofsson P et al. Increase of fetal hematocrit decreases the middle cerebral artery peak systolic velocity in pregnancies complicated by rhesus alloimmunization. J Matern-Fetal Med 1997; 6: 206–8.

29. Hernandez-Andrade E, Scheier M, Dezerega V et al. Fetal middle cerebral artery peak systolic velocity in the investigation of non-immune hydrops. Ultrasound Obstet Gynecol 2004; 23: 442–5.

30. Mari G, Deter RL, Carpenter RL et al. Noninvasive diagnosis by Doppler ultrasonography of fetal anemia due to maternal red-cell alloimmunization. N Engl J Med 2000; 342: 9–14.

31. Kush ML, Baschat AA, Weiner CP et al. When should you investigate elevated middle cerebral artery Doppler? Am J Obstet Gynecol 2004; 19: S149.

32. Bowman JM, Pollock JM. Transplacental fetal hemorrhage after amniocentesis. Obstet Gynecol 1985; 66: 749–54.

33. Bowman JM, Pollock JM, Peterson LE et al. Fetomaternal hemorrhage following funipuncture: increase in severity of maternal red-cell alloimmunization. Obstet Gynecol 1194; 84: 839–43.

34. Lee S, Bennett PR, Overton T et al. Prenatal diagnosis of Kell blood group genotypes: KEL1 and KEL2. Am J Obstet Gynecol 1996; 175: 455–9.

35. Bennett PR, Le Van KC, Colin Y et al. Prenatal determination of fetal RhD type by DNA amplification. N Engl J Med 1993; 329: 607–10.

36. Bennett PR, Warwick R, Vaughan J et al. Prenatal determination of human platelet antigen type using DNA amplification following amniocentesis. Br J Obstet Gynaecol 1994; 101: 246–9.

37. Liley AW. Liquor amnii analysis in the management of the pregnancy complicated by rhesus sensitization. Am J Obstet Gynecol 1961; 82: 1359–70.

38. Harman CR. Assessment of fetal health. In: Creasy RD, Resnick R, Iams JD (eds), Maternal Fetal Medicine, pp. 357–401. Saunders: Philadelphia, 2004.

39. Weiner CP. Human fetal bilirubin levels and fetal hemolytic disease. Am J Obstet Gynecol 1992; 166: 1149-54.

40. Weiner CP, Williamson RA, Wenstrom KD et al. Management of fetal hemolytic disease by cordocentesis. I. Prediction of fetal anemia. Am J Obstet Gynecol 1991; 165: 546–53.

41. Nicolaides KH. Studies on fetal physiology and pathophysiology in rhesus disease. Semin Perinat 1989; 13: 328–37.

42. Nicolini U, Santolaya J, Fisk NM et al. Changes in fetal acid base during intravascular transfusion. Arch Dis Child 1988; 63: 710–14.

43. Weiner CP, Williamson RA, Wenstrom KD et al. Management of fetal hemolytic disease by cordocentesis. II. Outcome of treatment. Am J Obstet Gynecol 1991; 165: 1737.

44. de Crespigny LC Robinson HP, Quinn M et al. Ultrasound-guided fetal blood transfusion for severe rhesus isoimmunization. Obstet Gynecol 1985; 66: 529–32.

45. Moise KJ Jr, Carpenter RJ Jr, Kirshon B et al. Comparison of four types of intrauterine transfusion: effect on fetal hematocrit. Fetal Ther 1989; 4: 126–37.

46. Moise KJ Jr, Deter RL, Kirshon B et al. Intravenous pancuronium bromide for fetal neuromuscular blockade during intrauterine transfusion for red-cell alloimmunization. Obstet Gynecol 1989; 74: 905–8.

47. Stefos T, Cosmi E, Detti L et al. Correction of fetal anemia on the middle cerebral artery peak systolic velocity. Obstet Gynecol 2002; 99: 211–15.

48. Harman CR, Bowman JM, Menticoglou SM et al. Profound fetal thrombocytopenia in rhesus disease: serious hazard at intravascular transfusion. Lancet 1988; 2: 741–2.

49. Segal M, Manning FA, Harman CR et al. Bleeding after intravascular transfusion: experimental and clinical observations. Am J Obstet Gynecol 1991; 165: 1414–18.

50. Harman CR, Biehl DR, Pollock JM et al. Intrauterine transfusion: kinetics of absorption of donor cells in fetal lambs. Am J Obstet Gynecol 1983; 145: 830–6.

51. Menticoglou SM, Harman CR, Manning FA et al. Intraperitoneal fetal transfusion: paralysis inhibits red cell absorption. Fetal Ther 1987; 2: 154–9.

52. Harman CR, Bowman JM. Intraperitoneal fetal transfusion. In: Chervenak FA, Isaacson GC, Campbell S (eds), Ultrasound in Obstetrics and Gynecology, vol. 2, pp. 1295–1313. Little, Brown: Boston, MA, 1993.

53. Harman CR, Bowman JM, Manning FA et al. Intrauterine transfusion intraperitoneal versus intravascular approach: a case control comparison. Am J Obstet Gynecol 1990; 162: 1053–9.

54. Harman CR, Manning FA, Bowman JM et al. Severe Rh disease – poor outcome is not inevitable. Am J Obstet Gynecol 1983; 145: 823–9.

55. Harman CR, Bowman JM, Menticoglou SM et al. Current technique of intraperitoneal transfusion: do not throw away the Renografin. Fetal Ther 1989; 4: 78–82.

56. Westgren M, Selbing A, Stangenberg M. Fetal intracardiac transfusions in patients with severe rhesus isoimmunization. BMJ 1988; 296: 885–6.

57. Baschat AA, Harman CR, Alger LS et al. Fetal coronary and cerebral blood flow in acute fetomaternal hemorrhage. Ultrasound Obstet Gynecol 1198; 12: 128–31.

58. Senat MV, Loizeau S, Couderc S et al. The value of the middle cerebral artery peak systolic velocity in the diagnosis of fetal anemia after intrauterine death of one monochorionic twin. Am J Obstet Gynecol 2003; 189: 1320–4.

59. Dembinski J, Haverkamp F, Maara H et al. Neurodevelopmental outcome after intrauterine red cell transfusion for Parvovirus B-19 induced fetal hydrops. Br J Obstet Gynaecol 2002; 109: 1232–4.

60. Klumper FJ, van Kamp IL, Vendenbussche FP et al. Benefits and risks of fetal red-cell transfusion after 32 weeks' gestation. Eur J Obstet Gynecol Reprod Biol 2000; 92: 91–6.

61. Sohan K, Billington M, Pamphilon et al. Normal growth and development following in utero diagnosis and treatment of homozygous alpha thalassemia. Br J Obstet Gynaecol 202; 109: 1308–10.

62. Remacha AF, Badell I, Pujol-Moix N et al. Hydrops fetalis-associated congenital dyserythropoietic anemia treated with intrauterine transfusions and bone marrow transplantation. Blood 2002; 100: 356–8.

63. Harman CR, Manning FA, Bowman JM et al. Use of intravascular transfusion to treat hydrops fetalis in a moribund fetus. Can Med Assoc J 1988; 138: 827–30.

64. Weiner CP, Pelzer GD, Heilskov J et al The effect of intravascular transfusion on umbilical venous pressure in anemia fetuses with and without hydrops. Am J Obstet Gynecol 1989; 161(6 pt 1): 1498–1501.

65. Bussel JB. Alloimmune thrombocytopenia in the fetus and newborn. Semin Thromb Hemost 2001; 27: 245–52.

66. Radder CM, Brand A, Kanhai HH. A less invasive treatment strategy to prevent intracranial hemorrhage in fetal and neonatal alloimmune thrombocytopenia. Am J Obstet Gynecol 2001; 185: 683–8.

67. Birchall JE, Murphy MF, Kaplan C et al. European collaborative study of the antenatal management of feto-maternal alloimmune thrombocytopenia. Br J Haematol 2003; 122: 275–88.

68. Detti L, Oz U, Guney I et al. Doppler ultrasound velocimetry for timing the second intrauterine transfusion in fetuses with anemia from red-cell alloimmunization. Am J Obstet Gynecol 201; 185: 1048–51.

69. Abdel-Fattah SA, Carroll SG, Kyle PM et al. The effect of fetal hydrops on the rate of fall of hemoglobin after fetal intravascular transfusion for red-cell alloimmunization. Fetal Diagn Ther 2000; 15: 262–6.

70. Egberts J, van Kamp IL, Kanhai HH et al. The disappearance of fetal and donor red blood cells in alloimmunised pregnancies: a reappraisal. Br J Obstet Gynaecol 1997; 104: 818–24.

71. Dildy GA, Smith LG Jr, Moise KJ Jr et al. Porencephalic cyst: a complication of fetal intravascular transfusion. Am J Obstet Gynecol 1991; 165: 76–8.

72. van Kamp IL, Klumper FJCM, Meerman RH et al. Treatment of fetal anemia due to red-cell alloimmunization with intrauterine transfusions in the Netherlands, 1988–1999. Acta Obstet Gynecol Scand 2004; 83: 731–7.

73. Farrant B, Battin M, Roberts A. Outcome of infants receiving in utero transfusions for haemolytic disease. N Z Med J 2001; 114(1139): 400–3.

74. Pessler F, Hart D. Hyporegenerative anemia associated with Rh hemolytic disease: treatment failure of recombinant erythropoietin. J Pediatr Hematol Oncol 2002; 24: 689–93.

8 Fetal reduction

Mark I Evans, David W Britt, Doina Ciorica, and †John C Fletcher

In the last 25 years, millions of babies have been born benefiting from infertility therapies, including more than 1 000 000 IVF babies. These positive family outcomes, however, have had serious side effects. The twin pregnancy rate, commonly quoted for decades to be 1 in 90, now has doubled to more than 1 in 45. All multiple pregnancies have continued to rise and the incidence of prematurity and related sequelae clearly correlate with fetal number (Figure 8.1; Table 8.1).[1] Infertility treatments are so pervasive that more than 70% of all twins and 99% of higher-order multiples derive from them (Table 8.2). With increasing public and professional attention, some of the very high-order multiples have diminished, particularly secondary to lower transfer numbers of embryos in IVF. There are some suggestions that the incidence of triplets and higher is slowly diminishing, but the incidence is still very high.

Appreciated pregnancy losses in multiple pregnancies are mostly related to how early in pregnancy one establishes the denominator.[2,3] Some reports by perinatologists are overtly optimistic because these physicians do not start counting until they begin to see patients at nearly 20 weeks, at which time most

losses have already occurred.[3,4] Many other articles have addressed those issues and will not be repeated here.[4–6]

In the 1980s, about 75% of multifetal pregnancy patients seeking reduction had pregnancies initiated with ovulation induction agents such as Pergonal.[7] However, even with the first month of the lowest dose of Clomid, quintuplets have occurred. Over the years, cases induced by assisted reproductive technologies (ARTs), such as IVF, have become increasingly common. Currently, about 70% of patients we see seeking reduction have pregnancies generated by ARTs (Table 8.3).[8]

Despite the increased utilization of ARTs,[8] the proportion of cases significantly hyperstimulated, and resulting in quintuplets or more has dramatically decreased to less than 10% of all cases seen by us. Nevertheless, the 2000 report of the

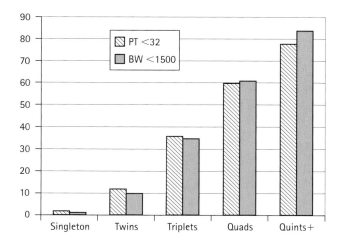

Figure 8.1 Risks of prematurity as a function of fetal number. Diagonal lines : preterm (PT) birth <32 weeks. Shaded area: birth weight (BW) <1500 g. Based on US Centers for Disease Control Data, 2002.

Table 8.1 Multiple births in the USA

Year	Twins	Triplets	Quadruplets	Quintuplets and higher multiples
2002	125 134	6898	434	69
2001	121 246	6885	501	85
2000	118 916	6742	506	77
1999	114 307	6742	512	67
1998	110 670	6919	627	79
1997	104 137	6148	510	79
1996	100 750	5298	560	81
1995	96 736	4551	365	57
1994	97 064	4233	315	46
1993	96 445	3834	277	57
1992	95 372	3547	310	26
1991	94 779	3121	203	22
1990	93 865	2830	185	13
1989	90 118	2529	229	40
% Change from 1989 to 2002	38.9%	172.8%	89.6%	72.5%

Data taken from National Vital Statitics Report, Vol. 52, no. 10, p. 22, 2003.

Table 8.2 Ratio of observed to expected multiples

Births	Observed	Expected	Ratio
Twins	125 134	44 686	2.80:1
Triplets	6898	496	13.9:1
Quadruplets	434	6	72.3:1
Quintuplets and higher multiples	69	0.07	985.7:1

Total births in 2002 – 4 021 726.

Table 8.3 Changes in etiology of multifetal pregnancies

Ovulation induction		Assisted reproductive technologies
1980s	75%	25%
1990s	50%	50%
2000s	30%	70%

Society of Assisted Reproductive Technologies (SART) suggested that, of all pregnancies achieved by ARTs, in the USA 58.5% are singletons, 28% twins, 7.5% triplets or higher, and 5.9% unknown.[9,10] In our experience with referred cases of ovulation stimulation, particularly those using follicle stimulating hormone (FSH) analogs, the proportion of cases that are quintuplets or more has fallen, but not as dramatically.[11]

Such data continue to emphasize the significant role of vigilance in the monitoring of infertility therapies. The vast majority of multifetal cases occur to physicians with the best of equipment and with the best of intentions who have an unfortunate and reasonably unpredictable or unpreventable maloccurrence. Despite this, clearly, some cases might have been prevented by increased vigilance.[11–13]

Patient issues

Over the past decade, the demographics of patients seeking multifetal pregnancy reduction (MFPR) have evolved considerably.[11,12] With the availability of donor eggs, the number of 'older women' seeking MFPR has increased dramatically. In our experience, over 10% of all patients seeking MFPR are over 40 years of age, and nearly half of them are using donor eggs. As a consequence of the shift to older patients, many of whom already had previous relationships and children, there is an increased desire by these patients to have only one further child. The number of experienced centers willing to do two to one reductions is still very limited, but we believe it can be justified in the appropriate circumstances.[11,13]

For patients who are 'older', particularly those using their own eggs, the issue of genetic diagnosis comes into play. By 2001, more than 50% of patients in the USA having ART

cycles were over 35 (Table 8.4).[1,9,10,14] In the 1980s and early 1990s, the most common approach was to offer amniocentesis at 16–17 weeks on the remaining twins. A 1995 paper suggested an 11% loss rate in these cases, which caused considerable concern.[15] However, the issue was settled by a much larger collaborative series in 1998 that showed that loss rates were no higher than comparable controls of MFPR patients who did not have amniocentesis.[16] The collaborative data showed a loss rate of 5%, which was certainly no higher than the post-MFPR group of patients who did not have genetic studies.

Since the centers with the most MFPR experience also happened to be the ones who also had the same accomplishments with chorionic villus sampling (CVS), combinations of the procedures were very logical. There are two main schools of thought as to the best approach to first-trimester genetic diagnosis; that is, should it be before or after the performance of MFPR? Published data in the early 1990s on doing the CVS first followed by reductions suggested a 1–2% error rate as to which fetus was which, particularly if the entire karyotype was obtained before going on to reduction.[17] Therefore, for the first 10–15 years, the approach we used was generally to do the reduction first at approximately 10.5 weeks in patients reducing down to twins or triplets, followed by CVS approximately 1 week later.[11,14] However, in patients going to a singleton pregnancy, essentially putting 'all of their eggs in one basket', we believed the best approach was to know what was in the basket before reducing the other embryos.[11,12] In these cases we performed CVS usually on all the fetuses or one more than the intended stopping number, and performed a fluorescent *in situ* hybridization (FISH) analysis with probes for chromosomes 13, 18, 21, X, and Y. Since about 30% of overall anomalies seen on karyotype would not be detectable by FISH with these probes,[18] there is always residual risk.[19] The absolute risk, given both a normal FISH and normal ultrasound, including nuchal translucency,[20] is only about 1/500. We believe that this risk is lower than the increased risk from the 2-week wait necessary to get the full karyotype. We have now commonly extended this approach to all patients who are appropriate candidates for prenatal diagnosis regardless of the fetal number. Over the past few years, more than half of our patients have combined CVS and MFPR procedures. With data now suggesting increased risks of chromosomal and other anomalies in patients conceiving by IVF and especially with intra cytoplasmic sperm injection

Table 8.4 Maternal age and ART (SART data – 2001)

All cases	81 915
Fresh nondonor	60 780
<35	28 778
35–37	14 416
38–40	11 301
41–42	4365
42+	2190

(ICSI) the utilization of prenatal diagnosis will likely increase even further.[21–26]

An alternative approach used by other investigators is to perform CVS and complete karyotype first and have the patient come back for the reduction. Although 'mistakes' may not have been uncommon 10 years ago, the chance of an error has been considerably reduced nowadays, and these investigators believe that the benefits of the full karyotype justify the wait. The question of which is the better of these two approaches is currently unsettled and would require a very large series to differentiate among small risks.

Procedures

MFPR is a clinical procedure developed in the 1980s when a small number of centers in both the USA and Europe attempted to reduce the usual and tremendously adverse sequelae of multifetal pregnancies by selectively terminating or reducing the number of fetuses to a more manageable number. The first European reports by Dumez,[27] and the first American report by Evans et al,[28] followed by a further report by Berkowitz et al,[29] and later Wapner et al,[30] described a surgical approach to improve the outcome in such cases.

Even these early reports appreciated the ethical dilemma faced by couples and physicians under such difficult circumstances.[13] In the mid-1980s, needles were inserted transabdominally and maneuvered into the thorax for the injection of potassium chloride mechanical destruction or air embolization despite relatively mediocre ultrasound visualization. Transcervical aspirations were initially tried, but with little success. Some centers used transvaginal mechanical disruption, but data suggested a significantly higher loss rate than with the transabdominal route.[31] Today, virtually all experienced operators perform the procedure by inserting needles transabdominally under ultrasound guidance.

Outcomes

Over more than a decade, several centers with the world's largest experience have collaborated to leverage the power of their data. In 1993, the first collaborative report showed a 16% pregnancy loss rate through 24 completed weeks.[17] While by today's standards, that was not a very satisfactory number, it did represent a major improvement for higher-order multiple pregnancies. Further collaborative papers have shown continued dramatic improvements in the overall outcomes of such pregnancies (Table 8.5).[11] The 2001 collaborative data demonstrated that the outcome of triplets reduced to twins, and that of quadruplets reduced to twins now perform essentially as if they started as twins.[11] Even with the tremendous advances in neonatal care for premature babies, the 95% take-home baby rate for triplets and the 92% take-home baby rate for quadruplets clearly represent dramatic improvements over natural statistics. Not only the pregnancy loss rate but also the rate of very dangerous early prematurity has been substantially lowered. Both continue to be correlated with the starting number. Data from recent years show that the improvements are, not surprisingly, greatest from the higher starting numbers (Figure 8.2).

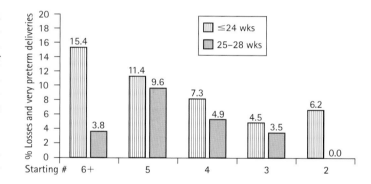

Figure 8.2 Multifetal pregnancy reduction: losses and very preterm deliveries by starting number. (Modified from Evans MI, Berkowitz R, Wapner R et al. Am J Obstet Gynecol 2001; 184: 97–103[11] with permission from Elsevier.)

Table 8.5 Multifetal pregnancy reduction – losses by years

	Total	Losses (weeks)		Deliveries (weeks)			
		% < 24	% > 24	% 25–28	% 29–32	% 33–36	% 37+
1986–90	508	13.2	4.5	10.0	21.1	15.7	35.4
1991–4	724	9.4	0.3	2.8	5.4	21.1	61.0
1995–8	1356	6.4	0.2	4.3	10.2	31.5	47.4

Modified from Evans MI, Berkowitz R, Wapner R et al. Am J Obstet Gynecol 2001; 184: 97–103[11] with permission from Elsevier

The lowest pregnancy loss rates are for those cases reduced to twins, with increasing losses for singletons followed by triplets. However, the rate of early premature delivery has been, not surprisingly, highest with triplets, followed by twins, and lowest with singletons. Mean gestational age at delivery was also lower for higher-order cases. Birth weights after MFPR decreased with starting and finishing numbers, reflecting increasing prematurity.[32]

While data in the literature are conflicting, our experiences suggest that triplets reduced to twins do much better in terms of loss and prematurity than do unreduced triplets. We believe that if a patient's primary goal is to maximize the chances of surviving children, that reduction of triplets to twins achieves the best live-born results. More recent analyses suggest that while mortality is lowest with twins, morbidity is lowest with remaining singletons.

Numerous papers have argued over the past few years whether triplets have better outcomes 'reduced' or not. Yaron, et al[33] compared triplets to twins data to unreduced triplets with two large cohorts of twins. The data show substantial improvement of reduced twins as compared to triplets. The data from the most recent collaborative series suggest that pregnancy outcomes for cases starting at triplets or even quadruplets reduced to twins do fundamentally as well as starting as twins. These data, therefore, support some cautious aggressiveness in infertility treatments to achieve pregnancy in difficult clinical situations. However, when higher numbers occur, good outcomes clearly diminish. A 2001 paper suggested that reduced triplets

did worse than continuing ones.[34] However, analysis of that series showed a loss rate after MFPR twice that seen in our collaborative series[11] and poorer outcomes in every other category for remaining triplets. Several other recent papers have likewise shown higher risks for 'unreduced' triplets than for reduced cases.[35–38] It is clear that one must use extreme caution in choosing comparison groups (Table 8.6). An ever increasing situation involves the inclusion of a monozygotic (MZ) pair of twins in a higher-order multiple.[39] Our experience suggests that, provided the 'singleton' seems healthy, the best outcomes are achieved by reduction of the MZ twins. Obviously, if the singleton is not healthy, keeping the twins is the next choice.

Pregnancy loss is not the only deleterious outcome. Very early preterm delivery correlates with the starting number. However, it has not been well appreciated that about 20% of babies born at less than 750 g develop cerebral palsy.[40] In Western Australia, Peterson et al showed that the rate of cerebral palsy was 4.6 times higher for twins than singletons per live births, but 8.3 times higher when calculated per pregnancy.[41] Pharoah and Cooke calculated cerebal palsy rates per 1000 first-year survivor at 2.3 for singletons, 12.6 for twins, and 44.8 for triplets.[42]

In the 2001 collaborative report, the subset of patients who reduced from two to one (not for fetal anomalies) included 154 patients. These data suggested a loss rate comparable to three to two, but, in about one-third of the two to one cases, there was a medical indication for the procedure, such as maternal cardiac disease, prior twin pregnancy with severe prematurity, or uter-

Table 8.6 Reduced vs 'unreduced' triplets comparison

Years	MFPR cases					
		Deliveries (weeks)				
	Losses <24	24–28	29–32	33–36	37+	
1980s	6.7%	6.1%	9.1%	36.9%	47.9%	
1990–4	5.7%	5.2%	9.9%	39.2%	45.2%	
1995–8	4.5%	3.2%	6.9%	28.3%	55.1%	
1998–2002	5.1%	4.6%	10.8%	41.8%	37.6%	
		Mean GA 35.5	PMR 10.0/1000)			
1998–2002(3–>l)	8.0%	4.0%	12.0%	4.0%	72.0%	
		Mean GA	39.5	PMR	0/1000	
	Nonreduced triplets					
1999 (Angel et al)[36]	8.0%	Mean GA 32.3		PMR 29/1000		
2000 (Leondires et al)[34]	9.9%	Mean GA 33.3		PMR 55/1000		
2001 (Lipitz et al)[35]	25.0%	Mean GA 33.5		PMR 109/1000		
2001 (Francois et al)[38]	8.3%	Mean GA 31.0		PMR 57.6/1000		

GA: gestational age; PMR: perinatal mortality rate
Reproduced from Evans MI, Krivchenia EL, Kaufman M, Zador IE, Birtt DW, Wapner RJ. The optimal management of first trimester triplets: reduce. Central Association of Obstetricians and Gynecologists. Annual Meeting, Las Vegas, Nevada, 27–30 October 2002.

ine abnormality.[11] In recent years, the demographics are changing and the vast majority of such cases are from women in their 40s, or even 50s, some of whom are using donor eggs, and who, more for social than medical reasons, want only a singleton pregnancy.[42,44] New data suggest that a singleton reduced from twins has a better prognosis than the original twins.[13] Consistent with the above, more women are desiring to reduce to a singleton. In a recent series of triplets, we found the average age of outpatients reducing to twins to be 37 years, and to a singleton, 41 years.[43] While the reduction in pregnancy loss risk for three to one is not as much as three to two (15% to 7% and 15% to 5%, respectfully), the gestational age at delivery for the resulting singleton is higher, and the incidence of neonates under 1500 g is 10 times higher for remaining twins than singletons.[1] These data have made counseling of such patients far more complex than previously (Figures 8.3 and 8.4). Not surprisingly, there are often differences between couples as to the desirability of twins or singleton.[45] There are also profound public health implications to these decisions, as US data from 2000 show that of $10.2 billion spent per year on initial newborn care, 57% of the money is spent on the 9% of babies born at under 37 weeks.[46] This issue is much more likely to rise than fall.

Societal issues

MFPR will always be controversial. In our experience, opinions on MFPR have never followed the classic 'pro-choice/pro-life' dichotomy.[2,7,11,14] We believe that the real debate over the next 5–10 years will not be whether or not MFPR should be performed with triplets or more. A serious debate will emerge over whether or not it is appropriate to offer MFPR routinely for twins, even natural ones for whom the outcome has commonly been considered 'good enough'.[43] Our data suggest that reduction of twins to a singleton actually improves the outcome of

the remaining fetus.[43] However, no consensus on the appropriateness of routine two to one reductions is ever likely to emerge. We do, however, expect the proportion of patients reducing to a singleton to increase steadily over the next few years.

The ethical issues surrounding MFPR will also always be controversial. Over the years, much has been written on the subject. Opinions will always vary substantially from outraged condemnation to complete acceptance. No short paragraph could do justice to the subject other than to state that most proponents do not believe this is a frivolous procedure, but see it in terms of the principle of proportionality, that is, as therapy to achieve the most good for the least harm.[13,47–49]

How patients 'hear' and internalize data and make decisions with respect to reduction have been fascinating to us over the years. Much of the literature on medical decision making has emphasized a rational choice model in which emotions, feelings, and values are treated as complications that must be considered as a second stage of an analysis that puts hard data regarding relative risks center stage.[50,51] Even in the literature on genuine alternative models of decision making (systematic versus heuristic, for example), a central assumption is that these are individual differences in style that can be identified through what people say.[52,53]

We have approached this problem from a different direction, arguing that where controversial, high-anxiety decisions are concerned, patients treat these decisions as an ongoing part of the social reality that they are creating to live in and raise a family.[54] These realities, composed of supportive people and institutions together with complexes of supportive values, norms, and attitudes, are the source of frames that the patients use to view the data.[47–49] The decisions they make and how they justify those decisions may help resolve incompatible elements in the realities in which they find themselves enmeshed.

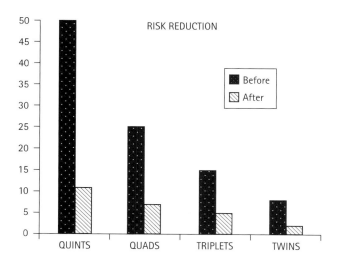

Figure 8.3 Risk reduction as a function of starting number. Numbers on left are risks for spontaneous pregnancy loss without reduction. Numbers on right are after reduction.

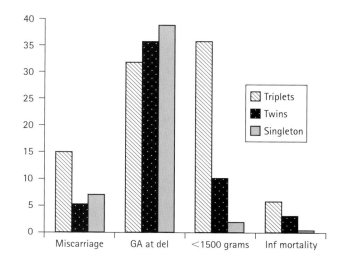

Figure 8.4 Risks and gestational age starting with triplets. Reduction of triplets to twins has lower pregnancy loss rates but higher incidence of prematurity, low birth weight, and infant mortality than reduction to a singleton. Numbers on left are risks with triplets, in the middle are risks with twins, and on the right are risks with a remaining singleton. GA: gestational age.

The one thing that all such patients have in common is a very strong desire to have a family (Table 8.7). But there does not appear to be a single set of supportive institutions, people, and norms that is conducive to going through the pain, stress, and resource expenditure of IVF and then to consider partial reduction as a pregnancy-management strategy. Rather, we think there are three viable alternative resolutions. The first of these, a rational medical model, looks superficially like what one would expect from the rational analysis model. But the commitment to factual analysis comes from patients having selected themselves into the hard sciences, medicine, dentistry, engineering, or the law – disciplines in which the 'facts' are crucial. Such women will want to see the numbers regarding the relative risk associated with different reduction choices and will want to engage in a rigorous discussion of the data and their implications. Very frequently, they will choose a final number for reduction that maximizes the chances of a take-home baby.

The lens of scientific objectivity is not the only frame through which women who have gone through IVF in order to have a child will examine these data. For those who have immersed themselves in a social reality that has a strong emphasis on norms against abortion and/or reduction – such that they themselves have such normative beliefs and are heavily involved in churches who reinforce similar beliefs – a detached examination of the 'facts' is simply not possible. These 'facts' hold no special moral authority. Their beliefs and those of the individuals and social institutions in which they have immersed themselves have a moral authority as well. The balance that such women will likely seek is one that reduces their relative risk to acceptable limits. So, unless the consequences are dire, they will not reduce or choose to reduce only to three. We labeled such a resolution the fundamentalist model.

Finally, there are those for whom the demands of career and/or existing children constitute powerful elements in their constructed realities. For such women – and this includes many of the older patients we encountered – the essential balance that they seek is a more secular one, a lifestyle model, one that emphasizes creating a family situation in which having a family can be balanced with having a career. Such women will more than likely choose reduction to two or even one embryo, depending on the number of other children they have and the level of resources that the family has.

Where women have selected themselves into and/or been trained to accept the legitimacy of rigorously determined statistics regarding relative risk (a medical frame), reduction choices *can* be straightforward – or at least they can appear to be relatively straightforward. This is usually not the case, however, for women who must forge a resolution among potentially incompatible elements, as for women who are struggling to reconcile the potentially oppositional elements of religious beliefs and involvement with risks associated with higher-level pregnancies (fundamentalist frame), or those who are struggling to reconcile the potentially conflicting identities of home and career (lifestyle frame). We have been able to examine some of these issues in a few studies to date. In one we were able to trace the extreme fluctuations in anxiety and stress as women progress through IVF and then must confront the painful choice of reduction.[48] In a second, we were able to show that the meaning of detecting a fetal anomaly changes depending on the needs of the patient and her spouse for some confirmation regarding their choice.[47]

Summary

Over the last two decades, MFPR has become a well-established and integral part of infertility therapy and the attempts to deal with sequelae of aggressive infertility management. In the mid-

Table 8.7 Frame comparison

	Medical frame	Fundamentalist frame	Lifestyle frame
Intensity of commitment to having children	High	High	High
Intensity of training in medicine, dentistry, hard sciences, and law	High	Low	Modest
Intensity of commitment to belief that life begins at conception	Modest	High	Modest
Intensity of commitment to career	High	Low	High
Source of moral authority for resolution	Relative survivability of fetuses	Minimization of damage to moral beliefs though a 'barely sufficient' reduction	Having a 'normal' life in a culture that values both careers and family for women

1980s, the risks and benefits of the procedure could only be guessed.[10-14] We now have very clear and precise data on the risks and benefits as well as an understanding that the risks increase substantially with the starting and finishing number of fetuses in multifetal pregnancies. The collaborative loss rate numbers, 4.5% for triplets, 8% for quadruplets, 11% for quintuplets, and 15% for sextuplets or more, are reasonable numbers to present to patients if the procedure is performed by an experienced operator. Our own experience and anecdotal reports from other groups suggest that less experienced operators have worse outcomes.

Pregnancy loss is not the only poor outcome. The other main issue with which to be concerned is very early preterm delivery and the profound consequences to such infants. Here again there is an increasing rate of poor outcomes correlated with the starting number. The finishing numbers are also critical, with twins having the best viable pregnancy outcomes for cases starting with three or more. Triplets and singletons do not do as well. However, an emerging appreciation that singletons have prematurity rates lower than twins is making the counseling far more complex. Finally, we continue to hope that MFPR will become obsolete as better control of ovulation agents and assisted reproductive technologies eliminate or make multifetal pregnancies uncommon.

References

1. Martin JA, Hamilton BE, Ventura SJ et al. Births: Final Data for 2001. National Vital Statistics Reports vol 51, no. 2. National Center for Health Statistics: Hyattville, MD, 2002.

2. Evans MI, Rodeck CH, Stewart KS, Yaron Y, Johnson MP. Multiple gestation: genetic issues, selective termination, and fetal reduction. In: Gleisher N, Buttino L Jr, Elkayam U, Evans MI, Galbraith RM, Gall SA, Sibai BM (eds), Principles and Practices of Medical Therapy in Pregnancy pp. 235–42 (3rd edition). Appleton and Lange: Norwalk, CT, 1998.

3. Evans MI, Ayoub MA, Shalhoub AG, Feldman B, Yaron Y. Spontaneous abortions in couples declining multifetal pregnancy reduction. Fetal Diagn Ther 2002; 17: 343–6.

4. Keith LG, Blickstein I (eds). Triplet Pregnancies. Parthenon Press: London, 2002.

5. Luke B, Brown MB, Nugent C, Gonzalez-Quintero VH, Witter FR, Newman RB. Risk factors for adverse outcomes in spontaneous versus assisted conception twin pregnancies. Fertil Steril 2004; 81: 315–19.

6. Anwar HN, Ihab MU, Johnny BR, Tarek SH, Abdallah MA, Antoine AA. Pregnancy outcomes in spontaneous twins versus twins who were conceived through in vitro fertilization. Am J Obstet Gynecol 2003; 189: 513–18.

7. Evans MI, Dommergues M, Wapner RJ et al. Efficacy of transabdominal multifetal pregnancy reduction: collaborative experience among the world's largest centers. Obstet Gynecol 1993; 82: 61–7.

8. Evans MI, Ciorica D, Britt DW, Fletcher JW. Multifetal pregnancy reduction. In: Blickstein I, Keith LG, eds. Multiple Pregnancy, second edition, pp. 535–43. Oxford: Taylor & Francis Medical.

9. Toner JP. Progress we can be proud of: U.S. trends in assisted reproduction over the first 20 years. Fertil Steril 2002; 78: 943–50.

10. Wright VC, Schieve LA, Reynolds MA, Jeng G, Kissin D. Assisted reproductive technology surveillance – United States, 2001. MMWR Surveill Summ 2004; 53: 1–20.

11. Evans MI, Berkowitz R, Wapner R et al. Multifetal pregnancy reduction (MFPR): improved outcomes with increased experience. Am J Obstet Gynecol 2001; 184: 97–103.

12. Adashi EY, Barri PN, Berkowitz R et al. Infertility therapy-assisted multiple pregnancies (births): an on-going epidemic. Reprod Med OnLine 2003; 7: 515–42.

13. Evans MI, Fletcher JC. Multifetal pregnancy reduction. In: Reece EA, Hobbins JC, Mahoney MJ, Petrie R (eds), Medicine of the Fetus and its Mother, pp. 1345–62. Lippincott Harper: Philadelphia. 1992.

14. Evans MI, Littman L, St Louis L et al. Evolving patterns of iatrogenic multifetal pregnancy generation: implications for aggressiveness of infertility treatments. Am J Obstet Gynecol 1995; 172: 1750–3.

15. Tabsh KM, Theroux NL. Genetic amniocentesis following multifetal pregnancy reduction twins: assessing the risk. Prenat Diagn 1995; 15: 221–3.

16. McLean LK, Evans MI, Carpenter RJ, Johnson MP, Goldberg JD. Genetic amniocentesis (AMN) following multifetal pregnancy reduction (MFPR) does not increase the risk of pregnancy loss. Prenat Diagn 1998; 18: 186–8.

17. Brambati B, Tului L, Baldi M, Guercilena S. Genetic analysis prior to selective termination in multiple pregnancy: technical aspects and clinical outcome. Hum Reprod 1995; 10: 818–25.

18. Evans MI, Henry GP, Miller WA, et al. International, collaborative assessment of 146,000 prenatal karyotypes: expected limitations if only chromosome-specific probes and fluorescent in situ hybridization were used. Hum Reprod 1999; 14: 1213–16.

19. Homer J, Bhatt S, Huang B, Thangavelu M. Residual risk for cytogenetic abnormalities after prenatal diagnosis by interphase fluorescence in situ hybridization (FISH). Prenat Diagn 2003; 23: 556–71.

20. Greene RA, Wapner J, Evans MI. Amniocentesis and choironic villus sampling in triplet pregnancy. In: Keith LG, Blickstein I, Oleszcuk JJ (eds) Triplet Pregnancy, 2003, pp. 73–84. Parthenon: London.

21. Zadori J, Kozinszky Z, Orvos H, Katona M, Kaali SG, Pal A. the incidence of major birth defects following in vitro fertilization. J Assist Reprod Genet 2003; 20: 131–2.

22. Pinborg A, Loft A, Schmidt L, Andersen AN. Morbidity in a Danish national cohort of 472 IVF/ICSI twins, 1132 non-IVF/ICSI twins and 634 IVF/ICSI singletons: health-related and social implications for the children and their families. Hum Reprod 2003; 18: 1234–43.

23. Place I, Englert Y. A prospective longitudinal study of the physical, psychomotor, and intellectual development of singleton children up to 5 years who were conceived by intracytoplasmic sperm injection compared with children conceived spontaneously and by in vitro fertilization. Fertil Steril 2003; 80: 1388–97.

24. Retzloff MG, Hornstein MD. Is intracytoplasmic sperm injection safe? Fertil Steril 2003; 80: 851–9.

25. Kurinczuk JJ. Safety issues in assisted reproduction technology. From theory to reality – just what are the data telling us about ICSI offspring health and future fertility and should we be concerned? Hum Reprod 2003; 18; 925–31.

26. Tournaye H. ICSI: a technique too far? Int J Androl 2003; 26: 63–9.

27. Dumez Y, Oury JF. Method for first trimester selective abortion in multiple pregnancy. Contrib Gynecol Obstet 1986; 15: 50.

28. Evans MI, Fletcher JC, Zador IE, Newton BW, Struyk CK, Quigg MH. Selective first trimester termination in octuplet and quadruplet pregnancies: clinical and ethical issues. Obstet Gynecol 1988; 71: 289–96.

29. Berkowitz RL, Lynch L, Chitkara U et al. Selective reduction of multiple pregnancies in the first trimester. N Engl J Med 1988; 318: 1043.

30. Wapner RJ, Davis GH, Johnson A. Selective reduction of multi-fetal pregnancies. Lancet 1990; 335: 90–3.

31. Timor-Tritsch IE, Peisner DB, Monteagudo A, Lerner JP, Sharma S. Multifetal pregnancy reduction by transvaginal puncture: evaluation of the technique used in 134 cases. Am J Obstet Gynecol 1993; 168: 799–804.

32. Torok O, Lapinski R, Salafia CM, Bernasko J, Berkowitz RL. Multifetal pregnancy reduction is not associated with an increased risk of intrauterine growth restriction, except for very high order multiples. Am J Obstet Gynecol 1998; 179: 221–5.

33. Yaron Y, Bryant-Greenwood PK, Dave N, et al. Multifetal pregnancy reduction (MFPR) of triplets to twins: comparison with non-reduced triplets and twins. Am J Obstet Gynecol 1999; 180: 1268–71.

34. Leondires MP, Ernst SD, Miller BT et al. Triplets: outcomes of expectant management versus multifetal reduction for 127 pregnancies. Am J Obstet Gynecol 2000; 183: 454–9.

35. Lipitz S, Shulman A, Achiron R et al. A comparative study of multifetal pregnancy reduction from triplets to twins in the first versus early second trimesters after detailed fetal screening. Ultrasound Obstet Gynecol 2001; 18: 35–8.

36. Angel JL, Kalter CS, Morales WJ et al. Aggressive prerinatal care for high-order multiple gestations: does good perinatal outcome justify aggressive assisted reproductive techniques? Am J Obstet Gynecol 1999; 181: 253–9.

37. Sepulveda W, Munoz H, Alcalde JL. Conjoined twins in a triplet pregnancy: early prenatal diagnosis with three-dimensional ultrasound and review of the literature. Ultrasound Obstet Gynecol 2003; 22: 199–204.

38. Francois K, SEARS C, Wilson R, Elliot J. Twelve year experience of triplet pregnancies at a single institution. Am J Obstet Gynecol 2001; 185: S112.

39. Yakin K, Kahraman S, Comert S. Three blastocyst stage embryo transfer resulting in a quintuplet pregnancy. Hum Reprod 2001; 16: 782–4.

40. Neonatal encephalopathy and cerebral palsy: defining the pathogenesis and pathophysiology. Task Force of American College of Obstetricians and Gynecologists, ACOG, Washington, DC, 2003.

41. Petterson B, Nelson K, Watson L et al. Twins, triplets, and cerebral palsy in births in Western Australia in the 1980s. BMJ, 1993; 307, 1239–43.

42. Pharoah PO, Cooke T. Cerebral palsy and multiple births. Arch Dis Child. Fetal and Neonatal Edition 1996; 75: F174–7.

43. Evans MI, Kaufman MI, Urban AJ, Krivchenia EL, Britt DW, Wapner RJ. Fetal reduction from twins to a singleton: a reasonable consideration. Obstet Gynecol 2004; 104: 102–9.

44. Templeton A. The multiple gestation epidemic: The role of the assisted reproductive technologies. Am J Obstet Gynecol 2004; 190: 894–8.

45. Kalra SK, Milad MP, Klock SC, Crobman WA. Infertility patients and their partners: differences in the desire for twin gestations. Obstet Gynecol 2003; 102: 152–5.

46. St John EB, Nelson KG, Oliver SP, Bishno, RR, Goldenberg RL. Cost of neonatal care according to gestational age at birth and survival status. Am J Obstet Gynecol 2000; 182: 170–5.

47. Britt DW, Risinger ST, Mans M, Evans MI. Devastation and relief: conflicting meanings in discovering fetal anomalies. Ultrasound Obstet Gynecol 2002; 20: 1–5.

48. Britt DW, Risinger ST, Mans M, Evans MI. Anxiety among women who have undergone fertility therapy and who are considering MFPR: trends and scenarios. J Maternal-Fetal Neonatal Med 2003; 13: 271–8.

49. Britt DW, Evans WJ, Mehta SS, Evans MI. Framing the decision: determinants of how women considering MFPR as a pregnancy-management strategy frame their moral dilemma. Fetal Diagn Ther 2004; 19: 232–40.

50. Redelmeier DA, Rozin P, Kahneman D. Understanding patients' decisions: cognitive and emotional perspectives. JAMA 1993; 270: 72–6.

51. Chapman GB, Elstein AS. Cognitive processes and biases in medical decision making. In: Chapman GB, Sonnenberg FA (eds), Decision Making in Health Care: Theory, Psychology and Applications, pp. 183–210. Cambridge University Press: New York, 2000.

52. Steginga SK, Occhipinti S. The application of the heuristic-systematic processing model to treatment decision making about prostate cancer. Med Decis Making 2004; 24: 573–83.

53. Hamm RM. Theory about heuristic strategies based on verbal protocol analysis: the emperor needs a shave. Med Decis Making 2004; 24: 681–6.

54. Britt DW, Campbell EQ. Assessing the linkage of norms, environments and deviance. Soc Forces 1977; December: 532–49.

9 Spontaneous and indicated abortions

Márta Gávai and Zoltán Papp

Definition and clinical picture

Abortion is the termination of a pregnancy, induced or spontaneous, before the conceptus is sufficiently developed to survive after delivery. The precise gestational age at which the infant is able to survive is difficult to define. Most authorities restrict the term 'abortion' to the first 20 weeks of pregnancy; or in retrospect, to the delivery of any infant weighing less than 500 g. In the following discussion, abortion is defined as expulsion of the products of conception before gestational week 20. Abortions taking place before week 12 are termed (first-trimester) abortions; those occurring at weeks 12–20 late (second-trimester, midtrimester) abortions. This subdivision into two different categories is important because of the different etiologies and types of treatment applied.

Threatened or threatening abortion

This is characterized by vaginal bleeding, ranging from bloody vaginal discharge or spotting to profuse, bright red bleeding. Pain may be present, either intermittent or constant, due to uterine contractions, at the loin or groin area, resembling menstrual cramps. Pelvic examination reveals the cervix intact and the os closed; the corpus uteri is soft, its size corresponding to the gestational age. This definition makes threatened abortion a common complication in early pregnancy, occurring in about one of four or five pregnancies, about one-half ending in spontaneous abortion. The bleeding and pain may be intermittent, may vary in intensity, and may persist for many days and even weeks.

Inevitable abortion

Inevitable abortion presents with bright red, often profuse, vaginal bleeding and uterine contractions. The cervix is shortened and dilating, and parts of the conceptus may be visible in the vagina or through the os. The uterus is hard and tender during contractions. With the dilating cervix, the membranes rupture and expulsion of the conceptus, in part or in whole, will invariably follow.

Incomplete abortion

In incomplete abortion, only parts of the conceptus have been expelled. The history will be that of passage of fragments of tissue together with bright red vaginal bleeding and uterine contractions. After the passage of products of conception, the bleeding will continue in varying intensity, ranging from bloody discharge, possibly accompanied by expulsion of bits of tissue, to profuse bleeding, occasionally leading to hypovolemic shock. Pain resulting from uterine contractions may be present periodically. At clinical examination, the cervix is dilated, and products of conception may be seen or felt through the os. The corpus uteri is enlarged, soft, subinvoluted, and possibly tender if infection has supervened.

Complete abortion

In complete abortion, the products of conception have been expelled completely. Its occurrence is more common in the first weeks of pregnancy due to the loose embedding of the ovum in the endometrium. After the passage of the products of conception, the hemorrhage and pain subside, but some vaginal discharge, usually blood-stained, may proceed for some days. On examination, the cervix is closed, and the corpus possibly enlarged, but firm and well involuted.

Missed abortion

Missed abortion designates the retention of the conceptus in the uterus after the death of the fetus. Before this occurs, the patient may have presented with the history of threatened abortion. The often scanty bleeding usually continues for several days or weeks, becoming a persistent brownish vaginal discharge. Pain is uncommon. With the death of the conceptus, the patient's impression of being pregnant disappears. The breasts become smaller, and the uterus fails to grow. It may even shrink in size as a result of the absorption of amniotic fluid and maceration of the fetus. With prolonged retention of the dead conceptus in the uterus, disturbances in the blood coagulation mechanism may occur (e.g., hypofibrinogenemia and prolonged or uncontrolled bleeding). Prior to the widespread use of ultrasound, not infrequently the fetus was retained *in utero* for a prolonged period of time. In the present period of medical technology, specific criteria have been established to diagnose fetal death *in utero* early, and to obviate this pathologic progression.

Septic abortion

Any type of abortion may be associated with infection, but retention of the products of conception or parts of them, such as missed and incomplete abortion, are particularly predisposing. Inadequately sterilized instruments used in criminally or self-induced abortions carry a high risk of infection. The infection usually takes the course of endometritis with chills and elevated body temperature; foul-smelling, purulent vaginal discharge; and lower abdominal and pelvic tenderness. Parametritis, tubo-ovarian abscess, peritonitis – localized or generalized – or life-endangering septic shock with cardiovascular collapse and renal failure may ensue.[1] A variety of microorganisms may cause septic abortion, but *Escherichia coli*, *Streptococcus pyogenes* and other hemolytic streptococci, *Staphylococcus aureus*, and *Bacteroides* are the most frequently encountered. Occasionally, the potentially serious clostridial bacteria are the causative agents.

Habitual (recurrent) abortion

Habitual abortion is the occurrence of three or more consecutive spontaneous abortions. Habitual abortions take the course of one of the above-described types of abortion.

Incidence

One of the problems in establishing the exact incidence of abortion is the various definitions used, with the lack of a definite date in pregnancy until which the expulsion of the conceptus or the death of the fetus can be called an abortion. It is generally estimated that at least 10–15% of all pregnancies terminate in spontaneous abortion. These figures are based upon abortions recognized clinically and by means of laboratory tests and histologic examination. An unexpected delay in the menstrual period followed by excessively heavy bleeding may in many instances result from early pregnancy wastage, where the fertilized ovum never was implanted properly. The number of these early 'occult' abortions cannot be accurately determined, since the evidence of pregnancy usually is missing. Hertig[2] has calculated a biologic rate of spontaneous abortion of approximately 28%, once the menstrual period was missed. From various data, it appears that the real incidence of spontaneous abortion is much higher than the 10–15% usually mentioned.

Etiology

The exact causes of most spontaneous abortions are considered unknown. In the early weeks of pregnancy, the expulsion of the conceptus is usually preceded by the death of the embryo. Later, the fetus frequently is expelled alive. The causes of abortion can be fetal or genetic, maternal, paternal, and combined factors.

Fetal or genetic factors

In their study of 1000 cases of spontaneous abortion, Hertig and Sheldon[3] found defects or abnormalities of the expelled conceptus in 62%. About one-half of the abortuses examined represented pathologic ova, with absent or defective embryos.[4] Embryos with localized anomalies were found in 3%, and placental abnormalities showed an incidence of 10%.

The exact causes of the anomalies are still unknown, but it has been presumed that the defective ovum resulted from 'germ-plasm defects'. Chromosome abnormalities are responsible for many early spontaneous abortions,[5] including cases which at histopathologic examination revealed blighted ova, placenta, and cord abnormalities (Figure 9.1).

Chromosome aberrations are present at conception in nearly 10% of zygotes. These are of reduced viability, and most of the affected embryos die and are expelled spontaneously. Chromosome aberrations are present in 60% of early abortions, 6% of midtrimester abortions, and 4–5% of stillborn fetuses.

Although there are exceptions, in general, additional chromosomal material is more compatible with life than a defi-

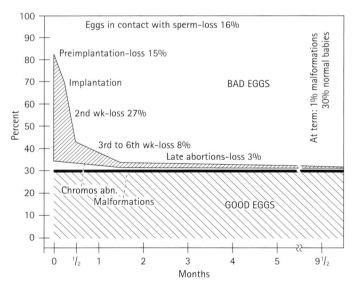

Figure 9.1 Emil Witschi's concept of the natural history of reproductive wastage. A large proportion of fertilized ova are lost soon after conception. These early losses are not apparent clinically. Many embryos and fetuses are lost because of early spontaneous abortion, others during the second trimester, and relatively few around term. Of all conceptions, only about 30% result in healthy, live-born babies.

ciency. In abortion material, mainly trisomies and triploidy can be found.[6] The monosomic zygotes usually die and are eliminated without any clinical sign of abortion. Among the monosomic zygotes, only those with 45,X monosomy are viable. About 2% of these survive the intrauterine period and are born with Ullrich–Turner syndrome. In samples from spontaneous abortions, trisomy for any of the chromosomes, except chromosomes 1 and 5, may be found. Trisomy 16 occurs most frequently and leads to abortion in every case. A small number of some of the other trisomies escape intrauterine selection, and their bearers may be born alive (1–2% of trisomy 13, 5–10% of trisomy 18, and 15–25% of trisomy 21).[7–9]

Autosomal trisomies are associated with advanced maternal age (e.g., trisomy 21), whereas monosomy X and polyploidy are not. Other mechanisms, such as the age of the gametes, virus infections, chemicals, drugs, or radiation, may possibly interfere with the chromosomal composition.

Maternal factors

The preliminary condition for *implantation* of the blastocyst is a properly prepared endometrium developed under the influence of the ovarian hormones. In the cells of the endometrial glands, it is possible to detect alkaline phosphatase from early in the follicular phase. When glycogen is released into the glandular lumina after ovulation, the alkaline phosphatase breaks down glycogen into glucose and fructose, which are needed by the trophoblast during implantation. When this metabolism is adequate, the environment for nidation, and further development of the embryo is created. Factors that adversely influence the carbohydrate metabolism, and thus the nourishment of the endometrial bed, may hinder the proper development of early pregnancy.

The human blastocyst normally implants in the fundal part of the uterus. However, occasionally, the implantation takes place in abnormal locations inside the uterus (e.g., close to the internal os). With such a low implantation, spontaneous abortion frequently occurs. If the pregnancy continues, it will present as a case of placenta previa.

Endocrine deficiencies

Endocrine deficiencies play a significant role in spontaneous abortions. The proper development of the endometrium and the maintenance of the decidua (the implantation, placentation, and embryonic development) rely on a proper hormonal function of the corpus luteum and the trophoblast. Estrogen and progesterone from the ovary stimulate and maintain the endometrium. With implantation, the trophoblast begins the production of chorionic gonadotropin, sustaining the corpus luteum of pregnancy, which in turn keeps the decidua alive and maintains the metabolic processes necessary for fetal growth. The corpus luteum and the trophoblast/early placenta are essential for further gestational development. If one of the two fails, a vicious cycle may ensue, ending in termination of the pregnancy. Inadequate progesterone production has been blamed for causing spontaneous, especially habitual, abortions. However, progestational hormone therapy seems to have a limited effect in preventing abortions. Whether deficient progesterone production is the cause or the effect of abortion is difficult to determine. The corpus luteum of pregnancy is the main site of progesterone production until gestational weeks 8–10. After this, the production in the ovary diminishes, and the placenta becomes the main source of progesterone. Bilateral oophorectomy in gestational week 10 does not interfere with the successful outcome of pregnancy.[10]

Uterine abnormalities

These may be *congenital*, arising from anomalies of müllerian fusion of various degree, and resulting in conditions such as uterus didelphys, uterus bicornis unicollis, uterus unicornis, or uterus subseptus. Among the *acquired* abnormalities, leiomyomas deforming the uterine cavity are especially likely to cause abortion. Uterine synechiae (Asherman's syndrome), resulting from previous infection, curettage, or the scarring of the uterine wall from previous surgery, may cause abortion. Malposition of the uterus is seldom an obstacle to proper progress of pregnancy. These uterine abnormalities, congenital or acquired, may interfere with the blood circulation in the decidua and the nutrition of the growing embryo/fetus. On the other hand, the pregnancy may be carried to term in spite of a malformed uterus. If uterine abnormalities are suspected in connection with repeated pregnancy wastage, proper investigational procedures, including hysterosalpingography and possibly hysteroscopy, should be performed and any detected anatomic defect corrected.[11]

A special entity of uterine abnormalities is cervical incompetence. This condition is discussed in Chapter 14.

Infections

Viral as well as bacterial infections have been suspected of causing abortions. Syphilis is the classic example of maternal infection, spreading across the placenta and causing fetal death and abortion in the second trimester. Various other microorganisms, such as herpes simplex virus, *Toxoplasma gondii*, *Listeria monocytogenes*, and *Mycoplasma* spp., have been associated with spontaneous abortion.[12]

Maternal diseases

Hypothyroidism and diabetes mellitus are conducive to the loss of early pregnancy, whereas chronic renal and cardiovascular diseases, such as nephritis and hypertension, are more likely to be associated with late fetal death or premature delivery.

Surgery during pregnancy and occupational exposure to inhalation anesthetics increase the risk of spontaneous abortion.[13] Disturbances in hemostasis, IUD failures, and physical and psychic trauma, as well as occupational and other socioeconomic factors (e.g., drinking alcohol or using illicit drugs during pregnancy, smoking, and nutritional and vitamin deficiency) are also of significance in the causation of abortion.[14–16]

Considerable interest has centered in recent years on the roles of antiphospholipid antibodies and the various types of thrombophilia syndromes in pregnancy losses during both early and advanced gestations.[17–19] Since the management of these complications is a medical, rather than surgical problem, their detailed discussion is outside of the scope of this chapter.

Other factors

Paternal factors

Semen quality is influenced by factors such as radiation, certain drugs, anesthetics, occupation, and infection. The greater the frequency of abnormal sperm heads, the higher the risk of spontaneous abortion. It has been reported[20] that the sperm concentration was significantly higher in repeated and habitual abortion groups, with a tendency to polyzoospermia (i.e., more than 200×10^6/ml sperm).

Combined (maternal and paternal) factors

The frequency of structural chromosomal anomalies among aborters is higher than in the general populations (0.8% vs 0.3%).[21] There are also some balanced carrier translocation karyotypes among habitual aborters.[22–24]

Pathology

Most pathologic changes are secondary to fetal death in early abortions. After this, 'live abortions' become more frequent. Following fetal death, the placental function gradually deteriorates, leading to the disintegration of the decidua by hemorrhage and necrosis. The ovum acting as a foreign body stimulates the uterus, causing expulsion of the products of conception or parts of them.

In cases of spontaneous abortion after gestational weeks 6–8, some chorionic tissue usually remains adherent to the uterine wall. During months 4 and 5 of pregnancy, the placenta is divided into cotyledons. Until this has been accomplished, any spontaneous abortion should be considered as incomplete.

At histologic examination, a frequent pathologic finding is hydropic swelling or degeneration of the chorionic villi. Hydropic degeneration may resemble hydatidiform mole.

Sometimes an ovum is surrounded by extravasated blood collecting between the decidua and the chorion, where it coagulates and forms layers. This is referred to as a blood or carneous mole. In some cases the appearance is nodular due to localized hematomas of varying sizes, and it is called a tuberous mole. In some cases of missed abortion, the amniotic fluid may be absorbed to such an extent that the fetus becomes compressed, forming a fetus compressus. Occasionally, this happens to such a degree that the fetal remnants resemble parchment, the so-called fetus papyraceus. This is not infrequently found in cases of twin pregnancy where one fetus died early in pregnancy and the other continued developing.[25]

Diagnosis

When the patient presents with vaginal bleeding in early pregnancy, the fetus may have been dead for some time. If parts of the chorionic tissue are still functioning, the pregnancy test may be positive. If spontaneous termination of pregnancy is awaited, many days of unnecessary delay and anxiety will result. Only in cases where expelled products of conception can be examined or when parts of the conceptus are visible through the os can the diagnosis of irreversible abortion be made with certainty on clinical grounds alone.

A number of diagnostic tests have been applied to the evaluation of early threatened pregnancy. With the development of accurate radioimmunoassays, a variety of hormonal parameters have become diagnostic tools. Unfortunately, there are no exact hormone values, levels, or trends that permit differentiation between the doomed pregnancies and those proceeding to viability.

In the assessment of the anatomic integrity of an early pregnancy, ultrasound plays the dominant role. The gestational sac may be first demonstrated 5–6 weeks after the last menstrual period. From gestational week 7 onward, it is possible to demonstrate fetal heart movements and even fetal motion. From approximately week 12, details of the fetal body can be detected.

In a case of early pregnancy complicated by vaginal bleeding, an ultrasound examination should include the evaluation of the appearance and size of the gestational sac, the presence of embryonic echoes and life signs, the measurement of crown–rump length, and the location of the placenta.[26] An echo-free area between the membranes and the uterine wall represents blood indicative of threatened abortion. The size of such hematomas is predictive of the outcome of the pregnancy.

In cases of unembryonic gestations, a gestational sac without echoes can be demonstrated. Absence of fetal life signs after 8 or 9 weeks' gestation is suggestive of an unsuccessful outcome for the pregnancy. The lack of growth of the embryo/gestational sac or degenerative change in the sac indicates missed abortion. A well-formed gestational sac, which on subsequent examination demonstrates fragmentation, also is evidence of a missed abortion.

Ultrasonic demonstration of fetal life signifies a successful outcome for the pregnancy in 80–90% of cases of threatened abortion.[27] In cases of incomplete abortion, it is possible to demonstrate retained conceptional products in the uterus with ultrasonography through the absence of the thin, midline echo seen in complete abortions.

Treatment

In cases of vaginal bleeding, thorough medical history should be taken, focusing on earlier pregnancies (abortions and deliveries), and a general physical and pelvic examination performed. If present and retrievable, an intrauterine contraceptive device should be removed. In cases of pronounced bleeding, blood should be drawn for blood indices, typing, and cross-matching. If infection is suspected, cultures should be taken from the cervical canal and the blood in order to identify any pathogens and their antibiotic sensitivity. Unless the medical history and/or pelvic examination indicates that abortion is inevitable or has taken place, adequate diagnostic procedures should be initiated to diagnose failing pregnancy. When elective termination of the pregnancy is a legally acceptable option, the patient is to be counseled about the prognosis of her pregnancy and the increased risk of fetal anomalies associated with threatening abortions.

The majority of spontaneous abortions are caused by conceptional defects; thus, therapeutic efforts rarely will prove effective. Coitus should be avoided during bleeding and for 1 or 2 weeks after its cessation.

Most trials have failed to demonstrate any benefit from progestional agents in the treatment of threatened and habitual abortions.[28,29] Progestogen therapy should be restricted to the very few instances where progesterone deficiency has been demonstrated (e.g., special cases of habitual abortion). In such cases, 17-OH-progesterone caproate should be used in order to avoid female masculinization or other teratogenic impact.

The frequency of miscarriage in cases of threatened abortion may approach 50%.[27] An increased incidence of premature deliveries (e.g., small-for-date infants, placental abruption and infarction, perinatal asphyxia, perinatal mortality, and congenital abnormalities) is anticipated in women whose pregnancies were complicated by vaginal bleeding during the first two trimesters.

Inevitable, incomplete, complete, habitual, and missed abortions involve hemorrhage that may require transfusion. The uncommon but serious disorders of coagulation mechanism (e.g., hypofibrinogenemia, disseminated intravascular coagulation) should be kept in mind.

In cases of septic abortion, bacterial cultures should be taken from the cervix and blood. Gram staining of the specimen may reveal the causative bacterial agent. Broad-spectrum antibiotics in large doses should be instituted, with therapy being individualized when bacterial sensitivity patterns are available. The central venous pressure and urinary output may need to be monitored, the fluid and electrolyte balance carefully studied, and blood-gas analyses performed for the purpose of correcting any deficits. The retained products of conception should be removed from the uterine cavity as soon as practical.

Surgical management in the first trimester

The selection of instruments for dilation and curettage should be based on the characteristics of each instrument.

Tenaculum

The employment of a single-toothed tenaculum will focus tension on a small area of the cervix, making laceration of that site more likely. The double-toothed tenaculum will lessen the effect. Some consider the bullet-type tenaculum efficient in preventing this complication. Several types of tenacula are presented in Figure 9.2. Multiple tenacula are of particular value when there is distortion of the cervix due to previous surgery or if a local lesion is present.

Dilator

A great variety of instruments are available to dilate the cervix. The choice will vary with the condition of the cervix, the available time, and the personal preference of the surgeon. If there is no medical condition (e.g., bleeding) requiring intervention, a medical rather than an instrumental approach may be considered. Injury to the cervix from dilation is positively related to the extent of dilation and inversely to the period of time over which the procedure is performed.

Hygroscopic dilators (laminaria, synthetic tents)

Removal of fluid from the cervix is primarily responsible for dilation of 0–12 mm. Hygroscopic dilators absorb water, sufficient to account for cervical dilation on the basis of volume reduction. The conventional dilator forces fluid from the cervix into the soft tissue of the lower uterine segment. Distention of tissues in this area can be detected. Dilators above 9 mm force fluid into the lower uterine segment in excess of available tissue space, resulting in displacement of the inner wall of this area of the uterus down into the path of the dilator. At higher levels of dilation, the fluid is forced farther up the uterine wall. The balloon dilator exerts uniform pressure on the entire area, not

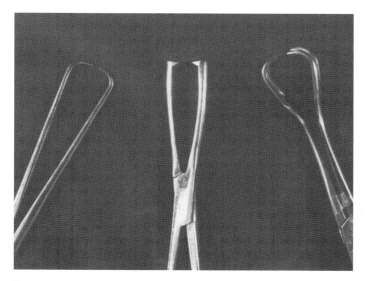

Figure 9.2 Various types of tenacula. From left to right: single-toothed, bullet-type, multiple-toothed.

allowing movement of fluid out of the cervix and is, therefore, less effective in causing dilation.

The laminaria is prepared from seaweed (*Laminaria digitata*) which is sterilized and rolled into a small, compact, tubular structure approximately 6 cm in length. It is prepared in three diameters: small (3–5 mm), medium (6–8 mm), and large (8–10 mm). Upon exposure to a moist environment, it will increase three to four times in diameter over a 6–8-hour period. Its use is not associated with injury to the cervix.

Synthetic dilators (e.g., Dilapan (polyacrylonitrile), Lamicel (magnesium sulfate sponge)) and, alternatively, *L. japonicum* are often used. These osmotic dilators serve to dilate the endocervical canal by absorbing cervical moisture. This uptake of water and the resulting expansion of the dilator produces both softening of the cervix and dilation of the endocervical canal in 4–6 hours.[30]

Artificial cervical dilator devices[31]
A variety of balloon-type devices have been used to dilate the cervix. The device is inserted into the cervical canal and inflated with fluid. It may be left in place up to 24 hours. A significant, immediate expulsion rate, as well as considerable pain, is associated with the instillation of the fluid.

Medical dilator
Cervical ripening in first-trimester abortion can be achieved with prostaglandins; progesteron agonists; prostaglandin analogs, such as sulprostone, gemeprost, and misoprostol; and a folic acid analog.

Prostaglandins
Prostaglandins (PG) are believed to play a critical biologic role in the control of cervical function. Various commercial PGE$_2$ formulations are currently available for cervical ripening (intravenous solutions, intravaginal tablets, intracervical gel, intravaginal gel, intravaginal insert with retrieval system, and vaginal suppositories).

Oral tablets and intravenous infusions were the first to be used but, because of side effects related to the systemic absorption of prostaglandins, their rapid inactivation in the circulation, and the consequent need for high doses, these methods have been largely supplanted by local administration of PGE$_2$. Intravaginal tablets are prone to a variety of influences which may affect absorption, and intracervical gels can be inconvenient to use. Intravaginal PGE$_2$ gels are convenient and effective; however, containment can be difficult as the gel tends to flow out of the vaginal canal. Hours after administration of PGE, circulating concentrations of PGE metabolite increase dramatically, indicating rapid absorption of exogenous PGE$_2$. Significantly, the pronounced increase in PGE metabolite concentrations occurs after 3–4 hours and coincides with the onset of uterine contractility. It has been proposed that PGE$_2$ does not stimulate contractions; they are mediated by the release of endogenous PGF. Consequently, the ideal PGE$_2$ formulation may be one that is capable of reproducing these changes *in vivo*;

is simple to administer and control; and is effective, safe, and convenient to use.

PG are local hormones since, with few exceptions, they exert their effects and are inactivated principally in the tissues or organs in which they are synthesized. Those found most abundantly in the uterus, and in the menstrual and amniotic fluid, are of the E and F types. Prostacyclin (PGI2) is confined largely to the uterine, umbilical, and fetal vasculature, where it may serve to ensure an adequate flow of blood and a patent ductus arteriosus. Clinical investigation for obstetric use has been limited almost entirely to PGE$_2$, PGF$_{2\alpha}$, and the synthetic derivative, 15-methyl PGF$_{2\alpha}$.[32]

Antiprogestins
Many processes in female reproductive physiology depend on progesterone. This hormone facilitates the action of estradiol in inducing the luteinizing hormone (LH) surge in the follicular cycle and supports the luteal phase. A compound action of progesterone plays an important role in the interruption of pregnancy. With the identification of the progesterone receptor came the realization that its antagonist was a potential candidate for such a compound.

Mifepristone is similar in structure to progesterone and glucocorticoids, but lacks the C19 methyl group and the 2-carbon side chain at C17 of these hormones and has a conjugated C9–C10 double bond. The chemical structures of other synthetic antiprogestins are similar to that of mifepristone.[33]

The antiprogestin action of mifepristone is mediated by the PR, a ligand-activated transcription factor with domains for DNA binding, hormone binding, and transactivation. Members of this nuclear receptor superfamily include androgen, estrogen, and mineralocorticoid receptors, as well as receptors for thyroid hormones, retinoids, and vitamin D. Mifepristone binds to the progesterone and glucocorticoid receptors.

Progesterone and mifepristone produce a conformational change in the form of progesterone receptor that permits it to bind to DNA. Its activation by progesterone or mifepristone is accompanied by a loss of associated heat-shock proteins and dimerization. The activated receptor dimer binds to progesterone-response elements in the promoter region of progesterone-responsive genes. In the case of progesterone, this binding will increase the transcription rate of these genes, producing progestin effects. In contrast, a receptor dimer complex that has been activated by mifepristone also binds to progesterone response elements, but an inhibitory function in the C-terminal region of the hormone-binding domain renders these DNA-bound receptors transcriptionally inactive. This is the basis for the progesterone-antagonistic action of mifepristone, underlying its abortifacient and contraceptive actions.

Misoprostol is a synthetic 15-deoxy-16-hydroxy-16-methyl analog of naturally occurring PG E1. It is a viscous oil susceptible to the same types of chemical degradation as natural PG E, stable at room temperature. This means that the drug is easily stored and transported. Misoprostol exhibits a wide range of biologic activities. It is protective of the gastric mucosa, and has vasodilator, immunosuppressive, and uterotonic effects. The uterotonic features of misoprostol are of value in pregnancy termination and in the medical management of miscarriage. Vaginal misoprostol provides safe and effective preoperative dilation.[34]

Methotrexate is a folic acid analog that competitively inhibits dihydrofolate reductase, an enzyme necessary for DNA sythesis. Methotrexate is approved for use in treating certain cancers, psoriasis, and rheumatoid arthritis. Treatment for ectopic pregnancy and early abortion represents off-label use of the drug.[35]

Types of surgical instruments used to dilate the cervix

The conventional type of dilator is pressed against the external os, causing dilation of the opening. Examples of this type are the Hegar, Pratt, Hank, or Hawkin-Ambler dilators. The Hegar dilator increases in 0.5-mm increments and has a rounded tip, unlike the modified types that have tapered ends (Figure 9.3). The latter types permit more gradual dilation of the cervix and require less force during use, and therefore the potential for injury to the cervix is less.

Curette

Curettes vary in size as well as in the structure of the curetting surface. The surface may be smooth and sharp, with one continuous 'cutting' surface, or serrated with teeth of varying sizes. Injury to the myometrium is more likely to occur with the latter (Figure 9.4). The zeal of the surgeon in performing the curettage can be a factor in the production of injury to the myometrium and resultant scarring.

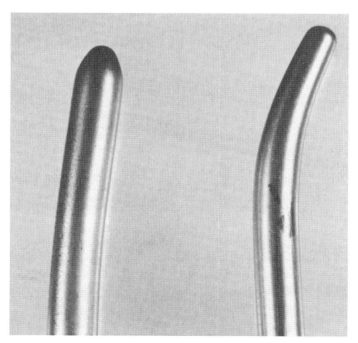

Figure 9.3 Pratt dilator (right) and Hegar dilator (left).

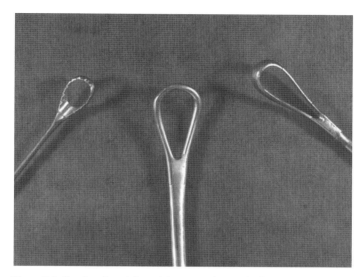

Figure 9.4 Curettes. From left to right: serrated, smooth, sharp, with one continuous cutting surface.

Other instrumentation

Other instruments include uterine sounds, ovum forceps, weighted speculum, right-angle retractors, and malleable probe.

Dilation and curettage (D & C) for incomplete abortion

The procedure can be inpatient or ambulatory. Various anesthetic techniques can be used, including paracervical block or general anesthesia. Anesthetic agents that promote uterine relaxation (e.g., halothane) should be avoided. Prior to curettage, the patient should be examined under anesthesia to determine the size and position of the uterus.

After proper placement of the patient on the operating table in the lithotomy position and induction of anesthesia, the vagina and perineum are cleansed in the usual manner. No shaving or clipping of vulva/perineal hair is necessary or desirable. The urinary bladder is emptied by catheterization. This step can be omitted if the bladder is not distended on the pelvic examination. Draping of the area is performed, more from tradition than from necessity.

A weighted speculum is placed in the vagina and a small, right-angle retractor is inserted anteriorly to expose the cervix. The cervix is grasped with a tenaculum placed on the midportion of the anterior lip. Traction is gently made downward to straighten the cervicouterine angle. While this is being done, the urethral meatus should be protected from pressure of the instrument. Any tissue present in the cervical canal can be removed with forceps.

A sound that has been shaped to conform to the position of the uterus may be passed through the cervical canal into the uterine cavity. This procedure will give confirmatory information on the uterus and the angle between the cervical canal and the uterine cavity.

The sound should pass easily due to the dilation of the cervical canal occurring with the abortion process. The fundus of the uterus will be detected by resistance to further gentle passage of the sound. The degree of resistance will vary and may be minimal in some instances. Oxytocic agents can be administered prior to this step, but are of questionable value at the early stages of gestation.

Dilation of the cervical canal is performed at this time. Frequently, this is not required and may be harmful, especially in the young, nulliparous woman. The dilator, preferably a tapered dilator (e.g., Hanks), is gently grasped with the thumb below the instrument and the index, middle, and ring fingers above it. The little finger of the operator's hand should be supported against the perineum to minimize uncontrolled advancement of the dilator into the uterus. The tip of the dilator is inserted into the cervical canal and is advanced just beyond the internal os, using steady but minimal force. Resistance may be encountered at the level of the internal os. This can be overcome if constant, steady pressure is applied, rather than forceful thrusts. The latter maneuver can result in uncontrolled advance of the instrument and uterine perforation. Each dilator should remain in the cervical canal for a time sufficient to allow adjustment to that size before its removal. The dilator should be removed easily from the cervix before proceeding to insertion of the next larger size. Dilation should proceed to a size sufficient for curettage or evaluation to be performed. Generally, a dilator size 1 mm greater than the number of weeks of gestation is necessary.

In second-trimester abortions, digital exploration and evacuation of the uterus may be performed. The uterus should be positioned anteriorly. The index finger and, if possible, also the middle finger are inserted through the cervix into the uterine cavity, while the other hand is placed on the patient's abdomen to depress the fundus of the uterus. Any tissue that is felt is detached with the examining fingers and removed. The procedure is repeated until no additional tissue fragments are encountered.

A curved or straight ovum forceps (or similarly structured instrument) is introduced into the uterine cavity and the cavity systematically explored for tissue masses that can be removed. It is important that the operator introduce each instrument into the uterus with gentleness and caution.

The position of the uterus may change during the procedure. A retroverted uterus that has been repositioned anteriorly may not remain in place. The direction of the cavity must be determined during passage of the ovum forceps and also before they are opened and closed.

A standard procedure for curettage should be utilized. All areas of the uterine cavity are explored. The instrument is laid on the palmar surface of four fingers and held with the opposing thumb. The curette is introduced into the cervical canal and moved to the uterine fundus, whose resistance is gently appreciated.

The curette should be pulled downward over the uterine wall while slight pressure is exerted on the inner surface of the instrument. The curette should be removed as each area is explored to collect the tissue that has been obtained. The operator should discontinue the procedure once the yield of tissue is significantly decreased. At that time, minimal or no bleeding should be present. The uterine cavity should not be curetted too vigorously, since this can lead to removal not only of the functional layer of the endometrium, but also of the basalis. A grating sensation indicates that the curettage of the area should be discontinued. The decision of whether to proceed with curettage, if evacuation with finger exploration and ovum forceps appears to have completed the process, depends on the judgment of the surgeon.

All tissues obtained should be collected in a gauze bag placed around the weighted speculum. It should be rinsed free of blood and clots prior to submitting the tissue to pathology. The surgeon should note any intrauterine irregularities at the time of curettage.

Following the abortion, Rho (D) immunoglobulin (RhoGAM) should be administered to Rh-negative mothers at risk. A dose of 50 µg appears adequate to prevent sensitization in abortions occurring prior to 13 weeks' gestation. For abortions occurring at 13 weeks' gestation or later, a standard 300-µg dose is recommended.

Women with incomplete abortion may present with local and systemic evidence of infection. Generally, the infection is confined to the uterus. Antibiotic coverage should be directed to bacteria generally encountered in pelvic infection. Gram-negative aerobic and anaerobic organisms are usually present.[16] Since it is not possible to await the results of culture, treatment should be instituted on admission to the hospital. The clinical response usually is rapid once the uterus has been evacuated. Antibiotic treatment is continued during the immediate postoperative period or beyond if there is evidence of spread of the infection beyond the uterus.[36]

Vacuum aspiration

In contrast to traditional curettage, it is the suction at the tip of the cannula, and not mechanical movement of the curette, that disrupts and separates the products of conception from their uterine attachment, facilitating removal. The relative vacuum created allows the pressure of the ambient atmosphere transmitted through the body of the mother to force the uterine contents into the collecting system. The vacuum may be considered in relative or absolute terms, depending on whether normal pressure (at sea level) is viewed as 0 or 760 mmHg. At higher elevations, there will be an associated decrease in atmospheric pressure, with resultant reduction in available theoretical maximum vacuum from the approximate 1.0 kg/cm^2. A suction of 45 mmHg (relative) is sufficient for completion of the procedure.

Although the details of specific systems may vary, the principle is the same. A suction curette with a distal opening is placed in the uterus. The negative pressure is controlled by occluding an aperture in the proximal part of the curette. In this system, this control is provided by a sliding ring, which can be moved over the opening. The curette is connected by plastic tubing to a collection bottle, which contains a gauze trap for the tissue. There is a second collection bottle to increase the capacity of the system. The collection bottles are connected to the vacuum source.

The curettes are usually constructed of plastic and may be rigid or flexible. Generally, they have a rounded tip with one or more side openings. Selection of a cannula depends on the preference of the surgeon.

The preparation of the patient is similar to that described under conventional D & C. The patient is examined to confirm previous findings. A speculum is placed in the vagina to expose the cervix. The anterior lip of the cervix is grasped with a tenaculum, and gentle, downward traction is made. Since the suction curette is not placed into the fundus of the uterus, but just beyond the internal os of the cervix, sounding of the uterus may not be necessary. The cervical canal must be dilated sufficiently to permit insertion of the cannula. The use of PGE_2 can facilitate the operation. A suppository containing 20 mg of dinoprostone is inserted high into the vagina. The patient remains recumbent for 10 minutes after insertion. Additional medication can be administered at 3–5-hour intervals until the desired effect is achieved. Uterine contractions are usually observed within 10–15 minutes after vaginal placement of the suppository. PG analogs may also be given intramuscularly. Cervical softening and effacement will accompany the contractions. The sequential use of suppositories may be necessary to obtain evacuation of the products of conception. The delivery of the placenta may be delayed for 1–2 hours. If bleeding is not evident, expectant management can be practiced. In 30–40% of patients, there will be retention of some products of conception, and D & C is necessary. Sonography may be used to confirm the completeness of the abortion (e.g., presence of a uterine midline echo). If there is a question of retained products, D & C should be performed.[37]

In missed abortion, there is usually sufficient time to dilate the cervix prior to suction cannula. The vacuum should not be instituted until the aperture of the cannula is just beyond the internal os of the cervix. When the cannula is withdrawn, similar precaution should be taken. Injury to the area of the internal os can occur when the suction cannula passes this area with the vacuum system operative.

The transparent tubing should be observed to ascertain the passage of the residual products of conception from the uterine cavity. The cannula should be slowly rotated to allow the aperture of the cannula to face all areas of the uterus. The cannula is not intended to 'scrape' or curette the walls of the uterus. The vacuum dislodges fragments of tissue and delivers them to the suction curette. The procedure can be considered complete when the yield of tissue is greatly decreased and foamy serosanguinous fluid appears within the suction tubing.

Management of missed abortion

During the first trimester and the early portion of the second one, missed abortion can be evacuated by suction curettage. When the size of the uterus is considered too large for safe evacuation by D & C, medical induction should be used. Intravenous oxytocin is less effective in the second trimester than later in pregnancy in producing effective uterine contractions, but its effectiveness is improved if the cervix has undergone effacement and dilation. The preferred method of treatment is surgery through the insertion of a hygroscopic dilator into the cervical canal the evening before surgery.

The vagina and cervix should be surgically cleansed and the cervix stabilized with a tenaculum or sponge forceps. The laminaria is grasped with a sterile uterine dressing forceps and is inserted into the cervical canal until its distal tip passes the internal os. It should slide easily into the cervical canal. If the upper margin of the laminaria is not placed at the level of the internal os, it will expel itself during swelling. Its proximal 5–10 mm should protrude from the external os. A folded sponge placed against the cervix will reduce the tendency for expulsion. The maximum swelling of the laminaria occurs over a 6–8-hour period. If further dilation is desired, it can be removed, and two small laminaria inserted in its place. It is preferable to use two small laminaria in parallel instead of a single large one.

The patient should remain recumbent after insertion to avoid vagal tone reaction and syncope. Most patients will have low abdominal cramps for a few minutes. These may recur, but are generally mild and can be relieved by analgesics. Failure of the laminaria to dilate the cervix occurs in a small percentage of patients due to its expulsion from the cervical canal. Fever and infection are infrequent complications of this procedure. Frequently, no further dilation of the cervix is required.

Complications

Complications relative to dilation and curettage of the uterus can be related to specific instrumentation. The cervix of the young nullipara, especially in early pregnancy, is resistant to dilation. This may predispose to injury of the cervix and perforation of the uterus. Signs and symptoms of the latter may not develop for several hours. Hemorrhage may be immediate or delayed. Trauma to the basal endometrium and myometrium may manifest at a later date as menstrual dysfunction or infertility (Asherman's syndrome).

Cervical

Laceration
The most common injury occurring during D & C is laceration of the cervix due to the tenaculum pulling free. It occurs more often with the single-toothed tenaculum. Lacerations that require repair occur in 1–2% of procedures. Surgical repair should be performed after the completion of the D & C. In most

instances, the lacerations are small and stop bleeding by the end of surgery.

Lacerations from the dilator may be more extensive, particularly in the young nullipara whose cervix is small and difficult to dilate. The amount of force exerted at the internal cervical os to produce dilation varies with stage of gestation, the type of dilator, and the extent of dilation. The cervix in the earlier stages of gestation requires greater force to produce dilation. As pregnancy progresses, less force is necessary. Age, race, and gravidity do not affect this finding. The cervix is most resistant to further dilation at 9 mm.

Only modest force is required to dilate the cervix sufficiently to accomplish evacuation. Gentle force is the least traumatic and most effective. When excessive effort is applied, the tenaculum may pull free from the cervix. If this happens, injury to the area of the internal cervical os may ensue.

False passage. When the sound or dilator is introduced without appropriate direction or control, a false cervical canal may be created. Persistence in dilation of this false passage may result in a significant laceration of the cervix, or in the formation of a canal which communicates with the vagina as a cervical fistula. Whenever there is difficulty in identifying the external cervical os (e.g., missed abortion), or if abnormal resistance is encountered during the passage of an instrument, the operator should reconfirm the position and direction of the cervical canal by gentle passage of a probe or sound.

Other effects. An increased incidence of cervical pregnancy after D & C for induced abortion has been reported.[38] In rare instances, cervical or paracervical implantation of fetal tissue with subsequent symptomatology has occurred.[39]

Late effects of cervical injury may be manifest as cervical stenosis due to synechiae, or reproductive failure due to cervical incompetency[40] (Figure 9.5).

Uterine hemorrhage

Bleeding during or after D & C for completion of an abortion is a frequent complication. Incomplete evacuation of the uterine contents is primarily responsible. The operative procedure should not be terminated until bleeding from the uterus is minimal and the organ is firmly contracted. Other causes of bleeding must be excluded. Generally, uterine bleeding is not associated with perforation. The cervix should be inspected carefully to determine any bleeding sites.[40]

Since the operative procedure to empty the uterus is a 'blind' one, it may not be possible to ascertain that all tissue has been removed. The symptoms caused by incomplete emptying of the uterus may be delayed, occurring after the patient has left the hospital. Bleeding and cramps, necessitate another D & C. Blood replacement should be provided as necessary. Sonography is capable of identifying retained products of conception *in utero* and is useful, therefore, for the diagnosis of incomplete evacuation.

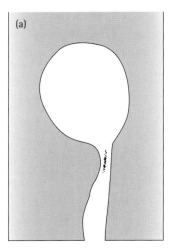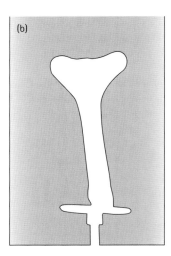

Figure 9.5 A schematic representation of cervical changes in nulliparous women following first trimester pregnancy termination. The original research rested upon cervicohysterographic studies performed immediately before (a) and 8 weeks after (b) the abortion procedures.[40] Note the loss of the original structure of the isthmus uteri. Also note that these abortions were done prior to the introduction of the suction apparatus into gynecologic practice.

Perforation

The quoted incidence of uterine perforation at time of D & C is derived primarily from data relating to elective termination of pregnancy. In these reports the rate of perforations varies from 0.75–15 per 1000 procedures. Some believe that the incidence of unrecognized perforations is many times higher. Perforation can result from any instrument, but it occurs most frequently during sounding of the uterus. For this reason many experts omit this step. Knowledge of the position of the uterus prior to instrumentation helps to avoid this complication. Not only anteroposterior uterine orientation should be determined, but lateral deviation as well. Inspection of the vaginal fornices may suggest lateral displacement when one fornix is much wider than the other. Confirmation can be obtained by observing the direction the sound or the smallest dilator takes when it is passed into the uterus. Downward traction with a tenaculum on the cervix will tend to straighten the cervicouterine angle and avoid perforation.

All instruments should be advanced slowly into the uterus. Dilators should be introduced just beyond the internal os. Suction cannulas also should be introduced to this depth and the products of conception aspirated with the cannula in this position. The cervix of early pregnancy (8 weeks or less) or of the young, nulliparous woman is most resistant to dilation. Forceful efforts must be avoided.

Perforation can be diagnosed when there is a sudden decrease in resistance to an instrument, or passage occurs to a depth greater than the measured size of the uterine cavity. This latter finding may not be reliable in lateral perforations where the structures of the intraligamentar space may limit the passage of the perforating tool. Perforation is definitely established with the recovery of obvious extrauterine tissue.

When the surgery is performed under local anesthesia, perforation may be suspected if the patient develops pain. If the perforation occurs in the midline of the uterus, she will experience severe midline pain that subsides rapidly; while with a lateral perforation, the pain is severe, persistent, and localized to the affected side.

Management will depend on circumstances, but discontinuation of the operative procedure is essential whenever perforation is suspected. The site of perforation should be noted, particularly in reference to the lateral or midline area of the uterus. The patient's vital signs must be closely monitored. A laparotomy is indicated if the perforation has resulted in removal of fat or other extrauterine tissue, if there is evidence of shock, if there has been extensive, previous abdominal surgery, if the patient is very obese, or if the urine is bloody.

If the perforation is midline and there is no urgent indication (e.g., bleeding) for completion of the evacuation, observation can be performed and the procedure completed somewhat later under laparoscopic guidance. The laparoscopist can guide the other operator away from the perforation site and observe contraction of the uterus as it is emptied. The perforation site is inspected for size, bleeding, and extrusion of the products of conception. Large lacerations with active bleeding and/or extruded products of conception require laparotomy.

When the perforation is in the lateral portion of the uterus, the uterus is empty, and there is no indication for laparotomy, ultrasound and in some instances laparoscopy should be performed. The broad ligament areas should be thoroughly inspected. If an extraperitoneal hematoma is observed, it should be watched for a change in size. An increase in size is an indication for laparotomy for control of the bleeding. The serosal surface of the bladder and bowel is inspected as completely as possible through the laparoscopy. If more than superficial injury is noted, laparotomy should be performed.

If none of the above-noted complications exist or develop and the patient is stable, she may be discharged after 24–48 hours of observation. Sonography should be utilized to define the hematoma and to observe its resolution.

Synechiae

Curettage of the pregnant or recently pregnant uterus is the primary antecedent factor for the development of intrauterine synechiae.[41] Elective termination of a pregnancy and D & C for incomplete abortion are the most commonly associated factors. The former group is at higher risk than the latter. The technique of sharp curettage is particularly traumatic to the endometrium. Trauma to the basal layer of the endometrium predisposes to adherence of the anterior and posterior uterine walls. Local infection also may play a role.

Prevention of spontaneous abortions

After one spontaneous abortion, the risk of another in the next pregnancy is not significantly higher than in the general population. The prevention of spontaneous abortion is mainly directed toward correcting etiologic factors conducive to recurrent abortion.[42] A detailed history of previous abortions must be taken; careful physical and pelvic examinations performed; and andrologic, immunologic, radiologic, and other relevant laboratory tests done.[43,44]

Prior to conception, maternal disorders such as diabetes mellitus and hypothyroidism should be adequately treated. In case uterine abnormalities, congenital or acquired, have been demonstrated, proper operative procedure (metroplasty) should be performed. (Anomalies connected with duplication of the uterus can be documented by hysterosalpingography and/or ultrasonography.)

Overripeness of the ovum, preovulatory or postovulatory or other anomalies in the mechanism of ovulation have been associated with an increased frequency of early spontaneous abortion.[45,46] In cases of recurrent abortions where ovopathies, abnormal ovulation or luteal phase defects are suspected, induction of ovulation may be considered.

If the second or even the third pregnancy also ends in abortion, without obvious cause, it is justifiable to search for genetic reasons – chromosome rearrangement or X-linked dominant inheritance.[9,46,47] Both parents should have peripheral blood cultures set up for chromosome analysis. There may be an opportunity to examine aborted products of conception.[21] If a parent is found to carry a balanced rearrangement, and there is as yet no healthy child, the outlook is unfavorable. When a parent carries a chromosome rearrangement, options include prenatal diagnosis (chromosome analysis), artificial insemination by donor (AID), in vitro fertilization, or adoption. The question of X-linked dominant inheritance can be answered by clinical and genealogical examination.[9] Also recommended are investigations for evidence of antiphospholipid and thrombophilia syndromes.[17–19]

Incarceration of the retroflexed uterus

This entity represents the only circumstance where an otherwise inevitable abortion can be prevented. On very rare occasions, a uterus in fixed retroflexion becomes trapped in the true pelvis. The patient is usually asymptomatic during the first trimester and, thus the condition remains unrecognized initially. However, around weeks 13–14 the gravida becomes symptomatic. Pelvic discomfort appears first. This is followed by urinary retention. If the condition remains unrecognized and, thus, untreated, the patient ends up in the emergency room on account of excruciating pelvic pain associated with inability to void. On account of the rarity of this complication, it may remain undiagnosed even at this point. If so, the bladder becomes immensely distended and its walls thickened due to edema. Portions of the mucous membrane may slough off and, in the same process, urinary tract infection develops and escalates into severe pyelonephritis. The distended bladder, particularly in connection with carelessly performed pelvic examination, may rupture. In the absence of timely surgical intervention, this complication can be fatal. The same is true of the alternative final outcome; development of ischemic necrosis in the uterine walls leading to pelvic and later generalized peritonitis.

For an examiner who is mindful of this clinical entity, the diagnosis is easy. The woman's excruciating pain, her inability to void, the extreme distension of the bladder, the tenderness of the lower abdomen to touch, and the associated guarding are almost diagnostic. A careful pelvic examination makes the diagnosis conclusive through the palpation of the uterus filling the posterior part of the pelvis. Not infrequently, the cervix is out of the examiner's reach as it points upward towards the ramus of the pubic bone.

Whereas probably most cases of incarceration could be prevented by the use of a Hodge pessary and by the mother spending the night in the prone position, because the retroflexed uterus only rarely becomes trapped, such measures are almost never taken prophylactically. Almost invariably, the diagnosis is made when the gravida becomes symptomatic and even then, sometimes with considerable delay. By that time, the correction of the complication no longer is simple.

The removal of the uterus from its entrapped position usually requires major anesthesia. Far too often, the patient's discomfort is so extreme, that she cannot cooperate with the somewhat time-consuming process of administering a spinal anesthesia. On this account, general anesthesia is probably the most suitable for this procedure.

With the patient in the lithotomy position, after catheterization of the urinary bladder, the operator introduces two or, if possible more, fingers into the posterior fornix of the vagina. Some degree of force is needed to lift the uterus out of its entrapped position and push it into the false pelvis. The external hand takes over at this point and holds the uterus in its new position in front of the promontory of the sacrum. Later this function is taken over by an assistant, while the operator packs the fornix with gauze in order to prevent the return of the organ into its previous position. When removed 24 hours later, the gauze pack may be replaced with a pessary. With or without such measures, once lifted out from the true pelvis, the uterus seldom returns to its entrapped position. When rarely it does, the same procedure needs to be repeated. Fortunately, the growth of the uterus precludes its later entrapment as the pregnancy progresses.

This technique permits the correction of uterine entrapment in the overwhelming majority of the instances. If it fails, it can be repeated with a finger introduced into the rectum. However, if this is still unsuccessful, the complication requires immediate laparotomy. Thus, manual correction is best performed under double setup. If attempts at emptying the bladder have been unsuccessful, its overdistension must be relieved by suprapubic puncture before the abdominal incision. Once the abdomen is open, manual elevation of the pregnant uterus from the posterior pelvis seldom entails significant difficulty. If it does, allowing air to enter the space behind the organ may facilitate the procedure. If everything fails, removal of some of the amniotic fluid by uterine puncture may prove helpful. Alternatively, or in combination with the latter, the use of an obstetric vacuum extractor may be warranted.[48]

If everything fails, and particularly in those cases where necrosis of the myometrium is a threat, hysterotomy and evacuation of the products of conception may be the ultimate solution. It has been suggested that in this eventuality antefixation of the uterus should be part of the surgical procedure.

Procedures for midtrimester indicated termination

With the development of genetic counseling, new information has become available to affected patients and families. Prenatal diagnosis with the option of termination of pregnancy provides important reassurance for couples at risk of genetic disorders.

Conventional techniques

In patients up to 12 weeks' gestation, conventional techniques are used, including cervical dilation, either instrumental or medical, followed by vacuum aspiration or curettage. Intracervical laminaria and PG induce fetal ejection: the embryo is usually delivered whole, thus permitting pathologic examination.[9,49]

After week 12, generally abortion is induced medically. However, dilation and evacuation (D & E) also is a common technique for second-trimester pregnancy termination.[50] During the induction, the fetus usually is expelled completely. Nonetheless, instrumental emptying of the uterus is often required, on account of incomplete expulsion of the placenta.

Ideally, induction of abortion should not damage the fetus, and should allow full histopathologic examination, and further investigations where appropriate.[51] It is often necessary to dilate the cervix and stimulate uterine contractions for the expulsion of the products of conception. These requirements are partly met by the use of (1) PG,[52] PG analogs, and antiprogesterones; (2) intra-, and extra-amniotic abortificiant (hypertonic saline, and other solutions);[9,53] (3) pretreatment with laminaria or synthetic dilators; and (4) concurrent intravenous oxytocin. In rare cases, abdominal hysterotomy may be considered.

Cervical ripening

The role of the cervix in pregnancy has been often oversimplified. It was thought that it simply acts as a sphincter in pregnancy which relaxed during delivery. In fact, although in early pregnancy the cervix is long and tight, it begins to shorten, open, and relax by midgestation, a process termed 'ripening'.

In the cervical connective tissue, biochemical and biophysical changes are initiated by estrogens and PG. Cross-bridges between collagen molecules are broken, and the glycosaminoglycan and proteoglycan content of the matrix increases. Cervical connective tissue fibroblasts synthesize PG in large amounts; these in turn stimulate collagen metabolism with diminished collagen synthesis and increased breakdown.[54]

Cervical ripening can be achieved with PG, progesteron agonits, and PG analogs. Various commercial PGE_2 formulations are currently available (intravenous solutions, intravaginal tablets, intracervical gel, intravaginal gel, intravaginal insert with retrieval system, and vaginal suppositories).

PG and PG analogs

PG are naturally occurring fatty acid derivatives with a wide range of applications in obstetrics, especially relating to midtrimester pregnancy termination.[55] Intravenous administration of PGF_α and PGE_2 causes side effects – erythema, nausea, vomiting, and diarrhea – that are very troublesome. Intra-amniotic injection of PG is an accepted method of termination. For this purpose, $PGF_{2\alpha}$ is the most suitable.[56] Results are somewhat better when PG are introduced extraamniotically. A blunt-tipped, flexible plastic or rubber cannula can be introduced between the uterine wall and the fetal membranes, for injection or infusion. Giving PG by this route requires a lower dosage, since the injected drug rapidly reaches the myometrium. Dosage for $PGF_{2\alpha}$ would be 750 μg every 2 hours; for PGE_2, 200 ng every 2 hours. Repeated injections must be given.[52,57]

Natural PG cannot be given intramuscularly, as they are highly irritating locally. However, PG analogs can. They have also been given in vaginal pessaries and jelly. $PGF_{2\alpha}$ should not be used in active cardiac, pulmonary, renal, or hepatic disease and is relatively contraindicated for patients suffering from bronchial asthma, hypertension or sickle cell disease. PG do not damage the fetus; thus the histopathologic examination is not interfered with. However, they have undesirable side effects, and even maternal death has occasionally been reported.[58] Preference should be given to PGE_2 as a local preparation for cervical ripening.

The mother's vital functions must be checked at regular intervals. The application can be repeated up to three times daily. The gel is preferable to the sponge. It rarely causes uterine hypertonus and is less likely to provoke premature rupture of the membranes. The membranes should be broken only when the internal os and the cervix appear sufficiently ripe. Oxytocin infusion can then be started, if desired.

The membranes should never be ruptured with an unripe cervix. In cases of gross hydrocephalus, or abdominal distension, with a nonviable fetus, cephalocentesis (ventriculocentesis) or abdominocentesis may be performed during labor, to preserve the birth canal and facilitate vaginal delivery.[59,60]

Rh-negative patients should be given anti-D gamma globulin at the time of any invasive procedure, or termination (200–300 μg, irrespective of gestational age).

Hypertonic saline

Intra-amniotic injection of hypertonic saline (50 ml of 20% sodium chloride) leads to abortion. Fetal death and expulsion result from dehydration. Although not without danger, this technique is still used sometimes for midtrimester termination.

Transabdominal amniocentesis is performed under local anesthesia (1% lidocaine) with a 1.2-mm diameter needle (thicker than that used in diagnostic amniocentesis). Amniotic fluid is withdrawn, approximately 10 ml for every week of gestation, and 50–100 ml of sterile 20% saline is injected. The injection must be given into the amniotic fluid. If given subcutaneously, intraperitoneally, or into the myometrium, it may cause pain and serious complications.

Uterine contractions are felt immediately after injection. The uterus becomes tense and enlarges. As the injected Na^+ and Cl^- ions reach the maternal circulation, the mother feels thirst.

Entry of saline into the maternal circulation provokes blushing, feeling of heat and nausea, falling blood pressure, bradycardia, and, occasionally, cardiac arrest. Saline induction must never be employed under general anesthesia or in the presence of hypertension, cardiac, or renal disease.

Late complications of hypertonic saline induction include various coagulopathies, especially drops in factor V and factor VIII levels. The platelet count may also fall, the prothrombin time increase, and fibrin degradation products appear. Such changes seldom emerge less than a few hours after injection. Most commonly, they present 10–24 hours later. Thus, women should not leave the hospital within 24 hours of the induction.

The fetal heart usually fails within 2 hours of the saline injection. Abortion occurs in about 24–36 hours. In 10% of the cases, the uterine contractions are poor and oxytocin needs to be given (5–30 IU in 500 ml 5% glucose infusion). This method has the advantage that the aborted fetus rarely shows signs of life.

As an alternative to hypertonic saline, intra-amniotic 50% glucose solution has been used. This avoids hypernatremia, but the induction is slow. Glucose is a good culture medium; thus, prophylactic antibiotics may have to be given.

Intra-amniotic hypertonic urea solution has also been used, but is an inefficient way of inducing abortion. All hypertonic injection techniques have the relative disadvantage that they damage the fetus; thus, histopathologic examination is difficult or impossible, although the placenta and membranes may still be suitable for cytogenetic and biochemical examination.

Decision making regarding the fate of pregnancy

Termination of pregnancy, with the aim of preventing the birth of a fetus with an incurable disorder, is a traumatic and unhappy option. However, this procedure is frequently performed.[61] When there is a hope of treatment for a prenatally diagnosed disorder, premature induction of labor may prevent *in utero* progression of the disease and/or permit prompt postnatal surgery (e.g., in case of omphalocele ruptured *in utero*). Between these two extremes there are a great number of disorders, very variable in severity, which demand individual judgment. It seems justified to outline some general principles relating to the decision-making process in the pregnancy situation.[9,62]

■ *Condition 1: correct genetic diagnosis.* The diagnosis, in affected child or adult, or in the fetus *in utero*, must be made with up-to-date methods and the results recorded in writing (*ethics of the clinician/the investigator; ethics of the laboratory*).
■ *Condition 2: adequately informed parents.* No matter what their level of education, every couple must be informed and, as far as possible, made to understand the nature of the disease in question, its severity, its prognosis, and the possibilities of cure or treatment (*ethics of the counselor; ethics of genetic counseling*).
■ *Condition 3: free decision by the parents.* The couple may choose to continue the pregnancy, or they may choose its termination (*ethics of the couple/the parents; ethics of the family*).
■ *Condition 4: actions taken are within the law.* Society creates laws that regulate the termination of pregnancy. These and the professional codes and regulations provide a framework within which each case must be evaluated individually (*ethics of society; public health ethics*).

Medical indications for termination

Risk to the mother's life
Termination of pregnancy may be permitted at any time when serious illness threatens the mother's life (e.g., heart failure, life-threatening obstetric complications). In such cases the doctor in charge documents the illness in the notes.

Risk of genetic disorder or teratogenic damage
When the risk of genetic disorder or teratogenic damage to the fetus is high, the disorder/damage is likely to be severe, and prenatal diagnosis is not available, termination up to week 12 of pregnancy in many countries is permitted.

Risk of genetic disease or malformation
When the risk of serious genetic disease or malformation in the fetus is 50–100%, and there is no possibility of treatment, termination may be permitted until week 20 in some countries and up to week 24 in others.

(1) The theoretical probability of fetal disease is 100%: a parent carries a homologous balanced translocation (e.g., 21/21; a female fetus from a father carrying an X-linked mutant gene of a dominant trait, etc.).
(2) There is 100% probability of a chromosome disorder associated with severe developmental retardation and physical

defects; enzymopathies, congenital malformations, and other pathologic conditions (prenatal diagnosis).
(3) The theoretical probability of a severe autosomal dominantly inherited disorder (e.g., Huntington's disease) is 50% or above.
(4) A mother carrying an X-linked recessive gene is pregnant with a male fetus, and fetal hemizygosity cannot be excluded.
(5) With prenatal exposure to rubella or cytomegalovirus infection, the fetal risk may reach the 50% level.

Occasionally, some serious fetal defect, likely to be fatal in the immediate postnatal period, is discovered. Such pregnancies, if continued, may be accompanied by obstetric complications threatening the mother's health (poly/oligohydramnios, placental abruption, uterine rupture, or uterine atony) and/or psychological disturbances (occasionally psychopathy).

Within the time limits permitted by the law, the mother must be given the option of pregnancy termination for a postnatally nonviable fetus, especially when her own health is endangered. Conditions considered incompatible with postnatal life include the following:[9]

(1) Severe central nervous system malformations (e.g., anencephaly and/or rachischisis with or without hydrocephalus, hydranencephaly, alobar holoprosencephaly, iniencephaly).
(2) Severe bilateral renal diseases (e.g., renal agenesis with Potter sequence, infantile-type polycystic kidney disease, multicystic kidney dysplasia).
(3) Severe chromosome aberrations (e.g., triploidy, trisomy 13).
(4) Neonatal lethal chondrodysplasia (e.g., thanatophoric dysplasia, achondrogenesis) and type II osteogenesis imperfecta.
(5) Severe multiple forms of the ADAM complex (e.g., craniofacial disruption, thoracoabdominal eventeration).

Selective termination in multiple pregnancy

Improved ultrasound technology and invasive prenatal diagnostic procedures have facilitated the detection of fetal abnormalities in multiple gestations. Advances in assisted reproductive technologies also have led to an increased incidence of multiple gestation, particularly as result of ovulation induction.

Fetal disease or disorder in a twin pregnancy may be concordant or discordant. In the former situation both fetuses are affected, and termination may be carried out as for a single pregnancy. In a discordant twin pregnancy, when only one of the fetuses is affected, the following three outcomes are possible:

(1) The couple may decide against any form of termination, and the pregnancy is continued. One should note that, in general, abnormal/affected fetuses have a much higher mortality *in utero* than normal ones (up to 75–85% for trisomy 21, and up to 90 to 95% for trisomy 18, between conception and term); continuation of a discordant twin pregnancy may often result in the 'natural' death of the affected twin, and survival of the healthy one.

(2) The parents may decide to lose both fetuses, the affected and the healthy one.

(3) Selective termination of pregnancy, bringing about the death of the affected twin while preserving the normal one, may be attempted.

Over the past 15 years, multifetal pregnancy reduction has become a well-established and integral part of infertility therapy for the sequelae of aggressive infertility management. In the mid-1980s, the risks and benefits of the procedure could only be guessed. We now have clear and precise data on the risks and benefits of the procedure and an understanding that the risks increase substantially with the starting and finishing number of fetuses in multifetal pregnancies. The collaborative loss rate numbers (i.e., 4.5% for triplets, 8% for quadruplets, 11% for quintuplets, and 15% for sextuplets or more) seem reasonable for the procedures performed by an experienced operator.[63,64]

If *selective termination* is chosen, the affected fetus can be removed by hysterotomy; however, there is little experience with this technique and no real information on its safety for the second twin. Induced cardiac arrest is another mode of selective termination; air, formaldehyde, or potassium solution is injected into the circulation of the affected fetus, either into the umbilical vein under fetoscopic control, or directly into the heart, guided by ultrasound. Alternatively, or in combination with the injection method, the affected fetus may be exsanguinated.[65,66]

The following procedure is probably the least dangerous for the normal twin.[25] A volume of 10 ml 20% NaCl solution is injected into the heart of the affected fetus. The fetus is not exsanguinated, to avoid possible bleeding from the unaffected fetus through any arteriovenous anastomoses. Presumably, the hypertonic saline acts directly on the myocardium. Within the circulation, the saline is diluted to such a degree that it will not damage the other fetus even if placental anastomoses are present.

Soon after injection, the affected fetus becomes bradycardic, and all cardiac activity ceases within a few hours. The mother is checked regularly in the clinic for several weeks, and further ultrasound examinations are made at 3–4-week intervals, to follow development of the surviving fetus and absorption of the other. At such times, maternal blood should also be examined for signs of diffuse intravascular coagulation. The dead fetus becomes a fetus papyraceus, but the other should develop normally.

Various technical procedures have been described, including transcervical minisuction to remove fetuses at 8–11 weeks. Another method is the transvaginal aspiration of the early embryo, usually at approximately 6–7 weeks. This technique is analogous in many respects to oocyte aspiration for *in vitro* fertilization.[67]

Disorders for which selective termination may be offered or requested can be divided into two groups. In the first one, the affected fetus might live for months or years, although severely handicapped (e.g., mental retardation), or only later develop neurologic problems (e.g., some enzymopathies). *In utero* development of the healthy twin would not be endangered in this situation. Intervention (selective termination) seems justifiable on grounds of the severe disorder in the affected fetus. The second group consists of congenital malformations incompatible with postnatal life. These are often associated with a progressive polyhydramnios, which may considerably disturb growth and development of the healthy twin. In this situation, intervention may be additionally justified: to ensure the development of the healthy fetus and to prevent obstetric complications. With or without intervention, the affected fetuses would not survive delivery.[9]

Embryopathology and fetal pathology

As a result of recent developments in prenatal diagnosis, many diseases and disorders previously accessible only after birth can be examined in the embryo or fetus. Morphologic investigation of induced or spontaneous abortions is termed 'embryopathology and fetal pathology'. With an induced abortion, the aims of investigation are (1) to check the accuracy of the prenatal diagnosis and (2) to identify any abnormalities that were not detected prenatally.[9] The aims of investigation in spontaneously aborted material are (1) to note anything suggestive of a high risk of recurrent abortion and (2) to identify any genetically significant pathology. Research into the etiology and pathology of acquired and genetic diseases and disorders is a further aim of embryo/fetopathology. To work in this field demands not only specialized embryologic and pathologic knowledge, but also experience and training in obstetrics and genetics.

Only fresh, unfixed material can be examined. If it is necessary to transport the abortus, it should be cooled (as in melting ice). For most purposes biopsies are useless or impossible to obtain once the fetus has been exposed to formalin. Fixative, if added, also upsets the external appearances, colors the skin, and, due to its slow rate of tissue penetration, may not preserve deep viscera anyway. Before fixation, the pathologist should be convinced of the presence or absence of contractures, limb or other deformities, dermal changes, anatomic congenital malformations, and injuries.

To detect enzymopathies, samples are taken from those tissues (usually liver, kidney, heart, skeletal muscle, brain, and placenta) in which the pathologic metabolite is likely to accumulate. The skin and the fascia lata are also useful for enzyme assay; fibroblasts can be cultured *in vitro*. Samples are taken with a sterile scalpel and slices are placed in sterile serum-free culture medium or normal saline. The samples are transported to the laboratory without freezing or warming, at room temperature.

Occasionally, the prenatal diagnosis (e.g., congenital nephrosis) can be confirmed by electron microscopy. For this purpose, the electron microscope laboratory protocol must be followed at the time of sampling.

For chromosome examination, blood can be obtained from the umbilical cord or by direct cardiac puncture. The sample is collected into a sterile tube containing heparin. The blood thus obtained is suitable for serum tests. Samples for culturing bacteria, viruses, fungi, and parasites must be taken under strictly aseptic conditions. Chromosome analysis can also be performed on cultured lung, spleen, gonad, or other tissues. While dissecting dead fetuses and embryos, precautions are to be taken in handling AIDS-infected material.

After external inspection, attempts are made to separate the decidual, chorionic, amniotic, and embryonal/ fetal elements. Special attention should be paid to the umbilical cord. The condition of the various tissues and membranes is noted, and any distortion, disintegration, or maceration that came about *in utero* is distinguished from any change or damage at the time of delivery or later. Histologic examination may help decide the exact nature and the timing of certain 'injuries'. The crown–rump and the crown–heel measurements are recorded.

Embryos may be sectioned sagittally, *in toto*, and examined microscopically. Fetuses are necropsied in detail. The face, eyes, nostrils, mouth, palate, and ears are inspected. The shape of the cranium is described and small encephaloceles are searched for. Pterygium and hygroma are looked for in the neck. The chest, the back, and the umbilical cord with its vessels are scrutinized thoroughly. One should remember that before gestational week 18 the clitoris of the female fetus is as large as the penis of the male; the labia majora develop later. The limbs, including the palms, fingers, soles, and toes, are examined. Special attention is paid to the placenta and the fetal membranes.[68]

Any detected abnormalities are described and measured carefully. The degree of maceration/autolysis is recorded. The intact embryo is photographed from the front, from the side, and from behind. Abnormalities are photographed in detail. Photographic documentation allows a retrospective review of the original findings and is useful for teaching, research, and publication.

External inspection is followed by autopsy. The organs are inspected *in situ*. For this purpose, scissors, forceps, a probe, and a magnifying lens are needed. The brain is fixed *in toto*, and later sliced, for examination. The placenta and the fetal membranes are thoroughly examined macroscopically and histologically. One should keep in mind the possibility of hydatidiform mole.

Histologic examination of lungs, liver, and kidney should be considered routine; that of other organs as appears appropriate. Buffered formalin is used as a fixative. Samples of material obtained from abortions terminated for nonmedical reasons may be used as controls.

Total body radiography is done to record skeletal disorders and to study some soft tissue disorders. Tape may be used to keep the embryo in a correct position. Anteroposterior and lateral views are taken, using 18×24-cm film. Skeletal abnormalities can be demonstrated convincingly with the alizarin red technique.

To obtain reliable postmortem ventriculograms, 10 ml of cerebrospinal fluid is withdrawn, and then 5 ml of buffered formalin is injected, followed by 5 ml of meglumine diatrizoate (Gastrografin). Postmortem angiography is valuable for study of vascular malformations.

Post-termination counseling

It is important to follow up women who have had termination for fetal abnormalities. They may become depressed immediately after the termination and may require support. They need to discuss what was wrong with the fetus, and the prospects for future pregnancies. It is the geneticist/obstetrician who should provide much of the support (trained nursing staff (health visitor, psychiatric social worker) attached to the genetics/obstetrics department), such as arranging for 'post-termination counseling'.

References

1. Boué J, Boué A, Lazar P. Retrospective and prospective epidemiological studies of 1500 karyotyped spontaneous human abortions. Teratology 1975; 12: 11–26.
2. Hertig AT. Implantation of the human ovum. In: Behrman SJ, Kistner RW (eds), Progress in Infertility, pp. 114 (2nd edn.) Little, Brown: Boston, 1975.
3. Hertig AT, Sheldon WH. Minimal criteria required to prove prima facie case of traumatic abortion or miscarriage. Ann Surg 1943; 117: 596.
4. Shepard TH, Fantel AG, Fitzsimmons J. Congenital defect rates among spontaneous abortuses. 20 years of monitoring. Teratology 1989; 39: 325–31.
5. Witschi E. Developmental causes of malformation. Experientia (Seperatum) 1971; 27: 1245–7.
6. Harris MJ, Poland BJ, Dill FJ. Triploidy in 40 human spontaneous abortuses: assessment of phenotype in embryos. Obstet Gynecol 1981; 57: 600–6.
7. Canki N, Warburton D, Byrne J. Morphological characteristics of monosomy-X in spontaneous abortions. Ann Genet 1988; 31: 4–13.
8. Dewald GW, Michels VV. Recurrent miscarriages. Cytogenetic causes and genetic counseling of affected families. Clin Obstet Gynaecol 1986; 29: 865–85.
9. Papp Z. Obstetric Genetics. Hungarian Academic Press: Budapest, 1990.
10. Diczfalusy E, Borrell U. Influence of oophorectomy on steroid excretion in early pregnancy. J Clin Endocrinol Metab 1961; 21: 1119.
11. Papp Z, Csécsei K, Tóth Z et al. Exencephaly in human fetuses. Clin Genet 1986; 30: 440.
12. Naessens A, Foulon W, Cammu H et al. Epidemiology and pathogenesis of *Ureaplasma urealyticum* in spontaneous abortion and early preterm labor. Acta Obstet Gynecol Scand 1987; 66: 513–16.
13. Axelsson G, Rylander R. Exposure to anaesthetic gases and spontaneous abortion: response bias in a postal questionnaire study. Int J Epidemiol 1982; 11: 250–6.
14. Csécsei K, Szeifert GT, Papp Z. Amniotic bands associated with early rupture of amnion due to an intrauterine device. Zentralbl Gynakol 1987; 109: 738–41.

15. Harlap S, Shiono PH, Ramcharan S. Spontaneous foetal losses in women using different contraceptives around the time of conception. Int J Epidemiol 1980; 9: 49–56.

16. Kline J, Stein Z, Susser M et al. Fever during pregnancy and spontaneous abortion. Am J Epidemiol 1985; 121: 832–42.

17. Gharavi AE, Pierangeli SS, Levy RA et al. Mechanisms of pregnancy loss in antiphospholipid syndrome. Clin Obstet Gynecol 2001; 44: 11–19.

18. Kujovich JL. Thrombophilia and pregnancy complications. Am J Obstet Gynecol 2004; 191: 412–24.

19. Vinatier D, Duefour P, Cosson M et al. Antiphospholipid syndrome and recurrent miscarriages. Eur J Obstet Gynecol Reprod Biol 2001; 96: 37–50.

20. Homonnai ZT, Paz GF, Weiss JN et al. Relation between semen quality and fate of pregnancy. Retrospective study of 534 pregnancies. Int J Androl 1980; 3: 574–84.

21. Kajii T, Ferrier A. Cytogenetics of aborters and abortuses. Am J Obstet Gynecol 1978; 131: 33.

22. Papp Z, Gardó S, Dolhay B. Chromosome study of couples with repeated spontaneous abortions. Fertil Steril 1974; 25: 713.

23. Simpson JL, Meyers CM, Martin AO et al. Translocations are infrequent among couples having repeated spontaneous abortions but no other abnormal pregnancies. Fertil Steril 1989; 51: 811–14.

24. Tharapel AT, Tharapel SA, Bannerman RM. Recurrent pregnancy losses and parental chromosome abnormalities. Br J Obstet Gynaecol 1985; 92: 899–914.

25. Papp Z, Tóth Z, Csécsei K. Ultrasound surveillance of pregnancies after metroplasty for septate uterus. Zentralbl Gynakol 1986; 108: 1307.

26. Simpson JL, Mills JL, Holmes LB et al. Low fetal loss rates after ultrasound-proved viability in early pregnancy. JAMA 1987; 258: 2555–7.

27. Jouppila P. Clinical and ultrasonic aspects in the diagnosis and follow-up of patients with early pregnancy failure. Acta Obstet Gynecol Scand 1980; 59: 405–9.

28. Berle P, Behnke K. Über Behandlungserfolge der drohenden Fehlgeburt. Geburtshilfe Frauenheilkd 1977; 37: 139.

29. Papp Z, Skapinyecz J, Gardó S et al. The value of hormone therapy in the treatment of threatened abortions. Med Gynaecol Androl Sociol 1975; 8: 19.

30. Lindelius A, Varli IH. Hammarstrom M. A retrospective comparison between lamicel and gemeprost for cervical ripening before surgical interruption of first-trimester pregnancy. Contraception. 2003; 67: 299–303.

31. Stubblefield PG, Frederiksen MC, Berek JS et al. Evaluation of a balloon dilator before second-trimester abortion by vacuum curettage. Am J Obstet Gynecol 1979; 135: 199–201.

32. Mitchell MD. Biochemistry of the prostaglandins. Baillieres Clin Obstet Gynecol 1992; 6: 687.

33. Robbin A, Spitz IM. Mifepristone: clinical pharmacology. Clin Obstet Gynecol 1996; 39: 436–50.

34. Fong YF, Singh KP. A comparative study using two dose regimens (200 μg or 400 μg) of vaginal misoprostol for pre-operative cervical dilatation in first trimester nulliparae. Br J Obstet Gynaecol 1998; 105: 413–17.

35. Creinin MD, Potter C, Holovanisin M et al. Mifepristone and misoprostol and methotrexat/misoprostol in clinical practice for abortion. Am J Obstet Gynecol 2003; 188: 664–9.

36. Larsson PG, Platz-Christensen JJ, Dalaker K et al. Treatment with 2% clindamycin vaginal cream prior to first trimester surgical abortion to reduce signs of postoperative infection: a prospective, double-blinded, placebo-controlled, multicenter study. Acta Obstet Gynecol Scand 2000; 79: 390–6.

37. Howie FL, Henshaw RC, Naji SA et al. Medical abortion or vacuum aspiration? Two year follow up of a patient preference trial. Br J Obstet Gynaecol 1997; 104: 829–33.

38. Shinagawa S, Nagayama M. Cervical pregnancy as a possible sequela of induced abortion. Report of 19 cases. Am J Obstet Gynecol 1969; 105: 282–4.

39. Ayers LR, Drosman S, Saltzstein SL. Iatrogenic paracervical implantation of fetal tissue during a therapeutic abortion. Obstet Gynecol 1971; 37: 755–60.

40. Arvay A. Gorgey M, Kapu L. La relation entre les avortements (interruptions de la grossesse) et les accouchements prématurés. Rev Franc Gynec Obstet 1967; 62: 81–6.

41. Taylor PJ, Cumming DC, Hill PJ. Significance of intrauterine adhesions detected hysteroscopically in eumenorrheic infertile women and role of antecedent curettage in their formation. Am J Obstet Gynecol 1981; 139: 239–42.

42. Houwert-de Jong MH, Eskes TKAB, Termijtelen A et al. Habitual abortion: a review. Eur J Obstet Gynecol 1989; 30: 39.

43. Glaser D, Wank R, Bartsch-Sandhoff M et al. Immunotherapy after recurrent abortions with a paternal chromosomal translocation. Geburtshilfe Frauenheilkd 1989; 49: 58–60.

44. Parke A, Maier D, Hakim C et al. Subclinical autoimmune-disease and recurrent spontaneous abortion. J Rheumatol 1986; 13: 1178–80.

45. Iffy L. Embryologic studies of time of conception in ectopic pregnancy and first trimester abortion. Obstet Gynecol 1965; 26: 490–8.

46. Mikamo K, Iffy L. Aging of the ovum. Obstet Gynecol Annu 1974; 3: 47–99.

47. Morton NE, Chiu D, Holland C et al. Chromosome anomalies as predictors of recurrence risk for spontaneous abortion. Am J Med Genet 1987; 28: 353–60.

48. Lancet M, Jakobovits A. Abnormalities of position, shape, and structure of the pregnant uterus. In: Iffy L, Kaminetzky HA (eds), Principles and Practice of Obstetrics and Perinatology, p. 1471 Wiley: New York.

49. Swahn ML, Bygdeman M. Termination of early pregnancy with RU 486 (Mifepristone) in combination with a prostaglandin analogue (Sulprostone). Acta Obstet Gynecol Scand 1990; 68: 293–306.

50. Autry AM, Hayes EC, Jaobson GF et al. A comparison of medical induction and dilation and evacuation for second trimester abortion. Am J Obstet Gynecol 2002; 187: 393–7.

51. Shulman LP, Ling FW, Meyers CM et al. Dilation and evacuation is a preferable method for mid-trimester genetic termination of pregnancy. Prenat Diagn 1989; 9: 741–2.

52. Klinte I, Hamberger L, Wiqvist N. 2nd-trimester abortion by extra-amniotic instillation of Rivanol combined with intravenous

administration of oxytocin or prostaglandin-F2-alpha. Acta Obstet Gynecol Scand 1983; 62: 303–6.

53. Uldbjerg N, Ekman G, Malmström A et al. Biochemical and morphologic changes of human cervix after local application of prostaglandin E2 in pregnancy. Lancet 1981; 1: 267–8.

54. WHO Task Force on the Use of Prostaglandins for the Regulation of Fertility. Prostaglandins and abortion. II. Single extra-amniotic administration of 0.92 mg of 15-methyl-prostaglandin F2a in Hyskon for termination of pregnancies in weeks 10 to 20 of gestation: an international multicenter study. Am J Obstet Gynecol 1977; 129: 593–6.

55. Hill NCW, MacKenzie IZ. 2308 second trimester terminations using extra-amniotic or intra-amniotic prostaglandin E2: an analysis of efficacy and complications. Br J Obstet Gynaecol 1989; 96: 1424–31.

56. Schneider D, Langer R, Golan A et al. Induced early midtrimester abortion in primigravid adolescents: comparison between laminaria dilatation-evacuation and extra-amniotic PGFi2a infusion. Isr J Obstet Gynecol 1991; 2: 170.

57. WHO Task Force on Prostaglandins for Fertility Regulation, Special Programme of Research, Development and Research Training in Human Reproduction. Vaginal administration of 15-methyl-PGF2a methyl ester for preoperative cervical dilatation. Contraception 1981; 23: 251–9.

58. Less A, Goldberger SB, Bernheim B et al. Vaginal prostaglandin E2 and fetal amniotic fluid embolus. JAMA 1990; 263: 3259–60.

59. Chervenak FA, McCullough LB. An ethically justified, clinically comprehensive management strategy for 3rd-trimester pregnancies complicated by fetal anomalies. Obstet Gynecol 1990; 74: 311–16.

60. Papp Z, Tóth Z, Szabó M et al. Prenatal screening for neural tube defects and other malformations by both serum AFP and ultrasound. In: Kurjak A (ed), The Fetus as a Patient, pp. 167–80. Elsevier: Amsterdam, 1985.

61. Cohen LG. Before Their Time: fetuses and Infants at Risk. American Association of Mental Retardation: Washington, D.C. 1990.

62. Papp Z. Genetic counseling and termination of pregnancy in Hungary. J Med Philos 1989; 14: 323.

63. Evans MI, Kramer RL, Yaron Y et al. What are the ethical and technical problems associated with multifetal pregnancy reduction? Clin Obstet Gynecol 1998; 41: 46–54.

64. Patkós P, Tóth-Pál E, Papp Z et al. Multiembryonic pregnancy reduction: the Hungarian experience. Am J Obstet Gynecol 2002; 186: 596–7.

65. Itskovitz-Eldor J, Drugan A, Levron J et al. Transvaginal embryonic aspiration (TEA) – a safe method for selective reduction in multiple gestation. Am J Obstet Gynecol 1992; 166: 3581–5.

66. Kerenyi TD, Chitkara Y. Selective birth in twin pregnancy with discordancy for Down's syndrome. N Engl J Med 1981; 304: 1525–7.

67. Evans MI, Krivchenia EL, Gelber SE et al. Selective reduction. Clin Perinatol 2003; 30: 103–11.

68. Ornoy A, Salamon-Arnon J, Ben-Zur Z et al. Placental finding in spontaneous abortions and stillbirths. Teratology 1981; 24: 243–52.

10 Percutaneous intrauterine fetal shunting

Sundeep G Keswani, R Douglas Wilson, and Mark P Johnson

In utero fetal surgery continues to develop with improved imaging, improved selection of candidates for fetal surgery, and the use of innovative fetal therapy. Imaging techniques such as fetal ultrasound (2-D, 3-D), fetal echocardiography, fetal Doppler assessment including the placenta, and magnetic resonance imaging (MRI) have allowed more accurate diagnosis and assessment to be utilized prior to *in utero* fetal therapy.[1] The broad categories of surgical *in utero* fetal therapy can be separated into either *open* uterine techniques or *closed* endoscopic/ultrasound guided techniques requiring only puncture of the uterus with single or multiple ports. The 'Achilles' heel' of open fetal surgery, due to its traumatic nature, is increased incidence of preterm labor and delivery. Conversely, the benefits of minimally invasive fetal intervention include decreased uterine irritability and decreased incidence of preterm labor. Current practice prior to maternal/fetal surgery must include a discussion with the parents of the risks and benefits to both mother and fetus. The ethical discussion will vary depending on whether the congenital malformation has a high likelihood of lethality compared with nonlethal fetal anomalies.[2]

Fetal abnormalities involving outflow obstruction of the bladder or fluid-filled, space-occupying lesions in the fetal chest result in severe morbidity and/or mortality depending on the severity of the abnormality.[3-8] Select patients with these disorders may benefit from *in utero* drainage of these fluid-filled lesions. This chapter aims to summarize the present status of closed *in utero* fetal therapy using a pigtail shunt to create vesicoamniotic or thoracoamniotic decompression of the fluid-filled space. The specific pathology involves lower urinary tract bladder neck obstruction, pleural effusion (PE), and macrocystic adenomatoid malformation of the lung (CCAM). Each of these conditions will be reviewed, looking at the pathophysiology, selection criteria for *in utero* therapy, operative shunt technique, perioperative complications, and perinatal/neonatal outcome.

Obstructive uropathy

Fetal obstructive uropathies are a diverse and heterogeneous group of developmental abnormalities that generally involve obstruction of the proximal urethra in the male fetus.[9-11] Megacystis or enlarged bladder may derive from two main etiologies.[12] In the first group, there may be an obstruction of the flow of urine out of the bladder. This is more common in the male fetus and is due to abnormal development of the urethra. The specific etiology for the obstruction may range from complete urethral atresia to the formation of urethral valves that develop within the proximal urethra. Bladder obstruction in the female fetus is usually due to complex cloachal developmental anomalies. In the second group, enlarged bladder is secondary to nonobstructive causes. This group is very heterogeneous, usually has normal amniotic fluid volumes, and is excluded from *in utero* therapy.

Pathophysiology of *in utero* urinary tract obstruction

Bladder neck obstruction[12-16] may be complete or partial, but the more complete the obstruction, the earlier in gestation is the onset of bladder enlargement. Complete urethral obstruction or significant restriction of urethral flow results in accumulation of urine within the fetal bladder, leading to megacystis (Figure 10.1). Prolonged obstruction results in smooth muscle hypertrophy and hyperplasia within the bladder wall and eventually impairment of contractual capacity, compliance, and elasticity. Bladder distention results in elevated intravesical pressures which may overcome the delicate physiologic valve mechanism at the ureterovesical junctions. Reflux eventually results, contributing to development of hydroureters and hydronephrosis. Hydronephrosis develops from both continued urine production and ureteral reflux from the distended and

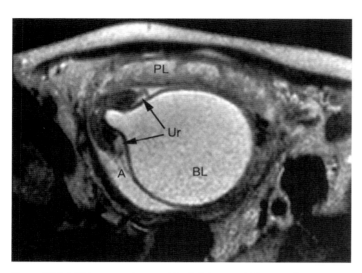

Figure 10.1 MRI transverse image of fetal abdomen with lower urinary tract obstruction (BL = bladder; Ur = hydroureters; A = ascites; PL = placenta).

obstructed bladder. The renal pelvises and calyces systems become progressively enlarged and compress the renal parenchyma against the distended renal capsule.[12–16] Histologic studies indicate a progressive dilation of the distal to proximal renal tubule associated with the development of peritubular and interstitial fibrosis. Ultrasound is able to identify these renal changes due to the increasing echogenicity of the renal parenchyma. This obstructive process leads to type IV cystic degeneration of the kidneys and renal insufficiency at birth.[12–16]

After 14 weeks' gestation, amniotic fluid volume is principally derived from fetal urine production. In cases of urinary tract obstruction, fetal urine cannot replenish amniotic fluid volume lost by membrane reabsorption, fetal swallowing, and fetal breathing, and the result is the development of progressive oligohydramnios. Subsequent severe oligo- or anhydramnios and massive megacystis lead to physical deformation and physiologic changes characteristic of the prune belly and Potter sequence, which include a markedly protuberant abdomen with apparent decrease in skeletal muscle present within the rectus sheath, joint contractures, compressive facial abnormalities, and pulmonary hypoplasia from intrathoracic pressure alterations and impaired fetal breathing that appears to have an important effect on lung development and maturation. The presence of severe oligohydramnios during the transition from the canalicular to the alveolar phase of development, which occurs at 18–24 weeks' gestation, results in severely underdeveloped lungs and respiratory insufficiency at birth.[15] Nakayama et al documented a 45% mortality rate in boys presenting at birth with posterior urethral valves (PUV), a defect directly attributable to pulmonary insufficiency.[17]

PUV are unique to the male fetus/newborn. The incidence is 1 in 8000 births.[18] PUV comprise three types,[19] the most common type I having folds extending from the verumontanum to the membranous urethra, type II (least common) having folds from the verumontanum up to the bladder neck, and type III

having a concentric diaphragm with the central lumen in the prostatic urethra. PUV occur sporadically, and do not have an increased risk of recurrence in future pregnancies. PUV usually occur in isolation without organ system involvement outside the urinary tract, but there may be secondary deformations due to oligohydramnios sequence including the face, limbs or lungs. Confirmation of prenatally suspected PUV occurs in 50% of cases, with typical findings of fetal hydroureteronephrosis, distended and thickened bladder, and dilated posterior urethra.[20] Multivariant analysis identified only two variables as independent predictors of fetal urethral obstruction: oligohydramnios and (odds ratio 5.95%, CI 1.5–15) megacystis (odds ratio 9.95, 95% CI 2–14).[21]

Urethral atresia is a condition that might present in a similar manner but is much less common.[12] Since the urethral obstruction is complete, it is usually associated with earlier onset of oligohydramnios than other etiologies.

Another megacystis diagnosis is prune belly syndrome,[13–15] which is described in boys with urinary tract dilation, and is associated with cryptorchidism and incomplete development of the abdominal wall muscles. The term 'prune belly syndrome' has been used for both obstructive and nonobstructive uropathies with this similar clinical appearance. There is some debate whether the condition represents a case of functional urinary flow impairment or results from a transient physical obstruction of the fetal urethra.

Prenatal selection criteria for vesicoamniotic shunting

Fetuses with isolated megacystis, bilateral hydronephrosis, decreased amniotic fluid volume, no other associated congenital anomalies, a normal 46 XY male karyotype, and serially improving urine hypotonicity (Table 10.1) are considered appropriate for therapy.[12–15,22–26] The diagnosis of renal impairment is more difficult at less than 20 weeks' gestation, since early in gestation fetal urine is almost isotonic with plasma due to the physiologic immature tubular function. Serial fetal urine samples allow a better assessment of renal function, and the recommendation is for three fetal urine specimens over a 5–7-day period.[13–15,22] Ultrasound findings and fetal urinary analysis are combined to identify appropriate fetal candidates for in utero therapy.[12–15,22,23] The sonographic appearance of the fetal bladder may help differentiate 'prune belly syndrome' from obstructive uropathies.[14,15] The bladder is always thick-walled and tense in the presence of obstruction. Ultrasound may not be able to differentiate between posterior urethral valves and urethral atresia.[23] Increased renal echogenicity with loss of cortical medullary differentiation and the presence of subcortical cysts indicates renal dysplasia and is a poor prognostic sign for fetal renal function.[23] The severity of oligohydramnios can be evaluated by quantitative ultrasound assessment (amniotic fluid index).

Table 10.1 Fetal urine parameters to assess renal function

Parameters associated with potential renal salvage

Sodium	≤ 100 mEq/l
Osmolality	≤ 200 mOSm/l
Chloride	≤ 90 mEq/l
Calcium	≤ 8 mg/dl
Total protein	≤ 40 mg/dl
B-2 microglobulin	< 6 mg/l

Amnioinfusion, vesicocentesis, and vesicoamniotic shunt technique

Amnioinfusion is generally required prior to shunt insertion because of the markedly diminished amniotic fluid volume surrounding the fetus.[15] The amnioinfusion allows improved visualization and access to the fetus. Amnioinfusion is done under continuous ultrasound guidance, using warmed, lactated Ringer's solution, and a 20-gauge spinal needle inserted as high in the fundus as possible to decrease the risk of fluid leakage. Color-flow Doppler can be used to avoid the umbilical cord, which is usually present in the small apparent fluid pockets in these cases. The volume of amnioinfusion is usually 300–500 cc, resulting in a normal amniotic fluid index for the gestational age of the fetus. Maternal oral broad-spectrum antibiotic prophylaxis is recommended after both amnioinfusion and shunt placement.

Vesicocentesis is performed under continuous ultrasound guidance to ensure appropriate needle position throughout. Using a 22-gauge needle, the fetal abdomen is approached just above the pubic rami and lateral to midline. Before entering the bladder, color-flow Doppler is used to ensure that the potential needle track does not pass through the umbilical vessels that course laterally about the bladder. The needle is then passed into the lower bladder and the urine completely emptied while constantly maintaining needle-tip placement within the cavity of the shrinking bladder. Needle placement too high in the megacystis will not allow complete drainage, as the bladder drains downward into the fetal pelvis. Paralyzing the fetus with intramuscular administration of pancuronium prior to the vesicocentesis or vesicoamniotic shunt placement procedures is generally not necessary.

Careful sonographic evaluation prior to attempted shunt placement is essential to identify the location and position of the fetus and placenta. It is preferable that the fetus be approached without having to pass the shunt trocar through the placenta, although, if necessary, this can be done without subsequent problems in most cases.

Once the appropriate approach is chosen after sonographic evaluation, the maternal skin is anesthetized with 1% lidocaine and a small 3–5-mm stab wound is made to allow easy passage of the shunt trocar. The shunt trocar is then carefully introduced into the amniotic space near the lower fetal abdomen. An adequate pocket of amniotic fluid needs to be present in which to drop the distal end of the vesicoamniotic shunt on exiting the fetal abdomen. If no such space is present, amnioinfusion to create such a fluid pocket can be done through the trocar or its side port. We routinely use the shunt apparatus offered by Rocket of London, as well as their Rodeck vesicoamniotic shunt catheters (Figure 10.2). The tip of the trocar is positioned in the same manner as the vesicocentesis needle, and color-flow

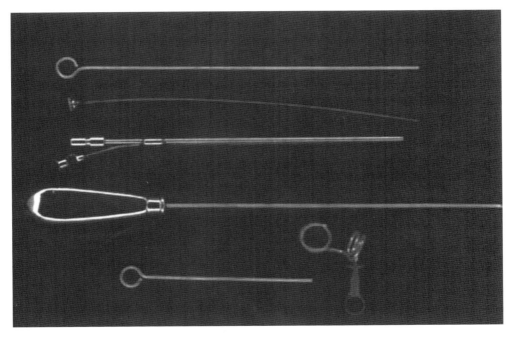

Figure 10.2 Rocket of London™ vesicoamniotic shunt apparatus and double pig-tail shunt.

Doppler used to confirm the absence of umbilical vessels at that position. The trocar is then quickly inserted into the bladder and positioned into a central location. At this point, the operative assistant should have carefully and gently straightened the vesicoamniotic catheter and passed it over the introducing guide wire. Once the catheter is loaded into the trocar sheath, the introducing wire is removed and the proximal end of the shunt is placed into the fetal bladder. The trocar is then backed out of the fetal abdomen deploying the straight segment of the shunt, and next the distal end of the pigtail shunt is deployed outside the abdomen into the amniotic space. The patient is then placed on external uterine monitoring for approximately 2 hours to rule out preterm contractions. Any indication of uterine irritability is aggressively treated with intravenous fluids and tocolytic medications. This is usually an outpatient procedure and rarely requires an overnight hospital stay.

Complications

Counseling the patient prior to any invasive needle or shunt procedure includes discussion of the risks of chorioamnionitis, premature rupture of membranes, direct trauma to the fetus, placental bleeding, and possible preterm labor.[12–15,22,24,27–36] Transient vesicoperitoneal fistulas occasionally occur after vesicocentesis, resulting in urinary ascites. These fistulas close spontaneously in 10–14 days with redevelopment of the megacystis. Displacement of the shunt is a fairly common complication, occurring in approximately 30–45% of reported cases. Appropriate fetal lower abdominal location decreases the risk of shunt displacement due to bladder decompression. Repeat shunt insertions may be necessary depending on the clinical situation. There are not good estimates for risk of pregnancy loss as a result of the shunt procedure. A recent review showed a 5% (9/169) intrauterine death rate following successful shunt placement.[23] Vesicocentesis pregnancy loss rates are considered to be similar to amniocentesis rates at 0.5–1.0%.

Outcome

Reviews of published studies[24,27–36] have indicated that limiting intervention to fetuses with good prognosis (i.e., adequate fetal renal function) appears to improve survival and results in a lower incidence of renal failure in survivors. Crombleholme et al[28] and Freeman et al[37] evaluated outcomes based on predicted prognosis as determined by fetal urine biochemistry. Forty-five patients underwent successful shunt intervention. In the group predicted to have good prognosis, 85% of survivors had normal renal function while in the group predicted to have poor prognosis this prognosis was confirmed in 88%. When amniotic fluid volume returned to normal, there was no postnatal respiratory compromise consistent with previous animal studies, indicating that correction of oligohydramnios prevents pulmonary hypoplasia.

Table 10.2 summarizes nine series with fetal obstructive uropathy evaluating treatment and outcome.[24,27–34] There may

be some duplication of cases in the early and later years of these center limited series, but the estimated incidence of renal impairment/failure in the treated survivors based on postnatal renal function is 46% (29/63). The length of follow-up is variable, so 46% is a minimal estimated of renal impairment and may be higher as overall survival for this population is only 44% (111/252).

More recently, we have reviewed our experience with vesicoaminiotic shunts.[38] Twenty fetuses were treated with vesicoamniotic shunts with an over-all survival rate of 90%. The follow-up of the survivors was nearly 6 years. Of these children, 44% had normal renal function, 22% had renal insufficiency, and a third required renal dialysis prior to renal transplant. Sixty percent had normal bladder function, and the majority of the children had minimal or no respiratory problems. These data with longer-term follow-up suggest that the use of vesicoamniotic shunts can salvage renal function and minimize long-term pulmonary complications in select patients.

Lastly, another small series demonstrated vesicocentesis at 10–14 weeks as a useful treatment option in some fetuses with early megacystis.[39] This could be considered in early onset presentation, but the personal experience of the authors has been that early megacystis may decompress spontaneously prior to 14 weeks' gestation.

Idiopathic pleural effusion

Fetal pleural effusions (PE) can present as isolated sonographic findings or as part of a more generalized picture of nonimmune fetal hydrops. They can be divided into primary and secondary causes.[5,40–44] Primary PE is a lymphatic malformation while secondary PE is usually due to associated abnormalities such as cardiac defects, anemia, infection, and aneuploidy. Primary PE occurs in approximately 1 in 12 000 pregnancies with a 2:1 male to female ratio.[40] Gestational age at presentation of less than 32 weeks and the presence of hydrops are associated with a high perinatal mortality rate of 36–46%.[40–44] Gender of the fetus, extent of the effusions, and mode of delivery are not significantly related to outcome. Isolated PE that does not progress to fatal fetal hydrops poses a threat to the developing fetus by acting as a space-occupying lesion with resulting intrathoracic compression of the developing lungs and potential disturbance of intrathoracic blood flow secondary to increased intrathoracic pressure and mediastinal shift of the heart and great vessels (Figure 10.3). The risk of deformation effects from the PE is directly related to the size of the space-occupying volume. There does not appear to be any significance to the laterality of the PE, but bilateral PE potentially will have more of a detrimental compressive effect.[44]

Table 10.2 Fetal obstructive uropathy: evaluation, treatment, outcome

Author	No.	Treatment groups			Outcomes				
		Open	Shunt	Other	Survivor	Survivor renal failure	TOP	IUD	NND
Elder et al[27] (1987)	57	2	21	47	6/28*	–	8/28	–	14/28
Crombleholme et al**[28] (1990)	24 (poor)	–	10	–	3	2/3	14	7	–
	16 (good)	–	9	–	13	2/13	1	2	–
Manning[29] (1991)	87	–	87	–	35	–	13	4	35
Lipitz et al[24] (1993)	25	–	14	–	9	7/9	9	–	7
Freedman et al***[30] (1999)	34	–	34	–	21	8/14		13	
Shimada et al[31] (1998)	6	–	6	–	6	1/6	–	–	–
Holmes et al[32] (2001)	14	2	9	3	8	5/8	–	–	6
McLorie et al[33] (2001)	12	–	9	–	6	3/6	3	3	–
Wilson[34] (unpublished)	6	–	3	3	4	1/4	2	–	–
			202		111/252 (44%)	29/63 (46%)			

* Review of literature article: management of 28 fetuses with megacystitis and oligohydramnios.
** Pretreatment renal prediction by urinary electrolytes: poor vs good.
*** Follow-up and greater than age 2 on 14 of 21 survivors.
TOP; termination of pregnancy; IUD; intrauterine death; NND; neonatal death.

Patient selection criteria for treatment of pleural effusion

Selection criteria for PE treatment by thoracoamniotic shunting requires primary PE etiology with normal karyotype, negative viral cultures, normal echocardiogram, no other significant congenital anomalies, rapid recurrence of the effusion after thoracocentesis, and gestational age of less than 32 weeks.[15,40,41] Minimal evaluation would include maternal infectious evaluation, but some reports suggest that cordocentesis is required for hematologic abnormalities (hematocrit and reticulocyte count), fetal infection IgG, IgM titers for specific infectious pathogens, and liver profile (enzymes, albumin, and total protein values).[15]

Thoracocentesis and thoracoamniotic shunt technique

Thoracocentesis utilizes a 22-gauge needle under continuous ultrasound guidance with insertion into the lower lateral aspect of the fetal hemithorax in the midaxillary line. This entrance point is important in that this is the most dependent portion of the thorax into which the effusion will collect as one aspirates, allowing the maximum amount of fluid to be removed while avoiding intrathoracic structures that may begin to return to their normal anatomic positions during the aspiration. Re-evaluation is then done in 24–72 hours, to look for recurrence of the effusion. Effusions which rapidly reaccumulate after thoracocentesis identify the fetus that will most likely benefit from chronic drainage through thoracoamniotic shunt placement as long as other causes of the effusions have been eliminated.

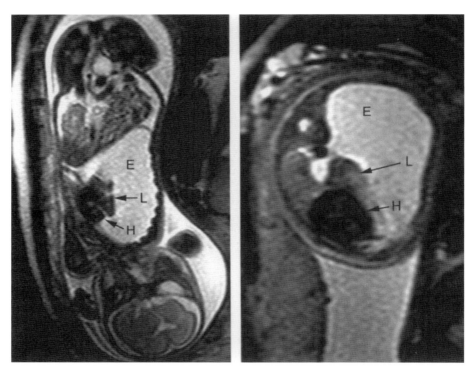

Figure 10.3 Sagittal and transverse MRI images of congenital pleural effusion (E). Notice the displacement and compression of the heart (H) and lungs (L), and the presence of hydrops (ascites and skin edema).

The technique of placing a thoracoamniotic shunt is similar to that used for bladder insertion, but the thoracic location of the shunt is a significant factor. Under ultrasound guidance, the appropriate approach to the fetal hemithorax is visualized. The maternal skin is then anesthetized with 1% xylocaine and a small, 3-mm incision through the skin is made to allow the insertion of the trocar apparatus. The sharp tip of the shunt trocar is anchored between the two chosen ribs at the entrance site. An appropriate position is at or just slightly posterior to the midaxillary line in the lower half of the thoracic cavity. By a gentle twisting action, the trocar is carefully advanced above the inferior rib through the chest wall such that the tip lies 3–5 mm within the chest cavity. The stylet is then removed and the double pig-tailed shunt inserted into the trocar sheath. At this point it is quite common for effusion fluid to flow quite briskly out the end of the catheter, and it is important to proceed quickly so that the effusion pocket does not drain, as draining would make catheter placement more difficult and the proximal end within the chest cavity would not be able to resume its original coiled shape.

Once the catheter has been fed into the trocar, a short push rod is introduced into and slowly advanced down the trocar sheath, displacing the proximal segment of the catheter into the intended cavity. The metal tip and high-density composition of the Rodeck catheter make visualization of its entrance into the fluid cavity quite straightforward. The catheter will begin to resume its original coiled configuration on exposure to the warm environment of the effusion cavity. The short push rod is then removed, and a long push rod inserted and advanced until the distal tip of the catheter is encountered within the trocar sheath. At this point the catheter needs to be stabilized with the push rod while the trocar sheath is backed out through the chest wall for a distance of approximately 1–1.5 cm, which represents the straight portion of the catheter. Once outside within the amniotic cavity, the tip of the trocar sheath is deviated slightly away from the entrance site, and the remainder of the catheter passed from the trocar using the long push rod. If the tip of the trocar sheath is not deviated slightly away from the entrance site, the catheter may be further advanced into the chest cavity instead of being dropped into the amniotic space. Once placed, the effusion can generally be noted to begin drainage, a process that begins rapidly because of the initial increased intrathoracic pressure, but may take 12–48 hours to complete. Again, prophylactic oral antibiotic therapy is recommended for these invasive fetal procedures.

If polyhydramnios is present, amnioreduction to normalize amniotic fluid volume and endovaginal assessment of the maternal cervix is required to assess the risk of preterm labor and delivery after the shunt procedure.

Complications

The most common complications of thoracic shunt procedures are related to displacement of the catheter into the amniotic cavity or less commonly into the thoracic cavity.[15,41,45–49] If the catheter has been in place for a period of time, it may not need replacement, as, occasionally, an epithelialized tract remains, which serves as a fistulous drainage tract. If the catheter is placed too high or too posterior in the chest cavity, it may result in incomplete drainage, as the catheter tip may become occluded by the fetal lung as it expands to fill the space created by draining the effusion. Additional malfunction of the catheter may be due to occlusion from the proteinaceous material within the effusion, or to thrombus if bleeding has occurred during the shunt placement. Pregnancy loss (prematurity, preterm delivery, or intrauterine fetal death from injury) as a result of the shunt insertion is estimated at 5%. Thoracocentesis risks for pregnancy loss are estimated at 0.5–1.0%.

Outcome

The benefit of thoracoamniotic shunting in fetuses with PE is dependent on the correct selection of those fetuses that would benefit by this treatment.[34,43,45–50] For fetuses with hydrops or significant risk of pulmonary hypoplasia secondary to the PE (gestational age less than 24 weeks, mediastinal shift with bilateral lung compression, or polyhydramnios), it has been shown that effective drainage of the PE with the prevention of chronic antenatal intrathoracic compression leads to improved antenatal lung growth. Aubard et al[41] identified hydrops as the only prognostic factor for outcome following multivariant analysis. Survival after thoracoamniotic shunts with and without hydrops was 67% and 100%, respectively, while without treatment survival was 21–23% in both groups. Table 10.3 summarizes the use of thoracoamniotic shunting for PE.[34,43,45–49] Thompson et al[50] reviewed 17 surviving infants who had under-

gone shunting for PE with a mean gestational age of 29 weeks and a range of 21–35 weeks. Twelve fetuses were hydropic at the time of shunting. Recurrent respiratory symptoms were identified in six infants, but this did not differ significantly from respiratory symptoms in a control group. More recently, we reviewed our 3-year experience with the use of thoracoamniotic shunts for PE.[51] There were nine hydropic fetuses with idiopathic PE that were shunted at an average age of 26 weeks, with a mean age at diagnosis at 22 weeks. The average length of shunt therapy was 7 weeks, and the average gestational age at delivery was 33 weeks. The perinatal survival rate was 69%. Given the poor prognosis of these hydropic fetuses, these data in conjunction with the studies in Table 10.3 suggest an improved outcome with the use of thoracoamniotic shunts for PE.

Congenital cystic adenomatoid malformation

Congenital cystic adenomatoid malformations (CCAM) are benign, space-occupying tumors due to overgrowth of terminal respiratory bronchioles. CCAMs are most often unilobar (80–95%) and may affect any lobe.[8,51–55] They are generally classified prenatally by ultrasound/magnetic resonance imaging (MRI) into microcystic (50%) or macrocystic (50%) types depending on the size of the cysts.[8] CCAMs can occasionally

Table 10.3 Pleural effusion and treatment by thoracoamniotic shunt: outcome

Author	No.	LB	SB	NND	TA/SA	Hydrops	Survival
Rodeck et al[45] (1988)	8	6	–	2	–	5	75% (hydrops 65%)
Nicolaides & Azar[46] (1990)	51	33	2	12	4	18 (LB 12/14 resolved)	65%
Lasser & Timor-Tritsch[47] (1991)	1	1				1	100%
Bernaschek et al[48] (1994)	9	3	4	1	1	9	33%
Wilkins-Haug & Doubilet[49] (1997)	2	2	–	–	–	2	100%
Aubard et al*[41] (1998)	80	57 (48 regression) (11 recurrence)	21		–	63	74% (hydrops 67%, no hydrops 100%)
Wilson[34]	3	1	1	1	–	1	33%

*Review article includes Rodeck et al[45] and Nicolaides & Azar[46].
LB = live birth; SB = stillbirth; NND = neonatal death; TA/SA = therapeutic abortion/spontaneous abortion.

contain a single or several dominant macrocysts, which fill with lung fluid, progressively enlarging until they form large, space-occupying lesions within the fetal lung. Large lesions can cause rapid mediastinal shift and compromise of the hemodynamic state of the fetus, with the development of nonimmune hydrops. Early development and enlargement of the lesions can result in significant compression of fetal lung tissues, which may result in lethal pulmonary hypoplasia if this occurs during critical lung transition from the canalicular to the alveolar stage at 18–24 weeks' gestation. Mediastinal shift can also lead to compression of the fetal esophagus, decreased fetal swallowing of amniotic fluid, and consequent development of polyhydramnios with the risk of preterm delivery. CCAMs have a communication with the tracheobronchial tree, and there is a potential risk of air trapping after birth with the macrocystic CCAMs.[8,52] The fastest rate of CCAM growth usually occurs at 20–25 weeks with a plateau in the growth beginning at 26 weeks.[52] The natural history of CCAMs with a dominant macrocyst is more unpredictable than microcystic lesions because the rate of growth of the cystic and solid component can be quite different.[52]

The goal of shunt therapy focuses on chronic drainage of large macrocysts. Early therapy is directed at preventing pulmonary hypoplasia, while later interventions are done for hemodynamic disturbance resulting in evolving hydrops or progressive polyhydramnios due to esophageal compression.

Patient selection criteria for shunt therapy of CCAMs

In utero surgical intervention should be considered only for those fetuses that have developed secondary complications that worsen their prognosis, such as early onset hydrops or progressive polyhydramnios, and in whom simple chronic drainage of a large dominant macrocyst would potentially correct the underlying physical disturbance that led to the secondary complications.

Potential shunt candidates should have the diagnosis of macrocystic CCAM confirmed by ultrasound and/or fetal MRI,

as fetuses with other potential lesions are not likely to benefit from shunt therapy and could be harmed by attempted interventions.

Initially, ultrasound-guided thoracocentesis should be utilized to drain the dominant macrocyst and then serial scanning to evaluate how rapidly the fluid reaccumulates and whether chronic shunt drainage may be required. Polyhydramnios may require amnioreduction to keep the amniotic fluid volume within normal gestational age limits. If polyhydramnios is present, maternal endovaginal cervical measurements are necessary to ensure preterm labor and delivery risks are not increased. As in the two other shunt therapy preoperative requirements, the fetus must have a normal karyotype and an otherwise negative workup for fetal hydrops, including hematologic, infectious, and cardiovascular etiologies.

Thoracocentesis and thoracoamniotic shunt technique

The technique for thoracocentesis and shunt insertion is similar to that described for PE, although there may be some minor variation related to the lobar involvement in the left or right lung. Additionally, the point of entrance into the fetal chest should be chosen with careful consideration given to how the cyst may shrink during the drainage process such that the cyst can be completely drained of essentially all its fluid while retaining the original postion of the needle insertion and eliminating the need for needle repositioning which could potentially increase the morbidity of the procedure (Figures 10.4 and 10.5). Maternal oral, broad-spectrum antibiotic prophylaxis is recommended for thoracoamniotic shunt placement.

Complications

Overall procedure complications are similar to those related to shunting for PE, although the risk of shunt malfunction due to occlusion may be increased.[48,56–61] A potential complication is the risk of injuring a major blood vessel when entering the chest and while traversing the pulmonary parenchyma before

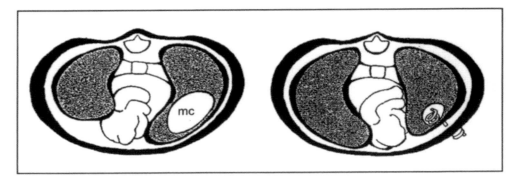

Figure 10.4 Drawing of a somewhat anteriorly positioned CCAM macrocyst (mc) before and after shunt placement. Prior fine-needle drainage of the macrocyst helped to determine the optimal position to enter the fetal chest for subsequent shunt placement.

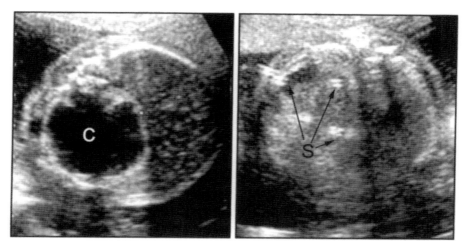

Figure 10.5 Ultrasound of a typical macrocystic CCAM with hydrops before and after shunt placement (C = macrocyst; S = shunt).

entering the macrocyst. This complication can be minimized if the shunt is placed while using color-flow Doppler to visualize major blood vessels. Although not directly contraindicated, all efforts should be made to avoid trocar passage through the placenta; this may result in hematoma formation or vascular damage to the placenta causing fetal demise or abruption. If a transplacental approach is necessary, color-flow Doppler to avoid large vessels should be employed.

As in all fetal therapies, the potential of uterine irritability exists. We therefore monitor patients for at least 2 hours and utilize aggressive tocolytic therapy as indicated.

Outcome

The natural history of CCAMs shows that fetal hydrops is a significant prognostic factor. Review of published reports[48,56–62] shows that hydrops was present in a live-born continuing group at 7% (8/117) and in a perinatal loss group at 52% (22/42) (Table 10.4). Laberge et al[61] reviewed 48 cases of CCAM and found that only hydrops was a significant prognostic factor. We have recently reviewed our experience with the use of thoracoamniotic shunts for macrocystic CCAMs[62] associated with fetal hydrpos or recurrent significant polyhydramnios. A total of 10 shunts were placed at a mean gestational age of 23 weeks after the initial diagnosis at 20 weeks. Insertion of the shunt resulted in a 50% reduction in the mass of the CCAM and the CCAM volume ratio.[52,62] The mean duration of the shunt was 10 weeks, and fetuses were delivered at an average of 33 weeks with a perinatal survival rate of 70%. These findings suggest an improved outcome in these otherwise critically ill fetuses.

Conclusions

Present-day obstetric care more frequently utilizes routine prenatal assessment by ultrasound at 18–22 weeks. Prenatal identification of renal and thoracic abnormalities are more common, and counseling regarding the medical and surgical options for these lesions continues to be developed. The key to success for the *in utero* therapy of bladder and thoracic abnormalities is appropriate evaluation to ensure correct diagnosis and prediction of the morbidity or mortality. The selection criteria for fetuses undergoing *in utero* therapy must be limited to those fetuses that are anticipated to benefit by the therapy. The preliminary data suggest that the use of vesicoamniotic and thoracoamniotic shunts can benefit this select group of fetuses with fluid-filled lesions of either the bladder or the chest, respectively. As the use of this therapeutic modality increases, prospective randomized trials will determine the utility, efficacy, risk, and benefits of intrauterine fetal shunting for the mother and the fetus.

Table 10.4 Cystic adenomatoid malformation of the lung (CCAM): outcomes after thoracoamniotic shunts placement

Author	No	Shunts	LB	SB	NND	TA/SA	Survival
Bernaschek et al[48] (1994)	4	4	3 (1 H)	–	1 (H)	–	75% shunt 3/4
Miller et al[56] (1996)	17	1 (PTD)	12	2 (2 H)	–	3 (2 H)	71% shunt 1/1
Dommergues et al[57] (1997)	33 (4BPS)	9 (H,P)	BPS 4 CCAM 23 (5 H)	–	3 (1 H)	3 (3 H)	79% Shunt 6/9
Monni et al[58] (2000)	26	0	17 (3 PTD)	–		9 (2H)	65%
Bunduki et al[59] (2000)	18	1	13 (2 H)	2 (2 H)	3 (3 H)	–	72% shunt 1/1
De Santis et al[60] (2000)	17	0	13	1 (H)	1 (H)	2	76%
Laberge et al[61] (2001)	48	1 (H)	36	0	4 (3 H)	8 (1 H)	75% shunt 0/1
Baxter et al[62] (2001)	10	10 (6H)	7 (4 H)	1 (H)	2 (H)	–	70% shunt 7/10
Total	169	26	124 (12H)	6 (6H)	14 (10H)	25 (8H)	73% shunt 18/26 (69%)

H = hydrops; P = polyhydramnios; PTD = preterm delivery; BPS = bronchopulmonary sequestration, LB = live birth, SB = stillbirth, NND = neonatal death, TA/SA = therapeutic abortion/spontaneous abortion.

References

1. Wilson RD. Prenatal evaluation for fetal surgery. Curr Opin Obstet Gynecol 2002; 14: 187–93.

2. Flake AW. Prenatal intervention: ethical considerations for life-threatening and non-life-threatening anomalies. Semin Pediatr Surg 2001; 10: 212–21.

3. Cromie WJ. Implications of antenatal ultrasound screening in the incidence of major genitourinary malformations. Semin Pediatr Surg 2001; 10: 204–11.

4. Cromie WJ, Lee K, Houde K et al. Implications of prenatal ultrasound screening in the incidence of major genitourinary malformations. J Urol 2001; 10: 204–11.

5. Santolaya-Forgas J. Opinion. How do we counsel patient carrying a fetus with pleural effusions? Ultrasound Obstet Gynecol 2001; 18: 305–8.

6. Farmer DL, Albanese CT. Fetal hydrothorax. In: Harrison MR et al, eds. The Unborn Patient, pp. 373–8. WB Saunders: Philadelphia, 2001.

7. Bunduki V, Ruano R, da Silva MM et al. Prognostic factors associated with congenital cystic adenomatoid malformation of the lung. Prenat Diagn 2000; 20: 459–64.

8. Adzick NS. Fetal cystic adenomatoid malformation of the lung: diagnosis, perinatal management and outcome. Semin Thorac Cardiovas Surg 1994; 6: 247–52.

9. Poucell-Hatton S, Huang M, Bannykh S et al. Fetal obstructive uropathy: patterns of renal pathology. Pediatr Develop Pathol 2000; 3: 223–31.

10. Housley HT, Harrison MR. Fetal urinary tract abnormalities. Natural history, pathophysiology, and treatment. Urol Clin North Am 1998; 25: 63–73.

11. Bianchi, DW, Crombleholme TM, D'Alton ME. Hydronephrosis: bladder outlet obstruction. In: Fetology, pp. 593–606. McGraw-Hill: New York, 2000.

12. McHugo J, Whittle M. Enlarged fetal bladders: aetiology, management and outcome. Prenat Diagn 2001; 21: 958–63.

13. Walsh DS, Johnson MP. Fetal intervention for obstructive uropathy. Semin Perinatol 1999; 23: 484–95.

14. Johnson MP, Freedman AL. Fetal uropathy. Curr Opin Obstet Gynecol 1999; 11: 185–94.

15. Johnson MP, Flake AW, Quintero RA et al. Fetal shunt procedures. In: Evans MI, Johnson MP, Moghissi KS (eds), Invasive Outpatient Procedures in Reproductive Medicine, pp. 61–89. Lippincott-Raven: Philadelphia, 1997.

16. Woolf AS, Thiruchelvam N. Congenital obstructive uropathy: its origin and contribution to end-stage renal disease in children. Adv Ren Replace Ther 2001; 8: 157–63.

17. Nakayama DK, Harrison MR, de Lorimier AA. Prognosis of posterior urethral valves presenting at birth. J Pediatr Surg 1986; 21: 43–5.

18. Cuckow PM. Posterior urethral valves. In: Stringer MD, Oldham KT, Mouriquand PDE (eds), Pediatric Surgery and Urology: Long Term Outcomes, pp. 487–500. Saunders: London, 1998.

19. Hill GS. Calcium and the kidney, hydronephrosis. In: Jennette JC, Olson JL, Schwartz MM (eds), Heptinstall's Pathology of the Kidney, pp. 891–936. Lippincott-Raven: Philadelphia, 1998.

20. Abbott JF, Levine D, Wapner R. Posterior urethral valves: inaccuracy of prenatal diagnosis. Fetal Diagn Ther 1998; 13: 179–83.

21. Oliveira EA, Diniz JS, Cabral AC et al. Predictive factors of fetal urethral obstruction: a multivariate analysis. Fetal Diagn Ther 2000; 15: 180–6.

22. Nicolini U, Spelzini F. Invasive assessment of fetal renal abnormalities: urinalysis, fetal blood sampling and biopsy. Prenat Diagn 2001; 21: 964–9.

23. Agarwal SK, Fisk NM. In utero therapy for lower urinary tract obstruction. Prenat Diagn 2001; 21: 970–6.

24. Lipitz S, Ryan G, Samuell C et al. Fetal urine analysis for the assessment of renal function in obstructive uropathy. Am J Obstet Gynecol 1993; 1: 174–9.

25. Nicolaides KH, Cheng HH, Snijders RJM et al. Fetal urine biochemistry in the assessment of obstructive uropathy. Am J Obstet Gynecol 1992; 3: 932–7.

26. Nicolini U, Fisk NM, Rodeck CH et al. Fetal urine biochemistry: an index of renal maturation and dysfunction. Br J Obstet Gynaecol 1992; 99: 46–50.

27. Elder JS, Duckett JW, Snyder HM. Intervention for fetal obstructive uropathy: has it been effective? Lancet 1987; 1007–10.

28. Crombleholme TM, Harrison MR, Golbus MS et al. Fetal intervention in obstructive uropathy: prognostic indicators and efficacy of intervention. Am J Obstet Gynecol 1990; 5: 1239–44.

29. Manning FA. The fetus with obstructive uropathy: the fetal surgery registry. In: Harrison MR et al (eds) The Unborn Patient, pp. 394–8. WB Saunders: Philadelphia, 1991.

30. Freedman AL, Johnson MP, Smith CA et al. Long-term outcome in children after antenatal intervention for obstructive uropathies. Lancet 1999: 354: 374–7.

31. Shimada K, Hosokawa S, Tohda A et al. Follow-up of children after fetal treatment for obstructive uropathy. Int J Urol 1998; 5: 312–16.

32. Holmes N, Harrison MR, Baskin LS. Fetal surgery for posterior urethral valves: long term postnatal outcomes. Pediatrics 2001; 108: E7.

33. McLorie G, Farhat W, Khoury AN et al. Outcome analysis of vesicoamniotic shunting in a comprehensive population. J Urol 2001; 166: 1036–40.

34. Wilson RD. British Columbia Women's Hospital, University of British Columbia, Vancouver, 1998, unpublished.

35. Herndon CD, Ferrer FA, Freedman A et al. Consensus on the prenatal management of antenatally detected urological abnormalities. J Urol 2000; 164: 1052–6.

36. Coplen DE. Prenatal intervention for hydronephrosis. J Urol 1997; 157: 2270–7.

37. Freedman AL, Bukowski TP, Smith CA et al. Fetal therapy for obstructive uropathy: specific outcome diagnosis J Urol 1996; 156: 720.

38. Biard JM, Johnson MP, Carr M et al. Long term outcomes in children treated by prenatal vesicoamniotic shunting for lower urinary tract obstruction (LUTO). Am J Obstet Gynecol 2003; 189: S220.

39. Carroll SGM, Soothill PW, Tizard J et al. Vesicocentesis at 10–14 weeks of gestation for treatment of fetal megacystis. Ultrasound Obstet Gynecol 2001; 18: 366–370.

40. Bianchi DW, Crombleholme TM, D'Alton ME. Hydrothorax. In: Fetology, pp. 313–21. McGraw-Hill: New York, 2000.

41. Aubard Y, Derouineau I, Aubard V et al. Primary fetal hydrothorax: a literature review and proposed antenatal clinical strategy. Fetal Diagn Ther 1998; 13: 325–33.

42. Hagay Z, Reece A, Roberts A et al. Reviews. Isolated fetal pleural effusion: a prenatal management dilemma. Obstet Gynecol 1993; 81: 147–52.

43. Laberge JM, Crombleholme TM, Longaker M. The fetus with pleural effusions. In: Harrison MR et al (eds) The Unborn Patient, pp. 314–19. WB Saunders: Philadelphia, 1991.

44. Weber AM, Philipson EH. Reviews. Fetal pleural effusions: a review and meta-analysis for prognostic indicators. Obstet Gynecol 1992; 79: 281–6.

45. Rodeck CH, Fisk NM, Fraser DI et al. Long-term in utero drainage of fetal hydrothorax. N Engl J Med 1988; 17: 1135–8.

46. Nicolaides KH, Azar GB. Thoraco-amniotic shunting. Fetal Diagn Ther 1990; 5: 153–64.

47. Lasser DM, Timor-Tritsch IE. In utero treatment of fetal hydrothorax with pleuro-amniotic shunting at 23 weeks' gestation. Am J Obstet Gynecol 1991; SPO Abstracts: 416.

48. Bernaschek G, Deutinger J, Hansmann M et al. Feto-amniotic shunting-report of the experience of four European centres. Prenat Diagn 1994; 14: 821–33.

49. Wilkins-Haug LE, Doubilet P. Successful thoracoamniotic shunting and review of the literature in unilateral pleural effusion with hydrops. J Ultrasound Med 1997; 16: 153–60.

50. Thompson PJ, Greenough A, Nicolaides KH. Respiratory function in infancy following pleuro-amniotic shunting. Fetal Diagn Ther 1993; 8: 79–83.

51. Wilson RD, Baxter JK, Johnson MP et al. Thoracoamniotic shunts: fetal treatment of pleural effusions and congenital cystic adenomatoid malformations. Fetal Diag Ther 2004, 19: 413–20.

52. Crombleholme TM, Coleman B, Hedrick HL et al. Cystic adenomatoid malformation volume ratio predicts outcome in prenatally diagnosed cystic adenomatoid malformation of the lung. J Pediatr Surg 2002; 37: 331–8.

53. Bianchi DW, Crombleholme TM, D'Alton ME. Cystic adenomatoid malformation. In: Fetology, pp. 289–97. McGraw-Hill: New York, 2000.

54. Osler AG, Fortune DW. Congenital cystic adenomatoid malformation of the lung. Am J Clin Pathol 1979; 70: 595–603.

55. Stocker JT, Madewell JER, Drake RM. Congenital cystic adenomatoid malformation of the lung: classification and morphologic spectrum. Hum Pathol 1977; 4: 155–171.

56. Miller JA, Corteville JE, Langer JC. Congenital cystic adenomatoid malformation in the fetus: natural history and predictors of outcome. J Pediatr Surg 1996; 31: 805–8.

57. Dommergues M, Louis-Sylvestre C, Mandelbrot L et al. Congenital adenomatoid malformation of the lung: when is active fetal therapy indicated? Am J Obstet Gynecol 1997; 177: 953–8.

58. Monni G, Paladini D, Ibba RM et al. Prenatal ultrasound diagnosis of congenital cystic adenomatoid malformation of the lung: a report of 26 cases and review of the literature. Ultrasound Obstet Gynecol 2000; 16: 159–62.

59. Bunduki V, Ruano R, Marquez da Silva M et al. Prognostic factors associated with congenital cystic adenomatoid malformation of the lung. Prenat Diagn 2000; 20: 459–64.

60. DeSantis M, Masini L, Noia G et al. Congenital cystic adenomatoid malformation of the lung: antenatal ultrasound findings and fetal-neonatal outcome. Fifteen years of experience. Fetal Diagn Ther 2000; 15: 246–50.

61. Laberge JM, Flageole H, Pugash D et al. Outcome of the prenatally diagnosed congenital cystic adenomatoid lung malformation: a Canadian experience. Fetal Diagn Ther 2001; 16: 178–86.

62. Baxter JK, Johnson MP, Wilson RD et al. Thoracoamniotic shunts: pregnancy outcome for congenital cystic adenomatoid malformation (CCM) and pleural effusion. Am J Obstet Gynecol 2001; 6: S245.

11 Cordocentesis

Carl P Weiner

Fetal blood sampling was originally performed at hysterotomy.[1] The subsequent development of fetoscopy in the 1960s allowed fetal vessel puncture under direct visualization. However, fetoscopy was cumbersome and risky since the procedure-related loss rates exceeded 5%. The development of high-resolution ultrasound made it possible to image clearly the umbilical cord. Spurred by a desire to diagnose accurately fetal toxoplasmosis, Daffos performed the first intentional percutaneous umbilical blood sampling under ultrasound guidance (cordocentesis) in the early 1980s.[2] The procedure rapidly gained favor with the demonstration of its safety[3–5] and directly spurred the development of fetal medicine. If necessary for technical reasons, fetal blood can also be obtained under sonographic guidance from either the fetal heart (cardiocentesis) or the intrahepatic umbilical vein (hepatocentesis).[6] A wide range of gestational appropriate fetal norms (hematologic, endocrinological, immunologic, biochemical, and biophysical)[7] were developed, a crucial step in the evolution of fetal medicine. While many early indications for cordocentesis have been supplanted by less invasive techniques, there remain several indications for fetal blood sampling. The most common now are the assessment and treatment of red cell and platelet alloimmunization, the antenatal diagnosis of inherited blood or metabolic diseases, rapid karyotyping of malformed or severely growth-restricted fetuses in some countries, and, rarely, the determination of fetal acid–base status (Table 11.1).[8]

Methods

Cordocentesis is performed in the outpatient setting by a single operator with or without an assistant. There is no benefit of maternal fasting, sedation, prophylactic antibiotics, or tocolysis. Cordocentesis can be performed as early as 12 weeks' gestation, though it is technically more difficult before 20 weeks, and the loss rate is much higher before 16 weeks' gestation. We encourage the patient's partner to attend both the counseling session preceding the procedure, and the procedure itself. The limitations and potential complications must be stated unambi-

Table 11.1 Indications for cordocentesis

Indication	%**
Rapid karyotype	50.7
Hemolytic disease	33.7
Severe, early-onset growth restriction	21.7
Congenital infection	16.9
Miscellaneous	4.2
Nonimmune hydrops fetalis	<1
Stuck twin syndrome	<1
Fetal drug therapy	<1
Maternal TSiG	<1
Alloimmune thrombocytopenia	<1

**Percentages taken from Weiner & Okamura.[8] Some patients had more than one indication.
TSiG = thyroid-stimulating immunoglobulin.

guously before written, informed consent is obtained, and a targeted ultrasound examination is performed.

Centers vary in style. There are two methods for performing cordocentesis: by freehand or by the use of a fixed-needle guide. Regardless of technique, the preferred location for umbilical cord puncture is the placental origin, where it is relatively fixed. The first few centimeters of the fetal origin of the umbilical cord are innervated; therefore, puncture may cause pain. The umbilical vein is the preferred target rather than the umbilical artery because of its lower association with complications. Like all percutaneous procedures, a 'no touch' philosophy is essential. If you do not touch the shaft of the needle, you cannot contaminate it.

The freehand technique typically employs a 20-gauge spinal needle 8–12 cm long.[2] The needle course is tracked by imaging the tip and shaft with the ultrasound transducer held either in the opposite hand of the operator or by the assistant. Since the needle is not fixed, the tip can move several centimeters in all axes should either the site of insertion be suboptimal or the fetus move during the procedure. Once the target is punctured, the operator secures the needle while the assistant

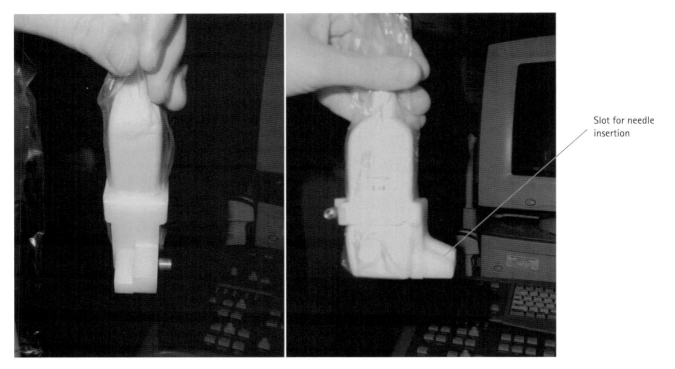

Slot for needle insertion

Figure 11.1 Typical example of a fixed-needle guide available for a variety of sector transducers from several accessory vendors. The one shown is from Protek Medical, Iowa City, Iowa, USA, made for Accuson. The guideline follows the on-screen software.

aspirates a series of 1-ml syringes. Larger syringes can create enough negative pressure to collapse the umbilical vein, leading to the erroneous conclusion the position has been lost. Preheparinization of the syringe is unnecessary unless fetal blood gases are needed. The sample is immediately placed into a specimen container prepared with the appropriate preservative. The freehand technique remains the most popular method for cordocentesis because of the flexibility it allows the operator.

Cordocentesis is also performed with a fixed-needle guide that is attached to the base of the ultrasound transducer (Figure 11.1).[3] Typically, the transducer is held by the operator's assistant. The predicted course of the needle, which can travel only in the vertical plane, is displayed on the ultrasound screen. This allows the operator to select in advance a precise target for puncture. Deviation from the predicted path occurs only when there is an abrupt change in the relationship between the puncture site in the maternal abdominal wall and the uterus as the needle traverses between the two. The most common causes are abrupt patient movement and failure of the assistant to hold the transducer surface flat against the maternal abdomen. Fetal movement is rarely an issue because of the speed of the procedure. Since lateral movement of the needle is not possible, a smaller gauge needle such as a 22 or 25 is used. It is important to line up the umbilical cord longitudinally rather than in cross section. It is preferable to target the 'easiest' location for a direct approach. In more than 50% of the cases, a free loop is targeted, and placental puncture is avoided if possible when the indication is alloimmunization (red blood cell or platelet), just as the

informed practitioner would do with amniocentesis. In contrast to the freehand technique, where there is a larger needle gauge and movement outside the vertical axis, local anesthesia is unnecessary for diagnostic procedures with a 22-gauge needle. A local anesthetic is placed subcutaneously independently of technique when the procedure is lengthy (e.g., intravascular transfusion). Prophylactic antibiotics are not indicated for either cordocentesis or intravascular transfusion. In my experience, amnionitis complicates less than 1 in 800 diagnostic procedures when the 'no touch' philosophy is rigorously adhered to and a needle guide is used (1 in 1200 procedures).

Fetal movement may either prevent a successful puncture or shorten the access time available, regardless of the technique used. Fetal movement while the needle is intraluminal increases the risk of umbilical cord trauma. Many operators administer a neuromuscular antagonist such pancuronium (0.3 mg/kg of estimated fetal weight) to eliminate fetal movement, especially when performing a midloop puncture. The pancuronium is given either intramuscularly into the fetal buttock, or, preferably, intravenously as soon as the vein is punctured; the effect here is evident within seconds. Vecuronium instead of pancuronium is preferred for simple diagnostic procedures because its shorter half-life allows a more rapid return of fetal movement and heart rate variability.[9] In contrast, pancuronium is preferred for fetal transfusion because it maintains fetal cardiac output despite the volume load.

The volume of blood removed depends on the gestation and indication for sampling. Five milliliters is typical and adequate for a karyotype, umbilical venous blood gases, and complete blood profile with Kleihauer–Betke testing, with 2 ml remaining for the remainder of the tests.

Major complications and risk factors for cordocentesis

The major complications of cordocentesis are listed in Table 11.2. They include all complications associated with amniocentesis plus fetal bradycardia, umbilical cord laceration, and thrombosis. Risk factors for cordocentesis are noted in Table 11.3.

Umbilical cord laceration and thrombosis are associated with freehand procedures. Such complications have not been reported when a needle guide was used.[8] Though bleeding from the umbilical puncture site is common, prolonged bleeding with sequelae is uncommon. Application of a 'no touch' technique and the use of disposable needles for a single puncture minimize the risk of amnionitis.

Bradycardia is the major complication of cordocentesis. Virtually all emergency cesarean deliveries and most perinatal losses are associated with fetal bradycardia. Umbilical artery puncture and hypoxia are the major risk factors for bradycardia (Figure 11.2). In the absence of profound anemia or fetal heart failure, fetal hypoxia is associated with an elevated umbilical artery resistance index, and it can be used as a risk marker. The incidence of bradycardia with absent and/or reversed diastolic flow approaches 25%. Umbilical artery puncture increases the risk of fetal bradycardia 5–10-fold.[10] The presence of either oligohydramnios or a two-vessel cord increases the risk of

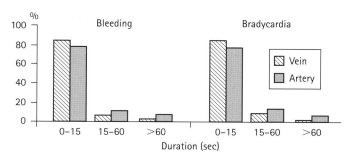

Figure 11.2 Fetal bradycardia and intra-amniotic bleeding occur more often and last longer when an umbilical cord artery rather than a vein is sampled.

arterial puncture. The observation that bradycardia may be associated with an elevated resistance index in one but not both umbilical arteries suggests that the cause is localized vasospasm. Pancuronium use is associated with a lower prevalence of bradycardia in appropriately grown but not growth-restricted fetuses.[9,10] It is likely that some episodes of bradycardia occur when fetal movement tugs on the umbilical cord, causing needle trauma and irritation to the underlying vascular smooth muscle. Bradycardia after umbilical vein puncture may reflect disruption of the adjacent umbilical artery smooth muscle as the tip traverses the cord. In the event of bradycardia, direct observation suggests that vigorous fetal stimulation by palpation is beneficial since the heart will speed up and then slow again if the manual stimulation is stopped too early. A variety of chronotropes (e.g., atropine) and bicarbonate have been given in an attempt for a fetal resuscitation without predictable effect.

Even when performed at a midloop, the fetus does 'react' to the cordocentesis. Umbilical artery resistance typically declines after either a diagnostic procedure or a fetal intravascular transfusion.[11] The higher the 'normal' baseline resistance index, the greater the decline. The decrease is associated with prostacyclin release from the vascular endothelium.[12] Endothelial adaptation to hypoxia may also explain why hypoxemia is a risk factor for bradycardia. Rizzo et al demonstrated that endothelin is released upon umbilical vein puncture of growth-restricted but not appropriately grown fetuses.[13] Fetuses who develop bradycardia release more endothelin, suggesting that the excess endothelin causes focal vasoconstriction at or near the puncture site.

Both techniques for cordocentesis have a learning curve. The learning curve is shorter when a needle guide is used. Until recently, it was generally accepted that the technique selected was a matter of operator preference and had no impact on outcome. However, there is a series of recent findings to challenge this concept.

The first line of evidence is indirect. The often stated 'advantage' of the freehand technique, its flexibility, may also increase risk. Analogously to a lever, a small movement at the hub of the needle amplifies the distance the tip moves. In association with this inescapable fact, freehand cordocentesis

Table 11.2 Complications of cordocentesis

(1) Bradycardia or asystole
(2) Premature rupture of membranes
(3) Premature labor
(4) Umbilical hemorrhage
(5) Placental hemorrhage
(6) Chorioamnionitis
(7) Umbilical thrombosis
(8) Fetal to maternal hemorrhage

Table 11.3 Risk factors for cordocentesis

(1) Umbilical artery puncture (associated with bradycardia)
(2) Fetal hypoxemia (associated with bradycardia)
(3) Technique (freehand vs needle guide)
(4) Gestational age before 20 weeks (both techniques)
(5) Number of punctures (freehand technique only)
(6) Duration of procedure (freehand technique only)
(7) Inexperience

produces a significantly greater incremental increase in the maternal serum α-fetoprotein concentration (MSAFP) than amniocentesis after controlling for placental puncture.[14] In contrast, the incremental change in MSAFP when a needle guide is used is similar to amniocentesis.[15] Further, the association between fetal thrombocytopenia and bleeding from the umbilical puncture site after freehand cordocentesis is high enough to have prompted a recommendation that all fetuses at risk of alloimmune thrombocytopenia receive a prophylactic platelet transfusion at cordocentesis.[16] Yet, there is no relationship between the fetal platelet count and the bleeding time from the puncture site when a needle guide is used.[17] The latter may reflect either less lateral movement of the needle after puncture or the thinner gauge needle, or both. The loss rates reported after second-trimester amniocentesis are lower when thinner needles are used.[18] In addition, reports suggest that amniocentesis performed with a needle guide is safer than one performed freehand.[19]

There is also a line of direct evidence favoring the use of a needle guide, though no single center has adequate volume for a randomized trial, and comparisons of loss rates sustained by groups using the freehand and needle guide techniques are problematic, since it is difficult to separate procedure-related losses from those secondary to the natural progression of disease. We sought to address the role of technique by combining our experience with another fetal medicine unit who shared in common the use of a fixed-needle guide for all procedures.[8] Over 25 operators with varying levels of experience performed 1260 diagnostic cordocenteses at a mean gestational age of 29 weeks. The umbilical vein (confirmed by the blood pressure reading) was punctured in 90% of the cases, demonstrating that the desired vessel can be targeted. A procedure-related loss was defined as any loss within 2 weeks of the procedure except those resulting from elective pregnancy termination. Overall, there were 12 losses (0.9%) (Table 11.4).

Though there are more recent studies, Ghidini et al provided adequate information for stratification.[20] All cordocenteses in this report were performed freehand except those from the University of Iowa, where a needle guide was used. After deleting the Iowa experience from analyses, the overall loss rate was 7.2% (96/1328) with the freehand method.[20] This rate was significantly higher than the overall loss rate when a needle guide was used (0.9%, 12/1,260; $p < 0.00001$). However, this is only a superficial comparison. To exclude the contribution of the underlying pathology to the loss rate, procedures should be divided into high and low risk, with the latter excluding chromosomal abnormalities, nonimmune hydrops, intrauterine growth restriction, and fetal infection. Such exclusions virtually eliminate all abnormal fetuses who might be at risk of a loss *unrelated* to the procedure. The perinatal loss rate for these low-risk procedures using the freehand technique was 3% (20/660). This rate is 15 times higher than the needle guide rate (0.2%, 2/1021; $p < 000001$), which *includes* fetuses with infection, hydrops, or structural malformations.

Donner et al reported 759 diagnostic cordocenteses *with a known outcome* using the freehand technique.[21] The study had some limitations. For instance, the final diagnoses were not reported in all cases, and 87% of the perinatal losses were excluded as being unrelated to the procedure; yet the loss rate was 0.8%, including 94 therapeutic terminations in the denominator. Subtracting the terminations from their total yields a loss of 1.1% (7/665). This rate is very similar to that of Nicolaides, as reported in the second edition of this textbook.[22] Of these pregnancies, 160 were sampled because of severe early-onset growth-restriction. One can estimate their low-risk group if the growth restricted fetuses are excluded and assuming that all fetuses with chromosomal abnormalities were in the growth restriction group, the therapeutic termination group, or the one fetus with trisomy 18 noted in the paper. This leaves a low-risk group of 504 in which there were six fetal/neonatal losses (1.2%). This rate is significantly higher than that achieved with a needle guide ($p = 0.03$).

These findings, both indirect and direct, strongly suggest that many of the procedure-related losses associated with cordocentesis are indeed technique dependent. A few skilled operators using the freehand technique may duplicate the results obtained with a needle guide. However, the majority of practitioners perform only a handful of cordocenteses per year; therefore, they would definitely benefit from using the needle guide.

Table 11.4 Frequency of major complications of cordocentesis when a needle guide is used

Final diagnosis	GA (weeks) at cordocentesis	*Percent emergency delivery	**Percent death within 2 weeks
RBC alloimmunization	28 ± 4	0.2	0.2
Uteroplacental dysfunction	32 ± 4	5.0	0.9
Chromosome abnormality	29 ± 6	7.7	9.9
All others	28 ± 6	0.3	0.2

*Weiner, unpublished.
**Weiner & Okamura.[8] Fetuses with a chromosome abnormality delivered by cesarean section were delivered before the karyotype was completed.

Indications and applications for cordocentesis

Antenatal diagnosis of blood disorders

The first indication for fetal blood sampling in the 1970s and early 1980s was the diagnosis of hemoglobinopathy and genetic defects affecting hemostasis.[1,23] However, in the 1990s, recombinant DNA techniques were introduced for the analysis of placental biopsy material or amniocytes for the diagnosis of many of these conditions in the first or second trimester of pregnancy.[23,24] Yet, cordocentesis is still needed for a phenotype diagnosis in those patients requiring confirmation of normality based on a linked probe, those who lack key affected relatives, those who are not informative by any of the available probes, and those in whom DNA analysis is not feasible because of late referral.

Antenatal diagnosis of metabolic disorders

There are more than 200 inherited, metabolic conditions for which the specific enzyme deficiencies are defined, and for which accurate diagnostic biochemical assays are available. Many of these conditions have no effective therapy and result in either early childhood death or serious disability. Prenatal diagnosis of over 100 of these disorders is now possible by the analysis of amniotic fluid, placental tissue, or fetal blood. Cordocentesis may be particularly useful when the gestational age is close to the local limit for abortion, as with late prenatal care, or after failed chorionic villus or amniotic fluid techniques.

Red blood cell (RBC) alloimmunization

Cordocentesis is not indicated in most cases of maternal RBC alloimmunization solely for fetal blood typing. Accurate typing can now be accomplished by applying polymerase chain reaction (PCR) to either trophoblast or amniocytes obtained in the early second trimester when the risk of exacerbating sensitization is lower.[25,26]

During the last 50 years, several therapeutic approaches were undertaken with the aim of ameliorating the severity of the condition and preventing intrauterine fetal death. Fetal blood sampling has made it possible to understand better the pathophysiology of the disease and has provided an improved method for assessment and treatment of fetal anemia.[27–32] The net result of better understanding is an improved perinatal outcome.

Previously, the severity of fetal hemolysis was estimated from (1) the history of previously affected pregnancies; (2) the level of maternal hemolytic antibodies in a first sensitized pregnancy; (3) the amniotic fluid bilirubin concentration; (4) the altered morphometry of the fetus and placenta; and (5) the presence of pathologic fetal heart rate patterns. However, there was a wide scatter of values around the regression lines describing

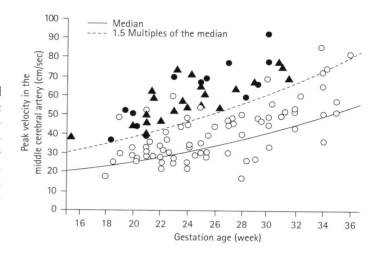

Figure 11.3 Nomogram for the prediction of fetal anemia based on the peak flow velocity in the fetal middle cerebral artery. Open circles: fetuses with no anemia or mild anemia; triangles: fetuses with moderate to severe anemia; solid circles: fetuses with hydrops. (Reproduced from Mari et al. N Engl J Med 2000; 342: 9–14. ©2006 Massachusetts Medical Society. All rights reserved.)

the associations between the degree of fetal anemia and the data obtained from these indirect methods of assessment.[33]

Perhaps the most important advancement in the noninvasive management of RBC alloimmune disease was the recognition that most anemic fetuses have elevated peak systolic velocities in the middle cerebral artery[34] (Figure 11.3). The vast majority of fetuses with moderate or severe anemia have elevated peak systolic velocity in the middle cerebral artery. However, some anemic fetuses may have normal velocities, and the relationship between velocity and the magnitude of the hemoglobin deficit may vary among fetuses.

The only accurate method for determining severity is blood sampling by cordocentesis with the measurement of fetal hemoglobin concentration, reticulocyte count, blood type, strength of the direct Coombs' test, and total bilirubin concentration. However, the overriding indication for, and the timing of, the first cordocentesis remains less than concrete. Invasive procedures should be minimized not only because of the fetal risk, but also because transplacental puncture enhances the risk of fetomaternal hemorrhage,[15,35] increases maternal antibody titer, and may worsen the disease. One approach is to avoid cordocentesis until the peak middle cerebral artery flow velocities are abnormal, especially in those pregnancies under 20 weeks' gestation. However, since some fetuses with mild to moderate anemia may have normal velocities, it is reasonable, depending on referral patterns and distances, to consider sampling all women with a history of severe disease, those with high antibody titers, and fetuses with pathologic heart rate patterns.

A fetal blood sample is obtained, the hemoglobin concentration measured, and an intravascular blood transfusion given as necessary (Figure 11.4).[36] The goal of the first transfusion is to correct the hemoglobin deficit completely unless

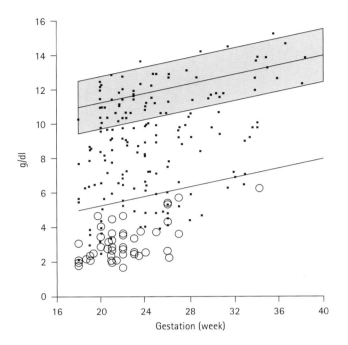

Figure 11.4 Fetal hemoglobin concentrations from RBC-isoimmunized pregnancies at the time of the first fetal blood sampling are plotted on the reference range (mean, 5th percentile, and 95th percentile; shaded area) for gestation. Hydrops fetalis (O) is associated with severe anemia.

there is evidence of hydrops. Immune hydrops is almost always secondary to high output heart failure characterized by an elevated umbilical venous pressure.[37] These fetuses tolerate poorly the first intravascular transfusion, and should be corrected initially to a hemoglobin level of no more than 8–9 gm/dl. In our institutions, we routinely monitor the fetal umbilical venous pressure to avoid overtransfusion. The sec-

ond transfusion is performed a few days later. The target hemoglobin for the second, as well as all subsequent transfusions, is approximately 18 gm/dl. Subsequent transfusions are given at 3–4-week intervals until 34–36 weeks' gestation, and their timing is based on the findings in the middle cerebral artery and the knowledge that after a fetal blood transfusion the mean rate of decrease in fetal hemoglobin is approximately 0.3 g/dl/per day (Figure 11.5).[36,37] Currently, the perinatal survival rate of RBC-isoimmunized pregnancies treated with cordocentesis exceeds 90% in experienced hands, and virtually all losses are associated with immune hydrops fetalis.[37] As far as long-term outcome, we have demonstrated normal long-term neurodevelopment even in the presence of profound anemia prior to treatment.[38,39]

The frequency of repeat cordocentesis in the affected fetus is determined by the change in the peak systolic velocity in the middle cerebral artery and by the 'hemolysis pattern' at the first sampling (Table 11.5).[39,40] This prospectively validated grading scheme is based on the reticulocyte count and the strength of the positive direct Coombs' test. Most fetuses do not require a second sampling. Sensitized fetuses with no severe anemia still remain at risk of postnatal hyperbilirubinemia, which is directly correlated with their antenatal bilirubin levels (Figure 11.6).[41]

Platelet alloimmunization

Immune thrombocytopenia (ITP) is not an indication for cordocentesis.[42] The procordocentesis argument is based on the assumed risk of fetal intracranial hemorrhage during labor. This fear is not supported by the aggregate experience of the last two decades. There is no more than one *fetal* loss documented in the literature secondary to intrapartum fetal hemorrhage.[43] Most losses attributed to ITP were associated with a

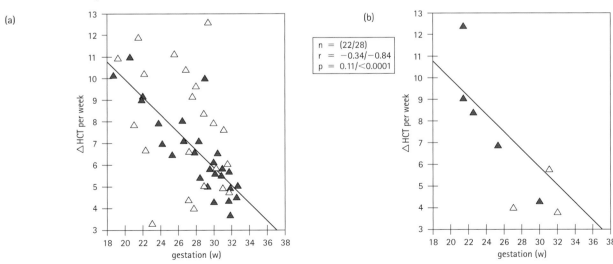

Figure 11.5 Rate of hematocrit decline after the first and subsequent transfusions. (a) Effect of gestational age on decline in hematocrit after transfusion. Open triangles, decline in hematocrit between first and second transfusions; closed triangles, decline for all subsequent transfusions. Regression line is based on all subsequent transfusions. HCT, Hematocrit. (b) Prospective confirmation of relationship shown in Figure 11.5(a) with new data. Open triangles, decline in hematocrit between first and second transfusions; closed triangles, decline for all subsequent transfusions. Regression line is from Figure 11.5(a). HCT, Hematocrit. (Reproduced from Weiner et al. Am J Obstet Gynecol 1991; 165: 1302–7[36] with permission from Elsevier.)

Table 11.5 Patterns of fetal hemolysis predictive of subsequent anemia

Pattern	Hematocrit	Reticulocytes	+/− Direct Coombs' test result	Interval for cordocentesis (wk)	Interval for scan (wk)	Comments
1	Normal	Normal	−/trace	–	4	Repeat if initial maternal indirect Coombs' test result < 128 and two-fold ncrease documented
2	Normal	Normal or < 2.5th percentile	1+/2+	5–6	2	Do not repeat after 32 wk if unchanged; delivery at term
3	Normal	>97.5th percentile	3+/4+	2	1	Continue through 34 wk if hematocrit value stable; deliver at 37–38 wk if not transfused
4	<2.5th percentile but >30%	Any	Any	1–2	1	Repeat, as long as hematocrit criteria fulfilled; deliver with pulmonary maturity if not transfused

Reproduced from Weiner et al. Am J Obstet Gynecol 1991; 165: 546–53[39] with permission from Elsevier.

maternal connective tissue disorder or a neonatal bleed. In almost all other instances of reported losses, either the cause of death or the timing of death was not stated or was unknown. Further, there is no direct or indirect evidence that cesarean section for auto-immune thrombocytopenia improves neonatal outcome.

The past decade has seen significant progress in the management of the fetus with severe alloimmune thrombocytopenia.[44,45] It is now clear that medical therapy consisting primarily of high doses of IV Ig (1–2 g/kg per week) with a prednisone rescue for suboptimal responders is effective treatment for the majority of affected pregnancies.[44] At-risk pregnancies begin their infusions at 10–20 weeks depending upon the past history. Most undergo a single cordocentesis around 28 weeks to confirm normal platelet counts. When secondary to Pl(A1) platelet antigen incompatibility, fetuses with platelet counts over 20 000 at the initiation of therapy are predicted to maintain their platelet count at the second fetal blood sampling at over 20 000. The characteristics of the previous sibling does not predict the initial fetal blood sampling, the second fetal blood sampling, or the response to treatment.[46] Even suboptimal fetal responders have a dramatic decrease in the risk of antenatal hemorrhage. Fetal platelet transfusion is associated with a high loss rate when used for primary therapy (up to 17%).[47] Today, platelet transfusions play a secondary role, and are usually indicated only for those fetuses with extremely low platelet counts or those with a count under 50 000 prior to a planned vaginal delivery. There is no relationship between the fetal platelet count and bleeding from the puncture site when a needle guide is used (Figure 11.7).[17]

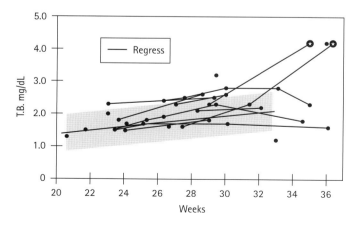

Figure 11.6 Relationship in pregnancies affected by RBC alloimmunization between fetal bilirubin and postnatal hyperbilirubinemia. (Reproduced from Weiner C. Am J Obstet Gynecol 1992; 166: 1449–54[41] with permission from Elsevier.)

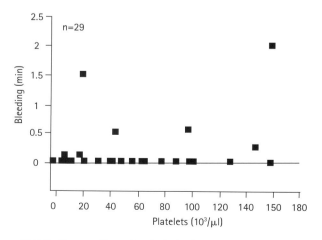

Figure 11.7 Scattergram illustrating the lack of a relationship between platelet count and the duration of bleeding from the umbilical cord puncture site in fetuses with ATP. (Reproduced from Weiner. Fetal Diagn Ther 1995; 10: 173–7 with permission from Karger.)

Rapid karyotype

The fetal lymphocytes can be stimulated to yield a rapid karyotype of high quality in less than 24 hours. This is especially useful for patients referred with severe early-onset fetal growth restriction at a potentially viable gestation or those with malformations detected just prior to the legal limit for pregnancy termination (Table 11.6).

Evaluation of nonimmune hydrops fetalis

The performance of cordocentesis is essential for a complete evaluation of nonimmune hydrops since it allows the separation of cardiac from noncardiac etiologies.[47] The umbilical venous pressure (UVP) is a surrogate for the central venous pressure. Recent studies of human fetuses[48] indicate that the UVP is very similar to right-sided heart pressure. An elevated UVP is consistent with myocardial dysfunction whether caused by anemia (e.g., Parvovirus infection, hemolytic disease), myocarditis, or obstructed cardiac return (thoracic mass effect) (Figure 11.8(a) and (b)). Successful treatment of cardiogenic hydrops is associated with normalization of the UVP before the hydrops

resolves. The UVP also predicts which fetus with hydrothorax and hydrops will respond to the placement of a thoracoamniotic shunt. If the hydrops is caused by a shift of the mediastinum, which obstructs cardiac return, shunting will be helpful. If the UVP neither is elevated nor normalizes after draining the chest, shunting will not help. In such cases, there is a different underlying etiology.

Severe early-onset growth restriction

Cordocentesis is no longer indicated solely for the measurement of the fetal acid–base status, especially in the presence of normal umbilical artery Doppler velocimetry. Assuming the mother is well ventilated and the vessel punctured is correctly identified, the blood gases are less likely to be abnormal than is the chance of a fetal loss. In over 1200 procedures, we have yet to identify a fetus with abnormal blood gases and a normal Doppler resistance index in the absence of either hydrops or fetal sepsis. Refinements in multivessel Doppler studies allow the safe exclusion of fetal hypoxemia, and the prediction of fetal hypoxemia and acidemia with reasonable clinical accuracy.[49–51]

Table 11.6 Malformations and associated chromosomal abnormalities of fetuses who had antenatal karyotyping (from 2nd Edition)

		Incidence of aneuploidy		
Defect	n	Isolated	Multiple	Common chromosomal defect
Brain		%	%	
Ventriculomegaly	185	3	27	Triploidy
Holoprosencephaly	52	<1	29	Trisomy 13
Posterior fossa cyst	45	<1	48	Trisomy 13, 18
Choroid plexus cyst	121	2	46	Trisomy 18
Face				
Cleft	64	<1	55	Trisomy 13, 18
Micrognathia	56	<1	66	Trisomy 18
Neck				
Nuchal edema	145	<1	40	Trisomy 21
Cystic hygromas	52	<1	71	Turner's syndrome
Chest				
Diaphragmatic hernia	79	<1	40	Trisomy 18
Heart defect	156	<1	65	Trisomy 13, 18, 21
Kidneys				
Hydronephrosis				
Mild	319	2	26	Trisomy 18, 13, 21
Severe	294	3	25	Trisomy 18, 21
Gut				
Esophageal atresia	24	<1	78	Trisomy 18
Duodenal atresia	23	17	53	Trisomy 21
Abdominal wall				
Exomphalos	116	<4	47	Trisomy 13, 18
Hydrops	209	7	17	Trisomy 21

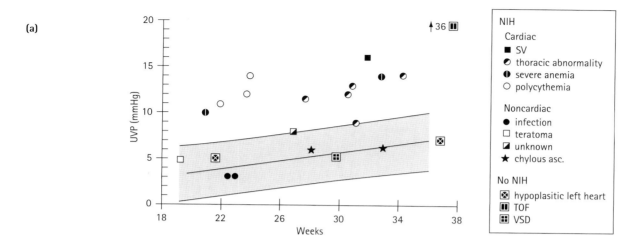

(a)

Figure 11.8(a) Umbilical venous pressure (UVP) measurements corrected for amniotic fluid pressure of 17 untreated fetuses with nonimmune hydrops (NIH) and four nonhydropic fetuses with major cardiac structural malformations plotted against 95% confidence interval for gestational age (shaded area). Data exclude nonimmune hydrops fetuses in whom only umbilical artery pressure had been measured. SVT, supraventricular tachycardia; TOF, tetralogy of Fallot; VSD, ventricular septal defect; chylous asc, chylous ascites.

(b)

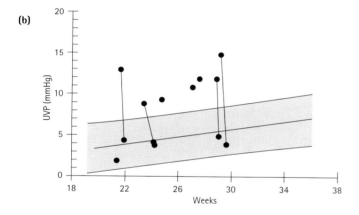

Figure 11.8(b) Umbilical venous pressure (UVP) measurements corrected for amniotic fluid pressure before first transfusion of eight fetuses with immune hydrops is plotted against gestational age. Umbilical venous pressure (where available) before second transfusion is shown for comparison. Seven of eight fetuses had high umbilical venous pressure. In each of these fetuses, umbilical arterial pressure returned to normal before the second transfusion and before resolution of hydrops. (Reproduced from Weiner C. Am J Obstet Gynecol 1993; 68: 817–23[47] with permission from Elsevier.)

The main problem with determining the timing for intervention in the severely growth-restricted fetus is the uncertainty of what causes neurodevelopmental damage (hypoxia vs acidemia). Moreover, very little is known about the impact of chronicity of the insult and gestational age on the final outcome. One study of children who were growth restricted as fetuses and had undergone cordocentesis suggests that it is the acidemia, not the hypoxemia alone, which is associated with compromised neurodevelopment.[52] More recently, we have followed with multivessel Doppler a group of severely growth-restricted fetuses delivered at less than 33 weeks' gestation until

2 years of age. For those delivered under 27 weeks, gestational age and birth weight remain the primary determinants of intact survival (unpublished).

Congenital infection

Preliminary reports suggest that cordocentesis for the diagnosis of fetal toxoplasmosis has been replaced by the application of PCR technology to samples of amniotic fluid, but this issue remains controversial. Although fetal blood sampling has been considered central to the diagnosis of fetal infection for all viruses other than CMV, it is very likely that this indication will also be supplanted by the application of PCR to amniotic fluid samples.

Miscellaneous

Not yet widely accepted but a valid indication for cordocentesis is presence of maternal thyroid-stimulating antibody (TSiG) or active maternal Graves' disease.[53–55] Emerging evidence suggests that even mild degrees of thyroid dysfunction may be associated with impaired long-term neurodevelopment.[56–58] While there is a relationship between the degree of maternal and fetal thyroid suppression with such agents as propylthiouracil (PTU), it is not uncommon for the fetus to be over- or undertreated despite the mother's being euthyroid. In the instance of fetal hyperthyroidism, the maternal PTU dose is increased and the woman should be given thyroxine replacement. In the instance of fetal hypothyroidism, the fetus can be given thyroxine intra-amniotically on a weekly basis.[58] Women with a history of Graves' disease who have undergone thyroid ablation should be screened for the presence of TSiG. The fetus is at minimal risk if the TSIG study is negative.

Conclusion

Cordocentesis is a useful and relatively safe technique. Its main usefulness is in the evaluation and management of RCB and platelet alloimmunization and also in all cases of suspected fetal anemia regardless of etiology. Its usefulness in the prenatal diagnosis of genetic diseases has been diminishing since the introduction of PCR techniques. There is no doubt that data obtained by cordocentesis have expanded greatly our understanding of the pathophysiology of fetal disease and have stimulated the development of fetal therapies.

References

1. Alter BP. Examination of fetal blood for hemoglobinopathies. In: Alter BP (ed.), Perinatal Hematology, pp. 13–29. Churchill Livingstone: New York, 1989.

2. Daffos F, Capella-Pavlovsky M, Forestier F. A new procedure for fetal blood sampling in utero: preliminary results of fifty-three cases. Am J Obstet Gynecol 1983, 146: 985–7.

3. Weiner CP. Cordocentesis for diagnostic indications – two years' experience. Obstet Gynecol 1987; 70: 664–8.

4. Daffos F. Access to the other patient [Review]. Semin Perinatol 1989; 13: 252–9.

5. Maxwell DJ, Johnson P, Hurley P, Neales K, Allan L, Knott P. Fetal blood sampling and pregnancy loss in relation to indication. Br J Obstet Gynaecol 1991; 98: 892–7.

6. Bang J, Bock JE, Trolle D. Ultrasound-guided fetal intravenous transfusion for severe rhesus haemolytic disease. BMJ 1982; 284: 373–4.

7. Ramsay MM, James DK, Steer PJ, Weiner CP, Gonik B (eds). Normal Values in Pregnancy (3rd Edition). WB Saunders: Philadelphia, 2005.

8. Weiner CP, Okamura K. Diagnostic fetal blood sampling – technique related losses. Fetal Diagn Ther 1996; 11: 169–75.

9. Mouw RJC, Hermans J, Brandenburg HCR, Kanhak HHH. Effects of atracurium or pancuronium on the anemic fetus during and directly after intrauterine transfusion (IUT): a double blind randomized study. Acta Obstet Gynecol Scand 1999; 78: 763–7.

10. Weiner CP, Wenstrom KD, Sipes SL, Williamson RA. Risk factors for cordocentesis and fetal intravascular transfusions. Am J Obstet Gynecol, 1991; 165: 1020–3.

11. Weiner CP, Anderson T. The acute effect of cordocentesis with or without fetal curarization and of intravascular transfusion upon umbilical artery waveform indices. Obstet Gynecol 73: 219–24, 1989.

12. Weiner CP, Robillard JE. Effect of acute intravascular volume expansion upon human fetal prostaglandin concentrations. Am J Obstet Gynecol 1989; 161: 1494–7.

13. Rizzo G, Capponi A, Rinaldo D, Arduini D, Romanini C. Release of vasoactive agents during cordocentesis: differences between normally grown and growth-restricted fetuses. Am J Obstet Gynecol 1996, 175: 563–70.

14. Nicolini U, Kochenour NK, Greco P et al. Consequences of fetomaternal hemorrhage after intrauterine transfusion. BMJ 1988; 297: 1379–81.

15. Weiner CP, Grant SS, Hudson J, Williamson RA, Wenstrom KD. Effect of diagnostic and therapeutic cordocentesis upon maternal serum alpha fetoprotein concentration. Am J Obstet Gynecol 1989; 161: 706–8.

16. Paidas MJ, Lynch L, Lockwood CJ, Alvarez MA, Bussel J, Berkowitz RL. Alloimmune thrombocytopenia: fetal and neonatal losses related to fetal blood sampling. Am J Obstet Gynecol 1995; 172: 475–9.

17. Weiner CP. Fetal blood sampling and fetal thrombocytopenia. Fetal Diagn Ther 1995; 10: 173–7.

18. Tabor A, Philip J, Bang J, Madsen M, Obel EB, Norgaard-Pedersen B. Needle size and risk of miscarriage after amniocentesis [Letter]. Lancet 1988; 1(8578): 183–4.

19. Weiner CP, Williamson RA, Varner MW, Grant S. Safety of second trimester amniocentesis. Lancet 1986; ii: 226.

20. Ghidini A, Sepulveda W, Lockwood CJ, Romero R. Complications of fetal blood sampling. Am J Obstet Gynecol 1993; 168: 1339–44.

21. Donner C, Simon P, Karioun A, Avni F, Rodesch F. Experience of a single team of operators in 891 diagnostic funipunctures. Obstet Gynecol 1994; 84: 827–31.

22. Nicolaides KH, Snijders RJM, Abbas A. Cordocentesis. In: Iffy L, Apuzzio J, Vintzileos (eds). Operative Obstetrics, 2nd edition. McGraw Hill: New York, 1999, pp 82–90.

23. Mibashan RS, Peake IR, Nicolaides KH. Prenatal diagnosis of hemostatic disorders. In: Alter BP (ed.), Perinatal Hematology, pp. 64–107. Churchill Livingstone: New York, 1989.

24. Boehm CD, Kazazian HH: Examination of fetal DNA for hemoglobinopathies. In: Alter BP (ed.), Perinatal Hematology, pp. 30–63. Churchill Livingstone: New York, 1989.

25. Yankowitz J, Li S, Murray JC. Polymerase chain reaction determination of RhD blood type: an evaluation of accuracy. Obstet Gynecol 1995; 86: 214–17.

26. Yankowitz J, Li S, Weiner CP. Polymerase chain reaction determination of RhC, Rhc, and RhE blood types: an evaluation of accuracy and clinical utility. Am J Obstet Gynecol 1997; 176: 1107–11.

27. Berkowitz RL, Chitkara U, Goldberg JD et al. Intrauterine transfusion in utero: the percutaneous approach. Am J Obstet Gynecol 1986; 154: 622–3.

28. Grannum PAT, Copel JA, Plaxe SC et al. In utero exchange transfusion by direct intravascular injection in severe erythroblastosis fetalis. N Engl J Med 1986; 314: 1431–4.

29. Nicolaides KH, Rodeck CH, Kemp J et al. Have Liley charts outlived their usefulness? Am J Obstet Gynecol 1986; 155: 90–4.

30. Nicolaides KH. Studies on fetal physiology and pathophysiology in rhesus disease. Semin Perinatol 1989; 13: 328–37.

31. Weiner CP, Robillard JE. Atrial natriuretic factor, digoxin-like immunoreactive substance, norepinephrine, epinephrine, and plasma renin activity in human fetuses and their alteration by fetal disease. Am J Obstet Gynecol 1988; 159: 1353–60.

32. Soothill PW, Lestas AN, Nicolaides KH et al. 2,3-Diphosphoglyc-erate in normal, anaemic and transfused human fetus. Clin Sci 1988; 74: 527–30.

33. Nicolaides KH, Sadovsky G, Cetin E. Fetal heart rate patterns in red blood cell isoimmunized pregnancies. Am J Obstet Gynecol 1989; 161: 351–6.

34. Mari G, Deter RL, Carpenter RL et al. Noninvasive diagnosis by Doppler ultrasonography of fetal anemia due to maternal red-cell alloimmunization. Collaborative Group for Doppler Assessment of the Blood Velocity in Anemic Fetuses. N Engl J Med 2000; 342: 9–14.

35. Nicolini U, Kochenour NK, Greco P. Consequences of fetomater-nal haemorrhage after intrauterine transfusion. BMJ 1988; 297: 1379–81.

36. Weiner CP, Williamson RA, Wenstrom KD et al. Management of fetal hemolytic disease by cordocentesis. II. Outcome of treatment. Am J Obstet Gynecol 1991; 165: 1302–7.

37. Weiner CP, Pelzer GD, Heilskov J, Wenstrom KD, Williamson RA. The effect of intravascular transfusion on umbilical venous pressure in anemic fetuses with and without hydrops. Am J Obstet Gynecol 1989; 161: 1498–1501.

38. Swingle HM, Harper DC, Bonthius D, Weiner CP, Widness JA, Aylward GA. Long-term neurodevelopmental follow-up and brain volumes of children following severe fetal anemia with hydrops. American Academy of Cerebral Palsy and Developmental Medicine, Los Angeles, 29 Sept–1 Oct 2004.

39. Weiner CP, Williamson RA, Wenstrom KD, Sipes SL, Grant SS, Widness JA. Management of fetal hemolytic disease by cordocen-tesis. I. Prediction of fetal anemia. Am J Obstet Gynecol 1991; 165: 546–53.

40. Weiner CP, Wenstrom KD. Outcome of alloimmunized fetuses managed solely by cordocentesis but not requiring antenatal transfusion. Fetal Diagn Ther 1994; 9: 233–8.

41. Weiner CP. Human fetal bilirubin levels and fetal hemolytic disease. Am J Obstet Gynecol 1992; 166: 1449–54.

42. Weiner CP. Why fuss over diagnosing fetal thrombocytopenia secondary to ITP? Contemp Ob Gyn 1995; 40: 45–50.

43. Bussel JB. Alloimmune thrombocytopenia in the fetus and newborn. Semin Thromb Hemost 2001; 27: 245–52.

44. Bussel JB, Berkowitz RL, Lynch L et al. Antenatal management of alloimmune thrombocytopenia with intravenous gamma-globulin: a randomized trial of the addition of low-dose steroid to intravenous gamma-globulin. Am J Obstet Gynecol 1996; 174: 1414–23.

45. Gaddipati S, Berkowitz RL, Lembet AA, Lapinski R, McFarland JG, Bussel JB. Initial fetal platelet counts predict the response to intravenous gamma-globulin therapy in fetuses that are affected by PLA1 incompatibility. Am J Obstet Gynecol 2001; 185: 976–80.

46. Overton TG, Duncan KR, Jolly M, Letsky E, Fisk NM. Serial aggressive platelet transfusion for fetal alloimmune thrombocy-topenia: platelet dynamics and perinatal outcome. Am J Obstet Gynecol. 2002; 186: 826–31.

47. Weiner CP. Umbilical venous pressure measurement in the evalu-ation of nonimmune hydrops. Am J Obstet Gynecol 1993; 168: 817–23.

48. Weiner Z, Efrat Z, Zimmer EZ, Iskovitz-Eldor J, Copel JA. Direct measurement of central venous pressure in human fetuses. Am J Obstet Gynecol 1997; 176: S19.

49. Baschat AA, Weiner CP. Umbilical artery doppler screening for detection of the small fetus in need of antepartum surveillance. Am J Obstet Gynecol 2000; 182(1 Pt 1): 154–8.

50. Baschat AA, Gembruch U, Reiss I, Gortner L, Weiner CP, Har-man CR. Relationship between arterial and venous Doppler and perinatal outcome in fetal growth restriction. Ultrasound Obstet Gynecol 2000; 16: 407–13.

51. Baschat AA, Gembruch U, Weiner CP, Harman CR. Qualitative venous Doppler waveform analysis improves prediction of critical perinatal outcomes in premature growth-restricted fetuses. Ultrasound Obstet Gynecol 2003; 22: 240–5.

52. Soothill PW, Ajayi RA, Campbell S, Ross EM, Nicolaides KH. Fetal oxygenation at cordocentesis, maternal smoking and child-hood neurodevelopment. Eur J Obstet Gynecol Reprod Sci 1995; 59: 21–4.

53. Wenstrom KD, Weiner CP, Williamson RA, Grant SS. Prenatal diagnosis of fetal hyperthyroidism using funipuncture. Obstet Gynecol 1990; 75: 1–5.

54. Yankowitz J, Weiner CP. Medical fetal therapy. Clin Obstet Gynaecol 1995; 9: 553–70.

55. Salerno M, Di Maio S, Militerni R, Argenziano A, Valerio G, Tenore A. Prognostic factors in the intellectual development at 7 years of age in children with congenital hypothyroidism. J Endocrinol Invest 1995; 18: 774–9.

56. Kooistra L, van der Meere JJ, Vulsma T, Kalverboer AF. Sustained attention problems in children with early treated congenital hypothyroidism. Acta Paediatr 1996; 85: 425–9.

57. Weber G, Siragusa V, Rondanini GF et al. Neurophysiologic stud-ies and cognitive function in congenital hypothyroid children. Pediatr Res 1995; 37: 736–40.

58. Van Loon AJ, Derksen JT, Bos AF, Rouwe CW. In utero diagnosis and treatment of fetal goitrous hypothyroidism, caused by maternal use of propylthiouracil. Prenat Diagn 1995; 15: 599–604.

12 Fetal endoscopic surgery and laser photocoagulation therapy

Ursula F Harkness and Timothy M Crombleholme

As prenatal diagnosis has become increasingly sophisticated, invasive therapies have been developed. The motivation for the development of *in utero* therapies springs from the realization that, with certain congenital anomalies, irreversible changes have already taken place by the time of birth, or, alternatively, may result in intrauterine fetal demise without *in utero* treatment. Several congenital anomalies have been successfully treated with open fetal surgery, but the indications for minimally invasive approaches are increasing. This chapter will review the current indications for minimally invasive fetal surgery, which have expanded significantly since the last edition of this book.

Fetoscopic treatment for congenital anomalies

Lower urinary tract obstruction

The most common etiology of chronic lower urinary tract obstruction in the male fetus is posterior urethral valves (PUV), which occur in approximately 1 in 4000 live births. In female fetuses, the most common cause of bladder outlet obstruction is urethral atresia. Complications associated with fetal lower urinary tract obstruction include progressive oligohydramnios, pulmonary hypoplasia, cystic renal dysplasia, and deformations of the face and extremities. Death ensues in up to 72% of fetuses with bladder outlet obstruction if left untreated.[1] Uncorrected oligohydramnios observed in the second trimester is particularly ominous; it has a perinatal mortality rate of 80–100%.

The initial approach to the fetus with suspected bladder-outlet obstruction should include a detailed ultrasound examination to rule out other associated anomalies and echocardiography. Lower urinary tract obstruction must be distinguished from other pathologic causes of fetal hydronephrosis. The presence of megacystis, thickened bladder wall, posterior urethral dilatation, bilateral hydronephrosis and ureterectasis characterizes the changes associated with PUV and urethral atresia, in contrast to the more common ureteropelvic junction obstruction, ureterovesical obstruction or vesicoureteral reflux. Since chromosomal abnormalities are found in up to 12% of fetuses with bladder outlet obstruction,[2] fetal karyotyping is indicated.

A major problem in the management of fetuses diagnosed with lower urinary tract obstruction is selecting those fetuses who are most likely to benefit from *in utero* intervention. Among cases of fetal urinary tract obstruction, a fetus with preserved renal function produces more hypotonic urine, whereas one with advanced renal dysfunction is a 'salt waster', producing more hypertonic urine. The usefulness of assessing urine chemistry in fetal obstructive uropathy lies in the separation of fetuses into 'good' or 'poor' prognostic categories based on the preservation of renal function reflected by the tonicity of the fetal urine. In one study, urine samples taken from fetuses who subsequently had a good outcome revealed levels of Na^+ less than 100 mEq/l, Cl^- less than 90 mEq/l, and osmolarity less than 210 mOsm/l.[3] These values were chosen because they were two standard deviations from the mean values of fetuses with a good prognosis. Fetuses with urine chemistries greater than these values had irreversible renal damage and suffered from severe oligohydramnios resulting in pulmonary hypoplasia. The efficacy of these proposed criteria was subsequently confirmed to reflect postnatal outcome and appropriately select fetuses for intervention.

Johnson et al modified this approach to include three sequential vesicocenteses at 24–hour intervals. This regimen permits a comparative analysis of stagnant urine (first sample) with fresh urine (third sample). Fresh urine samples are thought to reflect fetal renal function more accurately, and this approach increases the predictive value of fetal urinary electrolytes.[4] These authors suggest that excluding the following groups will improve the ability to select fetuses that will benefit from antenatal therapy: (1) those with associated anomalies, (2) those who are female or aneuploid, (3) those with kidneys which are echodense and small for gestational age or who have renal cortical cysts, and (4) those who fail to demonstrate sequential improvement of biochemical markers to below set cutoff values (Table 12.1).

There are no randomized trials regarding the use of amniotic shunts for prenatal bladder drainage for obstructive uropathies. In one meta-analysis which included nine case series (147 fetuses) and seven controlled series (195 fetuses), bladder drainage improved perinatal survival relative to no drainage in the controlled studies (odds ratio 2.5; 95% CI 1.1–5.9, $p = 0.03$).[5]

While prenatal intervention may help the fetus survive by correcting oligohydraminos and pulmonary hypoplasia, there is a growing appreciation that the long-term outcome of children after vesicoamniotic shunting may be complicated by renal insufficiency, bladder dysfunction, and growth problems. Freedman et al reported outcomes in 14 patients who survived beyond 2 years of age after having had *in utero* vesicoamniotic shunt placement.[6] Renal function was normal in only six (43%). Of the remaining eight patients, five had renal failure requiring kidney transplantation and three had chronic renal insufficiency. Three of the four whose obstructive uropathy was due to PUV required bladder augmentation. In addition, growth of these toddlers was a problem with 86% below the 25th percentile and 50% below the 5th percentile. In another study,[7] of patients who underwent various procedures with the majority being vesicoamniotic shunt, five of eight (63%) babies

born alive developed chronic renal disease. Two underwent renal transplant and another was awaiting transplant at the time of report. Five of eight babies underwent urinary diversion after birth. Although placement of a vesicoamniotic shunt seems simple, the procedure is technically challenging and carries an appreciable complication rate. Long-term shunt success is variable due in large part to shunt obstruction and displacement. Functional shunt failure has been reported to occur in 40–50% of cases after successful placement, mostly due to displacement of the shunt into the fetal abdomen or amniotic space. Other reported complications of vesicoamniotic shunt placement include preterm premature rupture of membranes, preterm labor, amnionitis, and iatrogenic gastroschisis. Another report described a case in which the shunt traversed the femoral triangle and inguinal ligament in the subcutaneous tissue before entering the bladder, raising the potential of extremity injury.[8]

The postnatal problems after vesicoamniotic shunting have been a catalyst for the development of alternative fetoscopic techniques to treat obstructive uropathy *in utero*. An endoscopic approach to the treatment of fetal obstructive uropathy is appealing because shunts can be placed under direct visualization, more accurate diagnosis can be made, and direct treatment of the urinary tract anomaly can be attempted. One approach involves cystoscopic identification of the underlying etiology and, in cases of posterior urethral valves, destruction of the membranous obstruction (Figure 12.1). Engineering and manufacturing advances have produced successive generations of smaller fiber-optic endoscopes that have made fetal cystoscopy a reality. Initially, using a variety of 1.7–2.2-mm endoscopes, Quintero et al were able to show that *in utero* diagnostic fetal cystoscopy is possible and later were able to identify proximal urethral obstructions.[9] Several attempts at laser ablation of posterior urethral valves were technical successes, but postoperative obstetric complications resulted in no long-term survivors from this early experience.[10] More recently, a 1-mm, semirigid, fiber-optic endoscopic system that allows a minimally invasive approach to diagnostic cystourethroscopy has been used. With a 1.2 × 2.4-mm, double-lumen trocar sheath, it is possible to pass wire probes or laser fibers to assist in diagnostic evaluation and offer the possibility of laser ablation of posterior urethral valves. Design modifications and refinements to this system have recently allowed us to visualize more reliably the source of proximal urethral obstruction and differentiate between urethral atresia and posterior urethral valves. The hope is that, by treating the source of the obstruction in midgestation, renal function will be preserved, and the need for postnatal urologic surgery to correct secondary anatomic bladder abnormalities may be eliminated. However, despite a compelling rationale for fetal cystoscopic treatments of posterior urethral valves and advances in fetoscopic techniques, this approach has yet to be shown to be a safe and effective treatment of lower urinary tract obstruction.

Table 12.1 Fetal urinary electrolyte and protein cutoff values for evaluation of renal function.

Sodium (mg/dl)	<100
Calcium (mg/dl)	<8
Osmolality (mOsm/l)	<200
β_2-Microglobulin (mg/l)	<4
Total protein (mg/dl)	<40

Values from Johnson MP, Bukowski TP, Reitleman C, et al. In utero surgical treatment of fetal obstructive uropathy: a new comprehensive approach to identify appropriate candidates for vesicoamniotic shunt therapy. Am J Obstet Gynecol 1994; 170: 1770–9.[4]

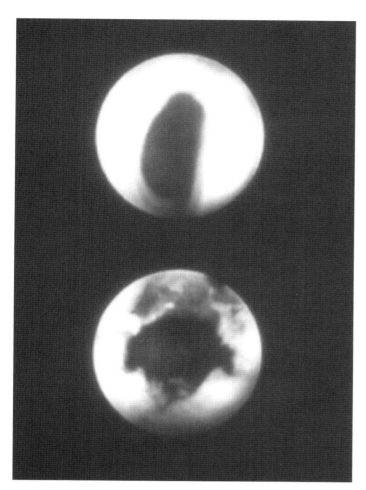

Figure 12.1 Cystoscopic evaluation of posterior urethral valve before treatment (above) and cystoscopic view of a posterior urethral valve after laser ablation (below).

Congenital diaphragmatic hernia

Congenital diaphragmatic hernia (CDH) is a defect in the diaphragm resulting from incomplete fusion of the primitive diaphragm. CDH occurs in approximately 1 in 2500–5000 live births and as frequently as 1 in 2200 prenatal ultrasound studies. Most commonly, the CDH is on the left (85–90%). The defect is on the right in approximately 10% of cases and may be bilateral in less than 5% of cases. Associated anomalies are seen in 25–57% of all cases of CDH and 95% of stillborns with CDH.[11,12] Chromosomal anomalies, including trisomy 21, 18, and 13, occur in association with CDH in 10–20% of cases that are diagnosed prenatally. The clinical spectrum of this anomaly ranges from fetuses who do very well with postnatal management to severely affected infants with profound pulmonary hypoplasia that precludes postnatal survival.

General indication of severity for left-sided diaphragmatic hernia is revealed by determining whether the liver is above or below the diaphragm[13,14] and also by the sonographic measurement of lung-to-head ratios (LHR).[15–17] Detection of liver posi-

tion is enhanced by magnetic resonance imaging (MRI). One study of 38 cases of CDH reported that MRI correctly diagnosed liver position in 37 (97%), whereas ultrasound correctly diagnosed liver position in 32 (84%).[18] In the most recent experience at the Children's Hospital of Philadelphia (CHOP), survival in left-sided CDH with liver in the abdomen was 91%, with only 24% requiring ECMO. Conversely, survival in left-sided CDH with significant herniation of the left lobe of the liver was only 51%, with 79% of patients requiring ECMO. The LHR is determined by taking the two-dimensional area of the right lung measured at the level of the four-chamber view of the heart (in mm) and dividing by the head circumference (in mm) to minimize the influence of gestational age on lung size (Figure 12.2). The LHR, although still useful, has proven less reliable in predicting survival than was previously thought, especially in the most severe category. LHRs greater than 1.4 are still associated with an excellent survival rate in the 80–85% range, with only 25% of patients requiring ECMO. An LHR of 1.0–1.4 is associated with survival of about 75%, with 69% requiring ECMO. The largest change has been the survival rate observed with patients with LHR less than 0.9, of whom up to 62% can be expected to survive, although almost all survivors require ECMO. It is not known whether the improved survival with LHR less than 1.0 reflects improved neonatal care, such as the use of 'gentilation' strategies, or whether greater experience with larger numbers of patients in this category of LHR is now giving a more accurate reflection of survival.

The degree of pulmonary hypoplasia is a critical determinant of survival in CDH. Herniation of viscera associated with CDH usually occurs during the pseudoglandular stage of lung development (5–17 weeks' gestation). Although the major bronchial buds are present, the number of bronchial branches

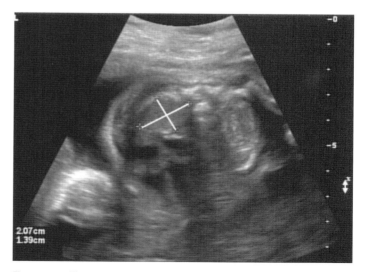

Figure 12.2 Ultrasound image demonstrating measurement of the right lung area at 25 weeks gestation. Calculation of the lung-to-head ratio (LHR) entails dividing the two-dimensional area of the right lung (longest length L1 × perpendicular length L2, both in mm) by the head circumference (in mm). Lung measurements are taken on axial images at the level of the four-chamber view of the heart.

is greatly reduced. If the herniation persists into later stages of lung development, the absolute number of alveoli is also reduced.[19] The pulmonary vascular bed is similarly abnormal, with both a reduction in the number of generations of vessels and an extension of muscularization to the preacinar capillary bed. These pulmonary vascular changes in preacinar capillaries are a histologic correlate of pulmonary hypertension. Although the diaphragmatic defect is easily corrected after birth, the pulmonary hypoplasia and pulmonary hypertension may not be.

This prenatal natural history of severe CDH has led to attempts to correct the diaphragmatic defect before birth, with some anecdotal reports of success. However, cases in which the fetal liver was herniated into the chest were uniformly unsuccessful since attempts to reduce the liver obstructed venous return from the placenta. Focus shifted to the use of other techniques that might correct the pulmonary hypoplasia before birth. Tracheal occlusion was applied in animal models of CDH, demonstrating that tracheal occlusion could correct the pulmonary hypoplasia associated with CDH.[20,21] The survival rate with an open fetal surgical approach, however, was disappointing, and fetoscopic techniques of tracheal occlusion were developed in hopes of avoiding the problems of preterm labor and complications from tocolytic agents associated with hysterotomy.

The fetoscopic techniques used for tracheal occlusion have evolved with growing experience by the University of California San Francisco (UCSF) group. In the initial fetoscopic approach using up to five ports, dissection of the fetal trachea with preservation of the recurrent laryngeal nerves proved difficult.[22] Two patients suffered bilateral vocal cord paralysis. In their initial approach with the 'fetendo' clip, Harrison et al reported a 75% survival rate compared with 15% in the open fetal surgical approach to tracheal occlusion and a 38% survival with standard postnatal therapy.[22] Not only did survival appear to be improved in this small series, but there was also a trend toward less preterm labor, less need for tocolysis, and shorter hospital stay. The UCSF group have now further refined their technique, eliminating the multiple ports and the neck dissection entirely by performing an endoluminal balloon tracheal occlusion.[23] A single port is used to introduce the hysteroscope into the amnion and the fetal oropharynx. The vocal cords are fetoscopically viewed for passage of a detachable balloon catheter through the vocal cords (Figure 12.3). The position in the trachea is determined sonographically before inflation and deployment of the balloon.

The National Institutes of Health (NIH) sponsored a prospective, randomized clinical trial comparing fetoscopic endoluminal balloon tracheal occlusion to conventional postnatal therapy.[24] This study enrolled 24 women at 22–28 weeks' gestation, all with isolated, severe, left-sided CDH with liver herniation and LHR below 1.4. Enrollment was terminated because of the unexpectedly high survival with standard care and the conclusion of the safety monitoring board that further recruitment would not result in significant differences between the groups. Survival at 90 days was 73% in the fetoscopic group

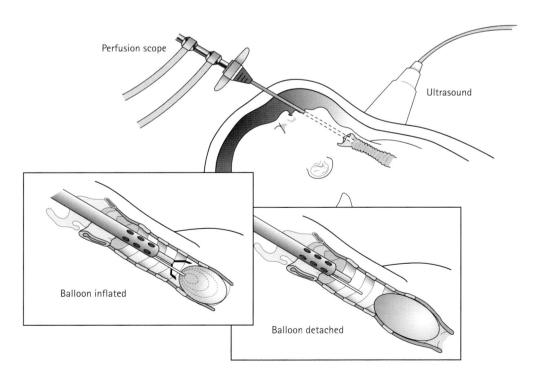

Figure 12.3 With sonographic and endoscopic guidance, the fetal trachea is cannulated with the telescope. After inflation, the balloon is detached 2 cm proximal to the carina (inset). (From Sydorak R, Albanese CT. Minimal access techniques for fetal surgery. World J Surg 2003; 27: 95–102 with permission from Springer.)

and 77% in the standard care group. There was also no significant difference in neonatal morbidities. Of note is that the average gestational age at delivery was 37.0 weeks in the standard care group and 30.8 weeks in the tracheal occlusion group. The pulmonary benefits of *in utero* tracheal occlusion may be counterbalanced by pulmonary complications of prematurity. One question that remains to be answered is whether fetoscopic tracheal occlusion will prove to be of benefit in the sickest babies, those with liver herniation and LHR of less than 0.9. The Belgian group led by Jan DePrest has been performing reversible fetoscopic tracheal occlusion in this high-risk group of fetuses, reporting a 90% survival rate. As yet, however, no randomized clinical trial has been conducted.

Sacrococcygeal teratoma (SCT)

A sacrococcygeal teratoma (SCT) is a congenital neoplasm composed of tissues from all three germ layers. Although these tumors are often benign, a subset of affected babies is at risk of intrauterine demise. The mortality rate for SCT diagnosed in the newborn period is only 5%, yet the mortality rate is 50% when the SCT is diagnosed prenatally.[25,26] When these tumors are diagnosed prior to 30 weeks' gestation, survival less than 10% has been reported, whereas the survival rate is 75% when the tumor is detected after 30 weeks' gestation.[27] The potentially lethal complications of SCT are vascular steal syndromes or exsanguinating tumor hemorrhage. These fetuses may develop high-output cardiac failure as a result of arteriovenous shunting through the tumor or fetal anemia.[25,28,29] Additionally, fetal SCT is sometimes associated with maternal, preeclampsia-like 'mirror syndrome' in association with hydrops. Fortunately, this is a rare fetal tumor, occurring in only 1 in 35 000–40 000 live births.

The uniformly dismal outcome in fetuses with SCT complicated by placentomegaly and hydrops has been the impetus for resection of this tumor *in utero*. The first successful resection of a fetal SCT with a long-term survivor was reported by Adzick et al.[30] Since this report, a total of five patients have undergone open fetal surgery for resection of an SCT in a hydropic fetus, with four survivors (Figure 12.4).

Attempts at treating fetal SCT with minimally invasive fetoscopic techniques have met with mixed results. Hecher and Hackeloer reported the successful treatment of an SCT by laser fetoscopy.[31] The base of this SCT was unusually narrow, without distortion of the anorectal sphincter complex by the mass. This is an important consideration, as most fetal SCTs distort the anorectal rectal sphincter complex, and such a laser fetoscopic approach, as described by Hecher and Hackeloer, might result in ischemic necrosis of the anorectal sphincter complex along with the SCT. In addition, the superficial vessels are the only ones accessible to the laser, while the deeper pelvic vessels may be more important in the development of high-output physiology. These difficulties are highlighted by the UCSF experience with the use of radiofrequency ablation (RFA).[32] The goal was the coagulation of the feeding vessels to the SCT that are responsible for the high-output state. The power of the

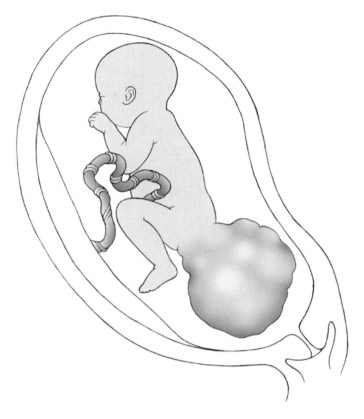

Figure 12.4 Schematic illustration of a fetal sacrococcygeal teratoma.

RFA in this ultrasound-guided technique could not be precisely controlled, and the fetus sustained necrosis of the anus, vagina, and bladder, with injury to the sciatic nerve. While RFA may hold promise for the future, many refinements in the use of this technique would need to be made before it could be recommended in the treatment of fetal SCT. Perhaps fetoscopic guidance would allow safer application of RFA, targeting vessels in areas remote from the anorectal sphincter complex.

Myelomeningocele

In recent years, fetal surgery has expanded from the treatment of life-threatening fetal anomalies, such as CDH, SCT, or hydropic congenital cystic adenomatoid malformations of the lung (CCAMs), to fetal anomalies that are severely debilitating but not life-threatening. Myelomeningocele may be the most controversial of the current nonlethal indications for fetal surgery. Fetoscopic repair of myelomeningocele by placement of a maternal split-thickness skin graft was first attempted by the group at Vanderbilt in four patients.[33] The two survivors in this small series did not appear to benefit from this procedure. A similarly disappointing experience with fetoscopic treatment of myelomeningocele was reported by the UCSF group. This approach has been abandoned in favor of an open surgical technique until advances in fetoscopic instrumentation make this a viable alternative approach.

Amniotic band syndrome (ABS)

Amniotic band syndrome (ABS) is another example of a usually nonlethal anomaly potentially treatable by fetoscopic surgery. This syndrome results from a rupture of the amnion during fetal development, which may subsequently attach to or encircle parts of the developing fetus. Constrictive bands most commonly affect the extremities but can also involve the craniofacial region, trunk, or umbilical cord. Involvement of the latter may result in fetal demise. The prenatal natural history of isolated extremity ABS is characterized by progression from distal edema owing to venous obstruction to in utero limb amputation secondary to vascular insufficiency. If diagnosed early enough in their course, these patients may benefit from in utero lysis of these fibrous bands.

Based on the experimental work by Crombleholme et al,[34] demonstrating the potential for functional recovery of banded extremities once released, Quintero et al performed the first fetoscopic lysis of amniotic bands in two human fetuses, using endoscissors in one fetus and YAG laser in the other.[35] Limb salvage was achieved, but one fetus suffered from serious facial deformities caused by ABS and the other had an incomplete release for fear of injury to the ankle. We recently performed fetoscopic laser release of three extremity amniotic bands in two fetuses, both with impending limb amputation.[36] Secondary lymphedema persisted postnatally in one fetus, while atrophy of the hand occurred in the other fetus. One lower extremity in which the band was released before irreversible damage occurred was completely normal at the time of delivery. The results of these few cases establish at least the feasibility of performing fetoscopic release of amniotic bands involving the extremities. In cases of umbilical cord involvement, this approach has the potential of being lifesaving.

Fetoscopic treatment for complications in monochorionic twins

Monochorionic twins discordant for anomaly

Perhaps the area where fetoscopic intervention has had its greatest impact is in the management of complications in monochorionic twins, such as anomalous cotwin with threatened fetal demise, twin reversed arterial perfusion sequence, and the twin–twin transfusion syndrome. A range of congenital malformations such as anencephaly, omphalocele, hydrocephalus, and atresia/stenosis of the gastrointestinal tract are more common in twin gestations. Congenital heart defects are twice as prevalent in monozygotic twins as in dizygotic twins or singleton pregnancies.[37] In addition, twins discordant for anomaly deliver earlier than the average twin delivery at 34 weeks.[38] Therefore, there are increased risks for the healthy cotwin, not only from intrauterine demise of the anomalous cotwin, but also from the risks attendant to premature delivery.

In a dichorionic pregnancy, it is possible to observe spontaneous intrauterine fetal demise or perform selective feticide by means of a potassium chloride injection, without significant risk to the healthy cotwin. This is not the case with monochorionic pregnancies in light of the vascular connections between the twins. The usual recommendation has been to manage these pregnancies expectantly, because alternative interventions, such as sectio parva (selective removal of the anomalous twin) or ultrasound guided embolization, have been unsuccessful. In monochorionic gestations, however, this strategy leaves the healthy cotwin at risk of simultaneous intrauterine fetal demise or severe neurologic morbidity. Fetoscopy provides a viable therapeutic option under these circumstances through fetoscopic cord ligation or coagulation. Crombleholme et al[39] reported the first use of fetoscopic cord ligation specifically to prevent neurologic injury in a surviving twin when death of a cotwin was imminent. This involved monochorionic diamniotic twins at 22 weeks' gestation; one twin was structurally normal and the other was diagnosed with hypoplastic left-heart syndrome complicated by severe right-ventricular dysfunction, marked left-ventricular endocardial fibroelastosis, severe tricuspid regurgitation, and early signs of hydrops, which together suggested imminent fetal demise. A fetoscopic cord ligation of the affected twin was successfully performed via a two-port technique. No central nervous system changes were noted in the surviving twin on follow-up sonograms, and a neurologically intact baby girl was subsequently delivered. Several groups have reported success with fetoscopic cord ligation or coagulation in instances where an anomalous cotwin may threaten the normal twin.

Twin reversed arterial perfusion (TRAP) sequence

Twin reversed arterial perfusion (TRAP) sequence occurs only in the setting of a monochorionic pregnancy. The incidence of this condition is about 1 in 35 000 births or 1% of monochorionic twin gestations. In the TRAP sequence, the acardiac/acephalic twin receives all of its blood supply from the normal or 'pump' twin (Figure 12.5). The term 'reversed perfusion' is used to describe this scenario because blood enters the acardiac/acephalic twin through its umbilical artery and exits through the umbilical vein. The grossly anomalous circulation whereby the parasitic acardiac twin is sustained by the normal 'pump' twin places increased demand on the normal baby's heart, resulting in cardiac failure. If left untreated, the 'pump' twin dies in up to 50–75% of cases. This is especially true when the acardiac/acephalic twin is greater than 50% of the size of the 'pump' twin by estimated weight.[40]

Quintero et al[41] reported the first successful umbilical cord ligation for TRAP sequence. A number of different techniques have since been used to treat TRAP sequence, including 40 cases of cord occlusion by embolization in five, ligation in 15, laser photocoagulation in 10, bipolar diathermy in seven, and monopolar diathermy in three (Figure 12.6). Intrafetal ablation

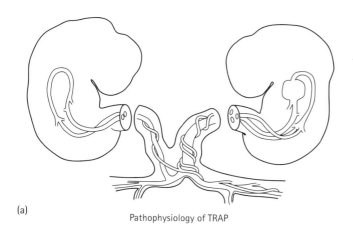

(a)

Pathophysiology of TRAP

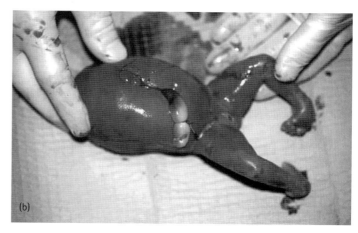

(b)

Figure 12.5 (a) Schematic illustration of pathophysiology of TRAP sequence. The circulation of the acardiac twin (left) is grossly anomalous, whereby this parasitic twin is sustained by the normal 'pump' twin (right). (b) Acardiac/acephalic twin delivered after cord ligation.

has also been performed by alcohol injection in five, monopolar diathermy in nine, interstial laser in four and radiofrequency in 13. Challis et al reported a failure rate for cord ligation of 10%, with fetal survival of 71% and risk of preterm premature rupture of membranes of 30%.[42]

We do not offer cord coagulation unless the acardiac twin to 'pump' twin ratio exceeds 70%. We have had nine patients where this ratio never exceeded 70%; expectant management

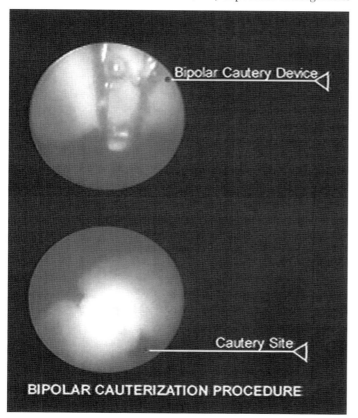

Figure 12.6 Fetoscopic images of umbilical cord occlusion by bipolar cautery (above) and the cord after successful cauterization (below).

was used, with all nine 'pump' twins surviving. One fairly consistent feature of the acardiac fetus is the presence of severe oligohydramnios in the acardiac sac, since most have no renal tissue to produce urine. We generally perform an amnioinfusion for the acardiac fetus at the beginning of the procedure, allowing better access for visualization of its anomalous two-vessel umbilical cord. A 4-mm operative trocar is then inserted into the expanded amniotic sac of the acardiac twin, and the anomalous cord is carefully evaluated with a 2-mm endoscope. A suitable membrane-free segment of cord is selected, the endoscope is removed, and the bipolar device is introduced under ultrasound guidance. The two-vessel cord is grasped and cauterized in two or three adjacent sites. The success of cauterization can be directly assessed fetoscopically. The absence of flow to the acardiac twin is then confirmed by a combination of power and color Doppler. Upon completion of the cauterization, amniotic fluid around the acardiac twin is removed through the operative trocar, and routine amnioreduction can be performed for the 'pump' twin. A single-port endoscopic procedure can be used up to 24 weeks' gestation. A two-port cord ligation may be necessary, however, at later gestational ages, since bipolar electrocautery may be inadequate to occlude completely the larger umbilical cord of these fetuses. With this approach, our experience shows a mean gestational age at delivery of greater than 33 weeks and an overall survival of 85%, with no significant maternal morbidity or mortality.

A newer alternative approach is unipolar radiofrequency ablation (RFA). This technique has the advantage of being an entirely sonographically-guided technique, using a 19-gauge unipolar radiofrequency device. The RFA needle is sonographically positioned near the umbilical artery as it enters the abdomen of the acardius (Figure 12.7). The advantage of this approach is that it is not limited by oligohydramnios in the acardiac sac or difficulty in gaining access to the short umbilical cord of the acardius. In addition, since this approach uses only a thin, 19-gauge device, there is decreased uterine irritability postoperatively. Tsao et al reported on the use of RFA in 13

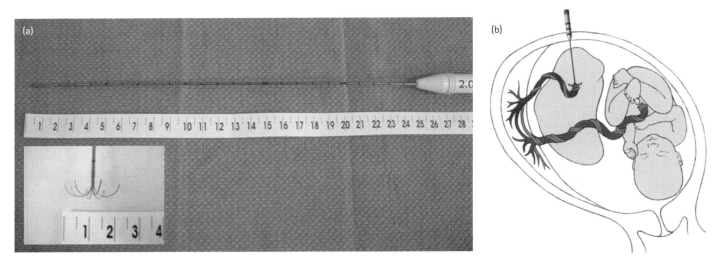

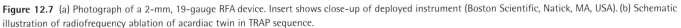

Figure 12.7 (a) Photograph of a 2-mm, 19-gauge RFA device. Insert shows close-up of deployed instrument (Boston Scientific, Natick, MA, USA). (b) Schematic illustration of radiofrequency ablation of acardiac twin in TRAP sequence.

monochorionic diamniotic twin gestations complicated by TRAP sequence.[43] The median gestational age at intervention was 20.1 weeks. Three of the pump twins had hydrops at presentation and eight had polyhydraminos. Blood flow to the acardiac twin was effectively obliterated in all cases. The median gestational age at delivery was 38.4 weeks. The only infant who died was born at 24.4 weeks due to PPROM and was already hydropic at the time of intervention. At the time of report, the 12 surviving infants were doing well and had normal neonatal neurodevelopmental assessments.

Twin–twin transfusion syndrome (TTTS)

Treatment options in TTTS
The natural history of severe TTTS is well established, with mortality approaching 100% if left untreated, especially when it presents at less than 20 weeks' gestation.[44,45] As a result, numerous treatments have been proposed, including selective feticide, cord coagulation, sectio parva, placental blood letting, maternal digitalis, maternal indocin, serial amnioreduction, microseptostomy of the intertwin membrane, and nonselective or selective fetoscopic laser photocoagulation. For decades in the USA, however, serial amnioreduction has been the most widely accepted therapy of TTTS.

Amnioreduction
Amnioreduction was first employed as a means to control polyhydramnios in the hope of prolonging the pregnancy. In uncontrolled series, amnioreduction appears to improve survival. Moise, in a review of 26 reports dating from the 1930s of 252 fetuses, found an overall survival of 49%.[46] Survival rates in more recent series, with more consistently aggressive serial amnioreduction to reduce amniotic fluid volume to normal, have ranged widely from as low as 37% to as high as 83%.[47–52]

However, these retrospective series comprised small numbers of patients from a range of gestational ages, as well as from a spectrum of severity of TTTS. Severity of TTTS and gestational age at diagnosis may have a profound impact on the observed mortality with any treatment strategy. The earlier in gestation TTTS presents, the worse the prognosis. Mari et al found that patients presenting with advanced TTTS prior to 22 weeks' gestation and absent end diastolic flow in the recipient umbilical artery had a survival rate with aggressive amnioreduction of only 13%; with absent end diastolic flow in the donor umbilical artery, survival was 33%.[53]

Microseptostomy
The paradoxical resolution of oligohydramnios after a single amnioreduction was first suggested by Saade et al to be due to inadvertent puncture of the intertwin membrane[54] (Figure 12.8). Intertwin septostomy was specifically proposed as a treatment for TTTS to restore amniotic fluid dynamics without the need for repeated amnioreduction. One objection to this approach is that it might result in a large septostomy, creating an essentially monoamniotic sac with the attendant risk of cord entanglement. For this reason, a fetoscopic 'microseptostomy' has been proposed to prevent this complication (Figure 12.9). In a small multicenter series of 12 patients, Saade et al reported an 81% survival with microseptostomy.[55] However, not only was this series small and uncontrolled, there was no report of neurologic or cardiac morbidity. In a direct comparison, albeit a small retrospective single-institution series, of serial amnioreduction versus microseptostomy, Johnson et al observed no survival advantage with either therapy.[56] This was confirmed by Saade et al, who recently reported the results of a multicenter, prospective, randomized clinical trial comparing amnioreduction to septostomy. The survival in each arm of the study was 65%.[57]

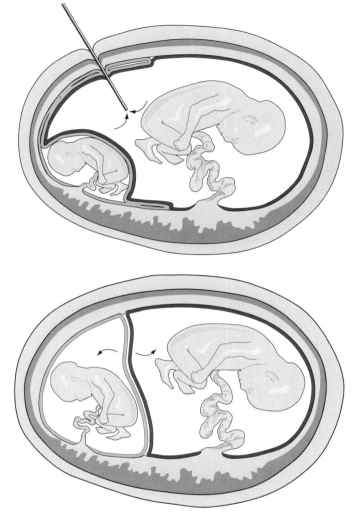

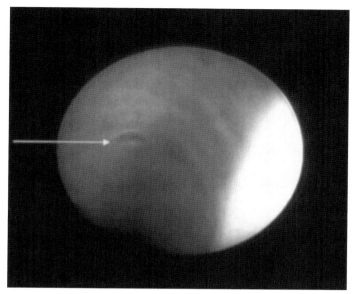

Figure 12.9 Endoscopic view of a laser microseptostomy.

Figure 12.8 Inadvertent intertwin septostomy has been suggested as the reason for the 'one-amnioreduction paradox', in which the signs of TTTS are corrected by a single amniocentesis. As this schematic drawing shows, the amniocentesis needle passes through the intertwin membrane (upper panel), which cannot be seen sonographically. This puncture of the intertwin membrane allows passage of fluid from one sac to the other (lower panel). (From Crombleholme TM. The treatment of twin–twin transfusion syndrome. Semin Pediatr Surg 2003; 12: 175–81 with permission from Elsevier.)

Fetoscopic laser photocoagulation

The first treatment for TTTS that attempted to treat the anatomic basis of the syndrome was reported by De Lia et al.[58,59] Fetoscopic laser was used to photocoagulate vessels crossing the intertwin membrane (Figure 12.10). In his first small series, De Lia reported a survival of 53% in 26 patients.[59] While survival was not significantly better than previous reports with serial amnioreduction, the neurologic outcome in 96% of survivors was 'normal' as assessed by head ultrasound. Other groups from Europe have reported similar survival with nonselective laser photocoagulation. Ville et al reported 53% survival with a fetoscopic laser technique which was better than the survival

observed with historical controls at the same center with serial amnioreduction (37%).[60] There also appeared to be an improvement in neurologic outcome in fetuses treated by laser, according to neonatal head ultrasound.

A nonselective fetoscopic laser technique photocoagulates all vessels crossing the intertwin membrane. This approach may be problematic, as the intertwin membrane often bears no relation to the vascular equator of the placenta. This nonselective laser photocoagulation of all vessels crossing the intertwin membrane may sacrifice vessels not responsible for the TTTS, resulting in a higher death rate of the donor twin from acute placental insufficiency.[61] More recently, a selective approach to fetoscopic laser photocoagulation in TTTS has been described.[61] Unlike the nonselective coagulation technique, initially described by De Lia et al, the selective technique does not photocoagulate every vessel crossing the intertwin membrane. Only direct, arterial-arterial and venovenous connections are photocoagulated, along with any unpaired artery going to a cotyledon, with the corresponding vein (and vice versa) going to the opposite umbilical cord. In a nonrandomized comparison of patients treated by serial amnioreduction at one center and selective laser photocoagulation at another, the overall survival was not statistically significantly different (61% for laser vs 51% for serial amnioreduction).[62] However, the survival of at least one twin with laser photocoagulation was 79%, while survival of at least one twin with serial amnioreduction was only 60% ($p < 0.05$).[62]

The Eurofoetus trial conducted by Senat et al[63] is thus far the only prospective, randomized trial that compares the efficacy and safety of treatment of twin-to-twin transfusion syndrome with laser therapy versus serial amnioreduction. Women presenting at 15–26 weeks' gestation with polyhydraminos in the recipient twin and oligohydramninos in the donor twin were allowed to participate. Enrollment was halted after a planned interim

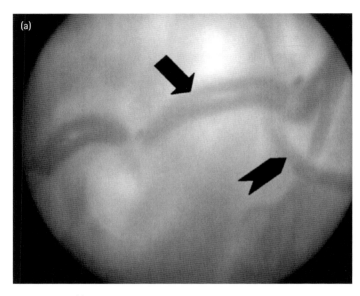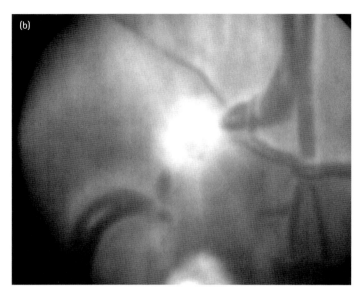

Figure 12.10 (a) Fetoscopic view of the placental surface shows an example of an arteriovenous connection via a placental cotyledon. The arrow indicates the artery from one twin leading to a cotyledon, with the venous drainage (arrowhead) leading to the other twin. (b) The appearance of the same vessel after laser photocoagulation. (From Crombleholme TM. The treatment of twin–twin transfusion syndrome. Semin Pediatr Surg 2003; 12: 175–81 with permission from Elsevier.)

analysis revealed a significantly higher likelihood of survival of at least one twin to 28 days of age (76% vs 56%; P = 0.009), and to 6 months of age (76% vs 51%; P = 0.002) in the laser group compared to the amnioreduction group. More infants were alive without neurologic abnormalities detected on neuroimaging studies in the laser group as well (52% vs 31%; P = 0.003). The overall survival in the laser arm was 57%. This is consistent with previous reports of nonselective fetoscopic laser (53%).[59,60] This is significantly lower, however, than the survival reported with selective fetoscopic laser (64–68%).[64,65] Of particular concern is the poor survival observed in the amnioreduction arm. The overall survival was only 39%, which is significantly lower than previously reported (60–65%).[53,57] Antenatal, peripartum, and neonatal care was provided by the referring hospital, and lack of standardization may explain some of these differences.[66] The decreased survival in the amnioreduction group may reflect the higher pregnancy termination rate in the amnioreduction group (16% vs 0% in the laser group). The terminations were requested after the diagnosis of severe fetal complications; it would be instructive to know whether these women were offered cord coagulation as a means of rescuing one baby.[66] Reliable assessment of neorologic outcome is critical when assessing efficacy of treatment for TTTS. While there was a lower rate of abnormality on neurologic imaging or clinical neurologic impairment in the laser group (7% vs 17%), there was no long-term neurodevelopmental assessment. The importance of this is highlighted by one study in which 6% of survivors after laser therapy had abnormalities on neonatal imaging, yet 11% had evidence of cerebral palsy at 1 year of age or older when neurodevelopmental assessment was performed.[67]

Crombleholme et al are currently conducting a NIH-sponsored, multicenter, prospective, randomized, controlled trial comparing aggressive amnioreduction with selective fetoscopic laser photocoagulation for severe TTTS prior to 22 weeks' gestation. Using blinded reviewers, this trial will correlate the results of serial prenatal ultrasound scans, fetal echocardiograms, and fetal magnetic resonance imaging (MRI) with treatment. In addition to the primary endpoint of recipient and donor twin survival, the NIH-sponsored trial will evaluate neonatal comorbidities and correlate neuroradiologic findings with neurodevelopmental outcomes at 18–22 months by evaluation at NICHD neonatal network centers.

Fetoscopic cord coagulation

Some centers have taken the view that the most definitive approach to treating TTTS is selective reduction by fetoscopic cord ligation or coagulation. The rationale for this approach is that cord occlusion and sacrifice of one twin arrests the syndrome, prolongs the gestation, and maximizes the outcome for the other twin.[68] We have reserved this approach for instances where advanced TTTS cardiomyopathy has irretrievably compromised the recipient twin with no hope for salvage. In such cases, due to unequal sharing between the donor and recipient, the selective fetoscopic laser procedure may result in the death of the donor twin from acute placental insufficiency within hours of the procedure, while the recipient twin dies from progressive TTTS cardiomyopathy. In this situation, fetoscopic cord coagulation may be the best option available. Cord coagulation preserves the vascular communications between the donor twin and the placenta in the recipient twin's domain. In 14 of 15 such cases, we have observed rebound fetal growth, restoration of amniotic fluid volume, and delivery of a neurologically intact donor twin at a mean gestational age of 34 weeks.

Sequential treatment

Our approach has been to offer sequential therapy tailored to the needs of a given set of twins according to gestational age at presentation and evidence of progression of hemodynamic compromise, based on Doppler velocimetry and echocardiographic changes.[69] In this approach, only those cases in which less invasive approaches have failed are offered the more invasive fetoscopic treatments. In patients who present later than 24 weeks' gestation, we have favored amnioreduction or microseptostomy in view of the much more favorable prognosis in these patients.[69] In patients presenting prior to 24 weeks without advanced cardiac changes in the recipient, we have tended toward microseptostomy as an initial therapy. As amniotic fluid dynamics are restored in both donor and recipient amniotic sacs with microseptostomy, serial amnioreductions are not necessary. This reduces the risk of chorioamniotic separation, which may preclude subsequent fetoscopic treatment. This group of patients presenting earlier in gestation tends to develop signs of hemodynamic progression of TTTS despite normal amniotic fluid dynamics. For this reason, all pregnancies undergo close serial sonographic and echocardiographic surveillance for progression in cardiac changes, hemodynamic changes, or progressive growth discordance, which would be indications for selective fetoscopic laser surgery. We reserve fetoscopic cord coagulation in TTTS for instances in which cotwin demise is imminent and fetoscopic laser surgery would adversely separate the placental mass in favor of the fetus with imminent demise, leaving the surviving donor fetus with placental insufficiency.

Complications of endoscopic fetal surgery

Preterm labor is the 'Achilles' heel' of fetal intervention.[70] It is, to some degree, a complication of all fetal surgery. Using a fetoscopic approach should decrease this risk but does not solve the problem. The etiology of preterm labor may be related to the disease process for which the surgery is indicated (i.e., associated with polyhydraminos or specific anomalies). Preterm labor may also be related to a fetal systemic inflammatory response that is a reaction to intervention.[71] A maternal inflammatory response to uterine trauma probably also plays a role in initiating preterm contractions. Unfortunately, as with spontaneous preterm birth, we still do not have adequate tocolytics available. For endoscopic laser procedures, our choice is to use magnesium sulfate, which is started in the operating room and continued for about 24 hours. We then switch to nifedipine for outpatient management.

Chorioamniotic separation is the most frequent complication of endoscopic fetal surgery, occurring in 36% of cases.[72] The incidence of chorioamniotic separation after fetal surgery is gestational age-dependent, occurring more frequently when the procedure is performed prior to 23 weeks' gestation.

Chorioamnioic separation is associated with an increased rate of preterm premature rupture of membranes (PPROM) and mortality[72] as well as chorioamnionitis. Estimates are that PPROM occurs in 6–10% of surgeries with one port[73] and up to 40–60% of surgeries with multiple ports.[22,74] Interestingly, the site of membrane rupture is often distant from the trocar site.[75]

Bleeding is not usually a major problem in endoscopic fetal surgery. It is well worth the time preoperatively to plan carefully with ultrasound an approach which allows room for manipulation of the endoscope while avoiding the placenta as well as the broad-ligament blood vessels. In the case of an anterior placenta, the patient may need to lie completely on one side. In all cases it is best to tilt the patient at least slightly to avoid vena caval obstruction.

References

1. Reuss A, Stewart PA, Wladimiroff JW et al. Non-invasive management of fetal obstructive uropathy. Lancet 1988; 2: 949–51.

2. Cusick EL, Didier F, Droulle P, et al. Mortality after an antenatal diagnosis of foetal uropathy. J Pediatr Surg 1995; 30: 463–6.

3. Glick PL, Harrison MR, Golbus MS et al. Management of the fetus with congenital hydronephrosis. II. Prognostic criteria and selection for treatment. J Pediatr Surg 1985; 20: 376–87.

4. Johnson MP, Bukowski TP, Reitleman C et al. In utero surgical treatment of fetal obstructive uropathy: a new comprehensive approach to identify appropriate candidates for vesicoamniotic shunt therapy. Am J Obstet Gynecol 1994; 170: 1770–9.

5. Clark TJ, Martin WL, Divakaran TG et al. Prenatal bladder drainage in the management of fetal lower urinary tract obstruction: a systematic review and meta-analysis. Obstet Gynecol 2003; 102: 367–82.

6. Freedman AL, Johnson MP, Smith CA et al. Long-term outcome in children after antenatal intervention for obstructive uropathies. Lancet 1999; 354: 374–7.

7. Holmes N, Harrison MR, Baskin LS. Fetal surgery for posterior urethral valves: long-term postnatal outcomes. Pediatrics 2001; 108: e1–e7.

8. Gatti JM, Kirsch AJ, Massad CA. Antenatal intervention: jeopardizing life or limb. Urology 2002; 60: viii–ix.

9. Quintero RA, Johnson MP, Smith C et al. In utero percutaneous cystoscopy in the management of fetal lower obstructive uropathy. Lancet 1995; 346: 537–40.

10. Quintero RA, Hume R, Smith C et al. Percutaneous fetal cystoscopy and endoscopic fulguration of posterior urethral valves. Am J Obstet Gynecol 1995; 172: 206–9.

11. Fauza DO, Wilson JM. Congenital diaphragmatic hernia and associated anomalies: their incidence, identification, and impact on prognosis. J Pediatr Surg 1994; 29: 1113–17.

12. Puri P. Congenital diaphragmatic hernia. Curr Probl Surg 1994; 31: 787–846.

13. Albanese CT, Lopoo J, Goldstein RB et al. Fetal liver position and perinatal outcome for congenital diaphragmatic hernia. Prenatal Diagn 1998; 18: 1138–42.

14. Guibaud L, Filiatrault D, Garel L et al. Fetal congenital diaphragmatic hernia: accuracy of sonography in the diagnosis and prediction of the outcome after birth. AJR Am J Roentgenol 1996; 166: 1195–202.

15. Lipshutz GS, Albanese CT, Feldstein VA et al. Prospective analysis of lung-to-head ratio predicts survival for patients with prenatally diagnosed congenital diaphragmatic hernia. J Pediatr Surg 1997; 32: 1634–6.

16. Landy JAM, Van Gucht M, Van Dooren MF, et al. Congenital diaphragmatic hernia: an evaluation of the prognostic value of the lung-to-head ratio and other prenatal parameters. Prenat Diagn 2003; 23: 634–9.

17. Metkus AP, Filly RA, Stringer MD et al. Sonographic predictors of survival in fetal diaphragmatic hernia. J Pediatr Surg 1996; 31: 148–52.

18. Hubbard AM, Crombleholme TM, Adzick NS et al. Prenatal MRI evaluation of congenital diaphragmatic hernia. Am J Perinat 1999; 16: 407–13.

19. Areechon W, Reid L. Hypoplasia of the lung associated with congenital diaphragmatic hernia. BMJ 1963; 1: 230–3.

20. DiFiore JW, Fauza DO, Slavin R et al. Experimental fetal tracheal ligation reverses the structural and physiological effects of pulmonary hypoplasia in congenital diaphragmatic hernia. J Pediatr Surg 1994; 29: 248–56.

21. Hedrick MH, Estes JM, Sullivan KM et al. Plug the lung until it grows (PLUG): a new method to treat congenital diaphragmatic hernia in utero. J Pediatr Surg 1994; 29: 612–17.

22. Harrison MR, Mychaliska GB, Albanese CT et al. Correction of congenital diaphragmatic hernia in utero. IX. Fetuses with poor prognosis (liver herniation, low lung-to-head ratio) can be saved by fetoscopic temporary tracheal occlusion. J Pediatr Surg 1998; 33: 1017–23.

23. Harrison MR, Albanese CT, Hawgood SB et al. Fetoscopic temporary tracheal occlusion by means of detachable balloon for congenital diaphragmatic hernia. Am J Obstet Gynecol 2001; 185: 730–3.

24. Harrison MR, Keller RL, Hagwood SB et al. A randomized trial of fetal endoscopic tracheal occlusion for severe fetal congenital diaphragmatic hernia. N Engl J Med 2003; 349: 1916–24.

25. Bond SJ, Harrison MR, Schmidt KG et al. Death due to high output cardiac failure in fetal sacrococcygeal teratoma. J Pediatr Surg 1990; 25: 1287–91.

26. Flake AW. Fetal sacrococcygeal teratoma. Semin Pediatr Surg 1993; 2: 113–20.

27. Flake AW, Harrison MR, Adzick NS et al. Fetal sacrococcygeal teratoma. J Pediatr Surg 1986; 21: 563–6.

28. Alter DN, Reed KL, Marx GR et al. Prenatal diagnosis of congestive heart failure in a fetus with a sacrococcygeal teratoma. Obstet Gynecol 1988; 71: 978–81.

29. Schmidt KG, Silverman NH, Harrison MR et al. High-output cardiac failure in fetuses with large SCT: diagnosis by echocardiography and Doppler ultrasound. J Pediatr 1989; 114: 1023–8.

30. Adzick NS, Crombleholme TM, Morgan MA et al. A rapidly growing fetal teratoma. Lancet 1997; 349: 538.

31. Hecher K, Hackeloer BJ. Intrauterine endoscopic laser surgery for fetal sacrococcygeal teratoma. Lancet 1996; 347: 470.

32. Paek BW, Jennings RW, Harrison MR et al. Radiofrequency ablation of human fetal sacrococcygeal teratoma. Am J Obstet Gynecol 2001; 184: 503–7.

33. Bruner JP, Richards WO, Tulipan N et al. Endoscopic coverage of fetal myelomeningocele in utero. Am J Obstet Gynecol 1999; 180: 153–8.

34. Crombleholme TM, Dirkes K, Whitney TM et al. Amniotic band syndrome in fetal lambs. I. Fetoscopic release and morphometric outcome. J Pediatr Surg 1995; 30: 974–8.

35. Quintero RA, Morales WJ, Phillips J et al. In utero lysis of amniotic bands. Ultrasound Obstet Gynecol 1997; 10: 316–20.

36. Keswani SG, Johnson MP, Adzick NS et al. In utero limb salvage: fetoscopic release of amniotic bands for threatened limb amputation. J Pediatr Surg 2003; 38: 848–51.

37. Burn J. The spectrum of genetic disorders in twins. In: Ward RH, Whittle M (eds), Multiple Pregnancy, pp. 74–83. RCOG Press: London, 1995.

38. Malone FD, D'Alton ME. Multiple gestation: clinical characteristics and management. In: Creasy RK, Resnik R (eds). Maternal-Fetal Medicine, pp. 598–615 (4th edition). WB Saunders: Philadelphia, 1999.

39. Crombleholme TM, Robertson F, Marx G et al. Fetoscopic cord ligation to prevent neurologic injury in monozygous twins. Lancet 1996; 348: 191.

40. Moore TR, Gale S, Benirschke K. Perinatal outcome of forty-nine pregnancies complicated by acardiac twinning. Am J Obstet Gynecol 1990; 163: 907–12.

41. Quintero RA, Reich H, Pruder KS et al. Brief report: umbilical cord ligation to an acardiac twin by fetoscopy at 19 weeks of gestation. N Engl J Med 1994; 330: 469–71.

42. Challis D, Gratecas E, Deprest JA. Cord occlusion techniques for selective termination in monochorionic twins. J Perinatal Med 1999; 27: 327–8.

43. Tsao K, Feldstein VA, Albanese CT et al. Selective reduction of acardiac twin by radiofrequency ablation. Am J Obstet Gynecol 2002; 187: 635–40.

44. Chescheir NC, Seeds JW. Polyhydramnios and oligohydramnios in twin gestations. Obstet Gynecol 1988; 71: 882–4.

45. Weir PE, Ratten GJ, Beischer NA. Acute polyhydramnios – a complication of monozygous twin pregnancy. Br J Obstet Gynaecol 1979; 86: 849–53.

46. Moise KJ Jr. Polyhydramnios: problems and treatment. Semin Perinatol 1993; 17: 197–209.

47. Rodestal A, Thomassen PA. Acute polyhydramnios in twin pregnancy. A retrospective study with special reference to therapeutic amniocentesis. Acta Obstet Gynecol Scand 1990; 69: 297–300.

48. Urig MA, Clewell WH, Elliott J. Twin–twin transfusion syndrome. Am J Obstet Gynecol 1990; 163: 1522–6.

49. Mahony BS, Petty CN, Nyberg DA et al. The 'stuck twin' phenomenon: ultrasonographic findings, pregnancy outcome, and management with serial amniocenteses. Am J Obstet Gynecol 1990; 163: 1513–21.

50. Elliott JP, Urig MA, Clewell WH. Aggressive therapeutic amniocentesis for treatment of twin–twin transfusion syndrome. Obstet Gynecol 1991; 77: 537–40.

51. Pinette MG, Pan Y, Pinette SG et al. Treatment of twin–twin transfusion syndrome. Obstet Gynecol 1993; 82: 841–6.

52. Reisner DP, Mahony BS, Petty CH et al. Stuck twin syndrome: outcome in 37 consecutive cases. Am J Obstet Gynecol 1993; 169: 991–5.

53. Mari G, Roberts A, Detti L et al. Perinatal morbidity and mortality rates in severe twin–twin transfusion syndrome: results of the International Amnioreduction Registry. Am J Obstet Gynecol 2001; 185: 708–15.

54. Saade GR, Olson G, Belfort MA et al. Amniotomy: a new approach to the 'stuck twin' syndrome. Am J Obstet Gynecol 1995; 172: 429–34.

55. Saade GR, Belfort MA, Berry DL et al. Amniotic septostomy for the treatment of twin oligohydramnios-polyhydramnios sequence. Fetal Diagn Ther 1998; 13: 86–93.

56. Johnson JR, Rossi KQ, Shaughnessy RW et al. Amnioreduction versus septostomy in twin–twin transfusion syndrome. Am J Obstet Gynecol 2001; 185: 1044–7.

57. Saade G, Moise K, Dorman K et al. A randomized trial of septostomy versus amnioreduction in the treatment of twin oligohydramnios polyhydramnios sequence (TOPS). Am J Obstet Gynecol (Society for Maternal–Fetal Medicine. Oral presentation, abstract 3): 2003; 187 (6).

58. De Lia JE, Cruikshank DP, Kaye WR. Fetoscopic neodymium: YAG laser occlusion of placental vessels in severe twin–twin transfusion syndrome. Obstet Gynecol 1990; 75: 1046–53.

59. De Lia JE, Kuhlmann RS, Harstad TW et al. Fetoscopic laser ablation of placental vessels in severe twin–twin transfusion syndrome. Am J Obstet Gynecol 1995; 172: 1202–11.

60. Ville Y, Hyett J, Hecher K, Nicolaides KH. Preliminary experience with endoscopic laser surgery for severe twin–twin transfusion syndrome. N Engl J Med 1995; 332: 224–7.

61. Quintero RA, Morales WJ, Mendoza G et al. Selective photocoagulation of placental vessels in twin–twin transfusion syndrome: evolution of a surgical technique. Obstet Gynecol Survey 1998; 53: 597–603.

62. Hecher K, Plath H, Bregenzer T et al. Endoscopic laser surgery versus serial amniocenteses in the treatment of severe twin–twin transfusion syndrome. Am J Obstet Gynecol 1999; 180: 717–24.

63. Senat MV, Deprest J, Boulvain M et al. Endoscopic laser surgery versus serial amnioreduction for severe twin-to-twin transfusion syndrome. N Engl J Med 2004; 351: 136–44.

64. Quintero RA, Dickinson JE, Morales WJ et al. Stage-based treatment of twin–twin transfusion syndrome. Am J Obstet Gynecol 2003; 188: 1333–40.

65. Hecher K, Diehk W, Zikulnig L et al. Endoscopic laser coagulation of placental anastomoses in 200 pregnancies with severe midtrimester twin-to-twin transfusion syndrome. Eur J Obstet Gynecol Reprod Biol 2000; 92: 135–9.

66. Fisk NM, Galea P. Twin–twin transfusion – as good as it gets? N Engl J Med 2004; 351: 182–4.

67. Banek CS, Hecher K, Hackeloer BJ et al. Long-term neurodevelopmental outcome after intrauterine laser treatment for severe twin-twin transfusion syndrome. Am J Obstet Gynecol 2003; 188: 876–80.

68. Crombleholme TM, Robertson F, Marx G et al. Fetoscopic cord ligation to prevent neurological injury in monozygous twins. Lancet 1996; 348: 191.

69. Milner R, Crombleholme TM. Troubles with twins: fetoscopic therapy. Semin Perinat 1999; 23: 474–83.

70. Harrison MR. Fetal surgery. Am J Obstet Gynecol 1996; 174: 1255–64.

71. Romero R, Gomez R, Ghezzi F et al. A fetal systemic inflammatory response is followed by the spontaneous onset of preterm parturition. Am J Obstet Gynecol 1998; 179: 186–93.

72. Harrison MR, Tsao K, Hirose S et al. Chorioamniotic membrane separation following fetal surgery. Am J Obstet Gynecol 2001; 184; S143.

73. Ville Y, Hecher K, Gagnon A, et al. Endoscopic laser coagulation in the management of severe twin-to-twin transfusion syndrome. Br J Obstet Gynaecol 1998; 105: 446–53.

74. Deprest JA, Van Ballaer PP, Evrard VA et al. Experience with fetoscopic cord ligation. Eur J Obstet Gynecol Reprod Bio 1998; 81: 157–64.

75. Danzer E, Sydorak RM, Harrison MR et al. Minimal access fetal surgery. Eur J Obstet Gynecol Reprod Bio 2003; 108: 3–13.

13 Fetal surgery

Robert H Ball and Michael R Harrison

The potential for the field of fetal surgery would not exist were it not for the ready availability of prenatal diagnosis. The opportunity for prenatal diagnosis is based primarily on the prevalence of routine ultrasound screening of pregnancies in the developed world. There is, however, a broad spectrum of detection rates for fetal malformations. Most malformations addressed with fetal surgery may be quite detectable as 'not normal' on routine screening but may not be accurately identified until a targeted examination is performed. It is self-evident that an accurate diagnosis is critical to determine the appropriateness of a fetal surgical intervention. Fetal malformations that are not isolated or are associated with aneuploidy or a syndrome have always been excluded as candidates for intervention. Great effort is therefore always made to confirm both an accurate diagnosis of a malformation and the fact that it is isolated. Ancillary techniques to ensure full and accurate assessment include fetal echocardiography, MRI, and karyotyping, depending on what additional problems the fetus is most at risk for. However, patients should always be counseled regarding the fallibility of the process.

The indications for fetal surgical interventions have expanded, as has the total number of procedures performed, the sites at which they are performed and the number of physicians performing them. Nevertheless overall these procedures remain very limited when compared to the number of pregnancies and even the number of fetuses with malformations. One of the responsibilities of physicians with an interest in prenatal diagnosis and intervention, over the next years, is to determine training needs and oversight for operators and centers involved in this field. It is unclear how many centers would be needed, given the rarity of malformations and the even smaller proportion of those with malformations that may need fetal intervention. We must decide whether ease of access is a substitute for volume of procedures performed. Certainly with access to the World Wide Web, patients in our experience have become savvy consumers who are readily able to contact us and provide us with the information necessary to make a preliminary assessment regarding their fetus's diagnosis. This, together with the increasing ease of large-volume electronic transfer of information, has, in our view, made geographic proximity less important.

Over the last decade, technological advances have allowed a transition towards less invasive procedures. Initial fetal surgical procedures pioneered by one of the authors (M.R.H.), at UCSF, depended on maternal laparotomy and hysterotomy. This approach evolved into laparotomy and uterine endoscopy, and, most recently, into percutaneous procedures using devices with diameters of 3 mm or less. Our experience suggests that the less invasive approaches are associated with a less complicated postoperative recovery for the mothers, but do not entirely eliminate morbidity.[1] Each of these approaches will be discussed in detail.

Open fetal surgery (hysterotomy)

The feasibility of performing hysterotomy and subsequent closure on the gravid human uterus was tested in the primate. The reason for using the primate model is because other gravid, large-animal models, such as the sheep, are much more forgiving. The sheep uterus is more thin-walled and has a multicotyledonary placenta. Closure is more straightforward, and preterm labor is rarely a significant problem. The safety profile in this series of primate fetal surgeries was reassuring, including subsequent fertility.[2] The human experience is now quite extensive, from both our own center and others,[1,3,4] primarily associated with a large number of fetal spina bifida repairs. We currently reserve maternal laparotomy/hysterotomy procedures for repair of spina bifida, resection of sacrococcygeal teratoma and other tumors, and lobectomy for congenital cystic adenomatoid malformation (CCAM) of the lung.

Risks and benefits

We have recently reviewed our experience at UCSF with maternal hysterotomy[1] (Table 13.1). Seventy-nine hysterotomies were performed between 1989 and 2003. There were significant immediate postoperative complications. In the early experience, pulmonary edema related to multiple tocolytic use, particularly nitroglycerin and aggressive fluid management, was a significant problem.[5] Almost 13% required transfusion for

Table 13.1 Maternal morbidity and mortality for 178 human fetal interventions at UCSF according to operative techniques

Operative technique	Open hysterotomy	Fetal endoscopic surgery (FETENDO)/Laparotomy-FETENDO	Percutaneous FIGS/Laparotomy-FIGS	All interventions
Patients with postoperative continuing pregnancy	79	68	31	178
Gestational age at surgery [weeks]	25.1	24.5	21.1	24.2
Range [weeks]	17.6–30.4	17.9–32.1	17.0–26.6	17.0–32.1
Gestational age at delivery [weeks]	30.1	30.4	32.7	30.7
Range [weeks]	21.6–36.7	19.6–39.3	21.7–40.4	19.6–40.4
Interval surgery to delivery [weeks]	4.9	6.0	11.6	6.5
Range [weeks]	0–16	0–19	0.3–21.4	0–21.4
Pulmonary edema	22/79 (27.8%)	17/68 (25.0%)	0/31 (0.0%)	39/178 (21.9%)
Bleeding requiring blood transfusion	11/87 (12.6%)	2/69 (2.9%)	0/31 (0.0%)	13/187 (7.0%)
Preterm labor leading to delivery	26/79 (32.9%)	18/68 (26.5%)	4/31 (12.9%)	48/178 (27.0%)
Premature rupture of membranes	41/79 (51.9%)	30/68 (44.1%)	8/31 (25.8%)	79/178 (44.4%)
Chorioamnionitis	7/79 (8.9%)	1/68 (1.5%)	0/31 (0.0%)	8/178 (4.5%)

UCSF: University of California at San Francisco; FIGS: fetal intervention guided by sonography.

intraoperative blood loss. Pregnancy outcomes were also significantly affected, with a premature rupture of membrane rate of 52%, and 33% having preterm labor refractory to maximal tocolytic management leading to delivery. The mean time from hysterotomy to delivery was 4.9 weeks (range 0–16 weeks). The mean gestational age at the time of delivery was 30.1 weeks (range 21.6–36.7 weeks). Others[6,7] have similar experiences with respect to an increased risk of preterm delivery after hysterotomy. Most of the morbidity associated with hysterotomy has decreased with experience. Nowadays, significant pulmonary edema or blood loss is rare, and the mean gestational age at the time of delivery for repair of fetal myelomeningocele (MMC) is around 34 weeks.

The practical aspects of hysterotomy and postoperative management have evolved since the initial years of experience. The following is a description of our current approach. Lengthy discussions regarding the risks, benefits, and alternatives of the procedure are important, including the experimental nature of the surgery. We generally differentiate the risks to the mother, the fetus, and the pregnancy in our counseling. The risks to the mother are similar to those of any major abdominal surgery, although in this case there is no direct physical benefit to her. In addition there are the risks associated with aggressive tocolytic therapy and bed rest in a hypercoagulable state. The risks to the fetus are primarily vascular instability and hypoperfusion intraoperatively leading to injury or death, and prematurity due to postoperative complications. The risks to the pregnancy are primarily preterm labor and premature rupture of

membranes and preterm delivery. Infectious complications are rare, except when premature rupture leads to prolonged latency. An important additional discussion point is that all subsequent deliveries, including the index pregnancy, must be delivered by cesarean section. Data regarding future fertility are reassuring, with no increased incidence of infertility in the UCSF experience in those patients attempting pregnancy.[8] Experience from CHOP suggests that the risk of uterine rupture in subsequent pregnancies may be as high as 17%, which would be considerably higher than the risk after previous low-transverse cesarean section (1% or less) or classical cesarean section (5%). Another potential risk in subsequent pregnancies is placenta accreta. The reason for this is that the site of a hysterotomy performed in the second trimester is never in the same area as a third-trimester cesarean section entry. There is an increased risk of placenta accreta in any case where implantation is in an area of uterine scarring. Multiple incisions will increase the likelihood of implantation in such an area. To our knowledge, there has not been a case of accreta in a fetal surgical patient of ours in a subsequent pregnancy.

Technique

Prior to surgery, the patients are premedicated with indomethacin and antibiotics. Compression stockings and pneumatic boots are placed on the lower extremities. General anesthesia is initiated with high levels of halogenated inhalational agents to maximize uterine relaxation. A Foley catheter is placed to drain the bladder. An epidural catheter is placed for postoperative pain control. After prepping and draping, ultrasound transducers with sterile covers are used to identify fetal lie and placental location. The latter will determine the need for exteriorization of the uterus to allow access to the posterior uterine aspect, in cases of anterior placenta. The transverse skin incision is generally a third of the way between the pubic symphysis and the umbilicus, but lower with an anterior placenta, so that the uterus can more easily be exteriorized. Usually, the rectus muscles need to be at least partially transected to allow appropriate exposure. Once the peritoneal cavity is entered, the ultrasound transducer is placed directly on the myometrium, and the edge of the placenta is identified and marked by cautery. The general strategy is to place the hysterotomy as far from the placenta as possible, with the direction of the incision parallel to its edge. This will minimize the risk of extension towards the placenta. The reason for this level of caution is that placental bed bleeding cannot be controlled. The additional

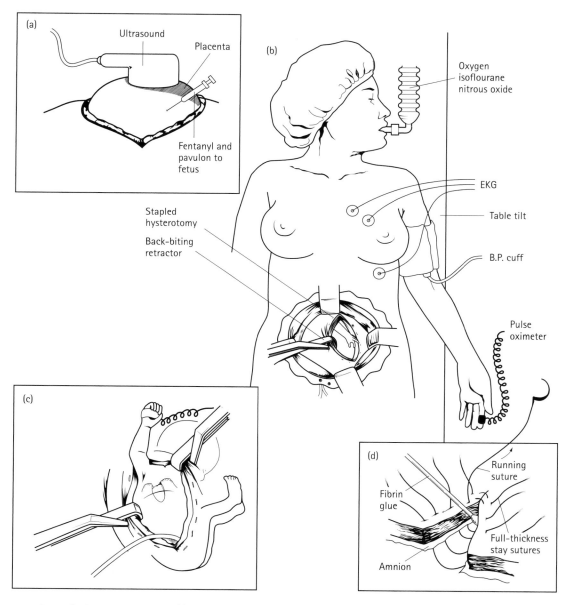

Figure 13.1 Summary of open fetal surgery techniques. (a) The uterus is exposed through a low, transverse abdominal incision. Ultrasonography is used to localize the placenta, inject the fetus with narcotic and muscle relaxant. (b) The uterus is opened with staples that provide hemostasis and seal the membranes. Maternal anesthesia, tocolysis, and monitoring are shown. (c) Absorbable staples and backbiting clamps facilitate hysterotomy exposure of the pertinent fetal part. A miniaturized pulse oximeter records pulse rate and oxygen saturation intraoperatively. (d) After fetal repair, the uterine incision is closed with absorbable sutures and fibrin glue. Amniotic fluid is restored with warm, lactated Ringer's solution.

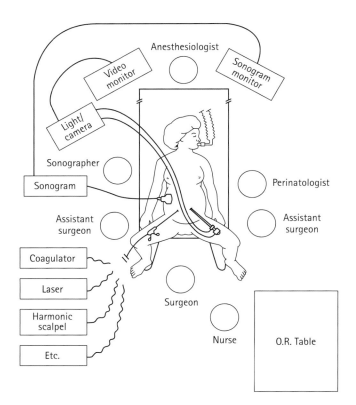

Figure 13.2 Drawing of the operating room setup. Note that there are two monitors at the head of the table: one for the fetoscopic picture and the other for the real-time ultrasound image.

determinant for the site of the hysterotomy is the fetal surgical site and fetal position. Frequently, transuterine fetal manipulation will become necessary.

Initial uterine entry can be performed either by the Bruner–Tulipan trocar or by direct cutdown. The initial entry is then extended with the Harrison uterine stapler. Use of ultrasound is critical to confirm that the stapler compresses no fetal part or loop of cord. The stapler fires a line of dissolvable staples 8 cm long and cuts in between them. This produces a hemostatic myometrial incision with the membranes tacked to the myometrium, minimizing the risk of dissection. Occasionally, bleeding from the myometrial edge requires placement of atraumatic clamps or a figure-of-8 stitch. Specially designed Harrison–Moran backbiting retractors provide further hemostasis and exposure (Figures 13.1 and 13.2).

Once the hysterotomy is appropriately hemostatic, attention can be turned to the fetus. Only that part of the fetus needed to perform the procedure should be exteriorized. This is important for fetal temperature control, dessication, and abruption secondary to uterine decompression. The fetus can be monitored either with a pulse oximeter or by sonographic surveillance of the fetal heart. During the surgery, continued relaxation of the uterus is monitored, and the serosal surfaces are irrigated with warm saline. If the uterus begins to contract, options include increasing inhalational agents, using nitroglycerin or loading with magnesium sulfate or all of the above measures.

After the procedure on the fetus, the uterine closure begins. This is usually the time we initiate the bolus of magnesium sulfate, followed by a maintenance dose. The uterus is closed in two layers of no. 0 polyglycolic monofilament suture. Full-thickness interrupted stay sutures are placed first, but not tied. Then, the continuous suture is placed. Prior to tying the continuous suture, a catheter is used to refill the amniotic cavity under ultrasound guidance. The fluid is replenished to a level of low normal fluid. Then, the stay sutures are tied. When it is certain that the suture line is hemostatic and watertight, the abdominal wall is closed in layers in the usual fashion.

Postoperative recovery in our unit is accomplished in the labor and delivery suite. For pain control, a preoperatively placed epidural catheter is used for the first 48 hours. Intravenous magnesium sulfate is continued for 24 hours, followed by oral nifedipine. Indomethacin is continued for a total of 48 hours, with ductal constriction surveillance performed by fetal echocardiography daily. The nifedipine is continued long term. Activity is limited to bed rest for the first 48 hours postoperatively and then liberalized. Upon discharge, patients are still encouraged to limit activity. Close outpatient follow-up with weekly visits and ultrasounds is our routine.

Indications for open fetal surgery

Myelomeningocele (MMC)

The most common indication for hysterotomy-based fetal intervention currently in our center is myelomeningocele. This is a devastating birth defect with sequelae that affect both the central and peripheral nervous systems. A change in cerebrospinal fluid (CSF) dynamics results in the Chiari II malformation and hydrocephalus. The abnormally exposed spinal cord results in lifelong lower extremity neurologic deficiency, fecal and urinary incontinence, sexual dysfunction, and skeletal deformities. This defect carries enormous personal, familial, and societal costs, as the near normal life span of the affected child is characterized by hospitalization, multiple operations, disability, and institutionalization. Although it has been assumed that the spinal cord itself is intrinsically malformed in children with this defect, recent work suggests that the neurologic impairment after birth may be due to exposure and trauma to the spinal cord *in utero*, and that covering the exposed cord may prevent the development of the Chiari malformation.[9]

Since 1997, more than 200 fetuses have had *in utero* closure of MMC by open fetal surgery. Preliminary clinical evidence suggests that this procedure reduces the incidence of shunt-dependent hydrocephalus and restores the cerebellum and brainstem to a more normal configuration. However, clinical results of fetal surgery for MMC are based on comparisons with historical controls, examine only efficacy and not safety, and lack long-term follow-up.

The National Institutes of Health (NIH) has funded a multicenter randomized clinical trial (Management of

Table 13.2 Fetal conditions that may benefit from treatment before birth

	Effect on development (rationale for treatment)		Result without treatment	Recommended treatment
Life-threatening defects				
Urinary obstruction (urethral valves)	Hydronephrosis	→	Renal failure	Percutaneous vesicoamniotic shunt
	Lung hypoplasia	→	Pulmonary failure	Fetoscopic ablation of valves
				Open vesicostomy
Cystic adenomatoid malformation	Lung hypoplasia–hydrops	→	Hydrops, death	Open pulmonary lobectomy
				Ablation (laser/RFA)
				Steroids
Congenital diaphragmatic hernia	Lung hypoplasia	→	Pulmonary failure	Open complete repair
				Temporary tracheal occlusion
				—Tracheal clip (open and fetoscopic)
				—Fetoscopic balloon (percutaneous/reversible)
Sacrococcygeal teratoma	High-output failure	→	Hydrops, death	Open resection of tumor
				Vascular occlusion – RFA, alcohol
				Radiofrequency ablation
Twin–twin transfusion syndrome	Donor-recipient steal through placenta	→	Fetal hydrops, death, neurologic damage to survivor	Fetoscopic laser ablation of placental vessels ⎫
				Amnioreduction ⎬ NIH trial
				Selective reduction ⎭
Acardiac/anomalous twin (TRAP)	Vascular steal	→	Death/damage to surviving twin	Selective reduction
	Embolization			Cord occlusion/division
				Radiofrequency ablation
Aqueductal stenosis	Hydrocephalus	→	Brain damage	Ventriculoamniotic shunt
Valvular obstruction	Hypoplastic heart	→	Heart failure	Balloon valvuloplasty
Congenital high-airway obstruction (CHAOS)	Overdistention by lung fluid	→	Hydrops, death	Fetoscopic tracheostomy
				Ex utero intrapartum treatment (EXIT)
Cervical teratoma	Airway obstruction	→	Hydrops, death	Open resection
	High-output failure			EXIT
				Vascular occlusion – alcohol/RFA
Non-Life-Threatening Defects				
Myelomeningocle	Spinal cord damage	→	Paralysis, neurogenic bladder/bowel, hydrocephalus,	Open repair (NIH trial)
				Fetoscopic coverage
Gastroschisis	Bowel damage	→	Malnutrition/short bowel	Serial amnio-exchange
Cleft lip and palate	Facial defect deformity	→	Persistent	Fetoscopic repair[†]
				Open repair

Table 13.2 Fetal conditions that may benefit from treatment before birth (continued)

	Effect on development (rationale for treatment)		Result without treatment	Recommended treatment
Metabolic and cellular defects				
Stem cell-enzyme defects	Hemoglobinopathy	→	Anemia, hydrops	Fetal stem cell transplant
	Immunodeficiency	→	Infection/death	Fetal gene therapy[†]
	Storage diseases	→	Retardation/death	
Predictable organ	Agenesis/hypolasia heart/lung/kidney	→	Neonatal heart/ lung/kidney failure	Induce tolerance for postnatal organ transplant[†] Tissue engineering[†]

RFA = radiofrequency ablation; TRAP = twin reversed arterial perfusion; EXIT = *ex utero* intrapartum treatment.
[†] Not yet attempted in human fetuses.

Myelomeningocele Study (MOMS)) of 200 patients that will be conducted at three centers: the University of California, San Francisco; the Children's Hospital of Philadelphia; and Vanderbilt University Medical Center (Nashville, TN), along with an independent data and study coordinating center, the George Washington University Biostatistics Center (Washington, DC).

The primary objectives of this randomized trial are to determine: (a) whether intrauterine repair of fetal MMC at 19–26 weeks' gestation using a standard multilayer closure improves outcome, as measured by death or the need for ventricular decompressive shunting by 1 year of life, compared with standard postnatal care; and (b) whether intrauterine repair of MMC can improve cognitive function as measured by the Bayley Scales of Infant Development at 30 months' corrected age as well as lower extremity motor and sensory function. There is a moratorium on performing this surgery outside the trial until the results are reported.

Cystic adenomatoid malformation (CCAM)
CCAM leading to hydrops is another indication for hysterotomy. Although congenital CCAM often presents as a benign pulmonary mass in infants and children, some fetuses with large lesions die *in utero* or at birth from hydrops and pulmonary hypoplasia.[10] The pathophysiology of hydrops and the feasibility of resecting the fetal lung have been studied in animals.[10,11] Experience in managing more than 200 cases suggests that most lesions can be successfully treated after birth, and that some lesions resolve before birth.[12] Although only a few fetuses with very large lesions develop hydrops before 26 weeks of gestation, these lesions may progress rapidly, and these fetuses die *in utero*. Careful sonographic surveillance of large lesions is necessary to detect the first signs of hydrops, because fetuses that develop hydrops can be successfully treated by emergency resection of the abnormal lobe *in utero*. Fetal pulmonary lobectomy has proven to be surprisingly simple and quite successful at two large fetal

surgery centers. For lesions with single, large cysts, thoracoamniotic shunting has also been successful.[13] Percutaneous ablation techniques are being investigated. We have seen regression of very large lesions with hydrops after maternal steroid treatment.

Sacrococcygeal teratoma (SCT)
Hysterotomy is the most common fetal surgical approach to treat fetuses in critical condition with large sacrococcygeal teratomas (SCT). Most neonates with SCT survive, and malignant invasion is unusual. However, the prognosis of patients with SCT diagnosed prenatally (by sonogram or elevated AFP) is less favorable. A subset of fetuses (fewer than 20%) with large tumors develop hydrops from high-output failure secondary to extremely high blood flow through the tumor. Because hydrops progresses very rapidly to fetal death, frequent sonographic follow-up is mandatory. Attempts to interrupt the vascular steal by sonographically guided or fetoscopic techniques have not yet been successful. Excision of the tumor reverses the pathophysiology if it is performed before the mirror syndrome (maternal preeclampsia) develops in the mother. Attempts to interrupt the vascular steal by ablating blood flow to the tumor by alcohol injection or embolization have not generally been successful. Hysterotomies in these cases may involve quite large incisions due to the large size of the masses.

Fetoscopic surgery (FETENDO)

With advances in technology and familiarity with endoscopic techniques, application of this technique to fetal surgery was natural. Common sense would suggest that the smaller the incision in the uterus, the lower the risk of subsequent pregnancy complications. At UCSF, endoscopic approaches were first applied to pregnancies complicated by diaphragmatic hernia, urinary tract obstruction, and twin-to-twin transfusion (laparotomy FETENDO or Lap-FETENDO).

The initial pioneering approach involved maternal minilaparotomies, with direct exposure of the uterus. Ultrasound is used to determine the point of entry and the laparotomy site, depending on placental location and fetal lie. Once the uterus has been exposed, stay sutures are placed, and a 3–5-mm step trocar is advanced into the amniotic cavity under direct ultrasound visualization. Initially, several trocars were required for *in utero* dissections, placement of staples, etc. Later, many procedures could be performed through a single trocar, using an endoscope with an operating channel. Initial caution regarding this approach led to perioperative management similar to that of hysterotomy cases. This included general anesthesia, use of multiple tocolytics, and prolonged hospitalization. One important difference even initially was that patients could labor after FETENDO procedures. Since that time, endoscopic procedures have become less invasive with very small instruments passed through 3-mm ports. This may explain why pregnancy outcomes were initially similar in the hysterotomy and endoscopy groups. When we reviewed this[1] (Table 31.1), pulmonary edema rates were similar, although transfusions were required less frequently (2.9% vs 12.6% for hysterotomy). The interval from procedure to delivery was also little changed (4.9 vs 6.0 weeks for hysterotomy), nor was the gestational age at delivery (30.4 vs 30.1 weeks for hysterotomy). In our experience, many of the deliveries were still by cesarean section as they were EXIT procedures.[14] This is essentially a cesarean section, in which the cord is not clamped until airway management is secure. It involves strategies similar to those used for open surgery, including uterine relaxation with general anesthesia, myometrial incision hemostasis with staples, and fetal monitoring. The endoscopic procedures that necessitated EXITs were balloon tracheal occlusions for congenital diaphragmatic hernias. This was also among the most frequent indication for an endoscopic fetal surgical approach at UCSF.

Percutaneous FETENDO

Currently, we rarely use the more invasive Lap-FETENDO and have since progressed towards a completely percutaneous approach, using a smaller 2.0-mm endoscope with an operating channel (Micro-FETENDO). We have used this technique for balloon tracheal occlusions, fetal cystoscopies and laser ablation in monochorionic twin gestations complicated by severe twin-to-twin transfusion. Based on our early experience and that of others[13] with percutaneous microendoscopy, we anticipate that the risk profile will be similar to percutaneous sonoguided procedures (see below). The perioperative management is very different. Patients are treated with prophylactic indomethacin and antibiotics. As uterine relaxation from inhalational agents is not required, we generally use spinal anesthesia. Ultrasound is again critical for safe uterine access to determine the best entry point. This is based on fetal position, placental location, membrane position in multiple gestations and uterine vascularity. Postoperative tocolytic therapy is usually based on uterine contraction activity. A 24–48-hour course of indomethacin or nifedipine is often all that is required. In cases where there are significant postoperative changes in uterine size, as with interventions for twin–twin transfusion syndrome, prophylactic intravenous magnesium sulfate may be helpful.

Indications for fetoscopic surgery (FETENDO)

Congenital diaphragmatic hernia (CDH)

The fundamental problem in babies born with congenital diaphragmatic hernia (CDH) is pulmonary hypoplasia. Research in experimental animal models and later in human patients over two decades has aimed to improve growth of the hypoplastic lungs before they are needed for gas exchange at birth. Anatomic repair of the hernia by open hysterotomy proved feasible, but it did not decrease mortality and was abandoned. Fetal tracheal occlusion was developed as an alternative strategy to promote fetal lung growth by preventing normal egress of lung fluid. Occlusion of the fetal trachea was shown to stimulate fetal lung growth in a variety of animal models. Techniques to achieve reversible fetal tracheal occlusion were explored in animal models and then applied clinically, evolving from external metal clips placed on the trachea by open hysterotomy or fetoscopic neck dissection to internal tracheal occlusion with a detachable silicone balloon placed by fetal bronchoscopy through a single, 5-mm uterine port, as described above.

Our initial experience suggested that fetal endoscopic tracheal occlusion improved survival in human fetuses with severe CDH. To evaluate this novel therapy, we conducted a randomized, controlled trial comparing tracheal occlusion with standard care. Survival with fetal endoscopic tracheal occlusion (73%) met expectations (predicted 75%) and appeared better than that of historic controls (37%), but proved no better than that of concurrent randomized controls. The higher than expected survival in the standard care group may be because the study design mandated that patients in both treatment groups be delivered, resuscitated, and intensively managed in a unit experienced in caring for critically ill newborns with pulmonary hypoplasia. Attempts to improve outcome for severe CDH by treatments either before or after birth have proven double-edged swords. Intensive care after birth has improved survival but has increased long-term sequelae in survivors, and is expensive. Intervention before birth may increase lung size, but prematurity caused by the intervention itself can be detrimental. In our study, babies with severe CDH who had tracheal occlusion before birth were born, on average, at 31 weeks, as a consequence of the intervention. The observation that their rates of survival and respiratory outcomes (including duration of oxygen requirement) were comparable to infants without tracheal occlusion who were born at 37 weeks suggests that tracheal occlusion improved pulmonary hypoplasia, but the improvement in lung growth was counterbalanced by pulmonary immaturity related to earlier delivery.

The current results underscore the role of randomized trials in evaluating promising new therapies. This is the second NIH-sponsored trial comparing a new prenatal intervention for severe fetal CDH. The first trial showed that complete surgical repair of the anatomic defect (which required hysterotomy), although feasible, was no better than postnatal repair in improving survival and was ineffective when the liver as well as the bowel were herniated.[15] That trial led to the abandonment of open complete repair at our institution and subsequently around the world. Information derived from that trial regarding measures of severity of pulmonary hypoplasia (including liver herniation and the development of the lung-to-head ratio (LHR)) led to the development of an alternative physiologic strategy to enlarge the hypoplastic fetal lung by temporary tracheal occlusion and to the development of less invasive fetal endoscopic techniques that did not require hysterotomy to achieve temporary, reversible tracheal occlusion.[16,17]

Our ability to diagnose accurately and assess the severity of CDH before birth has improved dramatically. Fetuses with CDH who have associated anomalies do poorly, whereas fetuses with isolated CDH, no liver herniation, and an LHR above 1.4 have an excellent prognosis (100% in our experience). In this study, fetuses with an LHR between 0.9 and 1.4 had a chance of survival greater than 80% when delivered at a tertiary care center. The small number of fetuses with lung head ratio below 0.9 had a poor prognosis in both treatment groups, and should be the focus of further studies.[18]

Since tracheal occlusion does work in enlarging hypoplastic lungs, approaches to tracheal occlusion other than that used here might be beneficial. Although the duration of occlusion in this study (36.2 ± 14.7 days) is comparable to that studied in animal models,[18–20] the optimal timing and duration of occlusion is not known in humans. Short-term occlusion later in gestation and earlier occlusion (with possible reversal in utero) have been studied in animal models[21,22] and applied in humans. It is also possible that the risk of premature rupture of membranes leading to preterm labor and delivery might be reduced by using smaller 2-mm fetoscopes percutaneuosly and by newly developed techniques to seal membranes. Fetuses with lung to head ratios less than 1.0 have poor survival and remain the focus for new treatment strategies either before or after birth.

Twin–twin transfusion syndrome (TTTS)

TTTS was one of the first entities to be treated endoscopically at UCSF. It is a complication of monochorionic multiple gestations resulting from an imbalance in blood flow through vascular communications, such that one twin is 'donating' blood (donor) to the other (recipient). It is the most common serious complication of monochorionic twin gestations affecting 4–35% of monochorionic twin pregnancies, or approximately 0.1–0.9 per 1000 births each year in the USA. Yet, despite its relatively low incidence, TTTS disproportionately accounts for 17% of all perinatal mortality associated with twin gestations.[23] The standard therapy has been limited to serial amnioreductions, which

appear to improve the overall outcome but have little impact on the more severe end of the spectrum in TTTS. In addition, survivors of TTTS treated by serial amnioreductions have an 18–26% incidence of significant neurologic and cardiac morbidity. Selective fetoscopic laser photocoagulation has emerged as an alternative treatment strategy with at least comparable, if not superior, survival to serial amnioreductions, as demonstrated in a randomized trial in Europe.[24] We are participating in an NIH-sponsored, prospective, randomized, multicenter trial comparing serial amnioreductions to selective fetoscopic laser ablation in improving survival and in improving cardiac, neurologic, and developmental outcomes in survivors.

Urinary tract obstruction

As a group at UCSF, we are particularly enthusiastic about the potential of fetal intervention in bladder outlet obstruction by percutaneous fetal cystoscopy. Fetal urethral obstruction produces pulmonary hypoplasia and renal dysplasia, and these often fatal consequences can be ameliorated by urinary tract decompression before birth. The natural history of untreated fetal urinary tract obstruction is well documented, and selection criteria based on fetal urine electrolyte and B_2 microglobulin levels and the sonographic appearance of fetal kidneys have been proven reliable.[25–28] Of all fetuses with urinary tract dilation, as many as 90% do not require intervention. However, fetuses with bilateral hydronephrosis and bladder distension due to urethral obstruction who subsequently develop oligohydramnios require treatment. Depending on the gestational age, the fetus can be delivered early for postnatal decompression. Alternatively, the bladder can be decompressed in utero by a catheter (Harrison vesicoamniotic shunt) placed percutaneously under sonographic guidance,[29] by fetoscopic vesicostomy,[30,31] or more recently by fetocystoscopic ablation of urethral valves.[29–32] Treatment with shunting has been relatively disappointing, as shunts often migrate or do not remain patent. Even when adequately decompressed, the obstructed bladder may not cycle correctly, resulting in severe bladder dysfunction requiring surgery after birth. We have now developed a percutaneous fetal cystoscopic technique to disrupt posterior urethral valves through a single 3-mm port.

Fetal intervention guided by sonography (FIGS)

The first fetal procedure, developed in the early 1980s, was percutaneous, sonographically guided placement of the Harrison fetal bladder catheter shunt. Many other catheter-shunt procedures have been developed and described.[33] More recently, we have developed percutaneous, sonographically guided radiofrequency ablation (RFA) procedures for management of anomalous multiple gestations. All these procedures we now group as 'fetal intervention guided by sonography' (FIGS). Very complicated procedures may still require laparotomy (Lap-FIGS).

Percutaneous or micro-FIGS is used to sample or drain fetal blood, urine, and fluid collection; to sample fetal tissue; to place catheter shunts in the fetal bladder, chest, abdomen, or ventricles; and to do RFA. The most common indication at UCSF is RFA for acardiac twins with twin reversed arterial perfusion (TRAP) sequence or monochorionic twins for selective reduction. Other operators have used bipolar coagulation or umbilical cord ligation for similar indications. Compared to the 17-gauge RFA needles we use, these techniques are more invasive, using at least 3-mm trocars. Additionally the length of the cord or its position may preclude use of these instruments. The perioperative management of these patients is similar to the current micro-FETENDO patients. The procedures are performed under spinal anesthesia, with prophylactic antibiotics and indomethacin. Postoperative tocolysis is rarely necessary and the patients frequently are discharged within hours of the procedure. Ultrasound is critical both for the planning and execution of the procedure. We attempt to avoid entry into the sac of a normal twin if at all possible. The RFA needle is guided into the abdominal cord insertion of the abnormal twin under ultrasound guidance. The tines are then deployed and energy delivered to the device to create thermal injury to the tissue. The device we currently use measures the temperature at the tines. This allows us to use an energy level to provide the quickest obliteration of the vascular communications possible. This is of benefit, as there are theoretical concerns regarding the differential obliteration of arterial and venous vessels, which might place the normal twin at risk of exsanguination. Ultrasound is also used to monitor the procedure and welfare of the normal twin. Thermal injury can be monitored by watching for the characteristic out-gassing. Once active energy delivery to the device has ceased, color-flow Doppler can be used to detect any residual flow, in both the cord and the abnormal fetus. Once absence of blood flow is confirmed, the tines are retracted and the device is withdrawn. We have not found an increased frequency of adverse outcomes with a transplacental approach. We have had good success with this approach, with a survival rate of close to 95% and a mean gestational age at delivery of over 35 weeks and an average time from procedure of over 11 weeks. There has been no maternal pulmonary edema or blood loss.

There are a few complicated FIGS procedures that may require maternal laparotomy to allow fetal positioning and sonography directly on the uterus (Lap-FIGS). A few simple structural cardiac defects that interfere with development may benefit from prenatal correction. For example, if obstruction of blood flow across the pulmonary or aortic valve interferes with development of the ventricles or pulmonary or systemic vasculature, relief of the anatomic obstruction may allow normal development with an improved outcome. For example, congenital aortic stenosis may lead to hypoplastic left heart syndrome. Stenotic aortic valves have been dilated by a balloon catheter placed by both FIGS and Lap-FIGS with some promising results.[34] The procedure is technically difficult. Several centers are developing experimental techniques to correct fetal heart defects.[35]

In summary, fetal surgery has evolved considerably since its birth at UCSF two decades ago. The indications remain quite limited, but have the potential to expand numerically as patients and providers become increasingly informed (Table 13.2). Recent advances in the development of less invasive fetal endoscopic (FETENDO) and sonography-guided techniques (FIGS) have extended the indications for fetal surgical intervention.

References

1. Golombeck K, Ball RH, Lee H et al. Maternal morbidity after fetal surgery. Am J Obstet Gynecol (submitted).
2. Adzick NS, Harrison MR, Glick PL et al. Fetal surgery in the primate. III. Maternal outcome after fetal surgery. J Pediatr Surg 1986; 21: 477–80.
3. Bruner JP, Tulipan N, Reed G et al. Intrauterine repair of spina bifida: preoperative predictors of shunt-dependent hydrocephalus. Am J Obstet Gynecol 2004; 190: 1305–12.
4. Johnson MP, Sutton LN, Rintoul N et al. Fetal myelomeningocele repair: short-term clinical outcomes. Am J Obstet Gynecol 2003; 189: 482–7.
5. DiFederico EM, Burlingame JM, Kilpatrick SJ, Harrison MR, Matthay MA. Pulmonary edema in obstetric patients is rapidly resolved except in the presence of infection or of nitroglycerin tocolysis after open fetal surgery. Am J Obstet Gynecol 1998; 179: 925–33.
6. Wilson RD, Johnson MP, Crombleholme TM et al. Chorioamniotic membrane separation following open fetal surgery: pregnancy outcome. Fetal Diagn Ther 2003; 18: 314–20.
7. Bruner JP, Tulipan NB, Richards WO, Walsh WF, Boehm FH, Vrabcak EK. In utero repair of myelomeningocele: a comparison of endoscopy and hysterotomy. Fetal Diagn Ther 2000; 15: 83–8.
8. Farrell JA, Albanese CT, Jennings RW, Kilpatrick SJ, Bratton BJ, Harrison MR. Maternal fertility is not affected by fetal surgery. Fetal Diagn Ther 1999; 14: 190–2.
9. Bouchard S, Davey MG, Rintoul NE, Walsh DS, Rorke LB, Adzick NS. Correction of hindbrain herniation and anatomy of the vermis after in utero repair of myelomeningocele in sheep. J Pediatr Surg 2003; 38: 451–8.
10. Adzick NS, Harrison MR, Glick PL et al. Fetal cystic adenomatoid malformation: prenatal diagnosis and natural history. J Pediatr Surg 1985; 20: 483–8.
11. Adzick NS, Harrison MR, Hu LM, Davies P, Reid LM. Compensatory lung growth after pneumonectomy in the fetus. Surg Forum 1986; 37: 648–9.
12. MacGillivray TE, Harrison MR, Goldstein RB, Adzick NS. Disappearing fetal lung lesions. J Pediatr Surg 1993; 28: 1321–4.
13. Blott M, Nicolaides KH, Greenough A. Postnatal respiratory function after chronic drainage of fetal pulmonary cyst. Am J Obstet Gynecol 1988; 159: 858–65.
14. Hirose S, Farmer DL, Lee H, Nobuhara KK, Harrison MR. The ex utero intrapartum treatment procedure: looking back at the EXIT. J Pediatr Surg 2003; 39: 375–80.

15. Harrison MR, Adzick NS, Bullard KM et al. Correction of congenital diaphragmatic hernia in utero. VII. A prospective trial. J Pediatr Surg 1997; 32: 1637–42.

16. Harrison MR, Adzick NS, Flake AW et al. Correction of congenital diaphragmatic hernia in utero. VIII. Response of the hypoplastic lung to tracheal occlusion. J Pediatr Surg 1996; 31: 1339–48.

17. Skarsgard ED, Meuli M, VanderWall KJ, Bealer JF, Adzick NS, Harrison MR. Fetal endoscopic tracheal occlusion ('Fetendo-PLUG') for congenital diaphragmatic hernia. J Pediatr Surg 1996; 31: 1335–8.

18. Lipshutz GS, Albanese CT, Feldstein VA et al. Prospective analysis of lung-to-head ratio predicts survival for patients with prenatally diagnosed congenital diaphragmatic hernia. J Pediatr Surg 1997; 32: 1634–6.

19. Papadakis K, De Paepe ME, Tackett LD, Piasecki GJ, Luks FI. Temporary tracheal occlusion causes catch-up lung maturation in a fetal model of diaphragmatic hernia. J Pediatr Surg 1998; 33: 1030–7.

20. VanderWall KJ, Bruch SW, Meuli M et al. Fetal endoscopic ('Fetendo') tracheal clip. J Pediatr Surg 1996; 31: 1101–3.

21. Luks FI, Wild YK, Piasecki GJ, De Paepe ME. Short-term tracheal occlusion corrects pulmonary vascular anomalies in the fetal lamb with diaphragmatic hernia. Surgery 2000; 128: 266–72.

22. Flageole H, Evrard VA, Piedboeuf B, Laberge JM, Lerut TE, Deprest JA. The plug–unplug sequence: an important step to achieve type II pneumocyte maturation in the fetal lamb model. J Pediatr Surg 1998; 33: 299–30.

23. Quintero RA. Twin-twin transfusion syndrome. Clin Perinatol 2003; 30: 591–600.

24. Senat MV, Deprest J, Boulvain M, Paupe A, Winer N, Ville Y. Endoscopic laser surgery versus serial amnioreduction for severe twin-to-twin transfusion syndrome. N Engl J Med 2004; 351: 136–44.

25. Adzick NS, Harrison MR, Glick PL, Flake AW. Fetal urinary tract obstruction: experimental pathophysiology. Semin Perinatol 1985; 9: 79–90.

26. Crombleholme TM, Harrison MR, Golbus MS et al. Fetal intervention in obstructive uropathy: prognostic indicators and efficacy of intervention. Am J Obstet Gynecol 1990; 162: 1239–44.

27. Manning FA, Harrison MR, Rodeck C. Catheter shunts for fetal hydronephrosis and hydrocephalus. Report of the International Fetal Surgery Registry. N Engl J Med 1986; 315: 336–4.

28. Nicolaides KH, Cheng HH, Snijders RJ, Moniz CF. Fetal urine biochemistry in the assessment of obstructive uropathy. Am J Obstet Gynecol 1992; 166: 932–7.

29. Glick PL, Harrison MR, Adzick NS, Noall RA, Villa RL. Correction of congenital hydronephrosis in utero. IV. In utero decompression prevents renal dysplasia. J Pediatr Surg 1984; 19: 649–5.

30. Johnson MP, Bukowski TP, Reitleman C, Isada NB, Pryde PG, Evans MI. In utero surgical treatment of fetal obstructive uropathy: a new comprehensive approach to identify appropriate candidates for vesicoamniotic shunt therapy. Am J Obstet Gynecol 1994; 170: 1770–6.

31. Crombleholme TM, Harrison MR, Langer JC et al. Early experience with open fetal surgery for congenital hydronephrosis. J Pediatr Surg 1988; 23: 1114–21.

32. MacMahon RA, Renou PM, Shekelton PA, Paterson PJ. In utero cystostomy. Lancet 1992; 340(8829): 123.

33. Wilson RD, Baxter JK, Johnson MP et al. Thoracoamniotic shunts: fetal treatment of pleural effusions and congenital cystic adenomatoid malformations. Fetal Diagn Ther 2004; 19: 413–21.

34. Allan LD, Maxwell D, Tynan M. Progressive obstructive lesions of the heart – an opportunity for fetal therapy. Fetal Ther 1991; 6: 173–6.

35. Hanley FL. Fetal cardiac surgery. Adv Cardiac Surg 1994; 5: 47–74.

14 Cervical insufficiency

Vincenzo Berghella, Jason Baxter, and Michele Berghella

Definition of cervical insufficiency (CI)

The concept of the cervix being 'so slack that it cannot rightly ... keep in the seed' was first hypothesized in the 1658 text *Practice of Physick* by Cole and Culpepper.[1] In the 1940s and 1950s, the term 'cervical incompetence' came into vogue, and surgical interventions were described to treat the 'weak' cervix. Only recently have properly controlled scientific studies on the subject been performed.

Cervical insufficiency (CI), formerly known as cervical incompetence, represents a subgroup of preterm birth (PTB). Its definition has been controversial, but the most accepted one is painless dilation leading to recurrent second-trimester losses.[2] The gestational age when these second-trimester losses (preceded by painless dilation) occur is usually 16–28 weeks. This definition implies that the PTB is caused by a cervical problem; that is, that the cervix is too weak to retain the pregnancy. Historically, cervical 'sufficiency' was viewed as a dichotomous variable: the cervix either is sufficient to retain the pregnancy to term, or is not, leading to painless dilation and second trimester loss. Recently, Iams et al have convincingly shown that cervical sufficiency (or competence) is a continuous variable.[3] This new concept has opened the way for new therapeutic approaches, in particular ultrasound-indicated cerclage, to attempt to alter cervical shortening in progress before it leads to PTB. In theory, this approach would obviate the clinical limitation of having to wait for two or more losses or PTB before therapeutic approaches are offered.

Incidence

Given the difficulties with diagnosis, the incidence of CI is difficult to ascertain. CI represents only a portion of all PTB under 32 weeks, which is 2% in the USA and 1% in other developed (e.g. European) nations. The best estimation of the incidence of CI is obtained by reviewing the incidence of cervical cerclage, the most commonly employed surgical intervention for CI. The best estimates report a range of 0.5–1% for the incidence of cerclage in the USA.[2] It should be noted that women with a prior second-trimester loss have a 70–90% chance of delivering at term in the subsequent pregnancy even without undergoing cerclage.[4]

Anatomy and physiology of the human cervix

The uterine cervix is derived from the fusion of the distal müllerian ducts and subsequent central atrophy. The cervix consists primarily (>70%) of fibrous connective tissue, mostly collagen types I and III, with most of the remainder consisting of smooth muscle. The percentage of smooth muscle is more prominent in the upper (29%) than in the lower (6%) parts of the cervix.[5] Only about 1% of cervical tissue is made of elastin. The upper limit of the cervix is difficult to distinguish from the uterine corpus in the nonpregnant woman. In pregnancy, the muscular lower segment of the corpus, or isthmus, distends and elongates, making its inferior border with the mostly fibrous cervix the functional internal cervical os. This sphincter-like region, not easy to discern to the millimeter histologically, helps keep the pregnancy *in utero*.

The strength of the cervix derives mostly from the connective tissue. The amount of connective tissue in the cervix is directly proportional to its strength, while the amount of smooth muscle tissue is inversely proportional to its strength.[5]

During pregnancy, the collagen bundles of the cervix become more dissociated, with fewer cross-links, and more soluble collagen fragments, with less hydroxyproline. Elastin is decreased in women with CI. Relaxin causes connective tissue remodeling and may play a role in CI. Elevated second-trimester serum relaxin has been related to decreased cervical length.

Table 14.1 Conditions associated with cervical insufficiency

Congenital

    Ehlers–Danlos syndrome
    Müllerian anomaly
    DES exposure

Acquired (usually traumatic and iatrogenic)

    Cone biopsy
        Cold knife
        Laser
        LEEP
    Multiple D & E*
    Obstetric cervical laceration

*For either spontaneous or voluntary terminations.

Associations and possible causes

A higher incidence of CI has been postulated in women exposed to diethylstilbestrol (DES) *in utero*[6] and those with Ehlers–Danlos syndrome or other connective tissue disorders. It is very rare for a woman to have a congenital cause of CI, and such associations have never been proven. Several historical factors have been associated with CI, as described in Table 14.1. The overwhelming majority of CI cases are associated with acquired factors. Most of the acquired factors involve surgery or trauma to the cervix and can be considered iatrogenic. Ablation of cervical intraepithelial neoplasia by cold-knife or laser cone biopsy or loop electrosurgical excision procedure (LEEP) could lead to CI based upon the amount of cervical tissue removed. Repeated dilation and curettage (D & C) or dilation and evacuation (D & E) for voluntary terminations, and sometimes even for spontaneous abortions, have been associated with CI. Gentle dilation of the cervix with laminaria before the D & C or D & E is recommended,[7] but seldom used in clinical practice except in the second trimester. Data definitively linking obstetric cervical lacerations with CI are not available.

More than just anatomic cervical defects, functional cervical deficiencies may play an important role. CI may represent a final common pathway of many causes of midtrimester pregnancy loss at the severe end of the spectrum of PTB. The main pathways leading to PTB include infectious, inflammatory, immunologic, uterine distention or structural factors (müllerian, DES, fibroids, etc.), and fetal abnormalities (genetic or structural/syndromic).

Diagnostic approaches

Obstetrical history

A history of painless dilation leading to recurrent second-trimester losses is the most accepted definition of CI.

Unfortunately, the requirement for recurrent second-trimester losses implies that a woman must lose at least two fetuses before a diagnosis is made and preventive measures implemented. Clinical characteristics of the second-trimester loss (whether the patient was symptomatic of painful contractions and/or bleeding, or not) do not seem to predict which women will have a recurrent second-trimester loss.[8]

CI should be diagnosed with caution when second-trimester loss occurs in a multiple-gestation pregnancy. We have shown that the incidence of recurrent PTB at ≤24 weeks after the early loss (mean 23 weeks) of a twin gestation when subsequently carrying a singleton gestation is 12%, with 88% delivering at ≥35 weeks.[9]

These limitations of diagnostic approaches based on obstetric history alone have prompted exploration of prepregnancy tests and diagnostic approaches during pregnancy in an attempt to diagnose CI before multiple losses occur.

Nonpregnant testing

Evaluation of the cervix in the nonpregnant state has been employed extensively in the past for evaluation of CI. Several screening tests have been proposed, including the ease of passage of a no. 8 Hegar dilator, catheter traction tests using Foley catheters, ease of leakage of fluid during hysteroscopy or hysterosalpingogram, measurement of the width of the upper cervical canal (by radiography or hysterography), and others. While most of these reports associate abnormalities of testing with *prior* pregnancy outcome, almost none of the studies report prediction of *future* pregnancy outcome. Based on a combination of these tests, cervical compliance scores have been proposed,[10] but do not appear to be very predictive or clinically useful. The prediction of CI in a future pregnancy based on pre- or interpregnancy tests is therefore very poor according to current evidence. This might be because the functionality of cervical tissues may be different in the nonpregnant from the pregnant state in the same woman. More research is needed in the area of nonpregnant testing before it can be of practical clinical use.

Testing during pregnancy

Transvaginal ultrasound cervical length

CI or early PTB is usually preceded by cervical opening, which begins to occur first at the internal os. This progressive opening of the cervix 'from the inside out' results in shorter functional length of the cervix and is not detectable by manual/digital evaluation of the cervix. Measurements of cervical length (CL) by transvaginal ultrasound (TVU) has been shown to be safe, well accepted by women, reproducible, and predictive of PTB. A recent review summarizes a large literature on this subject.[11] TVU is the reference standard for assessment of the cervix in pregnancy for prediction of PTB. No clinical decisions should be based on transabdominal (TA) ultrasound of the cervix alone, given its shortcomings.[11] TVU of the cervix has better predictive accuracy than manual/digital evaluation of the cervix.[12] Shortening and opening of the cervix starts at the internal os, and about three-fourths of women with asymptomatic short cervix on ultrasound have no appreciable changes by manual examination.[13] Screening of cervical changes in pregnancy to predict PTB or CI should be done with TVU, and *not* with manual examination or a different ultrasound technique. The technique of TVU has been well described (Figures 14.1–14.3).[11] While different parameters can be measured, CL is the most reproducible, with low (<10%) inter- and intraobserver variability. Other variables, such as funneling, do not add significantly to the prediction of PTB based on CL alone, (Figures 14.2 and 14.3).[14] The shortest best multiple CL measurements after spontaneous or transfundal-pressure changes should be used for PTB prediction. A CL of 25–50 mm is normal at 14–24 weeks in all pregnant women. In low-risk women, CL is a continuous variable, with a mean of 35–40 mm at 14–30 weeks, with the lower 10th percentile being 25 mm and the upper 10th (90th percentile) 50 mm.[15] Rarely do women have a short cervix under 25 mm before 14 weeks, and only those with a prior cone biopsy or second-trimester loss.[16] Early detection of short CL before 20 weeks can predict second-trimester losses and CI. The majority of women who will have PTB have a short cervix first around 18–22 weeks.[11] The earlier the short CL is detected by TVU, and the shorter the CL, the higher the risk of PTB. A cervix under 25 mm has a positive predictive value (PPV) of 70% for PTB under 35 weeks when detected at 14–18 weeks, and of 40% when detected at 18–22 weeks.[12] Therefore, it may be that patients at the highest risk of PTB (e.g., patients with possible CI, early PTB, or cone biopsies) may ben-

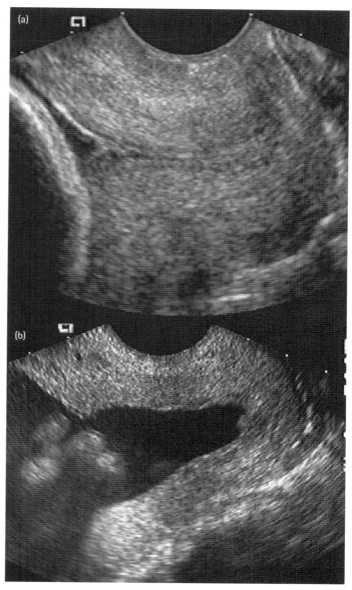

Figure 14.2 Transvaginal ultrasonography of closed normal cervix (a) and of a short cervix with significant funneling (b).

efit from early (i.e., 14–18 weeks) ultrasound examination to determine their need for intervention.

The benefit of repeated TVU examinations and the ideal interval for repeating TVU have not been clearly established. If a screening program were employed in relatively low-risk women, one TVU of the cervix at around 18–22 weeks would probably be most effective. It appears that one normal TVU CL at 14–18 weeks and another at 18–22 weeks is reassuring in most high-risk women.[17] In women at very high risk of PTB, such as those with prior second-trimester loss or very early spontaneous PTB, some clinicians have advocated TVU of the cervix every 2 weeks, at least at 14–24 weeks. The fact that TVU at 14–22 weeks is at least as predictive of PTB as TVU after 22 weeks is important, since interventions to prevent PTB

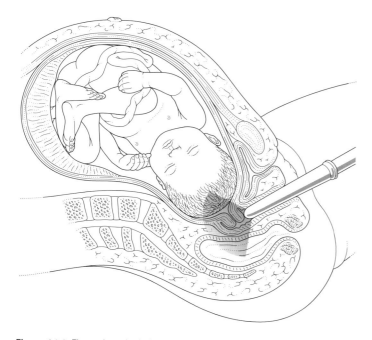

Figure 14.1 The endovaginal ultrasound probe is placed into the anterior fornix of the vagina to obtain the corresponding ultrasound image of the cervix.

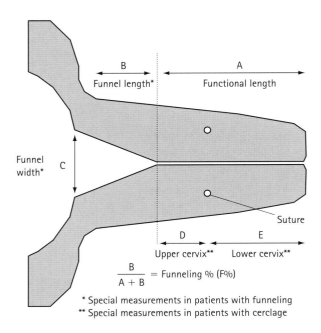

Figure 14.3 Schematic illustration of TVU cervical measurements.

are most effective when changes leading to PTB are detected early in the process.[11]

Many different populations have been screened, including asymptomatic women with singleton, twin, and triplet pregnancies and symptomatic women with preterm labor or premature preterm rupture of the membranes (PPROM). Studies have been done on low-risk women, high-risk populations, and women with a cerclage in place. The actual population screened has a tremendous effect on the significance of the TVU CL results. In low-risk women (cross-sectional studies) carrying singleton gestations, the sensitivity for PTB under 35 weeks of TVU CL under 25 mm at 22–24 weeks was only 37%, with a PPV of only 18%.[15] This means that 82% of these low-risk women who were found to have a short CL under 25 mm at 24 weeks delivered at $\geq$35 weeks. In women carrying singleton gestations but with a prior PTB under 32 weeks, the sensitivity of TVU CL under 25 mm at 16–24 weeks increased to 69%, with a PPV of 55%.[14] In twin gestations, TVU CL under 25 mm in the second trimester has a sensitivity of 30% and a PPV of 60%.[18] The low sensitivity may be due to the fact that multiple gestations have PTB not because of CI, but because of uterine overdistension.

The cervix may shorten in the second trimester, too early in pregnancy, for a variety of reasons. A short CL is a common final pathway, eventually leading to PTB. While some rare women can develop an early short CL because of an intrinsic weakness of the cervix due to a congenital disorder or a connective tissue disease, CI is more commonly due to prior traumatic or surgical damage. Other mechanisms leading to a short cervix include inflammatory, infectious, or immunologic processes, as well as simply contractions. Women with normal

CL have mechanical and immunologic protection against the ascent of lower vaginal microorganisms. Once shortened by these processes, the CL can provide easier access of potentially pathologic vaginal microorganisms to the intrauterine environment, leading to prolonged subclinical chorioamnionitis and subsequent CI or PTB. There is a strong association between a short CL on TVU and infection. High amniotic fluid interleukin (IL)-6, later development of chorioamnionitis, and acute inflammatory lesions of the placenta have all been associated with a short CL on TVU. A short CL leading to CI or PTB is often associated with PPROM instead of PTL, providing additional evidence for the role of infection in these women.

Usually, the cause and effect are unclear: did the short CL develop first and allow ascending infection, or did infection and inflammation develop first and cause shortening of the cervix?[19] Recent studies have shown that the majority of asymptomatic women with CL under 25 mm before 24 weeks have some contractions, more than controls with a normal cervix.[20,21] Again, it is unclear whether contractions cause the short CL or are a result of the short cervix, or whether these two factors work synergistically. A short CL probably develops due a combination of several of the above factors.

Some authors have considered a short CL in pregnancy as the pathognomonic sign of CI. We do not believe this to be accurate, since the short CL is just a common final pathway leading to PTB. For example, twin gestations that contract from overdistention develop a short CL, which in this case is a secondary, not a primary process. We postulate that a short CL might be confirmatory of CI only in the rare women with prior second-trimester losses who asymptomatically develop a short CL early in the second trimester in the next pregnancy.

Management

Avoidance of intervention (*primum non nocere*)

The negative predictive value of a CL of $\geq$25 mm in predicting PTB is relatively high if this length is obtained at 14–24 weeks in different populations. It is about 88–96% even in women at high risk of PTB such as those with a prior PTB or carrying twins. This information has been used by clinicians to avoid cerclage and other interventions in women in whom the obstetric history is poor but not clearly consistent with CI.

In fact, at least 60% of these high-risk women maintain a normal CL until after 24 weeks and deliver at term, and can be spared any intervention. Only about 40% develop a short CL, are at true risk of PTB, and should be offered intervention. One randomized trial and three case-control studies have compared management of women at high risk of PTB with prophylactic cerclage versus follow-up with TVU CL and cerclage only if indicated by development of a short CL on TVU. Most of the women included had a prior history consistent with possible CI, or at least prior second-trimester loss(es). Table 14.2 shows a summary of these four studies.[22–25] The incidence of PTB under

Table 14.2 Avoidance of prophylactic cerclage in high-risk populations

	n	PTB	PTB n(%)		OR
			HC	TVU	
Althuisius et al[*53]	67	<34weeks	3/23 (13)	6/44 (14)	NS
Kelly et al[25]	106	<35weeks	11/45(24)	13/61(21)	NS
Berghella et al[24]	177	<35weeks	15/66(23)	33/111(30)	NS
To et al[23]	84	<34weeks	6/41(15)	9/43(21)	NS
Total	434		35/175(20)	61/259(24)	0.81 (0.5–1.3)

HC, history-indicated cerclage; TVU, transvaginal ultrasound surveillance; OR, odds ratio.
*Randomized trial.

35 weeks was similar if the (over 400) women were managed with uniform prophylactic cerclage or careful follow-up with TVU CL. It is possible that a larger study would eventually show the 19% decrease in PTB to be statistically significant, but this would require 1700 women in each group. We have already stated that women who have had a prior PTB of a multiple gestation have a low (<12%) incidence of recurrent PTB if in the next pregnancy they carry a singleton gestation,[9] so that avoidance of multiple gestation should be the most important management strategy.

Nonsurgical interventions

Bed rest or modified activity
Best rest is commonly used for women with clear, possible, or even signs of CI. Unfortunately, no trials have been done to demonstrate its efficacy or detriment. Up to 1.5% incidence of thromboembolism has been reported in association with prolonged bed rest.[26]

Medical
17-Hydroxy progesterone 250 mg once a week IM from 16–20 weeks until 36 weeks has been shown to decrease PTB by about 33% in women with a prior PTB that occurred at 20–36 weeks.[27] The benefit is slightly higher for women with a prior PTB under 28 weeks and possible CI. In view of results from a prior meta-analysis[28] and another recent trial,[29] obstetricians may consider offering progesterone prophylaxis to all women with a prior PTB, including those with CI.

Indomethacin, antibiotics, omega-3 fatty acids, and other medical interventions have been postulated to be helpful in the management of women with CI or early PTB, but no evidence is available to demonstrate clear benefit. More research is needed.

Pessary
Minimal research has been done on the efficacy of a pessary to prevent CI or PTB. Women with a short CL may benefit from pessary placement,[30] but trials are necessary before clinical use.

Surgical intervention: cerclage

Cervical cerclage has been the traditional treatment for the diagnosis of CI. This intervention was originally devised by Lash and Lash,[31] and then refined by Shirodkar[32] and McDonald.[33] In their studies, cerclage was used for women with both a history of PTB or CI *and* recurrent manual cervical dilation. Over 35 different procedures for the treatment of CI have been reported in the world's literature.[34]

Transvaginal techniques
After adequate analgesia (typically with spinal anesthesia), the patient is placed in the dorsal lithotomy position, and surgical prep of the perineum and vagina is performed (gently in the vagina if the membranes are protruding from the cervix). We utilize a weighted speculum and right-angle retractors, as well as two or three sponge forceps (or DeLee cervical tenacula) on the cervix to optimize visualization of the surgical field (Figure 14.4).

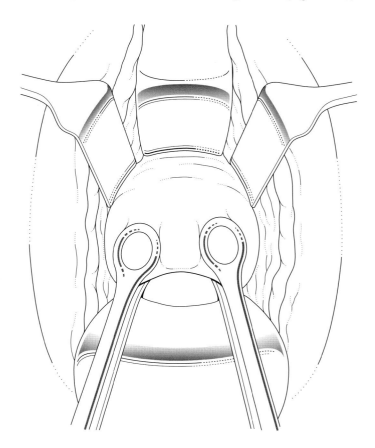

Figure 14.4 Transvaginal cerclage. A weighted speculum, right-angle retractors, and two or three sponge forceps on the cervix are used to optimize visualization of the surgical field.

The vast majority of cerclages performed today are modifications of the techniques described by Shirodkar and McDonald.

Shirodkar cerclage. First presented at a film festival in Paris in 1950, Shirodkar's procedure for the treatment of CI used human fascia lata as the suture material. After transverse incision of the cervicovaginal epithelium on both the anterior (at the reflection of the bladder) and posterior aspects of the cervix, the vesicovaginal and rectovaginal fascia is reflected cephalad to the level of the internal os, as when beginning a vaginal hysterectomy (Figure 14.5). Long Allis clamps are placed laterally with the jaws in the anterior and posterior incisions as high on the cervix as possible to maximize the cephalad dissection. The Allis clamps are used to place lateral traction on the submucosal tissue so that the cerclage can be effectively placed close to the medially located cervix while avoiding the laterally displaced uterine vessels (Figure 14.6). The suture is driven by two successive

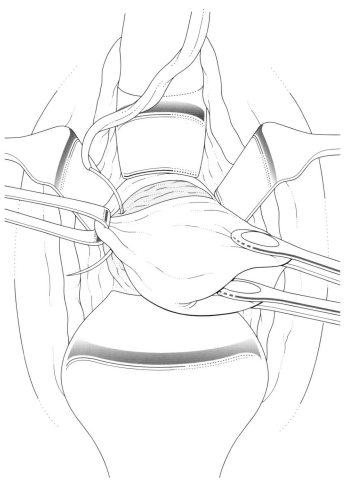

Figure 14.6 Modified Shirodkar cerclage. An Allis clamp is placed laterally with the jaws in the anterior and posterior incisions as high on the cervix as possible to maximize the cephalad dissection. Lateral traction is placed on the submucosal tissue to avoid the uterine vasculature.

passes with an atraumatic needle on each side (from posterior to anterior or vice versa) just distal to the Allis clamp above the insertion of the cardinal ligaments (Figure 14.7). After ensuring that the suture tape lies flat posteriorly, the suture is tied anteriorly, tight enough as to admit a fingertip at the external os, but closed at the internal os (Figure 14.8). Successive knots are placed to facilitate identification and later removal. The mucosal incisions are closed over (with the cerclage suture passing through) only if active bleeding is noted (Figure 14.9).

McDonald cerclage. In 1957, McDonald described a cerclage technique that requires no submucosal dissection. Just distal to the vesicocervical reflection (at the junction of the ectocervix and the anterior rugated vagina), a purse-string suture is placed in four to six passes circumferentially around the cervix (Figure 14.10). Each pass should be deep enough to contain sufficient cervic stroma to avoid 'pulling-through', but not so deep as to enter the endocervical canal (and risk rupture of the membrane).

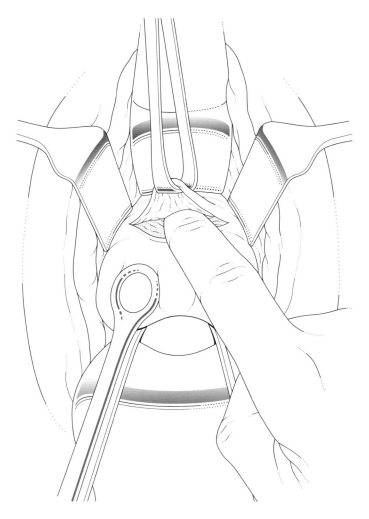

Figure 14.5 Modified Shirodkar cerclage. The initial transverse incision is made in the anterior cervicovaginal epithelium at the reflection of the bladder, and the vesicovaginal fascia is reflected cephalad to the level of the internal os, similarly to when beginning a vaginal hysterectomy.

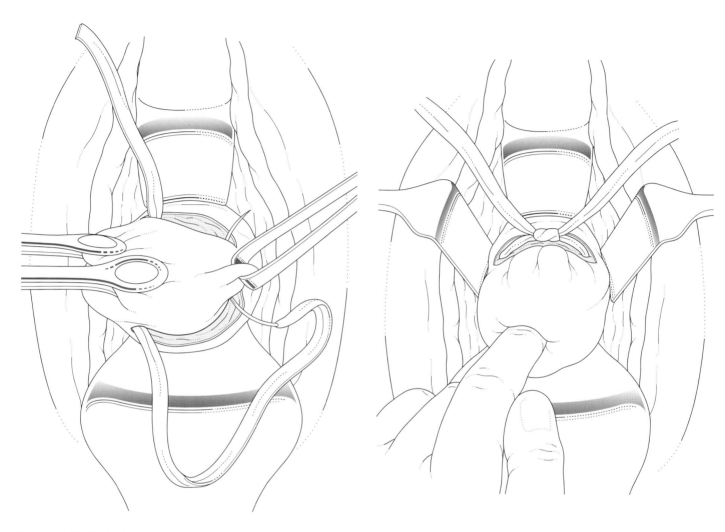

Figure 14.7 Modified Shirodkar cerclage. The suture is driven by successive passes with an atraumatic needle on each side just distal to the Allis clamp above the insertion of the cardinal ligaments.

Figure 14.8 Modified Shirodkar cerclage. After ensuring that the suture tape lies flat posteriorly, the suture is tied anteriorly, tight enough as to admit a fingertip at the external os, but closed at the internal os.

The uterine vessels should be avoided laterally (Figure 14.11). The suture should be placed high on the posterior aspect of the cervix, as this is the most likely site of suture displacement. The suture is tied anteriorly, successive knots are placed, and the ends are left long enough (2–3 cm) to facilitate later removal (Figure 14.12).

Transabdominal (TA) cerclage
Several techniques have been described to place the cerclage higher, closer to the internal os, including the TA cervicoisthmic cerclage. In our center, where over 100 of these procedures have been performed, a simple atraumatic technique under spinal anesthesia with a Pfannesteil incision is employed. After digital displacement of the uterine vessels bilaterally, a 5-mm Mersilene band is guided through the broad ligament at the level of the internal os by blunt perforation with a right-angle clamp (Figure 14.13).[35] The suture is tied anteriorly, and left in

place at the time of the necessary cesarean delivery at 38–39 weeks.

Laparoscopic cerclage. A laparoscopic approach has been described[36,37] as an interval procedure, but should not be attempted without appropriate laparoscopic suturing experience.

Medical and technical considerations for cerclage

Ultrasound
Before placing the cerclage, it is imperative to ensure fetal viability, and, as much as possible by gestational age, normal fetal anatomy. This is particularly important before TA cerclage.

Screening for infection
Before placing the cerclage, it is important to screen for infections when appropriate. Women with a prior PTB may be

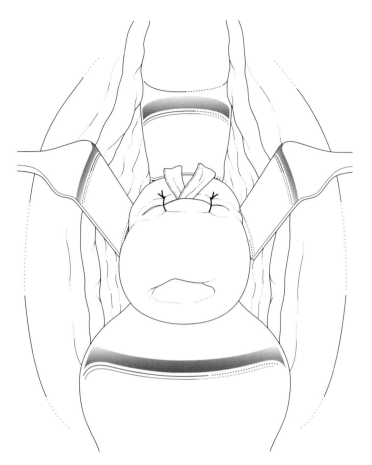

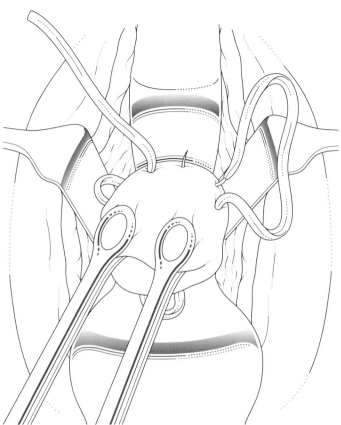

Figure 14.9 Modified Shirodkar cerclage. Successive knots are placed to facilitate identification and later removal. The mucosal incisions are closed over only if active bleeding is noted.

Figure 14.10 McDonald cerclage. Just distal to the vesicocervical reflection a purse-string suture is placed in four to six passes circumferentially around the cervix. The suture should be placed high on the posterior aspect of the cervix, as this is the most likely site of suture displacement.

screened for bacterial vaginosis and treated appropriately, since this may prevent recurrent PTB.[38] The incidence of intra-amniotic microbial infection is under 2% in women undergoing ultrasound-indicated cerclage,[39] and over 50% in those undergoing manual-indicated cerclage.[40] Therefore, strong consideration should be given to performing an amniocentesis before any manual-indicated cerclage, even if the risk of PPROM from this procedure might be high in this clinical setting.

Prophylactic antibiotics and tocolytics
'Prophylactic' antibiotics and tocolytics are commonly used at the time of cerclage, without any evidence of their benefit. Given the high success rate and early timing of history-indicated cerclage, when infection, inflammation, and contractions are rare, it is very doubtful that these adjunctive therapies would be shown to add benefit if studied properly. For ultrasound-indicated cerclage, indomethacin might have contributed to the benefit of cerclage in the one positive trial.[41] Since subclinical infection, inflammation, and uterine activity are more common at the time of manual-indicated cerclage, antibiotics and indomethacin therapy may be beneficial, but these interventions await confirmation from future research.

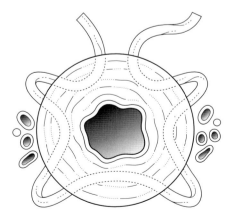

Figure 14.11 McDonald cerclage coronal section. Each pass should be deep enough to contain sufficient cervic stroma to avoid 'pulling-through', but not so deep as to enter the endocervical canal. The uterine vessels should be avoided laterally.

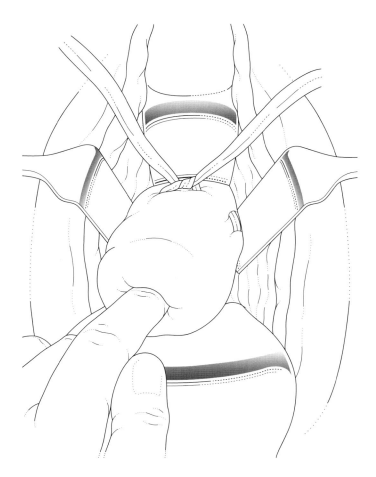

Figure 14.12 McDonald cerclage. The suture is tied anteriorly, tight enough to admit a fingertip at the external os, but closed at the internal os. Successive knots are placed, and the ends are left long enough to facilitate later removal.

Sutures

Several different suture materials have been employed for cerclage. The only controlled data on this subject do not show a difference between the efficacies of Mersilene, Tevdek, and Prolene. Tevdek was associated with a nonsignificant higher incidence of PPROM.[42]

History-indicated

Definition. A cerclage placed solely on the basis of prior obstetric or gynecologic history is often called a prophylactic or elective cerclage. The term 'elective' we believe to be misleading, since there is nothing elective about the procedure, which should be performed for specific indications only.

Indications. The only indication that has been confirmed by evidenced-based data is three or more second-trimester losses or PTBs.[43] The other clinical indication might include CI (again defined as prior painless cervical dilation leading to recurrent second-trimester losses). Other indications such as prior cone biopsy, müllerian anomaly, DES exposure, prior PTB not associated with CI, and Ehlers–Danlos syndrome, have occasionally

been used clinically, but have not been confirmed as indications that benefit from history-indicated cerclage.

Performed. History-indicated cerclage is usually performed at 12–15 weeks' gestation. This allows time to perform an early ultrasound to confirm viability and normal early anatomy (e.g., nuchal translucency) after the first-trimester spontaneous loss period has passed.

Efficacy. Prevention of PTB has been proven only for three or more prior second-trimester losses or preterm births[43] (Table 14.3). Trials on women at lower risk of PTB based on prior obstetric history have not shown benefit from history-indicated cerclage.[43–45] There are limited randomized data showing that history-indicated cerclage is not beneficial in other populations at high risk of PTB such as twins.[46] Unfortunately, there are very limited nonrandomized data showing that history-indicated cerclage is not beneficial in other populations at high risk of PTB such as patients with prior cone biopsy, müllerian anomaly, DES exposure, prior PTB not associated with CI, Ehlers–Danlos syndrome, etc. Given the paucity of data showing benefit from history-indicated cerclage, alternative management has recently moved to screening of high-risk pregnancies with TVU of the cervix to determine during pregnancy the risk of PTB, since the majority of women at high risk of PTB deliver at term even without intervention.[11]

Ultrasound-indicated

Definition. Ultrasound-indicated cerclage is defined as cerclage performed because a short cervix has been detected on TVU during pregnancy, usually in the second trimester. This cerclage has also been called therapeutic, salvage, or rescue cerclage. These terms cause confusion with emergency cerclage (defined below), and so the term 'ultrasound-indicated cerclage' seems the most appropriate.

Indications. As discussed previously, a short CL on TVU in the second trimester significantly increases the risk of PTB in all populations studied. Women with three or more second-trimester losses or PTBs should receive a history-indicated cerclage. Singleton gestations with prior PTB have been

Table 14.3 Randomized trials of phrophylactic cerclage

| | | PTB < 37w | | |
	n	Cerclage (%)	No cerclage (%)	P
Dor et al[46]	50	45	48	NS
Lazar et al[45]	506	7	6	NS
Rush et al[44]	194	34	32	NS
MRC/RCOG[43]	1292	26	31	NS
≥3STL*/PTB[43]	45	32	53	**

*STL, second trimester losses; ** RR 0.6, 95% CI 0.37–0.95

(a)

(b)

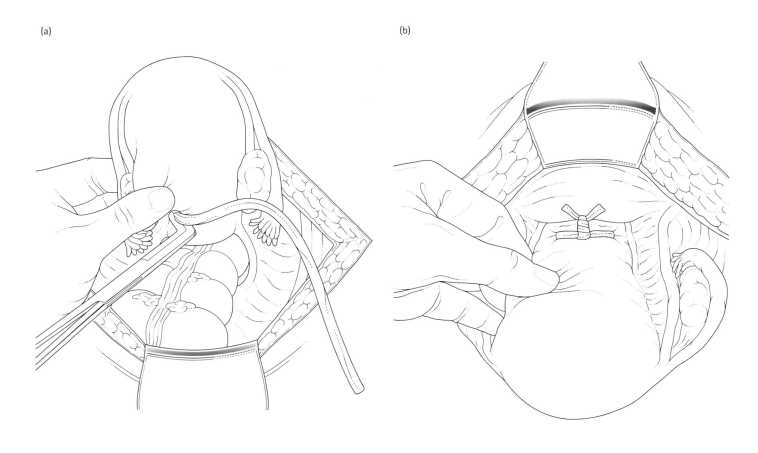

Figure 14.13 Transabdominal cerclage. After digital displacement of the uterine vessels bilaterally, a 5-mm Mersilene band is guided through the broad ligament at the level of the internal os by blunt perforation with a right-angle clamp. The suture is tied anteriorly.

suggested as candidates for ultrasound-indicated cerclage if the cervix shortens on TVU.[41] As a screening test, TVU CL has almost all the requisites for effectiveness, as it studies an important condition; detects a recognizable early asymptomatic phase; and is safe, well-accepted by women, reliable, and valid in its prediction. To be effective, however, when the test is positive (short CL), an early treatment (such as cerclage) must prevent the outcome (PTB).

Performed. As a short CL is usually not detected on TVU before 14 weeks, ultrasound-indicated cerclage is usually performed when the short CL is detected, usually at 14–24 weeks. Ultrasound-indicated cerclage is usually not offered at or after 24 weeks. This is because viability usually is possible at this gestational age, and the uterus is more sensitive to a foreign body, such as cerclage, at this gestational age. Some authors, especially in Europe, continue to offer ultrasound-indicated cerclage up to 27–28 weeks.[41, 47]

Efficacy. At least five *nonrandomized* studies have assessed the benefit of therapeutic cerclage when short CL is identified. Three employed screening in a cross-section of low-risk and high-risk patients,[48–50] and two screened only high-risk women.[17,51] Because cerclage was performed at the obstetrician's discretion in these studies, selection bias was present in all studies. Two[48,49] of the three cross-sectional and one[17] of the two high-risk studies reported no benefit from cerclage. In general, in these nonrandomized studies, obstetricians were more inclined to perform cerclages in women with the worst obstetric histories, and shorter and earlier-detected TVU CL than controls. A recent analysis of our nonrandomized data at Thomas Jefferson University (Philadelphia) showed that in 43 women without obstetric risk factors and a CL of under 25 mm, placement of cerclage did not decrease the incidence of PTB (relative risk (RR) 1.1; 95% CI 0.5–2.7). In contrast, in 73 women with prior PTB under 35 weeks and with a CL under 25 mm, placement of a cerclage reduced the incidence of recurrent PTB (< 35 weeks) by 40%, from 63% to 39% (RR 0.6; 95% CI 0.4–1.0). In 57 women with a prior second-trimester loss and CL under 25 mm, the incidence of PTB under 35 weeks was reduced from 65% without cerclage to 41% with cerclage (RR 0.6; 95% CI 0.4–1.0).

Randomized trials of cerclage are extremely difficult to perform, particularly when this procedure is believed by many patients and their doctors to be beneficial. The four randomized trials published so far on ultrasound-indicated cerclage to prevent PTB in women with a short CL have had different results, depending on the type of patients studied (Table 14.4).[17,41,47,52] Two trials that have focused on an *unselected population* showed no prevention of PTB in women who were randomized to receive cerclage. These included a study by Rust et al[39] of 113 women with either CL under 25 mm or funneling over 25%, and a study by To et al, who randomized 253 women with a CL of ≤15 mm at 23 weeks.[47] The 16% reduction of PTB under 33 weeks shown in the To trial was not statistically significant. The conclusion from these two studies including over 350 women mostly at low risk of PTB by history, is that ultrasound-indicated cerclage in unselected women with short CL on TVU does not prevent PTB. In contrast, a small trial (n = 35) by Althuisius et al, which included only patients at *high risk* of PTB, many of whom were suspected of having CI,[41] showed a decrease in PTB and neonatal morbidity and mortality with cerclage. Interestingly, when Rust et al[39] and To et al[47] analyzed a subgroup of their study population that had a prior PTB, again they did not find a benefit from cerclage. The last published trial, by our group, focused on women at high-risk of PTB. While overall results showed no benefit from cerclage for a short CL under 25 mm, in the small subgroup with a prior PTB under 35 weeks *and* a short CL under 25 mm there was a nonsignificant 48% decrease in recurrent PTB under 35 weeks. It is unclear whether this trend would have been significant with a larger sample size, or if this trend was due only to small numbers, and a larger sample would have shown no benefit from cerclage. Thus, even in high-risk women with a prior PTB and a short CL, it is unclear whether cerclage is beneficial in preventing recurrent PTB. All four studies included fewer than 100

women with prior PTB each, so that none are sufficiently powered to show a difference in this population even if there were one. A study by the National Institute of Child Health and Human Development (NICHD) now underway plans to recruit 300 women with prior PTB under 34 weeks and a CL under 25 mm, and would be able to determine with adequate power whether cerclage is beneficial or not in such high-risk women with a short CL. Before further trials and analyses are published, we agree with the American College of Obstetrics and Gynecology, which stated in November 2003 that 'the management of women who have ultrasound findings of a short cervix or funneling remains speculative, and the decision to proceed with cerclage should be made with caution'.[2]

Manual-indicated

Definition. Manual-indicated cerclage (that is, emergency or urgent) is a cerclage placed because of changes in the cervix (dilation, effacement, etc.) detected by manual examination.

Indications. Manual-indicated cerclage is performed for significant cervical changes detected on manual examination, often ≥2 cm dilation up to the internal os. Most of these changes are detected in women with risk factors for CI or PTB who are either examined serially or report vague symptoms such as an increase in discharge, back pain, or cramps.

Performed. Like ultrasound-indicated cerclage, manual-indicated cerclage is usually performed at 14–23 6/7 weeks. Bulging membranes, at or beyond the external os, are often encountered and Trendelenburg position, retrograde bladder filling, Foley catheter, sponge-on-a-stick, and/or amniocentesis may be necessary to reduce the membrane prolapse before adequate suture placement is possible.

Efficacy. Over 50% of women with cervical dilation of ≥2 cm have microbial invasion of the amniotic cavity.[40] Therefore amniocentesis should be considered before offering manual-indicated cerclage. Given the high incidence of infection and

Table 14.4 Ultrasound-indicated cerclage: randomized trials

Author	Group	n	History PTB (%)	GA studied (weeks)	CL cutoff (mm)	PTB (%) n
Althuisius et al[41]	Cerclage	19	74	16–27	<25	0 (0)*
	Control	16	75	16–27	<25	7 (44)*
Rust et al[39]	Cerclage	55	54	16–24	<25	19 (35)*
	Control	58	36	16–24	<25	21 (36)*
To et al[47]	Cerclage^	127	18	22–24	≤15	28 (22)**
	Control	126	18	22–24	≤15	33 (26)**
Berghella et al[52]	Cerclage	31	71	14–24	<25	14 (45)***
	Control	30	57	14–24	<25	14 (47)***

*PTB < 34 weeks; **PTB < 33 weeks; ***PTB < 35 weeks; ^used Shirodkar cerclage; all others used McDonald.

inflammation, the prognosis is usually guarded, with or without intervention.

Only one trial has evaluated the efficacy of manual-indicated cerclage.[53] Twenty-three women (seven with twins) with membranes at or beyond the external os at around 20–24 weeks were randomized to cerclage and indomethacin or usual care. All women received bed rest, thrombosis prophylaxis, and antibiotics. The 13 women in the cerclage group gained more days (54 vs 20 days ($p < 0.05$)) and delivered 4 weeks later than the control women (30 vs 26 weeks). The major limitations of this study are the small sample size and the inclusion of twins. The only other prospective (but not randomized) report on manual-indicated cerclage studied 43 women who had cervical dilation of ≥ 4 cm at 20–27 weeks and received cerclage or bed rest at the obstetrician's discretion.[54] Again, the cerclage group gained 4 more weeks versus controls (33 vs 29 weeks; $p = 0.001$). Over 25 retrospective observational series, mostly with no controls, have claimed benefit of manual-indicated cerclage. Clearly, a large, well-designed, prospective, randomized trial is needed to confirm benefit.

Transabdominal (TA)

Definition. As the word implies, 'transabdominal' (TA) cerclage is a cerclage placed around the cervix from an abdominal incision, and therefore 'from above', in contrast with transvaginal cerclage, which is placed from a vaginal approach, and therefore 'from below'.

Indications. TA cerclage has been performed for two main indications; that is, a prior failed history-indicated TV cerclage, or a cervix with no intravaginal portion. By 'prior failed cerclage', authors have usually meant that the woman had a history suggestive of CI, for which she received a history-indicated cerclage that failed to prevent another early PTB. Women with no or minimal intravaginal cervix usually have a history of large cone biopsies, surgical trauma, or cerclage complications, and also a history suggestive of CI.

Performed. TA cerclage is usually performed prophylactically at around 10–12 weeks. As with history-indicated cerclages, an early transvaginal ultrasound at 10–12 weeks should be performed to exclude gross fetal anomalies. Given the difficulty of operating around the pregnant uterus, TA cerclage should be performed by 12 weeks. If the woman presents after 12 weeks, TA cerclage can still be performed up to 18–20 weeks, but is increasingly technically difficult with each gestational week. About half of the case series have reported TA cerclage performed before pregnancy. The benefits of this approach are that technical difficulties with the pregnant uterus are avoided. The shortcomings of preconceptional TA cerclage placement are that spontaneous miscarriages and anomalous fetuses may necessitate more involved operating room procedures for management.

Efficacy. Over 22 observational case series have been published on the outcome of TA cerclage pregnancies. Almost all report excellent term delivery rates, usually over 80%. Unfortunately, almost all of these studies did not have controls for adequate comparison of less invasive management. The only adequately controlled study of TA cerclage compared women with a similar history of a failed (PTB under 33 weeks) transvaginal cerclage who received either a TA cerclage or another transvaginal cerclage (both at 10–15 weeks). The women who received TA cerclage had a better outcome than controls with transvaginal cerclage (PTB under 35 weeks, 18% vs 42%; $p = 0.04$; gestational age at delivery 36.3 vs 32.8 weeks, $p = 0.03$, respectively).[35] It should be noted that in this trial antibiotics and progesterone were uniformly given to the TA women. All data in the literature so far have been on TA cerclage performed on women with a singleton pregnancy for historical risk factors for PTB. There are no specific data on TA cerclage performed for cervical (manual or TVU) changes. Our limited experience has very poor results; therefore, we strongly advise against TA cerclage performed for TVU or manual cervical changes, unless as part of a research study. In contrast, our small series of twin pregnancies in which TA cerclage was performed for appropriate historical indications (as outlined above) had excellent outcomes (unpublished data).[5]

Management once cerclage is placed

TVU of the cervix has been evaluated for the follow-up of women with history-indicated, ultrasound-indicated, or manual-indicated cerclage in place. Most studies have shown that transvaginal cerclage is placed in the middle part of the cervix in the majority of cases, except for TA cerclage, always placed higher near the internal os (Figure 14.14).[55–57] Evaluation of pre- and postcerclage TVU CL has shown that CL usually increases postcerclage, and that an increase in CL is associated

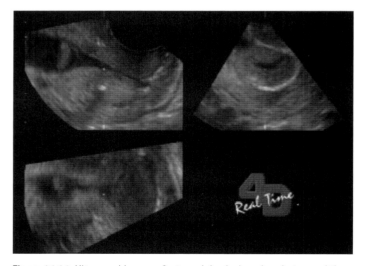

Figure 14.14 Ultrasound images of a transabdominal cerclage in two and three dimensions. Three-dimensional multiplanar display of a cervix with a cerclage in place. In 2DUS, we normally see just two bright dots representing the suture. In 3DUS in the axial plane, we can see the suture in its entirety. This view enables a complete assessment of the cerclage and its relationship with the cervical canal, which is 'fish-mouth'-shaped in the axial plane.

with a higher rate of term delivery.[58] Several studies have evaluated the accuracy of TVU for predicting PTB in patients with cerclage.[55–58] These studies all show that TVU cervical parameters are predictive of PTB. CL under 25 mm and upper cervix (the closed portion above the cerclage) under 10 mm are probably the two best predictive parameters. It is unclear what (if any) intervention would prevent PTB once the screening TVU of the cerclaged cervix is found to be abnormal. Limited data show that performing another reinforcing cerclage is not beneficial.[59]

Three-dimensional (3-D) ultrasound (3DUS) makes it possible to obtain an axial plane through the cervix at the level of the cerclage, demonstrating the entire stitch (Figure 14.14). This view is not obtainable with conventional 2-D ultrasound (2DUS). Whether 3-D imaging will improve clinical management in patients with or without a cerclage in place is unknown.

There are no controlled data to confirm that a decrease in activity is beneficial in women with a cerclage in place. It seems appropriate for women with cervical dilation to avoid intercourse. Transvaginal cerclage should be removed for persistent contractions to avoid cervical lacerations and evulsions. In cases of PPROM with a transvaginal cerclage in place, the cerclage should be removed immediately after 28–32 weeks to avoid the high rates of ensuing infection for both mother and fetus/neonate. Before 28 weeks, it might be advisable to consider removing the cerclage only after steroids for fetal lung maturity have been administered.[60] Transvaginal cerclage should always be removed around 36 weeks to avoid complications from term contractions. Removal of McDonald cerclage is usually straightforward as long as enough length has been left on the cut knot to be identified. Removal can almost always be done in the office without anesthesia with just a speculum, a pair of ring forceps, and long suture scissors. Occasionally (less than 10% of cases), a knot which is buried in tissue or a woman with low discomfort tolerance might necessitate removal in the operating room under regional anesthesia. Once it is removed, many women and their doctors anticipate cervical dilation, labor, and delivery to follow very soon. In fact, the mean interval between cerclage removal and spontaneous delivery is 16 days, with only 3% of women delivering within 48 hours of cerclage removal.[61] For women who have had a cerclage in their prior pregnancy for unclear indications, performing a cerclage in their next pregnancy has not been shown to be beneficial compared to close observation only.[62,63] Therefore, the saying, 'once a cerclage, always a cerclage', is misleading. This reinforces the importance of performing the initial cerclage only when appropriate.

Contraindications

Contraindications to cerclage placement include the presence of a lethal fetal abnormality, evidence of intrauterine infection (chorioamnionitis), active bleeding, preterm labor, and ruptured membranes. If resolved, prior bleeding and preterm labor can become relative contraindications. The minimum gestational age of fetal viability should serve as the maximum upper gestational age of cerclage placement. In developed countries this is 23–24 weeks' gestation, while it may be as high as 26–28 weeks in areas of the world with limited neonatal care capabilities. The increased sensitivity of the uterus and cervix to this surgical manipulation later in gestation should also limit later cerclage placement.

Complications

The most common major morbidities associated with cerclage placement are rupture of membranes, chorioamnionitis, and suture displacement.[2] The presence of the cerclage itself can lead to preterm contractions or labor and cervical lacerations. Intrapartum fever and endometritis occur more frequently in women with cerclage.[64] Cervical bleeding and contractions during and immediately after cerclage placement are common but not well studied. Some clinicians use indomethacin either prophylactically or therapeutically for the cramps and contractions that often occur after cerclage placement. Ultrasound-indicated and manual-indicated cerclages are associated with higher incidence of morbidity than history-indicated cerclage, probably due to the already ongoing inflammation/infectious labor process.

Bladder or urethra injuries at the time of cerclage placement have been reported;[65,66] they are extremely rare but increasing theoretical risks with attempts at 'higher' suture placement. Whether intraoperative ultrasound can minimize this theoretical risk has not been determined.

TA cerclage is associated not only with the increased risks of a laparotomy at the time of cerclage placement, but also with the increased risk of hemorrhage from inadvertent uterine vessel laceration. Furthermore, an additional laparotomy is necessitated for delivery of the fetus, whether this be (ideally) at term or in the second trimester soon after cerclage placement if membrane rupture or labor ensues. Laparoscopically placed TA cerclage holds the promise of decreasing this laporotomy-associated morbidity. Uterine rupture and maternal septicemia are extremely rare but life-threatening complications that have been reported in association with all types of cerclage.

Conclusions

CI, that is, painless dilation leading to recurrent second-trimester losses, occurs in 0.5–1% of pregnancies and probably represents the most extreme cases of the continuum of PTB. Diagnostic criteria are based on this history. Prepregnancy tests are unreliable, while TVU of the cervix during pregnancy may unmask a risk of recurrent PTB in women with a prior unclear CI or early PTB history by revealing a short CL in the second trimester.

Medical management is limited, but progesterone use starting at 16–20 weeks is possibly beneficial in preventing recurrent PTB in women with a prior PTB. Operative management involves cerclage, with modifications of the techniques described by Shirodkar and McDonald most commonly used today. Since no trials compare the efficacy of these two techniques, McDonald cerclage remains more popular given its simplicity. Randomized trials show evidence of benefit for history-indicated cerclage in women with clear CI; that is, three or more second-trimester losses or PTB. Women with unclear CI, such as those with just one PTB or second-trimester loss, DES exposure, müllerian anomaly, cone biopsy, or multiple D & E, can be followed with TVU of the cervix. In these women, ultrasound-indicated cerclage has not yet been shown to be beneficial, but holds promise, especially for women with prior PTB and a short CL. A recent small trial showed benefit of manual-indicated cerclage. In women who had a prior PTB under 33 weeks even with an early history-indicated transvaginal cerclage, TA cerclage decreases recurrent PTB compared to repeating a transvaginal cerclage.

References

1. Cole, Culpeper N. Practice of Physick. 1658.
2. ACOG Practice Bulletin. Clinical Management Guidelines for Obstetrician-Gynecologists. Cervical Insufficiency. 2003; 102: 1901–99.
3. Iams J, Johnson FF, Sonek J, Sachs L, Gebauer C, Samuels P. Cervical competence as a continuum: a study of ultrasonographic cervical length and obstetric performance. Am J Obstet Gynecol 1995; 172: 1097–1106.
4. Berghella V, Haas S, Chervoneva I, Hyslop T. Patients with prior second trimester loss: prophylactic cerclage or serial transvaginal ultrasounds? Am J Obstet Gynecol 2002; 187: 747–51.
5. Danforth DN. The fibrous nature of the human cervix, and its relation to the isthmic segment in gravid and nongravid uteri. Am J Obstet Gynecol 1947; 53: 541–60.
6. Ludmir J, Landon MB, Gabbe SG, Samuels P, Mennuti MT. Management of the diethylstilbestrol-exposed pregnant patient: a prospective study. Am J Obstet Gynecol 1987; 157: 665–9.
7. Harlap S, Shiono PH, Ramcharan S, Berendes H, Pellegrin F. A prospective study of spontaneous fetal losses after induced abortions. N Engl J Med 1979; 301: 677–81.
8. Berghella V, Gorski L, Talucci M. Painless vs symptomatic prior second-trimester loss: which is more predictive of subsequent preterm delivery? Am J Obstet Gynecol 2001; 184: S173.
9. Pelham J, Arvon R, Berghella V. Prior preterm birth of twins: risk of preterm birth in a subsequent singleton pregnancy. Am J Obstet Gynecol 2003; 101: 78S.
10. Zlatnick FJ, Burmeister LF. Interval evaluation of the cervix for predicting pregnancy outcome and diagnosing cervical incompetence. J Reprod Med 1993; 38: 365–9.
11. Berghella V, Bega G, Tolosa JE, Berghella M. Ultrasound assessment of the cervix. clinical obstetrics and gynecology. Clin Obstet Gynecol 2003; 46: 947–62.
12. Berghella V, Tolosa JE, Kuhlman KA, Weiner S, Bolognese R, Wapner RJ. Cervical ultrasonography compared to manual examination as a predictor of preterm delivery. Am J Obstet Gynecol 1997; 177: 723–30.
13. Berghella V, Kuhlman K, Weiner S, Teixera L, Wapner RJ. Cervical funneling: sonographic criteria predictive of preterm delivery. Ultrasound Obstet Gynecol 1997; 10: 161–6.
14. Owen J, Yost N, Berghella V et al. for the National Institute of Child Health and Human Development. Maternal-fetal medicine units network. JAMA 2001; 286: 1340–8.
15. Iams JD, Goldenberg RL, Meis PJ et al. The length of the cervix and the risk of spontaneous premature delivery. N Engl J Med 1996; 334: 567–72.
16. Berghella V, Talucci M, Desai A. Does transvaginal sonographic measurement of cervical length before 14 weeks predict preterm delivery in high-risk pregnancies? Ultrasound Obstet Gynecol 2003; 21: 140–4.
17. Berghella V, Daly SF, Tolosa JE et al. Prediction of preterm delivery with transvaginal ultrasonography of the cervix in patients with high-risk pregnancies: does cerclage prevent prematurity? Am J Obstet Gynecol 1999; 181: 809–15.
18. Goldenberg RL, Iams J, Miodovnik M et al. The preterm prediction study: risk factors in twin gestation. Am J Obstet Gynecol 1996; 175: 1047–53.
19. Odibo AO, Talucci M, Berghella V. Prediction of preterm premature rupture of membranes by transvaginal ultrasound features and risk factors in a high-risk population. Ultrasound Obstet Gynecol 2002; 20: 245–51.
20. Berghella V, for the NICHD MFMU Network. Frequency of uterine contractions in asymptomatic pregnant women with or without a short cervix on transvaginal ultrasound. Am J Obstet Gynecol 2003; 187: S127.
21. Lewis D, Pelham J, Sawhney H, Talucci M, Berghella V. Most asymptomatic pregnant women with a short cervix on ultrasound are having uterine contractions. Am J Obstet Gynecol 2001; 185: S144.
22. Althuisius SM, Dekker GA, van Geijn HP, Bekedam DJ, Hummel P. Cervical incompetence prevention randomized cerclage trial (CIPRACT): study design and preliminary results. Am J Obstet Gynecol 2000; 183: 823–9.
23. To MS, Palaniappan V, Skentou C, Gibb D, Nicolaides KH. Elective cerclage vs. ultrasound-indicated cerclage in high-risk pregnancies. Ultrasound Obstet Gynecol 2002; 19: 475–7.
24. Berghella V, Haas S, Chervoneva I et al. Patients with prior second-trimester loss: prophylactic cerclage or serial transvaginal sonograms? Am J Obstet Gynecol 2002; 187: 747–51.
25. Kelly S, Pollock M, Maas B, LeFebvre C, Manley J, Sciscione A. Early transvaginal ultrasonography versus early cerclage in women with an unclear history of incompetent cervix. Am J Obstet Gynecol 2001; 184: 1097–9.
26. Kovacevich GJ, Gaich SA, Lavin JP et al. The prevalence of thromboembolic events among women with extended bed rest prescribed as part of the treatment for premature labor or preterm premature rupture of membranes. Am J Obstet Gynecol 2000; 182: 1089–92.
27. Meis PJ, Klebanoff M, Thom E et al. Prevention of recurrent preterm delivery by 17 alpha-hydroxyprogesterone caproate. N Engl J Med 2003; 348: 2379–85.

28. Keirse MJNC. Progestogen administration in pregnancy may prevent preterm delivery. Br J Obstet Gynecol 1990; 97: 149–54.

29. da Fonseca EB, Bittar RE, Carvalho MH, Zugaib M. Prophylactic administration of progesterone by vaginal suppository to reduce the incidence of spontaneous preterm birth in women at increased risk: a randomized placebo-controlled double-blind study. Am J Obstet Gynecol 2003; 188: 419–24.

30. Broth R, Pereira L, Slepian J, Berghella V. Role of pessary in management of patients with cervical shortening. Am J Obstet Gynecol 2002; 187: S118.

31. Lash AF, Lash A. Incompetent internal os of the cervix – diagnosis and treatment. Am J Obstet Gynecol 1957; 79: 346.

32. Shirodkar VN. A new method of operative treatment for habitual abortions in the second trimester of pregnancy. Antiseptic 1955; 52: 299–300.

33. McDonald IA. Suture of the cervix for inevitable miscarriage. J Obstet Gynecol 1957; 64: 346–50.

34. Shortle B, Jewelewicz R. Clinical Aspects of Cervical Incompetence. Yearbook Medical Publishers: Chicago, 1989.

35. Davis G, Berghella V, Talucci M, Wapner RJ. Patients with a prior failed transvaginal cerclage: a comparison of obstetric outcomes with either transabdominal or transvaginal cerclage. Am J Obstet Gynecol 2000; 183: 836–9.

36. Scibetta JJ, Sanko SR, Phipps WR. Laparoscopic transabdominal cervicoisthmic cerclage. Fertil Steril 1998; 69: 161–3.

37. Gallot D, Savary D, Laurichesse H, Bournazeau JA, Amblard J, Lemery D. Experience with three cases of laparoscopic transabdominal cervico-isthmic cerclage and two subsequent pregnancies. Br J Obstet Gynaecol 2003; 110: 696–700.

38. McDonald H, Brocklehurst P, Parsons J, Vigneswaran R. Antibiotics for treating bacterial vaginosis in pregnancy. Cochrane Database Syst Rev 2004; 2.

39. Rust OA, Atlas RO, Reed J, van Gaalen J, Baldrucci J. Revisiting the short cervix detected by transvaginal ultrasound in the second trimester: why cerclage therapy may not help. Am J Obstet Gynecol 2001; 185: 1098–1105.

40. Romero R, Gonzalez R, Sepulveda W et al. Microbial invasion of the amniotic cavity in patients with suspected cervical incompetence: prevalence and clinical significance. Am J Obstet Gynecol 1992; 167: 1086–91.

41. Althuisius SM, Dekker GA, Hummel P, Bekedam DJ, van Geijn HP. Final results of the cervical incompetence prevention randomized cerclage trial (CIPRACT): therapeutic cerclage with bed rest versus bed rest alone. Am J Obstet Gynecol 2001; 185: 1106–12.

42. Pereira L, Llevy C, Lewis D, Broth R, Rust O, Berghella V. Effect of suture material on the outcome of emergent cerclage. Am J Obstet Gynecol 2004; 103: S35.

43. MRC/RCOG Working Party on Cervical Cerclage. Final report of the Medical Research Council/Royal College of Obstetricians and Gynaecologists multicentre randomized trial of cervical cerclage. Br J Obstet Gynaecol 1993; 100: 516–23.

44. Rush RW, Isaacs S, McPherson K, Jones L, Chalmers I, Grant A. A randomized controlled trial of cervical cerclage in women at high risk of preterm delivery. Br J Obstet Gynaecol 1984; 91: 724–30.

45. Lazar P, Gueguen S, Dreyfus J, Renaud R, Pontonnier G, Papiermik E. Multicentre controlled trial of cervical cerclage in women at moderate risk of preterm delivery. Br J Obstet Gynaecol 1984; 91: 731–5.

46. Dor J, Shalev J, Mashiach S, Blankstein J, Serr DM. Elective cervical suture of twin pregnancies diagnosed ultrasonically in the first trimester following induced ovulation. Gynecol Obstet Invest 1982; 13: 55–60.

47. To MS, Alfirevic Z, Heath VCF et al. Cervical cerclage for prevention of preterm delivery in women with short cervix: randomized controlled trial. Lancet 2004; 363: 1849–53.

48. Hibbard JU, Tart M, Moawad AT. Cervical length at 16–22 weeks' gestation and risk of preterm delivery. Obstet Gynecol 2000; 96: 972–8.

49. Hassan SS, Romero R, Maymon E et al. Does cervical cerclage prevent preterm delivery in patients with a short cervix? Am J Obstet Gynecol 2001; 184: 1325–31.

50. Heath VCF, Souka AP, Erasmus I, Gibb DMF, Nicholaides KH. Cervical length at 23 weeks of gestation: the value of Shirodkar suture for the short cervix. Ultrasound Obstet Gynecol 1998: 12; 318–22.

51. Guzman ER, Benito CW, Yeo L, Vintzileos AM, Walters C, Meirowitz N. Bed rest versus cervical cerclage in the treatment of cervical incompetence manifested by ultrasound around the time of fetal viability. Am J Obstet Gynecol 1999: 84; 40–6.

52. Berghella V, Odibo AO, Tolosa JE. Cerclage for prevention of preterm birth in women with a short cervix on transvaginal ultrasound: a randomized trial. Am J Obstet Gynecol 2004; 191: 1311–17.

53. Althuisius SM, Dekker GA, Hummel P, van Geijn HP. Cervical incompetence prevention randomized cerclage trial: emergency cerclage with bed rest versus bed rest alone. Am J Obstet Gynecol 2003; 189: 907.

54. Olatunbosun OA, al-Nuaim L, Turnell RW. Emergency cerclage compared with bed rest for advanced cervical dilatation in pregnancy. Int Surg 1995; 80: 170–4.

55. Andersen HF, Karimi A, Sakala EP, Kalugdan R. Prediction of cervical cerclage outcome by endovaginal ultrasonography. Am J Obstet Gynecol 1994; 171: 1102–6.

56. Berghella V, Davis G, Wapner RJ. Transvaginal ultrasound of the cervix in pregnancies with prophylactic cerclage. Am J Obstet Gynecol 1999; 180: S173.

57. Guzman ER, Houlihan C, Vintzileos A, Ivan J, Benito C, Kappy K. The significance of transvaginal ultrasonographic evaluation of the cervix in women treated with emergency cerclage. Am J Obstet Gynecol 1996; 175: 471–6.

58. Althuisius SM, Dekker GA, van Geijn HP, Hummel P. The effect of therapeutic McDonald cerclage on cervical length as assessed by transvaginal ultrasonography. Am J Obstet Gynecol 1999; 180: 366–9.

59. Baxter J, Airoldi J, Berghella V. Short cervical length history-indicated cerclage: is a reinforcing cerclage beneficial? Am J Obstet Gynecol 2005; 193: 1204–7.

60. Jenkins TM, Berghella V, Shlossman PA et al. Timing of cerclage removal after preterm premature rupture of membranes –

maternal and neonatal outcomes Am J Obstet Gynecol 2000; 183: 847–52.

61. Arvon R, Berghella V, Farrell C, Sawnhey H. Interval to spontaneous delivery after elective removal of cerclage. Am J Obstet Gynecol 2002; 187: S119.

62. Fejgin MD, Gabai B, Goldberger S, Ben-Nun I, Beyth Y. Once a cerclage, not always a cerclage. J Reprod Med 1994; 39: 880–2.

63. Pelham J, Lewis D, Farrell C, Berghella V. Prior cerclage: to repeat or not to repeat, that is the question. Am J Obstet Gynecol 2002; 187: S115.

64. Drakeley AJ, Roberts D, Alfirevic Z. Cervical stitch (cerclage) for preventing pregnancy loss in women. Cochrane Database Syst Rev 2003; 1: 1–27.

65. Ben-Baruch G, Rabinovitch O, Madjar I et al. Ureterovaginal fistula: a rare complication of cervical cerclage. Isr J Med Sci 1980; 16: 400.

66. Bates JL, Cropley T. Complication of cervical cerclage. Lancet 1977; 2: 1035.

15 Advanced extrauterine pregnancy

Armando E Hernandez-Rey and Gerson Weiss

An advanced extrauterine pregnancy (AEP) is defined as one that has implanted outside the endometrial cavity on any one of the surrounding reproductive or intra-abdominal organs and/or peritoneum, and has survived to 20 weeks of gestation. It is a rare complication, highly associated with maternal and fetal morbidity and mortality. Typically, AEP is classified by two factors: (1) the location of the gestation and (2) whether the site of implantation is primary or secondary. The latter most commonly occurs in the case of a tubal pregnancy that has extruded through the fimbriated end and implants itself on the parietal peritoneum.

The first description of an extrauterine gestation was by Albucasis (AD 936–1013), an Arab physician, in his treatise *At-Tasrif liman 'Ajiza 'an at-Ta'lif (The Method of Medicine)*,[1] and since then reports have abounded on the subject. The first operative delivery of an abdominal pregnancy was done by Jacob Nufer in the 1500s, wherein both the mother and the fetus survived.[2] A lithopedion, or 'petrified embryo' in the city of Sens (France) was reported by Cordaeus in the sixteenth century. In the eighteenth century, John Bard, surgeon to George Washington, reported the first successful operation of an ectopic pregnancy in the USA. Then, in 1903, Sir Edwin Craig championed the cause for early surgical intervention as a means of decreasing maternal mortality.[3]

During those early times, the only means of estimating gestational age was by the length of amenorrhea. Clinical signs such as Chadwick's sign (blue-purple hue of the cervix and congestion of the vaginal mucosa), Hegar's sign (softening of the isthmus),[4] and the eventual onset of fetal movements were presumptive evidence of pregnancy.

Today, refinements in sensitive human chorionic gonadotropin assays (β-hCG), and the increased resolution of ultrasonography and magnetic resonance imaging (MRI) allow precise estimation of the gestational age of the pregnancy and its location, making timely diagnosis possible. Further, these advances facilitate a better understanding of the natural evolution of AEP. For example, now we know that the progression of AEP past 20 weeks is dependent on specific characteristics inherent to the site of implantation, such as vascularity and its distensibility to accommodate the growing gestation. Fortunately, AEP is far rarer than it once was and is generally limited to abdominal, ovarian, or intraligamentary (within the broad ligament) sites.

Abdominal pregnancy

Abdominal pregnancy has a worldwide incidence ranging from 1:3300 to 1:10 200 and accounts for 1–4% of all ectopic gestations. Maternal and perinatal mortality rates of 0.5–18% and 40–95%,[5,6] respectively, have been reported in the literature. Rarely do these progress to advanced gestation; moreover, expectant management until viability is seldom an option.

Prior to the use of MRI's or ultrasound technology, diagnosis was often difficult, and the clinician had to rely on certain signs and symptoms, such as abdominal pain, gastrointestinal symptoms, painful fetal movements, abnormal presentations, an uneffaced and displaced cervix, vaginal bleeding, and palpation of a pelvic mass distinct from the uterus. Failure to induce uterine contractions during oxytocin infusion was also a well-established diagnostic technique.[7] Today, these imaging techniques can precisely locate the site of implantation of the pregnancy and help corroborate any clinical suspicion.

Although the most commonly reported sites of abdominal pregnancy are the pouch of Douglas and the posterior uterine wall, other sites include the uterine fundus, as well as extrapelvic sites such as the liver, spleen, lesser sac, and diaphragm.[8] In 1942, Studdiford suggested four diagnostic criteria for primary peritoneal pregnancy: (1) normal tubes and ovaries without evidence of injury; (2) no evidence of uteroperitoneal fistula; (3) pregnancy related exclusively to the peritoneal surface; and (4) pregnancy at an early enough stage of gestation to exclude the possibility of a secondary implantation, eliminating primary tubal nidation.[9] Secondary implantation occurs more commonly, but this fact has no clinical relevance since both primary and secondary AEP is managed in the same manner.

Treatment usually requires terminating the pregnancy with evacuation of all products of conception by laparotomy. In some instances, a patient may refuse termination due to religious or moral beliefs, and a more conservative approach is necessary. These cases mandate immediate hospitalization and continuous supervision of the fetal and, more importantly, maternal well-being. Patients must be informed of the 20–40% risk of malformation in living infants attributed to oligohydramnios and compression, such as facial asymmetry, torticollis, pulmonary hypoplasia, and joint deformities (Figure 15.1).[1] After resolution of the pregnancy when trophoblastic tissue has been left *in situ* for fear of excessive bleeding, anticipation of potential complications is imperative, including intra-abdominal or pelvic abscess, hemorrhagic shock, and fistula formation.

Tubal pregnancy

The ampullar region of the fallopian tube is by far the most common of all extrauterine sites for ectopic gestations. Early tubal pregnancies may end as tubal abortions, with extrusion of the pregnancy from the fimbriated end. Tubal pregnancies do not progress past 12–14 weeks. After this point of time, they rupture the tube, sometimes with catastrophic effects and do not become AEP. Further discussion of this topic is beyond the scope of this chapter and is usually reserved for general gynecology texts.

Cervical pregnancy

Cervical pregnancy occurs when implantation of placental tissue is established below the internal cervical os. Prior to the use of transvaginal sonography (TVUS), diagnosis was made in only 18% of cases preoperatively, and usually not until the time of dilation and curettage for a presumed incomplete abortion, with subsequently severe hemorrhagic complications. Today, a

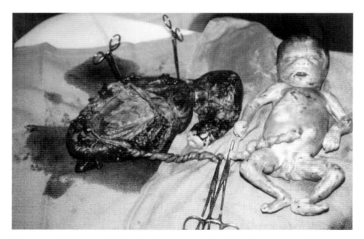

Figure 15.1 Advanced abdominal pregnancy. Fetal demise at 28 weeks' gestation with placental attachment to the right cornual region and to the broad ligament. Abdominal hysterectomy was performed without significant blood loss, and no postoperative complications were reported. (Image courtesy of Dr JJ Apuzzio.)

correct diagnosis is made 87.5%[10] of the time when β-hCG, ultrasound, and MRI are used together.

While estimates differ as to the true incidence of cervical ectopic pregnancies in the USA, it is clear that it is an extremely rare occurrence. Lipscomb et al found the incidence to be 1: 12 422.[11] The typical symptom is painless, first-trimester, vaginal (uterine) bleeding. On speculum examination, the cervix is hyperemic and considerably enlarged, creating the 'hourglass' (softened and significantly enlarged cervix equal to or larger than the uterine corpus) appearance on an abdominal ultrasound.

Cervical ectopic pregnancies with fetal cardiac activity at 10 or more weeks' gestation may be successfully managed with ultrasound-guided intrafetal injection of feticidal agents, but this form of ectopic pregnancy never reaches an advanced gestational age before the onset of symptoms.

Ovarian pregnancy

First reported in 1682 by Saint Maurice de Périgod, ovarian ectopic pregnancy is rarely seen; it constitutes only 0.5–3% of all ectopic pregnancies, and the incidence is only 1 out of every 7000–40 000 deliveries. There are 52 ovarian pregnancies recorded in the world literature as reaching viability; only 20% of them survived. Approximately 75% are terminated in the first trimester, 12% in the second trimester, and 12% in the third trimester.[12] Fertilization of the ovum inside the ovary and reverse migration of the embryo from the fallopian tube and implantation on the ovary are the accepted theories for its pathogenesis. Factors such as pelvic inflammatory disease, tubal surgery, and oophoritis have been associated with ovarian pregnancy. Several investigators have indicated that patients with ovarian pregnancies are younger, have higher parity, and have fewer fertility problems than the typical tubal pregnancy patients. Lehfeldt et al demonstrated that the incidence of ovarian pregnancy is disproportionately high in patients who use IUDs. According to their studies, the IUD is effective in preventing intrauterine pregnancy in 99.5% and tubal pregnancy in 95% of subjects, but it has little effect on ovarian pregnancy.[13] Shibahara et al postulate that blastocyst-stage embryo transfers may also be associated with ectopic implantation of embryos on the ovaries,[14] but the mechanism underlying this needs further elucidation.

Preoperative diagnosis of ovarian pregnancy is a challenge to clinicians. The findings are similar to those of a tubal pregnancy. Although TVUS may arouse suspicion, a definitive diagnosis is reached only by laparoscopy or laparotomy. Ultrasonographic signs specific for unruptured intrafollicular ovarian pregnancy are a thickened, uniformly echogenic wall of the sac, surrounded by ovarian stroma, and the absence of a pre-existing corpora lutea on either ovary, since the pregnancy grows within its confines.

In 1873, Spiegelberg established the following four criteria for an ovarian pregnancy, (1) the oviduct on the affected side must be intact; (2) the amniotic sac must occupy the position of the ovary; (3) the amniotic sac must be connected to the uterus by the ovarian ligament; (4) ovarian tissue must be present in the wall of the amniotic sac with concomitant histologic confirmation postoperatively.[15] Histology alone confirms the diagnosis. It can distinguish four distinct forms: intrafollicular, juxtafollicular, juxtacortical, and interstitial.

Conservative surgeries such as ovarian cystectomy or wedge resection are done in order to remove the products of conception when the diagnosis is made early or for those who may desire future childbearing. Usually, management is by laparotomy and unilateral salpingo-oophorectomy. Hemorrhage may occur in advanced cases, as in abdominal pregnancy. Methotrexate (MTX) is indicated as an adjunct only for organ-preserving operations with an incomplete resection or persistence of trophoblastic tissue.

Intraligamentary pregnancy

While some prefer to group this type of pregnancy within the broader category of abdominal pregnancies, it is a retroperitoneal pregnancy that occurs due to the rupture of the fallopian tube with subsequent implantation between the two leaves of the broad ligament. The similarities to an abdominal pregnancy include risk factors and clinical presentation. The reported incidence ranges between 1:75 and 1:613 of all extrauterine pregnancies.[16] It is usually not diagnosed before surgery because of the proximity to the uterine cavity and the rarity with which it occurs. MRI has proven to be very effective in confirming whether the pregnancy is retroperitoneal or intrauterine, and is used when ultrasound findings suggest a gestational sac separate from the uterus. Although rupture of the gestational sac can entail some bleeding, massive hemorrhage is not likely to occur due to the tamponade-like effect provided by the adjacent leaves of the broad ligament.[17] In fact, the broad ligament can expand to accommodate a pregnancy to viability. If diagnosed early, it can be treated laparoscopically, although laparotomy is usually warranted. There are no reports of the use of methotrexate in pregnancies confined to the broad ligament.

Diagnostic evaluation

Once an ectopic pregnancy has reached a viable gestational age, rarely are serum hormones or markers necessary to evaluate AEP. Nevertheless, a thorough understanding of their use within this clinical context is of the utmost importance so that an appropriate plan of care can be undertaken at an earlier gestational age when maternal morbidity is significantly reduced.

Hormonal assessment

Human chorionic gonadotropin (hCG)

Quantitative β-hCG measurements continue to be an important tool in the evaluation of extrauterine pregnancies. β-hCG measurements are used: (1) to make a diagnosis of an ectopic pregnancy in the setting of an empty uterine cavity and abnormal doubling of the hCG; (2) to assess the efficacy of either medical or surgical therapy with serial measurements.[10]

Under normal conditions, serum concentrations of hCG double approximately every 48–84 hours, in a curvilinear fashion, until reaching its maximum level, usually 100 000 mIU/ml, where it begins to plateau at around weeks 8–12 of gestation. Because the increase in hCG is essentially linear in early pregnancy, the rate of increase can be used to assess the viability of the pregnancy.[11,18] Tay et al state that there is no agreement as to what level of β-hCG is diagnostic of ectopic pregnancy.[19,20] In the presence of an ectopic mass or fluid in the pouch of Douglas, a cutoff point of 1500 mIU/ml is sufficient to identify a gestational sac by TVUS, versus levels of 2000 mIU/ml in the absence of these signs. As progression of the extrauterine pregnancy continues, titers will peak between 80 000 and 100 000 after 20 weeks, similar to the plateau seen in an intrauterine pregnancy gestation.

Serum progesterone

Several investigators have attempted to study the use of progesterone levels as a way to distinguish a viable from a nonviable pregnancy. Levels of at least 25 ng/ml are indicative of normal gestation. Conversely, serum progesterone levels less than 5 ng/ml are rarely associated with viability. In fact, the concomitant finding of low serum progesterone together with a rising hCG level is predictive of nonviable pregnancy, raising the level of suspicion for the presence of extrauterine pregnancy. Values of 5–25 ng/ml fall within the diagnostic 'gray zone'. Unfortunately, the routine use of progesterone alone in this clinical setting has not proven to be the panacea investigators had hoped for. A meta-analysis showed that the use of serum progesterone levels is insufficient to diagnose ectopic pregnancy.[21] Progesterone levels usually take 2–3 days to be reported, rendering it virtually useless in an acute setting.

Serum markers

Vascular endothelial growth factor (VEGF)

A well-known angiogenic factor, VEGF, has been implicated in the mechanisms involved in implantation and early pregnancy. It is also believed that this permeability factor is a critical regulator of amniotic fluid transport in the fetal membranes. Several investigators have reported that VEGF expression in the endometrium and corpus luteum is regulated by ovarian steroids and hCG. A positive correlation has been made between elevated levels of VEGF during the first trimester of normal intrauterine pregnancy and gestational age, β-hCG, estradiol, and progesterone levels. Abnormal implantation therefore further enhances the production of VEGF locally. Daniel and colleagues postulate that because VEGF production is dependent on hypoxia, and because implantation outside the endometrial cavity presents a hostile environment for the trophoblast, VEGF production must be elevated. To test their hypothesis, they compared serum levels in three groups: group I (normal intrauterine pregnancy), group II (abnormal intrauterine pregnancy), and group III (ectopic pregnancy). Each group was matched for gestational age as assessed by last menstrual period and ultrasound measurements. The serum level of VEGF was significantly higher in women with ectopic pregnancy (median, 226.8 pg/ml; range, 19.4–561.7 pg/ml) than in women with normal intrauterine pregnancy (median, 24.4 pg/ml; range, 2.7–196.8 pg/ml). Serum levels of VEGF in women with ectopic pregnancy was significantly higher than in women with abnormal intrauterine pregnancy (median, 59.4 pg/ml; range, 12.1–334.1 pg/ml), though this was not statistically significant. Serum VEGF level of over 200 ng/ml can distinguish an intrauterine from an extrauterine pregnancy with a specificity of 90% and a positive-predictive value (PPV) of 86%, and abnormal intrauterine from extrauterine pregnancy with a specificity of 80% and a PPV of 86%. In addition, combining progesterone levels with VEGF produces better results than using either marker alone – a reflection of their different sources. A serum VEGF level of over 200 pg/ml associated with a serum progesterone level of under 18 ng/ml can distinguish intrauterine from extrauterine pregnancy with a specificity of 95% and a PPV of 92%. It is even more significant that it can distinguish ectopic from abnormal intrauterine pregnancy with a specificity of 95% and a PPV of 92%, which is better than either marker alone.[22,23]

Serum creatine kinase (CK)
Because CK is an enzyme present in muscle cells, it has been hypothesized that injury to these cells would cause an increase in its levels. Several prospective studies have found that it is not specific for tubal muscle cells and therefore is not useful as a serum marker in this setting.[24]

Radiologic assessment

Radiography
With the advances made in ultrasonography in the last 20 years, the routine use of radiographic films in the evaluation of AEP has been relegated to medical anecdotes. In the past, it was used predominantly for both suspected abdominal and saccular (within a uterine horn, such as in uterus didelphys) pregnancies,[7] with the pathognomonic finding on lateral films of an overlapping of the maternal spine by fetal parts.[24] Similarly associated findings are (1) a persistent and unusual position of the fetus; (2) a transverse lie with the back up and high in the abdomen; (3) the position of the fetal head oddly placed in relation to the trunk; (4) the maternal gas pattern overlying the fetus; (5) an unusually clearly appearing fetus, due to the absence of an intervening uterine wall or 'uterine shadow'; and (6) in 2% of cases, after fetal death, the presence of calcifications, resulting in the formation of a lithopedion. In most cases, this is an incidental finding at autopsy, surgery, or imaging studies of the abdomen or pelvis, but it can also present with an acute abdomen secondary to a cecal volvulus or intestinal obstruction, a fistula, or even a pelvic abscess.

Ultrasonography
Since its inception, ultrasonography has revolutionized the management of ectopic pregnancy, and the combination of ultrasound and hCG levels is the diagnostic factor mainly responsible for the significant decrease in maternal morbidity and mortality rates in the last 25 years.[22] Standard protocols utilize a serum hCG concentration of 1500 mIU/ml as the minimum level necessary to visualize intrauterine gestation on TVUS. This level in the absence of intrauterine pregnancy predicts ectopic pregnancy with a sensitivity and specificity of 100% and 99%, respectively.[25] Since ectopic pregnancies are generally associated with lower β-hCG levels than intrauterine pregnancies at similar lengths of gestation, they can often be visualized with TVUS at far lower levels of hCG. By transabdominal ultrasound, the threshold of detection of extrauterine pregnancy is set higher at 6000–6500 mIU/ml. Kadar et al reported that, regardless of singleton or multiple gestation, a sac can be seen sonographically beyond 38 days from the last menstrual period.[26]

Undoubtedly, ultrasound has become extremely important in the diagnosis and management of AEP. Rarely is this more apparent than in the setting of abdominal pregnancy. Signs of abdominal pregnancy are a fetus separate from the uterus, and extrauterine placenta. Interestingly, many of the same radiologic signs found on plain film (anteroposterior/lateral views) are those that are seen on abdominal ultrasound, albeit with far superior resolution and clarity. For example, the close approximation of the fetal parts to the abdominal wall, malpresentation of the fetus found high in the abdomen, and fetal parts overlying the maternal spine on a lateral scan, as well as the absence of the uterine wall between the maternal bladder and fetus, are all signs of abdominal pregnancy.[27]

Improvements have also been made in the diagnostic capabilities of ultrasonography in the evaluation of cervical pregnancy. The most important one has been in differentiating cervical pregnancy from various forms of abortion.[10] For the diagnosis of ovarian or intraligamentary pregnancy, ultrasonographic assessment is not as reliable. Ultrasound echoes do not delineate clearly the site of implantation; therefore, MRI or direct visualization is necessary in these situations. Recently, color and pulsed Doppler has received much attention as an adjunct to TVUS for the initial evaluation of all forms of extrauterine pregnancy. It is believed that placental flow (or peritrophoblastic arterial flow) is related to the invasion of maternal tissues and vessels by trophoblastic villi, which accounts for the typically low-resistance flow noted.[28] Studies show that there is a 20% increase in blood flow in the presence of ectopic pregnancy when compared to only a modest 8% increase when intrauterine pregnancy is confirmed. Furthermore, sensitivity increases from 71 to 95% when ultrasound is used in combination with Doppler technology.[29]

Magnetic resonance imaging (MRI)

MRI is not a first-line method of radiologic evaluation. It is expensive and impractical to use in an emergency situation. However, it can aid in difficult cases when even the resolution by TVUS is insufficient. For instance, hemorrhagic ascites is often hypointense to water on T2-weighted images, and a gestational sac with hematoma shows heterogeneous signal intensity displaying areas of low signal.[30] By producing images in multiple planes, MRI clearly demarcates the area of implantation (Figure 15.2). Thus, pregnancy in the broad ligament can be distinguished from intrauterine pregnancy. MRI can also be employed to monitor the precise location, as well as the involution of remaining placental tissue during postoperative treatment with methotrexate. MRI is safe for both the mother and the fetus because it does not use ionizing radiation. This holds true even in the first trimester of gestation.[1]

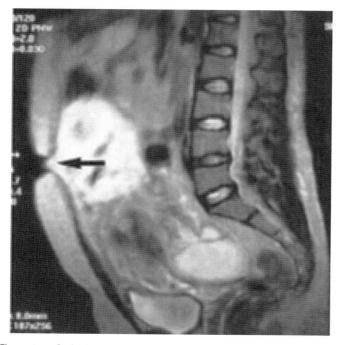

Figure 15.2 Sagittal fast spin echo T1–weighted MR scan, without fat suppression or contrast, shows possible placental attachment to the anterior abdominal wall. (From Cotter AM, Jacques EG, Izquierdo LA. Extended field of view sonography: a useful tool in the diagnosis and management of abdominal pregnancy. J Clin Ultrasound 2004; 32: 208. Reprinted with permission from John Wiley & Sons.)

Management

Management, whether medical or surgical, is dependent on the gestational age and the site of implantation. Abdominal pregnancy leaves no choice. Continuation of the pregnancy carries the possibility of fetal demise from inadequate perfusion at the placental site.[31] Occasionally, a patient desires conservative management despite the risks of continuing the pregnancy, and this situation requires immediate hospitalization and close monitoring of maternal and fetal well-being. Weekly ultrasound monitoring of fetal growth and, after the fetus reaches viability, nonstress tests twice per week are indicated in these situations. Shiu and Langer reported the delivery of two surviving infants at, respectively, 28.5 and 33 weeks' gestation.[2] Fetal assessment began in the early second trimester after the mothers refused to terminate the pregnancy.

The use of methotrexate (MTX) has changed our approach to the treatment of early extrauterine pregnancies. Surgical intervention is reserved for situations where hemodynamic instability or advanced gestation does not permit any alternative. Medical treatment in selected cases of early extrauterine pregnancy is as effective as laparoscopy. Both methods are equally effective in preserving tubal patency. MTX can be used to facilitate the involution of placental tissue left *in situ* at the time of laparotomy.

Surgical management

Although rare, AEP carries a maternal mortality rate eight times higher than that of early extrauterine pregnancy. Whether it is of abdominal, ovarian, or intraligamentary origin, surgical management is virtually the same. However, there are some important caveats that must not be forgotten.

Before proceeding with elective operative intervention, it is essential to localize the placenta and identify its blood supply by MRI or arteriography.[32] Adequate preoperative preparation is essential in anticipation of copious blood loss from unexpected placental detachment and inability to ligate the vascular supply to the placental bed (Figure 15.3). 'Cell saver' has proven to be important preemptively, but it is relatively contraindicated in the Rh-negative mother for fear of sensitization by an Rh-positive fetus.[2] Preoperative embolization of the placental bed has proven to be an effective method for reducing blood loss at the time of surgery and promotes the involution of trophoblastic tissue when the placenta is left *in situ*. Whether or not embolization is employed, the delivery should be performed with extreme caution to avoid the separation of trophoblastic tissue that may hemorrhage.[33]

Laparoscopy allows the diagnosis of ovarian pregnancy at an early gestational age and removal of the gestational sac while attempting to conserve as much ovarian tissue as possible by wedge resection. In case of advanced gestation, there is no alternative to the removal of the adnexa and other adjacent structures.[34]

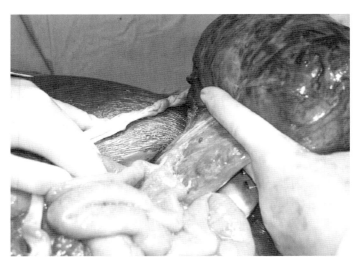

Figure 15.3 Placental attachment to the left infundibulopelvic ligament. (From Cotter AM, Jacques EG, Izquierdo LA. Extended field of view sonography: a useful tool in the diagnosis and management of abdominal pregnancy. J Clin Ultrasound 2004; 32: 208. Reprinted with permission from John Wiley & Sons.)

When a pregnancy is confined to the broad ligament, the ureter is an important consideration. Preoperative placement of a ureteral stent on the side the pregnancy is located is imperative for optimal visualization as it courses under the uterine artery, thereby minimizing the possibility of injury.

Once delivery of the fetus is complete, the placenta may be removed or left *in situ* and allowed to resorb after ligation of the umbilical cord. The residual placental tissue may be treated with methotrexate to accelerate absorption. When the latter two options are employed, sepsis, delayed hemorrhage, adhesions, and urinary or gastrointestinal obstruction are all complications that must be anticipated and prevented, if possible.

Medical management

MTX has a limited role in the management of AEP. In the early 1980s, Tanaka and Miyazaki pioneered its use in the treatment of ectopic pregnancy, based on Li's work some 30 years before, when using the same antimetabolite in the treatment of choriocarcinoma.[35–37] While this is primarily indicated for cases of unruptured tubal pregnancy in a hemodynamically stable patient, it can serve as an adjunct to surgical management or embolization in the treatment of AEP and is therefore mentioned in this chapter. MTX interacts with actively proliferating trophoblasts, as well as other cells with a high mitotic index,[38,39] by functioning as a folic acid analog that disrupts the synthesis and repair of DNA, and the multiplication of cells by inhibiting dihydrofolate reductase.[40] Initially, most cases were treated with MTX protocols similar to those used in gestational trophoblastic disease with intramuscular MTX 1 mg/kg on days 1, 3, 5, and 7 and folinic acid (leucovorin rescue) 0.1 mg/kg on days 2, 4, 6, and 8.[41]

Today, conversion to a single (50 mg/m^2 body surface area or approximately 1 mg/kg body weight) IM dose is most com-

monly used due to the efficacy and rare side effects compared to multidose regimens. The most common side effects associated with the administration of MTX are stomatitis, bone marrow depression, anorexia, and gastrointestinal disturbances, which, thanks to the modification in dosing regimens and addition of leucovorin to most extended protocols, are rarely reported today.[42]

There are no reports of the successful resolution of any gestation greater than 13 weeks treated with MTX alone. Lipscomb et al[11] found that a high serum hCG (>6500 mIU/ml) level is the most important factor associated with treatment failure, and because advanced gestations are usually associated with levels well above this threshold for eligibility, MTX is usually reserved for the treatment of trophoblastic tissue left *in situ*. For example, when dealing with abdominal pregnancy and after extraction of the fetus, the vexatious dilemma commonly encountered is whether to leave or remove the placenta. Separating it may lead to uncontrollable hemorrhage and leaving it *in situ* may predispose the patient to abscess formation.[43,44] By a very gentle technique so as not to dislodge the placenta, the cord should be cut close to its attachment on the placenta, and excess membranes should be trimmed away. Most placentas left in the abdomen will gradually undergo involution[42] and be absorbed uneventfully. A recent case report describes the natural course of placental involution without the use of MTX, after physicians elected to leave the placenta *in situ*. Placental involution was documented by serial β-hCG and ultrasound assessment. The dynamics of the regression in placental volume coincided with a reduction in vascularization. At 5 years, the placenta appeared as a small residual echogenic mass with no vascularity.[45] Unfortunately, this is not always the case. Abdominal pelvic abscess can be a very serious complication. When MTX is used, complete placental involution takes an average of 4–6 months. After cotreatment with arterial embolization, regression of trophoblastic tissue is seen in 3 months.[46]

Angiographic arterial embolization was initially developed for use in the gastrointestinal tract. Today, it is applied to other areas of the body for the control of hemorrhage.[47] Primarily reserved for abdominal and cervical pregnancy, this method is extremely effective in reducing the risk of hemorrhagic complications at the time of surgery for AEP. Rahaman et al reported a 29-year-old primigravida who had a 21-week abdominal pregnancy treated with preoperative arterial embolization before laparoscopically assisted fetal delivery. Postoperatively, four cycles of methotrexate were administered at 50 mg/m^2 IM every 3 weeks for the retained abdominal placenta. Transfusion was not required and serial ultrasound and β-hCG measurements demonstrated complete involution 13 weeks after the last dose of MTX. The patient delivered a full-term infant 2 years later.[48] In a similar case report, a 33-year-old woman presented abdominal pregnancy at 33 weeks' gestation with fetal death. The placental vasculature was embolized preoperatively. After operative delivery of the fetus, the placenta was left *in situ* in an effort to preserve fertility given its implantation on the reproductive organs. The patient suffered prolonged postoperative ileus but otherwise did well. Placental function ceased after 2 months.[49]

These two cases illustrate and highlight the importance of a combined approach using several therapeutic modalities in the treatment of AEPs.

Conclusion

In the last century, advances in medicine and technology have merged to help propel us into an era of significant decreases in maternal mortality. Nowhere is this more apparent than in the setting of AEP. Developments in bioassays such as those for measuring hCG and imaging techniques such as ultrasonography and MRI help clarify the pathogenesis and evolution of AEP by affording us the ability to deliver prompt and effective care without untoward consequences to the mother. Programs that promote early prenatal care make early intervention possible.

References

1. Costa SD, Presley J, Bastert G. Advanced abdominal pregnancy. Obstet Gynecol Surv 1991; 46: 515–24.
2. Shiu AT, Langer A. Advanced extrauterine pregnancy. In: Iffy L, Apuzzio JJ, Vintzileos AM (eds), Operative Obstetrics, pp. 144–53 (2nd edn.). McGraw-Hill: New York, 1992.
3. King G. Advanced extrauterine pregnancy. Am J Obstet Gynecol 1954; 67: 712–40.
4. Pritchard JA, MacDonald PC, Gant NF (eds). Williams' Obstetrics, pp. 85–89 (17th edn). Appleton-Century-Crofts: Norwalk, CT, 1985.
5. Atrash HK, Friede A, Hogue CJR. Abdominal pregnancy in the United States: frequency and maternal mortality. Obstet Gynecol 1987; 84: 1257–68.
6. Foster HW, Moore DT. Abdominal pregnancy. Report of 12 cases. Obstet Gynecol 1967; 30: 249–57.
7. Beacham WD, Hernquist WC, Beacham DW et al. Abdominal pregnancy at Charity Hospital in New Orleans. Am J Obstet Gynecol 1962; 84: 1257–72.
8. Martin JN, Sessums K, Martin RW et al. Abdominal pregnancy: current concepts of management. Obstet Gynecol 1988; 71: 549–56.
9. Studdiford WE. Primary peritoneal pregnancy. Am J Obstet Gynecol 1942; 44: 487–91.
10. Ushakov FB, Elchalal U, Aceman PJ et al. Cervical pregnancy: past and future. Obstet Gynecol Surv 1997; 52: 45–59.
11. Lipscomb GH, Stovall TG, Ling FW. Nonsurgical treatment of ectopic pregnancy. N Engl J Med 2000; 343: 1325–9.
12. Sandberg EC. Ovarian pregnancy. In: Langer A, Iffy L (eds), Extrauterine Pregnancy, pp. 245–53. PSG Publishing: Littleton, MA, 1986.
13. Lehfeldt H, Tietze C, Gorstein F. Ovarian pregnancy and the intrauterine device. Am J Obstet Gynecol 1970; 108: 1005–9.
14. Shibahara H, Funabiki M, Shiotani T et al. A case of primary ovarian pregnancy after in vitro fertilization and embryo transfer. J Assist Reprod Genetic 1997; 14: 63–4.
15. Spiegelberg O. Zur Casuistik der Ovarialschwangerschaft. Arch fur Gynakol 1873; 13: 73.
16. Vorapong P, Ruangsak L, Surang T et al. Pregnancy in the broad ligament. Arch Gynecol Obstet 2003; 268: 233–5.
17. Dorfman SF. Deaths from ectopic pregnancy, United States, 1979–1980. Obstet Gynecol 1983; 62: 344–8.
18. Braunstein GD, Rasor J, Adler D et al. Serum human chorionic gonadotropin levels throughout normal pregnancy. Am J Obstet Gynecol 1976; 152: 299–303.
19. Tay JI, Moore J, Walker JJ. Ectopic pregnancy. BMJ 2000; 320: 916–19.
20. Mol BWJ, Hajenius PJ, Engelsbel S et al. Serum human chorionic gonadotropin measurement in the diagnosis of ectopic pregnancy when transvaginal sonography is inconclusive. Fertil Steril 1998; 70: 972–81.
21. McCord ML, Muram D, Buster JE et al. Single serum progesterone as a screen for ectopic pregnancy: exchanging specificity and sensitivity to obtain optimal test performance. Fertil Steril 1996; 66: 513–16.
22. Lemus JF. Ectopic pregnancy: an update. Curr Opin Obstet Gynecol 2000; 12: 369–75.
23. Daniel Y, Geva E, Lerner-Geva L et al. Levels of vascular endothelial growth factor are elevated in patients with ectopic pregnancy: is this a novel marker? Fertil Steril 1999; 72: 1013–17.
24. Borlum KG, Blorn R. Primary hepatic pregnancy. Int J Gynecol Obstet 1988; 27: 427–43.
25. Bernhart K, Mennuti MT, Benjamin I et al. Prompt diagnosis of ectopic pregnancy in an emergency department setting. Obstet Gynecol 1994; 84: 1010–15.
26. Kadar N, Bohrer M, Kemmann E et al. The discriminatory human chorionic gonadotropin zone for endovaginal sonography: a prospective, randomized study. Fertil Steril 1994; 61: 1016–21.
27. Ombelet W, Vandermerve JV, Van Assche FA et al. Advanced extrauterine pregnancy: description of 38 cases with literature survey. Obstet Gynecol Surv 1988; 43: 386–92.
28. Ali V, Saldana LR, Balat IY et al. Pitfalls in sonographic diagnosis of abdominal pregnancy. South Med J 1981; 74: 4771–9.
29. Stenchever MA, Droegmuller W, Herbst AL, Mishell DR (eds). Comprehensive Gynecology pp. 443–78 (4th edn). Mosby: Norwalk, CT, 2001.
30. Nishino M, Hayakawa K, Iwasaku K et al. Magnetic resonance imaging findings in gynecologic emergencies. J Comput Assist Tomogr 2003; 27: 564–70.
31. Gilbert W, Moore J, Resnick R. Angiographic embolization in the management of hemorrhagic complications of pregnancy. Am J Obstet Gynecol 1992; 116: 43–9.
32. Tulandi T, Sammour A. Evidenced-based management of ectopic pregnancy. Curr Opin Obstet Gynecol 2000; 12: 289–92.
33. Strafford JC, Ragan WD. Abdominal pregnancy: review of current management. Obstet Gynecol 1977; 50: 548–58.

34. Tulandi T, Saleh A. Surgical management of ectopic pregnancy. Clin Obstet Gynecol 1999; 42: 31–8.

35. Li MC, Hertz A, Spencer DB. Effect of methotrexate therapy on choriocarcinoma and chorioadenoma. Proc Soc Exp Biol Med 1956; 93: 361–6.

36. Tanaka T, Hayashi H, Kutsuzawa T et al. Treatment of interstitial ectopic pregnancy with methotrexate: report of a successful case. Fertil Steril 1982; 37: 851–2.

37. Miyazaki Y, Shrina Y, Wake N et al. Studies on nonsurgical therapy of tubal pregnancy. Acta Obstet Gynaecol Jpn 1983; 35: 489.

38. Berkowitz RS, Goldstein DP, Bernstein MR. Ten years' experience with methotrexate and folinic acid as primary therapy for gestational trophoblastic disease. Gynecol Oncol 1986; 23: 111–18.

39. Gabbe SG, Niebyl JR, Simpson JL (eds). Obstetrics: Normal and Problem Pregnancies, pp. 745–6 (4th edn). Churchill Livingstone: London, 2002.

40. Takimoto CH. Antifolates in clinical development. Semin Oncol 1997; 24 (5 Suppl 18): S18-40–51.

41. Yankowitz J, Leake J, Hugguns G et al. Cervical ectopic pregnancy: review of the literature and report of a case treated by single-dose methotrexate therapy. Obstet Gynecol Surv 1990; 45: 405–14.

42. Maymon R, Shulman A, Maymon BBS et al. Ectopic pregnancy: the new gynecological epidemic disease: review of the modern work-up and the nonsurgical treatment option. Int J Fertil 1992; 37: 146–64.

43. Cagnazzi A, Landi S, Volpe A. Rhythmic variation in the rate of ectopic pregnancy throughout the year. Am J Obstet Gynecol 1999; 180: 67–71.

44. Babic D, Colic G, Mrden D. Complications after surgery for abdominal pregnancy due to retained placenta. Ginekol Obstet 1983; 23: 93–4.

45. Badria L, Amarin Z, Jaradat A et al. Full term viable abdominal pregnancy: a case report and review. Arch Gynecol Obstet 2003; 268: 340–2.

46. Valenzano M, Nicoletti L, Odicino F et al. Five-year follow-up of placental involution after abdominal pregnancy. J Clin Ultrasound 2003; 31: 39–43.

47. Nappi C, D'Ella A, Di Carlo C et al. Conservative treatment by angiographic uterine artery embolization of a 12 week cervical ectopic pregnancy: case report. Hum Reprod 1999; 14: 1118–21.

48. Rahaman J, Berkowitz R, Mitty H et al. Minimally invasive management of an advanced abdominal pregnancy. Obstet Gynecol 2004; 103: 1064–8.

49. Cardosi RJ, Nackley AC, Londono J et al. Embolization for advanced abdominal pregnancy with a retained placenta: a case report. J Reprod Med 2002; 47: 861–3.

16 Management of fetal malformations

Lami Yeo, Howard JA Carp, and Josef Shalev

Much to the dismay of parents, birth defects will unfortunately occur in human development. About 3% of all newborns have a recognizable major anomaly, and at least 5% will ultimately be diagnosed with a congenital defect.[1] Not only are birth defects the single most common cause of perinatal mortality in many countries, but they also evoke a wide range of emotions such as fear, anxiety, sadness, and regret. The subject of fetal malformations and their management is one of the most emotional and difficult challenges facing both clinicians and parents. In fact, one of the greatest fears in pregnancy is that an unhealthy child with abnormalities and deformities may be born. Factors which are crucial for adequate perinatal management include an accurate prenatal diagnosis of malformations, evaluation of associated abnormalities (structural and chromosomal) to delineate etiology and prognosis, delivery in the appropriate center, and appropriate counseling.

Depending on the gestational age and the type of diagnosis that is made, there are many options and decisions which parents have to consider. First and foremost, the management plan should always take into consideration the wishes of the parents. They need to understand which malformations are compatible with life, and if so, the potential for increased morbidity must be clearly understood along with the quality of life that will exist. In the second trimester (and even in the third trimester for some cases), the option of pregnancy termination exists, and the method (with its advantages and disadvantages) must be chosen. Invasive testing, such as amniocentesis, chorionic villus sampling, or percutaneous umbilical blood sampling, also must be considered, as the risks of aneuploidy increase when fetal malformations are present. Depending on the abnormality, other options that can be offered include genetic counseling, delivery at a tertiary care center, fetal surgery with the possibility of prenatal surgical correction or improvement, and consultation with other subspecialities such as pediatric surgery and neonatology. The diagnosis of fetal abnormality prenatally also requires an assessment of severity, an understanding of its pathophysiologic basis, differential diagnoses, risk of recurrence, and, naturally, management. One must keep in mind that malformations may not be isolated. There may be multiple anomalies present, and the possibility of genetic syndromes

should always be entertained, as they have important prognostic implications. It is clear that numerous requirements and challenges must be faced when dealing with fetal malformations.

In this chapter, we will discuss the diagnosis of fetal malformations, the role of pregnancy termination, psychological management, and the role of cesarean section in these abnormalities. We will also discuss some of the most common fetal malformations that carry a hopeless prognosis (anencephaly, alobar holoprosencephaly, hydranencephaly, ectopia cordis, and renal agenesis), as well as abnormalities that have increased perinatal morbidity, and where cesarean section may be indicated for dystocia or to improve neonatal outcome (hydrocephalus/spina bifida, encephalocele, large cystic hygroma, large fetal tumors, large nonsolid fetal masses, large omphalocele, and conjoined twins).

Diagnosis

In the era prior to the existence of prenatal diagnostic techniques, such as ultrasonography, managing fetal malformations prenatally was never an issue, because their existence was simply unknown and the diagnosis was not made prior to delivery. Malformations only became an issue after the neonate was born. In the past, however, even in these circumstances, because of the paucity of technology, surgical techniques, diagnostic imaging, and medical knowledge, how to treat and manage these abnormalities was often unclear and rudimentary. Naturally, in the current era, all of this has changed dramatically. Because of great technological advances such as prenatal ultrasonography, fetal abnormalities can and will be diagnosed prenatally, and parents will be faced with this issue ahead of time. The current goal, therefore, should be appropriate prenatal diagnosis and management based on current advances in diagnostic imaging, medical knowledge, the various techniques and resources available, and collaboration with other medical parties.

Because most anomalies are sporadic and uncommon, and often occur in otherwise low-risk women, identifying the true at-risk population causes considerable difficulty. In addition, despite dramatic improvements in our comprehension of congenital anomalies, the underlying cause is often unknown. Since most fetal abnormalities occur in the absence of known risk factors or family history, all pregnancies must be considered at risk of birth defects. Certain sections of the population, however, may be at higher risk than others. It is well known that patients with diabetes are predisposed to having congenital malformations involving the cardiac and the central nervous systems. Certain geographic regions and ethnicities can also predispose to abnormalities. For instance, the highest rates for open neural tube defects are reported in the UK and the lowest rates in Japan.[2] Some defects are multifactorial in origin, and increased risks of malformations in offspring are present if other family members are also affected, such as other siblings. Teratogens and the environment are also implicated in congenital defects, such as anticonvulsant medications leading to an increased risk of neural tube defects. Thus, it is apparent that many factors, including genetics, can play an important role in the etiology of fetal abnormalities.

The initial detection of fetal anomalies requires a method of systematic and thorough screening of all pregnancies at the appropriate time in gestation in order to be effective. This concept has fortunately led to great improvements in the efficacy of prenatal sonography. With current advances in technology, knowledge, and sonographic equipment, it is very feasible to diagnose an increasing number of fetal anomalies *in utero*. The key to accurate prenatal diagnosis is careful scanning of the fetus and knowledge of the abnormalities. Most importantly, this should be performed with a high level of expertise, since both false-positive and false-negative information can have a detrimental impact. Sonographers should be adequately and appropriately trained to ensure that examinations are performed at the highest level. In addition, in order to recognize malformations properly, one should be familiar with normal fetal anatomy, normal variants, and various sonographic landmarks. An appropriately performed systematic and targeted fetal anatomic survey should detect malformations in almost every organ system, such as central nervous, cardiac, skeletal, abdominal, and genitourinary. Amniotic fluid abnormalities can be associated with fetal anomalies; polyhydramnios may be indicative of gastrointestinal tract obstruction, and anhydramnios can be seen with bilateral renal agenesis or obstructive uropathy. Once a fetal abnormality is diagnosed sonographically, a careful and targeted survey should be performed on the rest of the fetus, to rule out the presence of additional anomalies.

The idea of utilizing sonography as a screening tool has gained widespread acceptance in some countries, while it remains controversial in others. Many in the USA still believe that fetal sonography should be limited to women with an indication. In the USA, approximately 60–70% of all pregnant women undergo ultrasound at various times in the gestation.[3] In contrast, many European countries perform ultrasound examinations routinely during pregnancy. However, the overall efficacy of routine sonographic screening for fetal abnormalities

varies widely. One of the first studies to determine the diagnostic accuracy of ultrasonography in high-risk pregnancies was performed in the UK during the late 1970s and early 1980s.[4] It was around this time that real-time imaging became widespread as a clinical tool. This study found that 95% of malformations were correctly diagnosed.[4] Other published sensitivities have ranged broadly anywhere from 13.3% to 82.4%,[5] with the average collaborative world experience being 50%.[6] After reviewing these extremely wide and different detection rates, it becomes apparent why the reliability and utility of sonographic screening for fetal abnormalities has become very controversial in some countries. Even for those who already advocate routine sonographic screening, when to perform scans and the number of sonographic examinations are debatable and inconsistent. We believe that all patients regardless of risk should have uniform routine access to obstetric sonography.

Obstetric ultrasonography should not be considered a 'prenatal test'. Rather, it should be regarded as a 'physical examination' of the fetus. Since the fetus has already been recognized as a 'patient', arguing against routine sonography is similar to arguing against performing a physical examination of the adult patient.

Other methods of screening for fetal malformations besides ultrasonography include biochemical modalities, such as triple or quadruple serum screening (for aneuploidy and neural tube defects) and maternal serum alpha fetoprotein. Of course, while screening is very useful, the accurate diagnosis of malformations requires more definitive testing, such as prenatal and postnatal testing, imaging studies after birth, neonatal examination, and genetic testing. In the presence of fetal anomalies known to be associated with an increased frequency of aneuploidy, fetal karyotyping is indicated. This may be done via amniocentesis, placental biopsy, or fetal blood sampling, depending upon the urgency of diagnosis. Amniocentesis can provide valuable information in a variety of circumstances. For instance, it can reveal karyotype, degree of amniotic fluid alpha fetoprotein elevation, presence of acetylcholinesterase, genetic data, and the presence of fetal infection. Performing fetal vesicocentesis when there is lower obstructive uropathy, such as bladder outlet obstruction, can provide chemical information regarding normal or abnormal renal function. Once chromosomal abnormalities are diagnosed because of the discovery of malformations (either prenatally or postnatally), the type of aneuploidy has the ultimate impact on prognosis. For instance, Down syndrome carries the potential for organ malformation and neurodevelopmental delay, but is still compatible with life. Trisomies 18 and 13, on the other hand, carry a uniformly poor prognosis; even in survivors, the morbidity is extremely high.

Fetal echocardiography is necessary when the sonographically detected fetal abnormality is one that is known to be associated with cardiac disease. Depending on the type and severity of fetal malformations, strong consideration should be given to delivery at a tertiary care center where neonatologists and appropriate pediatric subspecialists are immediately available. Prenatal counseling through a variety of medical venues and through a multidisciplinary combined team approach is extremely important and valuable, since it is often this information that will influence decision making. Patients need to understand which malformations are compatible with life and, for those that are, what type of quality of life is to be expected for their child. Parents will desire to know about the recurrence risk, their neonate's chances for survival, surgical correction, and resultant handicaps and morbidity. For instance, patients need to understand the implications of neural tube defects, and the increased morbidity that occurs with this diagnosis. Surgical procedures will need to be undertaken, and there will be an impact on physical performance and abilities. Consultation with pediatric neurosurgeons and other relevant specialists will offer invaluable information to prospective parents. Anencephaly, which is a lethal diagnosis, has very different implications from hydrocephalus, which may not be lethal but carries its own inherent morbidity. Other abnormalities (such as obstructive uropathy or spina bifida) may be amenable to fetal surgery in utero, while yet others, such as ectopia cordis, are not. When omphalocele is diagnosed prenatally, a combined team approach, involving consultation with the geneticist, the obstetrician, the neonatologist, and pediatric surgeons ahead of time, is often very valuable, sets expectations, and prepares patients for future surgery on their child.

Genetic counseling is also a vital component of the management process once fetal malformations are diagnosed. Depending on the mode of inheritance, patients may be at increased risk of having another child with abnormalities, and these risks can be discussed. If both parents are carriers of an autosomal recessive disorder, their offspring has a 25% chance of being affected with this disorder. Autosomal dominant abnormalities convey a much higher risk (50%) of recurrence. With multifactorial abnormalities such as neural tube defects, the risk of recurrence after one affected child is 2–3%, and after a second affected child the risk is approximately 6%.[7] Fortunately, the recurrence risk for most fetal anomalies is often minimal, and therefore the reassurance given through counseling offers invaluable and vital information for the parents.

Termination of pregnancy

While not all patients or clinicians would agree, some families will choose to terminate a pregnancy carrying a malformed fetus, while others would never consider this option. It is a decision wrought with moral, ethical, and emotional issues that are individualized for each family. Some may choose not to terminate their pregnancy in order to utilize organs of their fetus for transplantation. Once fetal abnormalities are diagnosed, appropriate management depends on the gestational age, the laws of the state or country, the type and severity of the anomaly, and the choices of the parents. Various techniques exist to accomplish termination, each carrying its own risks and benefits. For instance, some patients may specifically choose an induced

labor process with delivery, in order to have an autopsy performed for the purposes of delineating abnormalities further and confirming suspected malformations, establishing a diagnosis, and establishing recurrence risks. Karyotype analysis can also be performed on various fetal tissues. Induction of labor can be accomplished with laminaria, foley bulb catheter, prostaglandins, and/or oxytocin. Others, however, may choose to avoid going through labor in the second trimester, and instead have a surgical procedure (such as dilation and curettage, or dilation and evacuation) performed while under anesthesia. Undergoing this method may not make complete autopsy examination of the fetus feasible due to its destructive nature.

In any case, regardless of whether the neonate dies because of elective termination or a spontaneous event, a full postmortem autopsy should always be offered to determine the full extent of anomalies. If this is declined, at least a detailed external examination of the neonate should be offered. If not already performed, a full history of the mother should be taken, including possible environmental, drug, or radiation exposures. The family history should be discussed in detail, and photographs should be taken of all abnormalities found. Organ tissue biopsies (such as skin) may need to be taken for chromosomal analysis or other studies. Depending on the abnormality, more specialized testing such as radiologic studies or DNA testing may also be necessary, and karyotype analysis may also be performed on both parents. When available, it is often very valuable and beneficial to have a geneticist or someone who is experienced in dysmorphology examine the infant carefully and thoroughly in order to arrive at a detailed diagnosis, whether the neonate is alive or not.

It is important to remember that many women who choose termination as an option are riddled with feelings of guilt, sorrow, helplessness, failure, and resentment. They will often still experience feelings of mourning and may require further psychological assistance, support, or counseling.

Psychological management of parents

The birth of a severely deformed baby, whether viable or not, may lead to chronic symptoms such as ego disorientation, neurosis, and prolonged psychiatric treatment. Most severe malformations will require at least a thorough physical examination by the pediatrician, and possibly pediatric surgeon and geneticist in order to make a precise diagnosis. Any inaccurate information is liable to be counterproductive. Whether the anomaly has been diagnosed previously or not, the parents will ask the obstetrician soon after birth whether the baby is normal, or ask the extent of the anomalies. If the anomaly has not previously been diagnosed, it may be prudent to explain that the baby is having some difficulty which is causing enough concern to move him/her to the special care unit and that a full explanation will be given later. If the anomaly is expected, an initial assessment will be requested. It will then be necessary to give some explanation, and to explain that a detailed answer can be given only after a full assessment.

The full facts should be given in a sympathetic and understanding manner by an experienced practitioner, whether it be obstetrician, pediatrician, or geneticist. As psychiatric support may be necessary, a psychiatrist or psychologist should be involved. The parents should have the opportunity to question a team comprising the relevant disciplines about the risk of recurrence, the baby's chances of survival, surgical correction, and resultant handicaps.

The new parents may be resentful of their child and lost freedom. Both will often acknowledge a certain failure in the parental role. The parents will also have to be prepared for crises in the baby's health and understand his or her special needs. Hence, the parents must 'mourn' the normal baby they hoped for and lost. On being informed, both parents are likely to undergo an acute grief reaction.[8] Shock and disbelief are followed by waves of distress, emotional dyspnea, feelings of choking, guilt, and accusations of negligence. Later, there is a developing awareness that the pain and despair are associated with dread of this baby. A feeling of helplessness and identification with him or her, and a disorganization of personality may possibly follow. Then, there is resolution when the patient starts to cope. They reorganize, emancipate from the lost object, and form new object relationships. It may be helpful to meet similar parents and learn from their experience, in order to make decisions as to their baby's future. The patient or husband should be encouraged to see the baby, but only after a full explanation and accompanied by a physician or nurse.

After the patient's discharge home, obstetric management may cease, but this is a family at risk of psychiatric problems. The primary care physician, the social worker, and the community should be mobilized to provide the necessary support.

Role of cesarean section

At first, one might instinctively think that performing a cesarean section when lethal fetal malformations are present is an absurd notion. The traditional approach is often to avoid cesarean section when major congenital anomalies are present. Likewise, others may believe that performing a cesarean section when any fetal anomaly is present may improve neonatal outcome. However, in each case, the role of cesarean section must be carefully pondered, planned, and discussed. One must remember that cesarean sections are performed in any obstetric patient not only for fetal reasons, but also for maternal indications. For instance, a fetus with a large cervical teratoma may rotate through the birth canal in such a way that it is impossible to deliver vaginally. Significant hydrocephalus or encephalocele where the cranial size is very large may prevent a normal labor course with appropriate descent of the fetus.

Other fetal anomalies can predispose to obstructive labor patterns or can lead to difficult destructive procedures, such that cesarean section will be the optimal choice of delivery method.

The choice of cesarean section as an option ultimately depends on many factors, such as the patient's wishes, the experience of the obstetrician, the possibility of cephalopelvic disproportion, obstetric indications, maternal medical problems, prior operative procedures on the uterus, gestational age, the anomaly itself, the presence of associated abnormalities and overall prognosis, and whether damage, trauma, or increased morbidity to the mother (such as uterine rupture) will occur by delivering vaginally. With some fetal abnormalities, cesarean section may be indicated due to dystocia or to improve neonatal outcomes (hydrocephalus, sacrococcygeal teratoma, large omphalocele, etc.). In certain circumstances, elective cesarean section may clearly be preferable to vaginal delivery. However, in some cases of lethal malformations, a minor destructive procedure along with vaginal delivery may be preferred. Examples include cleidotomy in the case of shoulder dystocia with an anencephalic fetus, or cephalocentesis in a fetus with hydranencephaly to allow for a decrease in cranial size. In addition, when lethal abnormalities are present or the abnormality is thought to have a poor prognosis, the patient may choose a very conservative management, such as electing not to undergo cesarean delivery for fetal distress or a nonreassuring fetal heart tracing, and having no neonatal resuscitation performed at the time of delivery or afterwards. If chosen, this plan should be carefully and completely determined well before the patient undergoes labor. If the prognosis appears promising, the perinatal management should consist of antepartum serial fetal evaluation, cesarean section for fetal distress, and neonatal resuscitation.

In all cases, the situation should be discussed in detail thoroughly with the patient, so that she understands the risks and benefits of the delivery method chosen. Cesarean section itself carries an increased risk of maternal morbidity and mortality, such as thromboembolism, infection, or hemorrhage. In addition, one should always bear in mind that cesarean section does not always prevent an atraumatic or destructive delivery for the fetus and mother. There may still be difficulty in delivering the fetus despite an abdominal delivery, as in the case of large head size (hydranencephaly, hydrocephalus), fetal malpresentation/malposition, or an abnormal head to abdomen ratio (ascites, obstructive uropathy). One must consider the risks of extending the uterine incision or inevitably causing a tear versus morbidity caused to the fetus. Consideration of a low vertical or classical incision should be made and may be preferred in certain circumstances (vs low transverse) in order to facilitate extension of the uterine incision if necessary, keeping in mind the consequences for future pregnancies.

Fetal malformations with a hopeless prognosis

Anencephaly

This condition (Figure 16.1) does not give rise to the severe ethical problems associated with other fetal anomalies because it is incompatible with life. Anencephaly is a condition in which the alar plates of the cerebral segments of the neural plate fail to fuse. As the forebrain is composed mainly of alar plates, it is affected more than the hindbrain or midbrain. Failure of fusion disturbs the organization of the cranium; therefore, exencephaly and acrania follow. Forebrain elements such as the cerebral hemispheres fail to develop. Hence, the base of the brain is exposed or covered by membranes.

The incidence is roughly 3/1000 births, with a female to male ratio of 7:3.[9] The incidence has been decreasing in recent years, both in the USA[10] and in other countries.[11] This could be for two reasons: early diagnosis and the increasing acceptability of artificial abortion,[12] and folic acid supplementation.[10] Since folic acid supplementation has been increased, the incidence has been reported to have fallen by 16%.[10] However, although there is no question that folic acid supplementation has decreased the incidence of other neural tube defects, the beneficial effect on the incidence of anencephaly has been disputed.[13] A supplement of 400 µg is recommended, but a dose of 5 mg has also been suggested, particularly in high-risk patients (previously affected pregnancy, family history, or use of antiepileptic drugs).

Anencephaly may be suspected on the basis of known risk factors (a previous child with neural tube defect, antiepileptic drugs) and maternal serum alpha fetoprotein elevation, or may be diagnosed in a routine ultrasonographic examination (Figure 16.2). Most patients today undergo a midtrimester scan to exclude anomalies. If scanning is performed in the first trimester, the features have been well described on transvaginal scanning.[14] Since anencephaly is incompatible with life, the decision to perform abortion is relatively straightforward. If the pregnancy continues, the patient usually presents with hydramnios and a larger-than-expected uterus. Hydramnios may be secondary to the lack of cerebral tissue controlling swallowing, leading to accumulation of amniotic fluid. Some fetuses may be growth restricted due to poor growth potential. Electronic fetal heart rate monitoring may show signs of fetal distress. The pregnancy often continues beyond term and may be misdiagnosed clinically as a breech presentation.

Once the diagnosis is made, induction of labor may be considered. However, labor may be difficult to induce in these patients. When hydramnios causes respiratory difficulties, amniocentesis can be employed to drain up to several liters of fluid. This in itself may make the uterus more responsive to oxytocin. The presentation is often face or breech during labor. In cases of shoulder dystocia, gentle suprapubic pressure may help allow the shoulders to pass the pubic symphysis. Before applying such pressure, the bladder must be emptied. If not successful, cleidotomy may become necessary to reduce the fetal bulk. The procedure is performed by two fingers being passed along the ventral aspect of the fetus, and under their protection the clavicles are divided with scissors. There is danger, however, to maternal soft parts; therefore, the scissors must be guarded.

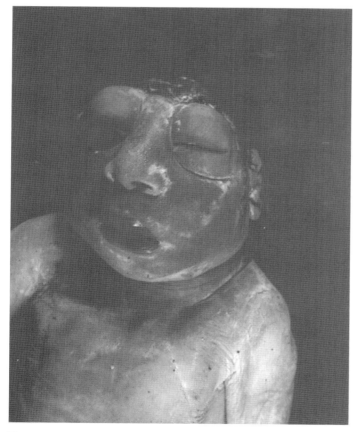

Figure 16.1. Gross features seen in a newborn with anencephaly. Note the absence of cerebral hemispheres.

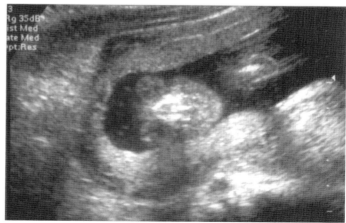

Figure 16.2 Coronal view of anencephalic fetus in the second trimester, showing absence of brain and calvaria above the prominent bony orbits.

There may also be difficulty in identifying the fetal ventral side, and the spine or the scapula might be divided by mistake.

The parents of anencephalic fetuses should undergo genetic counseling. Targeted ultrasound with the possibility of amniocentesis should be performed in subsequent pregnancies, as there is a 5% risk of another neural tube defect, including spina bifida. Anencephalic infants have been used as sources of organ transplantation, including heart,[15] kidney,[16] and even bladder.[17] However, the use of organs from anencephalic fetuses for transplantation involves complex ethical issues which have not been fully resolved.

Alobar holoprosencephaly

There are three major subtypes of holoprosencephaly, depending on the degree of anatomic abnormality: alobar, semilobar, and lobar. Overall, holoprosencephaly is uncommonly found at birth (1/16 000 neonates)[18] but is probably associated with a high intrauterine fatality rate, thus being more frequently seen prenatally. It is a genetically heterogeneous anomaly that can involve different chromosomes, with known holoprosencephaly-associated genes in existence. Salicylate ingestion in pregnancy has been reported in relation to this condition,[18] along with diabetes, ethanol use, and cytomegalovirus. Holoprosencephaly is a midline abnormality of the brain, resulting from failure of cleavage of the prosencephalon (forebrain) and formation of the midline structures. It is embryologically related to development of the midface, hence the common association with median facial anomalies involving the forehead, interorbital structures, nose, premaxilla, and upper lip. The prosencephalon gives rise to the cerebral hemispheres and diencephalic structures, including the neurohypophysis, third ventricle, and thalami.

The most severe form, alobar holoprosencephaly, is sonographically recognized in the fetus by the absence of the interhemispheric fissure and cerebral falx. There are a single monoventricle (Figure 16.3), fused thalami in the midline, absent third ventricle, and absent cavum septum pellucidum. The neurohypophysis (posterior lobe of the pituitary gland), olfactory bulbs and tracts are also absent. Normally, the roof of the ventricular cavity is enfolded within the brain; however, in alobar holoprosencephaly the roof may balloon out, forming a variable-sized cyst, known as the dorsal sac. A wide variety of midline facial anomalies (Figure 16.4) can be found on ultrasound, including cyclopia, anophthalmia, hypotelorism, proboscis, arhinia, and median cleft lip.[19] In general, the more severe facial malformations are associated with alobar holoprosencephaly, but there are exceptions. The face can rarely be normal.[18] In addition, microcephaly may be seen, and, less frequently, macrocephaly secondary to hydrocephalus.

Once alobar holoprosencephaly is diagnosed prenatally, karyotype testing should be performed, as chromosomal abnormalities are present in 50–60% of these fetuses. In particular, trisomy 13 is the most common aneuploidy, found in 50–75% of those with an abnormal karyotype.[20] However, there are a mul-

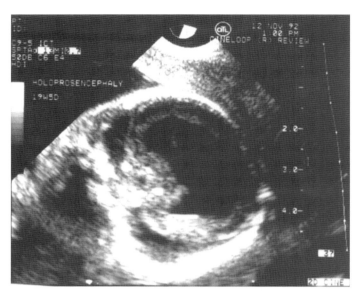

Figure 16.3 Coronal view of the fetal brain showing a single, sonolucent monoventricle in a second-trimester fetus with alobar holoprosencephaly.

titude of other karyotypic abnormalities that can be found. The rest of the fetus should be examined very carefully on ultrasound, as the risk of associated malformations (such as cardiac and renal) is increased, and, particularly when found, they increase the probability of an underlying chromosomal abnormality. Genetic counseling is also recommended, as the risk of nonaneuploid genetic syndromes is also increased with holoprosencephaly. Examples of these include the Kallman, Hall–Pallister, and Meckel syndromes.[20]

The prognosis for survival is dismal, as this is, for the most part, a lethal abnormality. Therefore, when it is identified prenatally, termination should be offered as an option. Some have estimated that only 3% of holoprosencephalic conceptions actually survive long enough to be considered a live birth.[21] If there is severe hydrocephalus and a trial of vaginal delivery is undertaken, cerebral decompression through cephalocentesis may be performed to avoid possible uterine rupture and the risk of dystocia. This procedure will be discussed under the section of hydranencephaly. In general, cesarean delivery should be considered only for maternal or obstetric indications. For infants who survive with alobar holoprosencephaly, aggressive resuscitation is usually not recommended. A complete physical examination and/or autopsy is recommended to determine whether the holoprosencephaly is isolated or part of a genetic syndrome. It is also important for patients to understand that hereditary forms of holoprosencephaly have been reported, including autosomal dominant with variable penetrance, autosomal recessive, and X-linked recessive modes of inheritance. This information may be important for future pregnancies. In addition, a detailed family history should be elicited, particularly inquiring about other family members with mental retardation, microcephaly, cleft lip/palate, eye abnormalities, etc.

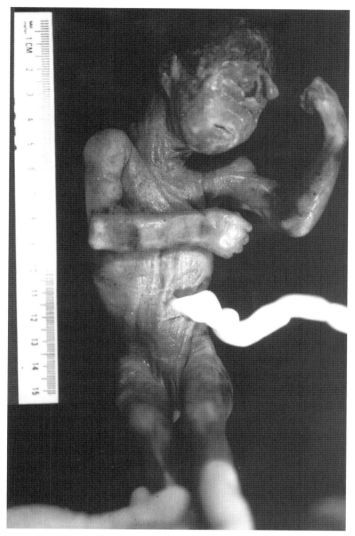

Figure 16.4 Gross pathologic features seen in the face of a neonate with alobar holoprosencephaly. A single eye globe (cyclopia) and a proboscis located above the median eye are visualized.

Hydranencephaly

Also known as hydrocephalic anencephaly, this condition occurs in 1.0–2.5 per 10 000 births.[22] In this condition, there are no cerebral hemispheres and an incomplete or absent falx. The inner two meninges (arachnoid and pia mater) form a sac-like structure that contains cerebrospinal fluid and surrounds the brain stem and basal ganglia. It is thought to be secondary to bilateral internal carotid artery occlusion and cerebral infarction, resulting in brain destruction that leads to liquefaction of the cerebral hemispheres. It is considered the most severe form of a spectrum of anomalies, which also includes porencephalic cysts and schizencephaly. Other possible associations include maternal exposure to carbon monoxide or butane gas, infections (such as congenital cytomegalovirus, herpes simplex, rubella, and toxoplasmosis), and intrauterine demise of a

cotwin in a monochorionic twin pregnancy. Therefore, serology and/or cultures for these infections should be offered. Hydranencephaly may be associated with other structural abnormalities, genetic syndromes, and aneuploidy; therefore, fetal karyotype testing should be considered. However, the typical scenario is that hydranencephaly is isolated, with no additional anomalies seen.

Due to the etiologic nature of hydranencephaly, early sonographic signs may reveal infarction and hemorrhage, and this is different from later findings, when it evolves to show a large cystic, sonolucent mass that fills the entire cranial cavity (Figure 16.5). Recent hemorrhage often appears echogenic, and with time, the appearance becomes more sonolucent. Therefore, serial sonograms may be indicated due to its evolving nature. One should remember that whenever massive intracranial hemorrhage is seen in a fetus sonographically, it should be followed for the subsequent development of hydranencephaly. Sonographically, there may be absent or discontinuous cerebral cortex; scattered and preserved areas of cortical tissue may be seen. The falx is often present (although it can be partially or completely absent), and the thalami and brainstem may be visualized protruding inside the cystic cavity. The cerebellum, midbrain, and brainstem are typically normal. Macrocephaly is usually present, and polyhydramnios may also be seen. Serial sonograms are indicated to follow for the development of macrocephaly. The differential diagnosis includes extreme and massive hydrocephalus, alobar holoprosencephaly, and porencephaly. With all three of these diagnoses, however, a thin rim of abnormal, but identifiable, cortical brain tissue remains persistent.

This disorder carries a very grim prognosis, since there has been destruction of the higher brain centers. Common signs include hyperreflexia and clonus, seizures, and irritability. If there is an intact hypothalamus allowing for thermoregulation, survival may last for several months, but most neonates will pass

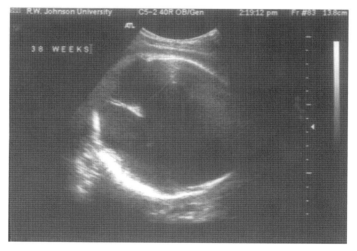

Figure 16.5 Axial scan of the fetal head at 38 weeks showing typical features of hydranencephaly (large cystic, sonolucent area) with no visible brain structure. A portion of the midline falx is evident.

away within the first year of life. On occasion, long-term survival has been reported. Pregnancy termination can be offered as an option, even as late as the third trimester. There is no increased recurrence risk since it is due to a destructive process in a previously normally formed brain (vs primary malformation). Autopsy should be offered to confirm the diagnosis.

Due to the dismal prognosis, vaginal delivery is preferred. If the diagnosis is sure, there is no necessity for delivery at a tertiary care center. Cesarean section for fetal distress is not recommended. In addition, neonatal resuscitative efforts are not required. Because macrocephaly is commonly associated with hydranencephaly, cephalocentesis may be necessary to allow for a successful vaginal delivery. Cephalocentesis is the performance of cerebral decompression by removing large amounts of intracranial fluid. This may be performed in instances of known hydranencephaly or alobar holoprosencephaly when the cranial size is very large, in order to avoid obstructed labor or the risk of uterine rupture. With a large-gauge needle, a maternal transabdominal or transvaginal approach can be undertaken with ultrasonographic guidance. The needle is inserted into the fetal head, and several liters of fluid may be withdrawn in one session. During labor, when the presentation is cephalic, the decompression is more easily performed vaginally. Simple aspiration (optimally through a fontanelle) using needle and syringe is usually sufficient to cause collapse of the fetal skull.

Ectopia cordis

This rare condition is a type of ventral wall defect, involving a thoracic defect of sternum and skin. Therefore, the dynamic fetal heart is uncovered by skin and is exposed outside the chest wall (extrathoracic). This must be distinguished from two conditions: absent sternum (dynamic heart is covered by skin) or failure of sternal fusion (wide separation of all sternal elements) in which the heart beats beneath the skin-covered gap, is within the chest, and is structurally normal. Normally, in embryologic development, the heart and pericardial cavity lie on the ventral surface of the embryo. Later, it is incorporated into the central chest with development of the lateral folds in the thoracic area. The heart gradually invaginates into the pericardial cavity. Therefore, the most common theory suggests that ectopia cordis results from failure of fusion of the lateral body folds in the thoracic region during the sixth postmenstrual week.[23] Mainly, there are two types of ectopia cordis, comprising 95% of all cases: thoracic (as described above) and thoracoabdominal, where the cardiac ventricles are displaced through a diaphragmatic defect into the abdomen. Thoracic ectopia cordis is the most common form.

Sonographically, the heart appears to be located outside the chest cavity and wall. The apex of the heart is usually deviated anteriorly, but may also be seen angled up toward the fetal chin. In some cases, only a portion of the heart herniates through the thoracic defect (Figure 16.6), making the prenatal diagnosis more difficult. It is associated with a high rate of cardiac and

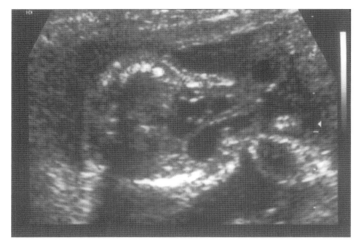

Figure 16.6 Transverse view of the fetal chest showing ectopia cordis, with a portion of the heart located outside the chest cavity and wall.

other abnormalities, such as omphalocele and craniofacial defects,[24] and therefore a complete, targeted sonographic examination should be performed. In particular, midline defects should be searched for. In one study, among eight fetuses with ectopia cordis seen, 63% also had omphalocele, and 75% also had structural cardiac defects.[24] A multitude of various cardiac anomalies have been reported, although they usually include a ventricular septal defect, with or without tetralogy of Fallot. Determining the cardiac anatomy is extremely important to establish prognosis; therefore, fetal echocardiography should also be performed. With thoracic ectopia cordis, the size and shape of the fetal chest should be assessed, as hypoplasia of the chest wall and lungs may be present. When ectopia cordis is seen in association with omphalocele, pentalogy of Cantrell should be suspected.

Because aneuploidy has been associated with ectopia cordis, fetal karyotype testing should be offered to the patient. Ectopia cordis has a severe prognosis and very high mortality rate, with most neonates passing away within a few days after birth, and few surviving more than a few months.[25] At best, the survival rate is 5–10%, and the presence or absence of underlying cardiac defects influences and is the main determinant of survival. When diagnosed prenatally, therefore, termination of the pregnancy as an option can be offered to the patient. The presence of cardiac defects portends an extremely poor prognosis, and patients should be counseled regarding this fact. Obviously, the more severe cardiac lesions will diminish the prognosis overall. In general, fetuses that survive with ectopia cordis are those lacking associated intracardiac defects.[26] No stillborn infants have had isolated ectopia cordis with normal heart anatomy. Even if the pregnancy goes to term and the neonate is born alive, there has never been a long-term survivor who underwent successful reconstruction and who had ectopia cordis associated with intracardiac defects.[26] While abdominal ectopia cordis is not incompatible with life, about ⅓ of fetuses are stillborn or die on the first day of life from severe cardiac malformations.[26] The presence of aneuploidy and other structural abnormalities also play a role in the overall prognosis.

If the patient continues the pregnancy, serial sonographic examinations are necessary to monitor fetal growth and well-being. Clearly, the patient should deliver at a tertiary care center where neonatologists, pediatric surgeons, and pediatric cardiac surgeons are available. Staging of the cardiac repair may be needed, and the surgical approach should be adjusted depending on the severity of the defect and other complicating issues.[25] The surgical repair can be quite difficult, due to the small thorax and the presence of various cardiac anomalies. Because in most cases of ectopia cordis there is absent skin covering the heart, immediate surgical closure of the defect is needed to prevent serious infection. Although in general the prognosis is serious for any neonate with ectopia cordis, for patients with normal cardiac anatomy, long-term survival is possible and has been reported.[26] In the presence of severe cardiac abnormalities where the prognosis is extremely poor, vaginal delivery is recommended without fetal monitoring or neonatal resuscitative measures. In the rare cases when the cardiac anatomy is normal and full resuscitation is the goal, cesarean delivery may be justified because of the potential adverse effects on venous return to the extrathoracic heart, and compromised fetal cardiac output during labor and delivery.[26] It also offers a planned delivery with preparations to have the surgical team available.

Bilateral renal agenesis

Bilateral renal agenesis is a lethal anomaly which causes death from pulmonary hypoplasia within hours or days after birth. Thus, early diagnosis is important and termination of pregnancy as an option can be offered. Potter first described this sequence with its characteristic facial appearance in 1946.[27] The incidence is 1/4500 births. The most common cause of this malformation is absence or malformation of the caudal end of the mesonephric duct, from which the ureteric bud arises. This ureteric bud must penetrate the metanephric blastema to induce the development of metanephric tubules and the subsequent kidney. This abnormality may arise unilaterally, but, if so, other features of the syndrome will be absent.

Potter sequence infants look prematurely senile, with an epicanthic fold extending into the cheek. The nose is turned down and the tip of the chin is prominent. The ears are usually distorted, while the legs are bowed and the feet clubbed. The skin is dry and loose, and the adrenals often are enlarged and fused. The lungs are hypoplastic. The diagnosis should be suspected in cases of oligohydramnios associated with absence of both kidneys and the urinary bladder. Prenatal sonographic diagnosis may be difficult due to severe oligohydramnios. Failure to demonstrate the fetal bladder during the first ultrasound scan is not pathognomonic for absent kidney function, because the fetus may have recently voided. However, with normal kidney function, the fetal bladder should be seen at some time over

approximately 1 hour. Bronstein has reported the possibility of normal amniotic fluid volume up to 16 weeks' gestation in cases of renal agenesis.[28] Since the fetal adrenals are frequently hyperplastic, they may be mistaken for kidneys. However, the absence of the renal pelvis and the lack of normal kidney architecture will aid in the differentiation of hyperplastic adrenals from normal kidneys. The absence of both renal arteries detected by color Doppler velocimetry on ultrasound will usually establish the diagnosis of renal agenesis.

Approximately 50% of these fetuses have associated major malformations.[29] These include cardiac defects (25%), cardiac defects and VATER (vertebral defects, anal atresia, tracheoesophageal, radial, and renal anomalies) (27%), digital anomalies (15%), and müllerian anomalies (20%), as well as neural tube defects, hydrocephalus, microcephaly, and gastrointestinal tract malformations (duodenal atresia, omphalocele).[30] As there is a disturbance of the distal mesonephric duct, it is not surprising that the müllerian duct often is involved, resulting in absence of the uterus and vagina. Renal agenesis may appear in approximately 30% of MURCS (müllerian hypoplasia/aplasia, renal agenesis, and cervicothoracic somite dysplasia) association. This severe, complex anomaly is also associated with absence of the uterus and tubes, which is almost impossible to diagnose prenatally by ultrasound.[31] Other syndromes associated with renal agenesis are branchio-otorenal syndrome, acrorenal-mandibular syndrome, cerebro-oculofacial skeletal syndrome, and Fraser's syndrome. The overall recurrence risk of bilateral renal agenesis is 3–6%. In cases of autosomal dominant and recessive inheritance, the recurrence risk is 50% and 25%, respectively.

Fetal anomalies where cesarean section is indicated (for dystocia or to improve neonatal outcome)

Hydrocephalus/spina bifida

Although these malformations may occur independently, they can often occur concurrently. Spina bifida is one of the more difficult congenital malformations to manage obstetrically, surgically, and ethically. The defect is mainly localized to the dorsal arch of the vertebrae (dorsal defects); in extremely rare cases, the defect splits the vertebral body (ventral defects). The incidence of the condition is approximately 1 per 1000; however, it varies geographically. In Wales, it is as high as 4/1000 live births,[32] whereas in Boston (USA) it is as low as 0.9/1000 live births, a decrease from 2.8/1000 live births in three to four decades.[33,34] The recurrence rate is approximately 6%.[35,36]

Prenatal diagnosis is made by ultrasound (Figures 16.7 and 16.8) with the help of associated abnormalities in the skull ('lemon sign', an inward displacement of frontal bones) and brain ('banana sign', an obliterated cisterna magna due to

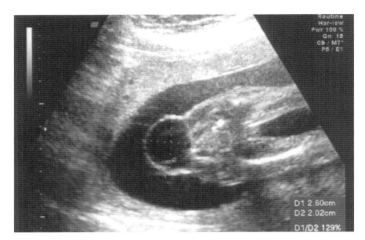

Figure 16.7 Transverse scan of fetal spine showing cystic myelomeningocele.

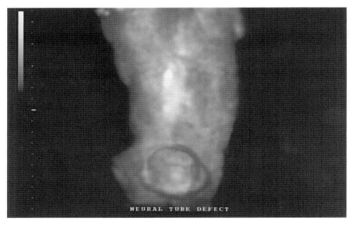

Figure 16.8 Three-dimensional sonogram showing the fetal back affected by a neural tube defect in the lumbosacral area.

downward traction of the cerebellum). The sensitivity of the cranial signs in identifying spina bifida is 99%.[37] The obliteration of the cisterna magna can also be visualized on MRI.[38] Ventricular enlargement is present in approximately 70% of open spina bifida cases during the midtrimester and in approximately 90% of cases at birth.[39] Spina bifida is usually associated with Arnold–Chiari malformation, type II. Displacement of the 4th ventricle and cerebellum may cause obstructive hydrocephalus. Spina bifida is also associated with deformities of the lower limbs, such as clubfoot, rocker bottom foot, and dislocation of the hip.

In open neural tube defects, alpha fetoprotein leaks from the cerebrospinal fluid to the amniotic fluid where it is found in high quantities. From here, it is absorbed into the maternal serum, where it can be detected in increased concentrations. Maternal serum screening is usually performed at 16–20 weeks'

gestation and often produces false-positive results.[40] Using a cutoff of 2.5 MoM, 80% of open spina bifida cases can be detected.[41] Due to the high false-positive results, however, follow-up of elevated maternal serum alpha fetoprotein should be performed by targeted ultrasound. Amniotic fluid alpha fetoprotein determination may be considered in cases of unexplained extremely high maternal serum alpha fetoprotein concentrations, or inability to perform a detailed fetal evaluation due to maternal obesity.

Meningocele causes little neurologic damage, is unassociated with hydrocephalus, and presents few problems to the obstetrician. However, meningomyelocele (Figure 16.7) presents a more serious problem. It is due to nondevelopment of the neural tube beyond the neural plate stage. It usually occupies several segments. Even with expert treatment, including a series of operations, these children display multisystem handicaps, including varying degrees of paralysis, multiple deformities of the lower limbs, and kyphoscoliosis. Approximately 20% of infants that undergo surgery die in the first year of life, and approximately 35% die within the first 5 years.[42] Only 13% ever learn to walk, while most remain chairbound. There is a lack of urine control, leading to retention with overflow; urinary infections; pyelonephritis; hydronephrosis; hypertension; and chronic renal failure. Only 17% have sphincter control.[43] In highly selected cases, prenatal fetal surgery in highly specialized centers may be considered as an option during the late second trimester.

Prenatal diagnosis of ventriculomegaly/hydrocephalus is based on enlargement of the atrium of the lateral ventricle of greater than 10 mm,[44] which is often associated with a relative 'shrinkage' (inability to fill entirely the width of the lateral ventricle) or dangling of the choroid plexus (Figures 16.9–16.11). Both shrinkage of the choroid plexus and enlargement of the lateral ventricular atrium over 10 mm are early signs of ventriculomegaly. In advanced hydrocephalus, the size of the lateral ventricles may increase ahead of the biparietal diameter (BPD).[45] Later, the BPD may increase above the expected average.

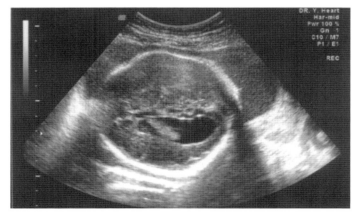

Figure 16.9 Axial scan at midgestation showing moderate ventriculomegaly with dangling choroid plexus.

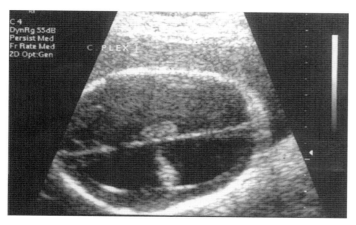

Figure 16.10 Marked dilation of both lateral ventricles with dangling choroid plexuses in a fetus with hydrocephalus.

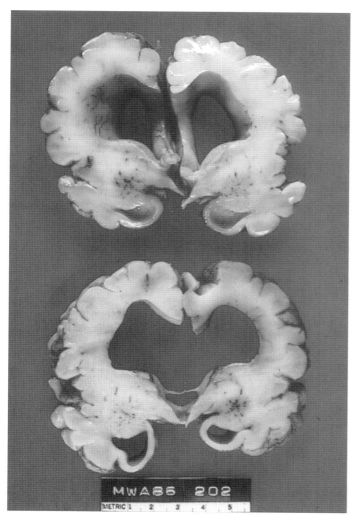

Figure 16.11 Gross coronal sections of a brain showing dilated lateral ventricles in a neonate affected with hydrocephalus.

If the diagnosis of fetal hydrocephalus is made early enough, abortion can be offered as an option. Oxytocin in intravenous infusion is often unsuccessful if the cervix is unfavorable. In some centers, prostaglandins are preferred for inducing labor. With significant fetal hydrocephalus, there may be a danger of uterine rupture in labor. In extreme degrees of hydrocephalus, the cranium may contain up to 10 l of fluid. In the absence of associated anomalies, cesarean section should be offered to improve outcome by avoiding traumatic delivery and instituting early neonatal treatment. However, in the presence of fetal hydrocephalus with other associated several fetal anomalies, hydranencephaly, alobar holoprosencephaly, or when chromosome abnormalities are diagnosed prior to the occurrence of labor, transabdominal cerebral decompression with a 17-gauge needle may be indicated to avoid obstructed labor or uterine rupture. This procedure is best performed under ultrasound guidance with an empty bladder. During labor, when the fetal presentation is cephalic, the decompression can also be performed transvaginally. Sonographically guided aspiration via an appropriately long needle is usually sufficient to cause collapse of the fetal skull.[46]

In the nineteenth century, various types of instruments were designed to extract the fetal head. The fetal scalp could be grasped with Willett's forceps and the skin incised first. Simpson's perforator, a specialized form of scissors, was especially designed for this role. Alternatively, the Drew-Smythe catheter could be used to destroy the vital centers of the medulla while performing the decompression.[47] However, these instruments can be used to extract only at full dilation. Few obstetricians today have experience with the use of these instruments, which have been largely relegated to the shelves of medical museums.

If the diagnosis of hydrocephalus is made during a breech delivery, the management may be difficult, particularly when the trunk has already been delivered and it is found impossible to deliver the head. In these cases, the diagnosis of fetal hydrocephalus or ventriculomegaly can be easily made by ultrasound. If the fetus is dead, the best management is decompression transabdominally with a needle. If a meningomyelocele is present, this can be perforated, releasing the cerebrospinal fluid.

Severe fetal hydrocephalus rapidly destroys the brain; therefore, the fluid must be drained postnatally by a unidirectional valve (such as the Holter or Pudenz type) to the heart or peritoneum. About 20% of all children with a valve die from its complications within 7 years.[48] However, approximately two-thirds of the survivors have normal or near-normal intelligence.[49,50] Fetuses with isolated hydrocephalus and no other associated anomalies, treated by early neonatal shunting, have an overall survival rate of 78.5%, and 82% of the survivors have IQs over 80. Head size and cortical thickness or thinness have no prognostic significance in cases of isolated fetal hydrocephalus.[50] Fetuses with isolated hydrocephalus and no associated anomalies should be managed by fetal surveillance and cesarean section, thus avoiding a traumatic delivery. However, in the presence of chromosome abnormalities, the prognosis for survival or meaningful survival is extremely poor. In these cases there may be an indication for cephalocentesis or termination.

Encephalocele

Otherwise known as cranial or occipital meningocele, this condition is diagnosed when intracranial structures and/or fluid protrude through a skull defect, typically midline. Usually, the sac contains brain tissue and meninges (encephalocele) or, less commonly, only meninges and cerebrospinal fluid (meningocele), and is not covered by bone. It is thought to be due to failure of closure of the rostral neural pore. Encephaloceles are also classified according to the location of the lesion (occipital, parietal, anterior). In 70% of encephaloceles, the location is occipital. Interestingly, the type and frequency of encephaloceles have a predilection for various geographic areas and population types. For instance, in Southeast Asia, the incidence is 1/5000 live births and frontal encephaloceles are more common; however, in the Western Hemisphere, the incidence is only 1–3/10 000 births.[51] Occipital encephalocele is also most common in European populations.

Occipital encephalocele (Figure 16.12) is generally considered part of the spectrum of neural tube defects, which tend to be multifactorial in etiology. It can be an isolated lesion which has not been shown to be familial with an increased incidence of affected siblings. This is in contrast to other types of neural tube defects, where the inheritance is multifactorial. However, there are multiple conditions and associations that can exist with encephalocele, such as genetic syndromes, chromosomal abnormalities, other fetal anomalies (hydrocephalus, central nervous system anomalies, spina bifida, facial defects, or renal and skeletal anomalies), and possible environmental causes. In 7–15% of cases, neural tube defects are present in association with encephalocele.[52] Importantly, one particular genetic syndrome that should be kept in mind is Meckel–Grubel syndrome

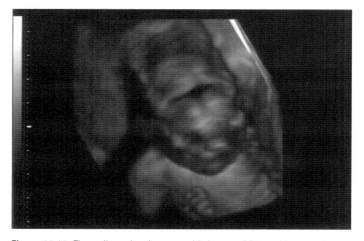

Figure 16.12 Three-dimensional sonographic image of fetus with a very large posterior encephalocele.

(polycystic kidneys, occipital encephalocele, and postaxial polydactyly), since this is an autosomal recessive disorder and has important implications for future pregnancies.

Sonographically, most encephaloceles are easy to diagnose by visualizing brain tissue protruding through a midline occipital defect. Their appearance may be diverse: purely cystic, solid mass with a gyral pattern continuous with the cranium, or a combined cystic and solid mass. The diagnosis is certain only if a bony defect in the skull is detected sonographically. One should remember that an encephalocele visualized in an asymmetric or atypical location can be related to amniotic-band syndrome or limb–body-wall complex. Small lesions and anterior encephaloceles may be more difficult to detect. Other sonographic signs may include distortion of normal brain landmarks, ventriculomegaly, frontal bossing, microcephaly (because intracranial structures protrude out of the skull), and obliteration of the cisterna magna. Encephaloceles may even show motion on real-time ultrasound as the fetus moves within the amniotic fluid. In addition, the prenatal sonographic appearance may change over time; both transient disappearances and transition from a solid to fluid pattern have been described.[53,54] Scalp hemangiomas or cysts can be misinterpreted as an encephalocele. They must also be differentiated from other lesions, such as cystic hygromas and teratomas.

Once an encephalocele is diagnosed, a careful and targeted sonographic examination of the rest of the fetal anatomy is indicated. Demonstrating other anomalies may contribute to diagnosing a genetic syndrome. It is important to realize that using alpha fetoprotein as an indirect sign is not helpful, since the lesions are covered with intact meninges. In general, the prognosis depends on location of the lesion, presence or absence of microcephaly, presence and amount of brain tissue in the herniated sac (perhaps the most important indicator), size of the defect, karyotype abnormalities, genetic syndromes, and the presence of other major fetal anomalies. Therefore, karyotype analysis should be offered. Moreover, the fact that brain tissue cannot obviously be seen within the sac on ultrasound does not always accurately predict the true pathology. In reported series, the overall mortality for encephalocele has been reported as 29–36%,[55] and there is an increased incidence of death *in utero*. In infants with microcephaly due to brain herniation, the prognosis is dismal. Posterior lesions tend to have a worse prognosis than anterior ones, because of the association with other anomalies (including intracranial), and possibly because frontal defects are usually smaller, or because loss of the frontal cortex may produce fewer neurologic defects. One report found that a favorable outcome correlated with an average head size at birth, a normal initial neurologic condition, operability of the condition, and an absence of disorders of neuronal migration.[55] Patients should be aware and counseled that even in cases of sonographically detected isolated encephaloceles without other associated abnormalities, there are still risks of significant neurologic defects. The prognosis is also much better for fetuses with meningocele than with meningoencephalocele. It is possible that fetuses having a meningocele containing only fluid or only a nubbin of brain tissue can survive with little or no disability.[56] The outcome for fetuses with demonstrable brain tissue in the mass is uniformly poor.

Therefore, many patients choose to terminate the pregnancy. Those who do not should meet with specialists in neonatology, genetics, and neurosurgery prenatally. In addition, the mode of delivery then becomes the issue and is determined by the sonographic findings. The patient should also deliver at a tertiary care center. In theory, especially when the encephalocele is isolated, cesarean delivery might improve prognosis and neonatal outcome by minimizing birth trauma and contamination of brain tissue by vaginal flora. Cesarean delivery has also been advocated in cases with pure meningocele and no other abnormalities, because almost half of these infants develop normally after surgery.[57] If there is a large amount of brain tissue seen within the sac (and thus a large-sized defect), microcephaly, associated fetal anomalies, or genetic syndromes, the chances for good outcome are remote, and cesarean delivery is generally not recommended. Discussions regarding cesarean for fetal distress and neonatal resuscitative measures should be made with the patient ahead of time. Cesarean delivery can also be considered in the following conditions: the encephalocele is large enough to cause cephalopelvic disproportion or dystocia, other obstetric considerations are present (prior classical cesarean), a coincidental viable twin is present, and the patient is aware of the risk of significant developmental defects in the infant and accepts it.[58] As previously discussed, because encephalocele may be associated with genetic syndromes, it is important to determine ultimately whether this is the case, as this may affect all future pregnancies.

Large cystic hygroma

This is an abnormal cystic mass of lymphatic origin usually occurring in the posterolateral area of the neck (Figure 16.13), although it can occur in other body areas. Large hygromas may extend around the face, over the vertex, and even down to the trunk, filling the amniotic cavity. They vary considerably in both size and appearance. They are thin-walled and fluid-filled, and internal septations may be seen sonographically, including a dense midline septum extending from the fetal neck across the full width of the hygroma. No bony defect in the skull is present nor is there microcephaly, thus distinguishing hygroma from encephalocele. When cystic hygromas resolve, the result may be redundant skin and the clinical appearance of a webbed neck, a common feature of Turner's syndrome.

Cystic hygromas have a high predisposition to aneuploidy. Overall, chromosomal abnormalities are found in more than 60% of fetuses with cystic hygroma. Interestingly, the frequency of aneuploidy and associated abnormalites varies with the gestational age, and the size and appearance of the hygroma. Large cystic hygromas (typically seen after 14 weeks) tend to have septations and carry a high risk of aneuploidy, especially Turner's syndrome (40–50%). However, for hygromas seen in the first trimester, the aneuploidy rate is different, since there is

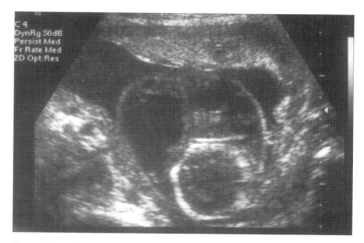

Figure 16.13 Transverse scan showing a very large, nuchal cystic hygroma with characteristic septations including a midline septum.

a higher proportion of Down syndrome and other chromosomal abnormalities. In a study of 56 first trimester fetuses with cystic hygromas, aneuploidy was found in 28.6%, including trisomy 18 (38%), Down syndrome (31%), Turner's syndrome (25%), and 47XXX (6%).[59] However, in fetuses with a normal karyotype, additional defects were diagnosed in 25% with cystic hygroma. Another study that compared 25 septated and 125 nonseptated cystic hygromas in the early second trimester[60] found that septated hygromas were more likely than nonseptated hygromas, to be associated with hydrops (40% vs 1.7%), aneuploidy (72% vs 6%), and other anomalies (52% vs 15%). Septated hygromas were also associated with a lower birth rate (12% vs 94%), and were less likely to be transient (44% vs 98%) than nonseptated hygromas. A recent study of 33 cystic hygromas (10–15 weeks) found that measurement of the volume (≥ 75 mm^3) may be a useful prognostic indicator in determining the risk of abnormal fetal karyotype, persistence of hygroma, and unfavorable pregnancy outcome; with this cutoff, there were sensitivities of 66.7%, 72.7%, and 90%, respectively.[61] Many fetuses with cystic hygroma visualized during the first trimester spontaneously die *in utero* before 20 weeks of gestation. Isolated cervical cystic hygromas that present late in gestation appear to be a completely different entity.[62] Reported cases have had hygromas located in the anterior and lateral location, and were not generally associated with hydrops or other anomalies. In such cases, overall mortality is very low.

Associated anomalies include cardiac, facial, vertebral, and genitourinary anomalies; diaphragmatic hernia; skeletal dysplasia; or nonaneuploid genetic syndromes. Therefore, a careful, targeted survey should be performed on the rest of the fetus. In addition, a fetal echocardiogram is recommended, along with karyotype testing. Occasionally, it may be difficult to sample the amniotic fluid due to the size of the hygroma; in these cases, aspirating the fluid from the hygroma itself can be successful, along with performing FISH (fluorescence *in situ* hybridization) studies to increase the success of karyotyping.

Besides aneuploidy, cystic hygromas are often associated with hydrops, fetal demise, or oligohydramnios. Even smaller, nonseptated cystic hygromas carry an increased risk of these complications. Therefore, once cystic hygromas are detected, signs of nonimmune hydrops (skin edema, ascites, and effusions) should be sought. When hydrops is associated with cystic hygromas, this combination is uniformly lethal and should be explained to the patient. A poor prognosis is also expected with the presence of other anomalies or aneuploidy. An important fact is that first-trimester cystic hygromas that do not lead to fetal demise tend to resolve spontaneously; they rarely persist throughout the entire gestation. If cystic hygromas have no other associated abnormalities, a normal karyotype, and no development of hydrops on serial ultrasound, an excellent outcome is expected.

Although some have undertaken *in utero* cyst aspiration of cystic hygromas[63] with the goal of preventing polyhydramnios, irreversible facial deformity, and progression to hydrops, there are few data to support routine *in utero* decompression. However, cyst aspiration to help secure an airway at birth may be indicated. In fetuses with isolated, large cystic cervical masses later in the pregnancy, there is a risk of airway compromise at birth, and they will often require delivery by the EXIT (*ex utero* intrapartum treatment) procedure. This procedure takes place during cesarean section, and involves placement of an endotracheal tube before the fetus is separated from the placenta. Delivery at a tertiary care center is necessary with neonatology and pediatric surgery standing by. Although a cervical mass of any size can certainly cause airway compromise, those masses sufficiently large enough to lead to polyhydramnios can obstruct the larynx/pharynx, and make intubation extremely difficult. Neonates with a large hygroma may have an unstable airway; therefore, surgical resection should be expedited as soon as feasible. Alternative treatments are also available, such as sclerosing agents and laser treatment.

Fetal tumors

Sacrococcygeal teratoma

Sacrococcygeal teratoma (Figure 16.14) is a mostly solid tumor in the fetus. Histologically, it is a congenital teratoma that arises from the caudal end of the primitive streak. These tumors may become malignant and are more common in females. Most sacrococcygeal teratomas are solid or mixed (85%), and are extremely vascular, as shown by color Doppler sonography. In 15% of cases, however, the tumor is entirely cystic. Polyhydramnios is frequent. High-output cardiac failure, due to hemorrhage into the tumor or arteriovenous shunting, may lead to hepatomegaly, placentomegaly, and hydrops fetalis. As the tumors tend to be large, obstetric complications such as dystocia and malpresentation may occur. Large tumors may rupture at delivery with considerable bleeding, causing fetal death. The high incidence of obstetric complications warrants close prenatal surveillance. Amnioreduction, cyst aspiration, and surgical debulking are potentially life-saving interventions.[64] Older

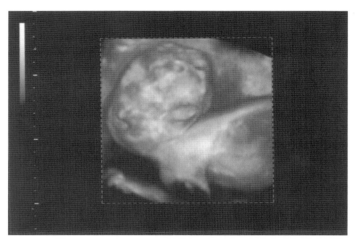

Figure 16.14 Three-dimensional image of fetus with a large sacrococcygeal teratoma.

publications describe operations designed to break up the tumor and allow easier extraction of the fetus. However, considering that the overwhelming majority of these teratomas are benign, the safest form of delivery is by cesarean section. On the other hand, with mainly cystic lesions, aspiration can decrease the tumor volume and potentially allow vaginal delivery.

Facial teratoma

Facial teratomas (or epignathus), which arise from the oral cavity and pharynx, are very rare. They may completely replace the brain as they grow into the cranium or fill the oral pharynx. Sonographically, this tumor appears as a complex, mostly solid mass that protrudes from the fetal mouth and nose. Facial teratomas may be confused with anterior cephaloceles. Associated findings with epignathus include aneuploidy, cardiac defects, hydrops, exophthalmos, and facial clefts. If the tumor is large, polyhydramnios may also be present. Even though most of these tumors are benign, for the most part, there is an extremely poor prognosis. Destruction or compression of adjacent structures and tumor size affect prognosis. A planned cesarean delivery is usually recommended in order to avoid fetal trauma and dystocia. Specialists in neonatology and pediatric surgery should be present at the delivery to provide immediate resuscitation, and establish the airway (intubation or tracheostomy); after this, surgical excision is performed.

Cervical teratoma

Cervical teratomas are extremely rare tumors arising from the fetal neck (usually the anterior neck). The vast majority found in fetuses and infants are benign, although they can be malignant. The problem with these tumors is that they can compress critical areas in the neck, cause hyperextension, and grow rapidly. Sonographically, they are asymmetric, unilateral, mobile, and well demarcated. Most are irregular masses with solid or mixed solid-cystic components. They can lead to pulmonary insufficiency secondary to mass effect *in utero*, with underdevelopment of the lungs. Fetuses are at risk of preterm delivery, death, polyhydramnios, malpresentation, and dystocia. Repeated sonographic examinations are recommended to monitor tumor size, fluid volume, and fetal well-being. Currently, fetuses with cervical teratomas are best managed at a tertiary care center by the EXIT (*ex utero* intrapartum treatment) procedure, where the neonate is delivered by cesarean section, but 'maintained' on placental support until the airway is established and secured.

Nonsolid masses

As in most of the anomalies previously described, ultrasound is invaluable in reaching a diagnosis. Whether caused by fetal ascites, distended bladder, or a common cloaca, the fluid can be withdrawn by abdominal paracentesis under sonographic guidance. In a case in 1980 of common cloaca with hydramnios,[65] there was difficulty in diagnosing this due to the rarity of persistent cloaca (1/200 000).[66] Today there are reports of the diagnostic features,[67] and therefore the diagnosis is less problematic than in the past. Transabdominal paracentesis yields a straw-colored acellular fluid. In the case of a persistent cloaca, mortality may be high, although there have been numerous survivors. However, a high incidence of both gynecologic and urologic problems has been reported.[68] The majority of patients born with cloacal malformation can achieve fecal and urinary control, although additional reconstructive surgery has been required in 46%.[68] Additionally, surgery is necessary to create a vagina for menstruation and sexual intercourse. If vaginal delivery is contemplated for the mother and there is gross fetal abdominal distention, fluid can be aspirated to allow vaginal delivery if there are other, associated severe anomalies. Cesarean section may be considered for fetuses with a good prognosis, and to avoid dystocia.

In cases of bladder distention possibly caused by a posterior urethral valve, there may be an indication for urinary paracentesis to prevent hydronephrosis and possibly fetal surgery.

Large omphalocele

An omphalocele is a central abdominal wall defect that results in herniation of intra-abdominal structures into the base of the umbilical cord, which is covered by a membrane. The umbilical cord insertion is thus situated on the apex of the herniated sac, and the size can be variable. It occurs in approximately 1/4000 births.[69] Omphaloceles may contain liver (extracorporeal liver) (Figure 16.15) and/or bowel, and therefore they differ in appearance sonographically. In bowel-containing omphaloceles, the amount of herniated bowel can be quite variable. It is important to distinguish omphalocele from umbilical hernia or gastroschisis, which is a periumbilical defect located to the right of the umbilicus that consists of bowel protruding through the defect into the amniotic fluid. Omphaloceles with intracorpo-

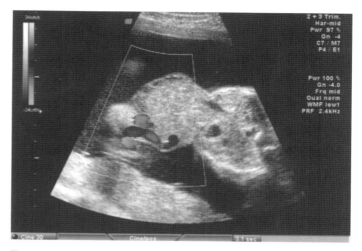

Figure 16.15 Transverse scan of the fetal abdomen showing a large omphalocele sac containing liver (extracorporeal). The umbilical cord insertion can be seen by color Doppler on the apex of the herniated sac.

real liver also cannot be diagnosed until after 12 weeks, when normal physiologic gut migration is complete (occurring at 8–12 postmenstrual weeks). However, unlike bowel, the fetal liver never normally follows a physiologic migration outside the abdominal cavity during development. Small omphaloceles can be missed and easily overlooked, especially if they contain only bowel. Occasionally, an omphalocele may rupture, where the abdominal contents float freely in the amniotic fluid as in gastroschisis. However, unlike gastroschisis, ruptured omphaloceles are usually large and have liver exposed also.

Approximately 1/3 of all omphaloceles have associated polyhydramnios and this is associated with a worse prognosis.[70] Hughes et al found that when fetuses with omphaloceles had abnormal fluid volume (polyhydramnios or oligohydramnios), the mortality rate was 88%, versus 25% in those with normal fluid volume.[70] Omphaloceles can also be a manifestation of many genetic syndromes, such as pentalogy of Cantrell, Beckwith–Wiedemann, amniotic band, OEIS (omphalocele, exstrophy bladder, imperforate anus, spinal abnormalities) complex, and limb–body-wall complex. Pentalogy of Cantrell is an association of cleft distal sternum, defect of apical pericardium with communication into the peritoneum, diaphragmatic defect, internal cardiac defect, and midline anterior ventral wall defect; the omphaloceles are typically supraumbilical or high.

Omphaloceles are associated with other fetal abnormalities and aneuploidy in more than half of the prenatally diagnosed cases. Therefore, a thorough evaluation of the fetal anatomy is indicated, and patients should be offered karyotype testing. When omphaloceles have been identified prenatally on ultrasound, the risk of additional malformations is 58–73%.[70–73] Organ system anomalies include the cardiac, central nervous, genitourinary, and gastrointestinal systems. Gilbert and Nicolaides found that the most frequent additional malformation was congenital heart disease (47%),[73] thus emphasizing the need for fetal echocardiography. Omphaloceles carry a high risk of aneuploidy, such as trisomy 18, trisomy 13, triploidy, and Turner's syndrome. In a recent study of 26 fetuses with omphalocele, overall 27% had an abnormal karyotype.[72] Another study found that of 35 cases of omphalocele diagnosed by ultrasonography, overall 54% had aneuploidy: trisomy 18 ($n = 17$), triploidy ($n = 1$), and Klinefelter's syndrome ($n = 1$).[73] The presence of additional anomalies will affect the actual risk of aneuploidy. Omphaloceles with intracorporeal liver (containing bowel) have a higher aneuploidy risk than those with extracorporeal liver.[74] In one study, the authors found an aneuploidy rate of 87% in omphaloceles with intracorporeal liver, versus 9% in extracorporeal liver.[74] Another study of 43 fetuses with omphalocele on prenatal ultrasonography found that aneuploidy correlated with the absence of liver in the omphalocele sac.[70] In general, when the omphalocele is extracorporeal and no other anomalies are identified, the risk of aneuploidy is very low.

The overall prognosis of omphaloceles depends on size, other associated abnormalities and their severity, presence of aneuploidy, and contents of the omphalocele sac. In fact, some have found that the presence of one or more concurrent malformations was associated with a perinatal mortality rate of 80%, and the presence of a major cardiac abnormality or aneuploidy increased the mortality rate to almost 100%.[70] The same authors found that in fetuses with normal fluid volume, no other anomalies, and extracorporeal liver, a favorable outcome could be expected.[70] Others have found, however, that omphaloceles with intracorporeal liver have a higher survival rate than those with extracorporeal liver (88% vs 48%), in spite of the significantly higher rate (16% vs 0%) of aneuploidy.[75] Once it is known that the fetus is chromosomally normal, smaller omphaloceles with intracorporeal liver are expected to have a favorable prognosis. A significant cause of increased morbidity and mortality in infants with omphalocele is respiratory insufficiency due to low lung volumes. In a group of 30 infants with omphalocele, one study found that 40% had severe respiratory distress at birth, including two who died within 2 days.[76] Of those infants with severe respiratory distress at birth, 67% ($n = 8$) had a giant omphalocele (liver-containing and/or omphalocele sac over 5 cm in diameter). Therefore, the worse prognosis seen for extracorporeal liver could be explained by the higher rate of respiratory failure in these infants, especially for giant omphaloceles (over 5 cm).[75,76] Chromosomally normal fetuses with omphaloceles and no life-threatening abnormalities may have an excellent outcome, since surgery can be performed after delivery.

Maternal serum alpha fetoprotein screening has a much higher sensitivity in detecting cases of gastroschisis than omphalocele. This is due to the presence of covering membrane with omphaloceles, as compared to direct exposure of the bowel to amniotic fluid in cases of gastroschisis. Once identified, the omphalocele should be measured, and the contents determined. Frequent sonographic examinations are recommended throughout the pregnancy to follow fetal growth and the omphalocele

size, since there may be a high incidence of intrauterine growth restriction. Examination for rupture of the omphalocele sac should be performed. Preterm labor is also a frequently associated finding. For isolated omphalocele cases, early prenatal consultation with pediatric surgeons and neonatologists should also favorably influence the perinatal outcome.

Pregnancies with omphaloceles can be allowed to go to term, and this should be the goal. While the delivery should certainly occur at a tertiary care center, the delivery mode is controversial. While many argue for cesarean section to decrease the potential risk of infection and avoid possible rupture of the sac and trauma in vaginal delivery, others have questioned the appropriateness and do not support routine cesarean section. Retrospective reviews do not support the idea that cesarean delivery is associated with an improved survival rate.[77] Some have found no evidence that vaginal delivery is safer than cesarean for fetuses with an isolated small omphalocele; however, those with giant omphaloceles (>5 cm) should be delivered by cesarean section to avoid dystocia.[78] One particular advantage of elective cesarean section is that it provides a planned delivery for the patient in a theoretically aseptic environment with the neonatal and surgical team ready for resuscitation and surgical correction. When the hernia is very small and the sac is intact, the fetus can probably be delivered vaginally, unless there are obstetric indications for cesarean delivery. Of course, for fetuses with coexisting life-threatening anomalies or aneuploidy with poor prognosis, the goal of vaginal delivery should be discussed with the patient.

After delivery, various options are available such as primary surgical closure or nonsurgical options. For very large omphaloceles, a staged reduction using a prosthetic silo is preferred. Nonsurgical management is recommended when respiratory distress is present, since this is worsened temporarily by closing the omphalocele defect.

Conjoined twins

Conjoined twins have been reported to occur in 1/40 000 deliveries and 1/100 000 live births.[79] The cause of this malformation is incomplete separation of blastomeres or the embryonic disk.[80] In most cases, this separation is complete, leading to identical twins. In incomplete division, the area remaining fused is usually the placenta or membranes, giving rise to the common finding of a single chorion surrounding two amniotic sacs, or anastomoses of both sets of fetal blood vessels within a common placenta. If, however, duplication of organizing areas occurs in the embryonic disk itself, conjoined twins may result. If two primitive streaks arise on the embryonic disk, the twins may be joined laterally (Figure 16.16a). If the primitive streak divides along its length cranially, two heads may form, leading to dicephalus (Figure 16.16c). If the cardiac area has already formed, the head fold duplicates, and syncephalus (Janiceps malformation) occurs with a fused face (Figures 16.16d). The development of one twin may also inhibit development of the other twin, leading to unequal conjoined twins, with one being

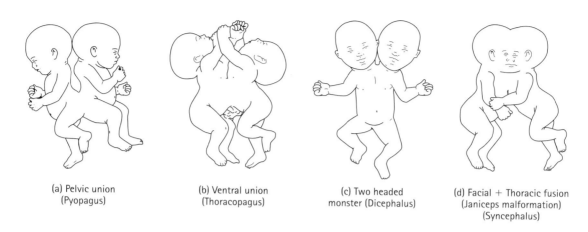

(a) Pelvic union
(Pyopagus)

(b) Ventral union
(Thoracopagus)

(c) Two headed
monster (Dicephalus)

(d) Facial + Thoracic fusion
(Janiceps malformation)
(Syncephalus)

Figure 16.16 Conjoined twins. (a) Pelvic union (pygopagus); (b) ventral union (thoracopagus); (c) two-headed (dicephalus); (d) facial and thoracic fusion (syncephalus) (janiceps malformation).

a parasite of the other. Infants joined at the head are known as craniopagus and account for 3% of all conjoined twins. A caudal union is known as ischiopagus (7% of conjoined twins). A dorsal union (pygopagus) constitutes 16% (Figure 16.16a), and a ventral union (thoracopagus), 74% (Figure 16.16b).[81]

In most parts of the world today, ultrasound scans are performed to diagnose fetal anomalies. Sonography has been able to diagnose conjoined twins in both the first[82,83] and second trimester.[84] It has the advantage of diagnosing shared organs, allowing parents to make an informed decision regarding continuation of the pregnancy. Prenatal ultrasonography has virtually replaced radiography for diagnosis; however, the latter has still been used to provide additional diagnostic criteria. Radiographic features include vertebral columns lying parallel and closer than usual, two heads at the same level lying face to face or obliquely, and no change in relative positions at subsequent examinations.

Due to the rarity of these malformations, few obstetricians have had experience in delivery of conjoined twins. If a definitive diagnosis is made early enough, the pregnancy can be aborted vaginally, but only if it is clear that the conjoined twins can be delivered without any maternal injury. This depends on gestational age and the size of the fetuses. Even at term, vaginal delivery can be accomplished for conjoined twins, as the union between the two is often pliable. There are recent reports in the literature describing that vaginal delivery can be accomplished;[85] however, it must be borne in mind that severe dystocia may occur. The older literature often describes the vaginal delivery of thoracopagus twins. If presenting as a breech, traction can be placed on the limbs, and the bodies then descend parallel to one another through the vaginal canal. After delivery of the shoulders and upper limbs, the bodies can be carried forward over the pubic symphysis, thus allowing the posterior head to engage. After delivery of this head, the anterior head can then be delivered. Thoracopagus can also be delivered with the heads presenting first. One head is expelled first, then the

second head, and then the two bodies. However, most of the reports described came from a time when cesarean section was still a relatively hazardous procedure. In addition, many of the conjoined twins were stillborn. In most cases, manipulative and destructive procedures had to be performed, such as version, decapitation, and evisceration. Currently, however, cesarean section has become a relatively safe procedure and undoubtedly less injurious to the mother than the aforementioned types of labor and delivery. If conjoined twins are present near or at term, cesarean section is indicated, even if the fetuses are already dead or have little chance of survival. Because some conjoined twins can be separated and live full and independent lives, there may also be a fetal indication for cesarean section.

Obstetric management should be directed to having a healthy mother and two salvageable infants.[86] Hence, it is our recommendation that if the pregnancy is not terminated and the pregnancy progresses to the stage of fetal viability, these infants are entitled to the best obstetric care available. After birth, a full neonatal and imaging assessment can be carried out,[87] which will allow both physician and parents to know the prognosis for later life. The decision regarding surgical separation can be made only when the full extent of organ sharing has been determined, and the subsequent chances for survival of one or both infants becomes apparent.

Today, there are many conjoined twins alive either as conjoined twins, or after surgical separation. In some cases where major organs were shared, only one twin survived. The decision to operate depends on the contemplated risks and the extent of the union. The literature abounds with reports about the problems of anesthesia,[88] and legal and ethical problems.[89] In the fifteenth century, dicephalus conjoined twins were born in Scotland. This pair had two heads and were joined from the shoulder downward. They possessed only two legs, one belonging to each of them. They lived until the age of 28. The more famous Siamese twin brothers, Chang and Eng Bunker, lived for 63 years and fathered 22 normal children in total. Postmortem examination showed them to be joined by only a band of fibro-cartilaginous tissue that could have been divided. Today, some contemplate the possibility of living as a conjoined twin so intolerable as to attempt separation even when the surgery may be life-threatening for one or both twins. In 2000, the UK courts ruled that a pair of ischiopagus conjoined twins were to be separated surgically against the wishes of their parents.[90] In this case, one twin named 'Mary' was acardiac and dependent on the stronger twin 'Jodie'. On hearing that 'Jodie's' life was endangered by the extracirculatory load of 'Mary', the court ordered surgery to be performed. Although 'Mary' had no chance of survival alone, the court's decision was obeyed. The ethical and legal aspects of this case are still being hotly debated.

Summary

It is clear that the management of fetal malformations can be quite complex, from the time of diagnosis to the mode of delivery. It poses numerous challenges for both clinicians and the parents. In order to manage these pregnancies adequately, an accurate prenatal diagnosis with proper counseling should be made, the etiology and prognosis must be determined, evaluation of associated anomalies must be performed, delivery should occur in an appropriate center, and consultation with other multispecialists should be carried out.

References

1. Nyberg DA, McGahan JP, Pretorius DH, Pilu G. Diagnostic Imaging of Fetal Anomalies, p. xiii. Lippincott Williams and Wilkins: Philadelphia, 2003.
2. Holmes LB, Driscoll SG, Atkins L. Etiologic heterogeneity of neural-tube defects. N Engl J Med 1976; 294: 365–9.
3. Ewigman BG, Crane JP, Frigoletto FD et al. Effect of prenatal ultrasound screening on perinatal outcome. RADIUS Study Group. N Engl J Med 1993; 329: 821–7.
4. Campbell S, Pearce JM. The prenatal diagnosis of fetal structural anomalies by ultrasound. Clin Obstet Gynecol 1983; 10: 475–506.
5. Levi S. Ultrasound in prenatal diagnosis: polemics around routine ultrasound screening for second trimester fetal malformations. Prenat Diagn 2002; 22: 285–95.
6. Skupski DW, Newman S, Edersheim T et al. Fetus–placenta–newborn: the impact of routine obstetric ultrasonographic screening in a low-risk population. Am J Obstet Gynecol 1996; 175: 1142–5.
7. Main DM, Mennuti MT. Neural tube defects: issues in prenatal diagnosis and counseling. Obstet Gynecol 1986; 67: 1.
8. Engel GL. Grief and grieving. Am J Nurs 1964; 64: 93–7.
9. Lorber J. Congenital malformations of the central nervous system. In: Chamberlain G (ed.), Contemporary Obstetrics and Gynecology. Northwood: London, 1977.
10. Centers for Disease Control and Prevention (CDC). Spina bifida and anencephaly before and after folic acid mandate – United States, 1995–1996 and 1999–2000. MMWR Morb Mortal Wkly Rep 2004; 53: 362–5.
11. Martinez de Villarreal L, Perez JZ, Vazquez PA et al. Decline of neural tube defects cases after a folic acid campaign in Nuevo Leon, Mexico. Teratology 2002; 66: 249–56.
12. Zlotogora J, Amitai Y, Kaluski DN et al. Surveillance of neural tube defects in Israel. Isr Med Assoc J 2002; 4: 1111–14.
13. Green NS. Folic acid supplementation and prevention of birth defects. J Nutr 2002; 132(Suppl): 2356S–60S.
14. Achiron R, Achiron A. Transvaginal ultrasonic assessment of the early fetal brain. Ultrasound Obstet Gynecol 1991; 1: 336–44.
15. Parisi F, Squitieri C, Carotti A et al. Heart transplantation on the first day of life from an anencephalic donor. Pediatr Transplant 1999; 3: 150–1.
16. Gomez-Campdera FJ, Robles NR, Anaya F et al. Kidney transplantation from anencephalic donors. Report of 5 cases and a review of the literature. Child Nephrol Urol 1990; 10: 143–9.
17. Gomez-Campdera FJ, Albertos J, Anaya F et al. En bloc kidney and bladder transplantation from an anencephalic donor into an adult recipient. J Urol 1988; 140: 1553–4.
18. DeMyer W. Holoprosencephaly. In: Vinken PJ, Bruyn GW (eds), Handbook of Clinical Neurology, p. 431. Elsevier: Amsterdam, 1977.
19. Pilu G, Reece EA, Romero R et al. Prenatal diagnosis of craniofacial malformations by sonography. Am J Obstet Gynecol 1986; 155: 45.
20. Nyberg DA, McGahan JP, Pretorius DH, Pilu G. Diagnostic Imaging of Fetal Anomalies, p. 236. Lippincott Williams and Wilkins: Philadelphia, 2003.
21. Cohen MM. Perspectives on holoprosencephaly. III. Spectra, distinctions, continuities, and discontinuities. Am J Med Genet 1989; 34: 271–88.
22. Dixon A. Hydranencephaly. Radiography 1988; 54: 12.
23. Heron D, Lyonnet S, Iserin L et al. Sternal cleft: case report and review of a series of nine patients. Am J Med Genet 1995; 59: 154–6.
24. Klingensmith WC III, Cioffi-Ragan DT, Harvey DE. Diagnosis of ectopia cordis in the second trimester. J Clin Ultrasound 1988; 16: 204–6.
25. Morales JM, Patel SG, Duff JA et al. Ectopia cordis and other midline defects. Ann Thorac Surg 2000; 70: 111–14.
26. Bianchi DW, Crombleholme TM, D'Alton ME. Fetology: Diagnosis and Management of the Fetal Patient, p. 469. McGraw-Hill: New York, 2000.
27. Potter EL. Bilateral renal agenesis. J Pediatr 1946; 29: 68–72.
28. Bronstein M, Amil A, Achiron R et al. The early prenatal diagnosis of renal agenesis: techniques and possible pitfalls. Prenat Diagn 1994; 14: 291–7.
29. Potter EL. Bilateral absence of ureter and kidneys: a report of 50 cases. Obstet Gynecol 1965; 25: 3–12.
30. Romero R, Cullen M, Graunum P. Antenatal diagnosis of renal anomalies with ultrasound. III. Bilateral renal agenesis. Am J Obstet Gynecol 1985; 151: 38–43.

31. Mahajan P, Kher A, Khungar A et al. MURCS association – a review of 7 cases. J Postgrad Med 1992; 38: 109–11.

32. Laurence KM, Carter CO, David PA. Major central nervous system malformations in South Wales. I. Incidence, local variations and geographical factors. Br J Prevent Soc Med 1968; 22: 212–22.

33. Davis CF, Young DG. The changing incidence of neural tube defects in Scotland. J Pediatr Surg 1991; 26: 516–18.

34. Naggan L. The recent decline in prevalence of anencephaly and spina bifida. Am J Epidermol 1969; 89: 154–60.

35. Carter CO, David PA, Laurence KM. A family study of major central nervous system malformations in South Wales. J Med Genet 1968; 5: 81–106.

36. Lorber J. The family history of spina bifida cystica. Pediatrics 1965; 35: 589–95.

37. Watson WJ, Cheschier NC, Katz VL et al. The role of ultrasound in the evaluation of patients with elevated maternal serum alfa-feto protein: a review. Obstet Gynecol 1991; 78: 123–8.

38. Poutamo J, Vanninen R, Partanen K et al. Magnetic resonance imaging supplements ultrasonographic imaging of the fossa, pharynx and neck in malformed fetuses. Ultrasound Obstet Gynecol 1999; 13: 327–34.

39. Nyberg DA, McGahan JP, Pretorius DH, Pilu G. Diagnostic Imaging of Fetal Anomalies, p. 307. Lippincott Williams and Wilkins: Philadelphia, 2003.

40. Ferguson-Smith MA, May HM, Vince JD et al. Accordance of anencephalic and spina bifida births by maternal serum alfa-feto-protein screening. Lancet 1978; 1: 1330–3.

41. Macri JN, Weiss RR. Prenatal serum alpha-fetoprotein screening for neural tube defects. Obstet Gynecol 1982; 59: 633–9.

42. Hunt GM, Poulton A. Open spina bifida: a complete cohort reviewed 25 years after closure. Dev Med Child Neurol 1995; 37: 19–29.

43. Lorber J. Results of treatment of meningomyelocele. An analysis of 524 unselected cases with special reference to possible selection for treatment. Dev Med Child Neurol 1971; 13: 279–303.

44. Jeanty P, Dramaix-Wilmet M, Delbeke D et al. Ultrasonic evaluation of fetal ventricular growth. Neuroradiology 1981; 21: 127–31.

45. Campbell S. Early prenatal diagnosis of neural tube defects by ultrasound. Clin Obstet Gynecol 1977; 20: 351–9.

46. Chayen B, Rifkin MD. Cephalocentesis: guidance with an endovaginal probe and endovaginal needle placement. J Ultrasound Med 1987; 6: 221–3.

47. Dewhurst CJ. Integrated Obstetrics and Gynecology for Postgraduates, Ch. 24. Blackwell Scientific: Oxford, 1976.

48. Lorber J. Spina bifida cystica: results of treatment of 270 consecutive cases with criteria for selection for the future. Arch Dis Child 1972; 47: 854–73.

49. McCullough DC, Balzer-Martin LA. Current prognosis in overt neonatal hydrocephalus. J Neurosurg 1982; 57: 378–83.

50. Vintzileos AM, Campbell WA, Weinbaum PJ. Perinatal management and outcome of fetal ventriculomegaly. Obstet Gynecol 1987; 69: 5–11.

51. Nyberg DA, McGahan JP, Pretorius DH, Pilu G. Diagnostic Imaging of Fetal Anomalies, p. 298. Lippincott Williams and Wilkins: Philadelphia, 2003.

52. Fleming AD, Vintzileos AM, Scorza WE. Prenatal diagnosis of occipital encephalocele with transvaginal sonography. J Ultrasound Med 1991; 10: 285–6.

53. Budorick NE, Pretorius DH, McGahan MC et al. Cephalocele detection in utero: sonographic and clinical features. Ultrasound Obstet Gynecol 1995; 5: 77.

54. Bronshtein M, Zimmer EZ. Transvaginal sonographic follow-up on the formation of fetal cephalocele at 13–19 weeks' gestation. Obstet Gynecol 1991; 78: 528.

55. Martinez-Lage JF, Poza M, Sola J et al. The child with a cephalocele: etiology, neuroimaging, and outcome. Childs Nerv Syst 1996; 12: 540–50.

56. Bannister CM, Russell SA, Rimmer S et al. Can prognostic indicators be identified in a fetus with encephalocele? Eur J Pediatr Surg 2000; 10: 20–3.

57. Chervenak FA, Isaacson G, Mahoney MJ et al. Diagnosis and management of fetal cephalocele. Obstet Gynecol 1984; 64: 86.

58. Bianchi DW, Crombleholme TM, D'Alton ME. Fetology: Diagnosis and Management of the Fetal Patient, p. 109. McGraw-Hill: New York, 2000.

59. Ville Y, Lalondrelle C, Doumerc S et al. First-trimester diagnosis of nuchal anomalies: significance and fetal outcome. Ultrasound Obstet Gynecol 1992; 2: 314–16.

60. Bronshtein M, Bar-Hava I, Blumenfeld I et al. The difference between septated and nonseptated nuchal cystic hygroma in the early second trimester. Obstet Gynecol 1993; 81: 683–7.

61. Rosati P, Guariglia L. Prognostic value of ultrasound findings of fetal cystic hygroma detected in early pregnancy by transvaginal sonography. Ultrasound Obstet Gynecol 2000; 16: 245–50.

62. Benacerraf BR, Frigoletto FD. Prenatal sonographic diagnosis of isolated congenital cystic hygroma, unassociated with lymphedema or other morphologic abnormality. J Ultrasound Med 1987; 6: 63–6.

63. Chen CP, Jan SW, Liu FF et al. Echo-guided lymphatic drainage by fine-needle aspiration in persistent isolated septated fetal nuchal cystic hygroma. Fetal Diagn Ther 1996; 11: 150–3.

64. Hedrick HL, Flake AW, Crombleholme TM et al. Sacrococcygeal teratoma: prenatal assessment, fetal intervention, and outcome. J Pediatr Surg 2004; 39: 430–8.

65. Frenkel Y, Atlas M, Horowitz A et al. Fetal common cloaca – a case report and review. Eur J Obstet Gynaecol Reprod Biol 1980; 11: 115–20.

66. Tank ES, Lindenauer SM. Principles of management of exstrophy of the cloaca. Am J Surg 1970; 119: 95–8.

67. Warne S, Chitty LS, Wilcox DT. Prenatal diagnosis of cloacal anomalies. Br J Urol Int 2002; 89: 78–81.

68. Warne SA, Wilcox DT, Creighton S et al. Long-term gynecological outcome of patients with persistent cloaca. J Urol 2003; 170: 1493–6.

69. Nyberg DA, McGahan JP, Pretorius DH, Pilu G. Diagnostic Imaging of Fetal Anomalies, p. 519. Lippincott Williams and Wilkins: Philadelphia, 2003.

70. Hughes MD, Nyberg DA, Mack LA et al. Fetal omphalocele: prenatal US detection of concurrent anomalies and other predictors of outcome. Radiology 1989; 173: 371–6.

71. Blazer S, Zimmer EZ, Gover A et al. Fetal omphalocele detected early in pregnancy: associated anomalies and outcomes. Radiology 2004; 232: 191–5.

72. Axt R, Quijano F, Boos R et al. Omphalocele and gastroschisis: prenatal diagnosis and peripartal management. A case analysis of the years 1989–1997 at the Department of Obstetrics and Gynecology, University of Homburg/Saar. Eur J Obstet Gynecol Reprod Biol 1999; 87: 47–54.

73. Gilbert WM, Nicolaides KH. Fetal omphalocele: associated malformations and chromosomal defects. Obstet Gynecol 1987; 70: 633–5.

74. Getachew MM, Goldstein RB, Edge V et al. Correlation between omphalocele contents and karyotypic abnormalities: sonographic study in 37 cases. AJR Am J Roentgenol 1992; 158: 133–6.

75. St-Vil D, Shaw KS, Lallier M et al. Chromosomal anomalies in newborns with omphalocele. J Pediatr Surg 1996; 31: 831–4.

76. Tsakayannis DE, Zurakowski D, Lillehei CW. Respiratory insufficiency at birth: a predictor of mortality for infants with omphalocele. J Pediatr Surg 1996; 31: 1088–90.

77. Moretti M, Khoury A, Rodriguez J et al. The effect of mode of delivery on the perinatal outcome in fetuses with abdominal wall defects. Am J Obstet Gynecol 1990; 163: 833–8.

78. Lurie S, Sherman D, Bukovsky I. Omphalocele delivery enigma: the best mode of delivery still remains dubious. Eur J Obstet Gynecol Reprod Biol 1999; 82: 19–22.

79. Edmonds LD, Layde PM. Conjoined twins in the United States, 1970–1979. Teratology 1982; 25: 301–8.

80. Benirschke K. The pathophysiology of the twinning process. In: Iffy L, Kaminetzky HA (eds), Principles and Practice of Obstetrics and Perinatology, p. 1165. Wiley: New York, 1981.

81. Robertson EG. Craniopagus parietalis: report of a case. AMA Arch Neurol Psychiatry 1953; 70: 189–205.

82. Barth RA, Filly RA, Goldberg JD et al. Conjoined twins: prenatal diagnosis and assessment of associated malformations. Radiology 1990; 177: 201–7.

83. Daskalakis G, Pilalis A, Tourikis I et al. First trimester diagnosis of dicephalus conjoined twins. Eur J Obstet Gynecol Reprod Biol 2004; 112: 110–13.

84. Grutter F, Marguerat P, Maillard-Brignon C et al. Thoracopagus fetus: ultrasonic diagnosis at 16 weeks. J Gynecol Obstet Biol Reprod 1989; 18: 355–9.

85. Agarwal U, Dahiya P, Khosla A. Vaginal birth of conjoined thoracopagus – a rare event. Arch Gynecol Obstet 2003; 269: 66–7.

86. Wittich AC. Conjoined twins: report of a case and review of the literature. J Am Osteopath Assoc 1989; 89: 1175–9.

87. Martinez L, Fernandez J, Pastor I et al. The contribution of modern imaging to planning separation strategies in conjoined twins. Eur J Pediatr Surg 2003; 13: 120–4.

88. Thomas JM, Lopez JT. Conjoined twins – the anaesthetic management of 15 sets from 1991–2002. Paediatr Anaesth 2004; 14: 117–29.

89. Tomasso JB. Separation of the conjoined twins: a comparative analysis of the rights to privacy and religious freedom in Great Britain and the United States. Rutgers Law Rev 2002; 54: 771–801.

90. Separation of conjoined twins. Lancet 2000; 356: 953.

17 Intrauterine fetal demise

Wendy Kinzler and Anthony Vintzileos

Intrauterine fetal death is a devastating and difficult experience for parents as well as health-care providers. A systematic, yet empathetic approach to the diagnosis, evaluation, and management, regardless of gestational age, is crucial.

Fetal death is defined by the World Health Organization (WHO) as 'death prior to the complete expulsion or extraction from its mother of a product of conception, irrespective of the duration of pregnancy; the death is indicated by the fact that after such separation the fetus does not breathe or show any other evidence of life, such as a beating heart, pulsation of the umbilical cord, or definite movement of voluntary muscles.'[1] Fetal deaths are classified as *early* if they occur at less than 20 weeks' gestation, *intermediate* if they occur at 20–27 weeks' gestation, and *late* if they occur at 28 weeks' gestation or greater. Approximately 16% of all pregnancies end in fetal death.[2] Although attempts have been under way to standardize reporting of fetal death after 20 weeks' gestation and to improve the quality of the National Center for Health Statistics (NCHS) fetal death data file, even within the USA there is underreporting.[3] Based on recent NCHS statistics, the fetal mortality rate after 20 weeks' gestation was 6.5 (per 1000 live births plus fetal deaths) in 2001, down from 7.0 in 1995. However, racial disparity is evident, with the fetal mortality rate in white women being 5.5 compared with 12.1 in black women. Late fetal deaths account for approximately half of the overall fetal mortality rate.[4]

Diagnosis of fetal death

With the widespread availability of real-time ultrasound equipment, the diagnosis of fetal death is simple and reliable, with 100% sensitivity and specificity. Fetal heart motion can be detected by 7–8 weeks' gestation by abdominal ultrasound and as early as 5½–6 weeks' gestation by high-frequency transvaginal probes.[5] Failure to detect cardiac activity is diagnostic of fetal death. Other sonographic signs of fetal death include absent fetal motion, abnormal head shape due to overlapping skull bones, and reduced or absent amniotic fluid. Prior to obtaining ultrasound confirmation, fetal death may be suspected from a variety of clinical signs and symptoms. These include decreased or absent fetal movements, decreased fundal height, vaginal bleeding, inability to auscultate the fetal heart by transabdominal Doppler, and possibly elevated maternal serum α-fetoprotein.

Fetal death is usually quickly evident to the person performing the ultrasound. There is a 'stillness' within the uterine cavity, with no motion other than the pulsation of the maternal aorta. After confirming the absence of cardiac activity, it is important that the mother be included in confirming the diagnosis of fetal death. She should be allowed to visualize the screen after localizing the fetal heart with the ultrasound transducer kept still so as not to create motion artificially. After several seconds, she, too, will be able to confirm the diagnosis. This helps to eliminate the doubt surrounding the diagnosis and to reduce subsequent denial. Often, women are immediately asked when the last time fetal movement was experienced. This question is likely to elicit strong feelings of guilt that she did not seek medical attention in a timely fashion and does little to assist the medical team in making a diagnosis; it should be avoided.

Evaluation of fetal death

There are many conditions associated with fetal death (Table 17.1). Chromosomal abnormalities, congenital anomalies, and hypoxia remain the major causes of fetal death in the USA. In general, the earlier the gestational age at which death occurs, the more likely there is chromosomal abnormality (Table 17.2).[6] Identification of the cause of fetal death, whenever possible, is important for several reasons. First, it aids the parents in understanding what led to the demise of their fetus, and in doing so often alleviates for them self-imposed guilt. Second, if the cause of death is found, the parents may be counseled appropriately as to the recurrence risks of the specific condition. Third, for conditions which may recur, subsequent pregnancies may be managed with closer fetal surveillance and possible therapeutic intervention. Because the causes of fetal death are many, a systematic approach addressing potential maternal, fetal, and placental factors is most beneficial (Table 17.3).

Table 17.1 Conditions associated with fetal death

Chromosomal
  Numerical abnormalities
    Autosomal trisomies
    X-chromosome monosomy
    Triploidy and tetraploidy
  Structural abnormalities
    Robertsonian translocations
    Unbalanced reciprocal
      translocations
Congenital malformations
  CNS abnormalities
    Neural tube defects
    Hydrocephalus
  Cardiac
    Structural defects
    Arrhythmia
  Abdominal wall defects
  Genitourinary
    Bilateral renal agenesis
    Obstructive uropathy
    Infantile polycystic kidney
      disease
  Skeletal abnormalities
    Dwarfism
    Arthrogryposis
Infectious causes
  Bacterial (*Listeria*, ascending
    polymicrobial)
  Mycotic
  Parasitic (toxoplasmosis)
  Viral
    Cytomegalovirus
    Rubella
    Parvovirus
    Herpes simplex
    Syphilis
Immunologic
  Isoimmunization
  Autoimmune
    Antiphospholipid antibodies
Maternal conditions
  Diabetes
  Hypertension
  Trauma
  Drug abuse
  Inherited thrombophilia
Placenta/umbilical cord
  Abruption/infarction
  Previa
  Umbilical cord
    knots/strictures
  Vasa previa
  Cord entanglement
  Cord hemangioma
  Cord prolapse
Other
  Fetal growth restriction
  Postmaturity

Table 17.2 Percentage of fetal losses associated with chromosomal abnormalities by gestational age

Gestational age (weeks)	With chromosomal abnormalities (%)
8–11	53.5
12–15	47.9
16–19	23.8
20–23	11.9
24–27	13.2
≥28	6.0

Adapted from Warburton.[6]

Table 17.3 Evaluation of fetal death

Ultrasonic evaluation of fetal death

- Confirm fetal death
- Assess gestational age at the time of death (long bones, cerebellum)
- If multiple gestation, look for evidence of
  - Chorionicity
  - Twin-to-twin transfusion syndrome
- Search for congenital anomalies
- Assess the intrauterine environment
- Placental localization
- Evidence of abruption
- Evidence of infection or erythroblastosis fetalis
- Amniotic fluid volume

Amniocentesis (or chorionic villus sampling) for karyotype and amniotic fluid cultures
Maternal tests (HgbA1c, TORCH titers, Parvovirus B19 serology, Kleihauer–Betke test, anticardiolipin antibodies, lupus anticoagulant, inherited thrombophilia testing, urine toxicology)
Placental cultures
Placental pathology
Autopsy

Maternal

A careful maternal history and physical examination is part of the diagnostic evaluation of fetal death. Women should be asked about potentially infectious exposures, illicit drug use, trauma, or underlying medical conditions. It is extremely important to question the mother carefully so as not to induce blame. Maternal blood should be screened for the presence of fetal cells (Kleihauer–Betke test). In addition, serum glycosylated hemoglobin (HgbA1c), antiphospholipid antibodies, Parvovirus B19 and TORCH titers, serologic tests for syphilis, and urine toxicology screens should be ordered. Inherited thrombophilias (deficiencies in protein C, protein S, and antithrombin III; factor V Leiden mutation; and prothrombin gene mutation) carry a two- to threefold increased incidence of stillbirth, and testing should be considered, especially in the setting of fetal growth restriction or preeclampsia.[7]

Fetal

Ultrasound plays a key role in the evaluation of potential fetal and placental factors contributing to fetal death. The approximate gestational age at which death occurred can be estimated by fetal long bone (e.g., femur, humerus) measurements, assuming that there is no early fetal growth restriction. While the calvarium and intracranial anatomy are assessed, the biparietal diameter is not used to date the age at death, since soon after death the head becomes quite compressible, resulting in underestimation of the gestational age. The long bones, on the other hand, will remain relatively unchanged for several weeks. Transcerebellar diameter can also be helpful in dating the pregnancy and assessing possible growth restriction. Congenital anomalies and the presence of hydrops should be sought in all cases of fetal death. However, care should be exercised not to confuse postmortem ultrasound findings (e.g., skin and scalp edema) with fetal congenital malformations. Since chromosomal abnormalities are significant causes of fetal death at all gestational ages, chromosomal analysis is indicated. This information is best obtained by amniocentesis at the time of diagnosis. Autolysis of fetal tissues occurs soon after death. For this reason, viable tissue may not be available at birth for cytogenetic analysis. On the other hand, fetal cells floating in the amniotic fluid may survive for days after fetal death,[8] making amniocentesis the preferred method of obtaining a specimen for cytogenetic analysis. In addition to fetal karyotype, the amniotic fluid specimen should be cultured for *Listeria*, and other aerobic and anaerobic organisms. The amniotic fluid can also be assessed for TORCH infections with the use of polymerase chain reaction studies. If amnio-centesis is not performed, chromosomal studies should be sent from fetal blood obtained by cardiac puncture or from tissue (skin) biopsy. In special circumstances, muscle biopsies or fetal urine may be required. For first-trimester cases, chorionic villus sampling can minimize the chances of maternal cell contamination when evacuated products of conception are sent for karyotype.

If the fetus is delivered intact, photographs and radiographs should be taken and kept on file, particularly if unusual or dysmorphic features are found. Consultation with a geneticist may also be helpful. Parents should be urged to consent to autopsy in all cases of fetal death. Once the benefits of such an examination are pointed out to them, consent can usually be obtained. Eighty-one percent of women surveyed in a study by Rankin et al[9] agreed to a postmortem examination, and 14% of those that declined regretted that decision. Even when a fetal anomaly has been identified by ultrasound, autopsy has been shown to add information affecting the risk of recurrence in 27% of cases.[10] This examination should ideally be performed by a pathologist who has experience and/or special interest in perinatal pathology.

Placental

Placental and umbilical cord abnormalities may offer clues as to the cause of fetal death. The placenta may be abnormally thickened in cases of erythroblastosis fetalis and certain infections (e.g., syphilis, Parvovirus B19). A retroplacental clot, increased placental thickness, subchorionic hematoma or intra-amniotic blood may be visualized in cases of abruption. After delivery, placental cultures, including *Listeria monocytogenes*, should be sent. The placenta should always be examined histologically for evidence of thrombi, infarcts, inflammation, villitis, parasitic infestation, etc. Gross examination of the umbilical cord and placenta can identify circumvallate placentation, velamentous cord insertions, abnormal twisting, and/or thrombosis of the umbilical cord.

Fetal death in multiple gestations

Death of one fetus in a multiple gestation deserves special attention. Although the exact incidence of this event is unknown, it complicates approximately 0.5%–6.8% of twin gestations.[11] Demise of both twins is less likely. Outcome is influenced by gestational age at the time of the demise and by chorionicity. First-trimester fetal demise does not appear to affect adversely the outcome of the surviving twin.[12] In the second and third trimesters, both dichorionic and monochorionic twins are at risk of prematurity. In addition, monochorionic gestations are at risk of multiorgan ischemic damage, multicystic encephalomalacia, and neurologic sequelae in the surviving cotwin. It is estimated to occur in 5–40%, and the timing of this insult is most likely at the time of the demise. For this reason, immediate delivery has not been shown to alter outcomes.[13,14]

Ultrasound assessment plays a key role in evaluating fetal death in multifetal gestations. Attempts should be made to determine chorionicity, as this determines the risk to the surviving fetus. The presence of a dividing membrane and signs of twin-twin-transfusion syndrome should also be evaluated if a monochorionic gestation is confirmed. Both twins should be examined for the presence of structural abnormalities, and karyotyping of both fetuses by amniocentesis should be considered.

At previable gestations, both expectant management and pregnancy termination are options. At term or once lung maturity has been established, delivery is recommended. At 24–34 weeks, close surveillance of the pregnancy, monitoring the surviving fetus for growth and well-being and watching for signs and symptoms of preterm labor, is recommended. The risk of maternal consumptive coagulopathy in a multiple gestation where one fetus has died is rare. Baseline hematologic studies are recommended, including prothrombin time, partial thromboplastin time, fibrinogen, and platelet count.

Management

Once confronted with a fetal demise, the parents and healthcare provider must decide upon subsequent management. Options include expectant management while awaiting spontaneous uterine evacuation, medical management, or surgical intervention. Variables taken into consideration in making these choices include gestational age and uterine size at diagnosis, pre-existing medical and obstetric conditions, provider experience, and the emotional aspects involved.

Expectant

Expectant management is more likely to be considered in the early first trimester. A major advantage is avoiding the potential risks of surgery. However, it may be emotionally difficult for the parents to wait an unpredictable duration of time for spontaneous resolution. Complete abortion rates in the first trimester are 47–54%, but may take 4–6 weeks, with up to 10%

requiring emergency curettage for heavy bleeding.[15–17] In the second half of gestation, a disadvantage is the potential risk of hypofibrinogenemia. Fortunately, coagulation abnormalities in association with fetal demise are uncommon. In the absence of placental abruption or uterine perforation, this risk is estimated at 3%.[18] In addition, most patients will deliver within 2 weeks of fetal death,[19] minimizing the risk of a coagulopathy developing with prolonged retention *in utero*.[20] Baseline fibrinogen levels followed by weekly assessment has been recommended if expectant management is chosen. If a coagulation defect is identified, steps should be taken to evacuate promptly the uterus of the retained products of conception and correct the coagulopathy with the appropriate blood products.

Surgical techniques

Dilation and evacuation
Surgical emptying of the uterus by dilation and evacuation (D & E) involves dilation of the cervix followed by evacuation of the products of conception by a combination of suction aspiration, sharp curettage, and forceps as needed. The two methods of sharp curettage and vacuum aspiration with either a flexible or rigid cannula have not been shown to differ in complication rates.[21] Since there is considerable discomfort involved, some form of anesthesia is required (intravenous sedation, regional block, or general anesthesia). Cervical dilation at under 11–13 weeks' gestation is generally performed mechanically in the operating room just prior to evacuation. At gestational ages greater than this, preoperative preparation with either prostaglandins (PG) or laminaria tents may be considered. Hackett et al reported greater preoperative cervical dilation when the balloon of a 14F Foley catheter inserted into the cervical canal was inflated with 25 ml water compared with 3 mg prostaglandin (PG) E$_2$ inserted into the posterior fornix.[22]

The most serious and significant complications of D & E are cervical lacerations, uterine perforation, hemorrhage, retained products of conception, infection, and intrauterine adhesion formation. These complication rates increase with advancing gestational age and are greatest after 20 weeks' gestation.[23] While the death/case ratio is 3/100 000 procedures at 13–15 weeks' gestation, it increases fourfold when performed at 21 weeks' gestation.[24]

Although D & E is generally very effective, occasional difficulty is encountered in completely evacuating the uterus, especially at more advanced gestational ages (>16 weeks). In particular, the fetal calvarium and thorax are most often retained. Inspection of fetal tissue at the time of the procedure should help to confirm that all the major fetal parts have been removed. If one recognizes that the evacuation is incomplete, the procedure can be completed under ultrasonic guidance. An alternative approach is to administer an intravenous oxytocin infusion for several hours before returning the patient to the operating room. By that time the retained fetal parts will usually be visible at the internal cervical os, where they can be grasped and removed. Either approach is preferable to blind attempts at locating and removing the retained tissue; such efforts are more likely to result in uterine perforation and hemorrhage. Some have even advocated performing all D & E procedures under continuous direct ultrasound guidance, which is associated with lower complication rates (3.7% vs 15.9%) and less operative time.[25]

Surgical management, in addition to being safe and effective, avoids the unpredictable and longer experience of expectant or medical management. However, pathologic evaluation of a fragmented D & E specimen may not provide the same information as an intact fetus and placenta. It is also impossible for the parents to see and/or hold the object of their profound grief when the fetus is not intact. Parents should be counseled about both the advantages and disadvantages of this option.

Hysterotomy, hysterectomy, and laparotomy
Hysterotomy and hysterectomy are rarely required or indicated in the management of fetal death. Although the mother often states that she wants the dead fetus removed from her uterus immediately, the physician must resist the temptation to accommodate her. Performing a hysterotomy in such cases subjects the mother to significant morbidity, increased chance of mortality, and a much longer recuperative period. Moreover, pregnancies after hysterotomies are frequently associated with thin scars,[26] thus increasing the likelihood of uterine rupture; for this reason, most subsequent pregnancies are delivered by elective cesarean section.

Under unusual circumstances, hysterotomy or hysterectomy may be the preferred method of uterine evacuation. If a coexisting condition requires laparotomy, such as abdominal trauma, suspected ovarian cancer, or invasive cervical cancer, hysterotomy or hysterectomy may be performed. Other potential indications include suspected placenta accreta, obstructed labor, abdominal pregnancy, or maternal hemorrhage. If hysterotomy is performed, the techniques employed should be those used in cesarean section, except that the uterine incision should be only as large as necessary to remove all products of conception. If the uterus is to be preserved for subsequent pregnancies, the uterine incision should avoid the fundus, and a careful layered closure should be performed. Failed induction of labor should raise the suspicion of a possible abdominal or cervical pregnancy. When abdominal pregnancy is diagnosed, laparotomy and removal of the fetus is indicated. The cord should be tied close to the placental insertion and the placenta should be left *in situ*, where gradual resorption will occur. Attempts at removal are associated with a significant risk of hemorrhage and should be avoided.

Because of the increased rate of cesarean delivery, it is not uncommon to be faced with the challenge of managing a woman with a fetal demise and a previously scarred uterus. Induction of labor in the second trimester appears to be safe and effective. Misoprostol at doses of 600–800 μg[27] or extra-amniotic PGE$_2$[28,29] lead to delivery in 11–15 hours with no cases of uterine rupture reported in a total of 122 women. Although uterine rupture has been reported at 23 weeks after one 200 μg dose of misoprostol, this patient had two prior low-transverse cesarean sections, preterm premature rupture of membranes, and chorioamnionitis.[30] Chapman et al reported on 79 women with a previous cesarean delivery at a mean gestational age of 20 weeks undergoing induction of labor.[31] Forty-four percent were induced with PGE$_2$, 29% with concentrated oxytocin, 14% with both, and 7.5% with dilute oxytocin infusion. Mean induction to delivery time was 15 hours. When compared with the control group of women with unscarred uteri, a greater risk of blood transfusion (11% vs 5%) and a greater risk of uterine rupture (3.8% vs 0.2%) was noted in the cesarean group. Although heterogeneous in the induction methods, risk factors for uterine rupture included multiparity, prolonged induction times (>24 hours), and oxytocin use for more than 12 hours. Caution should be exercised in the presence of these risk factors.

Medical techniques

Prostaglandin (PG) E$_1$

PGE$_1$ (misoprostol) is a safe and effective way to facilitate uterine evacuation. It is inexpensive and well tolerated, does not require special storage techniques, and can be administered in similar dosing by the oral, sublingual, vaginal, or rectal routes. Various regimens with or without the use of mifepristone have been utilized in the first trimester with success rates of 52–83% (Table 17.4). The most common side effects include transient pyrexia, nausea, and diarrhea, the last of which can be reduced with vaginal rather than oral dosing.[32] Premedication with antipyretics, antiemetics, and antidiarrheals will further minimize these side effects. Sublingual misoprostol has been found to have higher bioavailability with higher peak serum concentrations than oral and vaginal routes.[33] In addition, it avoids the first pass through the liver and uncomfortable vaginal examinations and should be considered as a reasonable alternative, along with the rectal route, particularly for patients experiencing bleeding that may interfere with vaginal absorption.

PGE$_2$

PGE$_2$ is an effective means of terminating a pregnancy at 12–28 weeks' gestation. Twenty-milligram suppositories are placed in the posterior vaginal fornix at 3–5 hour intervals. Seventy percent of women deliver within 12 hours and 93% deliver in 24 hours with this protocol.[34] Induction to delivery times may be shortened with the concomitant use of mechanical cervical dilators (laminaria tents or intracervical Foley balloon). The mechanism of action is not clearly elucidated, but it does induce myometrial contractions in the gravid uterus in a manner similar to that seen in term labor. They are contraindicated in patients with known hypersensitivity to PGE$_2$ and in patients with acute pelvic infection. They should not be used in patients with *active* cardiac, pulmonary, renal, or hepatic disease or when contraindications to labor are present. However, unlike PGF$_{2\alpha}$, they may be used in patients with a history of asthma.

The effects of PGE$_2$ are not specific to uterine smooth muscle, a fact which accounts for the frequently observed side effects. Approximately 67% of patients experience nausea and/or vomiting and 40% experience diarrhea.[34] For this reason, pretreatment with antiemetics such as prochlorperazine (Compazine) and diphenoxylate (Lomotil) is recommended. Transient pyrexia is also noted in one-third of patients and can be managed with acetaminophen. While serious complications are rare, they may occur. Uterine rupture and cervical lacerations requiring hysterectomy have been reported.[35,36] In general, these serious complications have occurred in the third trimester when concomitant oxytocin has been used. Approximately 15% of patients will have incomplete uterine evacuation requiring surgical curettage.[34] It is usually in this group of patients that blood loss may exceed 500 ml, with an overall blood transfusion rate of 3–5%.

Another means of administering PGE$_2$ is intrauterine but extra-amniotic. This method is effective and safe and compares favorably to PGE$_2$ vaginal suppositories.[36] When administered via this route, much lower doses of PGE$_2$ are necessary and the side effects are less. In addition, oxytocin augmentation is rarely required. The technique involves inserting a Foley catheter (16F) into the cervix after cleansing the vagina with Povidone-iodine. The balloon is inflated to 30–50 cc when the catheter tip has passed the internal cervical os. PGE$_2$ can be administered as 200-μg boluses every 2 hours[28] or as a continuous infusion (10 mg in 500 ml isotonic saline).[29] Mean delivery

Table 17.4 Medical regimens for uterine evacuation using misoprostol (prostaglandin E$_1$)

Dose of misoprostol	Route of administration	Frequency of dosing
400 μg	Vaginal	Every other day
600 μg	Vaginal	Every 4 hours × 2 doses
800 μg	Vaginal	Every 24 hours × 2 doses
800 μg	Oral or vaginal	Every 4 hours × 2 doses
800 μg, then 400 μg	Vaginal	48 hours after 200 mg of oral mifepristone, then every 3 hours × 2 doses
400 μg	Oral	48 hours after 400 mg of oral mifepristone

times with or without the subsequent use of oxytocin after catheter dislodgment vary between 11 and 13 hours. Fever and gastrointestinal side effects occur less often.

$PGF_{2\alpha}$

Carboprost tromethamine, a 15-methyl $PGF_{2\alpha}$ analog, is approved in the USA for use as an intramuscularly injected abortifacient. Precautions, contraindications, and side effects are similar to those noted for PGE_2, except that $PGF_{2\alpha}$ should not be used in a patient with a history of asthma due to its bronchoconstriction properties. After premedication with antiemetics and antidiarrheals, a dose of 250 μg (1 ml) is injected deep intramuscularly and repeated at 1.5–3.5-hour intervals, depending on the uterine response. The major disadvantage of this route of administration is the need for repetitive, painful injections. However, this route may be preferred in the presence of ruptured membranes or a significant vaginal infection when intravaginal absorption may be less predictable. The mean induction to delivery time and frequency of side effects is similar to that seen for the PGE2 vaginal suppositories. This method has been used to manage fetal death with success rates of 90–100% within 24 hours.[37–39]

Oxytocin

Since high-dose PG are not approved by the US Food and Drug Administration for management of fetal death over 28 weeks, many choose to induce labor with oxytocin beyond this gestational age. At or near term, especially if the cervix is favorable for induction, oxytocin administered intravenously is safe and effective. Infusion should be begun at a low rate (0.5–2.0 mU/min) and be increased at 15–30-minute intervals according to uterine response. Oxytocin should always be administered in a solution of lactated Ringer's solution rather than aqueous dextrose, since water intoxication may occur with prolonged use. Uterine activity should be monitored and uterine hyperstimulation avoided. If the cervix is unfavorable, pretreatment with laminaria tents, intracervical Foley catheter, or low-dose PG preparations may shorten the induction-to-delivery time.[40] Oxytocin should not be administered if contraindications to labor exist, such as previous classical uterine scar, transverse lie near term, frank cephalopelvic disproportion, or placenta previa.

Concentrated oxytocin protocols have also been utilized for midtrimester inductions of labor. One such protocol is pre-

sented in Table 17.5. This infusion is given along with PGE_2 vaginal suppositories (10 mg every 6 hours) and either laminaria (1–6 tents left in place for 12 hours) or Foley catheter insertion into the cervical canal (inflation of 30-ml balloon and isotonic saline infusion at 30 ml/hour × 12 hours or until the catheter becomes dislodged). The use of this protocol at 16–24 weeks' gestation results in delivery within 16–17 hours.[41]

The intra-amniotic route of administration for any abortifacient (urea, saline, or PG) is not recommended in cases of fetal death, since rapid absorption may occur and serious complications may result.

Emotional aspects of fetal demise

Death is not the expected outcome of pregnancy. It is now well understood that the emotional reactions a couple experiences on fetal demise are similar to those on the death of any loved one. These emotional responses occur not only after late fetal death, but also after early miscarriage,[42] loss of one twin,[43] and midtrimester termination of pregnancy because of fetal anomalies.[44] Although the grief response is complex, there are fairly consistent and characteristic phases that can be recognized.[45] There is considerable variation, however, in how each individual moves through and copes with these reactions. It is imperative that any health-care provider assisting a couple at the time of a fetal loss be familiar with these emotional responses. Only then can the need for appropriate support be recognized and provided.

Most women will first experience an intense, immediate emotional response.[46] The initial phase is characterized by shock, which may last from several hours to 2 weeks, and is often accompanied by denial. Some of this denial may be lessened by involving the mother in confirmation of the diagnosis by showing her the absent cardiac activity on ultrasound. Next occur feelings of grief, dysphoria, guilt, and anxiety. It is particularly important at this time to avoid questions and comments that may be misinterpreted and add to the self-blame which invariably exists. Minimizing feelings of guilt is important, as they are predictors of grief intensity, coping difficulties, and progression to depression.[46] From these first few moments, the situation should be handled in a compassionate, sensitive, and sincere manner. The next phase of the grief process is charac-

Table 17.5 Concentrated oxytocin infusion protocol for second-trimester labor induction[41]

50 units in 500 ml D5NS over 3 hours; maintenance fluids of D5NS × 1 hour
100 units in 500 ml D5NS over 3 hours; maintenance fluids for 1 hour
150 units in 500 ml D5NS over 3 hours; maintenance fluids for 1 hour
200 units in 500 ml D5NS over 3 hours; maintenance fluids for 1 hour
250 units in 500 ml D5NS over 3 hours; maintenance fluids for 1 hour
300 units in 500 ml D5NS over 3 hours

D5NS: isotonic sodium chloride solution with 5% dextrose.
Adapted from Hogg and Owen[41] with permission from Elsevier.

terized by a longer period of disorganization, often interrupted by feelings of grief.[45] By 3–4 months, resolution and reorganization should have occurred. The intensity and duration of these emotional reactions, however, may be heightened if there has been a history of pregnancy losses, if there are no living children, if the loss occurred late in the pregnancy, particularly in the absence of warning signs, and if there is a history of poor coping, depression, or lack of social support.[46] All couples should be provided with referrals to support groups, bereavement teams, social workers, and/or psychologists with special interest and experience in perinatal loss.

It is important to have an increased awareness of the emotional impact of perinatal loss on both the mother and the father. The outward response of the father may be quite different from that of the mother. Men often suppress their feelings of sadness and anger in their attempts to focus and support their partner. As a result of this restricted expression of grief, they tend to receive less support, feel very isolated, and are at increased risk of developing a chronic grief response.[47,48] These differences in grief reactions can subsequently strain a couple's relationship. Therefore, being supportive and communicating with both parents is essential.

By providing ongoing psychological support to parents experiencing a perinatal loss, significantly fewer depressive symptoms have been reported.[49] Supportive interventions for these couples exist on a variety of levels. As previously discussed, minimizing feelings of denial and guilt occur at the time of diagnosis. It is important that options of pregnancy management be discussed, but that the couple not be rushed into making decisions, as long as immediate hospitalization is not required for medical necessity. At the time of delivery, encouraging the parents to see and hold the baby and collect mementos (photographs, locks of hair, footprints, and identification bracelets) can aid in grief resolution. Kellner et al found that 92% of parents chose to see their baby and 54% chose to hold their baby after perinatal death.[50] This decision is not based on physical appearance, and even in severely macerated or anomalous fetuses, parents will benefit from this interaction. While those who see their baby never regret their choice, those who do not, often regret the decision. In addition, naming the baby helps in affirming his/her existence and should be encouraged.[51]

Regarding disposal of the body, all options available to the patient should be discussed. These may include hospital disposal, private burial, and private cremation. In cases of cremation, the ashes can be offered to the parents. While hospital disposal may be most convenient to the parents, a privately arranged memorial service or funeral has several benefits. Such a service offers a certain 'finality' to the fetal death, allowing progression of the normal grieving process. It also offers family and friends the opportunity to express their sorrow, and many find comfort in knowing where their baby is buried.[52]

Although parents should be given adequate privacy, they should not be isolated and abandoned. An expression of our own feelings and a discussion of potential reactions from family and friends will be of assistance. Under no circumstances,

regardless of gestational age at time of death, should comments be made such as 'you are young – you can have another' or 'you already have a healthy child – you should be grateful for that.' It has been estimated that over 50% of women experiencing a perinatal loss felt that health-care providers were insensitive and failed to provide the opportunity to talk about the loss, and these women sensed a lack of caring and sympathy. As a result, anger is fostered and women often seek the care of new providers in subsequent pregnancies.

Follow-up outpatient visits should address both the physical and emotional needs of the mother. The loss should be discussed openly and available information regarding etiology disclosed. The health-care provider should not only be familiar with the signs of normal grieving, but should also be able to recognize signs of pathologic grief reactions, including the development of depression, anxiety neuroses, psychosomatic reactions, or suicidal ideation. If these states are suspected, immediate psychiatric referral is warranted. More than half of women become pregnant within 1–2 years after a perinatal loss.[53] Although some studies have reported that patients who become pregnant within 6 months are more likely to suffer from a prolonged grief reaction,[52,54] other studies have not confirmed this.[55] Recommendations should be based on the individual couple's emotional functioning. Regardless of the time of delivery, a subsequent pregnancy is often marked by strong anxiety, which becomes most intense near the gestational age at which the previous loss occurred.[55]

Conclusion

Intrauterine fetal death is a devastating event in the lives of parents and distressful for health-care workers as well. The obstetrician must deal with the physical aspects of death – confirmation of the diagnosis, diagnostic work-up, and management of uterine evacuation – as well as the emotional needs of the parents. Physicians and parents may choose to await the spontaneous onset of labor or actively to effect uterine evacuation. The latter can be achieved by both medical and surgical methods. The method of choice as well as the timing of delivery is determined by the gestational age, the experience of the physician, and the medical and emotional needs of the patient. A thorough sonographic and pathologic evaluation of the fetus and placenta is indicated, and can assist in explaining the present loss, assessing recurrence risks, and determining the need for special interventions during subsequent pregnancies. Compassion, sensitivity, and openness are essential and help both parents and health-care providers through these difficult times.

References

1. World Health Organization. Manual of the International Classification of Diseases, Injuries and Causes of Death (9th rev.) WHO: Geneva, 1977; 1: 763.

2. National Center for Heath Statistics. National Survey of Family Growth, Cycle V, 1995. CD-ROM 23(3), 2000.

3. Goldhaber MK. Fetal death ratios in a prospective study compared to state fetal death certificate reporting. Am J Public Health 1989; 79: 1268–70.

4. Arias E, Anderson RN, Kung HC, et al. Deaths: final data for 2001. Natl Vital Stat Rep. 2003 Sep 18; 52(3): 1–115.

5. Goldstein SR, Timor-Tritsch IE. Ultrasound in Gynecology, p. 150. Churchill Livingstone: New York, 1995.

6. Warburton D. Chromosomal causes of fetal death. Clin Obstet Gynecol 1987; 30: 268.

7. Arkel YS, Ku DH. Thrombophilia and pregnancy: review of the literature and some original data. Clin Appl Thromb Hemost 2001; 7: 259–68.

8. Saal HM, Rodis JF, Weinbaum PJ et al. Cytogenetic evaluation of fetal death: the role of amniocentesis. Obstet Gynecol 1987; 70: 601.

9. Rankin J, Wright C, Lind T. Cross sectional survey of parents' experience and views of the postmortem examination. BMJ 2002; 324: 816–18.

10. Boyd PA, Tondi F, Hicks NR et al. Autopsy after termination of pregnancy for fetal anomaly: retrospective cohort study. BMJ 2004; 328: 137–40.

11. Cleary-Goldman J, D'Alton M. Management of single fetal demise in a multiple gestation. Obstet Gynecol Survey 2004; 59: 285–98.

12. Pompler HJ, Madjar H, Klosa W et al. Twin pregnancies with single fetal death. Acta Obstet Gynecol Scand 1994; 73: 205–8.

13. D'Alton ME, Newton ER, Cetrulo CL . Intrauterine fetal demise in multiple gestation. Acta Genet Med Gemellol 1984; 33: 43–9.

14. Fusi L, Gordon H. Twin pregnancy complicated by single intrauterine death. Problems and outcomes with conservative management. Br J Obstet Gynaecol 1990; 97: 511–16.

15. Wieringa-de Waard M, Vos J, Bonsel GJ et al. Management of miscarriage: a randomized controlled trial of expectant management versus surgical evacuation. Hum Reprod 2002; 17: 2445–50.

16. Acharya G, Morgan H. Does gestational sac volume predict the outcome of missed miscarriage managed expectantly? J Clin Ultrasound 2002; 30: 526–31.

17. Ngai SW, Chan YM, Tang OS et al. Vaginal misoprostol as medical treatment for first trimester spontaneous miscarriage. Hum Reprod 2001; 16: 1493–6.

18. Maslow AD, Breen TW, Sarna MC et al. Prevalence of coagulation abnormalities associated with intrauterine fetal death. Can J Anaesth 1996; 43: 1237–43.

19. Tricomi V, Kohl SG. Fetal death in utero. Am J Obstet Gynecol 1957; 74: 1092.

20. Prichard JA. Fetal death in utero. Obstet Gynecol 1959; 14: 573.

21. Kulier R, Fekih A, Hofmeyr GJ et al. Cochrane Database Syst Rev 2001; 4: CD002900.

22. Hackett GA, Reginald P, Paintin DB. Comparison of the Foley catheter and dinoprostone pessary for cervical preparation before second trimester abortion. Br J Obstet Gynaecol 1989; 96: 1432–4.

23. Peterson WF, Berry FN, Grace MR et al. Second trimester abortion by dilation and evacuation: an analysis of 11,747 cases. Obstet Gynecol 1983; 62: 185.

24. Grimes DA, Schulz KF. Morbidity and mortality from second trimester abortions. J Reprod Med 1985; 30: 505.

25. Acharya G, Morgan H, Paramanantham L et al. A randomized controlled trial comparing surgical termination of pregnancy with and without continuous ultrasound guidance. Eur J Obstet Gynecol Reprod Biol 2004; 114: 69–74.

26. Clow WM, Crompton AC. The wounded uterus: pregnancy after hysterotomy. BMJ 1973; 1: 321.

27. Herabutya Y, Chanarachakul B, Punyavachira P. Induction of labor with vaginal misoprostol for second trimester termination of pregnancy in the scarred uterus. Int J Gynecol Obstet 2003; 83: 293–7.

28. Debby A, Golan A, Sagiv R et al. Midtrimester abortion in patients with a previous uterine scar. Eur J Obstet Gynecol Reprod Biol 2003; 109: 177–80.

29. Shapira S, Goldberger S, Beyth Y et al. Induced second trimester abortion by extra-amniotic prostaglandin infusion in patients with a cesarean scar: is it safe? Acta Obstet Gynecol Scand 1999; 78: 511–14.

30. Chen M, Shih JC, Chiu WT et al. Separation of cesarean scar during second-trimester intravaginal misoprostol abortion. Obstet Gynecol 1999; 94: 840.

31. Chapman SJ, Crispens M, Owen J et al. Complications of midtrimester pregnancy termination: the effect of prior cesarean delivery. Am J Obstet Gynecol 1996; 175: 889–92.

32. Pang MW, Lee TS, Chung TKH. Incomplete miscarriage: a randomized controlled trial comparing oral with vaginal misoprostol for medical evacuation. Hum Reprod 2001; 16: 2283–7.

33. Zeiman M, Fong S, Benowitz N et al. Absorption kinetics of misoprostol with oral or vaginal administration. Obstet Gynecol 1997; 90: 88–92.

34. Southern EM, Gutknecht GD. Management of intrauterine fetal demise and missed abortion using prostaglandin E_2 vaginal suppositories. Obstet Gynecol 1976; 47: 602–5.

35. Sawyer MM, Lipshitz J, Anderson GD et al. Third trimester uterine rupture associated with vaginal prostaglandin E_2. Am J Obstet Gynecol 1981; 140: 710.

36. Scher J, Jeng D, Moshirpur J et al. A comparison between vaginal prostaglandin E_2 suppositories and intrauterine extra-amniotic prostaglandins in the management of fetal death in utero. Am J Obstet Gynecol 1980; 137: 769.

37. Boes EG. Missed abortion, hydatiform mole and intrauterine fetal death treated with 15-methyl-prostaglandin $F_{2\alpha}$. S Afr Med J 1980; 58: 878.

38. Tsalacopoulos G, Bloch B, Rush JM. Missed abortion treated with intramuscular 15-(s)-15-methyl-prostaglandin $F_{2\alpha}$. S Afr Med J 1982; 61: 828.

39. Ylikorkala O, Kirkinen P, Jarrinen PA. Intramuscular administration of 15-methyl-prostaglandin $F_{2\alpha}$ for induction of labour in patients with intrauterine fetal death or an anencephalic fetus. Br J Obstet Gynecol 1976; 83: 502.

40. Ekman G, Ulmstern U, Wingerup L. Intracervical application of PGE2 gel combined with early intravenous infusion of oxytocin

for induction of term labor in women with unripe cervix. Arch J Gynecol 1983; 61: 234.

41. Hogg BB, Owen J. Laminaria versus extra-amniotic saline solution infusion for cervical ripening in second-trimester labor inductions. Am J Obstet Gynecol 2001; 184: 1145–8.

42. Peppers LG, Knapp RJ. Maternal reactions to involuntary fetal/infant death. Psychiatry 1980; 43: 155.

43. Wilson AL, Fenton LJ, Stevens DC et al. The death of a newborn twin: an analysis of parental bereavement. Pediatrics 1982; 70: 587.

44. Adler B, Kushnick T. Genetic counseling in prenatally diagnosed trisomy 18 and 21: psychosocial aspects. Pediatrics 1982; 69: 94.

45. Parkes CM. Bereavement. Br J Psychiatry 1985; 146: 11.

46. Brier N. Understanding and managing the emotional reactions to a miscarriage. Obstet Gynecol 1999; 93: 151–5.

47. Murphy FA. The experience of early miscarriage from a male perspective. J Clin Nurs 1998; 7: 325–32.

48. Samuelsson M, Radestad I, Segesten K. A waste of life: fathers' experience of losing a child before birth. Birth 2001; 28: 124–30.

49. Carrera L, Diez-Domingo J, Montanana V et al. Depression in women suffering perinatal loss. Int J Gynecol Obstet 1998; 62: 149–53.

50. Kellner KR, Donnelly WH, Gould SD. Parental behavior after perinatal death: lack of predictive demographic and obstetrical variables. Obstet Gynecol 1984; 63: 809.

51. Peppers LG, Knapp RJ. Motherhood and mourning. Perinatal Death, p. 125. Praeger: New York, 1980.

52. LaRoche C, Lalinee-Michaud M, Engelsmann F et al. Grief reactions to perinatal death – a follow up study. Can J Psychiatry 1984; 29: 14.

53. Cuisinier M, Janssen H, de Graauw C et al. Pregnancy following miscarriage: course of grief and some determining factors. J Psychosom Obstet Gynaecol 1996; 17: 168–74.

54. Hughes PM, Turton P, Evans CDH. Stillbirth as risk factor for depression and anxiety in the subsequent pregnancy: cohort study. BMJ 1999; 318: 1721–4.

55. Cote-Arsenault D, Nomvuyo M. Impact of perinatal loss on the subsequent pregnancy and self: women's experiences. J Obstet Gynecol Neonat Nurs 1999; 28: 274–82.

18 Antepartum hemorrhage

Gábor Németh, Gerard Hansen, and György Bártfai

Antepartum hemorrhage (APH) has been defined as bleeding from the genital tract between week 22 of the pregnancy and the onset of labor. This complication occurs in about 10–15% of all pregnancies. Whatever the cause of the bleeding, the obstetrician is dealing with two patients. Obstetric hemorrhage is a significant threat to the fetus. Premature delivery and perinatal mortality rates are increased several-fold in connection with second- and third-trimester bleeding episodes.

The most frequent causes of APH are abruptio placentae and placenta previa. Vasa previa is a rare obstetric etiologic factor. Other causes, not directly related to the gestation, are cervical erosion, trauma, vulvovaginal varicosities, genital infections, and genital tumors. Hematuria and rectal bleeding may create an erroneous impression of obstetric hemorrhage. Because of the high mortality and morbidity rates that accompany APH, the establishment of a firm differential diagnosis is of utmost importance.

Abruptio Placentae

Etiology and epidemiology

Separation of the placenta from the implantation site is a dangerous obstetric complication for both the mother and the fetus.[1] It is generally believed that defective endometrial and placental vasculature are contributory factors in certain cases. The clinical picture ranges from mild, and thus innocuous, to severe and potentially fatal forms.

Abruption of the placenta occurs with increasing frequency in multiparous women and among the oldest and youngest primigravidas. This phenomenon is consistent with the observation that degenerative vascular changes in the decidua basalis of the endometrium predispose to placental separation from the implantation site.[2] The cause of the abruption cannot be determined in a considerable proportion of the cases. Furthermore, the roles of the various causative factors vary with time and geographic location.

Traditionally, most placental abruptions were attributed to maternal hypertension. Four decades ago, a study found a ninefold increase in its incidence among chronically hypertensive mothers.[3] With the ever increasing use of the automobile, abdominal trauma has become an important causative factor in the economically developed world. Unfortunately, intentional abdominal trauma, far too often inflicted by the father of the child, is a frequent cause of placental abruption. The effect of the trauma may not be immediately obvious. However, in the course of 24 hours, even relatively modest trauma may progress to a significant degree of abruption. External cephalic version and cordocentesis are infrequent but well-recognized etiologic factors.

Maternal tobacco use, both before and during pregnancy, has been linked to placental abruption. More recent and far more dangerous, however, is the recreational use of crack, a heat-stable, smokable cocaine alkaloid, which increasingly blights the lives of inner-city populations both in the USA and elsewhere. In some metropolitan medical centers, due to cocaine use, the rate of occurrence of this complication has doubled and even trebled. With both agents, there is a dose-response relationship between the intensity of use and the incidence of placental abruption. Smoking and hypertension synergistically pose a higher risk of placental abruption than would be expected through simple addition of their respective estimated risks.

When the site of placental attachment covers a uterine fibroid tumor, there is an increased risk of placental abruption. The risk is also increased in cases of multiple pregnancy and is maximum following the delivery of the first twin. The sudden uterine decompression that accompanies spontaneous or artificial rupture of the membranes may also lead to abruption. This is particularly threatening in cases of polyhydramnios.

Nutritional deprivation, particularly folic acid deficiency, has been suspected to predispose to placental separation. There is circumstantial evidence to suggest that some cases of abruption are associated with poor placentation. The finding of high midpregnancy levels of maternal serum alpha-fetoprotein (AFP), in the absence of fetal abnormality, predicts an increased risk of complications in advanced gestation, including placental abruption.

There is evidence to indicate the existence of a link between chorioamnionitis and detachment of the placenta.[4]

The increase of the risk has been estimated to be as much as threefold when prolonged premature rupture of the membranes becomes complicated by chorioamnionitis.[5]

Clinical presentation

Placental abruption varies widely in clinical presentation, from a small amount of vaginal bleeding to massive hemorrhage, leading to diffuse intravascular coagulation (DIC) and fetal demise. Commonly associated signs and symptoms are back pain, vaginal bleeding, fetal compromise evidenced by nonreassuring fetal heart rate tracings, and hypertonic or tetanic uterine contractions. Typically, the patient develops pain over the uterus that gradually increases in severity. Uterine contractions also increase in frequency and became tetanic in character. Faintness and syncope may occur, followed by signs of shock. The uterus becomes tender and hard, and it does not relax. The diagnosis of placental abruption may be delayed if the bleeding is concealed, but is readily obvious when it is revealed. In most instances, the diagnosis is made clinically. It is confirmed by the finding of clots attached to the placenta after delivery. Ultrasound is an insensitive and unreliable diagnostic tool. Negative findings are common even with clinically significant placental separations.

In severe abruptions, the rates of the maternal and perinatal complications are high. However, in contemporary obstetric practice, maternal death is rare. Severe hemorrhage is conducive to postpartum infection. The so-called Couvelaire uterus (hemorrhage among the myometrial fibers) predisposes to postpartum hemorrhage and may require hysterectomy in rare cases. When the abruption is moderate, the associated fetal morbidity is usually due to prematurity. Abruption exceeding 50% of the implantation site causes stillbirth. For the objective determination of the severity of placental abruption, the following grading system has been recommended:[6]

> Grade I. Slight vaginal bleeding and minimal uterine irritability. The maternal blood pressure, the fibrinogen level, and the fetal heart rate pattern remain within the normal range.
> Grade II. Mild to moderate bleeding. There are irritable uterus, strong uterine contractions, maternal tachycardia possibly with postural hypotension, reduced fibrinogen level (1.5–2.5 g/l), and evidence of fetal compromise on electronic monitoring.
> Grade III: Moderate to severe bleeding. There are tetanic and painful uterus, maternal hypotension, fibrinogen level under 1.5 g/l, and associated coagulation abnormalities. Fetal death has occurred.

In approximately 20% of the cases, placental abruption entails no vaginal bleeding (concealed hemorrhage). Indeed, in this entity, reliance upon the magnitude of visible bleeding may lead to serious underestimation of the actual blood loss.

Diagnosis

Conclusive prenatal diagnosis of abruption of the placenta is difficult. Since ultrasound examination may not reveal the retroplacental hematoma, the differential diagnosis essentially rests upon sonographic exclusion of low implantation of the placenta. The entity has been categorized according to the site of the placental detachment as retroplacental and marginal[7,8] (Figure 18.1). In a typical case, acute retroplacental separation probably derives from the rupture of an arteriole in the endometrium, secondary to the capillary changes caused by preeclampsia. It is generally assumed that the rupture of spiral arteries results in high-pressure bleeding that eventually expands and separates the placenta from the implantation site. In this process, much or most of the placenta may become separated. It has been suggested that this event causes increased coagulation activity as a result of release of thromboplastin from the decidua and the trophoblast.[9] In the same process, the decidua also releases prostaglandin precursors that cause uterine hypertonus.

Peripheral separation of the placenta, described in the old literature as marginal sinus rupture,[10] causes low-pressure bleeding that has little effect upon the maternal and fetal circulatory status. Nonetheless, it may cause premature labor or premature rupture of the membranes.

Careful examination of the placenta after delivery displays signs of infarction as well as detachment. These small impressions are covered by firm clots, the extent of which provides a clue to the severity of the abruption.

Traditionally, the vaginal bleeding associated with placenta previa was described as painless, whereas that deriving from abruption of the placenta was characterized as painful. Although the difference between the two symptoms was a helpful diagnostic tool in the past, contemporary obstetricians seldom need to rely on this distinction.

Consequences of placental abruption: epidemiology and diagnosis

In contemporary practice, abruption of the placenta is probably the most frequent cause of DIC. Other pathologic conditions conducive to DIC are amniotic fluid embolism, chorioamnionitis, septic abortion, HELLP syndrome, in utero fetal death with the products of conception retained for several weeks, and shock.[11] When it occurs against the background of obstetric hemorrhage, DIC originates from the release of thromboplastin and endotoxin into the maternal circulation. These activate thrombin, aggregating platelets and fibrin within the capillaries. The latter in turn releases fibrin degradation products that trigger consumption of platelets and coagulation factors (consumption coagulopathy). Microvascular bleeding can arise from areas subject to trauma. Damage occurs not only from blood loss but

Marginal abruption

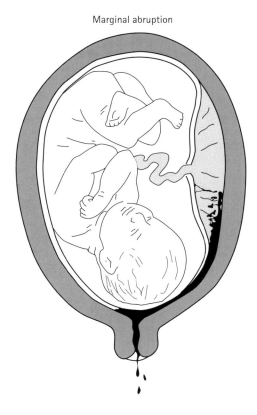

Retroplacental bleeding

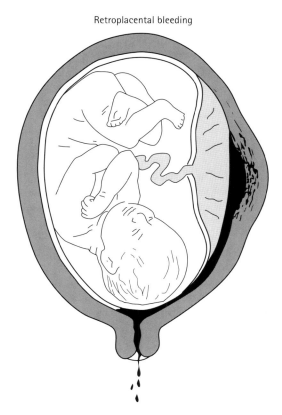

Figure 18.1 The two main types of placental separation: marginal and retroplacental. (This illustration was contributed to the first edition by Drs Kjell Haram, Per Bergsjo and Magnar Ulstein. ©2006 Leslie Iffy.)

also as a result of hypoxia and tissue ischemia from fibrin plugs in the microvasculature. This can result in renal and pulmonary failure and in Sheehan's syndrome (avascular necrosis of the anterior pituitary gland). DIC should be suspected when, despite administration of fresh frozen plasma (FFP), the fibrin degradation products and D-dimers remain abnormal. Treatment, including replacement of blood products, should depend on specific laboratory findings.

In the 1930s a maternal mortality rate of 1.7% was reported from the New York Lying-In Hospital in connection with APH presenting with external bleeding. With concealed hemorrhage, the rate of maternal losses was 11.8%.[12] By the 1970s maternal death from obstetric hemorrhage had become exceedingly rare.[13] In contrast, abruption of the placenta still entails a high perinatal mortality rate. Even in recent years one out of nine cases of abruption of the placenta entailed fetal or neonatal demise.[14] More than one-half of these were stillbirths. The tendency of abruptio placentae to recur in subsequent pregnancies has been reported with rates varying from 3.7 to 17.3%.[14] Of all cases, 20% involve concealed hemorrhage.[6] In these cases, the blood may be accumulating behind the placenta, held back by the presenting part, and sequestered in the amniotic fluid, or it may infiltrate the uterus and the broad ligaments. The amount of concealed retroplacental blood may be considerable.[8]

The symptoms of abruption include vaginal bleeding (usually dark, menstrual-like blood), abdominal discomfort, pain,

backache (especially when the placenta is in a posterior position), lack of fetal movements, and symptoms of shock.[2] Other classical signs include increased uterine tenderness and tonus (grade II or III abruption). In severe cases, the abdomen is hard, like wood, and tense. The clinical signs are more directly related to the extent of the placental separation than to the external blood loss. The newborn is often anemic after delivery.

Abruption of the placenta is to be suspected in the presence of the following signs:

■ bleeding after 20 weeks' gestation
■ uterine irritability manifesting in frequent uterine contractions (more than five contractions in 10 minutes) or uterine hypertonus
■ uterine tenderness or backache
■ evidence of fetal compromise on electronic fetal monitoring.

The presence of retroplacental hematoma is suggested by the finding on ultrasound examination of a thickened, heterogeneous placenta with rounded margins and intraplacental sonolucencies. The placenta may appear as much as 9 cm in thickness, compared to the normal 4–5 cm.[7] Ultrasound examination can exclude major congenital malformations. It markedly facilitates the differential diagnosis between abruption of the placenta and placenta previa. Advanced ultrasound equipment in the hands of an expert can contribute to a correct diagnosis of acute APH.

Prevention and treatment

Discontinuation or reduction of smoking and avoidance of street drugs provide considerable protection against abruption of the placenta. Appropriate treatment of chronic hypertension and timely delivery in case of preeclampsia also reduce the risk of placental separation substantially.

Rapid decompression of the overdistended uterus is an uncommon cause of abruption but may occur in patients with polyhydramnios. Placental separation occurs with relative frequency after the delivery of the first twin. Therefore, it has been recommended that the second twin should be delivered within 20 minutes after the birth of the first one.[16]

Proper use of automobile safety belts protects against abruption. It needs to be remembered that the belt itself can cause damage. It is important to use both shoulder and lap belts, with the latter applied low at the level of the pelvic bones. The shoulder belt should be worn at the level of the chest, and not over the uterus. The position of the patient in the car should be upright with the headrest adjusted to avoid whiplash injury.[8]

Placental abruption has a tendency to recur in subsequent gestations. Therefore, elective delivery at 37–38 weeks' gestation appears to be a reasonable policy for those who have had a previous abruption.

The management of antepartum bleeding in early pregnancy requires mature medical judgment. The viability of the fetus at a given gestational age must be measured against the likely impact of the bleeding upon maternal and fetal well-being and the long-range outlook for the pregnancy in the case of expectant management.

Patients with evidence of separation of the placenta must be hospitalized. Fresh blood was used in the past for blood replacement. In contemporary practice, blood component therapy, which reduces the risk of infection, is preferred. For the treatment of DIC, fresh-frozen plasma (FFP) is used to correct coagulation defects. FFP contains factors V and VIII, fibrinogen, and other coagulation factors. When the bleeding is severe, platelet and red cell concentrates may be needed along with albumin or plasma. The transfusion of packed red blood cells is ideal for increasing the oxygen-carrying capacity of the patient's blood.

FFP should be administered in the face of liver disease, coagulation defects, thrombotic and thrombocytopenic purpura, and antithrombin III deficiency. It should be given when the prothrombin time and/or activated partial thromboplastin time values are more than 1.5 times normal or when obvious small vessel bleeding is encountered. Two to four units are usually given at a time. One unit should increase each clotting factor by 2–3%.

Platelet transfusion is advised when the patient's platelets are deficient in number or function. Thrombocytopenia is likely to result when 1.5–2 times the woman's blood volume has been transfused, or in the case of consumptive or dilutional coagulopathy. Platelet transfusion is also indicated if the platelet count falls below 20 000, if operative intervention is planned, or if the blood loss continues with a platelet count of 50 000 or fewer. One unit of platelets per 10 kg body weight should be given. Cryoprecipitate is often given in case of declining fibrinogen levels out of proportion to other coagulation factors. Although it is tempting to try to restore hemoglobin levels to normal during resuscitation, a hematocrit of 30–35% represents a good compromise between oxygen-carrying capacity and blood viscosity.

The first fluid given should be crystalloid solution. The circulation parameters should show improvement after the infusion of 1–2 l. Thereafter, two units of cross-matched blood are customarily given. If sudden severe hemorrhage occurs, there is no reason for delaying resuscitation. The main fluid loss is from the circulation, since significant shift of fluid from the interstitial space could not yet have occurred. The fluid should be blood or colloid. Two to three milliliters of crystalloid solution should be given for each estimated milliliter of blood loss to maintain normovolemia. Prompt and vigorous treatment of shock is required to avoid insufficient renal perfusion and ensuing renal failure. Hypovolemic shock, when prolonged, may lead to DIC. The fluid therapy is to be based upon the following measurements:[11]

- blood pressure
- pulse rate
- blood indices
- urine output
- core-peripheral temperature difference
- serum electrolyte and acid–base levels
- clotting studies
- in selected cases, central venous pressure determinations.

Accurate intake-output recording is a critical aspect of the management. Adequate kidney function is indicated by a urine output of 30 ml/hour or more.

In severe preeclampsia, normal volume expansion with crystalloids may not be sufficient. Therefore, it is advisable to administer 500 ml 5% albumin with every 4 l crystalloid solution.

Dehydration and acidosis are frequent sequelae of severe hemorrhage from abruption. Adequate fluid replacement and provision of adequate calories are required to correct acidosis. Should these measures fail, intravenous administration of sodium bicarbonate may be required. If urine output is less than 30 ml/hour, the use of diuretics may need to be considered.[10]

Method of delivery

The management of abruption of the placenta depends upon the severity of the bleeding, the length of the gestation, and the maternal and fetal conditions. Cesarean section is the choice if the bleeding is severe and the fetus is still alive.[17] Only if the delivery is imminent can the vaginal route be considered. However, in case of mild abruption with no evidence of fetal compromise, a trial of labor is acceptable, provided the labor progresses according to Friedman's criteria[18] and is well tolerated by the maternal-fetal pair.[15]

The liberal use of cesarean section has decreased perinatal mortality substantially.[18] The time interval between the occurrence of the abruption and delivery has considerable bearing upon the prospect of neonatal survival.[19] It needs to be borne in mind that, in this clinical entity, the time between the first appearance of fetal distress and *in utero* fetal demise may be short.

Renal failure and clotting defects due to hemorrhage do not represent a contraindication to abdominal delivery. However, vigorous blood replacement is important when prompt surgical intervention is deemed necessary. When the outlook for vaginal delivery is favorable and a trial of labor is decided upon, amniotomy is recommended.[1] Continuous electronic fetal heart rate monitoring is critically important. Recurrent hemorrhage or sign of deterioration in the fetal condition requires abandonment of the original plan and delivery by the abdominal route without any delay. In view of this ever existing possibility, the operating room must be kept in emergency readiness whenever a patient is in labor against a background of abruption of the placenta.

After the abruption of the placenta, spontaneous onset of labor frequently ensues. In such cases, the progress of the labor tends to be rapid. If otherwise, uterine stimulation with oxytocin is required.

Whereas in the middle of the twentieth century most cases of placental abruption were managed by induction of labor and eventual vaginal delivery, by the 1980s, abdominal delivery was the treatment of choice in the USA.[20] This change in philosophies contributed to the dramatic reduction of perinatal mortality rates during the last decades of the twentieth century (Figure 18.2).

In case of *in utero* fetal death, the preferred management is amniotomy followed by oxytocin stimulation. Hysterotomy may be still necessary, however, when the attempt is unsuccessful, insofar as both placental abruption and the presence of a dead fetus predispose to coagulation defects.[21]

Postpartum hemorrhage frequently follows delivery in connection with abruption of the placenta as a result of a clotting defect or uterine atony. On this account, routine infusion of oxytocin during the third stage of labor is advisable. It is to be remembered that, once delivery has been effected and all products of conception have been removed from the uterus, spontaneous correction of the bleeding and clotting defects can be anticipated within hours.

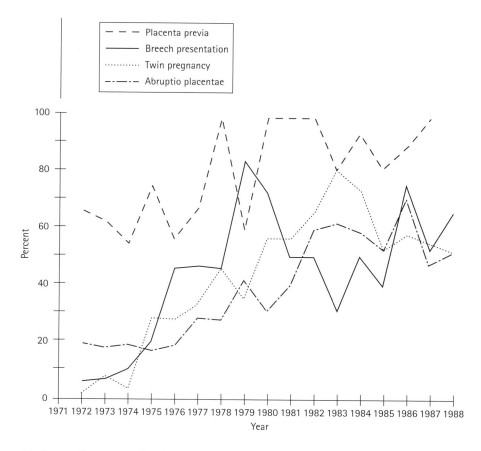

Figure 18.2 Trends with regard to the use of cesarean sections in various pathologic conditions of pregnancy between 1972 and 1988 (placenta previa, breech presentation, twin pregnancy, and abruption of the placenta) reported by Nimmo et al.[19] Note the increasing use of cesarean sections in connection with each of the quoted pathologic entities.

Placenta Previa

Next to abruption, placenta previa is the most frequent cause of APH. This phenomenon, which occurs only in menstruating primates, involves implantation of the placenta over or in the proximity of the internal os of the cervix. It occurs in about 1 out of 200 term pregnancies. It is a matter of interest that the majority of lower-segment implantations result in abortion, and only a minority progress beyond week 20 of the gestation.[15] Depending on the site of the implantation, various degrees of low implantation have been distinguished in the literature.[21]

(1) *Central placenta previa.* The placenta completely overlaps the internal os.
(2) *Partial placenta previa.* The edge of the placenta overlaps the internal os partially but not completely.
(3) *Marginal placenta previa.* The placenta reaches but does not overlap any part of the internal os.
(4) *Low-lying placenta.* This term has no generally accepted interpretation. It refers to a situation when the lowest margin of the placenta is close to the internal os of the cervix. It appears reasonable to consider the implantation low-lying when the distance between the lowermost limit of the placenta and the margin of the internal os is less than 2 cm.

During labor, in the process of cervical dilation, the relationship between the placenta and the cervical os changes. In this process, a previously central placenta previa may turn into a partial one. This distinction is more of academic than practical interest, insofar as the management is not significantly dependent upon the type of the implantation.

The placenta appears implanted over the lower segment with relative frequency on ultrasound examinations performed during the early second trimester. However, in about 90% of the instances, this impression turns out to be a technical error and the presumptive diagnosis of previa is ruled out by subsequent ultrasound examinations performed during the third trimester.[22] This phenomenon is often incorrectly referred to in the literature as 'placental migration'.

Under normal circumstances, the fertilized ovum implants on the endometrium of the uterine corpus. Whereas this is invariably the pattern of the implantation in lower animals, implantation in menstruating primates occurs with relative frequency on the lower uterine segment in the proximity of the internal os of the cervix. Eventually, in the process of its development, the placenta reaches or even overlaps with the internal os. This type of implantation represents the clinical entity of placenta previa. High maternal age, previous infertility, multiparity, and history of a variety of reproductive abnormalities, as well as previous occurrence of low implantation, predispose to the occurrence of placenta previa. Particularly strong predisposing factors are previous delivery by cesarean section and myomectomies that invade the uterine cavity.[6,15,23] Four centuries ago, Mauriceau proposed that placenta previa resulted from the fertilized ovum falling from the fundus of the uterus to its lower segment as a result of gravity.[23] This idea has been incorporated in the 'flux theory'. The latter interpretation offers the following mechanism: luteal phase defect, involving delayed ovulation, is followed by postconception ('placental sign') bleeding. The latter displaces the migrating blastocyst onto the lower segment of the uterus or, by an equal chance, to an ectopic site.[16] Then implantation occurs. The fact that the fertilized ovum tends to implant at the site of a previous cesarean section incision supports the theory that mechanical factors play a causative role in the occurrence of this entity. With the exploding cesarean section rate, that of placenta previa also increased substantially in recent years.

It has been reported that the incidence of fetal growth retardation is increased in connection with placenta previa.[24] In contrast, pregnancy-induced hypertension appears to be rare in the presence of low implantation of the placenta.[25]

Signs and symptoms

The typical manifestation of placenta previa is painless vaginal bleeding during the second half of the gestation. However, spotting or bleeding, interpreted as threatening abortion, can be discovered with relative frequency in the background of these cases.[26] The first episode of bleeding virtually never causes maternal demise, nor does it threaten the life of the fetus.[16] However, subsequent bleeding episodes can endanger the lives of both.

The magnitude of the bleeding is commensurate with the degree of detachment of the placenta from the implantation site. The hemorrhage tends to increase in severity episodically, and the time intervals between these episodes tend to be shorter and shorter. Eventually, after several recurrent bleeding incidents, both the mother and the fetus may lose enough blood to become anemic. This sequence of events is conducive to neonatal respiratory distress syndrome after delivery.

In the past, on rare occasions, patients with placenta previa remained asymptomatic, and thus undiagnosed, until the onset of labor at or near term. This is now rare, as the widespread use of ultrasound antepartum, leads to timely diagnosis in the overwhelming majority of the instances.[27] Placenta previa is to be included in the differential diagnosis whenever vaginal bleeding occurs during the second half of the pregnancy. On external examination, the uterus is usually found to be soft and non-tender. The presenting part is frequently above the pelvic inlet because the low-implanted placenta prevents engagement. For the same reason, breech presentation and transverse lie occur with relative frequency in connection with this pathologic entity.[28]

Digital vaginal examination in suspected placenta previa is absolutely contraindicated. The initial examination in APH must be limited to speculum examination. This usually reveals a normal-appearing closed cervix, often covered by blood or clots.

Until the mid-1970s, the differential diagnosis between placenta previa and abruption of the placenta largely rested upon radiologic studies. The arrival of ultrasonography made the radiologic investigations outdated.[29] The site of the implantation of an anteriorly implanted, low-lying placenta is easy to detect with contemporary ultrasound technology. On the other hand, the exact localization of the posteriorly implanted placenta may be difficult. Maternal obesity, distended bladder, and uterine activity may hinder the diagnosis in these cases. The rate of error with transabdominal sonography is in the range of 2–6%.[30] The visualization of the internal cervical os is facilitated by transvaginal sonography. In expert hands, such examination can be performed with relative ease without eliciting bleeding.

Management

As late as the mid-nineteenth century, the maternal mortality rate from placenta previa was at the range of 25%. The introduction of combined external-internal fetal version from vertex to breech by Braxton-Hicks intended to improve this sinister picture. However, unfortunately, it actually increased the rate of maternal mortality to 50% until, after almost two decades of routine use, this ill-advised intervention was abandoned. Irrespective of the method of delivery, the fetal mortality rate was almost 100% until the introduction of cesarean section into obstetric practice.

By the turn of the twentieth century, cesarean section could be performed with relative safety by obstetric surgeons. Soon it became the standard method of delivery in cases of placenta previa. As a result, the maternal mortality rate fell to 5% by the early 1900s, and the majority of babies could be delivered alive. By the 1920s, cesarean section was used liberally for the management of placenta previa. At that time, the maternal mortality rate was as low as 2%, despite the fact that blood transfusion and antibiotics were still more than a decade away.[30]

The general principles governing the management of bleeding from placenta previa in the late second and early third trimesters resemble those previously outlined in connection with abruption of the placenta, including laboratory investigations, fetal surveillance, and stabilization of the maternal circulatory status. The diagnosis having been established, the management decision rests upon the length of the gestation, the degree of the bleeding, and the fetal condition.

Recurrent and severe bleeding episodes often necessitate delivery long before term. The high incidence of premature delivery still translates into a relatively high rate of perinatal morbidity (up to 4–5% in contemporary practice). For the same reason, the rates of both short and long neonatal morbidity are increased. Neonatal anemia necessitating blood transfusion is a frequent complication.

The idea of delaying cervical dilation and, thus the occurrence of bleeding from placenta previa, by cerclage has emerged again and again during the last decades.[31–33] However, the results in the practices of most physicians have been less than convincing. Thus, there is no solid evidence to support its routine use.

When delivery is delayed for more than 24 hours after the establishment of the diagnosis of placenta previa, the management is labeled 'expectant'.[33] When this management pattern is feasible, liberal hospitalization of the patient is warranted. In some obstetric services, patients with placenta previa are kept in hospital from the time of the first episode of bleeding until delivery, since the magnitude of the hemorrhage is not predictable and 1 or 2 hours' delay may make the difference between fetal – and occasionally even maternal – life and death. Beginning in the 1930s, week 37 of gestation was considered the optimum time for abdominal delivery. However, against the background of modern neonatal life-supporting technology, it seems questionable whether delay beyond the 35th completed week is warranted in case of any significant degree of hemorrhage from placenta previa. Elective cesarean section may have lower maternal and fetal risks than emergency surgery performed against the background of life-endangering hemorrhage.

The occurrence of significant bleeding beyond week 20 of pregnancy is the harbinger of a poor prognosis. In the majority of these instances, termination of the pregnancy becomes inevitable before the completed week 28 of the gestation.[34]

The cornerstone of 'expectant management' is the maintenance of maternal blood indices above a hematocrit concentration of 30%. Therefore, with any type of APH, blood transfusion is used more liberally than in other types of blood loss. Maternal hypotension and hypovolemia tend to reduce uterine blood flow, leading to fetal hypoxia. Beta-mimetic agents increase these effects and, for this reason as well as for others, are not recommended for the suppression of the uterine activity that accompanies abruption of the placenta and, less frequently, bleeding from placenta previa. Magnesium sulfate has fewer adverse cardiovascular side effects, and may be given when APH is associated with preeclampsia.

Prophylactic corticosteroids for the acceleration of fetal lung and brain maturity are routinely used when, because of APH, the possible need for premature delivery emerges. It needs to be remembered, furthermore, that the occurrence of third-trimester bleeding warrants the administration of anti-D immunoglobulin in Rh-negative, nonimmunized mothers.

A minority of American obstetricians feel that patients with placenta previa can be managed on an outpatient basis if the blood indices of the gravida are favorable (hemoglobin 11 gm/dl and hematocrit above 35%). It this management is elected, the patient must rest at home under supervision and under circumstances that permit her immediate transfer to the hospital when the next bleeding episode occurs. According to one study, the delivery can be delayed longer when the patient is kept in a hospital environment and, as a result, of the two alternatives, the institutional care appears more cost-effective.[33]

Technique of delivery

Cesarean section should be performed when the fetus is deemed mature. The goal is delivery by week 36 or after fetal lung maturity has been demonstrated.

Cesarean section for placenta previa can be extremely difficult. The most commonly encountered problem is hemorrhage. The site of the uterine incision should be chosen cautiously in order to avoid, if possible, the necessity of cutting through the placenta before the delivery of the fetus. The surgical difficulties depend largely upon the site of the placental implantation. When the placental implantation is anterior, it may be necessary to cut through the placenta in order to reach the fetus *in utero*. This is a potentially dangerous procedure since the bleeding deriving from the incision of the placenta is fetal blood. Thus, significant delay may cause fetal exsanguination. As a rule of thumb, anterior implantation hinders the entry but, in the absence of invasion of the myometrium by the placenta, facilitates the surgical control of the bleeding that inevitably occurs. In contrast, when the implantation is posterior, entry into the uterine cavity and removal of the fetus entail little difficulty. However, since the posterior aspect of the lower segment of the uterus does not contract well, control of the hemorrhage arising from the implantation site may create difficulties. Whatever is done, it should be done quickly and efficiently in order to minimize blood loss.

For a variety of reasons, the degree of intraoperative hemorrhage is unpredictable. Therefore, the preparation for cesarean section in connection with placenta previa must be thorough and farsighted. The surgical team must be prepared to handle extreme difficulties that require exceptional measures. These may include uterine artery ligation, hypogastric artery ligation, or cesarean hysterectomy.

Because the lower uterine segment cannot contract efficiently, the degree of hemorrhage that follows the removal of the products of conception is dependent, to a great extent, upon the site of the implantation of the placenta. When the previa is central and thus covers the internal cervical os, profuse bleeding is the rule. Lesser degrees of previa described as 'partial, marginal and lateral', tend to bleed less and less (Figure 18.3). Since the placental bed lies directly on poorly contractile uterine muscle in these circumstances, the operative team should be prepared for massive hemorrhage at delivery of the placenta. The blood replacement must keep pace with the blood loss in such instances. Thus, close cooperation among the members of the team is essential. In order to minimize the risks that the entry into the uterus entails in case of incision of the placenta, some surgeons prefer classical cesarean section to the lower-segment transverse approach in connection with placenta previa. This approach may be particularly useful when the lower uterine segment is poorly developed (less than 34 weeks' gestation). With this approach, the time between the uterine incision and the removal of the fetus can be shortened.

The religious convictions of Jehovah's Witnesses lead them to refuse transfusion of blood and other blood components. In such cases, detailed discussion of the risks and benefits of the available alternatives is of particular importance. Since the relevant laws vary from state to state and because the state laws have changed with relative frequency in recent years, an all-inclusive policy with regard to the management of patients who refuse blood transfusion cannot be provided.[35] There are general policies in most institutions, however, with regard to the 'bloodless surgery' program. The implementation of the relevant policies often involves many facilities and disciplines, including the pharmacy, the administration, the hematologist, the surgeon, the anesthesiologist, and the blood bank, as well as other specialists and subspecialists.

The decision-to-delivery interval in case of emergency cesarean section is an important factor. Undue delay and hasty action both may entail risks.[36,37] In the USA, a 30-minute start-up time is generally considered feasible in the environment of a properly equipped obstetric unit. In the case of APH, the decision-to-incision time needs to be reduced further. It is not always possible to dictate precise guidelines. The obstetrician must decide when further attempts at less radical treatment will be futile and the decision to perform a cesarean section must be made.

Perinatal mortality

Maternal death in connection with placenta previa is extremely rare in contemporary practice. Exceptions are those instances where the low implantation of the placenta is complicated by chorionic invasion of the lower uterine segment. With this complication, the maternal mortality rate still may approach 5%.

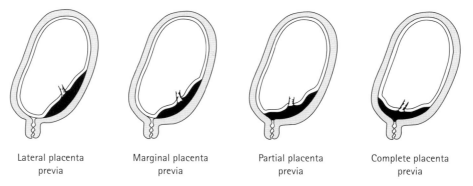

| Lateral placenta previa | Marginal placenta previa | Partial placenta previa | Complete placenta previa |

Figure 18.3 Various types of placenta previa according to the implantation sites. (This illustration was contributed to the first edition by Drs Kjell Haram, Per Bergsjo and Magnar Ulstein. ©2006 Leslie Iffy.)

The prospects for the fetus have changed vastly since the precesarean section days, when fetal death was the rule whenever the placental implantation involved the lower uterine segment. Before and during World War II, the perinatal mortality was still 25% in New York City. By the 1980s, the reported mortality rate ranged between 42 and 81 per 1000.[34,35] At the end of the same decade, the mortality rate was 67 per 1000 in Norway.[7] It is probably fair to say that during the first decade of the twenty-first century, the perinatal mortality rate does not exceed 5% in American centers.

Placenta accreta and percreta

When the chorionic villi invade the myometrium, the technical term is 'placenta accreta'. Deficient development of the endometrial decidua predisposes to deep penetration of the uterine wall by the chorionic villi. The extent of placental invasion appears to be influenced by the nature and condition of the uterine tissues at the implantation site. The invasion can be extensive enough to allow the placenta to burrow through the wall of the lower uterine segment and to invade the urinary bladder.[38] A previous cesarean section increases the risks of both placenta previa and placenta accreta exponentially.[39,40] This development has important clinical consequences. When placenta previa occurs in a scarred uterus, the need for hysterectomy, necessitated by severe hemorrhage, has been found to be as high as 16% compared with a 3.6% risk when placenta previa occurs in an unscarred uterus.[41] Over three decades ago, it was reported that when the complication of placenta previa-accreta was treated without the performance of hysterectomy, the maternal mortality rate was as high as 42%.[42]

Extensive preparations for any surgical procedure involving placenta previa after a previous cesarean section is of great importance as placenta accreta or placenta percreta may be encountered.[43] These preparations should include the placement of two intravenous lines as well as the availability of several units of cross-matched blood. It needs to be remembered that adhesions caused by the preceding surgery may hinder the performance of an emergency hysterectomy. It is necessary, therefore, to release all adhesions that may hinder quick removal of the uterus in an emergency situation.

Placenta percreta, that is, complete penetration of the entire thickness of the uterus, is a life-threatening obstetric complication. In this clinical entity, the placenta may invade the bladder as well as other pelvic structures. While a rare complication in the USA, it is a relatively frequent one (1 out of 540 deliveries) in Thailand. This high incidence is probably related to the high prevalence of trophoblastic disease in the Far East.[44]

Placenta percreta can present at any gestational age between week 8 and term. Predisposing factors include the scar of the previous cesarean section, previous dilation and curettage, advanced maternal age, retained products of conception, previous endometritis, and past trophoblastic disease.[21] Previous

cesarean sections also increase the risk of placenta previa-accreta. Recent trends favoring abdominal delivery in a variety of high-risk situations have already resulted in a sharp increase in the rate of occurrence of placenta previa-accreta.[45]

Early recognition of invasive growth of the placenta implanted over the lower uterine segment is conducive to favorable outcome because it provides an opportunity for the obstetrician to deal effectively with this complication. Since placenta accreta-percreta is asymptomatic throughout pregnancy, its early diagnosis requires a high level of suspicion and awareness of the predisposing factors. Early diagnosis may be possible with the use of real time ultrasound, Doppler studies, and magnetic resonance imaging. Ultrasound examination of all gravidas with a history of previous cesarean section is extremely important. One should determine the location of the placenta and search for venous lakes penetrating the myometrium. The ultrasound findings suggestive of placental invasion include absence of thinning of the myometrium, lacunar spaces or 'Swiss cheese' appearance in the placental parenchyma, abnormalities in the interface between the uterus and the bladder, and extension of the placental tissue beyond the uterine serosa. Management options for this entity include elective cesarean hysterectomy on the one hand and abdominal delivery with conservative management and retention of the placenta on the other.[46] Cesarean hysterectomy has been long regarded as the management of choice. However, it carries a high maternal morbidity rate, including both physical and psychological consequences, as well as the loss of fertility.[47] Conservative management leaving the placenta in situ is an attractive alternative, which frequently permits the avoidance of massive intraoperative hemorrhage as well as the loss of the uterus. A fast-growing opinion supports the view that the conservative approach, rather than cesarean hysterectomy, should be the first line of management in cases of placenta accreta-percreta.[48]

Bleeding from an aberrant vessel

Vasa previa is said to be present when fetal vessels, unsupported by placenta or umbilical cord, traverse the membranes on their way to a velamentous umbilical cord. A less frequent type of vasa previa involves the passage of vessels between lobes of the placenta (placenta bilobata and placenta succenturiata). Rupture of the membranes, whether spontaneous or artificial, may cause rupture of some of the vessels passing over the membranes, leading to rapid fetal exsanguination.[49] The reported fetal mortality rate in this condition is 33–100%.[50]

Velamentous insertion of the umbilical cord, which is a prerequisite for vasa previa, occurs in about 1% of singleton and 10% of multiple gestations.

On rare occasions, even in the absence of bleeding, compression of aberrant vessels may cause hypoxia and even fetal demise. Apart from artificial rupture of the membranes, bleeding from an aberrant vessel has been described in connection with the placement of a fetal scalp electrode. This complication is particularly lethal when it occurs in connection with a twin gestation.

Traditionally, the diagnosis of bleeding from an aberrant vessel rested upon the following triad:

(1) spontaneous or artificial rupture of the membranes
(2) occurrence of bleeding shortly after the rupture of the membranes
(3) evidence of fetal distress on electronic monitoring within seconds or minutes after events (1) and (2).

It is intuitive that prevention of perinatal mortality would depend on prenatal diagnosis of this condition and abdominal delivery before rupture of the membranes occurs. For this reason, standard obstetric ultrasound protocols should probably be modified to include screening for vasa previa. An attempt to identify placental umbilical cord insertion should probably be a routine part of second- and third-trimester, obstetric, ultrasound examinations. In women at increased risk (second-trimester, low-lying placenta pregnancies resulting from *in vitro* fertilization, and those with accessory placental lobes), a routine transvaginal color Doppler sonography of the region over the cervix, if vasa previa cannot be excluded by transabdominal sonography, could facilitate the diagnosis. Sonographic prenatal diagnosis has the potential to prevent fatal outcomes deriving from vasa previa.

Extrachorial placenta and APH

This anomaly describes a condition where the chorionic plate of the placenta is smaller than its basal plate. Thus, the villous tissue projects beyond the borders of the chorionic plate. When the placenta is 'circummarginata', the border between the villous and membranous chorion is provided by a flat ring of membrane. When the placenta is 'circumvallata', this marginal ring has raised edges. Between the extrachorial placenta and the fetal membranes, there is a decidual layer. The placenta is extrachorial in about 30% of all cases. The incidence of circumvallata is in the range 0.5–6.9%.[51] The diagnosis rests upon careful inspection of the placenta after delivery.

The clinical importance of placenta circummarginata is negligible. On the other hand, 25–50% of all patients with placenta circumvallata suffer APH secondary to separation of the placenta from the implantation site and bleeding from its margin. This hemorrhage often resembles the clinical manifestations of placenta previa. Although the bleeding is modest in most instances, it may occasionally result in second-trimester abortion, preterm delivery, and significant APH.

References

1. Green-Thompson RW. Antepartum haemorrhage. Clin Obstet Gynecol 1982; 9: 479–515.

2. Green JR. Placental abnormalities: placenta previa and abruptio placentae. In: Creasy RK, Resnik R (eds), Maternal-Fetal Medicine, p. 539. WB Saunders: Philadelphia, 1984.

3. Hibbard LT. Placenta previa. Am J Obstet Gynecol 1969; 104: 172–84.

4. Darby MJ, Caritis SN, Shen-Schwarz S. Placental abruption in preterm gestation: an association with chorioamnionitis. Obstet Gynecol 1989; 74: 88–92.

5. Gonen R, Hannah ME, Milligan JE. Does prolonged preterm rupture of the membranes predispose to abruptio placentae? Obstet Gynecol 1989; 73: 347–50.

6. Benedetti TJ. Obstetric hemorrhage. In: Gabbe SG, Niebyl JR, Simpson JL (eds), Obstetrics, p. 485. Churchill Livingstone: New York, 1986.

7. Nyberg DA, Finberg HJ. The placenta, placental membranes and umbilical cord. In: Nyberg DA, Mahony BS, Pretorius DH (eds), Diagnostic Ultrasound of Fetal Anomalies. Text and Atlas, p. 623. Yearbook Medical Publishers: Chicago, 1990.

8. Haram K, Bergsjo P, Ulstein M. Antepartum hemorrhage. In: Iffy L, Apuzzio JJ, Vintzileos AM (eds), Operative Obstetrics, p. 281. (2nd edition). McGraw-Hill: New York, 1992.

9. Pritchard JA. Haematological problems associated with delivery, placental abruption, retained dead fetus and amniotic fluid embolism. Clin Haematol 1973; 2: 563–86.

10. Harris BA Jr. Peripheral placental separation: a review. Obstet Gynecol Surv 1988; 43: 577–81.

11. Laros RK Jr. Coagulation disorders in pregnancy. In: Iffy L, Kaminetzky HA (eds), Principles and Practice of Obstetrics & Perinatology, p. 1121. Wiley: New York, 1981.

12. Stander HJ. Hemorrhage. In: Stander HJ, Henricus J (eds), Textbook of Obstetrics, p. 939 (3rd edition). Appleton-Century: New York, 1945.

13. Kaunitz AM, Hughes JM, Grimes DA et al. Causes of maternal mortality in the United States. Obstet Gynecol 1985; 65: 605–12.

14. Ananth CV, Wilcox AJ. Placental abruption and perinatal mortality in the United States. Am J Epidemiol 2001, 153: 332–7.

15. Hladky K, Yankovitz J, Hansen WF. Placental abruption. Obstet Gynecol Surv 2002; 57: 299–305.

16. Kelly JV, Iffy L. Placenta previa. In: Iffy L, Kaminetzky HA (eds), Principles and Practice of Obstetrics & Perinatology, p. 1105. Wiley: New York, 1981.

17. Barron SL. Antepartum haemorrhage. In: Turnbull A, Chamberlain G (eds), Obstetrics, p. 469. Churchill Livingstone: Edinburgh, 1989.

18. Friedman EA. Monitoring the labor process. In: Iffy L, Charles D (eds), Operative Perinatology, p. 477. Macmillan: New York, 1984.

19. Nimmo RA, Murphy GA, Adhate A et al. Factors affecting perinatal mortality in an urban center. Natl Med Assoc J 1991; 83: 147–52.

20. Hurd WW, Miodovnik M, Hertzberg V et al. Selective management of abruptio placentae: a prospective study. Obstet Gynecol 1983; 61: 467–73.

21. Breen JL, Neubecker R, Gregori CA et al. Placenta accreta, increta and percreta. Obstet Gynecol 1977; 49: 43–7.

22. Newton ER, Barss V, Cetrulo CL. The epidemiology and clinical history of asymptomatic midtrimester placenta previa. Am J Obstet Gynecol 1984; 148: 743–8.

23. Mauriceau F. Les Maladies des femmes grosses, et accouchées. Chez l'Auteur: Paris, 1968.

24. Gabert HA. Placenta previa and fetal growth. Obstet Gynecol 1971; 38: 403–6.

25. Nicolaides KH, Faratian B, Symonds EM. Effect on low implantation of the placenta on maternal blood pressure and placental function. Br J Obstet Gynaecol 1982; 89: 806–10.

26. Nyberg DA, Mack LA, Benedetti TJ et al. Placental abruption and placental hemorrhage: correlation of sonographic findings with fetal outcome. Radiology 1987; 164: 357–61.

27. Chapman MG, Furness ET, Jones WR et al. Significance of the ultrasound location of placental site in early pregnancy. Br J Obstet Gynaecol 1979; 86: 846–8.

28. Hibbard BM, Hibbard ED. Etiological factors in abruptio placentae. BMJ 1963; 2: 1430–6.

29. Farine D, Fox HG, Jakobson S, Timor-Tritisch IE. Vaginal ultrasound for diagnosis of placenta previa. Am J Obstet Gynecol 1988; 159: 566–9.

30. Bill AH. The treatment of placenta previa by prophylactic blood transfusion and cesarean section. Am J Obstet Gynecol 1927; 14: 523.

31. Lovset J. Preventive treatment of severe bleeding in placenta previa. Acta Obstet Gynecol Scand 1959; 38: 551–4.

32. Arias AG. Abdominal pain in pregnancy. In: Turnbull A, Chamberlin G (eds), Obstetrics, p. 605. Churchill Livingstone: Edinburgh, 1989.

33. Silver R, Depp R, Sabbagha RE et al. Placenta previa: aggressive expectant management. Am J Obstet Gynecol 1984; 150: 15–22.

34. McShane PM, Heyl PS, Epstein ME. Maternal and perinatal morbidity resulting from placenta previa. Obstet Gynecol 1985; 65: 176–82.

35. Loriau J, Manaouil C, Montpellier D et al. Surgery and transfusion in Jehovah's Witness patient. Ann Chir 2004; 129: 263–8.

36. Hillemanns P, Hasbargen U, Strauss A et al. Maternal and neonatal morbidity of emergency cesarean section with a decision-to-delivery interval under 30 minutes: evidence of 10 years. Arch Gynecol Obstet 2003; 268: 136–41.

37. MacKenzie IZ, Cooke I. What is a reasonable time from decision-to-delivery by cesarean section? Evidence from 415 deliveries. Br J Obstet Gynaecol 2002; 109: 498–504.

38. Weckstein LN, Masserman JSH, Garite TJ. Placenta accreta: a problem of increasing clinical significance. Obstet Gynecol 1987; 69: 480–2.

39. Clark SL, Koonings PP, Phelan JP. Placenta previa/accreta and prior cesarean section. Obstet Gynecol 1985; 66: 89–92.

40. Hung TH, Shau WY, Hsieh CC et al. Risk factors for placenta accreta. Obstet Gynecol 1999; 93: 545–50.

41. Nielsen TF, Hagberg H, Ljungblad U. Placenta previa and antepartum hemorrhage after previous cesarean section. Gynecol Obstet Invest 1989; 27: 88–90.

42. McHattie TJ. Placenta previa accreta. Obstet Gynecol 1972; 40: 795–8.

43. Piya-Anant M. Management of previous caesarean section presented with placenta previa. J Med Assoc Thailand 1987; 70: 673–7.

44. Cox SM, Carpenter RJ, Cotton DB. Placenta percreta: ultrasound diagnosis and conservative surgical management. Obstet Gynecol 1988; 71: 454–6.

45. Armstrong CA, Harding S, Matthews T et al. Is placenta accreta catching up with us? Aust NZ J Obstet Gynaecol 2004; 44: 210–13.

46. O'Brien JM, Barton JR, Donaldson ES. The management of placenta percreta: conservative and operative strategies. Am J Obstet Gynecol 1996; 175: 1632–8.

47. Bennett MJ, Sen RC. 'Conservative' management of placenta previa percreta: report of two cases and discussion of current management options. Aust NZ J Obstet Gynaecol 2003; 43: 249–51.

48. Panoskaltsis TA, Ascarelli A, De Souza N et al. Placenta increta: evaluation of radiological investigations and therapeutic options of conservative management. Br J Obstet Gynecol 2000; 107: 802–6.

49. Oyelese Y, Catanzarite V, Prefumo F et al. Vasa previa: the impact of prenatal diagnosis on outcomes. Obstet Gynecol 2004; 103: 937–42.

50. Schachter M, Tovbin Y, Arieli S et al. In vitro fertilization is a risk factor for vasa previa. Fertil Steril 2002; 78: 642–3.

51. Fox H. Pathology of the Placenta, p. 107, WB Saunders: Philadelphia, 1978.

19 Intrapartum fetal monitoring

Yinka Oyelese

Rationale for intrapartum fetal monitoring

The main objective of intrapartum fetal heart-rate (FHR) monitoring is to prevent stillbirth and hopefully fetal brain damage resulting from oxygen deprivation in labor. Until the nineteenth century, cerebral palsy was attributed mainly to childhood febrile convulsions.[1] In 1861, William John Little, a British orthopedic surgeon, presented 47 cases of cerebral palsy at the Obstetrical Society of London.[2] He noted that, in the majority of cases, the pregnancies had been complicated by prematurity, birth trauma, or asphyxia at birth.[2] As a result of his work, it was felt for much of the next century that cerebral palsy resulted almost exclusively from oxygen deprivation in labor.[1] While auscultation of the fetal heart was first reported in 1818 by the Geneva surgeon François Mayor, who distinguished it from the maternal pulse,[1] it was Kergaradec, in 1822, who first described the FHR, and asked, 'Will it not be possible to judge the state of health or disease of the fetus from the variations that occur in the beat of the fetal heart?'[1] However, it was not until the twentieth century that FHR monitoring for the purpose of evaluation of fetal well-being became a reality. This was probably because, prior to the twentieth century, there were no safe interventions for delivery should intrauterine fetal compromise be detected. As a result, all obstetric interventions were aimed at maternal rather than fetal well-being. However, by the mid-1950s, with the advent of blood transfusion, improved surgical techniques, advances in safe anesthesia and asepsis, and the introduction of antibiotics, cesarean delivery had become a relatively safe procedure. It became possible to deliver a living newborn with the expectation that the mother would survive the surgical procedure without life-threatening complications.

In the late 1950s, Hon and colleagues at Yale introduced the electronic FHR monitor.[3] A few years later, in 1962, Saling developed a technique for measuring the fetal scalp capillary pH, oxygen saturation, and P_{co_2}.[4] Together, these two advances provided the foundation for intrapartum assessment of the fetus.

Labor exposes the fetus to considerable stress. During contractions, the pressure in the myometrium exceeds that in the uterine vessels. As a consequence, uterine blood flow supplying the placenta is interrupted during each contraction. Therefore, the fetus depends on the blood flow between contractions. Normally, the fetus has sufficient oxygen reserves to cope with the temporary isolation from its oxygen supply during uterine contractions. If there is no break between contractions, there are inadequate oxygen reserves, or uterine blood flow between contractions is compromised, the fetus will lose its ability to cope with the stress of labor. The analogy can be made to a person holding his or her breath under water. While it is possible to hold one's breath for 30 seconds, and surface for a breath of air every 30 seconds or so for an indefinite period, holding one's breath continuously for more than about 3–5 minutes without the ability to take a fresh breath will eventually lead to brain damage in most people. Intrapartum fetal assessment aims primarily at early detection of situations in which the fetus is deprived of sufficient oxygenation.

Abnormalities and aberrations of the FHR have become accepted as surrogate markers of potential fetal oxygen deprivation that could lead to fetal death or brain damage. Identification of some of these abnormalities of the FHR may allow timely obstetric intervention – most frequently cesarean delivery – thereby removing the fetus from the hostile environment and the ongoing stress of labor, with the potential of preventing fetal death or injury.

Fetal oxygen deprivation, especially during labor, may result from reduction of blood flow from the maternal circulation to the placenta and from the placenta to the fetus. These are termed 'uteroplacental insufficiency' and 'fetoplacental insufficiency', respectively. Fetal oxygen deprivation, on a biochemical level, is brought about by failure to maintain the function of the Krebs cycle for the production of adenosine triphosphate (ATP), which involves a shift to the Embden–Meyerhof pathway. With sufficient oxygen deprivation, the production of lactic acid causes the brain cell protoplasm to swell, resulting in lysis of the cell wall, and cell death, ultimately ending in fetal damage or death.

Uteroplacental insufficiency may be caused by inadequate exchange of oxygen and carbon dioxide in the intervillous space brought about by an inadequate blood supply reaching the space. This may have its clinical origin in primary disease of the placenta, maternal hypotension, uterine hyperactivity during labor, severe maternal anemia, or severe maternal hypoxemia. Fetoplacental insufficiency is the most common form of acute intrapartum fetal oxygen deprivation. In the form of umbilical cord compression, the potential for fetoplacental insufficiency is present in 30–90% of all fetuses during labor. It usually does not represent a major problem except when it is repetitive or severe. Examples of conditions that can result in severe fetoplacental insufficiency include cord prolapse and true knots of the cord.

The primary techniques techniques used for the assessment of fetal oxygenation during labor include monitoring of the FHR, fetal scalp capillary sampling for pH, fetal stimulation, evaluation of amniotic fluid for the presence of meconium, and, more recently, fetal pulse oximetry and ST analysis of the fetal electrocardiogram.

While evaluation of fetal movements has been utilized as a marker of fetal life in the antepartum period, with the onset of labor, both fetal movements and the mother's perception of them tend to decrease, making this form of assessment impracticable for the intrapartum determination of fetal oxygen deprivation. The biophysical profile, while widely used in the antepartum setting, is rarely used intrapartum, though a recent study suggested that it may have a role in fetal assessment in labor.[5]

Intermittent FHR monitoring

Intermittent FHR auscultation, performed according to the guidelines of the American College of Obstetricians and Gynecologists (ACOG), is considered acceptable by some authorities for fetal evaluation in almost all low-risk labors as well as in appropriately selected labors of high-risk patients.[6] After palpation of the patient's abdomen to identify fetal lie and position, a DeLee fetal stethoscope or hand-held Doppler device is used to listen to the fetal heart tones. Listening is done over the fetal back at the fetal chest level. In selected high-risk pregnancies, the ACOG recommends that the FHR be monitored every 15 minutes after a contraction in the first stage of labor, and every 5 minutes in the second stage of labor. In low-risk pregnancies, the FHR may be monitored every 30 minutes in the first stage and every 10–15 minutes in the second stage. It is important that the examiner takes the maternal pulse so as not to record it as the FHR in error. The examiner should also palpate the uterus regularly for contractions, and listen to the heart rate for at least 1 minute after each contraction. The FHR and the timing, duration, and intensity of contractions should be recorded in the patient's chart on each occasion. Studies that have demonstrated good outcomes with intermittent FHR monitoring have usually had one-on-one continuous care of the patient by a nurse or midwife throughout labor. Needless to say, the demands on personnel and time make this impracticable in most modern obstetric settings in the USA. The most common indications for continuous FHR monitoring are listed in Table 19.1.

Table 19.1 Indications for continuous heart monitoring

Labor after a prior cesarean
Diabetes
Prematurity
Suspected fetal growth restriction
Preeclampsia
Bleeding in pregnancy
Induction of labor
Augmentation of labor with oxytocin
Twins

Electronic FHR monitoring

The most widely used form of intrapartum fetal assessment is continuous electronic FHR monitoring (EFM). Normal FHR findings are highly predictive of a healthy fetus and newborn. Generally, the FHR is monitored by a Doppler ultrasound transducer placed on the mother's abdomen and secured by a strap. The transducer is placed so that it overlies the fetal back at the chest level. Doppler ultrasound detects the Doppler shift that occurs with movement of the atrioventricular heart valves; this is then translated into a heart rate by a microprocessor. Because the particular valve movement used to calculate the heart rate varies from one beat to the next, errors may result in the rate counting of these monitors. Therefore, autocorrelation is used to attempt to improve the accuracy of heart rate counting. A separate monitor, the tocodynamometer, attached by another strap, records uterine contractions. The tocodynamometer provides quantitative data on the frequency of contractions, semiquantitative data on the duration of contractions, and nonquantitative data on the amplitude or strength of contractions. Thus, both FHR and uterine activity are recorded simultaneously, usually on a continuous paper roll. The paper speed in the USA is usually 3 cm/minute, although in Europe the speed is 1 cm/minute. On the vertical scale are recorded the FHR in beats per minute (bpm), while on the lower scale uterine contractions are recorded.

Where it is not possible to obtain a satisfactory FHR tracing, usually due to maternal obesity, excessive fetal or maternal movement, or descent of the fetus in the birth canal in the second stage of labor, a small spiral electrode may be passed through the cervix and attached to the fetal scalp or buttocks. In order to attach the electrode, the membranes must be ruptured, and there must be sufficient cervical dilation to permit the placement of the electrode on the fetal scalp or buttocks. The electrocardiographic signal from the fetus is calculated by the R–R interval; this is recorded each time the fetal heart beats. Besides allowing more accurate assessment of the FHR, signal loss, a problem with external monitoring, is overcome in most circumstances when internal monitoring is used. Complications are infrequent. Nonetheless, fetal scalp abscess, cranial osteomyelitis, ocular penetrating injury, and leakage of cerebrospinal fluid have been reported in association with fetal scalp electrode monitoring.[7-10] Transmission of the maternal pulse via a fetal scalp electrode in a situation where there is a dead fetus has been described.[11]

Similarly, the intrauterine pressure catheters (IUPC) may be used to monitor the force of uterine contractions as well as their frequency in an objective manner. These are soft, pliable silicone or plastic catheters. Quantitative data relating to the duration, frequency, and amplitude of contractions are displayed continuously. This is particularly helpful in situations where there is failure of progress despite oxytocin augmentation, or when monitoring of uterine contractions is considered essential and cannot be achieved externally due to maternal obesity or fetal movement. The IUPC may also be used to infuse saline into the uterine cavity for the relief of variable decelerations or to dilute thick meconium. Most modern IUPCs have a clear channel through which the color of the amniotic fluid may be observed. Complications are rare, but include placental abruption, cord injury, and, very rarely, uterine rupture. Contraindications to invasive monitoring include active genital herpes, human immunodeficiency virus infection, and maternal hepatitis B infection.

Definitions and pathophysiology of FHR patterns

In an attempt to standardize the interpretation of electronic FHR patterns, a National Institute of Child Health and Human Development research planning workshop was convened in 1995 and 1996.[12] This workshop defined normal and abnormal FHR patterns, and made recommendations of areas for further research. These definitions were based on visual interpretations of the tracings, and on the 3 cm/minute paper speed. The report was careful not to attribute any etiology to any of the patterns. Patterns were defined as baseline, periodic, or episodic. Periodic patterns were defined as those associated with uterine contractions, while episodic patterns were not associated with contractions.

The components of the fetal heart tracing are as follows:

(1) the baseline rate
(2) baseline variability
(3) presence of accelerations
(4) periodic or episodic decelerations
(5) changes or trends of the FHR over time.

Examples of some normal and pathologic FHR patterns are given in Figures 19.1–19.3.

Baseline rate

The baseline refers to the average heart rate between periodic changes (accelerations and decelerations). The normal baseline FHR is 110–160 bpm.[12] However, rates of 90–180 bpm are not necessarily pathologic in the absence of other heart-rate abnor-

malities.[13] The baseline drops with gestational age as a consequence of vagal maturation of the fetus.[14-16] A baseline above 160 bpm is called tachycardia, and one below 110 bpm is bradycardia.[12] Fetal tachycardia may result from fever, thyrotoxicosis, intra-amniotic infection, fetal anemia, fetal tachyarrhythmia, and maternal administration of certain drugs, including beta-sympathomimetic tocolytics, and parasympatholytic agents such as atropine or scopolamine. Finally, fetal tachycardia may be a sign of fetal hypoxia. Fetal bradycardia may be the consequence of maternal administration of beta-blockers, such as propranolol. Mothers with systemic lupus erythematosus can produce antibodies that can cross the placenta and damage the conduction system in the fetal heart, causing congenital heart block and resultant fetal bradycardia.

Baseline variability

This refers to the variation of the heart rate from the baseline. Normal variability is highly predictive of a nonacidotic fetus[17] (Figure 19.1). FHR variability represents an interplay between the cardioaccelerator and cardioinhibitor centers in the fetal brainstem, and is regulated by the autonomic nervous system.[18] Physiologically, there is variability on a beat-by-beat basis of 3–8 bpm around the average. Fluctuations in long-term variability occur in 3–5 cycles per minute. When no baseline amplitude changes are detectable, variability is said to be absent. Minimal variability is 0–5 bpm. Amplitude changes of 6–25 bpm represent moderate variability, while amplitude exceeding 25 bpm is marked variability.[12] Short-term variability can be appreciated only when the heart rate is continuously and instantaneously calculated and recorded on a beat-by-beat basis, using the fetal electrocardiographic R wave signal to trigger the cardiotachometer. Long-term variability can be recognized by using an external ultrasonographic Doppler system. A persistent loss of variability is one of the most ominous characteristics of a FHR tracing.[17,19,20] Short periods of reduced variability (30–45 minutes or less) may be associated with fetal sleep. Administration of narcotics or sedatives in labor can also reduce variability. Exaggerated or increased fetal heart-rate variability (>25 bpm) may indicate a shift in the P_{O_2}–P_{CO_2} relationship, which the barochemoreceptors mediate. Without the presence of significant repetitive FHR deceleration, there is no significant clinical change in fetal oxygenation. Increased FHR variability followed by loss of beat-by-beat variability may indicate fetal oxygen deprivation.

Accelerations

An acceleration is defined as an abrupt increase in heart rate of greater than 15 bpm above baseline, and lasting longer than 15 seconds and less than 2 minutes from its onset to return to baseline (Figure 19.1).[12] A prolonged acceleration lasts 2–10 minutes. A persistent increase in baseline over 10 minutes is considered a baseline change. Accelerations are often associated with fetal movement or contractions, and are generally accepted as evidence of fetal well-being.

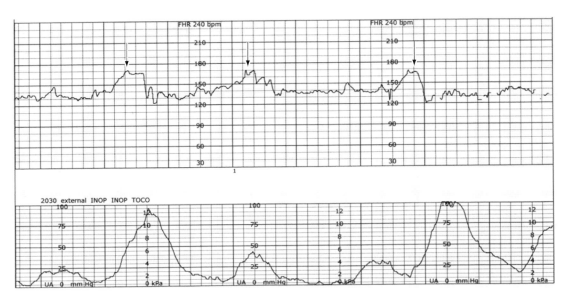

Figure 19.1 Normal reassuring intrapartum FHR tracing.

The upper tracing is of the FHR, while the lower tracing is of uterine contractions. The baseline heart rate of 135 is normal. There is good variability, accelerations are present (arrows), and there are no decelerations. Uterine contractions are occurring about every 1–2 minutes. FHR: fetal heart rate.

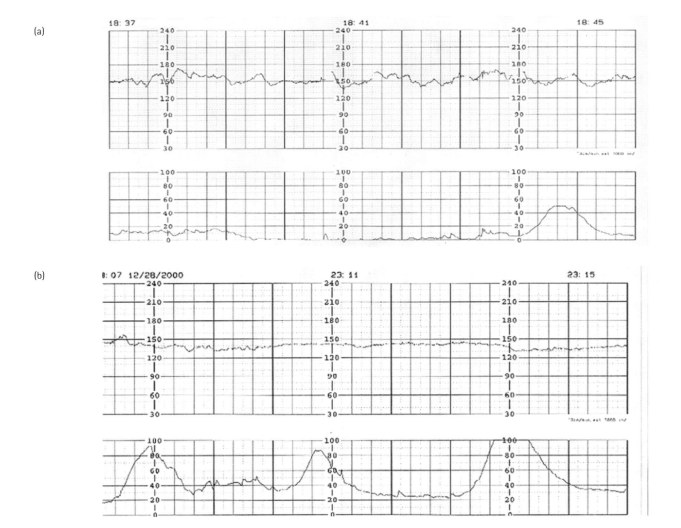

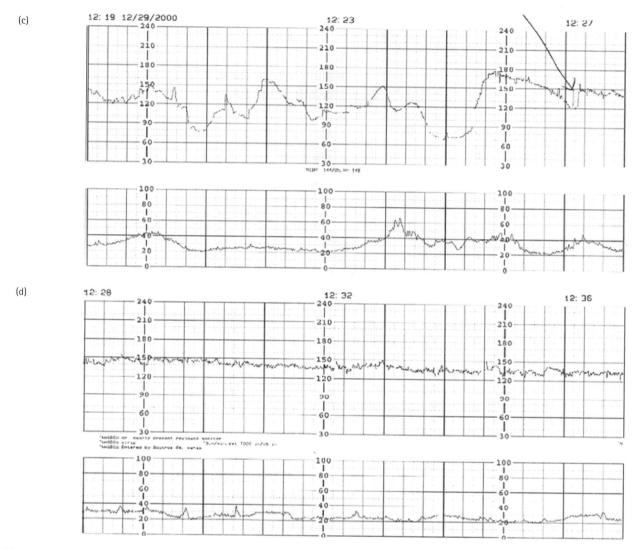

Figure 19.2. Normal and pathological FHR tracings

This series of fetal heart tracings demonstrates the progression of pathologic heart tracings in labor. They show the progression from a reassuring fetal heart tracing to one where variability is absent and where late decelerations occur. Subsequently, the baseline wanders and there are severe variable decelerations with a loss of variability. Finally, there is artifactual recording of the maternal heart. This case illustrates the need for vigilance when monitoring any patient in labor with a uterine scar. (a) The patient, a woman with a prior cesarean delivery for a breech at term, presented at term for a trial of labor. On admission, the fetal heart tracing was reassuring, with a normal baseline, good variability, no decelerations, and several accelerations. Uterine contractions were infrequent. (b) One and a half hours later. The FHR baseline is 130 bpm. Variability is absent to minimal. There are shallow late decelerations. Uterine contractions are occurring about every 3 minutes. (c) About 8 hours later. There are severe variable decelerations, with a loss of variability. The FHR baseline is wandering. A fetal scalp electrode was attached (arrow). Contractions are irregular. (d) The heart tracing recorded with a fetal scalp electrode attached to the fetal scalp. It appears that the FHR baseline is about 130, with an unusual pattern of variability. Accelerations are absent. There are no decelerations. At this time, the maternal pulse is also in the 130s. This heart rate pattern is of maternal origin. The infant was stillborn. At delivery, the uterus was found to be ruptured.

Decelerations

Decelerations refer to short-lasting decreases in FHR.

Late decelerations

A late deceleration is a *gradual* decrease and return to baseline FHR change associated with a uterine contraction where the nadir of the deceleration occurs after the peak of the contrac-tion.[12] Late decelerations are thought to represent uteroplacental insufficiency and decreased intervillous exchange between the fetus and the mother.[21,22] Initially, they may represent a vagally mediated reflex response, with normal heart-rate variability. However, late decelerations may be associated with fetal hypoxia, especially when there is an associated absence of variability.[17,22–25] They may occur with placental abruption,

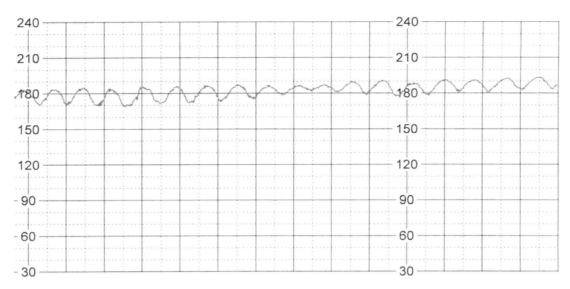

Figure 19.3 Sinusoidal fetal heart tracing.

excessive uterine activity (whether spontaneous or oxytocin-induced), maternal hypotension, anemia, or ketoacidosis. Even mildly repetitive late decelerations of only 5–10 bpm may indicate a sufficient degree of fetal oxygen deprivation to result in acidosis and brain damage. Persistent late decelerations may indicate fetal myocardial depression. At this point, loss of variability may occur along with reactive tachycardia. However, in a deteriorating or dying fetus, late decelerations may give way to marked bradycardia.

Early decelerations

An early deceleration is one in which there is a *gradual* decrease in FHR associated with a uterine contraction that is coincidental with the contraction (the nadir of the deceleration occurs simultaneously with the peak of the contraction). The FHR returns to the baseline promptly with the end of the contraction. Early decelerations are generally considered benign and are thought be caused by pressure on the fetal head during its descent down the birth canal in the active phase of labor, with a resultant reflex slowing of the heart rate mediated by the vagus nerve.

Variable decelerations

A variable deceleration is one where there is an *abrupt* decrease in FHR below the baseline, and where the decrease in FHR below the baseline is greater than 15 bpm, and lasts longer than 15 seconds and less than 2 minutes. Variable decelerations vary in timing, shape, depth, and duration. They are usually the result of cord compression.[26] The deceleration is mediated by the vagus nerve, and the degree of fall in heart rate is dependent on the degree of cord compression. Variable decelerations are frequently observed in breech presentations, with oligohydramnios, and when there is a nuchal cord, or the cord is around some other part of the fetus. As the umbilical cord is occluded, the fetal peripheral resistance increases, the fetal P_{O_2} falls, and the P_{CO_2} rises. Through the baroreceptors and chemoreceptors, a reflex release of acetylcholine at the sinoatrial node causes an almost instantaneous and somewhat erratic drop in FHR. Variable decelerations are the most common periodic FHR changes observed during labor. Often, they can be corrected by changing the maternal position.

With moderate and severe variable decelerations, a significant reduction in funic blood flow may occur with the accumulation of carbon dioxide in the fetal compartment, causing respiratory acidosis. With repetitive or prolonged variable decelerations, fetal metabolic acidosis may occur.[26] With marked oxygen deprivation, a delayed recovery in the FHR to the baseline level may develop. On occasion the FHR may fall below 60 bpm. Severe or deep variable decelerations should lead to a vaginal examination to rule out a cord prolapse or vasa previa.[27] Moreover, in patients undergoing a trial of labor after prior cesarean, variable decelerations may be the first sign of uterine rupture.[28] Finally, severe intrapartum variable decelerations may be a sign of intra-amniotic infection, especially in the premature fetus.[29]

Prolonged decelerations

Prolonged decelerations are decelerations that last more than 2 minutes, but less than 10 minutes. A deceleration greater than 10 minutes is a baseline change. Prolonged decelerations may unexpectedly occur during labor. The FHR may drop below 80 bpm; the deceleration may last for several minutes. These decelerations may be related to uterine hyperactivity, fetal manipulation, conduction anesthesia with maternal hypotension, supine hypotension, prolapse of the cord, uterine rupture, rupture of a vasa previa, placental abruption, or intravenous narcotic use. Prolonged decelerations have the potential to result rapidly in fetal hypoxia and acidemia.[30] The outcome depends primarily on the FHR variability prior to the onset of the deceleration.[30] If the deceleration has no apparent cause, corrective measures, including maternal evaluation of blood pressure, repositioning, hydration, and oxygenation, should be undertaken. If this fails to resolve the problem, operative delivery may be required.

Sinusoidal FHR patterns

Sinusoidal FHR patterns, first described by Manseau et al, in 1972,[31] in 11 severely affected Rh-sensitized fetuses, consist of a regular sine wave undulation about a baseline, with absent variability (Figure 19.3). These patterns have been associated with fetal anemia resulting from rhesus isoimmunization, ruptured vasa previa, fetomaternal hemorrhage, placental abruption, uterine rupture, twin-to-twin transfusion, fetal hypoxia, fetal cardiac malformations, or maternal cardiopulmonary bypass.[32] Similar patterns, termed pseudosinusoidal, may result from administration of opiates in labor. Modanlou and Murata defined a sinusoidal heart rate pattern as one with a stable baseline of 120–160, oscillation of the sinusoidal heart rate above and below the baseline, a frequency of 2–5 cycles per second with an amplitude of 5–15 bpm, and absent short-term variability with no areas of normal variability[32] (Figure 19.3). A true sinusoidal fetal heart tracing should be regarded as an ominous sign of fetal compromise, associated with a significant risk of fetal mortality or severe morbidity. Such a pattern demands immediate evaluation and intervention.[32] While pseudosinusoidal patterns are most often associated with normal neonatal outcome, careful fetal assessment is indicated when such patterns are detected.

Fetal arrhythmia

Certain irregularities of the heart rate, on auscultation, or on FHR monitoring, should lead to suspicion of fetal arrhythmia. When this occurs, the obstetrician, using an electrocardiographic monitor, may evaluate the presence of P, QRS, and T waves of the fetal signal. Although most fetal cardiac arrhythmia are transient and of little clinical significance, some are important. Fetal supraventricular tachycardia may evoke heart failure and hydrops. A persistent rate of 50–70 bpm may represent a complete heart block. Approximately 40% of these fetuses will have congenital heart disease, including ventricular septal defects. Fetal heart failure and hydrops have been associated with congenital heart block.

Clinical application of FHR patterns

The ACOG divides intrapartum FHR patterns into reassuring and nonreassuring patterns.[6] A reassuring FHR pattern is one where the baseline is normal, there is good variability, accelerations are present, and there are no decelerations or other nonreassuring features (Figure 19.1).[6] While there is almost

universal consensus that a normal FHR tracing is highly predictive of normal fetal oxygenation and acid–base status, and most experts agree that certain patterns are associated with poor outcomes (recurrent late decelerations associated with absent variability, true sinusoidal heart rate patterns, and persistent fetal bradycardia), there is little agreement on the significance of FHR patterns between these two extremes.[22,33,34] Skupski et al carried out a survey of maternal fetal medicine specialists regarding their approach to the management of various FHR abnormalities.[33] There was consensus that a cesarean delivery should be performed after 30 minutes of repeated late or severe variable decelerations, after 10 minutes of bradycardia, and in all cases of prolonged absent FHR variability. However, these specialists had a variety of approaches to other FHR patterns.

The following patterns should be considered nonreassuring and require further action:

(1) baseline tachycardia or bradycardia, especially when persistent
(2) absent baseline variability
(3) change in baseline
(4) recurrent late decelerations
(5) recurrent deep variable decelerations, especially when accompanied by a lack of variability
(6) sinusoidal heart-rate patterns.

There are a number of possible responses to a nonreassuring FHR pattern. The first is to perform another test that is more specific for fetal hypoxia than a nonreassuring FHR tracing. The second is to initiate actions aimed at removing or relieving the insult that caused the abnormal FHR pattern. The third is to deliver the fetus. When the cervix is not fully dilated and vaginal delivery is not imminent, this action is usually cesarean delivery. The final possible response is to allow labor to continue, without reassurance about fetal status. Needless to say, this is imprudent, and fraught with danger of fetal injury or death. A decision tree indicating appropriate actions for nonreassuring FHR patterns is given in Figure 19.4.

Intrapartum management and therapy

When the FHR monitoring pattern is reassuring, generally no further intervention is required. However, when there is nonreassuring FHR pattern, some further evaluation or intervention is indicated. For persistent variable decelerations, typically the result of compression of the umbilical cord, or when there is postural maternal hypotension, changes in maternal position may lead to resolution of the decelerations. Amnioinfusion may relieve variable decelerations associated with cord compression from oligohydramnios.[35] When nonreassuring fetal FHR patterns occur, especially when these are the result of excessive uterine activity, stopping an oxytocin infusion if one is running may

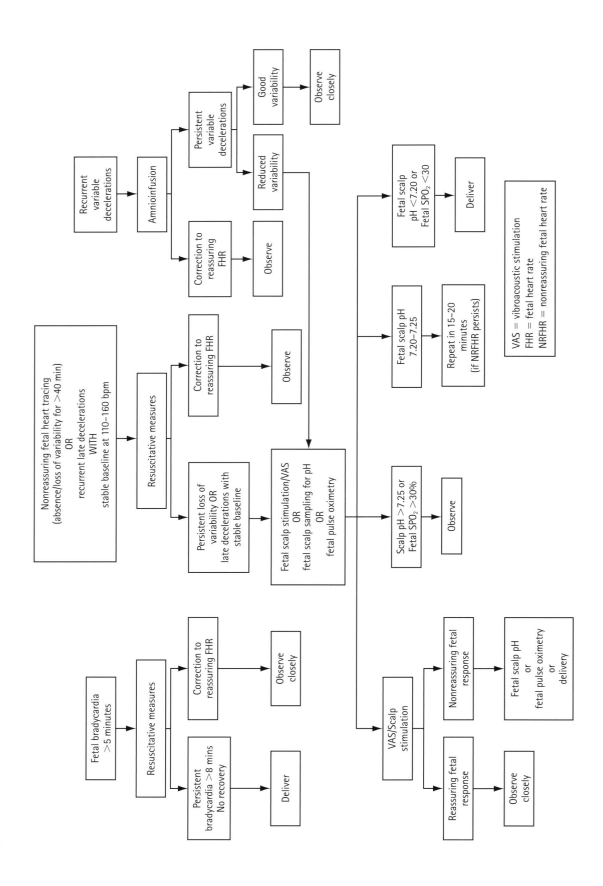

Figure 19.4. Decision tree for the management of nonreassuring FHR patterns.

solve the problem. Alternatively, tocolytic therapy to stop contractions may be beneficial, thereby allowing restoration of uterine blood flow.[36,37] The tocolytic that is most commonly used for this purpose is 0.25 mg subcutaneous terbutaline. Tocolytics should not be used as the only treatment but only with simultaneous preparations for operative delivery. Under these circumstances, tocolytic therapy is associated with vaginal delivery in 20% of the cases. Intravenous fluid therapy may relieve fetal bradycardia or decelerations associated with hypotension after administration of epidural anesthesia. Where the FHR pattern is nonreassuring, further tests to confirm fetal well-being are indicated. These may include fetal scalp stimulation or vibroacoustic stimulation, scalp capillary sampling to determine pH, fetal pulse oximetry or, more recently, ST analysis of the fetal electrocardiogram.

Fetal scalp acid–base evaluation

Intrapartum fetal scalp blood sampling for evaluation of the fetal condition was introduced by Saling in 1960.[4] While the fetal scalp capillary pH gives a fairly accurate estimate of fetal oxygenation and acid–base status, it provides only a snapshot of fetal status at the time of the sampling. Thus, often, repeated scalp sampling is necessary until delivery occurs. The main indication for scalp sampling is a nonreassuring fetal heart tracing. Fetal pH values are used because of the somewhat erratic P_{O_2} levels in the fetal scalp capillary blood and the relative instability of P_{O_2} electrodes. When fetal oxygen deprivation is sufficient to cause the utilization of the anaerobic (Embden–Meyerhof) pathway for energy production, lactic acid is generated and the pH level falls. Fetal blood pH and respiratory gas evaluation may signal fetal jeopardy prior to damage and permit timely delivery. Fetal scalp capillary pH values of 7.25 or greater are considered normal; with these values, labor may be allowed to proceed. Values of 7.20–7.24 are considered preacidotic, and warrant close continued re-evaluation, with the scalp sampling repeated in 20–30 minutes. Values of 7.19 or less are indicative of fetal acidosis and necessitate immediate delivery. While fetal damage rarely occurs unless the pH is less than 7.0, not effecting expeditious delivery may result in a further drop in pH.[38] In a study of 64 fetuses with Apgar scores of 9 and 10 at 1 and 5 minutes after birth, respectively, Weber and Hahn-Pedersen found the mean fetal scalp pH values to fall from 7.38 in early labor to 7.28 at delivery.[39] Normal values for umbilical cord arterial and venous blood gases prior to and after the onset of labor have been described by Vintzileos et al (Table 19.2).[40]

On occasion, maternal acidosis may result in fetal acidosis secondary to the equilibration of hydrogen ions across the placenta. When combined maternal and fetal acidosis is found, the comparison of maternal and fetal base excess can be used to distinguish between a hypoxic fetus and one that receives an excessive amount of hydrogen ions from the mother. When maternal acidosis is observed, efforts should be made to determine the etiology, such as sepsis, ketoacidosis, or dehydration, and correct the problem. With maternal respiratory alkalosis associated with hyperventilation, falsely elevated fetal pH values may occur.

The base deficit (excess) is an indicator of fetal buffer reserves available to neutralize hydrogen ions or fixed acids. The longer the fetus is exposed to recurrent stress, the more likely its acid–base status is suddenly to deteriorate. With recurrent stress, stable pH values, and a rising base deficit, the temporal interval before deterioration of the fetal condition becomes progressively shorter. Thus, the judicious clinical use of base excess-deficit as an indicator of fetal well-being, especially when there are equivocal or nonreassuring FHR patterns, should be encouraged. The ACOG recommends that fetal scalp sampling be considered before cesarean delivery for nonreassuring FHR patterns. Goodwin et al examined the pattern of fetal scalp sampling over 7 years at their institution, where an average of 16 330 births took place annually.[41] The rate dropped from 1.76% to 0.03%. There was no associated increase in cesarean deliveries for nonreassuring fetal status, meconium aspiration syndrome, or low Apgar scores necessitating neonatal intensive care unit admission. These authors questioned the role of fetal scalp sampling. While scalp pH sampling is widely performed in several countries, the procedure has fallen out of favor in the USA. Chauhan et al examined the compliance of obstetricians with the ACOG guidelines for cesarean delivery for nonreassuring FHR patterns.[42] They found that scalp pH was determined in only 5% of 1128 cesareans for nonreassuring fetal heart tracings, and tocolytics were utilized for intrauterine resuscitation in 16% of 261 cesareans.[42] When cesarean delivery was performed for nonreassuring fetal heart tracings and umbilical cord pH was performed after delivery, the pH was greater than 7.0 in 90% of cases.[42]

Technique for fetal scalp sampling

To perform fetal scalp capillary sampling, the membranes must already be ruptured and the cervix dilated at least 2–3 cm in order to expose the fetal scalp. With the patient in a dorsal

Table 19.2 Normal newborn umbilical cord acid–base values after labor at term[40]

	pH	P_{O_2}	P_{CO_2}	Base excess
Umbilical artery (mean ± s.d.)	7.28 (± 0.07)	17.6 (± 6.0)	48.5 (± 8.8)	− 3.6 (± 3.9)
Umbilical vein (mean ± s.d.)	7.32 (± 0.07)	27.6 (± 8.4)	46.2 (± 8.4)	− 2.7 (± 2.8)

lithotomy or lateral Simm's position, the vulvar area is cleaned and draped. An amnioscope (a truncated cone) is inserted through the vagina and dilated cervix so that the smaller end of the endoscope rests against the fetal presenting part. Meconium, blood, mucus, and amniotic fluid should be wiped away. A small amount of silicone is sprayed over the exposed area in order to facilitate the visualization of the scalp and provide a smooth surface upon which a drop of blood can form. With a specially designed 2-mm microscalpel set in a plastic guard, the presenting part is punctured. A long, heparinized, glass capillary tube is introduced through the endoscope and touched to the fetal scalp. The blood runs into the tube by capillary pressure. Only 20 μl of blood is necessary to determine pH.

After the collection of a blood sample, pressure is applied to the puncture site and held for two contractions. Then it is observed for bleeding through a third. If bleeding continues, additional pressure may be required. The blood sample should be analyzed immediately. Ideally, equipment to analyze the sample should be present in the obstetric or neonatal suite. It is crucial that the equipment be calibrated regularly and that labor personnel are familiar with the equipment and can perform these analyses quickly.

Fetal stimulation

Because fetal scalp pH sampling is invasive, and may be technically difficult, alternative methods of further fetal assessment for an equivocal or nonreassuring FHR tracing have been explored. Clark et al retrospectively analyzed 200 fetal heart tracings where the fetuses had undergone fetal scalp sampling for pH.[43] They found that in no case where the fetal pH was less than 7.20 was there a FHR acceleration in response to the scalp sampling. However, 142 of 144 fetuses with a scalp pH greater than 7.28 responded with heart rate acceleration. Fetuses with scalp pH values of 7.21–7.28 exhibited a variable response (some had accelerations while others did not). In a further prospective study, they demonstrated that an acceleration in response to application of a nontraumatic clamp to the fetal scalp was invariably associated with a fetal scalp pH greater than 7.19.[44] However, 61% of fetuses who did not have heart rate acceleration had a pH over 7.19. Thus, these authors concluded that a positive scalp stimulation test could replace fetal scalp pH sampling for evaluation of fetal well-being in labor, and that performance of this test would make 50% of scalp pH samplings unnecessary. Other stimuli, including injections of cold, sterile water through an intrauterine pressure catheter,[45] pinching of the fetal scalp, physical movement of the fetus, or vibroacoustic stimulation of the fetus,[46] have gained popularity in recent years. Vibroacoustic fetal stimulation with an artificial larynx placed on the maternal abdomen has also been used to bring about FHR acceleration.[46] Skupski et al performed a meta-analysis of fetal stimulation tests and found that they were beneficial in reducing the rate of unnecessary cesarean deliveries.[47] However, they determined that the absence of FHR accel-

erations in response to scalp stimulation was not necessarily predictive of an acidotic fetus. If an acceleration is not achieved in response to scalp or auditory stimulation, fetal blood sampling for pH and base-excess determination, fetal pulse oximetry or cesarean delivery should be seriously considered.

Fetal pulse oximetry

Electronic FHR monitoring (EFM), in an indirect manner, attempts to evaluate fetal oxygenation, and detect fetal hypoxia and acidemia. While EFM has excellent sensitivity for these outcomes, it is severely limited by its high false-positive rate, which has led to countless unnecessary interventions and cesarean deliveries.[48] Pulse oximetry was recently introduced into adult and pediatric medicine, and has been used extensively, especially in the fields of anesthesiology, neonatology, and adult intensive care.[49] It has resulted in a reduction in anesthesia-related deaths and related lawsuits.[49] Pulse oximetry measures arterial oxygen saturation and thus may produce a more objective measurement of oxygenation in the fetus, resulting in fewer interventions for nonreassuring fetal heart tracings, without increasing the rate of hypoxic fetal injury.[50–57] However, pulse oximetry in the rather inaccessible fetus presents formidable problems. Extensive work on animals preceded the evaluation of pulse oximetry in the human fetus.[58] Ranges of normal and abnormal fetal oxygen saturation in labor have now been defined; the normal range of intrapartum fetal oxygen saturation (SP_{O_2}) is 35–65%.[59] Fetal SP_{O_2} above 30% is considered to be compatible with a good neonatal outcome; only when the fetal SP_{O_2} drops below this level for greater than 10 minutes does significant metabolic acidosis occur.[59] Carbonne et al performed a multicenter observational study of fetal pulse oximetry and found (1) that fetal pulse oximetry was successful in 95% of women; (2) that there was a significant association between low fetal SP_{O_2} (<30%) and poor neonatal condition; and (3) that at a threshold fetal SP_{O_2} of 30% or a fetal scalp pH of 7.20, the predictive values of fetal pulse oximetry and fetal blood analysis for an arterial umbilical pH less than 7.15 and for an abnormal neonatal outcome were similar.[53]

Garite et al carried out a multicenter, randomized, controlled trial of fetal pulse oximetry in 1010 women at nine centers.[56] They demonstrated a greater than 50% reduction in cesarean sections for nonreassuring FHR tracings in the study group. They found no increased neonatal mortality or morbidity among fetuses in the pulse oximetry arm of the study, concluding that fetal pulse oximetry is both accurate and safe. However, they did not find the expected overall reduction in cesarean delivery rates, because in the study group there was an increase in deliveries for labor dystocia.

A more recent, randomized, controlled trial demonstrated a 50% reduction in operative deliveries for nonreassuring FHR patterns with no increase in adverse fetal outcomes when fetal pulse oximetry was used.[60] However, again, an increase in cesarean delivery rate for dystocia was observed; however, the overall rate of cesarean delivery was not increased in the study group.[60]

Currently, fetal pulse oximetry is performed by the introduction of a flexible sensor through the cervix until it lies alongside the fetal cheek. This sensor has, on its surface, electrodes that detect contact, a photodetector, and two photoemitters that emit far-red (735 nm) and near-infrared (890 nm) light. The sensor is attached to a monitor that processes the signals. Fetal pulse oximetry has been approved by the US Food and Drug Administration as an adjunct to continuous FHR monitoring. However, as of 2004, fetal pulse oximetry has not been endorsed by the ACOG.[61]

Vintzileos et al recently reported their experience with transabdominal, continuous-wave, near-infrared spectroscopy on six nonlaboring women.[62] They found oxygen saturation levels of 50–74%, consistent with levels of oxygen found by transcervical intrauterine pulse oximetry. They suggested that this technology may provide a method for noninvasive, fetal pulse oximetry assessment.

ST analysis of the fetal electrocardiogram

More recently, attention has been directed at using the fetal electrocardiogram (ECG) for intrapartum monitoring of the fetus.[63–65] Data from animal experiments have indicated that the ST segment pattern of the fetal ECG reflects the ability of the myocardium to respond to hypoxia. Fetal hypoxia results in elevation of the ST segment and of the T-wave.[63,64] This elevation is quantified by an increase in the T/QRS ratio, and is the result of a surge in the level of catecholamines, beta-adrenoceptor activation, and glycogenolysis in the fetal myocardium.[63,64] This pattern identifies a fetus that is experiencing hypoxia, but whose coping mechanisms are adequate to deal with the insult. When ST depression occurs (identified by a negative ST–T segment), it probably reflects a myocardium unable to respond adequately to the hypoxic insult.

As a consequence of these findings, a CTG (cardiotocography) plus ST waveform analyzer (STAN®) was developed. There have been two randomized, controlled trials comparing traditional intrapartum fetal monitoring using CTG alone with CTG and ST analysis of the fetal ECG.[63,64] One of these, the Plymouth trial, demonstrated a 46% reduction in the rate of operative deliveries for 'fetal distress' when compared with traditional FHR monitoring alone.[63] Another study, the Swedish multicenter trial, which included 4966 women, showed a 53% reduction in umbilical artery metabolic acidosis (defined as a pH under 7.05 and base deficit over 12.0 mmol/l) at birth in the group monitored by CTG and ST analysis when compared with CTG alone.[64] An important finding of both these studies was that physicians were inclined to intervene on the basis of traditional fetal monitoring (CTG), ignoring ST analysis, thereby violating the study protocols. Interestingly, a randomized

controlled trial evaluating the use of the P–R interval in the fetal ECG along with CTG failed to demonstrate a reduction in operative deliveries or neonatal academia when compared with labors monitored by CTG alone.[65] Overall, it appears that the use of STAN combined with traditional CTG may lead to a significant reduction in both operative deliveries for fetal distress and metabolic acidosis at birth. However, at the present time, ST analysis requires an internal fetal scalp electrode, making it invasive. Consequently, it may be best used selectively on fetuses who have demonstrated abnormal FHR patterns on conventional monitoring, rather than routinely on all laboring patients. Further research and training of physicians, midwives, and nurses are required before this promising technology achieves widespread usage in obstetric practice.

Evaluation of meconium

Meconium has long been considered a marker of fetal status.[66] Without a doubt, the hypoxic fetus in labor often does pass meconium. While early experimental studies on animals suggested that meconium passage could be induced by fetal hypoxia, such as that caused by cord occlusion, at least one recent study has disputed this.[67] The rate of meconium passage increases with increasing gestational age, with meconium present in 26% of postdate births.[68] Meconium passage is dependent on maturation of the fetal parasympathetic nervous system. In a preterm fetus, it is extremely uncommon and should be viewed as pathologic. Green-stained amniotic fluid in the very preterm fetus may be an indication of intra-amniotic infection. If the labor is otherwise uncomplicated, and the fetal heart tracing is reassuring, the presence of meconium may carry little import. However, when there is evidence of impaired fetal oxygenation, as manifested by abnormal FHR patterns, the presence of meconium, particularly when it is thick, should prompt thorough evaluation for evidence of hypoxia, and appropriate management should be taken to relieve that insult or remove the fetus from the hostile environment. While 7–22% of live births are complicated by the presence of meconium, the incidence of meconium aspiration syndrome is only 2 per 1000 live births.[66] Katz and Bowes[66] and Ghidini and Spong[69] postulated that meconium is not the cause of severe meconium aspiration syndrome. Rather, they suggest that the syndrome is caused by fetal lung damage resulting from fetal hypoxia. Katz and Bowes also state that good outcomes in the presence of thick meconium probably result from avoidance of perinatal asphyxia rather than suctioning of the fetus.[66] In fact, neonatal outcomes of pregnancies complicated by intrapartum meconium with normal FHR patterns are similar to those with normal FHR patterns in labor where the amniotic fluid is clear.[66] Likewise, outcomes of infants where meconium staining and abnormal FHR patterns complicated labor are similar to those where there was no meconium with similar FHR patterns.[66] Miller and Read[70] demonstrated that thick meconium in prolonged gestation is associated with reduced pH and abnormal respiratory gas values. When clear amniotic fluid is noted early during a high-risk labor and thick meconium is found later, careful attention to FHR and acid–base balance is mandatory. Several randomized studies have demonstrated improved perinatal outcomes when thick meconium is treated by amnioinfusion.[71–75] These improved outcomes may be from relief of cord compression and variable decelerations, resulting in prevention or relief of hypoxia. In a study of 8394 'low-risk' women, Greenwood et al demonstrated that in half of the cases where meconium is passed in labor, the meconium is not noticed until after the delivery of the fetal head.[76] These authors concluded that clear amniotic fluid is an unreliable sign of fetal well-being. The presence of meconium in the amniotic fluid in labor should lead to further assessment and extreme vigilance. In the presence of a nonreassuring FHR pattern, further evaluation is indicated.

Amnioinfusion

The term 'amnioinfusion' refers to the introduction of sterile fluid into the amniotic cavity. The use of this procedure for the relief of variable decelerations in labor was first described by Miyazaki and Nevarez in 1985.[77] The rationale for this intervention was based on the observation that variable decelerations frequently are the consequence of cord compression. In labor, after rupture of the membranes, some degree of oligohydramnios is not uncommon. Consequently, the cord may become compressed between the fetus and the uterine wall. Instillation of sterile fluid into the uterine cavity produces a 'cushion' between the fetus and the uterine wall, relieving these decelerations. Spong et al demonstrated that whether or not amnioinfusion relieved variable decelerations depended on the amniotic fluid index prior to the amnioinfusion.[78] When variable decelerations were associated with a normal amniotic fluid index, amnioinfusion was frequently not beneficial, suggesting that in these cases the cord compression was due to the cord's being wrapped around a fetal part, such as the neck or a limb, or to a true knot of the cord.[78] Initial studies suggested that prophylactic amnioinfusion for oligohydramnios in labor was associated with fewer cesarean deliveries, improved neonatal Apgar scores, and reduced neonatal morbidity when compared with a policy of no amnioinfusion. However, in the control groups in these studies, no amnioinfusion was performed, even when variable decelerations occurred. More recent studies, including a meta-analysis, indicate that amnioinfusion is of benefit only when there are variable decelerations associated with oligohydramnios; therefore, it is therapeutic as opposed to prophylactic amnioinfusion that is beneficial.[79] Amnioinfusion is frequently used when thick meconium is detected in labor. Amnioinfusion significantly decreases the thickness of the meconium, and has been associated with lower cesarean delivery rates and improved Apgar scores. It is also associated with reduced rates of meconium below the vocal cords, decreased rates of meconium-aspiration syndrome and hypoxic-ischemic neonatal encephalopathy, neonatal ventilation, and admission to neonatal intensive care.[75] Finally, there is a trend to reduced perinatal mortality.[75] However, while several randomized studies have demonstrated that prophylactic amnioinfusion in labor complicated by thick meconium improves neonatal outcomes, Spong et al have argued that this is by relief of coexistent variable decelerations rather than by dilution of meconium.[73] Another mechanism may be by the relief of oligohydramnios.

Amnioinfusion may be performed by two routes. The one almost universally used is via a transcervical catheter (usually the intrauterine pressure catheter). Much more infrequently, amnioinfusion may be performed via the transabdominal approach with a spinal needle. A number of protocols are used for amnioinfusion. Generally, 500–1000 ml saline is given as a bolus, after which a continuous infusion is given, typically at a rate of about 100–200 ml per hour. The use of saline at room temperature has been demonstrated to be as effective as when warmed to body temperature. Amnioinfusion does not lead to longer labor.[80] Intermittent bolus amnioinfusion has been shown to be as effective as continuous amnioinfusion.[81] Amnioinfusion is regarded as safe in the trial of labor of a woman with a prior cesarean.[82] Fetal shivering with amnioinfusion has been described.[83]

Special situations

Twins

The monitoring of twins in labor presents a particular diagnostic dilemma. Bakker et al examined 172 twin pregnancies in labor and found that the FHR signal was suboptimal in 26–33% of twins in the first stage and 41–63% of twins in the second stage.[84] It is not uncommon for the same twin's FHR to be recorded twice, with the observer mistakenly believing that two separate fetal hearts are being traced. It is important to make sure that two different fetal heart traces are obtained, and that they do not persistently follow the same pattern of accelerations and decelerations. Monitoring of twins in labor may be facilitated by rupturing the membranes of the leading twin as soon as cervical dilation and station safely allows this, and to attach a scalp electrode to that fetus.

Trial of labor after previous cesarean

Labor after a prior cesarean carries a risk of uterine rupture. Abnormalities of the FHR tracing are the most consistent clinical sign of uterine rupture, occurring in about 87% of cases.[85–88] In particular, bradycardia and recurrent late or severely variable decelerations may indicate uterine rupture. Sinusoidal FHR tracing is another pattern that may occur. Early recognition of these FHR anomalies, and immediate cesarean delivery may prevent severe fetal morbidity and mortality (Figure 19.2). For these reasons, early intervention is indicated when there are persistent FHR abnormalities in a woman undergoing trial of labor after a previous cesarean delivery. It was believed that when the uterus ruptured, there would be a loss of intrauterine pressure that could be picked up by the intrauterine pressure catheter (IUPC). However, studies have indicated that uterine pressures after uterine rupture are neither predictable nor consistent, limiting the use of the IUPC in the detection of uterine rupture.[88]

Congenital heart block and fetal arrhythmia

Fetal arrhythmia, especially heart block, presents significant problems for intrapartum monitoring. Because of the abnormal FHR patterns, traditional monitoring methods may be of minimal value. The use of intrapartum fetal pulse oximetry for this purpose is ideal, and, indeed, it has been described.[89,90]

The impact of intrapartum FHR monitoring on perinatal outcomes

It was believed that the advent of intrapartum, continuous electronic FHR monitoring (EFM) would lead to the disappearance of stillbirth and cerebral palsy. Early reports, including a review of nearly 47 656 electronically monitored patients, noted a substantial reduction in the rates of intrapartum and neonatal deaths.[91] After a few years, however, it became clear that these initial lofty expectations were unduly optimistic, and that there was no change in the rate of cerebral palsy, while the cesarean section rates for 'fetal distress' skyrocketed.[48] Several randomized, controlled studies failed to show any reduction in intrapartum death rates in women who had continuous EFM when compared with those monitored by intermittent fetal auscultation.[92–99] The best known of these, the Dublin trial, was a randomized, controlled study of 12 964 women in whom continuous EFM was compared with intermittent auscultation.[99] Fetal scalp pH assessment was allowed as indicated. Women who had EFM had shorter labor and had fewer analgesia requirements. Cesarean and forceps delivery rates, Apgar scores, and neonatal intensive care admissions were similar in both groups. There were 14 stillbirths or neonatal deaths in each group. While there were twice as many seizures in the intermittently auscultated group as in the EFM group, the neurologic deficit at 1-year follow-up was not different between the two groups. Follow-up at 4 years of age of the children who had had neonatal seizures revealed no differences in the rate of cerebral palsy between the two groups.[100]

In a further study from Dublin, Impey et al carried out a randomized, controlled trial of 8580 low-risk women, comparing a labor ward admission, 20-minute FHR tracing or intermittent FHR auscultation only, with the option of continuous fetal monitoring if indicated. There was no significant difference in adverse perinatal outcomes or operative delivery rates. The authors concluded that admission FHR tracing offered no advantage over intermittent auscultation.[101]

In 1993, Vintzileos et al[102] published the results of a randomized controlled trial of 1428 pregnant women, comparing intrapartum EFM with intermittent auscultation. They demonstrated reduced perinatal mortality in the EFM group; however, there was a higher rate of interventions in that group. These authors carried out a further analysis of the same study, and the primary outcome measure was the prediction of fetal acidemia at birth, defined as an umbilical arterial pH under 7.15.[103] The sensitivity of EFM for acidemia was 97% compared with 34% for auscultation ($p < 0.001$). The positive-predictive value of EFM was 37% versus 22% ($p < 0.05$), while the negative predictive value was 99.5% versus 95% ($p < 0.001$). Thus, this study did show a significant reduction in intrapartum deaths due to asphyxia in women who had continuous, intrapartum electronic fetal surveillance. While this study was at variance with previous studies, it was the only study at the time that had used strict criteria for defining normal and abnormal FHR patterns. Subsequently, a meta-analysis by Vintzileos et al[104] examining nine randomized, controlled studies indicated that the perinatal mortality due to fetal hypoxia was reduced by EFM when compared with intermittent auscultation (odds ratio (OR) 0.41). However, in the EFM group, there was an increased rate of cesarean (OR 2.55), forceps, and vacuum deliveries (OR 2.50) for fetal distress. A year later, another meta-analysis by Thacker et al examined 12 randomized, controlled trials, and found that EFM was associated with fewer neonatal seizures (relative risk (RR) 0.5) and fewer neonates with a 1-minute Apgar score less than 4 (RR 0.82), again at the cost of an increased cesarean delivery rate (RR 1.33).[105]

It is not clear why electronic FHR monitoring has failed to make an impact on the rates of cerebral palsy. Parer and King[34] offered a number of explanations. First, probably only 10% or less of cases of cerebral palsy can be attributed to intrapartum asphyxia. Therefore, intrapartum fetal monitoring could not be expected to prevent the other 90% of cases of cerebral palsy. Second, some episodes of fetal asphyxia are so rapid and catastrophic that even prompt delivery may not prevent fetal brain damage. Finally, there is considerable variability in the interpretation of FHR patterns, and in the responses of physicians to these patterns.

Assessment of acid–base status in the neonate

The umbilical cord pH and blood gases give objective information about oxygenation in the infant at the time of delivery and therefore are indicative of whether or not labor has resulted in hypoxia. Immediately after delivery, a segment of the cord should be double clamped and put aside. Ideally, samples should be taken from both the artery and the vein. The samples are drawn in heparinized syringes. The ACOG has recommended that cord gases be obtained only in cases where labor and delivery or the pregnancy have been complicated.[106] However, some authorities recommend obtaining cord blood gases at all deliveries.[107] The argument for this is that less than 10% of all cases of cerebral palsy result from intrapartum events, and several of these cases occur in vigorous newborns. These authorities argue that cord gases may determine, in an objective manner, whether the brain damage was the consequence of an intrapartum hypoxic insult. They also argue that routine cord pH determinations are advisable from a medicolegal standpoint, and would help understand the pathophysiology of the brain damage, excluding birth asphyxia as the cause of neonatal depression in 80% of cases. Certainly, there is consensus that cord gases should be obtained in all high-risk and complicated pregnancies, and when neonatal depression occurs.

Helwig et al used a perinatal database to determine normal values of umbilical cord pHs in 16 060 vigorous newborns.[108] Median values for arterial pH, P_{O_2}, P_{CO_2}, and base excess were 7.26, 177 mmHg, 52 mmHg, and -4 mEq/l, respectively. The abnormal cutoff values for these parameters were similar to those described by Vintzileos et al.[40]

Conclusion

Intrapartum fetal assessment is performed with the goal of preventing stillbirth or brain damage due to intrapartum fetal oxygen deprivation. Continuous EFM, the most widely used form of intrapartum fetal assessment, has failed to live up to its initial promise. Although its use has reduced the number of stillbirths, and, under certain settings, the number of perinatal deaths due to hypoxia, it has not led to a reduction in the rate of cerebral palsy. In addition, its routine use has resulted in the skyrocketing of cesarean section rates. Yet, continuous EFM will continue to be the method of choice for the evaluation of the fetus in labor, at least for the foreseeable future. This is primarily because it makes relatively few demands on manpower, is easy to use, allows documentation that can be reviewed in the future, and has found almost universal acceptance. The alternative, intermittent auscultation, requires one-on-one nursing care, which is probably impractical and uneconomical by today's standards. While fetal scalp capillary sampling for pH provides a snapshot of fetal well-being, it has fallen into relative disfavor, at least in the USA. Fetal pulse oximetry and ST segment analysis both hold great promise for assessing fetal well-being, but neither have, at the present time, had widespread acceptance in the USA. They are both likely to be used as adjuncts to EFM rather than as a primary method of fetal assessment. In the future, it is possible that, with advances in technology, noninvasive fetal pulse oximetry will be used as an adjunct to FHR monitoring, and may eventually replace EFM. Meanwhile, more standardized interpretation of the FHR may lead to a reduction in cesarean delivery rate, and may then show an improvement in outcomes of pregnancies where intrapartum EFM is utilized. Computer-assisted interpretation of FHR may also increase the specificity of FHR interpretation.[109]

The twentieth century brought the ability to view the fetus as a patient in its own right. Advances in the twenty-first century may help us better understand in utero physiology, and may lead to the development of technologies that will bring about further reduction in perinatal and infant morbidity resulting from insults during pregnancy and labor.

References

1. Baskett TF. On the Shoulders of Giants; Eponyms and Names in Obstetrics and Gynaecology. RCOG Press: London, 1988.
2. Little WJ. On the influence of abnormal parturition, difficult labours, premature birth, and asphyxia neonatorum, on the mental and physical condition of the child, especially in relation to deformities. Trans Obstet Soc London 1861; 3: 293–344.
3. Hon EH. The electronic evaluation of the fetal heart rate: preliminary report. Am J Obstet Gynecol 1958; 77: 1084–99.
4. Saling E: Neues Vorgehen zur Untersuchung des Kindes unter der Gebrut: Einführung, Technik, und Grundlagen. [New technique for examining the fetus during labor: introduction, technique and basics]. Arch Gynakol 1962; 197: 108–22.
5. Kim SY, Khandelwal M, Gaughan JP et al. Is the intrapartum biophysical profile useful? Obstet Gynecol 2003; 102: 471–6.
6. Fetal heart rate patterns: monitoring, interpretation and management. Technical Bulletin. No. 207, 1995 American College of Obstetricians and Gynecologists: Washington, DC.
7. Cordero L, Anderson CW, Zuspan FP. Scalp abscess: a benign and infrequent complication of fetal monitoring. Am J Obstet Gynecol 1983; 146: 126–30.
8. McGregor JA, McFarren T. Neonatal cranial osteomyelitis: a complication of fetal monitoring. Obstet Gynecol 1989; 73(3 Pt 2): 490–2.
9. Nieburg P, Gross SJ. Cerebrospinal fluid leak in a neonate associated with fetal scalp electrode monitoring. Am J Obstet Gynecol 1983; 147: 839–40.
10. Miyashiro MJ, Mintz-Hittner HA. Penetrating ocular injury with a fetal scalp monitoring spiral electrode. Am J Ophthalmol 1999; 128: 526–8.
11. Ramsey PS, Johnston BW, Welter VE et al. Artifactual fetal electrocardiographic detection using internal monitoring following intrapartum fetal demise during VBAC trial. J Matern Fetal Med 2000; 9: 360–1.
12. Electronic fetal heart rate monitoring: research guidelines for interpretation. National Institute of Child Health and Human Development Research Planning Workshop. Am J Obstet Gynecol 1997; 177: 1385–90.
13. Sherer DM, Onyeije CI, Binder D, Bernstein PS, Divon MY. Uncomplicated baseline fetal tachycardia or bradycardia in postterm pregnancies and perinatal outcome. Am J Perinatol 1998; 15: 335–8.
14. Pillai M, James D. The development of fetal heart rate patterns during normal pregnancy. Obstet Gynecol 1990; 76: 812–16.
15. Park MI, Hwang JH, Cha KJ et al. Computerized analysis of fetal heart rate parameters by gestational age. Int J Gynaecol Obstet 2001; 74: 157–64.

16. Renou P, Warwick N, Wood C. Autonomic control of fetal heart rate. Am J Obstet Gynecol 1969; 105: 949–53.

17. Williams KP, Galerneau F. Intrapartum fetal heart rate patterns in the prediction of neonatal acidemia. Am J Obstet Gynecol 2003; 188: 820–3.

18. Kozuma S, Watanabe T, Bennet L et al. The effect of carotid sinus denervation on fetal heart rate variation in normoxia, hypoxia and post-hypoxia in fetal sheep. Br J Obstet Gynaecol 1997; 104: 460–5.

19. Low JA, Victory R, Derrick EJ. Predictive value of electronic fetal monitoring for intrapartum fetal asphyxia with metabolic acidosis. Obstet Gynecol 1999; 93: 285–91.

20. Murata Y, Martin CB Jr, Ikenoue T et al. Fetal heart rate accelerations and late decelerations during the course of intrauterine death in chronically catheterized rhesus monkeys. Am J Obstet Gynecol 1982; 144: 218–23.

21. Martin CB, de Haan J, van der Wildt B et al. Mechanisms of late decelerations in the fetal heart rate. A study with autonomic blocking agents in fetal lambs. Eur J Obstet Gynecol Reprod Biol 1979; 9: 361–73.

22. Freeman RK. Problems with intrapartum fetal heart rate monitoring interpretation and patient management. Obstet Gynecol 2002; 100: 813–26.

23. Gaziano EP, Freeman DW. Analysis of heart rate patterns preceding fetal death. Obstet Gynecol 1977; 50: 578–82.

24. Hadar A, Sheiner E, Hallak M et al. Abnormal fetal heart rate tracing patterns during the first stage of labor: effect on perinatal outcome. Am J Obstet Gynecol 2001; 185: 863–8.

25. Sheiner E, Hadar A, Hallak M et al Clinical significance of fetal heart rate tracings during the second stage of labor. Obstet Gynecol 2001; 97: 747–52.

26. Ball RH, Parer JT. The physiologic mechanisms of variable decelerations. Am J Obstet Gynecol 1992; 166: 1683–8.

27. Cordero DR, Helfgott AW, Landy HJ et al A non-hemorrhagic manifestation of vasa previa: a clinicopathologic case report. Obstet Gynecol 1993; 82: 698–700.

28. Sheiner E, Levy A, Ofir K et al. Changes in fetal heart rate and uterine patterns associated with uterine rupture. J Reprod Med 2004; 49: 373–8.

29. Salafia CM, Ghidini A, Sherer DM et al. Abnormalities of the fetal heart rate in preterm deliveries are associated with acute intra-amniotic infection. J Soc Gynecol Invest 1998; 5: 188–91.

30. Williams KP, Galerneau F. Fetal heart rate parameters predictive of neonatal outcome in the presence of a prolonged deceleration. Obstet Gynecol 2002; 100: 951–4.

31. Manseau P, Vaquier J, Chavinie J et al. Sinusoidal fetal cardiac rhythm. An aspect evocative of fetal distress during pregnancy. J Gynecol Obstet Biol Reprod (Paris) 1972; 1: 343–52.

32. Modanlou HD, Murata Y. Sinusoidal heart rate pattern: reappraisal of its definition and significance. J Obstet Gynaecol Res 2004; 30: 169–80.

33. Skupski DW, Chervenak FA, McCullough LB et al. Cesarean delivery for intrapartum fetal heart rate abnormalities: incorporating survey data into clinical judgment. Obstet Gynecol 1996; 88: 60–4.

34. Parer JT, King T. Fetal heart rate monitoring: is it salvageable? Am J Obstet Gynecol 2000; 182: 982–7.

35. Hofmeyr GJ. Amnioinfusion for umbilical cord compression in labour. Cochrane Database Syst Rev 2000; 2: CD000013.

36. Kulier R, Hofmeyr GJ. Tocolytics for suspected intrapartum fetal distress. Cochrane Database Syst Rev 2000; 2: CD000035.

37. Afschar P, Scholl W, Bader A et al. A prospective randomised trial of atosiban versus hexoprenaline for acute tocolysis and intrauterine resuscitation. Br J Obstet Gynaecol 2004; 111: 316–18.

38. Neonatal Encephalopathy and Cerebral Palsy: Defining the Pathogenesis and Pathophysiology. American College of Obstetricians and Gynecologists: Washington, DC, 2003.

39. Weber T, Hahn-Pedersen S. Normal values for fetal scalp tissue pH during labour. Br J Obstet Gynaecol 1979; 86: 728–31.

40. Vintzileos AM, Egan JFX, Campbell WA et al. Asphyxia at birth as determined by cord blood pH measurements in preterm and term gestations: correlation with neonatal outcome. J Matern Fetal Med 1992; 1: 7–13.

41. Goodwin TM, Milner-Masterson L, Paul RH. Elimination of fetal scalp blood sampling on a large clinical service. Obstet Gynecol 1994; 83: 971–4.

42. Chauhan SP, Magann EF, Scott JR et al. Emergency cesarean delivery for nonreassuring fetal heart rate tracings: compliance with ACOG guidelines. Obstet Gynecol Surv 2004; 59: 422–3.

43. Clark SL, Gimovsky ML, Miller FC. Fetal heart rate response to scalp blood sampling. Am J Obstet Gynecol 1982; 144: 706–8.

44. Clark SL, Gimovsky ML, Miller FC. The scalp stimulation test: a clinical alternative to fetal scalp blood sampling. Am J Obstet Gynecol 1984; 148: 274–7.

45. Wax JR, Flaherty N, Pinette MG et al. Small-volume amnioinfusion: a potential stimulus of intrapartum fetal heart rate accelerations. Am J Obstet Gynecol 2004; 190: 380–2.

46. Lin CC, Vassallo B, Mittendorf R. Is intrapartum vibroacoustic stimulation an effective predictor of fetal acidosis? J Perinat Med 2001; 29: 506–12.

47. Skupski DW, Rosenberg CR, Eglinton GS. Intrapartum fetal stimulation tests: a meta-analysis. Obstet Gynecol 2002; 99: 129–34.

48. Banta DH, Thacker SB. Historical controversy in health technology assessment: the case of electronic fetal monitoring. Obstet Gynecol Surv 2001; 56: 709–19.

49. Dildy GA, Clark SL, Loucks CA. Intrapartum fetal pulse oximetry: past, present, and future. Am J Obstet Gynecol 1996; 175: 1–9.

50. Gorenberg DM, Pattillo C, Hendi P et al. Fetal pulse oximetry: correlation between oxygen desaturation, duration, and frequency and neonatal outcomes. Am J Obstet Gynecol 2003; 189: 136–8.

51. Luttkus AK, Friedmann W, Homm-Luttkus C et al. Correlation of fetal oxygen saturation to fetal heart rate patterns. Evaluation of fetal pulse oximetry with two different oxisensors. Acta Obstet Gynecol Scand 1998; 77: 307–12.

52. Dildy GA 3rd. Fetal pulse oximetry: a critical appraisal. Best Pract Res Clin Obstet Gynaecol 2004; 18: 477–84.

53. Carbonne B, Langer B, Goffinet F et al. Multicenter study on the clinical value of fetal pulse oximetry. II. Compared predictive

values of pulse oximetry and fetal blood analysis. The French Study Group on Fetal Pulse Oximetry. Am J Obstet Gynecol 1997; 177: 593–8.

54. Goffinet F, Langer B, Carbonne B et al. Multicenter study on the clinical value of fetal pulse oximetry. I. Methodologic evaluation. The French Study Group on Fetal Pulse Oximetry. Am J Obstet Gynecol 1997; 177: 1238–46.

55. Dildy GA, Clark SL, Loucks CA. Preliminary experience with intrapartum fetal pulse oximetry in humans. Obstet Gynecol 1993; 81: 630–5.

56. Garite TJ, Dildy GA, McNamara H et al. A multicenter controlled trial of fetal pulse oximetry in the intrapartum management of nonreassuring fetal rate patterns. Am J Obstet Gynecol 2000; 183: 1049–58.

57. Yam J, Chua S, Arulkumaran S. Intrapartum fetal pulse oximetry. II. Clinical application. Obstet Gynecol Surv 2000; 55: 173–83.

58. Nijland R, Nierlich S, Jongsma HW et al. Validation of reflectance pulse oximetry: an evaluation of a new sensor in piglets. J Clin Monit 1997; 13: 43–9.

59. Seelbach-Gobel B, Heupel M, Kuhnert M et al. The prediction of fetal acidosis by means of intrapartum fetal pulse oximetry. Am J Obstet Gynecol 1999; 180: 73–81.

60. Kuhnert M, Schmidt S. Intrapartum management of nonreassuring fetal heart rate patterns: a randomized controlled trial of fetal pulse oximetry. Am J Obstet Gynecol 2004; 191: 1989–95.

61. American College of Obstetricians and Gynecologists Committee on Obstetric Practice. ACOG Committee Opinion, No. 258, September 2001. Fetal pulse oximetry. Obstet Gynecol 2001; 98: 523–4.

62. Vintzileos AM, Nioka M, Lake M, et al. Transabdominal fetal pulse oximetry with near-infrared spectroscopy. Am J Obstet Gynecol 2005; 192: 129–33.

63. Westgate J, Harris M, Curnow JS et al. Plymouth randomized trial of cardiotocogram only versus ST waveform plus cardiotocogram for intrapartum monitoring in 2400 cases. Am J Obstet Gynecol 1993; 169: 1151–60.

64. Amer-Wahlin I, Hellsten C, Noren H et al. Cardiotocography only versus cardiotocography plus ST analysis of fetal electrocardiogram for intrapartum fetal monitoring: a Swedish randomised controlled trial. Lancet 2001; 358: 534–8.

65. Strachan BK, van Wijngaarden WJ, Sahota D et al. Cardiotocography only versus cardiotocography plus PR-interval analysis in intrapartum surveillance: a randomised, multicentre trial. FECG Study Group. Lancet 2000; 355: 456–9.

66. Katz VL, Bowes WA Jr. Meconium aspiration syndrome: reflections on a murky subject. Am J Obstet Gynecol 1992; 166: 171–83.

67. Westgate JA, Bennet L, Gunn AJ. Meconium and fetal hypoxia: some experimental observations and clinical relevance. Br J Obstet Gynaecol 2002; 109: 1171–74.

68. Eden RD, Seifert LS, Winegar A et al. Perinatal characteristics of uncomplicated postdate pregnancies. Obstet Gynecol 1987; 69: 296–9.

69. Ghidini A, Spong CY. Severe meconium aspiration syndrome is not caused by aspiration of meconium. Am J Obstet Gynecol 2001; 185: 931–8.

70. Miller FC, Read JA. Intrapartum assessment of the postdate fetus. Am J Obstet Gynecol 1981; 141: 516–20.

71. Hofmeyr GJ. Amnioinfusion for meconium-stained liquor in labour. Cochrane Database Syst Rev 2002; 1: CD000014.

72. Rathor AM, Singh R, Ramji S et al. Randomised trial of amnioinfusion during labour with meconium stained amniotic fluid. Br J Obstet Gynaecol 2002; 109: 17–20.

73. Spong CY, Ogundipe OA, Ross MG. Prophylactic amnioinfusion for meconium-stained amniotic fluid. Am J Obstet Gynecol 1994; 171: 931–5.

74. Mahomed K, Mulambo T, Woelk G et al. The Collaborative Randomised Amnioinfusion for Meconium Project (CRAMP). II. Zimbabwe. Br J Obstet Gynaecol 1998; 105: 309–13.

75. Pierce J, Gaudier FL, Sanchez-Ramos L. Intrapartum amnioinfusion for meconium-stained fluid: meta-analysis of prospective clinical trials. Obstet Gynecol 2000; 95: 1051–6.

76. Greenwood C, Lalchandani S, MacQuillan K et al. Meconium passed in labor: how reassuring is clear amniotic fluid? Obstet Gynecol 2003; 102: 89–93.

77. Miyazaki FS, Nevarez F. Saline amnioinfusion for relief of repetitive variable decelerations: a prospective randomized study. Am J Obstet Gynecol 1985; 153: 301–6.

78. Spong CY, McKindsey F, Ross MG. Amniotic fluid index predicts the relief of variable decelerations after amnioinfusion bolus. Am J Obstet Gynecol 1996; 175: 1066–7.

79. Hofmeyr GJ. Prophylactic versus therapeutic amnioinfusion for oligohydramnios in labour. Cochrane Database Syst Rev 2000; 2: CD000176.

80. Macri CJ, Schrimmer DB, Greenspoon JS et al. Amnioinfusion does not affect the length of labor. Am J Obstet Gynecol 1992; 167: 1134–6.

81. Ouzounian JG, Miller DA, Paul RH. Amnioinfusion in women with previous cesarean births: a preliminary report. Am J Obstet Gynecol 1996; 174: 783–6.

82. Rinehart BK, Terrone DA, Barrow JH et al. Randomized trial of intermittent or continuous amnioinfusion for variable decelerations. Obstet Gynecol 2000; 96: 571–4.

83. Petrikovsky B, Silverstein M, Schneider EP. Neonatal shivering and hypothermia after intrapartum amnioinfusion. Lancet 1997; 350: 1366–7.

84. Bakker PCAM, Colenbrander GJ, Verstraeten AA et al. Quality of intrapartum cardiotocography in twin deliveries. Am J Obstet Gynecol 2004; 191: 2114–19.

85. Ridgeway JJ, Weyrich DL, Benedetti TJ. Fetal heart rate changes associated with uterine rupture. Obstet Gynecol 2004; 103: 506–12.

86. Ayres AW, Johnson TR, Hayashi R. Characteristics of fetal heart rate tracings prior to uterine rupture. Int J Gynaecol Obstet 2001; 74: 235–40.

87. Sheiner E, Levy A, Ofir K et al. Changes in fetal heart rate and uterine patterns associated with uterine rupture. J Reprod Med 2004; 49: 373–8.

88. Rodriguez MH, Masaki DI, Phelan JP et al. Uterine rupture: are intrauterine pressure catheters useful in the diagnosis? Am J Obstet Gynecol 1989; 161: 666–9.

89. Dildy GA, Loucks CA, Clark SL. Intrapartum fetal pulse oximetry in the presence of fetal cardiac arrhythmia. Am J Obstet Gynecol 1993; 169: 1609–11.

90. van den Berg PP, Nijland R, van den Brand SF et al. Intrapartum fetal surveillance of congenital heart block with pulse oximetry. Obstet Gynecol 1994; 84: 683–6.

91. Yeh SY, Diaz F, Paul RH. Ten-year experience of intrapartum fetal monitoring in Los Angeles County/University of Southern California Medical Center. Am J Obstet Gynecol 1982; 143: 496–500.

92. Haverkamp AD, Thompson HE, McFee JG et al. The evaluation of continuous fetal heart rate monitoring in high-risk pregnancy. Am J Obstet Gynecol 1976; 125: 310–20.

93. Haverkamp AD, Orleans M, Langendoerfer S et al. A controlled trial of the differential effects of intrapartum fetal monitoring. Am J Obstet Gynecol 1979; 134: 399–412.

94. Luthy DA, Shy KK, van Belle G et al. A randomized trial of electronic fetal monitoring in preterm labor. Obstet Gynecol 1987; 69: 687–95.

95. Thacker SB. The efficacy of intrapartum electronic fetal monitoring. Am J Obstet Gynecol 1987; 156: 24–30.

96. Kelso IM, Parsons RJ, Lawrence GF et al. An assessment of continuous fetal heart rate monitoring in labor. A randomized trial. Am J Obstet Gynecol 1978; 131: 526–32.

97. Shy KK, Luthy DA, Bennett FC, et al. Effects of electronic fetal-heart-rate monitoring, as compared with periodic auscultation, on the neurologic development of premature infants. N Engl J Med 1990; 322: 588–93.

98. Herbst A, Ingemarsson I. Intermittent versus continuous electronic monitoring in labour: a randomised study. Br J Obstet Gynaecol 1994; 101: 663–8.

99. MacDonald D, Grant A, Sheridan-Pereira M et al. The Dublin randomized controlled trial of intrapartum fetal heart rate monitoring. Am J Obstet Gynecol 1985; 152: 524–39.

100. Grant A, O'Brien N, Joy MT et al. Cerebral palsy among children born during the Dublin randomised trial of intrapartum monitoring. Lancet 1989; 2(8674): 1233–6.

101. Impey L, Reynolds M, MacQuillan K et al. Admission cardiotocography: a randomised controlled trial. Lancet 2003; 361(9356): 465–70.

102. Vintzileos AM, Antsaklis A, Varvarigos I et al. A randomized trial of intrapartum electronic fetal heart rate monitoring versus intermittent auscultation. Obstet Gynecol 1993; 81: 899–907.

103. Vintzileos AM, Nochimson DJ, Antsaklis A et al. Comparison of intrapartum electronic fetal heart rate monitoring versus intermittent auscultation in detecting fetal acidemia at birth. Am J Obstet Gynecol 1995; 173: 1021–4.

104. Vintzileos AM, Nochimson DJ, Guzman ER et al. Intrapartum electronic fetal heart rate monitoring versus intermittent auscultation: a meta-analysis. Obstet Gynecol 1995; 85: 149–55.

105. Thacker SB, Stroup DF, Peterson HB. Efficacy and safety of intrapartum electronic fetal monitoring: an update. Obstet Gynecol 199; 86: 613–20.

106. ACOG technical bulletin. Umbilical artery blood acid-base analysis. No. 216, November 1995. American College of Obstetricians and Gynecologists: Washington, DC.

107. Thorp JA, Rushing RS. Umbilical cord blood gas analysis. Obstet Gynecol Clin North Am 1999; 26: 695–709.

108. Helwig JT, Parer JT, Kilpatrick SJ et al. Umbilical cord blood acid-base state: what is normal? Am J Obstet Gynecol 1996; 174: 1807–12.

109. Devoe L, Golde S. Kilman Y et al. A comparison of visual analyses of intrapartum fetal heart rate tracings according to the new National Institute of Child Health and Human Development guidelines with computer analyses by an automated fetal heart rate monitoring system. Am J Obstet Gynecol 2000; 183: 361–6.

20 Normal vaginal delivery

Morton A Stenchever and Lisa N Gittens-Williams

The role of the operator conducting delivery is to guide the fetus through the lower portion of the birth canal without injury to the mother or infant. To achieve this goal, the attendant must have an understanding of the preceding events. He or she must have the ability, furthermore, to perform interventions that either facilitate delivery or prevent unwanted complications.

Most modern obstetric suites provide for delivery of the mother in the dorsal lithotomy position. The legs may be placed in stirrups or leg holders, but should never be fixed into position as they may need to be removed in the event that shoulder dystocia occurs. Care should be taken to avoid injury to maternal nerves. Draping of the perineum serves to protect both the mother and the operator from infection.

Delivery of the head

After the fetal head descends, flexes, and rotates to the occiput anterior position, the labia minora will distend, and crowning will occur. At this time, an opening of approximately 3–4 cm will be seen at the introitus. Should episiotomy be deemed necessary, it should be preformed at this time.

As the occiput passes under the pubic arch, the operator should be facing the perineum with a towel draped over the dominant hand. As the fetal head delivers by extension, the birth attendant will use the toweled hand to support the perineal body, palpating the fetal chin. The opposite hand is placed flat with fingers extended and partially separated over the vertex. As the vertex delivers under the symphysis, the lower hand guides the head over the perineum, while the upper one ensures that sudden expulsion and rapid extension do not occur with maternal pushing or uterine contractions. The operator should have a direct view of the perineum, so as to observe for and prevent tearing or extension of an episiotomy. The fetal head can be controlled and delivery facilitated through the use of a modification of the original maneuver described by von Ritgen in 1828.[1] This maneuver is accomplished by palpating the fetal chin and applying traction in the anterior-inferior direction, which will reduce the perineal body over the fetal head and chin (Figure 20.1).

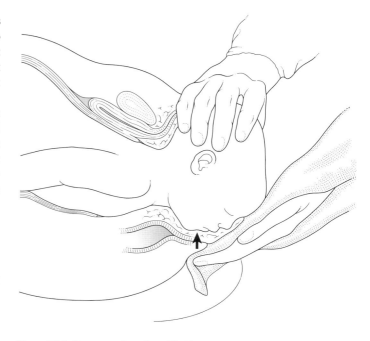

Figure 20.1 Demonstration of modified Ritgen's maneuver.

As soon as the head is delivered, the operator should discard the towel, as it may be contaminated with fecal material. The head will restitute to its previous position (i.e., LOA, ROA, etc.). The baby's mouth and nasopharynx should be suctioned. Bulb suctioning is generally performed when there is no meconium staining of the amniotic fluid noted. When meconium staining is present, the De Lee suction device attached to a mechanical vacuum source is used to clear the fetal airway.

After clearing the fetal mouth and nasopharynx, the operator should inspect and palpate the fetal neck for the presence of a nuchal cord. Any identified nuchal cord should be reduced, if possible, by gently slipping it over the infant's head. Management of the tight nuchal cord which cannot easily be reduced is controversial. Many textbooks suggest that such a nuchal cord should be doubly clamped and cut. However such a practice is unwise and should be avoided unless absolutely necessary, because, if the operator encounters difficulty with the extraction of the body, irreversible damage to the fetus can result. Several such cases were reported by Iffy et al, who concluded that the practice of severing the cord prior to full delivery of the baby is very dangerous.[2]

Delivery of the body

After restitution of the fetal head, the operator should place his or her hands on either side of the fetal head along the parietal bones with the fingers pointing towards the occiput. The operator should avoid placing hands on the fetal neck, as this can result in nerve injury. In many cases, spontaneous delivery of the fetal shoulders will immediately follow the delivery of the fetal head; however, frequently, a delay occurs. A 2–4-minute pause before the rotation and passage of the shoulder through the pelvis at the peak of the next contraction is a natural physiologic phenomenon. In the absence of complications such as cord prolapse or abruptio placentae, this delay creates no risk. If the shoulders are not spontaneously delivered, the operator should wait for the next contraction, and then encourage the mother to push.[3] The application of continuous gentle downward traction on the fetal head, directed towards the floor, should result in the delivery of the anterior shoulder at this time (Figure 20.2a). The operator should then visualize the perineum and next lift the body upward to deliver the posterior shoulder (Figure 20.2b). Once both shoulders are delivered, the accoucheur guides the body along his or her arm (Figure 20.3). Once the baby is delivered, it is held so that the head is lower than the body, and the oral and nasal passageways are suctioned once again.

Cutting of the cord

There has been controversy about when the cord should be clamped. Proponents of immediate clamping believe that infusing additional volume into the fetus may result in excessive red cell destruction or hypervolemia. The opposite argument states that the fetus may benefit from the extra volume contained in the placenta. A volume of up to 80 cc has been reported to shift into the neonate if the cord is not clamped during the first 3 minutes of life.[4] It is to be remembered, however, that the baby loses blood if held under the level of the uterus. In one study a reduction in need for blood and albumin transfusion was noted in those infants whose cord clamping had been delayed by 20 seconds after delivery, compared to those who had immediate clamping.[5] A reasonable approach is to cut the cord after the nasopharynx has been suctioned.

The umbilical cord should be cut between two clamps placed approximately 4–5 cm from the fetal abdomen. A plastic cord clamp is placed later 1–2 cm from the fetal abdomen and the cord is cut again. If assessment of cord pH is indicated,

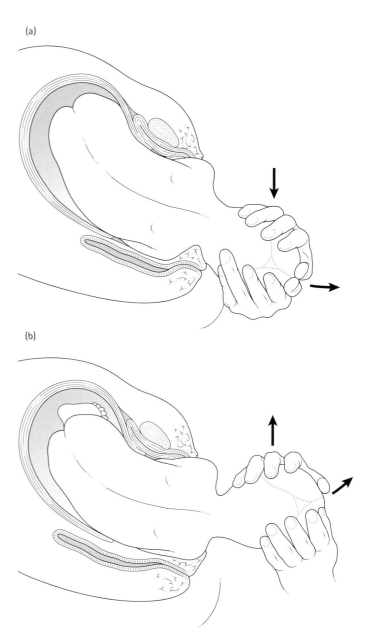

Figure 20.2 Delivery of shoulders. (a) Anterior and (b) posterior.

a segment of the remaining cord can be clamped, cut, and sent for blood gas analysis.

Delivery of the placenta

After severing the cord, appropriate blood samples are taken from the placental side of the cord. With this completed, the operator looks for signs of placental separation. Signs of placental separation include elongation of the cord, a palpable globular mass on the maternal abdomen, and a sudden gush of blood with protrusion of the placenta through the cervix into the vagina.

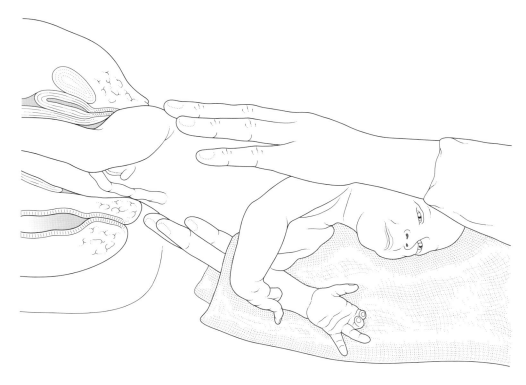

Figure 20.3 Delivery of body.

The average duration of the third stage of labor is 8 minutes. Placental separation occurs within 30 minutes after the delivery of the fetus in 95% of parturients. Once signs of separation are noted, the attendant may assist in the delivery of the placenta. This is achieved by placing the extended fingers of one hand on the maternal abdomen, just above the symphysis pubis and then moving the fingers over the uterine fundus. With the opposite hand the attendant may apply gentle traction on the cord (Brant–Andrews maneuver) (Figure 20.4a and b).[6] The mother may then be asked to bear down.

In delivering the placenta, the operator must not force placental separation. The practice of holding the fundus with the abdominal hand may be continued until the placenta is delivered.[7] An alternative method, Credé's maneuver, in which the cord is fixed with the lower hand while the uterine fundus is gently compressed by the abdominal hand, may also be used.

Occasionally, the placenta delivers but the membranes do not rapidly separate and remain, extending up into the uterus. Such membranes may be grasped with ring forceps and twisted to achieve removal. The trailing membranes may be grasped with another ring forceps placed higher up on the membranes. This process is repeated until all membranes are removed. The placenta and its membranes should be inspected immediately to ensure that they are intact.

A succenturiate placenta may inadvertently be left in the uterus. A ruptured vessel near the placental margin or a jagged edge to the placenta may alert the operator to the possibility of retained cotyledon. If retained products are suspected, the uterus should be explored manually with or without a gauze sponge. The inspection of the placenta should also include evaluation of the cord for the presence of two arteries and one vein. The presence of a single artery suggests an up to 50% possibility of fetal anomaly or growth restriction. This finding should be reported to the pediatric attendant.[8]

After removal of the placenta, the uterine fundus should be assessed for firmness. To achieve this, the operator places his hand on the maternal abdomen and gently massages the fundus while oxytocin is administered.

Use of oxytocics

Oxytocin (Pitocin) and methylergonovine maleate (Methergine) are widely used to control blood loss after delivery. They have been shown to be superior to placebo or no prophylaxis. Uterine contractions are critical in the control of blood loss.[9] The contractions close the vessels in the uterine wall. Oxytocin causes rhythmic uterine contractions that affect primarily the fundal portion. It has little or no secondary effect on blood pressure when administered as a continuous infusion. Methergine can cause uterine spasm that involves the lower uterine segment and has a hypertensive effect in many women. It is associated with increases in femoral arterial pressure, pulmonary arterial pressure, and wedge pressure.[10,11]

15-Methyl-F-prostaglandin (Prostin 15 M) is a potent uterotonic agent which can be injected intramuscularly or directly

(a)

(b)

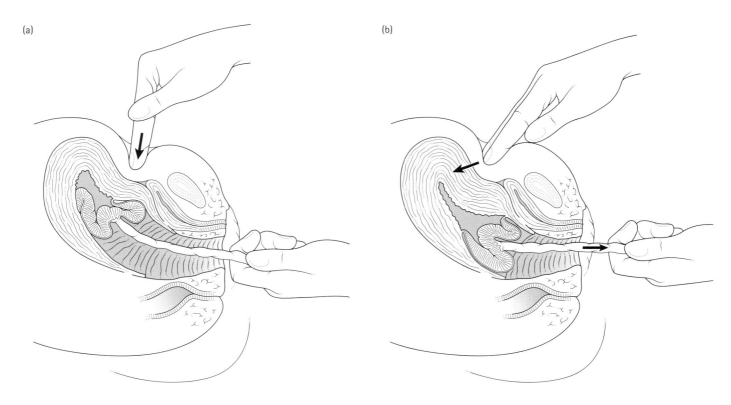

Figure 20.4 Brandt–Andrews maneuver for delivery of placenta. (a) Positioning of abdominal hand; (b) performance of the maneuver.

into the myometrium. It is used primarily in cases of postpartum hemorrhage, as is the E1 prostaglandin, Misoprostol. However, the literature does not support their superiority to conventional injectable oxytocics for routine management of the third stage of labor.[12,13]

Active management of the third stage with oxytocics plus cord traction has been reported. The cord was not clamped and the placenta was delivered with maternal expulsion. The patients had shorter third stage of labor but no reduction in blood loss.[14]

While some trials suggest that oxytocin plus ergotmetrine is superior to oxytocin alone for the management of the third stage, others show that ergometrine often causes nausea vomiting and raised blood pressure.[15] In most obstetric units in the USA, oxytocin is administered by adding 20 units to 1 l of fluid and adjusting the infusion rate to achieve the desired uterine contractile effect.

Although most experts agree that the management of the third stage of labor should include the administration of oxytocics to reduce maternal blood loss, the timing of administration varies among institutions.[16] The administration of oxytocin and ergonovine before the placental delivery will reduce blood loss.[9,17] However, this practice may entrap an undiagnosed twin. Most trials report decreased blood loss with active management.[7,18] In patients at low risk of postpartum hemorrhage, however, delaying the administration of oxytocin after the placental delivery does not significantly increase the risk of maternal hemorrhage.[14]

Management of the retained placenta

Retained placenta affects 0.5–3% of women after delivery. Dynamic visualization of the uterus during the third stage of labor by radiography and ultrasound has shown that placental separation depends upon contraction of the myometrium and subsequent detachment and expulsion.[19] The risk of retained placenta and hemorrhage is increased in gestations less than 26 weeks and when the duration of the third stage is prolonged.

Regardless of gestational age, the frequency of hemorrhage peaks 40 minutes after the delivery. About 90% of placentas at term will be delivered by 15 minutes and only some 2% will still be undelivered at 30 minutes.[20] If the placenta is not expelled after 30 minutes, it may be abnormally adherent, or may be entrapped by the contracted cervix. Under such circumstances, manual placental removal is indicated.

The prerequisites for manual removal include the following. An IV line should be placed and fluids administered. A tube of maternal blood should be sent for type and screen or cross-match. The necessity for the procedure should be explained to the patient and her consent obtained. Adequate anesthesia, regional, general, or IV sedation, should be given.

The operator should wear fresh sterile gloves. A sterile sleeve should be placed over the dominant arm. The field should be redraped. The operator then holds the umbilical cord with the assisting hand and introduces the dominant hand into the uterine cavity. The outside hand is then placed on the uterine fundus. The operator uses his fingers to locate the plane between the uterine wall and the placenta. When this plane is identified, gentle motion of the fingertips is used to separate the placenta from the uterine wall (Figure 20.5). The operator should resist the urge to exert undue traction on the cord as this may tear the placenta or cord and result in retained fragments. The operator should also resist the urge to scoop out fragments of the placenta in pieces. Generally, separation occurs with ease. The process should be continued until the placenta is completely detached. The opposite hand assists in the placental delivery by lifting the fundus towards the examining hand and giving counter pressure. Once the placenta is removed, with or without a sterile piece of gauze placed over the operator's hand, manual curettage is performed. The goal is to remove an intact placenta.

After the placenta has been removed, it should be inspected for completeness. If it does not appear intact or if it has been removed in fragments, the operator should re-explore the uterus and remove remaining fragments and membranes. Exceptionally, if remaining placental fragments cannot be removed manually, a large blunt curette may be introduced to remove them. Sharp curettage should be avoided. Routine use of antibiotics for manual exploration is not beneficial.

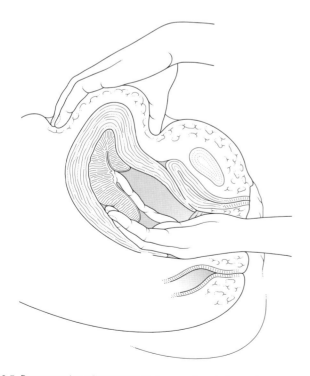

Figure 20.5 Demonstration of maneuver to remove placenta from uterus manually.

Management of the fourth stage of labor

The fourth stage of labor includes the time when inspection of the birth canal and repair of lacerations and episiotomy take place. During this immediate postpartum period, the mother is observed for stability and postpartum hemorrhage.

Inspection of the birth canal involves a systematic evaluation of lacerations and bleeding. The first step is to inspect the episiotomy, if one has been performed, and determine whether extension has occurred or other perineal damage exists. Blood loss related to episiotomy should be noted. If excessive, it may require immediate intervention. The vagina is then inspected for lacerations. The operator should place one hand into the vagina, and inspect its deep areas, using a ring forceps with a large sponge. Lacerations of the vagina should be noted and repair performed with 2–0 chromic catgut or a comparable synthetic absorbable suture. In some cases, for repair of a deep vaginal laceration, an assistant has to provide adequate exposure.

After the vagina, the cervix should be checked. It may be visualized by the operator placing his hand onto the pelvic floor, to facilitate its direct inspection. If the entire cervix cannot be seen, a useful technique is to place ring forceps onto the anterior and posterior cervical lips, and, with gentle traction, lift and observe the cervix. Alternatively, ring forceps may be used to grasp the anterior cervical lip, and the cervix may be grasped with a second forceps in a circumferential fashion, to 'walk around the cervix' until all areas are visualized. Any laceration noted on the cervix must be repaired.

Routine manual uterine exploration is not indicated. Exploration should be reserved for those women where bleeding is excessive, or placental separation is thought to be incomplete.

Use of episiotomy

A relaxing incision known as episiotomy is frequently performed to protect the maternal soft tissue from unduly stretching or lacerating. Although a decrease in episiotomy rates has been noted between 1985 and 2000, it is still performed in up to 40% of vaginal deliveries in the USA.[21,22] It is most commonly indicated in association with instrumental delivery or to hasten delivery in cases of fetal compromise.

Two types of episiotomy are commonly performed. A median (midline) episiotomy refers to a vertical incision made from the posterior fourchette towards the rectum.[23] This incision in the midline severs the skin, the subcutaneous tissue, and the central junction of the paired bulbocavernosus, ischiocavernosus, and superficial transverse perineal muscles; the area known as the perineal body.

A mediolateral episiotomy may be done if room is required and the operator does not wish to risk a fourth-degree laceration. Extra room may be needed in the case of a large fetus or for an instrumental delivery. The incision will include some muscle bundles.

Since the mediolateral incision protects against posterior perineal trauma, it has long been recommended as the preferred incision for women with inflammatory bowel disease, prior rectovaginal fistula, or prior posterior perineal repair, where protection of the rectum is critical.

Satore et al evaluated puerpural pelvic floor strength and dysfunction among women who underwent mediolateral episiotomy and compared this to others who had either intact perineum or spontaneous first- and second-degree lacerations after vaginal delivery. These investigators concluded that mediolateral epsiotomy did not protect against urinary and anal incontinence or genital prolapse, and was conducive to dyspareunia and pain.[24]

The role of prophylactic episiotomy has been long debated. Early proponents of this practice argued that the repair of a straight surgical incision is easier than that of an irregular, jagged injury. Proponents additionally argued that episiotomy could prevent perineal trauma and pelvic floor relaxation. In one study, midline episiotomy carried a fourfold increase in third- and fourth-degree lacerations in primiparas and a 13-fold increase in mulitparas when compared to mediolateral or no episiotomy.[25]

Recent studies have confirmed that routine episiotomy is associated with increase in anal and rectal tears,[26–28] and is not contributory to a decreased frequency of severe perineal tears.[23] When comparing women who had an episiotomy to those who had either spontaneous laceration or no laceration, those who had an episiotomy had more postoperative fecal incontinence.[29] While repair of an episiotomy may be easier than that of a laceration, the belief that pain is less and healing is better with an episiotomy than a tear has proven to be false.[30] In an evaluation of data from six trials, the latter was associated with less posterior perineal trauma, less need for repair, and fewer healing complications. Based on risks of complications, the evidence does not support its routine use.[28,31] The decision for episiotomy should be individualized and take into account the complications and morbidity associated with it.[28,32] Some investigators suggest that an episiotomy rate of greater than 30% is excessive.[22]

Technique of episiotomy

A midline episiotomy should be made when the fetal head is crowning and has distended the vulva to 2–3 cm. If a regional block is in place, no additional anesthesia may be required; alternatively, local anesthesia should be given. The operator should place his or her fingers inside the perineum to protect the fetal head. Using a straight scissors, a downward incision is made from the midpoint of the posterior fourchette, towards the rectum, through approximately half of the perineal body. The incision can be extended further vertically up the vaginal mucosa for a length of approximately 2–3 cm.

A mediolateral episiotomy is made by cutting from the midpoint of the posterior fourchette through the vaginal mucosa at a 45° angle. The incision may be made to the right or to the left. The direction usually depends upon the operator's dominant hand. The length of the median incision should be adequate to allow delivery of the head.

Complications of episiotomy

In addition to increased incidence of third- and fourth-degree lacerations, episiotomy can be associated with excessive blood loss, particularly if the incision is made before the fetal head distends the vulva. Midline episiotomy is associated with more perineal and pelvic floor damage than no episiotomy or spontaneous lacerations.[33] Those episiotomies that are complicated by extension to third- and fourth-degree lacerations may be associated with anal sphincter incontinence, pelvic floor injury, rectovaginal fistula, and pelvic prolapse.[34]

The mediolateral incision is associated more commonly with poor cosmetic results and greater blood loss. There is, however, no evidence to indicate that the mediolateral episiotomy is associated with more pain than the midline incision.[35] Both types of episiotomy can be complicated by infection, hematoma, and dehiscence.

Repair of episiotomy

Repair of episiotomy is generally delayed until after delivery of the placenta. This practice avoids the disruption of the repair should the placenta be retained and manual exploration of the uterus be required. Midline episiotomy is generally repaired with 2–0 or 3–0 chromic catgut or a comparable synthetic absorbable suture.[36,37]

Repair of the episiotomy begins with the identification of the apex of the incision. The first suture is placed above the apex and tied. Suturing should progress in a continuous running fashion to approximate the vaginal mucosa. The first stitch should be locked to aid in hemostasis at the apex, but not the remainder of them unless the edges of the incision are bleeding. Locking the sutures in this region may invert the vaginal mucosa and lead to inclusion cysts. When the vaginal suture reaches the hymenal ring, it should be brought inside the vaginal mucosa and completed by the placement of a deep suture which approximates the two bulbocavernous muscles in the midline. The suture is then tied and the knot buried (Figure 20.6a). Next, two to three interrupted sutures are placed to approximate the deep layers of the perineum (Figure 20.6b). Lastly, a continuous subcutaneous suture is begun at the vaginal edge of the perineum, leaving the end tied for later use. This end may be held temporarily by a hemostat. The subcutaneous sutures are placed in a continuous running fashion to the lower perineal edge of the wound (Figure 20.6c), and then returned in a subcuticular pattern back to the vaginal perineal margin (Figure 20.6d). The suture is then tied to the original hemostat end. This allows for burying of the final knot so that no suture will remain exposed.

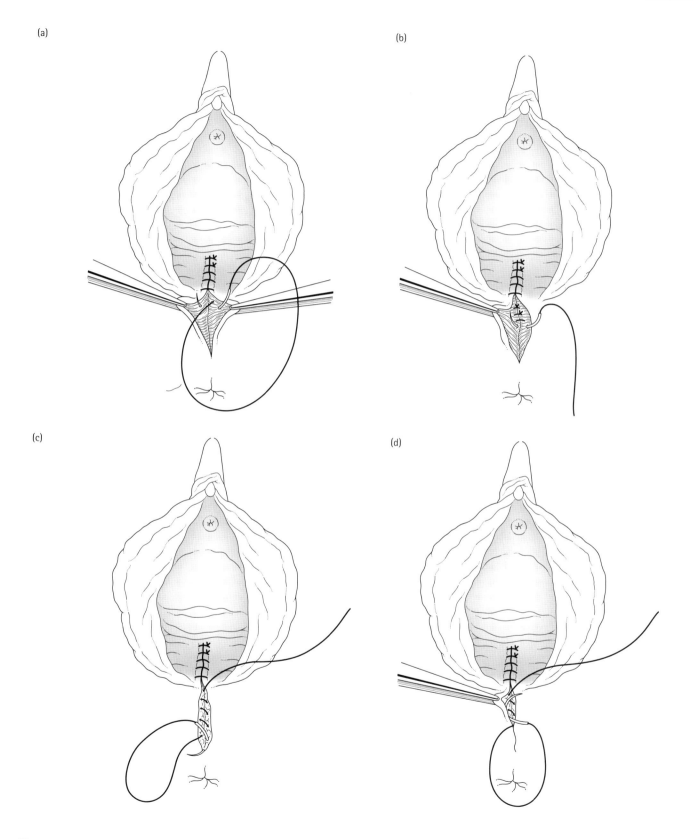

Figure 20.6 Repair of median episiotomy. (a) Closure of vaginal and bulbocavernosal muscles, (b) closure of deep layers, (c) subcutaneous closure, (d) subcuticular closure.

Postepisiotomy pain and swelling can be managed with ice packs and oral or topical analgesia. When fourth-degree lacerations have occurred, stool softeners may be prescribed. Postepisiotomy infectious morbidity is uncommon, but prophylactic antibiotics may reduce infectious morbidity in high-risk patients. Since primary repair after third- and fourth-degree lacerations may prove inadequate, patients who had extensions of their episiotomy to third- or fourth-degree tears should be counseled about symptoms of fecal incontinence and sexual dysfunction.[31]

Delivery of the malpresenting fetal head

Face presentation

The incidence of face presentation is 0.1–0.3% of all vertex deliveries. Cesarean delivery is indicated for cases of suspected cephalopelvic disproportion, large infants, desultory labor, or failure to progress. If the mentum is posterior, cesarean section should be performed, since this position does not allow for natural expulsion of the fetus.

Overall, there is a 50% cesarean rate associated with face presentation. In a review of 50 300 deliveries, 40 cases of face presentation were examined. Thirty percent of the operative deliveries were for fetal distress; the rest were performed for failure to progress in labor. Vaginal delivery occurred in 88% with mentum anterior, 45% with the mentum transverse, and 2.5% of those with mentum posterior rotations. Twenty-seven percent of mentum posterior spontaneously rotated to mentum anterior. Fetal distress was particularly common in the mentum posterior presentation.[38] Appropriate management of face presentation is to allow spontaneous labor unless indications for abdominal delivery are present. If the pelvis and the uterine contractions are adequate, vaginal delivery may ensue.

After descent, as the face appears at the vulva, the chin will be under the symphysis and the operator can deliver the head by assisted flexion (Figures 20.7a and b). Performance of a deep episiotomy is helpful in these cases. The shoulders are then delivered as in a cephalic presentation.

Manual conversion of the face presentation to a vertex or rotation of the posterior mentum anteriorly, manually or with forceps, should not be attempted, although successful bimanual conversion of mentoposterior to occipitoanterior presentation has been described.[39]

Brow presentation

Brow presentation represents a fetal position midway between the full flexion of the occiput presentation and the full extension of the face presentation (Figure 20.8). Except in the case of a very small fetus or a very large pelvis, engagement of the fetal head in the brow presentation is impossible. Since there is cephalopelvic disproportion and because a great deal of molding has taken place, thereby locking the head into a fixed position, cesarean delivery is indicated. If during the course of labor, the brow presentation persists, the prognosis for vaginal delivery is poor. If the brow converts to smaller presenting fetal head diameter, delivery may occur as in the occiput presentation.

Malrotations of the fetal head

Occiput posterior rotation has been reported in 10–25% of the cases in the early stage of labor and in 10–15% in the active phase. Persistent fetal occiput posterior position occurs in

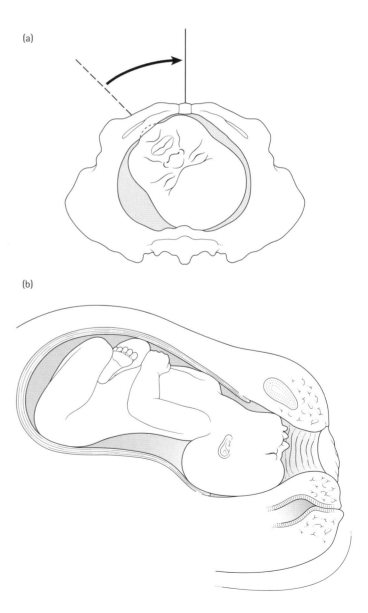

Figure 20.7(a,b) Face presentation with the mentum anterior.

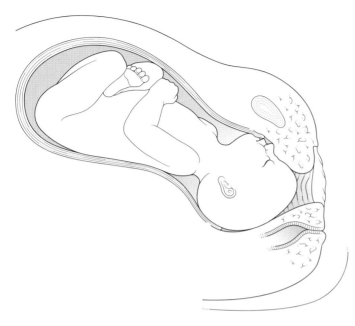

Figure 20.8 Brow presentation.

approximately 5% of all deliveries. The incidence is higher in primiparas than in multiparas. Persistent occiput posterior is rotation associated with prolonged labor, and need for induction, oxytocin augmentation, and epidural use. Persistent occiput posterior rotation is associated with short maternal stature and prior cesarean delivery.[40,41]

The majority of occiput posterior positions change to anterior during labor even at full cervical dilation.[42] With good flexion of the head, its presenting diameter is minimized; with less flexion, the large occipitofronatal diameter is presenting. In either case, the head is delivered by further flexion. The face should be expelled to the chin before one attempts to deliver the rest of the head. A large episiotomy is often required.

A variety of maneuvers, including positioning the mother in the knee to chest position and pelvic rocking, have been described to facilitate rotation of the fetus. These efforts have not proven to be effective.[43] Occiput posterior rotation is also associated with high rates of third- and fourth-degree perineal lacerations, excessive blood loss, and postpartum infections when compared to delivery in the occiput anterior position.[41]

While malrotation occurs more commonly in anthropoid and android pelves, transverse arrests tend to occur in the flat (platypelloid) pelvis. It is important that the operator recognize these malpositions so that appropriate assistance to the delivery of the head can be given to minimize maternal trauma.

Vaginal birth after caesarean

Before allowing vaginal birth after cesarean section, the operator should obtain informed consent and review the risks and benefits of the procedure. The actual delivery of the patient

undergoing vaginal birth after cesarean is not different from that of patients without a uterine scar. Epidural anesthesia and use of oxytocics intrapartum and postpartum are not contraindicated. Routine exploration of the uterus to assess for dehiscence of the uterine scar is not necessary. If there is excessive bleeding or signs of hypovolemia, complete assessment of the previous uterine scar and the entire lower genital tract is in order.[44]

Vaginal delivery of the premature infant

Delivery of the premature infant presenting by the vertex is a variation of normal vaginal birth. Because of the small fetal size relative to the maternal pelvis, malpresentation, asynclitism, and compound presentations are relatively common. These are managed in the same way as for the term fetus. The operator must be vigilant in observing for a loop of cord or other fetal part that may present alongside the fetal head. If a hand or arm accompanies the head into the pelvis, watching and waiting are the best approach. If the compound presentation persists, gentle maneuvering of the arm or hand towards the pelvis may be attempted.

If the fetus is small relative to the pelvis, even in compound presentation it may be delivered without difficulty. Most studies have shown that for the low-birth-weight fetus without signs of fetal compromise, vaginal delivery is preferable.[45] Reducing trauma to the premature fetus at delivery and optimizing neonatal care are paramount in the management. Personnel for the resuscitation of the infant should be immediately available. Often a bulging bag of water is presenting as the cervix dilates. The operator must remember that the cervical dilation may prove incomplete, once the membranes are ruptured. A portion of cord or a small fetal part may be in advance of the vertex. Use of ultrasound may be helpful to clarify this situation. Artificial rupture of the membranes in these circumstances must be approached judiciously, and should be attempted only when the cervix is approaching full dilation. The membranes may then be needled, allowing slow decompression of the amniotic sac and safe descent of the vertex into the pelvis. Spontaneous delivery can then be allowed with focus on controlling the delivery of the head to prevent rapid expulsion. Episiotomy may be used as indicated.

References

1. Speert H. Obstetrical and Gynecologic Milestones, p. 577. Macmillan: New York, 1958.

2. Iffy L, Varadi V, Papp E. Untoward neonatal sequelae deriving from cutting of the umbilical cord before delivery. Med Law 2001; 20: 627–34.

3. Iffy L, Ganesh V, Gittens L. Obstetric maneuvers for shoulder dystocia. Am J Obstet Gynecol 1998; 179: 1379–80.

4. Yao AC, Lind J. Placental transfusion. Am J Dis Child 1974; 127: 128–41.

5. Ibrahim H, Krouskop RW, Lewis DF et al. Placental transfusion: umbilical cord clamping and preterm infants. J Perinatol 2000; 20: 351–4.

6. Brandt MI. The mechanism and management of the third stage of labor. Am J Obstet Gynecol 1933; 28: 266.

7. Prendiville WJ, Harding JE, Elbourne DR et al. The Bristol third state trial: active versus physiological management of third stage of labour. BMJ 1988; 297: 1295–300.

8. Heifetz SA. Single umbilical artery: a statistical analysis of 237 autopsy cases and review of the literature. Perspect Pediatr Pathol 1984; 8: 345–78.

9. Prendiville WJ, Elbourne DR, Chalmers I. The effects of routine oxytocic administration in the management of the third stage of labour: an overview of the evidence from controlled trials. Br J Obstet Gynaecol 1988; 95: 3–16.

10. Hendricks CH, Brenner WE. Cardiovascular effects of oxytocic drugs used postpartum. Am J Obstet Gynecol 1970; 108: 751–60.

11. Secher NJ, Arnsbo P, Wallin L. Haemodynamic effects of oxytocin (syntocinon) and methyl ergometrine (methergin) on the systemic and pulmonary circulations of pregnant anaesthetized women. Acta Obstet Gynecol Scand 1978; 57: 97–103.

12. Gulmezoglu AM, Forna F, Villar J et al. Prostaglandins for prevention of postpartum haemorrhage [Review]. Eur J Obstet Gynecol Reprod Biol 2003; 3: 1.

13. Khan RU, El-Refaey R. Pharmacokinetics and adverse-effect profile of rectally administered misoprostol in the third stage of labor. Obstet Gynecol 2003; 101: 968–74.

14. Thilaganathan B, Cutner A, Latimer J et al. Management of the third stage of labour in women at low risk of postpartum haemorrhage. Eur J Obstet Gynecol Repod Biol 1993; 48: 19–22.

15. Mitchell GG, Elbourne DR. The Salford Third Stage Trial. Oxytocin plus ergometrine versus oxytocin alone in the active managment of the third stage of labor. Online J Curr Clin Trials 1993; 83.

16. Khan GQ, John IS, Wani S et al. Controlled cord traction versus minimal intervention techniques in delivery of the placenta: a randomized controlled trial. Am J Obstet Gynecol 1997; 177: 770–4.

17. Sorbe S. Active pharmacologic management of the third stage of labor. A comparison of oxytocin and ergemetrine. Obstet Gynecol 1978; 52: 694–7.

18. Prendiville WJ, Elbourne D, McDonald S. Active versus expectant management in the third stage of labour. Cochrane Library 2004; vol (3).

19. Herman A, Weinraub Z, Bukovsky I et al. Dynamic ultrasonographic imaging of the third stage of labor: new perspectives into third stage mechanism. Am J Obstet Gynecol 1993; 168: 1496–9.

20. Dombrowski MP, Bottoms SF, Saleh AA et al. Obstetrics: third stage of labor: analysis of duration and clinical practice. Am J Obstet Gynecol 1995; 172: 1279–84.

21. Goldberg J, Holtz D, Hyslop T et al. Has the use of routine episiotomy decreased? Examination of episiotomy rates from 1983 to 2000. Obstet Gynecol 2002; 99: 395–400.

22. Weber AM, Meyn L. Episiotomy use in the United States, 1979–1997. Obstet Gynecol 2002; 100: 1177–82.

23. Anthony S, Buitenjijk SE, Zondervan KT et al. Episiotomies and the occurrence of severe perineal lacerations. Br J Obstet Gynaecol 1994; 101: 1064–7.

24. Sartore A, De Seta F, Maso G et al. The effects of mediolateral episiotomy on pelvic floor function after vaginal delivery. Obstet Gynecol 2004; 103: 669–73.

25. Shiono P, Klebanoff MA, Carey JC. Midline episiotomies: more harm than good? Obstet Gynecol 1990; 75: 765–70.

26. Angioli R, Gomez-Marin O, Cantuaria G et al. Severe perineal lacerations during vaginal delivery: the University of Miami experience. Am J Obstet Gynecol 2000; 182: 1083–5.

27. Carroli G, Belizan J. Episiotomy for vaginal birth. Cochrane Database Syst Rev Issue 2, 2004.

28. Eason E, Labrecque M, Wells G et al. Preventing perineal trauma during childbirth: a systematic review. Obstet Gynecol 2000; 95: 464–71.

29. Signorello LB, Harlow BL, Chekos AK et al. Midline episiotomy and anal incontinence: retrospective cohort study. BMJ 2000; 320: 86–90.

30. Larsson PG, Platz-Christenson JJ, Bergman B, Wallstersson G. Advantage or disadvantage of episiotomy compared with spontaneous perineal laceration. Gynecol Obstet Invest 1991; 31: 213.

31. Gjessing H, Backe B, Sahlin Y. Third degree obstetric tears; outcome after primary repair. Acta Obstet Gynecol Scand 1998; 77: 736–40.

32. Combs CA, Robertson PA, Laros RK Jr. Risk factors for third-degree and fourth-degree perineal lacerations in forceps and vacuum deliveries. Am J Obstet Gynecol 1990; 163: 100–4.

33. Klein MC, Gauthier RJ, Robbins JM et al. Relationship of episiotomy to perineal trauma and morbidity, sexual dysfunction, and pelvic floor relaxation. Am J Obstet Gynecol 2004; 171: 591–8.

34. Poen AC, Felt-Bersma RJF, Strijers RLM et al. Third-degree obstetric perineal tear: long-term clinical and functional results after primary repair. Br J Surg 1998; 85: 1433–8.

35. Coats PM, Chan KK, Wilkins M et al. A comparison between midline and mediolateral episiotomies. Br J Obstet Gynaecol 1980; 87: 408–12.

36. Grant A. The choice of suture materials and techniques for repair of perineal trauma: an overview of the evidence from controlled trials. Br J Obstet Gynaecol 1989; 96: 1281.

37. Mahomed K, Grant A, Ashurst H et al. The Southmead perineal suture study: a randomized comparison of suture materials and suturing techniques for repair of perineal trauma. Br J Obstet Gynaecol 1989; 96: 1275.

38. Benedetti TJ, Lowensohn RI, Truscott AM. Face presentation at term. Obstet Gynecol 1980; 55: 199–201.

39. Neuman J, Beller U, Lavie O et al. Intrapartum bimanual tocolytic-assisted reversal of face presentation: preliminary report. Obstet Gynecol 1994; 84: 146–8.

40. Fitzpatrick M, McQuillan K, O'Herlihy C. Influence of persistent occiput posterior position on delivery outcome. Obstet Gynecol 2001; 98: 1027–31.

41. Ponkey SE, Cohen AP, Heffner LJ, Lieberman E. Persistent fetal occiput posterior position: obstetric outcomes. Obstet Gynecol 2003; 101: 915–20.

42. Akmal S, Tsoi E, Howard R et al. Investigation of occiput posterior delivery by intrapartum sonography. Ultrasound Obstet Gynecol 2004; 24: 425–8.

43. Kariminia A, Chamberlain ME, Keogh J et al. Randomised controlled trial of effect of hands and knees posturing on incidence of occiput posterior position at birth. BMJ 2004; 328: 490.

44. Scott JR. Avoiding labor problems during vaginal birth after cesarean delivery. Clin Obstet Gynecol 1997; 40: 533–41.

45. Bauer J, Hentschel R, Zahradnik H et al. Vaginal delivery and neonatal outcome in extremely-low-birth-weight infants below 26 weeks of gestational age. Am J Perinat 2003; 20: 181–8.

21 Shoulder dystocia

Joseph Ramieri and Leslie Iffy

Shoulder dystocia has no generally accepted definition. According to the most widely used interpretation, the diagnosis is applicable 'when, in the absence of spontaneous expulsion of the fetus, the standard delivery procedure of gentle downward traction of the fetal head has failed to accomplish delivery'.[1] Based on the traditional British concept of midwifery, the definition of this entity is different in certain European countries[2,3] and some services in the USA.[4] According to this interpretation, interruption of the birthing process following the delivery of the head is a physiologic phenomenon which requires no intervention. Arrest of the shoulders is not deemed to have occurred, therefore, until and unless the next uterine contraction, that usually follows the emergence of the head within 2–3 minutes, has failed to expel the shoulders and the rest of the fetal body. Intrinsic to this concept is the understanding that retraction of the shoulders against the perineum ('turtle sign') is a part of the physiologic delivery process and only seldom a harbinger of arrest of the shoulders. The difference between these concepts is far reaching both conceptually and in terms of clinical implications. However, when the next contraction fails to expel the body, the diagnosis is considered established by all criteria. From that point on, there is little disagreement about the actions to be taken.[5–9]

Rate of occurrence

The reported incidence of shoulder dystocia is 0.15–1.7% of all deliveries.[4,8–12] The more than 10-fold difference in range is an indication of the fact that the diagnosis is subjective and depends upon the training, experience, emotional stability, and state of mind of the person conducting the delivery. In those services where nonintervention until the next uterine contraction is the preferred approach, the reported incidence is low.[4]

Although the rate of cesarean sections has increased in the USA about fivefold during the last 50 years,[13,14] that of shoulder dystocia has not decreased. Instead, fetal injuries associated with this complication became the leading medicolegal threat for obstetricians.[12] Currently, approximately 40% of all mal-practice litigations in the specialty involve claims associated with brachial plexus injuries.[15] Thus, along with premature delivery, fetal damage associated with arrest of the shoulders at birth is probably the most important unresolved problem in contemporary obstetrics.

Etiology

A broad variety of conditions and circumstances conducive to arrest of the shoulders at birth have been identified. They can be divided into three categories (Tables 21.1–21.3).

Inadequacy of the pelvis can make vaginal delivery difficult or impossible. Reduction of the anteroposterior diameter (platypelloid pelvis), is particularly important. However, excessive size of the fetus may preclude its passage even through a pelvis which is adequate by definition. Fetopelvic disproportion may be caused by the fact that, under certain circumstances, the width of the shoulders exceeds the greatest diameter of the head. This situation may lead to arrest of the shoulders in the process of delivery.

Small maternal stature is often associated with diminished pelvic dimensions. By predisposing to increased fetal size, excessive weight gain during pregnancy is conducive to the inability of the shoulders to pass through the birth canal.[16] With regard to the role of pre-existing maternal obesity, literature data differ.[5,16,17] Although relatively seldom mentioned in the

---

Table 21.1 Preconceptional risk factors for shoulder dystocia

Small maternal stature
Narrow pelvis
Gross obesity
Large maternal birth weight
Past birth of child large for gestational age
Past history of shoulder dystocia
Family history of diabetes
Personal history of diabetes
Age above 35 without past childbirth

Table 21.2 Prenatal risk factors for shoulder dystocia

Gestational diabetes
Borderline glucose tolerance
Fetus large for gestational age
Weight gain of 35 lbs (15.5 kg) or more during pregnancy
Postdatism or postmaturity
Preeclampsia

Table 21.3 Intrapartum risk factors for shoulder dystocia

Protracted or arrested first stage of labor
Protracted or arrested second stage of labor
Prolonged second stage
Use of extraction instrument
Use of oxytocin
Conduction anesthesia

literature, the mother's own birth weight is a useful predictor of that of her child and, thus, of the risk of arrest of the shoulders at delivery.[18]

Previous delivery of a large child is a risk factor for shoulder dystocia rather than reassurance about the woman's ability of giving birth to another big baby uneventfully. High recurrence rates have been reported after a preceding shoulder dystocia.[1] Family history of diabetes is a predisposing factor for gestational diabetes and, thus, another unfavorable prognostic factor.

It is a widespread misconception that the increased rate of postoperative complications in obese women warrants preferential delivery of morbidly obese gravidas by the vaginal route. In fact, there are data to indicate that the incidence of shoulder dystocia among grossly obese women may be almost 10-fold higher than in the general population.[19] Therefore, morbid obesity is a consideration for, rather than against, abdominal delivery.

Although it is a routine procedure in most teaching institutions, the need to screen all pregnant women by a glucose-loading test late in the second trimester of the pregnancy is still disputed.[20] As a result, a disturbingly high proportion of shoulder dystocia-related fetal injuries can be traced back to undiagnosed, uncontrolled, or inadequately controlled maternal diabetes.[21,22] There seems to be little justification, therefore, to replace routine testing of gravidas' glucose tolerance by some complex formula and calculate diabetic predisposition based on maternal age, race, body mass index, family history, and previous pregnancy outcome.

Minor degrees of glucose intolerance that do not fulfill the criteria for gestational diabetes still predispose to fetal macrosomia and its consequences.[23] Vice versa, excessive fetal weight gain can be avoided in the majority of diabetic patients by strict diet and, if necessary, by the use of insulin.[24]

It has been suggested that maternal weigh gain exceeding 35 lbs (15.5 kg) may increase the risk of large for gestational age

fetal status by as much as 10-fold.[1] According to most, but not all[17] authorities, prolongation of the pregnancy beyond the expected date of confinement increases the fetal risk exponentially, since fetal weight exceeding 4000 g is almost twice as frequent at week 42 of the gestation as at week 40.[25] The fetal risk further increases because the rate of growth of the fetal body exceeds that of the head at and beyond term gestation. A difference of 1.6 cm or more between the chest and head circumferences and a ≥4.8-cm discrepancy between those of the shoulders and the head identify a kind of fetal macrosomia which is highly conducive to shoulder dystocia at birth.[26,27] A discrepancy of ≥1.4 cm or more between the diameters of the fetal trunk and the head (biparietal diameter) has been found more predictive of a fetal weight exceeding 4000 g than the actual demonstration of such fetal weight by the customary techniques.[28]

Although arrest of the shoulders may occur after a normal labor process and even with precipitated delivery, intrapartum complications predispose to shoulder dystocia. Protraction or arrest disorder during the first stage[29] can be found in its background with relative frequency. Even more important is a prolonged second stage or one associated with protraction or arrest disorder.[5,6,21,22]

Uterine stimulation with oxytocin is a suspected predisposing factor.[5,21] However, since its use is frequently prompted by the occurrence of protraction or arrest disorder, its role is difficult to determine with certainty. The same applies to conduction anesthesia, the administration of which frequently leads to the use of oxytocin.[1]

There is a close relationship between the delivery of the fetus by forceps or vacuum extractor and arrest of the shoulders at birth.[5,21,30,31] Since an important early paper specifically referred to 'midpelvic extractions',[5] contemporary papers frequently imply that only the, by now largely abandoned, midforceps and midvacuum extraction operations are predisposing. In fact, at the time of the publication of the quoted paper, the term 'midpelvic extraction' incorporated those procedures that, on the basis of a recent reclassification,[32] are now referred to as low-forceps and low-vacuum extractions. Similar confusion has derived from the redefinition of the term 'macrosomia',[33] indicating a birth weight of 4500 g versus the traditional definition of 4000 g.[34] Papers published after this reclassification usually interpreted the term as a body weight exceeding 4500 g. Actually, writers who referred to 'macrosomia' prior to 1992 implied a weight exceeding 4000 g.[5] These misleading byproducts of well-intentioned innovations need to be kept in mind. Contemporary authors often misinterpret old literature data.

There is general agreement that the use of extraction instruments increases the risk of shoulder dystocia. However, opinions vary with regard to the magnitude of the increase of the risk from as little as 1.4-fold[17] to as much as 10–17-fold.[6,21,31] The wide difference among various estimates may be due to the fact that they are often used in cases of protracted or arrested second stage, complications that are conducive themselves to arrest of the shoulders at birth. Whereas the use of any kind of extraction instrument predisposes to shoulder dystocia, sequential application of vacuum extractor and forceps, in any order, increases the risk exponentially.[21,31] Since they are conducive to protracted labor, malrotation, deflexion, and asynclitism of the fetal head have similar effect.

Pathologic mechanisms of arrest of the shoulders

The introduction of radiographic pelvimetry into clinical practice contributed to the understanding of the fetopelvic relationship during the labor process.[35] Recognition of the fetal risks associated with exposure to irradiation largely removed diagnostic radiographic techniques from contemporary obstetric practice. An untoward effect of this development has been the loss of obstetricians' interest in the physiology of the labor and delivery process.[36]

Rarely, the natural forces fail to accomplish the expulsion of the body because, after its rotation, the anterior shoulder comes into collision with the pubic bone. Various technical procedures, to be described later, have been designed to overcome this particular situation, the classical clinical picture of shoulder dystocia. The use of traction or any other maneuver prior to the external rotation of the head is counterproductive, since the shoulders are not yet ready to pass through the midpelvis. Aware of the above described mechanism, British obstetricians refrain from intervention until the rotation of the shoulders has been completed. This often requires one more contraction and, thus, waiting for about 2–3 minutes.[2,3]

Some obstetricians, unmindful of the normal mechanism of labor, equate the turtle sign with the diagnosis of shoulder dystocia. Thus, they utilize traction under the erroneous impression that, once the head has been delivered, the fetus is in immediate danger. Actually, the child is not imperiled at this time.[37,38] If left alone, babies delivered by the process of 'two-step delivery'[36] are born in excellent condition. Cord around the neck, even if wrapped twice,[39] is less of a problem than complete disruption of the fetoplacental circulation. Therefore, clamping and cutting of the umbilical cord prior to the delivery of the shoulders is strongly discouraged. Implementation of this technique entailed catastrophic consequences in those instances when, following the severance of the cord, arrest of the shoulders had prevented prompt extraction of the body.[40]

Meconium staining of the amniotic fluid is not an indication for rapid extraction of the fetus from the birth canal. The next uterine contraction that follows the delivery of the head, before expelling the body of the child, squeezes a large amount of fluid out of the lungs[39] (Figure 21.1). Therefore, 'two-step delivery' may prevent or reduce the severity of meconium aspiration.

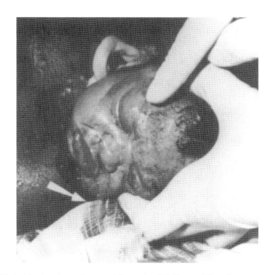

Figure 21.1 Mechanism of normal 'two-step' delivery. After the emergence of the head, the cord around the neck was loosened. No attempt was made to deliver the body until the occurrence of the next uterine contraction. The picture was taken during the onset of the next contraction. It depicts an important effect of the contraction: the expression of a substantial amount of mucus (arrow) from the respiratory tract. The cord complication was anticipated because of variable fetal heart rate decelerations documented on external fetal monitoring. (By the courtesy of Dr Vivic Johnson.)

Prediction and prevention

Over 10 years ago, the problem of shoulder dystocia was summarized in a publication as follows: 'Most of the traditional risk factors for shoulder dystocia have no predictive value, shoulder dystocia itself is an unpredictable event, and infants at risk of permanent injury are virtually impossible to predict. Thus, no protocol should serve to substitute for clinical judgment.'[41]

This defeatist philosophy was repeated in some publications,[42–44] often with the implication that the terms 'prediction' and 'prevention' are interchangeable. Actually, preventive medicine has seldom relied on prediction. The elimination of devastating diseases, such as smallpox, tuberculosis, and puerperal fever, and the teratogenic effects of drugs did not hinge upon prospective identification of individuals who would contract a particular infection or would suffer from the untoward effect of a potentially teratogenic agent. Thus, the numerous publications that confirmed and reconfirmed the unpredictability of shoulder dystocia have not helped to decrease the number of fetal injuries. Instead, orthopedic centers specializing in the surgical repair of Erb's palsy have mushroomed in the USA in recent years.

The fatalistic belief in the unpredictability of shoulder dystocia appears to have derived from two major considerations:

(1) The perceived difficulty of detecting macrosomia reliably by sonography.
(2) Mathematical calculations that claimed that an inordinate number of cesarean sections would be needed to reduce the rate of brachial plexus injuries.[45,46]

Intrinsic to the first argument has been the concern that sonography may overestimate the fetal weight, coupled with lack of attention to the fact that, by an equal chance, it can underestimate it. The philosophy that sonographic assessment of fetal weight at term is unacceptably unreliable is not shared by many prominent experts. Langer and associates calculated that, using an estimated fetal weight threshold of 4250 g as an indication for abdominal delivery for diabetic women, 76% of diabetes-related brachial plexus injuries could be prevented.[47] It is interesting, furthermore, that, with due recognition of its limitations, sonographic estimation of the fetal weight has been relied upon in many clinical situations, ranging from the determination of the expected date of confinement to detection of fetal growth retardation and the diagnosis of discordance between twins.

As for the mathematical calculation suggesting that 2335 cesarean sections would be needed to prevent one brachial plexus injury,[45,46] one need only remember that the generally quoted rate of arrest of the shoulders at birth is about 1% in the USA.[6,12] Of these babies, approximately 7% die or suffer permanent injury.[5,48] Thus, out of 1500 infants delivered vaginally, one becomes damaged due to arrests of the shoulders. Accordingly, one does not have to be a statistician to recognize that the quoted calculation is grossly inaccurate. Besides, this and other estimations ignore the fact that what needs to be prevented is not the shoulder dystocia but the fetal injuries deriving from it.

Management of delivery

The delivery of the head without the rest of the body does not cause immediate fetal compromise. Textbooks and other publications have emphasized for decades that delivery in the course of two separate uterine contractions is not a pathologic phenomenon.[2–4,37,39,49,50] The fact that the face of the fetus turns blue during the intervening time may be unnerving for the uninitiated.[49] The anxiety soon evaporates, however, when the next contraction expels the child in vigorous condition.[39]

Contemporary practice standards permit the use of manipulative techniques to facilitate the delivery of the fetal body. However, they must be used with due attention to the physiology of the birthing process. Actions that are not in synchrony with the latter are counterproductive. It is critically important to avoid strong traction. The majority of brachial plexus injuries involve extraction of the child's body within 3 minutes of the delivery of the head, that is, before the end of the next uterine contraction.[22] Traction is not useful until the external rotation of the head has been completed. Thereafter, if utilized at all, it must be unerringly gentle. It is a useful technique to give support to the posterior parietal bone as pulsion is made upon the anterior mandibular region. This method maintains the axis of the cervical spine as close as possible to that of the thoracic spine, thus avoiding stretching of the brachial plexus.

Ideally, the preparations for possible shoulder dystocia should begin before the delivery of the head. If the patient is not already in the lithotomy position, or if the delivery begins with the mother on a labor bed, the patient must be placed immediately at the edge of the table or that of the bed with her legs held in stirrups or supported by two assistants, as circumstances permit. After the emergence of the head, intravenous infusion, or increase of the rate of flow, of oxytocin is contributory to development of effective uterine contractions for the expulsion of the body from the birth canal.

Sharp hyperflexion of the patient's legs against her abdomen had been found useful for facilitating the delivery long before McRoberts re-emphasized its importance.[50,51] Traditionally, it was used only during contraction. Thus, cooperative parturients, laboring without conduction anesthesia, could implement it without any assistance (Figure 21.2). Under the circumstances of threatening or existing shoulder dystocia, this position needs to be maintained for a prolonged period of time. Therefore, it requires two assistants. The position aligns the sacrum with the lumbar spine and rotates the symphysis pubis to a blunt angle, thus facilitating the passage of the shoulder underneath. According to one report, in the course of more than 5000 deliveries, the McRoberts maneuver alone resolved all cases of shoulder dystocia without the use of any other technique.[52] Essentially, this finding confirms that nonintervention until the next uterine contraction drastically reduces the occurrence of serious shoulder dystocia.[4.36]

Often, the uterine contraction continues after the delivery of the head. If so, it rotates the shoulders into the anteroposte-

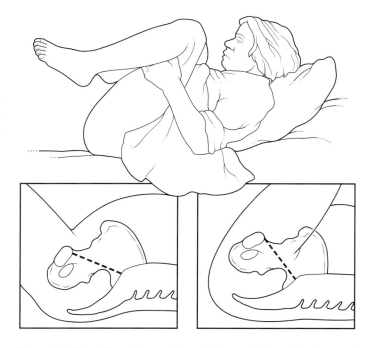

Figure 21.2 Before the routine use of conduction anesthesia, self-implemented hyperflexion of the legs by the parturient was a routine delivery position. In contemporary practice, when used for the management of shoulder dystocia, the legs must be supported by two assistants. (From O'Leary JA. Shoulder Dystocia and Birth Injury. McGraw-Hill: New York, 1992.)

rior diameter of the pelvis. At this point, gentle traction at an angle of about 30° under the horizontal, supported by suprapubic pressure, may facilitate the delivery of the body. Suprapubic pressure is generally applied by an assistant. With one or two fists or the palms of the hands immediately over the symphysis pubis, the anterior shoulder is depressed with a lateral bias toward the infant's face to facilitate rotation of the shoulders into the oblique diameter in order to allow its passage under the pubic arch. For effective use of this approach, the bladder must be empty. Ideally, bearing-down effort by the mother, suprapubic pressure by the assistant, and light traction by the accoucheur should be applied simultaneously. This well-orchestrated effort must be pursued with awareness of the fact that delivery of the head and the body during the same uterine contraction is not necessary.

After the delivery of the head, the next uterine contraction may be slightly delayed. This time offers an opportunity for optimizing the effect of the next one. The mother can be placed into a favorable position for delivery and the assistants can move to the sides of the parturient. Meanwhile, the accoucheur can suction the mouth and nose of the child and check for nuchal cord. When present, it should be eased around the head of the fetus if it can be done without difficulty. Causing avulsion of the cord at its umbilical insertion can lead to catastrophe. Besides, its handling can reduce the still existing circulation through the umbilical vessels. Facilitated by the McRoberts maneuver, with suprapubic pressure (Figure 21.3) and gentle downward traction, but most of the time even without, the next contraction expels the shoulders and then the body of the fetus.

Fundal pressure has been shown to be counterproductive and detrimental to the fetus.[53] Therefore, with one bizarre exception,[54] the contemporary literature discourages its use for the purpose of overcoming shoulder dystocia.[1,6,7,55]

A strong consensus supports the view that extensive episiotomy is one of the most effective measures for overcoming shoulder dystocia.[1,6,55] This opinion is not inconsistent with the expediency that delivery of the shoulders can be accomplished over an intact perineum or a routine episiotomy in the majority of the instances.[7] However, the cutting of a deep (third-degree mediolateral or fourth-degree median) episiotomy should precede strong traction invariably.

The corkscrew maneuver, introduced by Woods,[56] was designed to overcome the collision between the symphysis and the anterior shoulder. Since rotational movement is more likely to allow easy removal of a cork from a neck of the bottle than simple pull, he recommended manual rotation of the shoulders. In this process, pressure is applied against the clavicle and the scapula or against the anterior aspect of the upper arm (Figure 21.4). This effort should remove the shoulder from its locked position and allow its passage somewhat laterally under the ramus pubis. Rubin's modification implies rotation from back to front with the opposite hand.[57] This author attributed significance to the fact that, whereas the Woods maneuver causes abduction of the posterior shoulder, his technique induces adduction, thus diminishing the transverse diameter of the shoulders.

Opinions vary about the efficacy of these rotational techniques. It is widely accepted, on the other hand, that delivery of the posterior arm, if performed successfully, is conducive to the passage of the shoulders within a short period of time. The critical and probably most difficult part of this technique is the insertion of the hand of the operator into the birth canal. Some authors consider general or conduction anesthesia necessary for

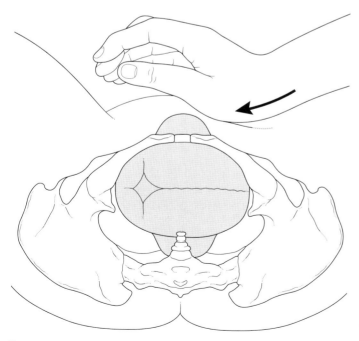

Figure 21.3 Application of suprapubic pressure. (From O'Leary JA. *Shoulder Dystocia and Birth Injury*. McGraw-Hill: New York, 1992.)

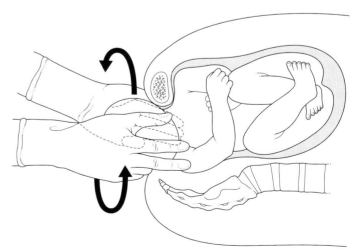

Figure 21.4 The corkscrew maneuver. The shoulders are rotated by applying pressure on the scapula and the clavicle. The head is not to be rotated! (From O'Leary JA. *Shoulder Dystocia and Birth Injury*. McGraw-Hill: New York, 1992.)

this maneuver. When the fetal back is turned to the left side, the operator's left hand is to be used. Vice versa, the right hand is needed if the back is turned to the right. Inserting the index finger around the elbow or the wrist, the operator grasps the lower arm of the child and delivers it in front of the chest. The delivery of the rest of the body is usually easy. If other-wise, the accoucheur may rotate the body of the child until the previously anterior shoulder is located posteriorly. Then, the same maneuver follows with the other hand.

The limiting time factor for safe vaginal delivery after the collision of the shoulder with the symphysis is the inevitable detachment of the placenta from its implantation site after much of the uterine contents has been expelled. When the placental separation will take place is impossible to predict. The experience with twin deliveries may be a practical guide, noting that abruption of the placenta seldom occurs less than 20 minutes after the delivery of the first twin, that is, after the expulsion of about one-half of the uterine contents. In the absence of intervention, the fetal condition does not change for a few minutes after the emergence of the head.[37] The rapid decline of the fetal blood pH described some decades ago[58] probably resulted from coincidental stressful manipulations. Nonetheless, since the subject does not offer itself to experimentation, there is no solid ground for challenging the belief that retention of the body for 10 or more minutes after the emergence of the head carries a substantial risk of neonatal death or neurologic damage. Rather than relying on any arbitrary time limit, it appears reasonable to place a scalp electrode onto the head of the fetus if shoulder dystocia persists and to avoid forceful intervention as long as the fetal heart rate remains reassuring, since physical trauma is conducive to shock.

In Australia and Africa, symphysiotomy (described elsewhere in this volume) is used routinely for the treatment of shoulder dystocia. Because injury to the maternal urethra and bladder is associated with this operation with relative frequency, it has gained little acceptance in the USA. In contrast, cephalic replacement, generally referred to as the Zavanelli maneuver, has created some interest. Having been promoted by O'Leary in recent years,[1] the technique is best described by his own words:

(1) The head is replaced by utilizing constant but firm pressure on the occiput with the palm of the right hand so as to flex the head while depressing the posterior vaginal wall with the left hand; (2) the vertex is pushed as far cephalad as possible, usually to zero station, where it will remain without assistance; and (3) insertion of a Foley catheter is recommended after completion of the maneuver.

As for the role of the Zavanelli maneuver in contemporary obstetrics, the same author made the following recommendations:

As a last resort in the management of shoulder dystocia, with cephalic replacement, tocolysis and abdominal delivery seem to offer the best outcome. This technique should only be used when continued persistence at vaginal manipulation would lead to a predictably poor outcome. If the infant has been damaged, the placenta separated, or profound hypoxia has occurred, it should not be attempted. At present, the technique is not recommended for routine use until more traditional procedures had failed.

It should be noted, however, that delay until the infant is moribund may be partially responsible for many of the poor outcomes associated with this maneuver.

Purposeful fracturing of the clavicle on the side of the impaction has been described as a practical technique for overcoming shoulder dystocia. While sound theoretically, the technique is difficult and particularly so in a macrosomic fetus whose bones are strong. Thus, it remains an approach which only a few practitioners dare to utilize.

An analysis by McCall, based on over 100 cases of shoulder dystocia-related birth injuries, drew attention to the fact that the fetal damage deriving from this complication is not restricted to brachial plexus injuries.[48] He found that 7% of the babies involved died and 20% suffered brain injury secondary to hypoxia or intracranial hemorrhage. Several later publications, based on fewer cases, denied the relationship between shoulder dystocia and central nervous system damage. However, more recent research, based on more than 200 shoulder dystocia-related birth injuries, found the rate of central nervous system injuries comparable to that reported by McCall. In this series, the rate of brachial plexus injuries was in excess of 90%.[21,22]

Most brachial plexus lesions noted at birth heal by the age of 6 months. However, when the neurologic deficit persists for 12 months, the damage is probably permanent.[59]

The frequency of injuries involving the upper trunk of the brachial plexus (segments C 5–7), often referred to as Erb–Duchenne palsy, is far higher than damage to the lower branches (C 7–T 1) (Klumpke type of palsy). The latter injury is unlikely to occur without the coincidental involvement of the upper trunks. Recently developed surgical techniques, often requiring multiple operative interventions, can bring about improvement in the function of the involved extremity, but no cure. Consequently, the injury predictably restricts the professional and vocational opportunities of the affected individual later in life.

Controversies concerning etiology

Apart from being devastating for many of its victims, cases of shoulder dystocia have affected the professional lives of obstetricians also. Consequently, this entity has often been discussed in the medicolegal context.[6,17,21,22,41,42,44,45,54] In this process, a series of papers appeared recently, suggesting that, in many cases, brachial plexus injury is a prenatal event, unrelated to the arrest of the shoulders at birth.[60–65] Based on the information that evidence of denervation in adult subjects is not detectable by electromyography until 10–14 days after the insult, evidence of denervation within a few days after birth in affected newborns was interpreted as proof that the injuries had been sustained *in utero* before the onset of labor. This concept had to be discarded when a pertinent study showed that neuromuscular deficits develop much faster in fetal than in adult pigs.[66] An alternative hypothesis, namely, that brachial plexus injury is frequently caused during the labor process by uterine forces, still prevails. However, since the maternal forces mobilized during labor and delivery are expulsive in nature, it is difficult to perceive a natural mechanism which could imitate the effect of traction injuries. The latter have been proven to be associated with forceful extraction of the shoulders.

Rare cases of brachial plexus lesion, attributed to spontaneous *in utero* injury, have been reported.[64,67,68] However, if *in utero* acquired Erb's palsy is relatively frequent, it should occur often among neonates delivered abdominally, since the rate of cesarean sections has been at the range of 25% during the last two decades. It is a matter of interest, therefore, that in a published series of over 200 brachial plexus injuries, only one of the affected children was delivered by (a repeat) cesarean section.[15] The delivery of a macrosomic baby had been preceded by two failed extraction attempts in that case and involved the Zavanelli maneuver. Thus, there is doubt whether even this single case can be attributed to forces other than those utilized during the delivery attempts. It appears reasonable to conclude, therefore, that, if it occurs at all, brachial plexus injury unrelated to the process of delivery is a rare phenomenon with little bearing upon the overall problem of shoulder dystocia at birth.

Intrauterine malposition has also been posited as a cause of brachial plexus injury. However, such an etiology would necessarily result in atrophic changes in the muscle innervated by the plexus at the time of birth.

Prediction and prevention

The knowledge that most cases cannot be predicted[41] should not stop physicians from preventing as many incapacitating fetal injuries, deriving from shoulder dystocia, as possible. In most instances, this complication is not lightening out of the blue but the last stage of a process which can often be influenced by early recognition and careful elimination of factors conducive to this complication. An algorithm designed to show a path that offers a chance for preventing shoulder dystocia-related birth injuries is shown in Table 21.4.

While calculating the risk of shoulder dystocia in relation to birth weight in nondiabetic and diabetic women, various authors utilized a broad variety of approaches, endpoints, and interpretations.[69–72] The most extensive and probably most reliable data were published by Nesbitt et al[72] and were based upon the combined material of over 300 hospitals, involving more than half a million deliveries in the year 1992 (Table 21.5). In this material, diabetic mothers giving birth to 4000–4250-g babies experienced shoulder dystocia in about 8% of all instances. The rate increased to over 20% when the birth weights exceeded 4500 g. In nondiabetic patients, the fetal risks were comparable to those of infants of diabetic mothers who weighed 250 g less. The use of an extraction instrument increased the risk of arrest of the shoulders by approximately 40%.

Another study found that of those infants delivered under conditions of shoulder dystocia, 20% sustained injuries.[30] Among these, 30% suffered permanent neurologic or other deficits. These results are comparable with data deriving from other sources.[11] They permit the calculation, therefore, that approximately one out of 13 cases of shoulder dystocia entails permanent fetal sequelae.

The view that in macrosomia shoulder dystocia is not the only mechanism of fetal damage[69] needs to be remembered.

Table 21.4 Algorithm for the prevention of shoulder dystocia

First encounter	History about the mother's own birth weight, personal and family history of diabetes, past delivery of child large for gestational age, and birth injury. (Glucola screening test if positive history is obtained.)
Examination	Attention to maternal weight (diet). Detailed pelvic assessment (to be documented in detail).
Prenatal visits	Close attention to weight gain. Involve nutritionist if needed. (In case of glucosuria: diabetic screening at any gestational length.)
26–28 weeks	Routine diabetic screening (glucola test). If 135 mg/dl or more at 1 hour, arrange 3-hour glucose tolerance test promptly. If the blood glucose level is 190 mg/dl after 1 hour, the patient is gestational diabetic. No more testing is needed.
36–40 weeks	Estimate fetal weight clinically at every visit. If large for gestational age fetus at term (≥3800 g) is suspected, double-check fetal weight with ultrasound.
Term	If estimated fetal weight is 4000 g or more, discuss delivery risks with the mother.*

*See Table 21.5.

Table 21.5 Incidence of shoulder dystocia in relation to fetal weight and maternal diabetic or nondiabetic status*

Fetal weight extraction	Spontaneous delivery non-diabetic	Spontaneous delivery diabetic	Instrumental extraction nondiabetic	Instrucmental diabetic
3500–3750 g	0.5%	2.5%	1.5%	4%
3750–4000 g	2.5%	5%	3.5%	8%
4000–4250 g	5%	8%	7.5%	12%
4250–4500 g	8%	13%	12%	16%
4500–4750 g	13%	23%	20%	27%
4750–5000 g	21%	29%	23%	35%

*Based on data published by Nesbitt et al.[72]

Through multiple mechanisms, large fetal size is conducive to death and injury in a variety of ways.[73] Some of them are the consequence of protracted or arrested labor due to relative fetopelvic disproportion. In such cases, the maternal morbidity rate also is increased, as are the risks associated with those cesarean sections performed after arrested labor. Thus, the conflict between maternal and fetal interests is not always clearcut.

A widely cited interpretation of the prevailing consensus,[74] quoting the investigations of Nesbitt et al,[72] concluded that elective cesarean section is only indicated in case of an estimated fetal weight of 5000 g. The data shown in Table 21.5 provide no basis for this opinion. Even less do they support the conclusion that 'suspected fetal macrosomia is not a contraindication to attempted vaginal birth after prior cesarean delivery'.

In the twenty-first century, the medical profession recognizes the right of women to choose delivery by elective cesarean section even in the absence of a medical indication. There is little justification, therefore, to substitute the preferences of medical practitioners or organizations for the choice of a well-informed patient. What kind of risk a mother is willing to accept for herself and for her child is a decision which only she can make. Doctors can guide the mother toward a reasonable choice but cannot be the final decision-making authority. Once the risks and benefits have been truthfully explained, most patients can and are willing to contribute to the formulation of a reasonable management plan.

Conclusions

As previously stated, there are several risk factors that increase the chance of encountering shoulder dystocia. Most of these are associated with macrosomia, by far, the greatest single factor associated with this problem. It must be understood, however, that the majority of shoulder dystocias are unpredictable. Arrest of the shoulders may occur even in the absence of any attendant risk factor. Therefore, the obstetrician must always maintain vigilance with respect to its occurrence.

Because of the low incidence of this complication, very few graduating residents have seen or handled more than a few cases. When presented with a case of shoulder dystocia, the inexperienced obstetrician may panic and become confused, exerting unacceptable and maldirected forces upon the infant's head, and thus producing permanent brachial plexus injury.

The only cogent and practical way of developing experience is to use 'release' maneuvers and to practice these maneuvers over and over in cases where no shoulder dystocia is extant. Residents do not wait until they assist in surgical procedures to learn to tie knots, nor do they wait until a victim of a heart attack is encountered to practice cardiopulmonary resuscitation. The analogy is clear.

We recommend that both residents and experienced attending physicians have a 'drill' in mind, remembering that no single release maneuver has been proven superior to any other. Each maneuver has its place in a given situation and none can accomplish safe delivery in every case. We offer the following approach when the turtle sign presents itself, portending shoulder dystocia:

(1) Never clamp or cut the cord before the shoulders are released.
(2) Wait for the next contraction after the one that delivered the head. Very often, this contraction with exhausting effort will effect delivery because the shoulders have had a chance to rotate to the oblique or anteroposterior diameter. The obstetrician also has the time to take a deep breath and mentally rehearse his or her drill.
(3) If delivery is not forthcoming after the next contraction, maneuvers should be instituted:
   (a) *McRoberts*. The maternal thighs are flexed sharply toward the abdomen with personnel actively assisting on each side.
   (b) *Suprapubic pressure*. (Fundal pressure is to be avoided.) Suprapubic pressure should be executed by a nurse or an

assistant, using the heel of the hand or the fist. The anterior shoulder should be directed toward the infant's face. This Rubin modification of suprapubic pressure will help rotate the shoulder into the larger oblique diameter.

(c) *Rubin modification of Wood's maneuver.* Two fingers are inserted behind the anterior scapula, and rotation pressure exerted such that the anterior shoulder is being rotated toward the face while the assistant continues to apply lateral suprapubic pressure in the same direction.

(d) *Perform a generous episiotomy or episioproctotomy.* This alone will suffice to solve the problem in many situations. It will also give adequate room to insert the fingers posteriorily to effect the next maneuver.

(e) *Deliver the posterior arm.* This maneuver may be effected more efficaciously if the opposite hand is inserted along the infant's back until the elbow is reached. Posterior fingers involved beyond the elbow to the forearm may then be flexed to put the hand of the infant within reach of the obstetrician's grasp on the anterior side of the infant.

(f) *Hibbard maneuver.* While the posterior aspect of the infant's head is supported by the obstetrician's hand, strong pressure is exerted upon the junction of the anterior trapezoid muscle with the neck toward the hollow of the sacrum in an attempt to pass the anterior shoulder. A second rotational maneuver with suprapubic pressure should then be attempted.

(g) Unless the anterior shoulder has been freed, there should be no attempt to use traction upon the head in an attempt to release the shoulder. Once it is released, care must be taken to support the posterior aspect of the head with mild traction at an angle not to exceed 30º or, preferably, by pulsion from above made upon the infant's mandible and neck.

(4) If you do not have adequate assistance, ask for help! If a more experienced obstetrician is nearby, do not hesitate to seek his/her support!

These maneuvers must be executed deliberately but expeditiously. If all are ineffective, immediate transition to the Zavanelli maneuver may be considered. The infant's head is manually rotated to the OA position. Pressure is put upon the occiput with the dominant hand while the opposite is used as assistance to flex fully the infant's head. The vertex is then pushed up into the pelvis as high as possible and a Cesarean section performed as soon as possible. A tocolytic agent (we suggest terbutaline 0.25 mg) should be given as soon as the obstetrician has determined that the maneuver will be employed.

Points to remember:

(1) Wait for the contraction after the delivery of the head.
(2) Never exert downward traction upon the infant's head in the face of suspected shoulder dystocia.

(3) Perform each maneuver in a sequence which has been memorized and practiced many times.
(4) If it is utilized, incorporate the Zavanelli maneuver before severe hypoxia is present.
(5) Practice, practice, practice!

References

1. O'Leary JA. Shoulder dystocia: prevention and treatment. In: Iffy L, Apuzzio JJ, Vintzileos AM (eds), Operative Obstetrics, p. 234–43. (2nd edition), McGraw-Hill: New York, 1992.
2. Roseveas SK, Stirrat GM. Handbook of Obstetric Management, pp. 251. Blackwell Science: Oxford, 1996.
3. Papp Z. A Szülészet-Nögyógyászat Tankönyve, p. 432. Semmelweis Kiadó: Budapest, 1999.
4. Iffy L. Shoulder dystocia. Am J Obstet Gynecol 1987; 156: 1416.
5. Benedetti TJ, Gabbe SG. Shoulder dystocia. A complication of fetal macrosomia and prolonged second stage of labor with mid-pelvic delivery. Obstet Gynecol 1978; 52: 526–9.
6. O'Leary JA. Shoulder Dystocia and Birth Injury. McGraw-Hill: New York, 1992.
7. Cunningham FG, Gant FN, Leveno K et al. Williams' Obstetrics (21st edition). McGraw-Hill: New York, 2001 pp. 459–64.
8. Lanni SM, Seeds JW. Malpresentations. In: Gabbe SG, Niebyl JR, Simpson JL (eds), Obstetrics p. 473 (4th edition). Churchill Livingstone: New York, 2002.
9. Bowes WA Jr. Clinical aspects of normal and abnormal labor. In: Creasy RK, Resnik R (eds), Maternal-Fetal Medicine, p. 532 (4th edition). WB Saunders Co: Philadelphia, 1999.
10. Hardy AE. Birth injuries of the brachial plexus. J Bone Joint Surg 1981; 63: 98–101.
11. Hopwood HG. Shoulder dystocia: fifteen years' experience in a community hospital. Am J Obstet Gynecol 1982; 144: 162–6.
12. Gross TL, Sokol RJ, Williams T et al. Shoulder dystocia: a fetal-physician risk. Am J Obstet Gynecol 1987; 156: 1408–18.
13. Nimmo RA, Murphy GA, Adhate A et al. Factors affecting perinatal mortality in an urban center. Natl Med Assoc J 1991; 83: 147.
14. ACOG Committee Opinion No. 179, November 1996.
15. Iffy L, Djordjevic MM, Apuzzio JJ et al. Diabetes, hypertension and birth injuries: a complex interrelationship. Bull Isr Soc Obstet Gynecol 2004; 2: 36.
16. Sama J, Iffy L. Maternal weight and fetal injury at birth. Med Law 1998; 17: 61–8.
17. Robinson H, Tkatch S, Mayes DC et al. Is maternal obesity a predictor of shoulder dystocia? Obstet Gynecol 2003; 101: 24–7.
18. Klebanoff MA, Mills JL, Berendes HW. Mother's birth weight as a predictor of macrosomia. Am J Obstet Gynecol 1985; 153: 353–7.
19. Johnstone NR. Shoulder dystocia: a study of 47 cases. Aust N Z J Obstet Gynaecol 1979; 19: 28–31.
20. ACOG Technical Bulletin. Fetal macrosomia. 1991; No. 159.
21. Iffy L, Váradi V, Jakobovits A. Common intrapartum denominators of shoulder dystocia related birth injuries. Zentralbl Gynakol 1994; 116: 33–7.

22. Iffy L, Váradi V. A vállak elkadásával kapcsolatos magzati sérülések kóroki tényezöi. Magy Noorv Lap 2001; 64: 365.

23. Lindsay MK, Graves W, Klein L. The relationship of one abnormal glucose tolerance test value and pregnancy complications. Obstet Gynecol 1989; 73: 103–6.

24. Coustan DR, Imrah J. Prophylactic insulin treatment of gestational diabetes reduces the incidence of macrosomia, operative delivery, and birth trauma. Am J Obstet Gynecol 1984; 150: 836–42.

25. Boyd ME, Usher RH, McLean FH. Fetal macrosomia: prediction, risks, proposed management. Obstet Gynecol 1983; 61: 715–22.

26. Modanlou HD, Komatsu G, Dorchester W et al. Large for gestational age neonates: anthropometric reasons for shoulder dystocia. Obstet Gynecol 1982; 60: 417–23.

27. Harris BA Jr. Shoulder dystocia. Clin Obstet Gynecol 1984; 27: 106–11.

28. Wladimiroff JW, Bloemsma CA, Wollenburg HCS. Ultrasonic diagnosis of the large-for-dates infant. Obstet Gynecol 1978; 52: 285–8.

29. Friedman EA. Labor: Clinical Evaluation and Management (2nd edition). Appleton-Century-Crofts: New York, 1978.

30. Benedetti TJ: Managing shoulder dystocia. Contemp Ob Gyn 1979; 14: 33.

31. Benedetti TJ. Birth injury secondary to shoulder dystocia. In: Report of the 93rd Ross Conference, Columbus, Ohio, Ross Laboratories, 1987.

32. ACOG Technical Bulletin. Operative vaginal delivery. No. 196, August 1994.

33. ACOG Technical Bulletin. Fetal macrosomia. No. 159, September 1991.

34. Manning S. General principles and applications of ultrasonography. In: Creasy RK, Resnik R (eds), Maternal-Fetal Medicine, pp. 169, 183 (4th edition). W.B. Saunders: Philadelphia, 1999.

35. Mengert WF. Pelvic measurements of 4144 Iowa women. Am J Obstet Gynecol 1938; 36: 260.

36. Iffy L, Apuzzio J, Ganesh V. A randomized controlled trial of prophylactic maneuvers to reduce head-to-body delivery time in patients at risk for shoulder dystocia. Obstet Gynecol 2003; 102: 1089–90.

37. Stallings SP, Edwards RK, Johnson JWC. Correlation of head-to-body delivery intervals in shoulder dystocia and umbilical artery acidosis. Am J Obstet Gynecol 2001; 185: 268–74.

38. Harris DA Jr. Shoulder dystocia. The Female Patient. 1990; 15: 69–76.

39. Bottoms SF, Sokol RJ. Mechanisms and conduct of labor. In: Iffy L, Kaminetzky HA (eds), Principles and Practice of Obstetrics & Perinatology, p. 815. Wiley: New York, 1981.

40. Iffy L, Váradi V, Papp E. Untoward neonatal sequelae deriving from cutting the umbilical cord before delivery. Med Law 2001; 20: 627–34.

41. Nocon JJ, McKenzie DK, Thomas LJ, Hansell RS. Shoulder dystocia: an analysis of risks and obstetrics maneuvers. Am J Obstet Gynecol 1993; 168: 1732–7.

42. ACOG Practice Bulletin. Fetal macrosomia. No. 22 (November) 2000.

43. Bryant DR, Leonardi MR, Landwehr JB, Bottoms SF. Limited usefulness of fetal weight in predicting neonatal brachial plexus injury. Am J Obstet Gynecol 1998; 179: 686–9.

44. Donnelly V, Foran A, Murphy J et al. Neonatal brachial plexus palsy: an unpredictable injury. Am J Obstet Gynecol 2002; 187: 1209–12.

45. ACOG Practice Patterns: Shoulder dystocia. No. 7 (October) 1997.

46. Rouse DJ, Owen J, Goldenberg RL et al. The effectiveness and costs of elective cesarean delivery for fetal macrosomia diagnosed by ultrasound. JAMA 1996; 276: 1480–6.

47. Langer O, Berkus MD, Huff RW et al. Shoulder dystocia: should the fetus weighing ≥4,000 gm be delivered by cesarean section? Am J Obstet Gynecol 1991; 165: 831–7.

48. McCall JO Jr. Shoulder dystocia. A study of after effects. Am J Obstet Gynecol 1962; 83: 1486.

49. Eastman NJ, Hellman LM. Williams' Obstetrics, p. 423 (11th edition). Appleton-Century-Crofts: New York, 1961.

50. Greenhill JP. Obstetrics, p. 278 (11th edition). WB Saunders: Philadelphia, 1955.

51. McRoberts WA. Maneuvers for shoulder dystocia. Contemp Obstet Gynecol 1984; 24: 17.

52. Smeltzer JS. Prevention and management of shoulder dystocia. Clin Obstet Gynecol 1986; 29: 299–308.

53. Gross SJ, Shime J, Farine D. Shoulder dystocia: predictors and outcome. Am J Obstet Gynecol 1987; 156: 334–6.

54. Sandmire HS. From Green Bay a game plan for shoulder dystocia. OBG Management (April) 1997, p 15.

55. Benedetti TJ. Shoulder dystocia. In: Pauerstein CJ (ed.), Clinical Obstetrics, p. 871. Wiley: New York, 1987.

56. Woods CE. A principle of physics as applicable to shoulder delivery. Am J Obstet Gynecol 1943; 45: 796–804.

57. Rubin A. Management of shoulder dystocia. JAMA 1964; 189: 835–7.

58. Wood C, Ng KH, Hounslow D et al. Time: an important variable in normal delivery. J Obstet Gynaecol Br Commonw 1973; 80: 295.

59. Volpe JJ. Neurology of the Newborn, p. 781 (3rd edition). WB Saunders: Philadelphia, 1995.

60. Jennett RJ, Tarby TJ. Disuse osteoporosis as evidence of brachial plexus palsy due to intrauterine fetal maladaptation. Am J Obstet Gynecol 2001; 185: 236–7.

61. Gonik B, Zhang N, Grimm NG. Prediction of brachial plexus stretching during shoulder dystocia using a computer stimulation model. Am J Obstet Gynecol 2003; 189: 1168–72.

62. Ouzounian JG, Korst LM, Phelan JP. Permanent Erb palsy: a traction-related injury? Obstet Gynecol 1997; 89: 139–41.

63. Gherman RB, Ouzounian JG, Miller DA et al. Spontaneous vaginal delivery: a risk factor for Erb's palsy? Am J Obstet Gynecol 1998; 178: 423–7.

64. Dunn DW, Engle WA. Brachial plexus palsy: intrauterine onset. Pediatr Neurol 1985; 1: 367–9.

65. Koenigsberger MR. Brachial plexus palsy at birth: intrauterine or due to delivery trauma? Ann Neurol 1980; 8: 228.

66. Gonik B, McCormick EM, Verweij BH et al. The timing of congenital brachial plexus injury: a study of electromyography findings in the newborn piglets. Am J Obstet Gynecol 1998; 178: 688–95.
67. Dunn DW, Engle WA. Brachial plexus palsy: intrauterine onset. Pediatr Neurol 1985; 1: 376.
68. Eng GE. Neuromuscular disease. In: Avery GB, Fletcher MA, MacDonald MG. Neonatology, pp. 1164, 1166 (4th edition). JB Lippincott: Philadelphia, 1994.
69. Modanlou HD, Dorchester WL, Phorosian A et al. Macrosomia – maternal, fetal, and neonatal implications. Obstet Gynecol 1980; 55: 420–4.
70. Spellacy WN, Miller S, Winegar A et al. Macrosomia – maternal characteristics and infant complications. Obstet Gynecol 1985; 66: 158–61.
71. McFarland LV, Raskin M, Daling JR et al. Erb/Duchenne's palsy: a consequence of fetal macrosomia and method of delivery. Obstet Gynecol 1986; 68: 784–8.
72. Nesbitt TS, Gilbert WM, Herrchen B. Shoulder dystocia and associated risk factors with macrosomic infants born in California. Am J Obstet Gynecol 1998; 179: 476–80.
73. Sack RA. The large infant. Am J Obstet Gynecol 1969; 104: 195–204.
74. American Academy of Pediatrics and the American College of Obstetricians and Gynecologists: Guidelines for Perinatal Care (5th edition). Washington, DC, 2002.

22 Postpartum hemorrhage

Akos Jakobovits and Jahir C Sama

Definition and classification

Traditionally, postpartum hemorrhage is defined as blood loss in excess of 500 ml. Severe hemorrhage occurs after less than 1% of deliveries and is a major contributor of maternal morbidity and mortality. It is classified as immediate if it occurs within 24 hours after the completion of the third stage; and as delayed if it occurs beyond this time and within 6 weeks of the puerperium.

The definition of blood loss in excess of 500 ml as abnormal is arbitrary. According to data from France, 58% of all obstetric bleedings develop after delivery. Of these, 51% follow instrumental vaginal deliveries, 19% spontaneous vaginal births, and 30% cesarean sections. The authors found that in cases of severe bleeding, patients had often received inadequate care due to late recognition of the severity of the hemorrhage. They considered 90% of the maternal deaths preventable.[1-3]

The postpartum blood loss exceeds 500 ml in 5% and 1000 ml in 1–2% of all childbirths.[4] In developed countries, the rate of maternal mortality due to postpartum bleeding is about one in 100.[5] Appropriate instruction of the delivery unit personnel and strict adherence to prearranged protocols can reduce the incidence of life-endangering blood loss significantly.[6]

In cases of twin pregnancy, the postpartum blood loss exceeds 500 ml in 38.2% and 1000 ml in 6.6% of the cases. The zygocity and gender of the twins have no identifiable effect upon the amount of the bleeding.[7]

The difficulty in estimating blood loss accurately[8] makes the diagnosis of postpartum hemorrhage imprecise. Methods to quantitate blood loss are cumbersome, time-consuming, and require complicated laboratory analysis; they are, therefore, seldom employed. For the most part, clinical estimation of blood loss is subjective. This explains the wide range in reported incidence.[9] A drop in hematocrit from the intrapartum to postpartum period of more than 5% reflects blood loss in excess of 500 ml and may be a useful guide, provided the determination is made on the third day postpartum and there has been no significant late bleeding. The shifts in fluids and diuresis that occur in the first few days postpartum make the drop in hematocrit less reliable during the first 24 hours after delivery, when the calculation of blood loss is most crucial. From a practical stand-point, because of the increase in blood volume during pregnancy and the hemodynamic changes that occur in the postpartum period, most patients can tolerate hemorrhage up to 1500 ml, provided they are in good health and not anemic to begin with.[10]

Risk factors and prevention

Advanced maternal age, parity, and previous postpartum hemorrhage are historical risk factors. The likelihood of recurrence is nearly 25% after one past episode, and rises to 50% after three previous hemorrhagic events.[11] Existing complications during the pregnancy, such as hypertensive disorders, diabetes, anemia, blood disorders, uterine anomalies and myomas, third-trimester bleeding, and overdistended uterus, predispose to hemorrhage. During labor chorioamnionitis, the use of tocolytic agents such as magnesium sulfate or ritodrine, precipitate or unduly long labor, cephalopelvic disproportion, and prolonged second stage also increase the risk of postpartum hemorrhage. During the delivery, the use of deep, prolonged general anesthesia and operative procedures such as midforceps, Dührssen's incision, or large episiotomy predispose to excessive blood loss. Finally, improper delivery of the placenta significantly increases the risk of postpartum hemorrhage (Table 22.1).

When risk factors are present, preventive measures may be instituted. These include correction of anemia before the onset of labor, the placing of a large-caliber needle to permit rapid infusion of fluids, typed, cross-matched blood being readily available, replacement of coagulation factors with bleeding disorders, and the prophylactic use of oxytocic agents after delivery. Postpartum uterine involution is hindered by a full bladder. This difficulty can be overcome by catheterization.

Diagnosis

Massive blood loss is readily apparent, especially during the first hour after the completion of the third stage of labor. Immediately after the delivery of the placenta, there is heavy and continuous

Table 22.1 Risk factors for postpartum hemorrhage

Historical	Antepartum	Intrapartum	Miscellaneous
Advanced maternal age	Overdistended uterus	Rapid labor	Preeclampsia
Multiparity	Macrosomia	Prolonged labor	Hypertension
Previous postpartum hemorrhage	Multiple gestation	Oxytocin use	Saline abortion
Previous uterine rupture	Hydramnios	General anesthesia	Sepsis
Previous uterine surgery	Placenta previa	Instrument delivery	Fetal demise
Previous placenta accreta	Abruptio placentae	Forceps	Thromboembolic disease
Previous placenta previa	Amnionitis	Podalic version	
Known uterine malformation	Magnesium sulfate	Duhrssen's incision	
Leyomyomata/adenomyosis	Drugs	Genital tract trauma	
Coagulation disorders	Aspirin, NSAID	Lacerations	
ITP	Antibiotics	Hematomas	
TTP	Thiazide diuretics	Ruptured uterus	
Hemophilia	Sedatives	Placenta accreta	
von Willebrand's disease	Tranquilizers		

ITP, immune thrombocytopenic pupura; TTP, thrombotic thrombocytopenic pupura.

blood flow from the vaginal introitus that quickly soaks the drapings and pools in the floor basins. Large clots form below while blood continues to gush from above. A sense of urgency envelopes everyone caring for the patient. Within a short period of time, she becomes pallid, tachycardic, tachypneic, and hypotensive, and if blood loss has exceeded critical levels, she goes into shock. The diagnosis may be less obvious if the bleeding is intermittent or protracted, mild to moderate, and the vital signs remain stable. It may be a few days later, when the significant drop in hematocrit is observed and the patient feels weak and dizzy upon walking, looks pallid, and has a fast and thready pulse, that the magnitude of blood loss is recognized.

It is practical to classify postpartum hemorrhage according to the pathophysiologic mechanism involved (Table 22.2). The major causes of immediate postpartum hemorrhage include uterine atony, genital tract trauma, and retained placental tissue. The major causes of delayed postpartum hemorrhage include subinvolution of the placental site, retained placental fragments, and chronic endometritis.

General principles of management

Severe hemorrhage can be dramatic and immediately life-threatening. It can lead to serious complications and sequelae. These include shock, renal shutdown, hypopituitarism (Sheehan's syndrome), postpartum amenorrhea (Asherman's syndrome),

and transfusion-related complications such as hepatitis and isoimmunization.

With prompt recognition of its development, correct identification of its cause, and aggressive therapy, the outcome is good in most cases.

A systematic sequence of therapeutic measures to control the bleeding must be followed. These include aggressive treatment of causative factors, maintenance of effective circulating intravascular volume by adequate replacement of blood and crystalloids, and prompt recognition and correction of coagulopathy. Blood should be transfused as quickly as it is lost. Typed and cross-matched fresh whole blood is ideal, followed by banked whole blood or packed red blood cells. If typed and cross-matched blood is not available, group O Rh-negative

Table 22.2 Causes of postpartum hemorrhage

Immediate	Delayed
Uterine atony	Subinvolution
Retained products	Retained placental tissue
Genital tract trauma	Chronic endometritis
Uterine inversion	Placental polyp
Coagulation disorders	

blood may be used. The use of equipment to pump blood under pressure expedites rapid transfusion. Until blood becomes available, plasma or blood substitutes can be used as a means of restoring circulating volume and oncotic pressure. More than one intravenous line may be necessary. The placement of a central venous pressure catheter as well as a Foley catheter may be useful to monitor fluid therapy. Adequate crystalloids include Ringer's lactate or saline, while plasma substitutes include dextran 40, gelatin solution, and plasminate. One must keep in mind that when massive hemorrhage has occurred and multiple transfusion of whole blood is employed, coagulation disorders and metabolic derangements can occur. Consequently, in these circumstances, coagulation profile, platelet and calcium levels, and blood gases should be determined. A quick and easy test for coagulopathy is to draw an extra tube of blood, tape it to the bed or wall, and observe for clot formation in 5–7 minutes after it is drawn. Two units of fresh frozen plasma and four units of platelets for every five units of whole citrated blood should be given to prevent this type of coagulopathy. If hypofibrinogenemia is found, fresh frozen plasma and cryoprecipitate are the best sources for fibrinogen replacement.

Although the use of blood may be lifesaving, it is not without its dangers. Excessive blood transfusion can lead to pulmonary edema. Other potential dangers include the risk of hepatitis, isoimmunization, hemolytic reactions, homologous serum jaundice, allergic and anaphylactic reactions, febrile reactions, citric acid intoxication, and cardiac arrest.[12] Although routine testing of blood donors for human immunodeficiency virus (HIV) has reduced the risk of its transmission to an extremely low level, it is nonetheless a danger.[13] For these reasons, transfusion should only be employed if significant hemorrhage occurs and the patient is in danger.

Successful management of postpartum hemorrhage depends on a team approach. Nurses, obstetricians, anesthesiologists, and blood-bank and laboratory personnel must work in concert to effect the systematic and orderly implementation of therapeutic measures.

Management of the third stage of labor

The conduct of the third stage of labor has a major influence on the development of postpartum hemorrhage. Placental separation usually occurs within a few minutes after the delivery of the fetus and is thought to result from the shearing mechanical force of the ensuing uterine contractions. The signs of placental separation include a gush of fresh vaginal bleeding, descent of the umbilical cord, and a change in the shape and position of the uterine fundus. However, these may be signs of placental descent, so that the clinical differentiation between separation and expulsion is difficult. Data from Fleigner[14] and Hibbard[15] showed that when minimal manipulation of the fundus and cord was performed, and the placenta was expressed only after

signs of descent were evident, 90% of the placentas were delivered within 15 minutes, and only 2–3% were retained after 30 minutes.

There is a broad spectrum of opinion and practice regarding the routine management of the third stage of labor. Early administration of oxytocic drugs at the delivery of the shoulders enhances uterine contractility and expedites placental separation.[16,17] In one published series, expression of the placenta by a combination of traction of the umbilical cord with the Brandt maneuver, reduced the frequency of postpartum hemorrhage from about 5% to 2%.[18]

Most studies have not demonstrated a clear benefit from active intervention.[19] Forceful traction on the cord can result in uterine inversion, retained secundines, and cord avulsion, with the consequent necessity to remove the placenta manually. Immediate manual removal increases the risk of bleeding by 30% as compared to management designed to facilitate spontaneous expulsion of the placenta by intravenous administration of oxytocin.[20]

Since existing data do not demonstrate a clear benefit from active intervention, probably the best approach is that once the cord has been clamped and cut, no attempt to deliver the placenta is made until there are signs of placental separation or 15–30 minutes have elapsed, provided there are no circumstances which call for earlier intervention. At this point, some assistance is required. The Brandt maneuver is a safe and popular method. It consists of placing the fingers of one hand externally against the contracted fundus above the symphysis pubis and applying pressure upward while simultaneous gentle traction on the cord causes descent of the placenta from the lower uterine segment. Then the direction of the pressure is reversed (downward). This will force the placenta out of the upper vagina and introitus. Strong traction on the cord and forceful fundal pressure should never be employed. Unless there is active bleeding or some other complication, there is no need to hurry. On the other hand, delaying the expression may cause uterine distention or trapping of the placenta if the cervix constricts; thus, this is not recommended either.

Routine administration of oxytocic agents after the placenta is delivered is almost universal practice in the USA. Oxytocin is customarily given by adding 10–20 U to 1000 ml IV fluid and running it at 10 ml/min. When given this way or intramuscularly, it has little or no adverse side effect. Ergonovine maleate (Ergotrate) and methylergonovine (Methergine) although equally effective, because of their vasopressor activity, can lead to acute pulmonary edema, cerebrovascular accident, and retinal detachment.[21] In an overview of 27 controlled trials on the effects of routine oxytocic administration in the management of the third stage of labor, a 40% reduction in the risk of postpartum hemorrhage was calculated for the study group.[22]

It is standard practice to examine the placenta routinely and confirm that it is intact. Routine postpartum digital exploration of the uterine cavity had been advocated, but several, more recent studies have refuted its utility.[23]

Uterine atony

Uterine atony results from failure of the myometrium to contract and/or stay contracted after the expulsion of the placenta, thereby allowing blood loss to continue at the implantation site. If any predisposing factor is present, the potential for excessive blood loss should be anticipated, a large-bore intravenous catheter should be placed, and blood should be readily available. The anesthesiologist should also be aware of the potential problem and consulted regarding the need to avoid deep anesthesia and uterine-relaxant drugs.

The diagnosis of uterine atony is suggested by the presence on abdominal examination of a large, boggy uterus that rises above the umbilicus. On this basis, a stepwise sequence of maneuvers designed to reverse uterine atony should be implemented (Table 22.3). The first step is firm abdominal massage of the uterine fundus with one hand. As uterine massage is performed, 20 U of oxytocin diluted in 1 l of normal saline or Ringer's lactate should be infused at a rate of 500–1000 ml/h. Intravenous bolus administration of oxytocin should be avoided because it can lead to sudden and profound hypotension, hypertension cardiac compromise,[24] and even death.[25]

Bleeding that has failed to respond to uterine massage, and uterotonic therapy calls for exploration of the birth canal. With the patient under adequate anesthesia, the lower genital tract should be carefully examined to rule out lacerations of the vulva, vagina, and cervix. The uterine cavity should be explored next with a hand and any retained cotyledon be removed.

If bleeding continues and the uterus is still atonic, the administration of prostaglandins (PG) has been shown to be successful in 60–80% of patients unresponsive to standard oxytocic therapy. The use of PG of the $F_{2\alpha}$ and E series has added a new dimension to the treatment of postpartum hemorrhage.[26] A 0.25-mg dose of the 15-methylated analog of $PGF_{2\alpha}$ is more potent and has a longer duration of action than its parent compound.[27] It can be injected intramuscularly, intravenously, or intramyometrially with equal effectiveness. Peak blood levels occur 15–60 minutes after intramuscular injection. Depending on the clinical situation, repeated injections can be made at 15–90-minute intervals. Most patients respond to one or two doses. The total dose should not exceed 1–1.5 mg. Side effects of PG therapy include gastrointestinal symptoms, such as diarrhea and vomiting, which occur in 10–25%, and fever, which occurs in 5% of the cases. Although blood-pressure elevation occurs rarely, the drug is contraindicated in women with cardiovascular and pulmonary disease because of its potential hypertensive and bronchoconstrictive effects.[28] Cardiovascular collapse with pulmonary edema after an overdose of intramyometrially injected $PGF_{2\alpha}$ has also been reported.[29]

The use of intrauterine packing may deserve a last attempt before resorting to surgical or angiographic modalities. If successful, it may temporarily control the bleeding and offer time for preparations for surgery and blood replacement. Uterine packing is seldom used in modern obstetric practice, and its effectiveness remains a controversial issue. Before the procedure is carried out, it is essential to ensure that there is no retained placental tissue, uterine rupture or inversion, genital tract trauma, or untreated coagulopathy. Equipment for packing, anesthesia, assistance, and lighting must be available. The preferred material is a 2- or 4-inch (5.08–10.16 cm) plain packing gauze. Oxidized cellulose can also be used. The actual method of packing can be either inserting the gauze with a long dressing forceps or using a facilitating packing device. With either method, the cervix is exposed and maintained in position by ring forceps placed on the anterior lip. The fundus of the uterus is grasped through the anterior abdominal wall and the packing instrument or device is introduced through the cervix until it is felt to be in contact with the fundus to ensure that the packing starts at the very top. Usually, 15–20 yards (13.716–18.288 m) of gauze are required to pack tightly a postpartum uterus.

Effective hemostasis should be observed within a few hours after packing. However, if bleeding continues through the pack, repacking should not be done. Rarely should it be left in for more than 24 hours. Preparations for surgery should be made in case bleeding recurs. The use of prophylactic antibiotics while the packing is in place may be beneficial in controlling infectious morbidity.

If the uterine packing is not tight enough and blood can collect above it, accumulation of blood in the space thus produced can result in considerable concealed blood loss, leading to consumption coagulopathy. A new device, the tamponade balloon catheter, has been designed to overcome this danger.[30] Essentially, a giant-size Foley catheter, the instrument can be inflated to fill the uterine cavity and apply pressure against the uterine walls from inside. Meanwhile, its catheter tip drains any blood accumulating in the dead space above it.

Hemorrhagic coagulopathy is a threat. Therefore, quick replacement of blood and coagulation factors must precede sophisticated hematologic diagnostic studies.[31]

Table 22.3 Steps to control uterine atony*

Abdominal uterine massage

Oxytocin infusion 20–40 U/l

Prostaglandins 15–methyl analog $PGF_{2\alpha}$, 0.25 mg IM, IV, MYOM

Uterine tamponade

Uterine cavity exploration/curettage

Uterine packing

Angiographic embolization

Hypogastric/uterine artery ligation

Hysterectomy

*IM = intramuscularly; IV = intravenously; MYOM = intramyometrially.

In cases of severe postpartum bleeding, the following course of action has been recommended:[20]

(1) Detailed documentation.
(2) Asking for help.
(3) Typing and cross-matching 6 units of blood.
(4) Transfusion through a thick cannula.
(5) Placement of a foley catheter.
(6) Fluid replacement with crystalloids and colloids until blood becomes available.
(7) Attention to signs of developing hemorrhagic coagulopathy. In case of suspicion, administration of fresh frozen plasma. Quick bedside fibrinogen test may be helpful. If the level is low, clotting takes more than 6 minutes and lysis less than 30 minutes.
(8) Consult hematologist.
(9) Initiate central venous pressure monitoring.
(10) Give O Rh-negative blood if fully compatible blood is not available.
(11) Warm the blood if it needs to be infused rapidly.
(12) Implement treatment in the environment of the intensive care unit.

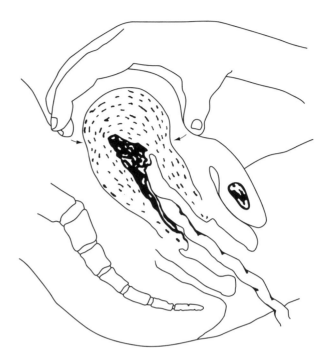

Figure 22.1 Manual removal of placenta. The fingers of the vaginal hand will dissect the cleavage plane between the uterine wall and placental margin until the placenta is completely detached.

Retained placenta

The incidence of retained secundines is 4–8% of all deliveries.[23,32] The spectrum varies from complete retention of a separated or still attached placenta to retention of placental fragments, cotyledons, or membranes. A retained placenta which is partially or completely separated is characteristically associated with early postpartum hemorrhage, whereas retained placental fragments relatively commonly lead to late postpartum bleeding. Retained fragments of membranes are rather common and do not cause postpartum hemorrhage.

Failure of the placenta to be delivered may be due to entrapment by a contracted lower uterine segment; failure of separation; or placenta accreta, increta, or percreta. In addition, the injudicious conduct of the third stage of labor may result in cord avulsion, or retention of a succenturiate lobe or fragmented placental pieces. Entrapment of a separated placenta is common.

Manual removal

Manual removal is indicated if the placenta is still retained 30 minutes after the delivery of the fetus, or if significant bleeding mandates earlier intervention. The procedure must be carried out under general anesthesia or spinal block to minimize patient discomfort. Aseptic principles should be adhered to. While the uterine fundus is held firm by one hand placed abdominally (Figure 22.1), the other hand is introduced into the uterine cavity along the cord until the placenta is reached and its margin is identified. A cleavage plane between the placenta and the uterine wall is then developed by deliberate digital separation .

If a cleavage plane cannot be developed, undue force should not be used. Pulling on the body of the placenta prior to digital separation is not advisable. Forceful attempts at removal can result in retention of placental fragments, uterine inversion, colporrhexis, or uterine rupture. Once the placenta has been removed, it should be carefully examined for the site of cord insertion, margins, abruptly terminating vessels, missing cotyledons, or retention of succenturiate lobes. When incomplete removal is apparent, the uterine cavity should be re-explored and any remaining placental tissue removed by gentle digital manipulation. Throughout these procedures, the external hand holds the fundus in a firm grasp and serves as a guide for the internal hand. Rarely, gentle and careful curettage using a large banjo-type curette may need to be employed to remove any remaining placental fragments. Failure of these measures to effect complete delivery of the placenta or to control bleeding calls for immediate additional measures. These include uterine packing, vessel ligation, and hysterectomy. Oxytocic drugs are administered to ensure that the uterus remains contracted. If the placenta cannot be separated, placenta accreta should be suspected and further attempts to remove the placenta should be abandoned. Instead, immediate preparation for laparotomy must be initiated.

Placenta accreta, increta, and percreta

Rarely, the placenta implants on an area without an intervening layer of decidua basalis, and invades the myometrium (accreta). This abnormal invasion of the myometrium may involve the whole (total) or part (partial/focal) of the placenta. The depth of penetration may be deep myometrial (increta) or may extend through the entire musculature to the serosa (percreta). Various degrees of placenta accreta occur in connection with 1/500 to 1/70 000 deliveries.[33] Predisposing factors include multiparity; advanced maternal age; implantation on a submucous myoma; and endometrial scarring from previous curettage, myomectomy, cesarean section incision, or Asherman's syndrome. Of particular note is the association with placenta previa when the latter occurs overlying a previous uterine incision. The current rate of cesarean deliveries will therefore increase the frequency with which placenta accreta occurs. Although the diagnosis can by confirmed only by histologic examination, it should be suspected whenever the placenta fails to separate and a distinct cleavage plane cannot be developed while attempting manual removal.

Miscellaneous etiology

Uterine rupture or dehiscence of a uterine scar is a major cause of obstetric hemorrhage. The risk of rupture is eight times higher after a preceding abdominal delivery than when the uterus is intact. Transverse incision placed at a relatively high level of the lower uterine segment is more prone to antepartum rupture than one at a low level. Other risk factors are multiparity, twin pregnancy, and instrumental deliveries.[7,34,35]

Arteriovenous malformations[36] are a rare cause of bleeding postpartum.[37] However, this unusual alternative needs to be kept in mind when blood flow is demonstrated on sonographic examination. The anomaly can be congenital or acquired. In case of bleeding associated with this anomaly, uterine curettage can cause catastrophic bleeding. Previous curettage, pregnancy termination, septic abortion, and gestational trophoplastic disease appear to predispose to such anomalies. High blood flow velocity (>96 cm/second) and low resistance to blood flow are suggestive of arteriovenous shunt or trophoplastic disease. High human chorionic gonadotropin concentrations are indicative of the latter alternative.[38]

For the identification of arteriovenous connection, the use of three-dimensional, color-Doppler technology is helpful. This permits the recognition and localization of increased vascularity. It also generates wave forms that permit the measurement of systolic and diastolic blood flow velocities.[39,40] Color-Doppler or gray-scale sonography facilitates the distinction between the vascular uterine wall and the retained product of conception. On gray-scale sonography, the placental tissue occupies the uterine cavity. In contrast, arteriovenous malformations often involve both the myometrium and the uterine cavity. The arteriovenous communications may regenerate; therefore, they can be managed expectantly.[41,42] When the bleeding is severe, uterine embolization usually permits the avoidance of hysterectomy.[30]

Retroperitoneal hematoma is an infrequent but dangerous form of postpartum bleeding. It is concealed and thus difficult to diagnose. The blood loss can be severe enough to cause hemorrhagic shock. The source of the bleeding may be difficult to find; thus, the involvement of a vascular or oncologic surgeon is desirable. When the bleeding vessel escapes detection, hypogastric artery ligation may be helpful.

Angiographic embolization

Selective angiography to locate the bleeding site and angiographic embolization have been shown to be efficacious in controlling bleeding when other measures have failed.[43] This procedure should be carried out only by skilled and experienced personnel in facilities where proper equipment is available. In addition, the patient should be hemodynamically stable and able to tolerate a 1–2-hour procedure. It should be considered if the patient does not want extirpative surgery and cannot medically tolerate anesthesia, and in cases of postpartum hemorrhage not amenable to surgical therapy, such as a deep vaginal hematoma.[44] It should also be resorted to in cases where bleeding has not been adequately controlled by surgical means, such as hysterectomy or hypogastric artery ligation. However, the technique is not foolproof.[45]

The technique involves the passage under fluoroscopic control of an intravascular catheter through the femoral artery, and advancing the catheter cephalad while performing an arteriogram of the bleeding site. Knowledge of the pelvic collateral vessels is important during angiography in order to identify all possible bleeding sites. The catheter should be advanced to a level just below the renal arteries in order to opacify all collateral vessels. After embolization, aortography should be done to confirm cessation of bleeding. If bleeding continues after embolization of the major artery, collateral branches can be individually identified and occluded.

Various embolic and vasoconstrictive agents have been used. These include autologous blood clot; Gelfoam pledgets or powder; Doinosil fluid; and a variety of vasoconstrictors such as vasopressin, dopamine, and norepinephrine. The use of vasoconstrictors (e.g., vasopressin) has the advantage of reducing the risk of ischemic complications. With regional vasoconstriction, bleeding from collateral reconstitution is also reduced. However, because the dose of these drugs needs to be tapered over 24 hours, it requires leaving the catheter in situ for an extended period of time. This requires intensive physician and nursing care to monitor the infusion.

A major potential complication of pelvic embolization is ischemia, resulting in nerve injury or infarction of the areas affected by the vascular supply. Embolization of both the anterior and posterior branches of the internal iliac artery can obstruct the vascular supply of the sciatic and femoral nerves, resulting in paresis of the lower limbs.[46] This complication is more likely to occur with the smaller particles of Gelfoam powder and if central surgical ligation had preceded embolization of the collateral vessels. Short-lived emboli such as blood clot can also be used; however, Gelfoam may be easier to prepare and its particle size easier to control. Arterial recanalization with subsequent pregnancy has been reported.[47]

Aortic compression

Aortic compression is an often overlooked yet simple adjuvant method in the management of postpartum hemorrhage while other surgical or medical therapies are being prepared. The maneuver consists of compressing the aorta by pushing on the abdominal wall with a closed fist at the level of the lumbosacral junction, which is just above the bifurcation and below the level of the renal arteries. The postpartum patient is an ideal candidate for this maneuver, since the abdominal wall is lax and the rectus muscles are diastatic. If the abdomen is opened, direct aortic compression can be an effective initial step in controlling the bleeding until uterine or hypogastric artery ligation is done or the bleeding site identified. If compression is needed for an extended period of time, an aortic compression device such as the Harris instrument can be utilized.[48]

Antishock trousers

The antishock trousers or MAST suit evolved primarily from military applications.[49,50] Although the MAST suit has a variety of medical applications, its primary use is in patients with severe intra-abdominal bleeding either preoperatively or postoperatively when surgical intervention has failed to control bleeding.[51] In the latter circumstances, the use of the MAST suit has successfully allowed stabilization of vital signs and control of bleeding, and has obviated the need for surgery.[50] The reported uses in obstetrics have been to manage uncontrollable postpartum hemorrhage due to ischiorectal hematoma and disseminated intravascular coagulation.[49,50]

The device is made of one piece of double-layered, polyvinyl fabric, and resembles a pair of wraparound trousers. It encloses the body from the lower margin of the ribs to the ankles. There are three separate chambers for inflation – one abdominal and two leg compartments. When inflated, it is capable of sustaining an internal air pressure up to 104 mmHg indefinitely. With foot pumps, the legs are inflated first, followed by the abdominal compartments. The pressure is measured by a manometer or gauge placed in the circuit. Beginning as low as 10 mmHg, it is increased by 5–10-mmHg increments until the vital signs are stabilized and adequate perfusion is established. Most venous bleeding is halted by pressures of 40–60 mmHg. Pressures up to 100 mmHg have been applied in patients with arterial bleeding, but such high pressures should

not be maintained for long periods of time. The suit should remain inflated at moderate pressures for a period of 12–24 hours after the bleeding has stopped. Deflation should be done gradually with decrements of 5 mmHg. The abdominal compartment is to be deflated before the legs.[50] When successful, the blood pressure is increased rapidly and blood loss is decreased. Blood pressure is improved by increased peripheral resistance secondary to the direct pressure effect on the vessels, shunting of blood flow from the lower body to the more vital upper body, improving venous return to the central circulation, and increasing cardiac output. Bleeding is reduced because the pressure applied to the exterior of the vessels results in a significant reduction of both the venous and arterial diameters. The MAST suit is also useful in decreasing the intravenous crystalloid requirements, and it allows valuable time for safe and complete cross-matching of blood for transfusion.

Potential adverse effects include hypoventilation, hypercarbia, and hypoxia, especially if the increased intra-abdominal pressure is so high as to compromise diaphragmatic excursion. If the inflation pressure is greater than the systolic pressure, reduction of blood flow to the lower extremities can result in lactic acid production and hyperkalemia. Decreased urinary output, skin breakdown, and deepening of cardiogenic shock are additional dangers. Most potential adverse effects are preventable if the trousers are positioned correctly and if only moderate pressures are used for not more than 48 hours. Initial concern about air embolism,[52] prompted by a case of postpartum bleeding without placental separation, has not been confirmed subsequently.

Surgical treatment

In the face of uncontrollable bleeding, such as from a ruptured uterus, one must proceed directly to surgical exploration. If the patient is desirous of future childbearing and is hemodynamically stable, elective or therapeutic pelvic vessel ligation or suturing of the identified bleeding site may be attempted first. The choice of uterine artery ligation versus hypogastric artery and/or ovarian artery ligation depends upon the site and cause of bleeding and the surgeon's expertise with each procedure. The higher success rate with uterine artery ligation would make this the initial procedure of choice.[53] However, if proper criteria are not met, pelvic vessel ligation should not be attempted and hysterectomy should be promptly performed.

Hypogastric artery ligation

Hypogastric artery ligation will control otherwise intractable obstetric hemorrhage and permit uterine conservation, usually without major complications. Higher success rates are reported for uterine atony and placenta accreta, and lower rates with uterine or broad ligament lacerations. Hypogastric artery ligation reduces distal blood flow and decreases distal pulse pressure. Thus, it converts the hemodynamics of the arterial system to those of a venous system amenable to hemostasis by simple clot formation.[54]

Knowledge of the anatomic location and relationship to neighboring structures facilitates their identification, dissection, and ligation. The aorta bifurcates at the level of the fourth lumbar vertebra into the common iliac arteries. These in turn bifurcate at the level of the sacral promontory into the external iliac artery, which courses laterally to the leg, where it becomes the femoral artery, and into the hypogastric artery, which descends medioinferiorly along the border of the psoas muscle into the pelvis. The ureter is attached to the undersurface of the peritoneum and crosses the hypogastric artery from a lateral to medial direction at its origin. Posterolaterally lie the external iliac vein and the obturator nerve. Posteromedially lies the internal iliac vein. Lateral to the hypogastric artery are the psoas muscles, major and minor. The hypogastric artery divides into anterior and posterior branches. The anterior branches supply blood to the pelvic viscera. The posterior division supplies blood to the fascia, buttocks, and medial surfaces of the thigh. An extensive network of anastomoses occurs in each hemipelvis vertically, ipsilaterally, and horizontally across the midline. This abundant collateral blood supply ensures that reproductive function is preserved and term pregnancies can follow even the ligations of both hypogastric and ovarian arteries.[55]

Since the hypogastric artery is a retroperitoneal structure, the first step is to enter this space. This can be done by an extraperitoneal or transperitoneal approach, depending on the source of the bleeding, the skill of the surgeon, and the condition of the patient. If there is any question as to whether intra-abdominal bleeding is present, the transperitoneal route should be utilized.

For the extraperitoneal operation, a Gibson incision is usually performed. The latter represents an inguinal incision starting from the pubic tubercle of the symphysis pubis and extending approximately 8 cm in a curvilinear fashion medial to the anterior superior iliac spine. The fat and subcutaneous fascial layers are dissected. The aponeurotic sheath of the external and internal oblique muscles are next transected in a conventional fashion. On lateral retraction, the rectus abdominis comes into view, exposing the extraperitoneal space. Only after identification of the ureter, infundibulopelvic ligament, common iliac artery, hypogastric artery, and external iliac artery is the ligation performed. A Babcock clamp may be applied on the hypogastric artery and a gentle attempt made to elevate it from the anterior surface of the iliac vein. Usually, however, this is not satisfactory. The areolar tissue joining the posterior wall of the internal iliac artery with the anterior wall of the vein needs to be carefully separated by blunt dissection. A right-angle clamp is then passed below the hypogastric artery. Next, a suture is placed in the tip of the clamp and passed under the hypogastric artery, usually from the medial to the lateral side to avoid the junction of right and left common iliac veins forming the inferior vena cava. The suture must be placed at the bifurcation of the common iliac artery to prevent thrombus formation proximal to the tie. Chromic suture material is preferred, and the artery is not transected. Closure of the abdominal incision is anatomically the reverse of the opening steps. A drain should be placed in the extraperitoneal space and removed in 24–48 hours.

For transperitoneal hypogastric ligation, the essential steps are as follows. Initially, the uterus is pulled forward over the symphysis pubis and held in place with moist sponges by an assistant. The intestines are packed away from the operative field. In case of uterine rupture or lesion of a uterine vessel, the site of the injury is to be dealt with initially. The round and infundibulopelvic ligaments are visualized. The peritoneum between the two ligaments is tented with tissue forceps and incised parallel to the infundibulopelvic ligament (Figure 22.2a). The index finger palpates through the rent in search of a pulsating vessel (i.e., the external iliac artery) and bluntly separates the areolar tissue above it. The artery is then traced cephalad to identify the bifurcation of the common iliac artery. At this point, one will notice the ureter passing across the bifurcation in a lateromedian direction. The ureter remains attached to the posterior leaf of the peritoneum of the broad ligament. The ureter with its peritoneum is retracted medially. This maneuver exposes the bifurcation of the common iliac artery, which can usually be identified by the presence of a bulge in the diameter of the vessel. At the bifurcation, the hypogastric artery, which is directed posteriorly, is picked up with a Babcock clamp (Figure 22.2b) and its course traced distally. Next, the hypogastric is dissected by blunt dissection for a distance of 2–3 cm, thus freeing it from its attachment by areolar connective tissue to the underlying iliac vein. A tonsil tip sucker, right-angle clamp, or peanut-type of sponge may be used for this blunt dissection. Great caution must be taken at this point to avoid injury to the vein.

No. 0 silk is threaded into the open right-angle clamp under the internal iliac artery (Figure 22.2c). The clamp with the thread is then withdrawn. The maneuver is repeated with the same thread to form a loop. The latter is then tied as close to the bifurcation as possible, thus avoiding the opportunity for clot formation in the blind segment of the vessel (Figure 22.2d). It is to be noted that the artery is not cut in the course of the operation. The procedure is concluded by closing the overlying peritoneum.

The ligature of one of the hypogastric (internal iliac) arteries having been completed, a similar procedure is carried out on the opposite side. When left-sided ligation is performed, the sigmoid usually needs to be drawn to the right by appropriate packing with moist sponges.

The use of absorbable sutures will allow for subsequent canalization of vessels, although ultimate uterine blood flow is not compromised if permanent suture material is used.[56]

The incidence of serious complications associated with hypogastric artery ligation is low if proper identification and careful dissection of landmark structures are carried out. Complications include misidentification and accidental ligation of the external iliac artery, laceration of the internal and exter-

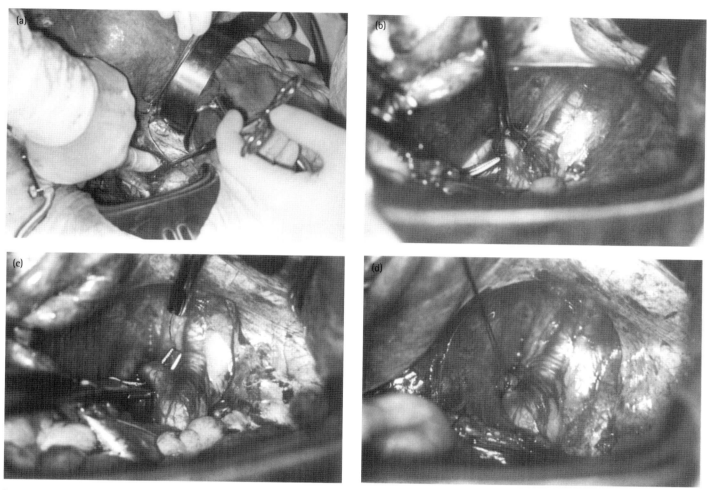

Figure 22.2 (a) Palpating for the pulsating external iliac artery through the opening of the peritoneum. (b) The Babcock clamp is picking up the right internal iliac artery at its origin from the common iliac artery. A right-angle clamp is to be passed under the vessel in a mediolateral direction. (c) The right-angle clamp having been passed under the internal iliac artery, a no. 0 silk thread is being fed into it. (d) The internal iliac artery has been ligated close to its origin from the common iliac artery.

nal iliac veins, ureter injury, retroperitoneal hematoma, and ischemic sequelae.[57] Accidental ligation of the external iliac artery, if unrecognized, can lead to loss of vascular supply to the ipsilateral leg. It is essential that the femoral pulse be palpated before and after artery ligation. Laceration of the thin-walled iliac vein occurs when too vigorous dissection of areolar tissue surrounding the artery is carried out or when the right-angle clamp is improperly passed beneath the hypogastric artery. Such laceration results in severe hemorrhage and is difficult to repair. Elevation of the artery with a Babcock clamp and passing the tip from lateral to medial may avoid injury to the iliac vein.

Ureteral injury may be avoided by properly identifying the ureter and retracting it manually out of the field before dissecting the areolar tissue surrounding the hypogastric artery. Retroperitoneal hematoma is prevented by meticulous hemostasis in the retroperitoneal space. Ischemic sequelae are rare because of the extensive collateral circulation, but can result in central pelvic ischemia, breakdown of the perineal skin and epi-

siotomy site, and paresis of the lower extremities from lower motor neuron damage.

Uterine artery ligation

The uterine artery originates as a branch from the anterior hypogastric artery. After coursing along the lateral wall of the pelvis, it arches over the ureter about 2 cm lateral from the uterus as the ureter runs beneath the cardinal ligament in its fascial tunnel. At this point, it gives off a descending branch to the cervix, which anastomoses with vaginal branches and the more important ascending branch. The ascending branch runs its course along the medial aspect of the broad ligament upward to anastomose with the ovarian vessels at the upper inner angle of the broad ligament. During pregnancy, the uterine artery elongates, hypertrophies, and carries 90% of uterine blood flow. Return flow is provided predominantly by the uterine veins and the hypertrophied ovarian veins.

Bilateral ligation of the ascending branch of the uterine artery was first suggested by Waters in 1952 as a method to manage postpartum hemorrhage when more conservative methods failed. He considered it a procedure to be used as an initial step to precede all extirpative methods.[58] Proponents of this technique recommend it over hypogastric artery ligation because the latter takes longer to perform, requires more dissection, and has lower success and higher complication rates. O'Leary found the procedure effective 95% of the time, with a 1% complication rate.[53] Despite favorable reports, the technique of uterine artery ligation is still not used frequently in the management of uncontrollable postpartum hemorrhage, partly due to a lack of surgical experience and partly due to insecurity regarding the exact position of the ureters.

The procedure can be used to control or prevent postpartum hemorrhage. The technique entails mass ligation or individual ligation. The early descriptions[58] stressed the importance of dissecting the uterine artery and vein, and ligating only the artery. Recently, mass ligation of both the artery and vein has been advocated as a simple, effective, and more rapidly performed procedure.[59] To ligate the left uterine artery, the uterus and fallopian tubes are elevated and moved to the right. The fingers of one hand compress the leaves of the broad ligament and run down to the level of the internal os or, in cases of cesarean section, just below the standard transverse uterine incision. Without dissecting the broad ligament, the pulsations of the ascending branch of the left uterine artery are palpated. Then, with a large Mayo needle, a no. 1 chromic catgut suture is passed at this level into and through the myometrium from anterior to posterior, 2–3 cm medial to the uterine vessel. Once the needle is extracted from the posterior myometrium, it is redirected from posterior to anterior through an avascular area in the broad ligament lateral to where the uterine vessel is palpated, and the suture is then securely tied (Figure 22.3).

The procedure to ligate the right uterine vessel consists of the following. The uterus is elevated and pushed to the left. Next, the needle is passed from anterior to posterior in an avascular area of the right broad ligament, lateral to the uterine vessel. It is then passed through the myometrium from posterior to anterior, 2–3 cm medial to the right uterine vessel, and tied.[59] Only absorbable suture should be used, and a figure-of-8 suture should be avoided.

Uterine artery ligation produces an immediate blanching of the uterus with resultant hypoxia and causes the uterus to contract and remain firm. It is important to include a significant amount of myometrium in the suture and to obliterate intramyometrial ascending arterial branches, because the degree of uterine ischemia is directly related to the amount of myometrium in the suture. Even if the uterus remains atonic, bleeding usually comes under control. Higher failure rates have been reported in cases of placenta previa/accreta, especially if the implantation of the placenta was over the scar of a previous lower segment cesarean section; in cases where the source of bleeding is from vessels supplied by the vaginal artery; and in those due to a clotting defect. Complications of uterine artery

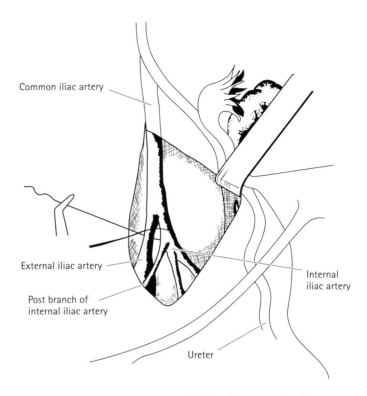

Figure 22.3 Technique of uterine artery ligation. Sutures are placed to encompass the ascending uterine arteries, as well as anastomotic branches from the ovarian arteries. (Courtesy CA Apuzzio.)

ligation are rare. Vein damage from multiple passages with the needle can result in broad-ligament hematoma. Anteriovenous sinus[60] formation has also been reported, but this complication can be prevented by using absorbable suture material, avoiding figure-of-8 sutures, and including a substantial amount of myometrium in the ligature.

Despite successful reports, transvaginal ligation of the uterine arteries is hazardous and bloody. It should not be attempted.

No long-term adverse effects of bilateral uterine artery ligation have been reported. Recanalization uniformly occurs with resumption of normal menstrual flow and subsequent pregnancies.[61]

Ovarian artery ligation

Bilateral ovarian artery ligation can be a valuable adjunct to hypogastric or uterine artery ligation.[62] The ovarian artery is a branch of the aorta and travels retroperitoneally in the infundibulopelvic ligament. It enters the mesovarium at the fimbriated end of the fallopian tube, where it courses above the ovary, giving off numerous branches to the fallopian tube. During pregnancy, it contributes 5–10 percent of the blood supply to the uterus. Due to the enlargement of all the vessels, the ovarian vessels are easy to palpate and visualize in the mesovarium. The area for ligation should be at the junction of the

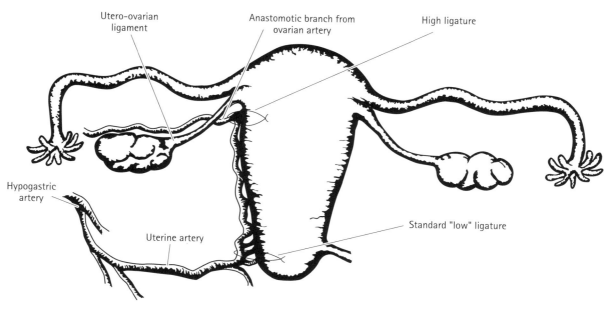

Figure 22.4 Ovarian arterial anatomy. Figure-of-8 represents area for ligation. (Courtesy CA Apuzzio.)

utero-ovarian ligament and the ovary, which is where the ovarian artery anastomoses with the uterine artery (Figure 22.4). Ligation at this site will allow maintenance of adequate blood flow to the ovary and the fallopian tube. At this point in the mesovarium, an avascular area above the artery should be identified and a 0-strength polyglycolic suture passed directly or through a window formed by a Kelly clamp. The ligature is then similarly passed through an avascular area below the artery and tied. Two simple ligatures can be used and there is no need to divide the vessel.

B-Lynch suture

If, after uterine exploration, the atony fails to resolve in response to medication and uterine massage, the B-Lynch suture may be effective.[63] The procedure requires laparotomy and separation of the bladder peritoneum from the cervix. Despite a reported adverse experience, involving ischemic necrosis associated with it,[64] this procedure has gained considerable popularity in recent years.[62] Typically, the operation is performed in connection with a cesarean section prior to the closure of the lower segment transverse uterine incision. Utilizing a 70–80-mm, round-bodied, hand needle with no. 2 plain or chromic catgut, Lynch recommends the placement of the suture 3 cm below the right end of the incision. Having penetrated the uterine cavity, the needle emerges 3 cm above the upper incision margin. At this point, the suture is carried over the body of the uterus at a distance of about 4 cm from its lateral border (Figure 22.5a). While an assistant compresses the uterus, the suture is carried to the posterior aspect of the organ and secured approximately at the level of the anterior incision

by driving the needle through the posterior aspect of the lower uterine segment (Figure 22.5b). Then, once again, the suture is carried through the fundus of the uterus and passed through the uterine cavity at the left angle of the uterine incision in the same manner as previously described. Depending upon the circumstances, the uterine incision can be closed either before or after the placement of the suture, which, in the end, is to be secured by a double-throw knot in order to prevent slipping. When the operation is performed after vaginal delivery, Lynch recommends the opening of the lower segment of the uterus in the same manner as in case of a cesarean section in order to ensure that the anteriorly placed suture enters the uterine cavity.[63]

Postpartum hysterectomy

Removal of the uterus postpartum or in the course of a cesarean section requires essentially the same technical steps as what gynecologic textbooks describe in connection with routine abdominal hysterectomy. However, since the former is usually performed under emergency conditions and on a patient who has already endured major blood loss, the surgeon is compelled to work under pressure and against narrow time limitations. A circumstance which needs to be remembered is that the uterine arteries, which follow a spiral course in the nonpregnant state, are stretched out in advanced pregnancy. If severed, they tend to spring back to their original shape and, as a result, move away from the operative field. This fact makes ligation and cutting of the arteries a precarious and somewhat risky undertaking under certain emergency situations. The technical details described in connection with uterine artery ligation should generally be followed when the uterus is to be removed.

(a)   (b)

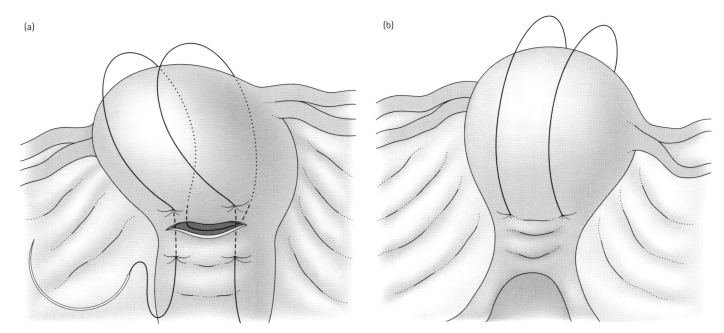

Figure 22.5 Illustration of the various steps of the B-Lynch operation. For details, consult the text.

Under many, if not most, circumstances, a total hysterectomy is not necessary for achieving hemostasis. Sober judgment is needed to decide in the context of the prevailing circumstances the risk-benefit ratios of the available operative options. Dilated blood vessels frequently hinder effective hemostasis and ongoing bleeding often obscures the surgical field. Therefore, in the absence of significant cervical pathology, subtotal hysterectomy is the safest alternative for this lifesaving intervention.

Because the cervix is usually effaced in case of cesarean hysterectomy, its removal entails less difficulty than in the nonpregnant state. On the other hand, after a presumed total removal, the seemingly effaced cervix may re-emerge at the time of the postpartum examination as a cervical stump.

Uterine rupture

Extremely rare in modern obstetrics in connection with an intact uterus, uterine rupture occurs with relative frequency after cesarean section, occasionally even before the onset of labor. The risk is particularly high after a classical incision and after surgical uterine reconstructive procedures. The most common and usually unrecognized type of rupture is dehiscence of a lower segment scar. When it is recognized during a repeated section, the opening of the separated wound edges needs to be extended to allow the delivery of the fetus. Thereafter, it is repaired in the usual fashion.

After a previous cesarean section, rupture of the uterus usually, but not invariably, involves the area of the incision. It creates a potentially catastrophic surgical emergency when the rupture extends to the parametrium and disrupts major blood vessels. Another serious potential injury is extension of the rupture to the cervix, not infrequently with coincidental damage to the bladder. The critical issues in this situation are the following:

(1) awareness of the retroperitoneal pelvic anatomy
(2) identification of the ureter
(3) hemostasis after visual identification of the bleeding vessel
(4) dissection of the bladder from the uterine isthmus and determination of the extent of the bladder injury
(5) decision about the optimum surgical management with due attention to the patient's realistic reproductive potential.

If the uterus is considered salvageable after full control of the hemorrhage, repair is to be performed as circumstances permit, using a late-absorbing suture material.

In the event of bladder injury requiring repair, the surgical correction must be established in such a manner that the organ remains watertight. This can be achieved by suturing the freshened edges of the musculature in one or more layers. To ensure adequate healing, the bladder must be kept empty using an indwelling Foley or suprapubic catheter for at least 8 days.

After conservative surgery, the patient is to be instructed about the high risk of recurrent uterine rupture in case of a future pregnancy.

Coagulation disorders

Genetic and systemic diseases that interfere with the coagulation process may cause or contribute to postpartum hemorrhage. These include von Willebrand's disease, blood dyscrasia, leukemia, and disseminated intravascular coagulopathy. The diagnosis is usually known prior to delivery on the basis of past personal or family history, or abnormal coagulation studies done upon admission to the labor and delivery suite. Usually, difficulty with bleeding is not encountered unless the coagulation abnormality is quite severe. Definitive management consists of replacement of the specific deficient coagulation factors. von Willebrand's disease is best treated with administration of factor VIII concentrate. If cryoprecipitate is not available, fresh frozen plasma or fresh whole blood can be used. Platelet deficiency can be corrected by the administration of platelet concentrate. Consumptive coagulopathy may result from severe obstetric hemorrhage itself or from other underlying causes, such as abruptio placentae, amniotic fluid embolism, fetal death, and severe infection. Treatment of the underlying disease coupled with the usual measures to combat hemorrhage and shock, including replacement of blood and coagulation factors, make up the corrective therapy.

Blood loss and blood replacement

The consequences of acute blood loss may be immediate or delayed. Hypovolemic shock is an immediate threat. However, bleeding also reduces the patient's natural resistance and aggravates the risk of infection. Since the overall blood volume increases during gestation by an average of 60%, women's tolerance of blood loss is better in the pregnant than in the nonpregnant state.

Hypovolemia causes reduced cardiac output. This leads to a sympathetic reaction with increased vascular resistance and tachycardia. Major degrees of hypovolemia, sufficient to cause shock, also involve fluid deficit in the vasculatory space. Damage to the capillary endothelial layer increases permeability and permits the migration of fluid to the intercellular space and the cells. When hypovolemia prevails, the circulation of blood is diverted from nonvital organs (intestines, kidneys, and musculature) to vital ones (brain and heart). Oliguria is an early sign of hypovolemia. The severity of the latter is reflected in the degree of reduction of urine output. For this reason, insertion of a Foley catheter for continuous quantitative assessment of the same may be desirable. It is important to keep the output at least 30 ml/hour. Administration of oxygen may help in maintaining adequate tissue oxygenation and, thus, preventing organ failure.

Acute hypovolemia may be overcome by the administration of lactated Ringer's or normal saline solution; 1–2 l delivered intravenously in the course of 30–60 minutes, until the blood pressure improves. As soon as practical, the blood loss is to be replaced by blood in commensurate amounts. Administration of crystalloids and blood in 3:1 ratio is conducive to rapid restoration of the circulatory equilibrium. The former is quickly removed from the circulation, improving diuresis. Administration of colloids (dextran and albumin) helps in maintaining adequate intravascular osmotic pressure.

Transfusion is indicated if the bleeding is severe clinically or if the hematocrit level falls to 25%. When it becomes necessary to infuse blood at a rate exceeding 100 ml/minute, it is important to warm the blood to body temperature in order to avoid hypothermia.

The purpose of transfusing packed red blood cells is to improve the oxygen-carrying capacity of the blood and to overcome orthostatic hypotension. It is necessary to check the coagulability of the patient's blood after the transfusion of 5–10 units of blood.[65] Frozen fresh plasma is to be given in case of liver disease, coagulation defect, disseminated intravascular coagulation, thrombotic and thrombocytopenic purpura, and antithrombin 3 deficiency, and in association with massive transfusions. It contains all clotting factors, including factors V and VIII. It needs to be Rh compatible with the patient's blood. It is customary to give 2–4 units at a time. Each unit increases the amount of clotting factors by 2–3%.[65]

Concentrated cryoprecipitate is prepared from fresh frozen plasma. It contains factor VIII, von Willebrand factor and fibrinogen in high concentrations.

In case of inadequate number or function of the patient's own platelets, thrombocyte transfusion is indicated. Transfusion is required if the platelet count falls under 20 000 or if, with a count of less than 50 000, major operation is contemplated. Critical thrombocytopenia predictably develops if the transfused blood exceeds the patient's own original blood volume by 50–100%. The usual amount of platelet transfusion is one unit for each 10 kg body weight. If the blood group of the donor or donors is unknown, RhoGAM is to be given to Rh negative women since red blood cells do occur among the platelets. The risk of infection is reduced if only one donor's platelets are used.

The appearance of thromboplastin and endotoxin in the circulation leads to disseminated intravascular coagulation (DIC). The quoted substances activate thrombin and aggregate platelets and fibrin in the capillaries. Fibrin degradation products consume thrombocytes and activate coagulation factors (consumption coagulopathy). Aggressive fluid replacement is conducive to coagulopathy but usually not before 80% of the original fluid volume has been replaced. As a result, even minor trauma results in microvascular hemorrhage. Apart from the blood loss itself, tissue hypoxia and ischemia contribute to the development of fibrin plugs in the capillary system. This leads to renal failure, pulmonary damage, and, occasionally, Sheehan's syndrome. The diagnosis of DIC is to be entertained if the laboratory parameters, including fibrin degradation products and D-dimers, remain abnormal after the administration of fresh frozen plasma. The optimum treatment for intravascular thrombosis is low-molecular-weight heparin.

Even after the patient has been stabilized after major blood loss, attention must be paid to the potential side effects deriving from the infusion of blood products. These include hemolytic febrile reactions, allergic manifestations, and pulmonary damage. Other untoward sequelae are renal insufficiency, cortical blindness, and adult respiratory distress syndrome. Naturally, these complications require the involvement in the management of a variety of specialists and subspecialists.

Delayed postpartum hemorrhage

Delayed postpartum hemorrhage can manifest at any time in the puerperium. In most instances, it occurs 7–14 days after delivery. Common causes are subinvolution of the placental site, retained fragments of placenta, and endometritis.

Subinvolution results from failure or delay of the endometrium to return to its normal state after separation of the placenta. Noninvoluted vessels have been found to be filled with thrombus, without endothelial lining, and with perivascular trophoblasts in the walls.[66] Uterine atony and submucous myomas have also been implicated in the pathogenesis. The diagnosis is confirmed when curettage fails to recover placental fragments.

Subinvolution of the uterus or retained placental tissue cause bleeding when the necrotic tissue sloughs off the endometrium and opens previously thrombosed vascular channels. Patients with late postpartum hemorrhage may present with a sudden gush of blood or intermittent spotting prior to an episode of profuse bleeding. On physical examination, the uterus usually appears large and boggy. If there is an associated infection, there is uterine tenderness, fever, and foul-smelling lochia. The diagnostic workup includes routine blood and coagulation studies for the assessment of the extent and nature of the blood loss, a thorough pelvic examination for old hematomas or lacerations, and sonographic study to detect retained placental parts.[67] The treatment depends upon the clinical presentation. In case the bleeding is profuse, hospital admission is mandatory and blood replacement is indicated. If endometritis is a suspected contributory factor, cervical-uterine cultures must be obtained and antibiotics prescribed. If the bleeding continues or retained tissue is suspected, curettage should be performed. The procedure itself may cause severe blood loss; therefore, several units of blood should be available before it is performed. The operation may be performed with local or paracervical block, or under general anesthesia. The size, location, and consistency of the uterus must be assessed prior to the initiation of the procedure. The cervix usually is dilated enough to permit the insertion of instruments with relative ease; if not, it should be dilated to 12–13 mm in the usual manner. Ovum or sponge forceps may be used to remove placental tissue. A large, serrated curette can be utilized to empty the uterine cavity. Great care must be exercised so as to not perforate the uterine wall or curette too zealously. Oxytocin is to be administered during the procedure.

Bleeding usually ceases within a short time after the completion of the curettage. Packing of the uterus or other surgical procedures are rarely required. Nonetheless, arrangements should be made for emergency hysterectomy, should uncontrollable hemorrhage occur. Consent for the same should be obtained from the patient before the operation, with due emphasis upon the fact that the need for such an intervention does arise on rare occasions. Of particular concern is the case when the patient arrives in the emergency room already exsanguinated or in, or near to, a state of shock. Under such circumstances the clinical picture may already be complicated by consumption coagulopathy, thus establishing a vicious circle with regard to the life-threatening hemorrhage. Even the most vigorous blood and fluid replacement may not keep the balance with the torrential blood loss that may prevail in this eventuality. Curettage of the uterus, as described above, may exaggerate the bleeding and drive the patient into irreversible shock. Some obstetricians feel that in case of late postpartum bleeding it may be judicious to perform uterine (or hypogastric) artery ligation prior to the evacuation of the uterus by curettage, the latter performed with the abdomen open and the operating surgeon ready for any further action that may be required. Needless to say, the availability of large amounts of blood and close cooperation with the blood bank are critically important under these, fortunately rare, set of circumstances.

The postoperative follow-up should give due attention to some worrisome complications, such as Sheehan's syndrome and Asherman's syndrome. It deserves mention that the former is not necessarily associated with severe shock and can occur even if the blood pressure was successfully maintained above shock levels.

References

1. Bouvier-Colle MH, El-Joud DO, Varnoux N et al. Evaluation of the quality of of care for severe obstetrical haemorrhage in three French regions. Br J Obstet Gynaecol 2001; 108: 898.

2. Bouvier-Colle MH, Péquignot F, Jougla F. Mise au point sur la mortalité maternelle en France: fréquence, tendances et causes. J Gynecol Obstet Biol Reprod 2001; 30: 768.

3. Bouvier-Colle MH, Varnoux N, Bréart G. Maternal Deaths in France. editions INSERM: Paris, 1994.

4. Stones RW, Paterson CM, Saunders NJ. Risk factors for major obstetric hemorrhage. Eur J Obstet Gynecol 1993; 50: 1443.

5. Why Mothers Die. Report of Confidential Inquiries into Maternal Deaths in the United Kingdom 1994–1996.

6. Rizvi F, Mackey R, Barrett T et al. Successful reduction of massive postpartum haemorrhage by use of guidelines and staff education. Br J Obstet Gynaecol 2004; 111: 496.

7. Powers WF, Kiely JL. The risk confronting twins: a national perspective. Am J Obstet Gynecol 1994; 170: 456.

8. Pritchard JA, Baldwin RM, Dickey JC et al. Blood volume changes in pregnancy and the puerperium. II. Red blood cell loss and changes in apparent blood volume during and following vaginal delivery, cesarean section, and cesarean section plus total hysterectomy. Am J Obstet Gynecol 1962; 84: 1271.

9. Brant HA. Precise estimation of postpartum hemorrhage: difficulties and importance. BMJ 1967; 1: 398.

10. Robson SC, Boys RJ, Hunter S et al. Maternal hemodynamics after normal delivery and delivery complicated by postpartum hemorrhage. Obstet Gynecol 1989; 74: 234.

11. Dewhurst CJ, Dutton WAW. Recurrent abnormalities of the third stage of labor. Lancet 1957; 2: 764.

12. Miller RD. Complications of massive blood transfusions. Anesthesiology 1973; 39: 82.

13. Friedland GH, Klein RS. Transmission of the human immuno-deficiency virus. N Engl J Med 1987; 317: 1125.

14. Fliegner JR. Third stage management: how important is it? Med J Aust 1978; 2: 190.

15. Hibbard BH. The third stage of labour. BMJ 1964; 1: 1485.

16. Golan A, Lidor AL, Wexler P et al. A new method for the management of retained placenta. Am J Obstet Gynecol 1983; 146: 708.

17. Reddy VV, Carey JC. Effect of umbilical vein oxytocin on puerperal blood loss and length of the third stage of labor. Am J Obstet Gynecol 1989; 160: 206.

18. Fliegner JR, Hibbard BM. Active management of the third stage of labour. BMJ 1966; 2: 622.

19. Hendricks CH, Eskes TK, Saameli K. Uterine contractility at delivery, and in the puerperium. Am J Obstet Gynecol 1962; 83: 890.

20. Jutchon SP, Martin WL. Intrapartum and postpartum bleeding. Curr Obstet Gynecol 2002; 12: 250.

21. Moir DD, Amoa AB. Ergometrine or oxytocin? Blood loss and side effects at spontaneous vertex delivery. Br J Anaesth 1979; 51: 113.

22. Prendiville W, Elbourne D, Chalmers I. The effects of routine oxytocic administration in the management of the third stage of labour: an overview of the evidence from controlled trials. Br J Obstet Gynaecol 1988; 95: 3.

23. Epperly TD, Fogarty JP, Hodges SG. Efficacy of routine postpartum uterine exploration and manual sponge curettage. J Fam Pract 1989; 28: 172.

24. Weis RF, Markello R, Mo B et al. Cardiovascular effects of oxytocin. Obstet Gynecol 1975; 46: 211.

25. Hendricks CH, Brenner WE. Cardiovascular effects of oxytocic drugs used postpartum. Am J Obstet Gynecol 1970; 108: 751.

26. Bigrigg A, Chuni D, Chissell S et al. Use of intramyometrial 15-methyl prostaglandin F_2 alpha to control atonic postpartum hemorrhage following delivery and failure of conventional therapy. Br J Obstet Gynaecol 1991; 98: 734.

27. Buttino L Jr, Garite TJ. The use of 15-methyl F_2 alpha prostaglandin (Prostin 15M) for the control of postpartum hemorrhage. Am J Perinatal 1986; 3: 241.

28. Hayashi RH, Castillo MS, Noah ML. Management of severe postpartum hemorrhage with a prostaglandin F_2 alpha analogue. Obstet Gynecol 1984; 63: 806.

29. Douglas MJ, Farquharson DF, Ross PL et al. Cardiovascular collapse following an overdose of prostaglandin F_2 alpha: a case report. Can J Anaesth 1989; 36: 466.

30. Bakri NY, Amri A, Abdul Jabbaar F. Tamponade ballon for obstetric bleeding. Int J Gynecol Obstet 2001; 74: 139.

31. Boehlen F, Morales MA, Fontana P et al. Prolonged treatment of massive postpartum hemorrhage with recombinant factor VIIa: case report and review of the literature. Br J Obstet Gynaecol 2004; 111: 284.

32. Doolittle HH. Routine manual inspection of the postpartum uterus. Study of the late effects. Obstet Gynecol 1974; 9: 422.

33. Breen JL, Neubecker R, Gregori CA et al. Placenta accreta, increta, and percreta. A survey of 40 cases. Obstet Gynecol 1997; 49: 43.

34. Phelan JP. Uterine rupture. Clin Obstet Gynecol 1990; 33: 432.

35. Sebire NJ, Jolly M, Harris J et al. Risk of obstetric complications in multiple pregnancies: an analysis of more than 400,000 pregnancies in the UK. Prenat Neonat Med 2001; 6: 89.

36. Wiebe ER, Switzer P. Arteriovenous malformations of the uterus associated with medical abortion. Int J Gynaecol Obstet 2000; 71: 155.

37. Chang F-W, Ding B-C, Chen D-C et al. Heavy uterine bleeding due to uterine arterio-venous malformations. Acta Obstet Gynecol Scand 2004; 83: 899.

38. Huang MV, Muradeli D, Thurston WA et al. Uterine arteriovenous malformation: gray scale and Doppler US features with MR imagining correlation. Radiology 1998; 206: 115.

39. Jain KA, Feffrey RB, Sommer FG. Gynecologic vascular abnormalities: diagnosis with Doppler US. Radiology 1991; 178: 549.

40. Kwon JH, Kim GS. Obstetric iatrogenic arterial injuries of the uterus: diagnosis with US and treatment with transcatheter arterial embolization. Radiographics 2002; 22: 35.

41. Nizzard J, Pessel M, Keersmaecker D et al. High-intensity focused ultrasound in the treatment of postpartum hemorrhage: an animal model. Ultrasound Obstet Gynecol 2004; 23: 262.

42. Timmerman D, Van den Bosch T, Peeraer K et al. Vascular malformations of the uterus: ultrasonographic diagnosis and conservative management. Eur J Obstet Gynecol Reprod Biol 2000; 92: 171.

43. Gilbert W, Moore T, Resnick R et al Angiographic embolization in the management of hemorrhagic complications of pregnancy. Am J Obstet Gynecol 1992; 166: 493.

44. Heffner LJ, Mennuti MT, Rudoff JC et al. Primary management of postpartum vulvovaginal hematomas by angiographic embolization. Am J Perinatol 1985; 2: 204.

45. Chu YJ, Cheng YF, Shen CC et al. Failure of uterine artery embolization: placenta accreta with profuse postpartum hemorrhage. Acta Obstet Gynecol Scand 2004; 83: 688.

46. Hare WSC, Holland CJ. Paresis following internal iliac artery embolization. Radiology 1983; 146: 47.

47. Ito M, Matsui K, Mabe K et al. Transcatheter embolization of pelvic arteries as the safest method for postpartum hemorrhage. Int J Obstet Gynecol 1986; 24: 373.

48. Harris LJ. A new instrument for control of hemorrhage by aortic compression: a preliminary report. Can Med Assoc J 1964; 91: 128.

49. Cutler BS, Daggett WM. Application of the 'G suit' to the control of hemorrhage in massive trauma. Ann Surg 1971; 173: 511.

50. Pearse CS, Magrina JF, Finley BE. Use of MAST suit in obstetrics and gynecology. Obstet Gynecol Surv 1984; 39: 416.

51. Hall M, Marshall JR. The gravity suit: a major advance in management of gynecologic blood loss. Obstet Gynecol 1979; 53: 247.

52. McBride G. One caution in pneumatic antishock garment use. JAMA 1982; 247: 1112.

53. O'Leary JA. Stop obstetric hemorrhage with uterine artery ligation. Contemp Obstet Gynecol 1986; 28: 13.

54. Burchell RC. Physiology of internal iliac artery ligation. J Obstet Gynaecol Br Commonw 1968; 75: 642.

55. Mengert WF, Burchell RC, Blumstein RW et al. Pregnancy after bilateral ligation of the internal iliac and ovarian arteries. Obstet Gynecol 1969; 34: 664.

56. Dubay ML, Holshauser CA, Burchell RC. Internal iliac artery ligation for postpartum hemorrhage: recanalization of vessels. Am J Obstet Gynecol 1980; 136: 689.

57. Evans S, McShane P. The efficacy of internal iliac artery ligation in obstetric hemorrhage. Surg Gynecol Obstet 1985; 160: 250.

58. Waters EG. Surgical management of postpartum hemorrhage with particular reference to ligation of uterine arteries. Am J Obstet Gynecol 1952; 64: 1143.

59. O'Leary JL, O'Leary JA. Uterine artery ligation for control of post cesarean section hemorrhage. Obstet Gynecol 1974; 43: 849.

60. Howard V. Iatrogenic arteriovenous sinus of a uterine artery and vein. Obstet Gynecol 1968; 31: 255.

61. O'Leary JL. Pregnancy following uterine artery ligation. Obstet Gynecol 1980; 55: 112.

62. Cruikshank SH, Stoelk EM. Surgical control of pelvic hemorrhage: ovarian artery ligation. Am J Obstet Gynecol 1983; 147: 724.

63. B-Lynch C. The B-Lynch suture for control of massive postpartum hemorrhage. Contemp Ob Gyn 1998; 43: 93.

64. Joshi VM, Shrivistava M. Partial ischemic necrosis of the uterus following a uterine brace compression suture. Br J Obstet Gynaecol 2004; 111: 279.

65. Shevell T, Malone FD. Management of obstetric hemorrhage. Semin Perinatol 2003; 27: 86.

66. Aziz N, Lenzi TA, Jaffrey RB Jr et al. Postpartum uterine arteriovenous fistula. Obstet Gynecol 2004; 103: 1076.

67. Khan A, Muradeli D. Imaging acute obstetric and gynecologic abnormalities. Semin Roentgenol 2001; 36: 165.

23 Forceps delivery

Joseph J Rovinsky and Anthony Caggiano

Obstetric forceps, for almost 400 years the hallmark of the obstetrician, probably have saved more maternal and fetal lives than any other surgical instrument extant. Yet, progress in other areas of obstetric management may have relegated these instruments to obsolescence. Delivery by obstetric forceps exacts a price from both mother and infant. Modern obstetric management, offering other alternatives,[1] calls into serious question whether the benefits justify the risk of such an instrumental delivery.[2] In this climate, teaching the use of obstetric forceps becomes increasingly difficult.[3,4] This can only accelerate the end of this era in obstetrics. The profession may be in the twilight zone of the age of forceps delivery.

History of obstetric forceps

The fascinating history of the development of obstetric forceps has been reviewed in great detail.[5–7] The following précis is based upon these sources.

The need for intervention in difficult and prolonged labors, often to save the life of the parturient, was recognized in antiquity. Ancient writings contain a number of passages dealing with the problems of obstructed labor. Instruments described primarily were intended for the extraction of fetuses already dead or for whom all hope of successful delivery had been abandoned. The Japanese employed fillets of whale bone placed over the fetal head. Sanskrit manuscripts antedating by far the Christian era referred to a knife and hook for perforation and extraction of the fetus. This concept of embryotomy persisted for centuries, and was described by Hippocrates in 400 BC Celsus (AD 25) reported a method of extraction by use of a hook if version failed. Specimens of such hooks, some with cutting edges, were found in the ruins of Pompeii. In the early second century AD, Soranus, a contemporary of Galen, described no fewer than seven instruments for use in embryotomy, including sharp instruments for opening the fetal head, forceps for breaking bones, and forceps for extracting fragments of bones from the uterus.

Hints that the delivery of a living child was possible appeared only infrequently. There is a suggestion in a marble bas-relief, dating from the second or third century AD and discovered in the early twentieth century near Rome, of the use of forceps in the delivery of a living infant. Avicenna (AD 980–1037), an Arab physician surnamed 'The Prince of Physicians', discussed the possibility of an instrument that would deliver a living infant. He wrote that if manual traction was not successful, it would be followed by the use of the fillet – a thin, narrow strip of dry leather applied around the circumference of the fetal head which, when moistened, shrunk and permitted traction without slipping off. He continued that if the use of the fillet was unsuccessful, 'let the forceps be applied, and let it be delivered by them'. He added that if the use of forceps was unsuccessful, the infant must be extracted by incision, 'as in the case of a dead fetus'. His contemporary, Albucasis (AD 936–1013), the most prolific Arab writer on surgery, described several obstetric instruments, including a prehensile instrument equipped with teeth; none of these could conceivably be used on a living child. The idea of an instrument that would successfully deliver a living fetus continued to occupy the attention of physicians dealing with obstetric complications. Rueff (AD 1554) described a pair of forceps without teeth. Pare (1549) presented a complicated instrument for extracting the fetus; this had three or four curved hooks which could be forcibly brought together by means of a screw, grasping the fetal head and permitting traction to be made upon it. However, Mauriceau, in his compendium of obstetric lore published as late as 1694, did not present any instrument for use upon a living child.

The weight of the evidence points to the invention of the short, straight obstetric forceps which introduced the modern forceps era by some member of the Chamberlen family, probably Peter the elder (1560–1631). Chamberlen's forceps, several models of which were discovered in 1813 and now rest in the museum of the Royal College of Medicine in London, was a simple but effective instrument. The forceps consisted of two branches, each about 12 inches long, having a fenestrated blade and a cephalic curve. The major innovation of these forceps was that the branches were separable and could be inserted singly; once applied to the fetal vertex, the branches were rejoined near the handles with a leather thong or a rivet. The forceps then functioned as a first-class lever, and extraction of the fetus without damage was possible.

The history and genealogy of the Chamberlen family, whose members practiced midwifery in England for three generations, constitute a fascinating example of professional life and ethics in the seventeenth century. The forceps were kept as a family secret for over 100 years. Hugh Chamberlen the elder did attempt to sell the family secret to Mauriceau in France in 1670; Mauriceau's interest waned when Chamberlen's forceps failed his critical test – the vaginal delivery of a rachitic dwarf after 3 hours of struggle; the poor woman died 24 hours later of a ruptured uterus. Nevertheless, the 'secret' of Chamberlen's forceps was difficult to conceal over such a long interval, and similar instruments began to appear on the Continent. Around 1730, Hugh Chamberlen sold his family secret to Roonhuysen, a Dutch obstetrician; unfortunately, Roonhuysen purchased only a single branch of the forceps! The first publication of the 'secret' in the medical literature was by Rathlaw of Holland in 1732. By the mid-eighteenth century, the form and use of the obstetric forceps had become public knowledge in England and on the Continent, and modifications of the original had begun to appear, the first of over 800 varieties of forceps that were described during the next 200 years.

In retrospect, the principles of forceps design seem simple. Most of the modifications in design or material introduced were elaborate but nonfunctional innovations. For example, in an effort to decrease the pressure of the forceps on the fetal head, Smellie (1754) recommended covering the forceps blades with leather (Figure 23.1); this suggestion was attacked almost immediately (fortunately) as 'conveying humors which are infectious . . . from one patient to another'. The concept reappeared in the twentieth century with the introduction of foam rubber and sterilizable 'booties' that could be placed on the forceps blades.

A small number of significant design advances can be singled out. In 1734, Dusée described a movable, interlocking mechanism for joining the two branches of the forceps. Levret (1744) and Pugh (1954) independently designed forceps with a pelvic curve, which facilitated traction when the fetal head was arrested at a high station in the pelvis (Figure 23.2). This solved some of the mechanical problems of the 'straight' forceps, but did not eliminate all of the difficulties associated with high and midforceps operations. It remained for Tarnier (1877) to develop a type of forceps traction in which the line of pull coincided with the pelvic axis (Figure 23.3). This 'axis traction' was the first substantive modification in over 100 years, and its principles still are employed today not only in technique but also in axis traction handles[8,9] and in the addition of a pelvic curvature.[10] A return to a modified straight forceps,[11,12] specifically designed for application to an asynclitic head and permitting a new application technique to a vertex in transverse arrest, became possible with the development of improved anesthetic techniques (Figure 23.4). An instrument designed specifically for application and traction in the anteroposterior diameter of the maternal pelvis was Barton's elegant solution to a problem over 300 years old.[13,14] Solid forceps blades were introduced in an attempt to reduce maternal vaginal trauma in forceps rotation, and the resultant problem of slippage on the fetal vertex was addressed by a semifenestrated modification.[15] There has been some interest in forceps designed solely for rotation of the fetal

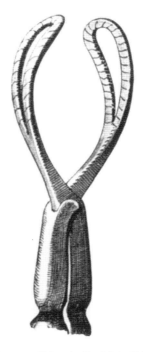

Figure 23.1 Smellie's forceps utilizing the 'English lock'. (Reproduced from Burger K. Operative Obstetrics. Franklin: Budapest, 1927.)

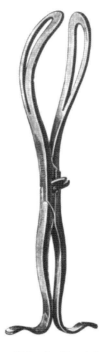

Figure 23.2 Levret's forceps utilizing the 'French lock'. (Reproduced from Burger K. Operative Obstetrics. Franklin: Budapest, 1927.)

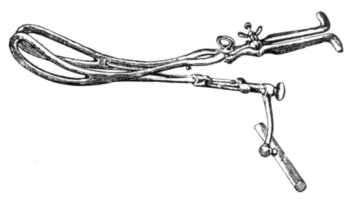

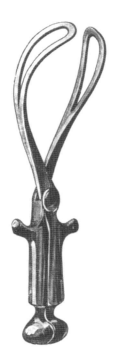

Figure 23.3 Tarnier's axis traction forceps. (Reproduced from Burger K. Operative Obstetrics. Franklin: Budapest, 1927.)

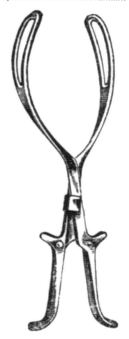

Figure 23.5 Naegele's forceps with 'German lock'. (Reproduced from Burger K. Operative Obstetrics. Franklin: Budapest, 1927.)

Figure 23.4 Kielland's forceps with 'sliding lock'. (Reproduced from Burger K. Operative Obstetrics. Franklin: Budapest, 1927.)

vertex.[16] More recently, the use of parallel or divergent (rather than crossed) forceps was recommended to minimize fetal head compression, an inevitable concomitant of traction.[17,18]

Types of forceps

Obstetric forceps consist of two branches or blades that are labeled right or left, according to the side of the maternal pelvis in which they lie after application. The rule of forceps is as follows: left blade, left hand, to left side of pelvis; right blade, right hand, to right side of pelvis.

Forceps may be characterized by the relationship of their blades. Converging forceps are not in use today. The vast majority of obstetric forceps are of the crossed type. Forceps with overlapping shanks and slightly smaller blades are typified by Elliott's forceps. Forceps with separated parallel shanks and

slightly longer blades are designed after Naegele's and Simpson's forceps (Figure 23.5). Regardless of their design, all forceps have the same parts: the blade, which fits the fetal head and the maternal pelvis; the shank, which is the portion between blade and handle; and the handle, with which the instrument is manipulated. The blade has two curves: the cephalic curve permits the instrument to fit the fetal head accurately when applied to its lateral aspects; the pelvic curve adapts the instrument to the curved axis of the pelvis. Specialized forceps such as Kielland's have no pelvic curve. In all forceps except Barton's, the cephalic curve and pelvic curve are at right angles to each other; in Barton's forceps, the pelvic curve and cephalic curve are parallel. The blades themselves may be solid, fenestrated, or semifenestrated. The shanks may be short (as for outlet forceps) or long (for manipulation higher in the pelvis), parallel, or overlapping, and straight or with a perineal curve to facilitate axis traction.

After application, in the X-type of forceps, the two blades cross and articulate with each other, the articulation being known as the 'lock'. In the English lock (Figure 23.1), the articulation is composed of shoulders and flanges; in the French lock (Figure 23.2), of a notch in one branch into which fits a pin or screw of the other branch; and in the German lock (Figure 23.5), the most rigid of the three, a combination of both principles. The sliding lock was introduced by Kielland (Figure 23.4). It permits accurate application to an asynclitic head.

The handles of most forceps are similar. They are hollow (to reduce weight), have transverse projections at their junction with the shanks, and may or may not have lateral indentations to enhance the grip. Kielland's forceps handles are solid, narrow, and kept apart by a metal bar. Some forceps handles have a screw mechanism to prevent inadvertent compression during traction. The divergent forceps terminate in finger grips rather than handles.

The multiple forceps available, their minor differences, and the reasons therefore have been described in great detail.[6,10,19,20] There was always a reason for each modification that was introduced. Longer blades and separated shanks were deemed better for the grasp of a severely molded fetal head, but they distended and often tore the perineum prematurely. Overlapping shanks avoided this problem, but increased the probability of fetal head compression. Fenestrated blades permitted a good grip on the fetal head, but often left significant marks on the baby; in doing a forceps rotation, the fenestrated blades offered more opportunities for vaginal lacerations. Solid blades reduced these problems, but more frequently slipped on the vertex during difficult rotations; semifenestrated blades (indented toward the fetus, smooth toward the maternal side) were an attempt to alleviate this problem. Whether or not the forceps handles should be indented (Simpson's forceps) or smooth (DeLee's forceps) seems, in retrospect, insignificant and purely a matter of personal preference. Today, most of these variations are of little clinical importance.

Traditional classification of forceps deliveries

Based upon well-considered publications which analyzed both personal experience and reports in the obstetric literature,[7,21,22] the following definitions for classification of forceps operations have been accepted:[23]

Outlet forceps

The application of forceps when the scalp is visible at the introitus without separating the labia, the skull has reached the pelvic floor, and the sagittal suture is in the anteroposterior diameter of the maternal pelvis (Figure 23.6).

Midforceps

The biparietal diameter of the vertex has passed the plane of the pelvic inlet. This is the application of forceps when the head is engaged, but the conditions for outlet forceps have not been met. In the context of this term, any forceps delivery requiring artificial rotation, regardless of the station is designated as a midforceps delivery. The term 'low midforceps' is disapproved (Figure 23.7).

High forceps

The application of forceps prior to the full engagement of the head is termed a 'high-forceps' application. A high-forceps delivery is never justifiable (Figures 23.8 and 23.9).

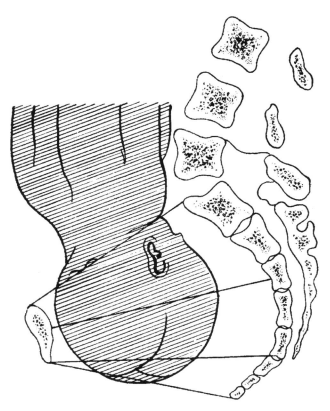

Figure 23.6 The head is deeply engaged. The sagittal suture has rotated into the anteroposterior diameter with the small fontanel directed toward the symphysis. Outlet forceps procedure can be performed at this point. (Reproduced from Burger K. Operative Obstetrics. Franklin: Budapest, 1927.)

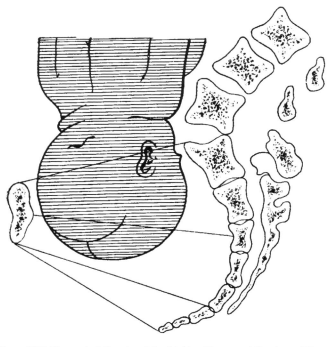

Figure 23.7 The greatest diameter of the fetal head has passed the plane of the pelvic inlet. By definition, a forceps procedure utilized at this point is 'midcavity forceps'. (Reproduced from Burger K. Operative Obstetrics. Franklin: Budapest, 1927.)

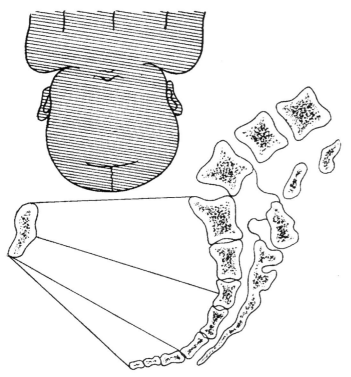

Figure 23.8 The head is high above the pelvic inlet (about − 5 station). Attempt at forceps delivery would require high-forceps procedure, which is absolutely contraindicated. (Reproduced from Burger K. Operative Obstetrics. Franklin: Budapest, 1927.)

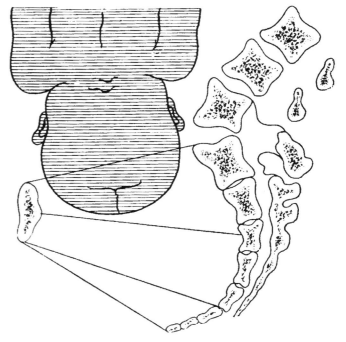

Figure 23.9 The greatest diameter of the fetal head is just entering the pelvis; according to British terminology, it is 'engaging'. The use of the forceps is still contraindicated at this point, and it would be, by definition, a 'high-forceps' procedure.

New classification

Despite the fact that issues of both maternal and fetal safety had by no means been resolved definitively;[24–32] and that a marked difference in outcome for both patients is reported between forceps used only for traction to effect delivery or for rotation of more than 45° plus traction,[33–35] in 1989, the Committee on Obstetrics: Maternal and Fetal Medicine of the American College of Obstetricians and Gynecologists[36] revised the definitions of forceps deliveries:

(1) *Station*: the relationship of the estimated distance, in centimeters, between the leading bony portion of the fetal head and the level of the maternal ischial spines. In classifying midforceps procedures, the level of engagement of the fetal head must be stated as precisely as possible. Engagement of the vertex occurs when the biparietal diameter has passed through the pelvic inlet, and is clinically diagnosed when the leading bony portion of the fetal head is at or below the level of the ischial spines (station 0 or more).

(2) *Outlet forceps*: the application of forceps when (a) the scalp is visible at the introitus without separating the labia, (b) the fetal skull has reached the pelvic floor, (c) the sagittal suture is in the anteroposterior diameter or in the right or left occiput anterior or posterior position, and (d) the fetal head is at or on the perineum. According to this definition, rotation cannot exceed 45°. There is no documented difference in perinatal outcome when deliveries involving the use of outlet forceps are compared with similar spontaneous deliveries, and there are no data to support the concept that rotating the head on the pelvic floor 45° or less increases morbidity. Forceps delivery under these conditions may be desirable to shorten the second stage of labor.

(3) *Low forceps*: The application of forceps when the leading point of the skull is at station +2 or more. Low forceps has two subdivisions: (1) rotation 45° or less (e.g., left occipitoanterior to occiput anterior, left occipitoposterior to occiput posterior), and (2) rotation of more than 45°.

(4) *Midforceps*: The application of forceps when the head is engaged but the leading point of the skull is above station +2. Under very unusual circumstances, such as the sudden onset of severe fetal or maternal compromise, application of forceps above station +2 may be attempted while simultaneously initiating preparations for a cesarean delivery in the event that the forceps maneuver is unsuccessful. Under no circumstances, however, should forceps be applied to an unengaged presenting part or when the cervix is not completely dilated.

This change in nomenclature in no way modifies the risks inherent in these procedures. On the one hand, the relatively lower risk of forceps used for traction (with rotation limited to 45° from the vertical axis), now called 'low forceps', is recognized and distinguished from 'true' midforceps operations.

(Note that this distinction was not permitted in the older definition, when the term 'low midforceps' was disapproved.) On the other hand, probably undue approval is given to rotational forceps maneuvers by including them as a subcategory of 'low forceps'.

Indications of forceps deliveries

Indications for the application of obstetric forceps may be fetal or maternal. Fetal indications primarily are related to fetal compromise – bradycardia, falling fetal scalp blood pH, or evidence of abruptio placentae. Maternal indications are more numerous, most frequently based upon failure to progress in labor because of secondary uterine inertia, failure of internal rotation, or maternal disease requiring shortening of the second stage of labor (e.g., cardiac disease). Other uses of forceps are of historical interest only.[37]

Conditions for the use of obstetric forceps

It is the responsibility of the obstetrician who contemplates the use of forceps to ensure that the conditions for the safe use of these instruments have been fulfilled. These conditions are as follows:

(1) The maternal pelvis must be adequate, with no evidence of cephalopelvic disproportion.
(2) The fetal vertex must be engaged.
(3) The cervix must be completely dilated and retracted.
(4) The fetal position and station must be known.
(5) There must be no bony or soft tissue obstruction (such as tumor previa).
(6) The membranes must be ruptured.
(7) The bladder and rectum must be empty.
(8) Adequate and appropriate anesthesia must be available.

Of equal if not greater importance are the following *contraindications* for the application of forceps:

(1) hydrocephalic infant
(2) fetal position uncertain or unknown
(3) mentum posterior face presentation
(4) brow presentation
(5) fetal vertex not engaged.
(6) incomplete cervical dilation
(7) contracted maternal pelvis (or gross fetal macrosomia)
(8) *lack of experience of the operator!*

Forceps procedures

Outlet forceps

To avoid the omission of essential steps, the obstetrician should carry out forceps operations in accord with a specific and unvarying routine. In time, this routine becomes automatic. This routine will be detailed here and not repeated subsequently.

The indications and conditions should be reviewed to be certain that the forceps operation is appropriate. The patient should be placed on the delivery table in lithotomy position, with her buttocks a little past the lower end of the table. She should be anesthetized, cleansed, and draped in routine fashion for an aseptic delivery. The position and station of the fetal vertex should be rechecked by vaginal examination. In an outlet forceps procedure, the presentation will be cephalic; the sagittal suture will be in the anteroposterior diameter of the maternal pelvis, or no further than 45° in either direction. The occiput and posterior fontanel should be under the symphysis pubis. The head should be visible at the introitus without separating the vulva, and the presenting part should be at station +4 (e.g., 4 cm below the plane of the maternal ischial spines).

The locked forceps should be held outside the vagina, in front of the perineum, in the same position that they will occupy once applied to the fetal vertex (Figure 23.10); in the occipitoanterior position, both a perfect cephalic and an ideal pelvic application are possible. The forceps blades will be applied to the fetal vertex over the parietal bones bilaterally in an occipitomental application, with the concave edges of the blades toward the occiput. The left blade will be next to the left sidewall of the pelvis, and the right blade near the right side wall, with the concave edges pointing toward the pubis. The diameter of the forceps will be perpendicular to the sagittal suture, and in (or almost in) the transverse diameter of the pelvis (Figure 23.11).

The left forceps is inserted first. The handle is held in the left hand, near the mother's right groin. The fingers of the right hand are placed in the vagina between the fetal head and the left vaginal wall (Figure 23.12). The left blade is then inserted gently into the space between the fingers and the fetal head at about the 5 o'clock position. The handle is lowered slowly to the horizontal and toward the midline, while the blade is moved up by the vaginal fingers over the left side of the fetal vertex toward an occipitomental application. When the vaginal fingers are removed, the forceps blade lies between the left parietal bone and the left pelvic wall. The forceps should be released by the operator and held in place by an assistant (Figure 23.13).

The right forceps blade is grasped in the right hand and held with the handle near the mother's left groin. The fingers of the left hand are inserted in the right side of the vagina between the fetal head and the vaginal wall. The right blade is inserted over the left blade, between the fingers and the fetal vertex, at about the 7 o'clock position (Figure 23.14). The handle is lowered to the horizontal and toward the midline, while the blade

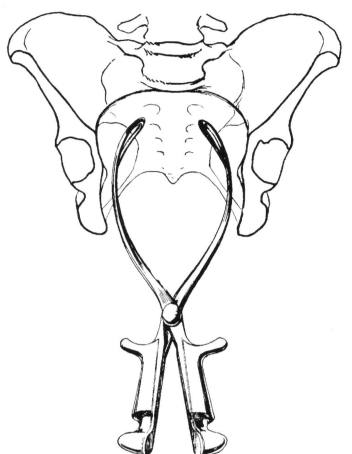

Figure 23.10 Contemplated application of the forceps in the transverse diameter of the pelvis. (Adapted from the original work of Ernst Bumm.)

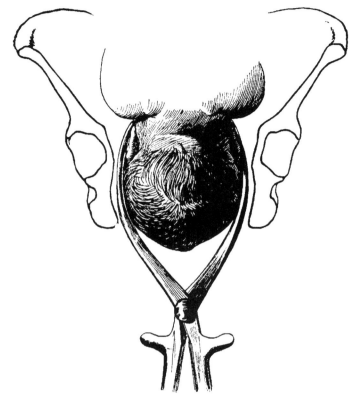

Figure 23.11 Actual application of the forceps in the transverse diameter of the pelvis. (Adapted from the original work of Ernst Bumm.)

is moved up by the vaginal fingers to an occipitomental position. When the vaginal fingers are removed, the forceps blade lies between the right parietal bone and the right pelvic wall (Figure 23.15). The forceps blades now are locked (Figure 23.16); if applied correctly, locking is easy; the handles must never be forced together (Figure 23.17).

As a routine, the fetal heart rate should be checked. The patient should be re-examined vaginally to be certain that nothing lies between the forceps and the fetal head, including umbilical cord, cervix, or fetal membranes. The application of the forceps must be rechecked. If the blades are a little off center, with one blade nearer the occiput and the other closer to the fetal face, the forceps must be unlocked and the blades repositioned. Now a gentle pull on the forceps should result in a slight advance of the vertex (Figure 23.18).

A complete reassessment must ensue if any of the following occur:

(1) Locking is difficult or impossible.
(2) Trial traction fails to advance the head.
(3) Vaginal examination reveals as incorrect application.

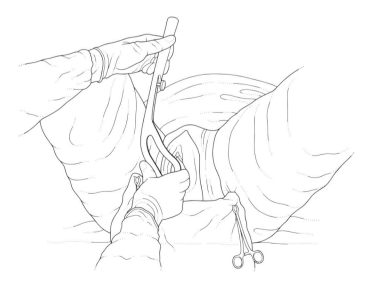

Figure 23.12 Introduction of the left blade in the course of application of the forceps. (Reproduced from Burger K. Operative Obstetrics. Franklin Co: Budapest, 1927.)

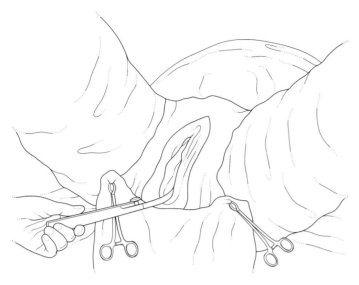

Figure 23.13 The left blade is in position and is held by an assistant. (Reproduced from Burger K. Operative Obstetrics. Franklin Co: Budapest, 1927.)

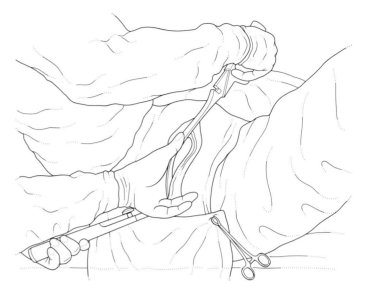

Figure 23.14 Introduction of the right blade. (Reproduced from Burger K. Operative Obstetrics. Franklin Co: Budapest, 1927.)

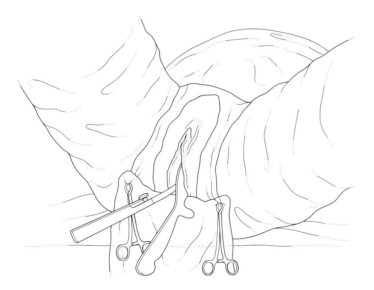
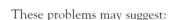

Figure 23.15 The position of the right blade following introduction and before the locking of the forceps. (Reproduced from Burger K. Operative Obstetrics. Franklin Co: Budapest, 1927.)

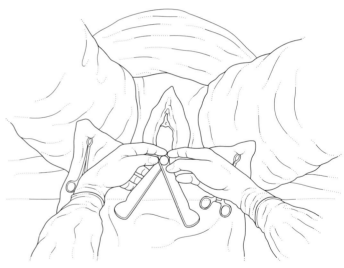

Figure 23.16 Locking the forceps after the two planes have been brought into the same plane. (Reproduced from Burger K. Operative Obstetrics. Franklin Co: Budapest, 1927.)

These problems may suggest:

(1) wrong diagnosis of position
(2) incorrect application of forceps
(3) previously unrecognized cephalopelvic disproportion (including fetal macrosomia – the point to anticipate and prevent subsequent shoulder dystocia)
(4) cervical tissue between the blades and the fetal head (and cervix incompletely dilated)
(5) uterine constriction ring.

If the foregoing criteria are satisfied, the operator may proceed to extract the head. The operator may sit on a stool and grasp the forceps with both hands, one on the handles and the other on the shanks. The ends of the handles must never be compressed. Traction is applied intermittently at about 1–2-min intervals for about 30 seconds. Between periods of traction, the forceps blades must be unlocked to relieve compression on the fetal head. The fetal heart should be auscultated after each traction. If possible, traction should be made during a uterine contraction and with the patient bearing down. The direction of traction must follow the birth canal (Figure 23.19). Initially, the pull should be out-

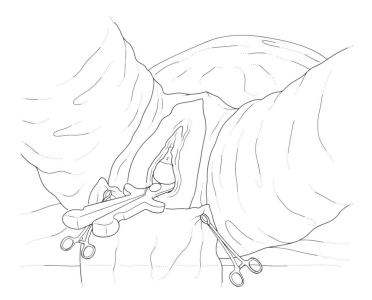

Figure 23.17 With the blades applied in the biparietal diameter, the forceps have been locked. (Reproduced from Burger K. Operative Obstetrics. Franklin Co: Budapest, 1927.)

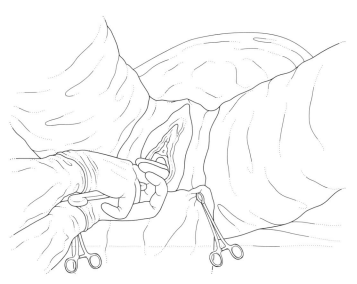

Figure 23.18 Traction is applied. Note the positions of the hands. (Reproduced from Burger K. Operative Obstetrics. Franklin Co: Budapest, 1927.)

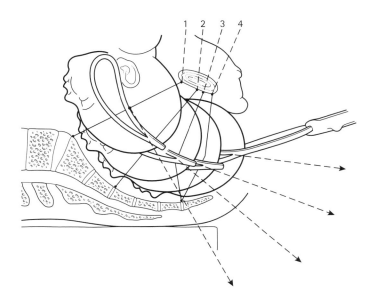

Figure 23.19 Direction of the traction in various forceps procedures. (From Dennan[73].)

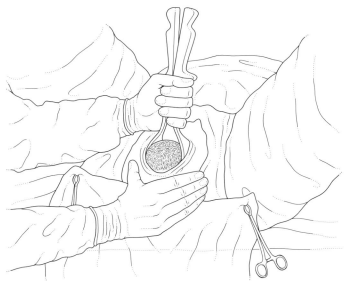

Figure 23.20 Delivery of the head with the use of forceps. In most clinical situations, this maneuver is preceded by episiotomy. (Reproduced from Burger K. Operative Obstetrics. Franklin: Budapest, 1927.)

ward and toward the rectum until the occiput comes under the symphysis and the nape of the neck pivots in the subpubic angle. In this maneuver (Saxtorph-Pajot's maneuver), the operator's hand on the forceps handles makes the traction in an outward direction while the hand on the forceps shanks exerts pressure posteriorly. After the occiput is under the symphysis, the birth of the head follows by extension and can be guided by the forceps before removal (Figure 23.20). Once the face has cleared the perineum, the forceps slip off easily. As an alternative, the forceps may be removed once the head is under the symphysis by revers-

ing the maneuvers of application, taking off the right blade first; the head then can be delivered by a modified Ritgen's maneuver; removing the forceps early reduces the circumference of the part passing through the introitus by 0.50–0.75 cm, which may be of significance occasionally. In all primigravidas and most multiparas, episiotomy is performed before forceps delivery.

At the conclusion of any forceps delivery, the vagina, cervix, and uterus must be examined to rule out the presence of lacerations; if any are detected, they must be repaired. To evaluate further the success of the forceps delivery, the operator should examine the newborn infant and record in the medical record any evidence of trauma.

Low and mid-forceps

Delivery from any position when the fetal vertex is above the pelvic floor, but particularly when rotation of the vertex is required, carries a degree of fetal and maternal risk which is a quantum jump removed from delivery by outlet forceps. A different type of analysis of the problem is required.

Assessment of pelvic dimensions and architecture

Pelvic capacity and configuration are critical determinants of obstetric management,[38] even when clinical evidence suggests weak uterine contractility (e.g., secondary uterine inertia). In the presence of relative cephalopelvic disproportion, the arrest in labor usually will occur with the head at the +2 station or higher. If there has been considerable molding, the position of the presenting part may be obscured, and the level of the leading point not helpful. In such cases, even with the leading point of the vertex at station +2, the biparietal diameter still may be above the pelvic inlet and the fetal head not engaged. The pelvic architecture may determine the position of the vertex and dictate the options for delivery. In a platypelloid (flat) pelvis, the transverse position may be the normal mechanism of delivery until the vertex is crowning. In an android pelvis, the persistent straight sacrum and converging pelvic side walls may inhibit anterior rotation of the occiput. It would be folly to attempt to rotate the vertex into pelvic diameters that are even less suitable for passage. In the anthropoid pelvis, on the other hand, rotation to an occipitoanterior position brings the fetal vertex into an alignment with pelvic dimensions best suited for vaginal delivery.[38] In all types of pelvic architecture, it is important to remember that convergence of the pelvic side walls and/or the anteroposterior diameters may result in relative cephalopelvic disproportion in the midpelvis even though the pelvic inlet was adequate; in combination with the tendency for a parturient to deliver babies of increasing weight in successive pregnancies, this results in the infamous 'multiparous trap'. These points must be clarified before the obstetrician takes instruments in hand for a forceps delivery.

Assessment of uterine and abdominal forces

Once the question of cephalopelvic disproportion has been eliminated, failure to progress in labor – to accomplish internal anterior rotation and to descend in the pelvis – results primarily from weak expulsive forces, stemming either from a secondary uterine inertia or inability of the abdominal musculature to contribute to the expulsive efforts. Failure of abdominal expulsive efforts may be the result of inborn or acquired conditions (e.g., poliomyelitis, spinal cord transection) or iatrogenic intervention (e.g., excessive maternal sedation, conduction analgesia). In such circumstances, stimulation of uterine con-

tractions by an intravenous solution of oxytocin, with all of the precautions and stipulations ordinarily followed in such cases, is preferable to forceps delivery. In most cases, this will accomplish the desired results – anterior rotation of the occiput, and descent of the vertex in the pelvis – ending either with spontaneous vaginal delivery or delivery by outlet forceps with minimal rotation.

In some patients, the resistance of the pelvic floor (the levator ani muscle) is diminished because of inborn or acquired maternal neuromuscular defects, prior overdistention as in the grand multipara, or injudicious iatrogenic intervention. In such patients, full flexion and internal anterior rotation of the occiput may be delayed until the vertex is at the pelvic floor and crowning. Pelvic floor inadequacy, in addition to pelvic architecture, may also result in rotation of the occiput into a direct posterior position. Delivery by forceps or spontaneously as a direct occiput posterior is preferable to any forceps rotation.

Delivery in occipitoanterior position

Delivery from an occipitoanterior position requires maneuvers similar to those described under outlet forceps (Figures 23.21 and 23.22). Because the vertex is higher in the pelvis, the risk to both infant and maternal tissues is increased – compression of the vertex resulting from traction and laceration of undistended maternal structures. The actual delivery will take longer; thus, the fetal heart rate must be monitored after each tractive effort. With the head above the pelvic floor, it is more difficult manually to apply traction in the direction of the pelvis axis (e.g., the curve of Carus) consistently. Saxtorph-Pajot's maneuver, described above under outlet forceps, may not suffice, and the utilization of a mechanical method of providing axis traction is helpful. Such instruments include the Bill handle,[8] which can be attached to any standard forceps possessing transverse projections at the junction of the handles with the shanks; forceps such as the DeWees, in which the axis traction handle is a structural part of the forceps themselves; or forceps such as the Hawk-Dennen, in which the shape of the instrument's shanks places the handles in the axis of the maternal pelvis.

Delivery from an occipitotransverse position

Except when the maternal pelvis has an anthropoid or android configuration, the fetal vertex engages in and descends through the maternal pelvis most frequently in an occipitotransverse position. On abdominal examination, this position is suggested by the presence of a longitudinal fetal lie, with the vertex at or in the pelvis; the fetal back is directed laterally, toward the mother's flank; the fetal small parts are palpable on the opposite side of the maternal abdomen; the cephalic prominence (forehead) is on the same side as the fetal small parts; and the fetal heartbeat is heard on the same side of the maternal abdomen as the fetal back. On vaginal examination, the sagittal suture is in the transverse diameter of the maternal pelvis (or within a few degrees thereof). The small posterior fontanel is on the same side as the fetal back – toward the mother's left in a left occiput

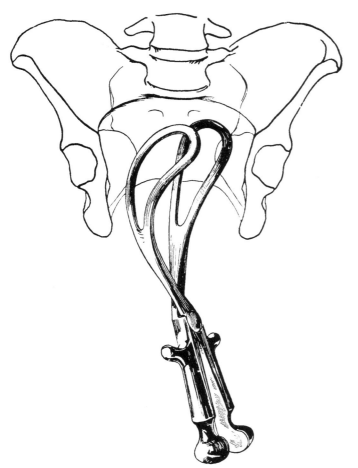

Figure 23.21 Orientation of the forceps before its application in the left oblique pelvic diameter. (Adapted from the original work of Ernst Bumm.)

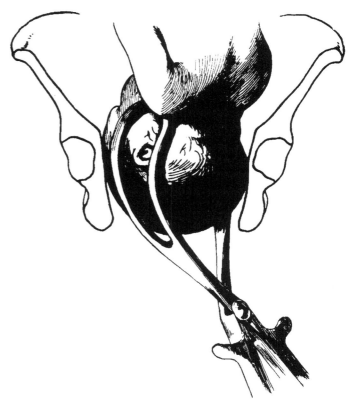

Figure 23.22 Actual application of the obstetric forceps in the left oblique diameter of the maternal pelvis. The position of the fetal head is left occipitoanterior (LOA). (Adapted from the original work of Ernst Bumm.)

transverse (LOT) position, and toward the mother's right in a right occiput transverse (ROT) position. The anterior fontanel and bregma lie on the opposite sides of the maternal pelvis. If the vertex is well flexed, the occiput is lower than the brow; if flexion is poor, the occiput and sinciput lie almost at the same level in the pelvis.

The normal evolution of an occiput transverse position is a result of the resistance of the pelvic floor to further downward descent of the vertex; there is an anterior rotation of the occiput of 90° (clockwise for ROT, counterclockwise for LOT), followed by delivery as an occiput anterior. Occasionally, no rotation occurs, and the vertex is arrested with the sagittal suture in the transverse diameter of the pelvis; infrequently, the occiput rotates posteriorly by 90° into an occiput posterior position. The diagnosis of transverse arrest can be made when there is a failure to rotate from the transverse position and to descend further in the pelvis for approximately 1 h in the primigravida and for 30 min in the multipara. At this point, the patient and the labor must be re-evaluated (see above).

In patients in whom relative cephalopelvic disproportion has been ruled out, there are no problems of pelvic architecture,

and stimulation of uterine contractions has not resulted in spontaneous evolution of the transverse position, manual maneuvers may facilitate anterior rotation of the occiput. Classically, persistent transverse arrest has been the major obstetric indication for forceps delivery.

Deep transverse arrest can be managed by any conventional type of forceps. Since rotation must be accomplished, instruments with long, overlapping shanks are preferable; forceps with separated and parallel shanks may unduly stretch or tear the maternal perineal and vaginal tissues. An instrument with a sliding lock is useful if any degree of asynclitism is present. The anterior forceps blade must be applied first to prevent elevation of the fetal vertex, which may result in encroachment of the more limited space in the anterior pelvic segment and possibly significant loss of station. A cephalic application is achieved by wandering the anterior blade over the face, and applying the posterior blade directly into the hollow of the sacrum. The handles of the forceps then are locked, and the application checked against the landmarks of the fetal skull. Rotation is performed by sweeping the handles in a wide arc of 90° to the symphysis (clockwise in the ROT position, counterclockwise in the LOT position). Rotation of the forceps handles through this wide arc is essential because of the pelvic curve of the conventional instrument. If the handles were merely twisted on their axis, the toes of the forceps blades would describe a wide and potentially injurious arc; moving the handles in a wide arc instead makes the toes of the blades the central axis of rotation (Figure 23.23). Once rotation is accomplished, the position of the fetal head must be rechecked to be certain that the sagittal suture has remained in the midline of the forceps; if necessary, the forceps application may be readjusted. Traction and extraction of the infant then are carried out as described previously.

Rotation of the fetal vertex must be achieved without the use of undue force. A well-molded vertex jammed forcefully into the deep pelvis may require slight elevation to facilitate easier rotation (Bill's maneuver), but care must be taken not to lose station significantly or to disengage the head. Resistance to rotation also may result from lack of full flexion of the vertex. Forceful rotation introduces shearing forces upon the fetal skull, whose deleterious effects are impossible to judge. It is the height of clinical acumen and experience to understand when excessive force is required for rotation and/or traction, to desist from further forced manipulation (trial forceps), and to move to delivery by cesarean section.

Special instruments have been designed to deal with special problems in transverse arrest.[11,39] The *Kielland's forceps* were designed specifically to facilitate biparietal application to the fetal vertex in any pelvic diameter and for rotation. Kielland's design eliminated the pelvic curve and provided a sliding lock for correction of asynclitism. They are the forceps of choice in cases of deep transverse arrest in the patient with a gynecoid or anthropoid pelvis. They should not be used in a patient with an android or platypelloid pelvis where further descent of the vertex in the transverse position is desirable. Kielland's forceps must never be used for traction before rotation in an occipitotransverse position! In such an instance, the anterior blade of the forceps rests directly against the base of the bladder, and vesicourethral injuries are easily produced.

The classic inversion technique of applying the anterior blade of the forceps was described originally by Kielland himself[11] and was designed to utilize the advantage in a tight pelvis of the triangular space in the lower uterine segment between the fetal shoulder and the vertex. The forceps must be oriented externally in the final position they will assume after application; markers on the forceps handles point toward the occiput. The anterior branch then is inverted and, with manual guidance, the blade is inserted along the anterior parietal bone inside the cervix and uterus, the cephalic side of the blade superior. (Since the blade is inverted, at this step the directional marker on the handle points toward the anterior fontanel.) The blade is inserted gently into the uterus until resistance is met and the forceps branch begins to turn spontaneously. Rotation of 180° toward the face, taking advantage of the curve of the blade, is performed by rotating the handle; the shank of the blade is in the axis of rotation. After rotation is completed, the blade drops against the anterior parietal bone in cephalic application. The posterior blade is inserted against the hollow of the sacrum, again with manual, intravaginal guidance to be certain there is no cervix between the blade and the vertex. Once a biparietal application is attained, the branches are locked; in the process, any asynclitism present is corrected. The application is checked with the landmarks of the fetal skull. Since Kielland's forceps have no significant pelvic curve, rotation can be performed in a limited arc, turning the vertex 90° to an occipitoanterior position. Once rotation is completed, Kielland's forceps have fulfilled their primary function, and the delivery may be completed by removal of the Kielland's forceps and application of a conventional instrument. Traction and extraction may be completed with Kielland's forceps if it is recognized that the forceps have no pelvic curve, and that extraction from midpelvis requires traction directed 45° or more below the horizontal plane of the pelvis.

Potential problems with this classic insertion technique include trauma to maternal tissues (especially the lower uterine segment), placental insertion site, and the umbilical cord. There must be no attempt to move the forceps during insertion against resistance. During the inverted insertion and rotation of the anterior blade, the arc traversed by the toe of the blade against the anterior lower uterine segment easily is palpable just above the symphysis of the mother. Problems such as this have resulted in the preference of some obstetricians for application of the anterior blade with the wandering technique (as with conventional forceps). Although this avoids the risks of intrauterine insertion and manipulation of the anterior blade, it sacrifices the very advantage that Kielland proposed in cases of deep transverse arrest which have occurred because of reduced transverse diameters of the pelvis.

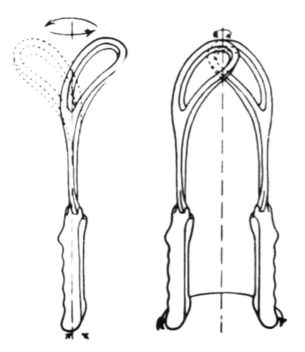

Figure 23.23 Wide arc circumscribed by handles allows for a small arc at the toes. (From Dennen[73].)

The remaining problem in the occipitotransverse position is the case of transverse arrest in a platypelloid pelvis, in which the normal evolution of labor requires descent of the vertex in the transverse position to the introitus. *Barton's forceps* are the only obstetric instrument extant that can be used to apply traction to the vertex in a transverse position (Figure 23.24). The anterior blade, which is hinged to facilitate application to the anterior parietal bone under the symphysis pubis, is introduced into the hollow of the sacrum and wandered over the occiput to a position over the anterior parietal bone. If there is marked posterior asynclitism, the anterior blade may be inserted directly over the anterior parietal bone. The posterior blade then is inserted, with manual intravaginal guidance, along the hollow of the sacrum, and the branches are locked. Traction with Barton's forceps can be applied safely only with the use of Barton's traction handle, which is an integral part of the forceps, and which ensures that the resultant forces applied will be in the direction of the pelvic axis and not against the base of the bladder. In some patients, the vertex actually may deliver in the transverse position. Usually, when the vertex is under the pubic arch and beginning to crown, spontaneous rotation toward an occiput anterior position begins and can be assisted by a 90° rotation of the forceps handles in a wide arch. At this low level in the pelvis, spontaneous delivery usually ensues as soon as the forceps blades are removed.

Delivery from an occipitoposterior position

Occipitoposterior positions occur in about 15% of vaginal deliveries. Cephalopelvic disproportion is a frequent and serious complicating factor. Persistent occipitoposterior position may occur in any pelvis with a reduced transverse diameter and may be the normal mechanism of labor and delivery in an anthropoid and android pelvis. An occipitoposterior position also may result from the presence of prominent ischial spines, reduced capacity of the forepelvis, convergence of the lateral

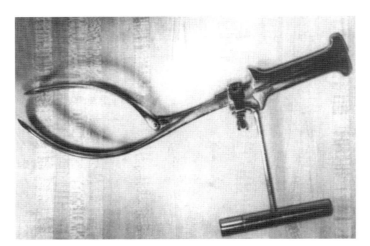

Figure 23.24 Barton's forceps with hinged anterior blade and traction handle. (From Thompson JP. Forceps. In: Iffy L, Kaminetzky HA (eds), Principles and Practice of Obstetrics and Perinatology. Wiley: New York, 1981.)

pelvic side walls, and a straight sacrum – all factors that inhibit anterior rotation. On abdominal examination, the presence of an occipitoposterior position is suggested by the presence of the fetal back in the maternal flank, often not clearly defined; fetal small parts filling the anterior maternal abdomen; a cephalic prominence which cannot be appreciated clearly; and a fetal heart that is auscultated most clearly on the side of the maternal abdomen opposite to the fetal back. On vaginal examination, the sagittal suture is in an oblique diameter of the maternal pelvis. The small fontanel is posterior, either to the right (ROP) or to the left (LOP); the anterior fontanel and bregma are in the opposite quadrants of the pelvis. Because failure of deep flexion is a concomitant of persistent occipitoposterior positions, the fontanels usually are at about the same level in the pelvis. In occipitoposterior positions, molding of the vertex results in some shortening of the occipitofrontal diameter and lengthening of the mentobregmatic diameter as the vertex becomes elongated. The diagnosis of position on vaginal examination may be obscured by molding and caput formation that mask the landmarks of the fetal skull; confirmation of position may require locating and identifying the pinna of the fetal ear.

The natural evolution of an occipitoposterior position in nine of ten cases is spontaneous internal anterior rotation of 135° to an occipitoanterior position, which occurs after the pelvic floor is reached and deep flexion established. In 10% of cases, the occiput rotates in a small arc of 45° into the hollow of the sacrum, becoming a direct occipitoposterior position. Spontaneous delivery or extraction by forceps can occur from either position.

Indications for intervention in patients with persistent occipitoposterior position[40] of the fetus include fetal distress, absence of descent, and prolonged second stage of labor. If there is evidence of cephalopelvic disproportion, cesarean section is indicated. For attempted vaginal delivery, the pelvic morphology must be known,[38] and a plan for extraction laid out in advance. When the transverse diameters of the pelvis are reduced, as in an anthropoid or android pelvis, the vertex must not be rotated into or through less favorable pelvic dimensions but should be extracted as an occipitoposterior position. Techniques of manual rotation of the vertex are useful only when the head has reached the pelvic floor and the pelvis has adequate dimensions.

A greater variety of instruments and procedures have been devised for the management of occipitoposterior positions than for any other malposition; only a few remain applicable in a modern context.[39,41–45] The simplest procedure is to deliver the vertex in a direct occipitoposterior position without any attempt at rotation. If the head is on the pelvic floor and beginning to distend the introitus, conventional forceps may be used. A biparietal application of the forceps is accomplished, with the concave edges of the blades directed toward the face. Forceps with long, tapering blades and an ovoid cephalic curve can best accommodate the accentuated molding of the skull; Simpson's or Elliott's forceps are well suited for this purpose. Traction is made posteriorly to draw the sinciput beneath the pubic arch. As the handles of the forceps are raised, the occiput is borne over the perineum by increased flexion of the vertex. A deep episiotomy is necessary to permit passage of the larger diameters of the head which present in this position. The nose, face, and chin then are borne under the symphysis by extension of the head.

Kielland's forceps have a special utility as a rotator. The directional markers on the handles must point toward the fetal occiput, so the forceps are applied in an inverted position with respect to the maternal pelvis. The blades are inserted with a wandering technique, the posterior blade always being applied first to prevent further posterior rotation of the occiput. The shanks of the blade form the axis of rotation, which is accomplished with pronation or supination of the forearm. Once an occipitoanterior position is attained, delivery may be carried out by substitution of a conventional forceps or by exerting traction with Kielland's forceps, bearing in mind that the forceps have no pelvic curve and that traction must be directed 45° or more below the horizontal plane of the pelvis.

Midforceps

Under the new definitions of forceps deliveries, midforceps are forcep operations in which the leading point of the head is above station +2. By implication, since the leading point of the unmolded vertex is 3 cm ahead of the largest plane of the head, the biparietal diameter, that diameter has barely entered the bony pelvic inlet. With any significant degree of molding, there exists the probability that the fetal vertex is not truly engaged, and that this represents a 'high forceps' maneuver, which must be proscribed. In these cases, the margin for error is very small. If any chance of a 'high-forceps' situation exists, a more prudent course of action is to proceed directly to abdominal delivery.

Forceps delivery of an aftercoming head in breech presentation
The problems, in general, of vaginal delivery of a breech presentation in a current context have been reviewed in detail elsewhere.[46–48]

Any obstetric forceps can be employed for the delivery of the aftercoming head. However, classic forceps, such as Simpson's or Elliott's, lack the advantage of a perineal curve and therefore tend to accentuate extension of the fetal body and neck, increasing the risk of fetal injury. Forceps that have a perineal curve, such as the Hawks–Dennen instrument, or that have a compensated pelvic curve, such as Kielland's forceps, can be employed for this purpose. However, since its introduction, the standard instrument for delivery of the aftercoming head has been the forceps designed by Piper.[49] This instrument is longer than the usual forceps, its handles are depressed below the arch of the shanks, the pelvic curve is reduced, and the shanks are long and curved. The tapered, shallow blades, with a springlike quality, make for an easy application and a good fit to the vertex. More recently, the modified Piper's forceps were introduced; the newer instru-

ment is somewhat shorter, and the conventional handles are replaced by a pivot lock and finger grips.[50]

Forceps can be applied to the aftercoming head only after the shoulders and arms have been delivered and the head, with chin posterior, is well in the pelvis; the forceps must never be applied to a vertex above the pelvic brim. The principles of forceps delivery of an aftercoming head are three: the forceps are inserted and applied from below upward; the application is pelvic rather than purely biparietal; and the mechanism of extraction is flexion of the fetal head, which is accomplished by elevating the handles of the forceps.

Once the shoulders have been delivered, the baby's body is supported by an assistant and elevated slightly, but not to an extent that would hyperextend the neck. Vaginal examination should reveal the vertex deep in the pelvis, with the long axis of the head in the anteroposterior diameter of the pelvis; the occiput is anterior and the face is posterior. The lower and upper limbs and the umbilical cord are kept out of the way. The left branch of Piper's forceps always is inserted first; this will permit locking of the branches without recrossing. The obstetrician assumes a position below the plane of the pelvic outlet, often kneeling on one knee. The handle of the left blade is grasped in the left hand, and the right hand is introduced between the hand and the left posterolateral wall of the vagina. The left blade is then inserted between the head and the fingers into a mento-occipital application, with the concave edge of the blade toward the occiput and the convex edge toward the face. The handle of the left blade is steadied by the assistant. The handle of the right blade is grasped in the right hand, and the left hand is introduced into the vagina between the head and the right posterolateral wall of the vagina. The right blade is inserted between the head and the fingers into a mento-occipital application. The forceps then are locked, and the application checked. Traction is outward and posterior until the nape of the neck is in the subpubic angle. The direction of force is then changed to outward and anterior, and the face and forehead are borne over the perineum by a process of flexion. Delivery usually is completed with the forceps still applied as the handles rise above the horizontal plane. Care must be exercised to prevent the head from dropping from between the blades as it is extracted.

Forceps delivery in modern obstetrics

Alternatives to forceps delivery

The utilization of obstetric forceps easily can be justified in an historic context. When obstetric forceps first were introduced, they aided delivery in cases of desultory, obstructed, or prolonged labor. They were employed primarily to salvage the mother, often with the recognition that fetal demise would result. There was no acceptable alternative to delivery.

Today, the risk of maternal mortality at cesarean section is less than the mortality rate associated with appendectomy; the operation is safer the earlier in labor it is performed; and it is incontrovertible that the safest method of delivery for the infant (eliminating iatrogenic errors of prematurity with modern diagnostic techniques) is an elective cesarean section before the onset of labor or rupture of the membranes.[47,51]

Risk of forceps delivery

Maternal risk

The maternal risks of injudicious forceps delivery were recognized from the start. Maternal injuries may include vaginal lacerations, episiotomy extensions, perineal and anal sphincter damage[2,52] bladder or urethral injuries, cervical tears, uterine rupture, and/or ureteral disruption. The primary cause of the most severe of these injuries, the high-forceps application and extraction, has been proscribed for 60 years. The major problem area remains the low-forceps operation. Attempts have been made to distinguish in advance between 'easy' and 'difficult' procedures,[19] not always successfully.

Fetal risk

The fetal risks of delivery by obstetric forceps are acceptable only in the context of greater maternal harm from any alternative. It is clear that these fetal risks, including facial bruising and lacerations, cephalhematomas, facial nerve paralysis, skull fractures, and intracranial tears and hemorrhages,[35,53–64] occur primarily in low-forceps operations with rotations and in midforceps operations.

There is a consensus that outlet forceps delivery imposes no burden on the infant.[22,23] The assumed benefits of routine, so-called prophylactic forceps originally proposed by DeLee are not pertinent in this modern era.[65] In contrast, forceps applied to the aftercoming head in breech delivery may be conducive to a reduction of perinatal mortality and morbidity,[55] probably because traction is applied to the skull rather than the shoulders or neck of the infant, and sudden decompression injury is prevented by a gradual and controlled delivery.

Current status of forceps delivery

Fifty years ago, a trend toward the elimination of delivery by midforceps was already under way.[66] Although there have been dissenters to this transformation in obstetric practice,[67,68] the trend continued and has increasingly been accepted.[4,69–71] Midforceps operations carry definite hazards for mother and infant. The risks for the mother of abdominal delivery probably are not greater and may be reducible by earlier intervention and improvements in clinical procedures. There is no comparison as to the safety of the infant at cesarean section. The process is becoming more inevitable with the disappearance of opportunities for training in forceps techniques. Maximum safety for mother and infant rests in the hands of experienced obstet-

ricians. In today's climate, the application of forceps in nonindicated cases purely as a training exercise cannot be countenanced. Even obstetricians already adequately trained in forceps delivery will lose their proficiency with the markedly reduced number of opportunities for such deliveries.

The changing parameters of obstetric management must be recognized, and should be accepted for the progress they denote.[72] The rational application of obstetric forceps today should be reserved for the operations of outlet forceps, low forceps without rotation, and, occasionally, forceps delivery of the aftercoming head. High-forceps deliveries were proscribed many decades ago. Midforceps delivery is disappearing, rightly, from obstetric practice today. Low-forceps operations involving more than 45° rotation from the vertical axis probably will follow into oblivion shortly, its disappearance hastened by our litigious contemporary society.

References

1. Brandstrup E, Lange P. Clinical experience with the vacuum extractor. Proceedings of the Third World Congress of Obstetrics and Gynecology (Vienna) 1960; 1: 80.
2. Glavind K, Bjork J. Incidence and treatment of urinary retention postpartum. Int Urogynecol J Pelvic Floor Dysfunct 2003; 14: 119–21.
3. Leslie II, Kepasquale-Lehnerz P, Smith M. Obstetric forceps training using the isometric strength testing unit. Am J Obstet Gynecol 2005; 105: 377–82.
4. Vacca A. Current obstetrics training programs are unlikely to provide registrars with sufficient skill in the safe use of Kielland forceps. Austr N Z J Obstet Gynecol 2000; 40: 226–7.
5. Das K. Obstet Forceps: Its History and Evaluation. CV Mosby: St Louis, Mor, 1929.
6. Laufe LE. Obstetric Forceps. Hoeber Medical Division, Harper & Row: New York, 1968.
7. Speert H. The obstetric forceps. Clin Obstet Gynecol 1960; 3: 761–6.
8. Bill AH. A new axis traction handle for solid blade forceps. Am J Obstet Gynecol 1925; 9: 606.
9. DeWees WB. New axis traction obstetric forceps. JAMA 1892; 19: 32.
10. Dennen EH. A new forceps with a traction curve. Am J Obstet Gynecol 1931; 22: 258.
11. Kielland C. Über die Anlegung der Zange am nicht notierten Kopf mit Beschriebund eines neuen Zangermodelles und einer neuen Anlegungsmethode. Monatsschr Geburtshilfe Gynak 1916; 43: 48.
12. Laufe LE. Divergent and crossed obstetric forceps. Comparative study of compression and traction forces. Obstet Gynecol 1971; 38: 885–7.
13. Barton LG, Caldwell WE, Studdiford WE Sr. A new obstetric forceps. Am J Obstet Gynecol 1928; 15: 16.
14. Parry-Jones E. Barton's Forceps. Williams & Wilkins: Baltimore, MD, 1972.

15. Luikart R. A modification of the Kielland, Simpson, and Tucker-McLane forceps to simplify their use and improve traction and safety. Am J Obstet Gynecol 1937; 34: 686.

16. Dyack C. Rotational forceps in midforceps delivery. Obstet Gynecol 1980; 56: 123–6.

17. Laufe LE. A new divergent outlet forceps. Am J Obstet Gynecol 1968; 101: 509–12.

18. Seidenschnur G, Koepcke E. Fetal risk in delivery with the Shute parallel forceps. Analysis of 1,503 forceps deliveries. Am J Obstet Gynecol 1979; 135: 312–17.

19. Davidson AC, Weaver JB, Davies P et al. Relation between ease of forceps delivery and speed of cervical dilatation. Br J Obstet Gynaecol 1976; 83: 279–83.

20. Quilligan EJ, Zuspan F. Douglas-Stromme's Operative Obstetrics (4th edition). Appleton-Century-Crofts: New York, 1982.

21. Dennen EH. A classification of forceps operations according to station of the head in the pelvis. Am J Obstet Gynecol 1969; 103: 470.

22. Nyirjesy L, Pierce WF. Perinatal mortality and maternal morbidity in spontaneous and forceps vaginal deliveries. Am J Obstet Gynecol 1964; 89: 568–78.

23. American College of Obstetricians and Gynecologists. Technical Bulletin. Operative vaginal delivery. No. 196, August 1994.

24. Acker D. Instrumental delivery in the 1990's: a commentary. Contemp Obstet Gynecol 1990; 35: 58.

25. Broman SH, Nelson KB. Perinatal risk factors in children with serious motor and mental handicaps. Ann Neural 1977; 2: 371.

26. Cardozo LD, Gibb DMF, Studd JW, Cooper DJ. Should we abandon Kielland's forceps? BMJ 1983; 287: 315–17.

27. Dierker LJ, Rosen MG, Thompson K et al. The midforceps: maternal and neonatal outcomes. Am J Obstet Gynecol 1985; 152: 176–83.

28. Healy DL, Quinn MA, Pepperell RJ. Rotational delivery of the fetus: Kielland's forceps and 2 other methods compared. Br J Obstet Gynaecol 1982; 89: 501.

29. O'Grady JP. Modern Instrumental Delivery. Williams & Wilkins: Baltimore, 1988.

30. O'Grady JP. A role exists for vaginal instrumental delivery. Contemp Obstet Gynecol 1990; 35: 49.

31. Richardson DA, Evans MI, Cibils LA. Mid forceps delivery; a critical review. Am J Obstet Gynecol 1983; 145: 621–32.

32. Traub Al, Morrow RJ, Ritchie JWH, Dornan KJ. A continuing use for Kielland's forceps? Br J Obstet Gynaecol 1984; 91: 894–8.

33. Nilsen ST. Boys born by forceps and vacuum extraction examined at 18 years of age. Acta Obstet Gynecol Scand 1984; 63: 549–54.

34. Chow SLS, Johnson CM, Anderson TD et al. Rotational delivery with Kielland's forceps. Med J Aust 1987; 146: 616–19.

35. Hughey MJ, McElin TW, Lussky R. Forceps operations in perspective. I. Midforceps rotation operations. J Reprod Med 1978; 20: 253–9.

36. Committee on Obstetrics. Maternal and Fetal Medicine: Obstetric Forceps. ACOG: Washington, 1988, 1989.

37. DeLee JB. The prophylactic forceps operation. Am J Obstet Gynecol 1920; 1: 34.

38. Caldwell WE, Moloy HC, Swenson PC. The use of roentgen ray in obstetrics. III. The mechanism of labor. Am J Radiol 1939; 41: 719.

39. Krivak TC, Drewes P, Horowitz GM, Kielland VS. Nonrotational forceps for the second stage of labor. J Reprod Med 2003; 44: 511–17.

40. Feldman DM, Borgida AF, Somer F et al. Rotational versus non-rotational forceps: maternal and neonatal outcomes. Am J Obstet Gynecol 1999; 181: 1185–7.

41. Bill AH. The treatment of the vertex occiput posterior position. Am J Obstet Gynecol 1931; 26: 215.

42. DeLee JB. The treatment of the occiput posterior position after engagement of the head. Surg Gynecol Obstet 1928; 46: 696.

43. King EL, Herring JS, Dyer I, King JA. The modification of the Scanzoni rotation in the management of persistent occipitoposterior positions. Am J Obstet Gynecol 1951; 61: 872–80.

44. Maughan GB. Safe and simple delivery of persistent posterior and transverse positions. Am J Obstet Gynecol 1956; 71: 741.

45. Reddoch JW. Management of occipitoposterior positions with special reference to the Scanzoni maneuver. South Med J 1934; 27: 615.

46. Milner RDG. Neonatal mortality of breech delivery with and without forceps to the aftercoming head. Br J Obstet Gynaecol 1975; 82: 783–5.

47. Rovinsky JJ. Abnormalities of position, lie, presentation, and rotation. In: Iffy L, Kaminetzky HA (eds), Principles and Practice of Obstetrics and Perinatology. Wiley: New York, 1981 p. 907.

48. Swartjes JM, Bleker OP, Schutte MF. The Zavanelli maneuver applied to locked twins. Am J Obstet Gynecol 1992; 154: 623.

49. Piper SB, Bachman C. The prevention of fetal injuries in breech delivery. JAMA 1929; 92: 217.

50. Laufe LE. An improved Piper forceps. Obstet Gynecol 1967; 29: 284–6.

51. O'Driscoll K, Foley M. Correlation of decrease in perinatal morbidity and increase in cesarean section rate. Obstet Gynecol 1983; 61: 1–5.

52. Ballard RC, Gardiner A, Duthie H et al. Anal sphincter fecal and urinary incontinence: a 34 year follow-up after forceps delivery. Dis Colon Rectum 2003; 46: 1083.

53. Chiswick ML. Forceps delivery – neonatal outcome. In: Beard RW, Paintin DB (eds), Outcome of Obstetric Intervention in Britain, pp. 33–41. Royal College of Obstetricians and Gynaecologists: London, 1980.

54. Chiswick ML, James DK. Kielland's forceps: association with neonatal mortality and morbidity BMJ 1979; 1: 7–9.

55. Cook WAR. Evaluation of the midforceps operation. Am J Obstet Gynecol 1967; 99: 327.

56. Curran JS. Birth-associated injury. Clin Perinatol 1981; 8: 111–29.

57. Egge K, Lyng G, Maltau JM. Effect of instrumental delivery on the frequency and severity of retinal hemorrhages in the newborn. Acta Obstet Gynecol Scand 1981; 60: 153–5.

58. Gei AF, Smith RA, Hankins GD. Brachial plexus paresis associated with fetal neck compression from forceps. Am J Perinat 1999; 20: 289–91.

59. Hellmann J, Vannucci RC. Intraventricular hemorrhage in premature infants. Semin Perinatol 1982; 6: 42–53.

60. Hepner WR. Some observations on facial paresis in the newborn infant: etiology and incidence. Pediatrics 1951; 8: 494–7.

61. Mann LL, Carmichael A, Duchin S. The effect of head compression on fetal heart rate, brain metabolism, and function. Obstet Gynecol 1972; 39: 721–6.

62. O'Driscoll K, Meagher D, MacDonald D, Geoghegan F. Traumatic intracranial haemorrhage in firstborn infants and delivery with obstetric forceps. Br J Obstet Gynaecol 1981; 88: 577–81.

63. Painter MJ, Bergman I. Obstetrical trauma to the neonatal central nervous system and peripheral nervous system. Semin Perinatol 1982; 6: 89–104.

64. Rubin A. Birth injuries: incidence, mechanisms, and results. Obstet Gynecol 1964; 23: 218–21.

65. Cohen WR. Influence of the duration of second stage of labor on perinatal outcome and puerperal morbidity. Obstet Gynecol 1977; 49: 266–9.

66. Taylor ES. Can midforceps operations be eliminated? Obstet Gynecol 1953; 2: 302–7.

67. Danforth DD, Ellis AH. Midforceps delivery: a vanishing art? Am J Obstet Gynecol 1963; 86: 29–37.

68. Dunlop DL. Midforceps operations at the University of Alberta Hospital, 1965–1967. Am J Obstet Gynecol 1969; 103: 471–5.

69. Bowes WA Jr, Bowes C. Current role of the midforceps operation. Clin Obstet Gynecol 1980; 23: 549.

70. Ingardia CJ, Cetrulo CL. Forceps – use and abuse. Clin Perinatol 1981; 8: 63–77.

71. Nimmo RA, Murphy GA, Adhate A et al. Factors affecting perinatal mortality in an urban center. Natl Med Assoc J 1991; 83: 147–52.

72. Park JS, Robinson JN, Norwitz ER. Rotational forceps: should these procedures be abandoned? Semin Perinat 2003; 27: 112–20.

73. Dennen EH. Forceps Deliveries (2nd edition). FA Davis: Philadelphia, 1964.

24 The vacuum extractor (Ventouse) for obstetric delivery

David N Dhanraj and Michael S Baggish

History

The use of a vacuum device to assist delivery was first attempted by James Yonge in 1706, who attached a 'cupping glass' to the fetal scalp by creating suction with an air pump.[1] Simpson, in Edinburgh[2] (1849), constructed a more practical suction instrument. His invention consisted of a pump that terminated in a metal cup over which a layer of leather was fitted. A double-valved piston pump working back and forth created the necessary vacuum. Although this 'suction tractor' was used by Simpson for both vertex and breech deliveries, it never gained much popularity, and it was later abandoned in favor of the forceps. McCahey, in Philadelphia[3] (1890), described an 'atmospheric tractor' in which metal cups were attached to an air pump by tubing. He reported success in using the device for the delivery of five infants.

Using a rubber suction cup reinforced with metal, Kuntzsch[4] delivered two infants; he was the first to introduce a pressure gauge into the system. Torpin (1938) developed a rubber-plunger type of suction cup, to which he attached a hollow rubber tube leading to a vacuum pump.[5] The inner surface of this appliance was studded with rubber projections to prevent the fetal scalp from being sucked into the tubing and to aid the attachment of the rubber hemisphere to the fetal head. Castallo[6] produced a similar working model; however, both he and Torpin used the instruments sparingly and never achieved great success with them. Couzigou (1947) described *la ventouse eutocique*, which used aluminum cups ranging in diameter from 40 to 65 mm.[7] His apparatus included a bottle between the vacuum cup and the pump to trap blood and amniotic fluid. Finderle's horn-shaped instrument with traction handles was introduced in 1955.[8] The cup was inserted into the vagina, and a terminal rubber cup was attached to the fetal head. Negative pressure of approximately 6 lbs (2.72 kg) was produced by means of a 200–300-ml syringe. Between 1953 and 1957, Malmström developed a modification of the device. This represents the current standard by which other vacuum extractors (VE) must be measured.[9,10] Shallow cups, varying in diameter, were constructed of stainless steel. The cups were flanged outward above the mouth so that the largest diameter is not at the opening proper, but, rather, higher in the interior of the cup. In Malmström's department, the VE virtually took the place of the forceps. The experiences in other Continental European, British, and Australian institutions were similar.[11–14] Bird[15] modified the Malmström system by attaching the suction tube eccentrically, at the side of the cup dome, to allow for greater maneuverability and more efficient traction by locating the traction chain at the center independently. An extensive review of the historical development of the VE may be found in Chalmers' monograph[16] and in Sjostedt's review.[13]

Although the metal cup was quite successful in effecting vaginal delivery, concerns arose regarding the occurrence of serious lacerations to the scalp. This decreased the popularity of the VE in the USA. The development of soft cups was an attempt to decrease scalp injuries. Between 1969 and 1973, two plastic cups were introduced. The Kobayashi silastic cup is flexible and wide and almost completely covers the occiput.[17] This device does not require the formation of a chignon. The silastic cup has been proved to be less injurious to the fetal scalp;[18] however, it is associated with an increased failure rate,[19] especially in the setting of asynclitism or severe molding.

Component instrumentation

All current devices are based to a large degree on Malmström's instrument. The Ventouse,[7] or VE, consists of several component parts. The cups are disk-shaped. The convex surface of the disk is fitted with a hollow stem, which in turn communicates with the concave cavity (fetal surface) (Figure 24.1). The smooth shape of the cup diminishes the risk of trauma to the fetal scalp and facilitates sealing and the formation of an artificial caput succedaneum. This chignon, or button, is maximal

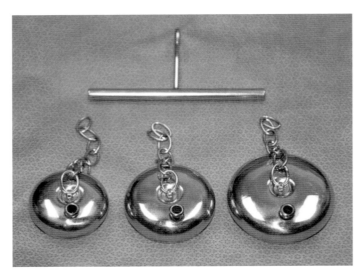

Figure 24.1 Malmström vacuum cups measure 4, 5, and 6 cm. The cups shown are made of stainless steel with the Bird modification, that is, eccentric fitting for suction tube attachment. The traction handle with hook couples directly to the cup chain.

inside the hemispheric walls above the cup edge (Figure 24.2). Rubber tubing attaches onto the stem located on the slightly convex surface of the cup (Figure 24.3). The second segment of rubber tubing extends to the inflow connection of the suction (trap) bottle. The third (final) section connects the outflow spigot of the suction bottle to the vacuum pump (Figure 24.4).

A traction chain passes directly from the cup and is hooked onto a traction bar. The vacuum tubing connects independently and eccentrically to a short stem outlet built into the cup (Figure 24.3).

A glass bottle is placed between the suction cup and the pump in order to collect blood, amniotic fluid, and other debris. The bottle is sealed with a rubber stopper. The stopper is perforated by a gauge to record negative pressure (Figure 24.4).

Current apparatuses use small hand pumps that connect disposable plastic cups and tubing with a filter that replaces the glass bottle. The Mityvac® device is an example of this (Figure 24.5). A disadvantage of this device is that the stem and cup are one piece that is not very flexible, making proper application difficult at times. The Kiwi Omnicup® is a further modification; it is a disposable 'all-in-one' instrument (Figure 24.6). The plastic cup is connected to a handle by tubing and a steel cable that runs through the tubing (Figure 24.7). This allows for flexibility and mobility of the cup similar to Bird's modification. The handle is integrated with a trigger that allows the operator to pump to a desired negative pressure. The pump on the handle contains the gauge and a pressure-release mechanism. There are several advantages of this device:

(1) It is much faster to employ since there is no assembly.
(2) It allows the obstetrician to perform the operation without assistance.
(3) It requires no maintenance since it is disposable.

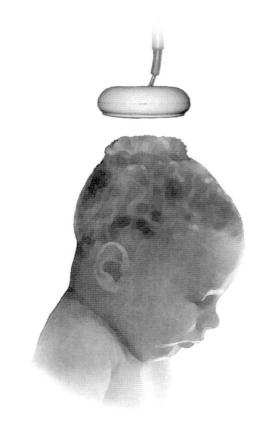

Figure 24.2 As suction is applied, a chignon, or button of scalp, is sucked into the cup. Since the edge-cup diameter is less than the interior-cup diameter, the greater volume of chignon is firmly fixed into the interior of cup.

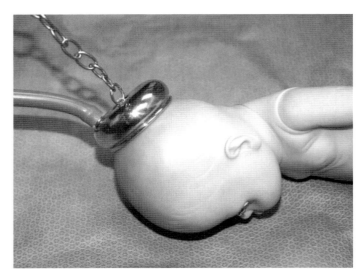

Figure 24.3 The 60-mm (6-cm) vacuum cup is attached to the head of a mannequin. The heavy-gauge tubing (left of image) is attached to a hollow stem on the convex surface of the cup. Traction is applied by the attached traction handle and transmitted to the chain and vacuum cup.

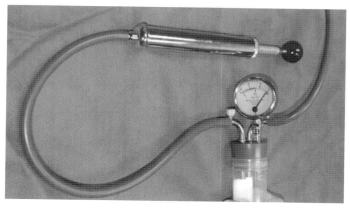

Figure 24.4 The tubing (Figure 24.3) attaches to one of three fittings on a stopper, which in turn is plugged into a collecting jar. The three metal tubular fittings are as follows: (1) inlet that couples with tubing from the vacuum cup; (2) outlet with vacuum relief valve that couples with tubing leading to the hand vacuum pump; (3) outlet to the vacuum-recording gauge.

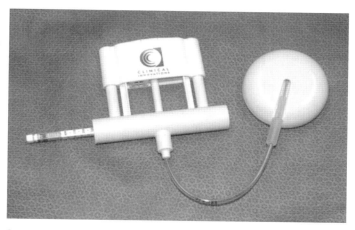

Figure 24.6 The Kiwi device has a Malmström-like cup attached to a combination handle and vacuum pump. The attachment is by flexible steel cable.

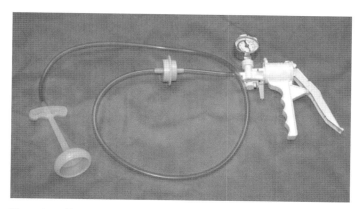

Figure 24.5 The Mityvac consists of a handle-cup, tubing, filter, and vacuum pump-gauge. Its disadvantage relates to the rather unwieldy fusion of the cup and handle as compared to the Malmström device.

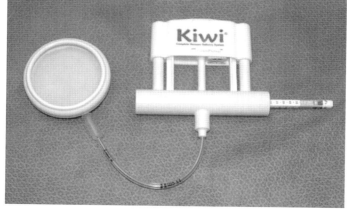

Figure 24.7 Same device as shown in Figure 24.6 with the cup reversed to show the interior. The cups, other than being constructed of plastic, are similar to Malmström cups. The vacuum pump-handle of the Kiwi assembly is very convenient and includes a vacuum relief valve.

(4) There is no chance of interpatient exposure as with reusable equipment.
(5) The design allows more precise application of the cup to the fetal scalp, since the connecter cable-tubing is completely flexible.

Vacuum use in the USA

Although forceps remain the instrument of many obstetricians, vacuum use now exceeds that of forceps in the USA. In the 1970s, forceps were the predominant instrument for operative vaginal delivery. Vacuum use exceeded forceps use by 1992. Vacuum is now utilized in about 6% whereas forceps are used in less than 3% of all deliveries. Currently, almost 50 000 vacuum extractions are performed per year.[20]

Indications

Several reports have suggested that the VE may have sufficient advantages over forceps to replace them for instrumental delivery.[13,21–25] Other authors[26,27] note that the indications for the use of the two instruments are similar. Some authors[28,29] consider both instruments independently important. The prerequisites for the use of the vacuum extractor are similar to those of forceps and are listed in Table 24.1.

Table 24.2 lists the indications for the use of the VE. A significant advantage over the obstetric forceps is that the vacuum instrument does not take up additional space in the vagina. The Ventouse allows the fetal head to 'seek its own space' rather than forcing its rotation, as is the case with the forceps. This 'autorotation' is conducive to delivery of the fetus under the

Table 24.1 Prerequisites for vacuum extraction

- Cephalic presentation
- Full cervical dilation
- Ruptured membranes
- Station 0 or lower (engaged head)
- Presence of experienced operator
- Operator certainty about position of fetal head
- Capability to perform a cesarean delivery
- Empty urinary bladder
- Adequate pelvis

Table 24.2 Indications for the use of the vacuum extractor

- Prolonged second stage of labor
- Maternal conditions where voluntary expulsive efforts are contraindicated or impossible, such as cardiac, cerebrovascular, or neuromuscular disorders
- Overly dense epidural anesthesia
- Fetal compromise

best circumstances since the fetal head accommodates itself to the pelvis where the greatest space exists for exit.

Maternal conditions that require shortening of the second stage are benefited by vacuum extraction. The instrument is particularly useful in situations where no anesthesiologist is available. Another important advantage of the VE over the forceps is that local infiltration or pudendal block anesthesia is more often adequate for delivery.

Solomons[30] reported the successful use of the VE for delivery of the fetal head at cesarean section. He cited a decreased risk of extension of the uterine incision, diminished bleeding from the wound, and reduced trauma to the fetal head as significant advantages.

Many authors consider the VE to be the instrument of choice for delivery of persistent occiput posterior and occiput transverse positions.[12,14,19,31–33] Bird considers proper positioning of the cup by the operator imperative for promoting flexion. The flexion is usually followed by anterior rotation of the occiput. Since the VE does not take up additional space within the pelvis, relatively more room is available for maneuvering the fetal head. 'Autorotation' usually occurs as traction is applied.[21,33] A fetus in occiput posterior position, in a gravida with an anthropoid pelvis (often associated with ample space posteriorly), can rotate either anteriorly or posteriorly depending upon which area has the larger capacity. Attempts to rotate the head manually with the vacuum cup as a lever invariably lead to scalp trauma and should be avoided.

Several reports[34–36] from the USA have confirmed that the VE makes delivery of the second twin exceptionally easy, and the reports suggest that it will eliminate the need for internal podalic version or breech extraction. The VE has frequently been employed for multiple deliveries.[16,29,35,36] It is advantageous

to use the VE for the second twin, according to some, even when the head is at a high level and without full cervical dilation.[37]

Contraindications

Contraindications to the use of the VE are listed in Table 24.3. They include fetopelvic disproportion, unengaged head, and malpresentations. Gestations of less than 34 weeks may be considered a contraindication to application of the VE, although the device was once used freely for such deliveries.[14,22,23] There are no data in the literature that satisfactorily establish a safe lower limit of gestational age for use of the vacuum, since no randomized trials have enrolled patients pregnant for less than 34 weeks. The use of vacuum in patients with incompletely dilated cervices has been described.[38] However, this is not recommended in current practice, as maternal deaths associated with cervical lacerations have been reported.[39]

Techniques and maneuvers

Adequacy of training

Strict limitations should be imposed upon trainees who use this apparatus. Too many poor results have been reported because of inadequate technical control.[36,40–42] Obvious mistakes, such as application to the face, forcing of delivery through an incompletely dilated cervix, lack of utilization of maternal forces, and attempts to deliver from too high a station, yield a high percentage of failure, as well as maternal and fetal trauma. Novices must be supervised. Criteria for VE applications include a completely dilated cervix, descent of the vertex to at least from 0 to +1 station, application over the posterior fontanelle, and avoidance of undue haste.

Table 24.3 Contraindications for the use of the vacuum extractor

- Operator inexperience
- Fetal prematurity (<34 weeks although some recommend no less than 36 weeks)
- Fetal scalp trauma
- Incomplete cervical dilation
- Uncertain fetal head position
- Active bleeding or suspected fetal coagulation defects
- Fetus with bone demineralization conditions
- Suspected macrosomia
- Inability to achieve proper application
- Prior failed forceps delivery
- Nonvertex presentation or other malpresentation
- Cephalopelvic disproportion
- Delivery requiring rotation or excessive traction
- Inadequate anesthesia

As sufficient experience is gained, more difficult procedures may be attempted, including use for malpositions, emergency deliveries, extraction at cesarean section, and delivery of the second twin. Understandably, the largest numbers of complications occur early in training. In the case of forceps, it would be inappropriate to do rotational procedures before acquiring expertise in outlet techniques. The same logic should apply to the VE.

Anesthesia

Because maternal cooperation is needed, the best results are obtained when uterine contractions and maternal bearing-down efforts are combined with traction. Spinal or epidural anesthesia can be used but have the potential disadvantage of blocking maternal bearing-down reflexes. Local or pudendal blocks are usually adequate, and in emergencies the vacuum has been used successfully even in unanesthetized patients.

Application

With the patient in lithotomy position, the cup is introduced into the vagina in the same fashion as one would insert a ring pessary (Figure 24.8). The cup is inserted sideways at the introitus. Simultaneously, strong pressure is exerted backward against the perineum. The cup is maneuvered to the sagittal suture and just anterior to the posterior fontanelle (Figure 24.9). The properly applied VE enhances flexion and maximizes the tendency for anterior rotation, thus presenting a smaller diameter of the fetal head for delivery. Bird[15] points out that the application of traction to a VE cup promotes complete flexion if the center of the cup is on, or directly behind, the posterior end of the mentovertical diameter. An ideal application would locate the center of the cup two finger breadths anterior to the posterior

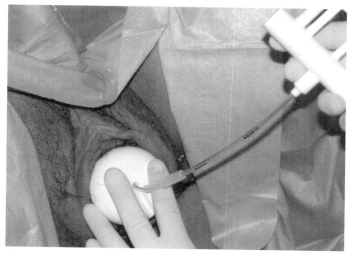

Figure 24.8 The vacuum cup is placed into the vagina and is correctly positioned. The left fingers of the obstetrician are swept along the periphery of the cup as the vacuum is created in order to ensure that no vaginal mucosa or cervical rim is sucked into the cup.

fontanelle, positioned equidistant over the sagittal suture.[11,21] This location is often referred to as the median flexion point. Good results with the VE, as with the forceps, depend upon proper application. Therefore, it is essential that the position of the occiput and the sagittal suture be determined accurately. An application away from the median flexion point leads to deflexion and/or lateral flexion, which result in a larger diameter being presented to the pelvic outlet and an increased failure rate[22,43–49] (Figure 24.10).

Once the operator ensures that no maternal tissue is covered by the cup, he or she can apply negative pressure. The recommended negative pressure is 450–600 mmHg. The immediate effect of the vacuum is the production of a large artificial caput succedaneum that fills the cup. The cup and the caput form a mechanical unit which allows traction to be applied. For the right-handed practitioner, the left hand remains in the vagina, maintaining contact with the cup. In the past, most authors advocated a stepwise increase in suction over several minutes to achieve an adequate chignon beneath the vacuum. Two randomized, controlled trials, however, have since dismissed the need for this.[50,51]

Traction

In addition to ensuring that no maternal tissues are caught in the cup, the operator's vaginal hand helps to maintain the contact of the instrument with the fetal scalp. Traction should always be intermittent and synchronous with the uterine contractions and the maternal bearing-down efforts. Unremitting traction will increase the risk of fetal injury and/or unintended detachment.[52] If traction is created with one hand, the middle and index fingers of the other exert pressure toward the concavity of the sacrum to enhance flexion. The inner hand also follows the movement of the fetal head. Coordination of activity between the right and left hands is of great importance in avoiding detachment of the cup, following the descent and rotation of the vertex, and adjusting the direction of the traction. The traction force must be applied in the direction of the pelvic axis and perpendicular to the cup.[53] Traction applied obliquely may lead to cup detachment and fetal scalp trauma.

Some have suggested that a traction force of 22.7 kg is the upper limit for fetal safety.[51] The average traction force with forceps is 16 kg in nulliparous and 12 kg in multiparous patients. In contrast, the average traction force with the vacuum is 8–15 kg.[54] Vacca showed that the maximum traction force required to facilitate delivery with the Kiwi Omnicup is 10 kg.[55]

In the past, detachment of the vacuum with traction, or 'pop-off', was considered a safety mechanism, assuming that this would occur before a dangerous force was applied. The Kiwi Omnicup is capable of generating as much as 23.2 kg traction force before detachment; therefore, pop-offs must be viewed with caution.[55] Many recommend that two to three detachments be the limit before the procedure is abandoned.[19,56–61] However, the operator should reassess whether to proceed even after the first detachment, especially if no descent occurs.

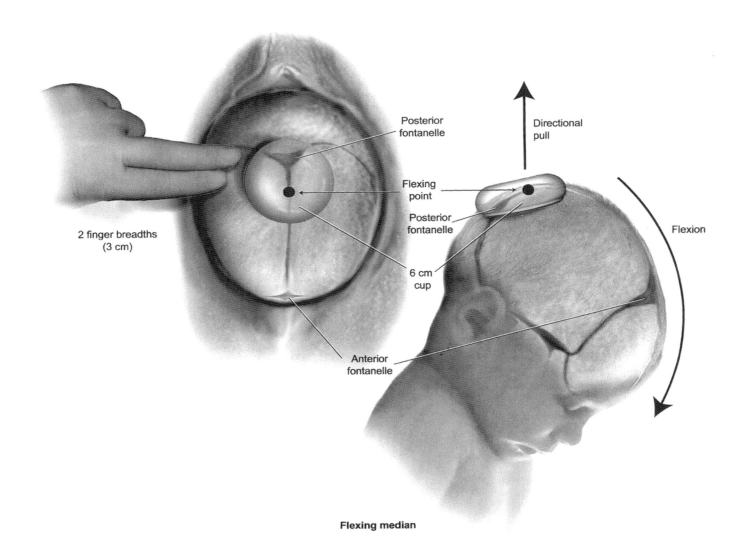

2 finger breadths
(3 cm)

Posterior
fontanelle

Directional
pull

Flexing
point

Posterior
fontanelle

Flexion

6 cm
cup

Anterior
fontanelle

Flexing median

Figure 24.9 The cup is placed in the midportion of the sagittal suture and overlaps the posterior fontanelle. The center of the cup is two finger breadths forward of the posterior fontanelle. If the cup is properly positioned, traction will automatically produce flexion of the fetal head.

It has been calculated that a pull of 10 kg perpendicular to the plane of the mouth of the cup results in a traction force of 59 kg/cm^2 at the rim of the cup.[14] The intracranial pressure produced by this force is roughly 75 kg/cm^2. The pressure created inside the skull by obstetric forceps with a similar 10-kg traction approaches 1400–1500 kg/cm^2. The explanation for the 20-fold difference lies in the coefficient of friction between skin and forceps blade. Theoretical estimates of the compression forces of the vacuum and of the forceps are 75 and 1500 gm/cm^2, respectively.[14] Mishell and Kelly[62] have found that the forceps exerted a 40% greater traction force upon the fetal skull than did the VE.

The interval between vacuum application and delivery time is of great importance if fetal complications are to be minimized. According to several series,[22,26,33] if a time limit of 30 minutes is observed, scalp damage will be minimal. If vaginal delivery cannot be accomplished by five pulls within the above time frame, abdominal delivery must be considered. In Bird's series,[11] 92% of the cases utilizing the VE had an application-delivery interval of less than 31 minutes. Although there is agreement that vacuum attempts should not exceed 30 minutes, many authorities recommend 15–20 minutes to limit further the risk of complications.[11,19,57,63]

Delivery

Delivery may occur over an intact perineum or may proceed after episiotomy and should be controlled with the VE. A valve on the suction pump immediately relieves the vacuum and allows quick detachment of the cup. All infants will retain a characteristic chignon or caput (Figures 24.11–24.13).

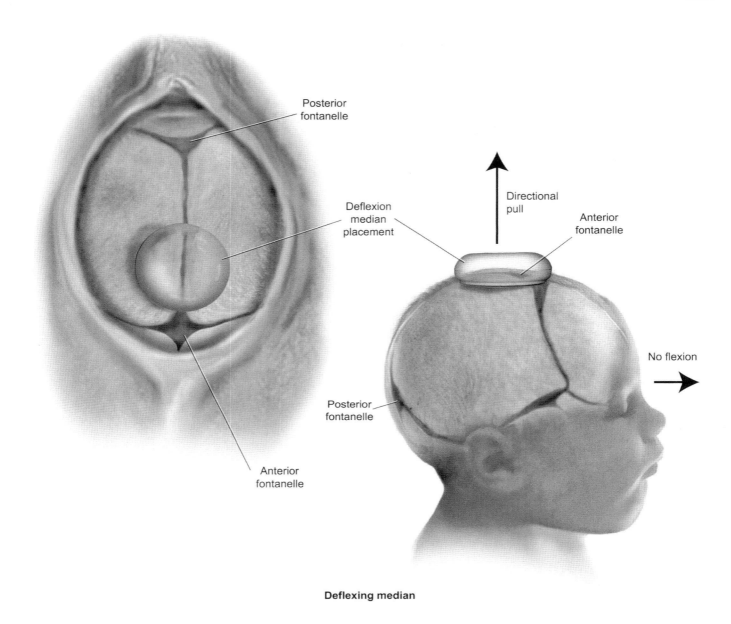

Deflexing median

Figure 24.10 A cup placed too far anteriorly either in the midsagittal suture or farther toward the anterior fontanelle will with traction result in a deflexed or extended head.

Vacuum failure

Several studies have confirmed that vacuum is associated with a higher rate of failure to effect delivery than forceps.[19,56,57,59,64] Johanson and Menon showed a vacuum failure rate of 11.6% compared to a forceps failure rate of 7.2%.[64] The soft cup is associated with an even higher incidence of failure. Although fewer scalp injuries occur with the soft cup, no other reduction in neonatal complications has been observed.[65] A meta-analysis showed a 9.5% failure rate with rigid cup and a 14.8% failure rate with soft cup.[66] The soft cup takes up more space, and its less flexible stem often prevents accurate placement, limiting its use to outlet deliveries.

Sequential use of forceps

Because of the failure rate associated with vacuum, one may be tempted to complete the delivery with forceps. Several studies show the success rate to be high. Towner et al[67] reviewed California delivery data of 583 340 births occurring between 1992 and 1994. One in three of these births were delivered by operative techniques. They found significantly more neonatal trauma associated with sequential instrument use, including a higher rate of intracranial hemorrhage, facial nerve injury, and brachial plexus injuries. Demisse et al[68] reported data from a cohort of over 350 000 deliveries and showed an increase in need for neonatal mechanical ventilation and increased

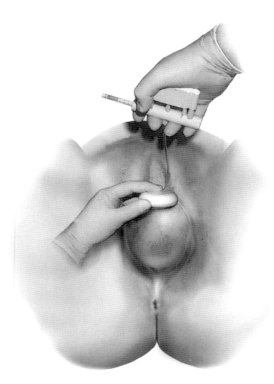

Figure 24.11 The vacuum has been applied. The operator's hand maintains contact with the vacuum cup and the infant's head especially during traction.

incidence of third- and fourth-degree perineal lacerations. Although the evidence is not entirely conclusive, most obstetricians would recommend cesarean section after failed vacuum. Proceeding to forceps is reasonable in some cases, such as technical problems with equipment, or where the fetal head is at the perineum and no macrosomia is suspected.

Special situations

The vacuum instrument has special advantages, particularly for selected obstetric circumstances, including malpresentation, delivery of the second twin, and delivery at cesarean section.

Malpresentation

In a large series of occipitoposterior and occipitotransverse positions delivered by VE, the failure rate was 4% in each group.[21] Posterior positions rotated to the anterior in 96% of the cases and persisted in the remaining ones. For occipitotransverse positions, 96% also rotated anteriorly, 2% delivered face up, and 2% persisted in the transverse. In a few cases, after VE rotation, forceps were used for delivery. The VE imposes no constraint on rotation, especially in the anthropoid pelvis. In the anthropoid pelvis, approximately one-third of the heads rotate posteriorly when traction is applied. In cases of occiput-transverse position, the VE achieves rotation with natural forces by promoting movements that forceps tend to inhibit.

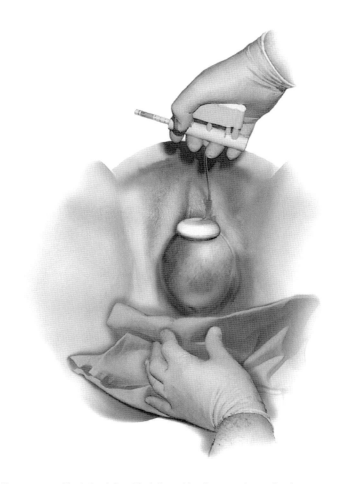

Figure 24.12 The infant's head is delivered by slow, steady traction in concert with the mother's pushing efforts. Note the towel utilized for the Ritgen maneuver.

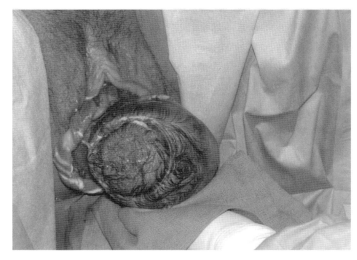

Figure 24.13 The cup has been removed. The cord has been released from around the baby's neck. Note the caput. The mother should be informed that the button is an expected result of the use of the vacuum device and will rapidly recede over 2–3 days.

While some authors do not view the vacuum favorably and prefer Barton's or Kielland's forceps for malpositions of the fetal head,[35] others contend that, if strict criteria are followed, the complication rate should approach zero when the VE is used.[25] In case of a borderline cephalopelvic disproportion, excessive traction is likely to result in detachment of the cup.

Cesarean section

The VE can be an effective adjunct to cesarean delivery. The resistance of the uterine wound is less than that of the tissues of the birth canal, and the device takes up less space than the operator's hand or the forceps blades. This minimizes the incidence of extensions of the uterine incision. None of the 20 babies delivered by Solomons[30] showed any evidence of caput 48 hours after delivery.

Twins

For the delivery of the second twin, the VE may be lifesaving, especially in cases where the cervix is not fully dilated.[35] In such instances, the VE can be used to help dilate the cervix for the delivery of the second infant. Some experts consider this method to be the procedure of choice for extracting the second twin. The VE is particularly useful in managing a delayed second twin, especially one with a high head. The use of the instrument is preferable to internal version and breech extraction.

Complications

Maternal injury

Maternal complications associated with the use of the VE are rare.[11,16,25,27,28,31,44] The use of the VE is precluded when maternal bearing-down effort is contraindicated. Injury to the vagina and cervix can result when these tissues enter the suction cup. They may be avulsed when traction is applied. Cervical injury with resultant hemorrhage may also be caused by vacuum extraction through an incompletely dilated cervix.

Incidences of third- and fourth-degree lacerations are increased with the use of vacuum versus spontaneous delivery; however, the risk is lower than that of forceps. A meta-analysis in 2000 showed a 6% decrease in anal sphincter injury when vacuum was used over forceps.[69] Thus, one anal sphincter injury is avoided for every 18 women delivered by VE instead of forceps. Demisse et al[68] showed the incidence of severe perineal laceration to be 5.8% in spontaneous delivery, 22% with forceps, 15% with vacuum, and 29% with forceps after failed vacuum.

Fetal injury

In the USA, much controversy with regard to the use of the VE relates to the extent and frequency of damage to the fetal head. In virtually every case of VE use, a prominent artificial caput is produced. The caput is greatly diminished a few hours after delivery, but persists to some extent for 5–7 days. According to Malmström,[22] ecchymoses are present on the fetal scalp 24 hours after delivery in 17% of the cases. Scalp necrosis and ulceration are more serious injuries but are rather uncommon. Instrumental vacuum misuse may cause scalp necrosis, which is sometimes followed by cerebral hemorrhage and alopecia. In one series, superficial scalp avulsions occurred in three of 91 infants without evidence of brain damage in any of them.[43] In another report of 100 infants delivered by VE, only one escaped scalp lesions.[41] An artificial caput was observed in 86 infants. In 10 neonates, the caput left a deep mark, and in three babies, avulsion of the skin was seen.

Cephalhematoma is a localized collection of blood under the periosteum. The amount of blood that can accumulate is limited by periosteal attachments at the periphery of each bone plate. Swelling does not cross the midline. It is self-limited and of little clinical importance[70] (Figure 24.14). On the other hand, subgaleal hematoma, where the blood is located between the galea and the vault of the skull, is a serious complication (Figure 24.14). This occurs when emissary veins are damaged and blood accumulates in the potential space between the galea aponeurotica (epicranial aponeurosis) and the periosteum of the skull (pericranium). Since the subaponeurotic space has neither containing membranes nor boundaries, the subgaleal hematoma may extend from the orbital ridges to the nape of the neck. This condition is dangerous because of the large potential space for blood to collect, resulting in hypovolemia, shock, and death.[71] The general signs associated with this catastrophe are pallor, muscle hypotonia, and hypotension, as well as various neurologic findings. Most recent studies estimate the incidence at 0.5–0.7%. Of all subgaleal hemorrhages diagnosed, vacuum was associated with 48.8%, spontaneous vaginal delivery (SVD) 28.4%, forceps 13.8% and caesarian section (C/S) 8.9%.[72] In a Malaysian study[73] the incidence of subgaleal hemorrhage was 41.4/1000 in vacuum-assisted vaginal delivery (VAVD) infants, with the highest incidence in neonates delivered with vacuum and weighing over 4000 g (66.3%).

Brandstrup and Lange[46] in 1961 compared autopsy findings in infants delivered by forceps and VE. Nine tentorial tears were found in the forceps group compared with none in the VE group. Among 264 VE deliveries, the perinatal mortality rate was 1.5%. Neurologic studies, including 1-year EEG follow-up, indicated that VE-assisted deliveries resulted in better outcomes than did spontaneous deliveries associated with a prolonged second stage of labor. In another study, all infants delivered by VE showed some evidence of scalp trauma. The 25.7% incidence of cephalhematoma seemed to be unrelated to the length of the suction time. However, skin abrasions and hemorrhages resulted when the suction was maintained for 20 minutes or longer. In this same series, the VE was erroneously applied to a face, resulting in an orbital hematoma and a subscleral hemorrhage.

Munsat et al[74] compared neonatal complications in 407 infants born spontaneously or delivered by VE. None of the

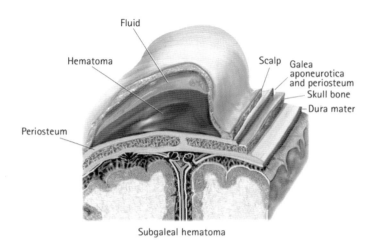

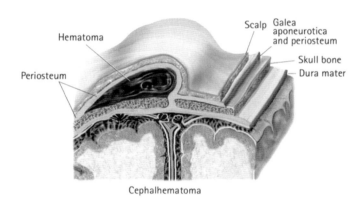

Figure 24.14 Subgaleal hematoma is a serious injury. Blood collects between the galea and the table of the skull. Large volumes of blood can accumulate, leading to hypovolemia. In contrast, cephalhematoma occurs under the tough, well-attached periosteum and is therefore self-limited.

VE cases showed persistence of ecchymoses or loss of skin integrity. There were no neurologic differences in the study groups during the first 6 weeks of life. However, fetal morbidity and mortality were increased when the VE was used prior to full cervical dilation.[31] Among 100 cases investigated by Lillie,[28] there were only two cephalhematomas. Among 7886 infants delivered in another series,[14] there were 152 fetal deaths. Of the 409 VE infants, two or three deaths could possibly be related to the use of the instrument. A recent report[29] cites a 10.6% incidence of cephalhematoma, a 1.3% incidence of perinatal mortality, and an 8.3% incidence of abrasions requiring treatment. The failure rate in this study was high at 10% (3.5% mechanical and 6.5% technical). Fetal death is usually due to brain damage or massive hematoma resulting from cephalopelvic disproportion.[25]

Fetal injuries are often due to overpersistence with the method and bad selection of cases. Investigators compared 336 newborns delivered by VE with 98 delivered by forceps and 915 born spontaneously.[75] They examined all babies on the first and fifth days of life, and 75% were re-examined again at 1 year of age. The VE children, just like the controls, sat up, crawled, exhibited no increased incidence of neurologic or psychologic disorders, and showed no difference in motor development.

In 1998, the US Food and Drug Administration issued a warning regarding vacuum extraction.[76] There were 12 neonatal deaths over 4 years associated with vacuum delivery whereas in the preceding 11 years there were only four deaths. From 1989 to 1995, vacuum use increased from 3.5% to 5.9% of deliveries, explaining some, but not all of the increased mortality. Although no clear etiology was given, the following recommendations were issued to attempt to decrease adverse outcomes:

- Use the device only when indicated.
- Ensure that the operator has been well trained in its use, indications, and contraindications.
- Understand the use of the particular device and that torque and rocking motions are potentially dangerous.
- Alert nurses and pediatricians that vacuum was used so that infants can be monitored for complications.

Long-term outcomes

Most data show good long-term outcomes in children delivered by vacuum. Blennow et al[77] studied a prospective cohort of 40 after born by VAVD and 40 infants born by SVD, and found that 42% of vacuum-delivered infants had cerebrospinal fluid (CSF) evidence of hemorrhage suggestive of intraventricular hemorrhage (IVH), as compared to 10% of those born by SVD. However, no difference in neurologic status was found at 14 months. A population-based retrospective cohort study of 50 000 subjects with over 1700 vacuum deliveries showed no difference in physical and cognitive impairment at age 17.[78]

Prospectus

Although the VE was slow in gaining acceptance in the USA, it has become the instrument of choice for many obstetricians. The hazards to the fetus, coupled with a general lack of expertise in performing complex forceps maneuvers, have furthered the case of the VE. The fact that it can be used easily without regional block anesthesia is another important advantage. With the increasing concern regarding pelvic floor dysfunction and anal sphincter disruption associated with the use of forceps, VE would appear to be the most acceptable method when obstetric intervention is required. Its ease of use, however, has led to its misuse by those who are not adequately trained and who fail to treat the instrument with the same respect given to forceps. As with any medical device, one must follow established guidelines to minimize the risk of injury to mother and infant when using VE. When utilized properly, it is an effective and important tool in the obstetrician's armamentarium.

References

1. Yonge J. Philos Trans R Soc Lond 1706–7; 25: 2387.

2. Simpson JY. On a suction-tractor, or new mechanical power, as a substitute for the forceps in tedious labours. Edinb Mon J Med Sci 1849; 32: 556.

3. McCahey P. Atmospheric tractor, a new instrument and some new theories in obstetrics. Med Surg Reporter 1890; 43: 6319.

4. Kuntzsch D. Über geburtshilfische Extraktionen mit meinem Vakuumbelm. Zentralbl Gynakol 1912; 36: 893.

5. Torpin R. Preliminary report of obstetric device. J Med Assoc Ga 1938; 27: 96.

6. Castallo MA. Extractor instead of forceps. Am J Obstet Gynecol 1955; 70: 1375.

7. Couzigou Y. La Ventouse eutocique. Bull Soc Med Paris 1947; 152: 34.

8. Finderle V. Extractor instead of forceps. Am J Obstet Gynecol 1955; 69: 1148–53.

9. Malmström T. Vacuum extractor – an obstetrical instrument. Acta Obstet Gynecol Scand 1954; 33 (suppl 4).

10. Malmström T. Vacuum extractor: indications and results. Acta Obstet Gynecol Scand 1964; 43 (suppl 1).

11. Bird GC. The use of the Malmström vacuum extractor in operative obstetrics. Aust N Z J Obstet Gynaecol 1966; 6: 242.

12. Chalmers JA. The vacuum extractor. Proc R Soc Med 1960; 53: 753.

13. Sjostedt JE. The vacuum extractor and forceps in obstetrics, a clinical study. Acta Obstet Gynecol Scand 1967; 46 (suppl 10). 1–208.

14. Snoeck J. The vacuum extractor (ventouse), an alternative to the obstetric forceps. Proc R Soc Med 1960; 53: 749.

15. Bird GC. Modification of Malmström's vacuum extractor. BMJ 1969; 3: 526.

16. Chalmers JA. The Ventouse, the Obstetric Vacuum Extractor. Year Book Publishers: Chicago, 1971.

17. Paul R, Saisch K, Pine S. The 'new' vacuum extractor. Obstet Gynecol 1973; 41: 800–2.

18. Kuit J, Eppinga H, Wallenburg H, Huikeshoven FJ. A randomized comparison of vacuum extraction delivery with a rigid and a pliable cup. Obstet Gynecol 1993; 82: 280–4.

19. Chenoy R, Johanson RB. A randomized prospective study comparing delivery with metal and silicone rubber vacuum extractor cups. Br J Obstet Gynaecol 1992; 99: 360–3.

20. Curtin SC, Park MM. Trends in the attendant place and timing of births, and in the use of obstetric interventions: United States, 1987–1997. Natl Vital Stat Rep 1999: 47: 1–12.

21. Bird GC. The importance of flexion in vacuum extractor delivery. Br J Obstet Gynaecol 1965; 83: 893.

22. Malmström T, Jansson I. Use of the vacuum extractor. Clin Obstet Gynecol 1965; 8: 893.

23. Chalmers JA, Fothergill RJ. Use of a vacuum extractor (ventouse) in obstetrics. BMJ 1960; 1: 1684–9.

24. Fothergill RJ. The safety of Malmström's vacuum extractor. Dev Med Child Neurol 1962; 4: 154.

25. Simons EG, Philpott RH. The vacuum extractor. Trop Doct 1973; 3: 34–7.

26. Barth WH, Newton M. The use of the vacuum extractor. Am J Obstet Gynecol 1965; 9: 403–6.

27. Weisberg HM, Burton GV. A study of vacuum extractor deliveries. J Can Med Assoc 1961; 85: 815–19.

28. Lillie EW. The use of the vacuum extractor in labour. Ir J Med Sci 1962; 1: 309–16.

29. Planché WC. Vacuum extraction, use in a community hospital setting. Obstet Gynecol 1978; 52: 289.

30. Solomons E. Delivery of the head with the Malmström vacuum extractor during cesarean section. Obstet Gynecol 1962; 19: 201–3.

31. Huntingford PJ. The vacuum extractor in the treatment of delay in the first stage of labour. Lancet 1961; 1: 1054–7.

32. Chalmers JA. The management of malrotation of the occiput. J Obstet Gynaecol Br Commonw 1968; 75: 889–91.

33. Ott WJ. Vacuum extraction. Obstet Gynecol Surv 1975; 30: 643–9.

34. Baggish M. Vacuum extraction. In: Iffy L, Kaminetzky HA (eds), Principles and Practice of Obstetrics & Perinatology, p. 1509. Wiley: New York, 1981.

35. Nyirjesy I, Hawks BL, Falls HC et al. A comparative clinical study of the vacuum extractor and forceps. Am J Obstet Gynecol 1963; 85: 1071.

36. Tricomi V, Hall JE. A report on the use of the Malmström vacuum extractor in obstetrics. Proceedings of the 3rd World Congress of Obstetrics and Gynecology, Vienna. 1961; 1: 95.

37. Meniru GI. An analysis of recent trends in vacuum extraction and forceps delivery in the United Kingdom. Br J Obstet Gynaecol 1996; 103: 168–70.

38. Johanson RB. Instrumental vaginal delivery. Guidelines and Audit Committee of the Royal College of Obstetricians and Gynaecologists, London, 2001.

39. Weiland A, Langer H. Hyperbilirubinamien bie Neugeborenen nach Vakuum Extraktion. Geburtshilfe Frauenheilkd 1965; 25: 320.

40. Guardino AN, O'Brien FB. Preliminary experiences with Malmström's vacuum extractor. Am J Obstet Gynecol 1962; 83: 300–6.

41. Aguero O, Alvarez H. Fetal injury due to the vacuum extractor. Obstet Gynecol 1962; 19: 212–17.

42. Spritzer TD. Use of the vacuum extractor in obstetrics. Am J Obstet Gynecol 1962; 83: 307–10.

43. Grossbard P, Cohn S. The Malmström vacuum extractor in obstetrics. Obstet Gynecol 1962; 19: 207–11.

44. Smedley GT. The vacuum extractor. Proc R Soc Med 1960; 53: 756.

45. Planché WC. Subgaleal hematoma. A complication of instrumental delivery. JAMA 1980; 244: 1597.

46. Brandstrup E, Lange P. Clinical experience with the vacuum extractor. Proceedings of the 3rd World Congress of Obstetrics and Gynecology, Vienna. 1961; 1: 80.

47. Planché WC. Fetal cranial injuries related to delivery with the Malmström vacuum extractor. Obstet Gynecol 1979; 53: 750.

48. Vacca A. The trouble with vacuum extraction. Curr Obstet Gynaecol 1999; 9: 41.

49. Miksovsky P, Watson J. Obstetric vacuum extraction: state of the art in the new millennium. Obstet Gynecol Surv 2001; 56: 736–51.

50. Bofill JA, Rust OA, Schorr SJ. A randomized trial of two vacuum extraction techniques. Obstet Gynecol 1977; 89: 758.

51. Lim FTH, Holm JP, Schuitemaker NW, et al. Stepwise compared with rapid application of vacuum in ventouse extraction procedures. Br J Obstet Gynaecol 1997; 104: 33–6.

52. Dhiraj U, Arulkumaran S. Neonatal subgaleal hemorrhage and its relationship to delivery by vacuum extraction. Obstet Gynecol Surv 2003; 58: 692.

53. Lancet M, Kessler I, Zosmer A. The vacuum extractor. In: Iffy L, Apuzzio JJ, Vintzileos AM (eds), Operative Obstetrics, p. 324 (2nd edition). McGraw-Hill: New York, 1992.

54. Moolgaoker AS, Ahamed SO, Payne PR. A comparison of different methods of instrumental deliveries based on electronic measurements of compression and traction. Obstet Gynecol 1979; 54: 299–309.

55. Vacca A. Operative vaginal delivery: clinical appraisal of a new vacuum extraction device. Aust N Z J Obstet Gynaecol 2001; 41: 156–60.

56. Bofil JA, Rust OA, Schorr SJ et al. A randomized prospective trial of the obstetric forceps versus the M-cup vacuum extractor. Am J Obstet Gynecol 1996; 175: 1325.

57. Johanson RB, Rice C, Doyle M et al. A randomized prospective study comparing the new vacuum extractor policy with forceps delivery. Br J Obstet Gynaecol 1993; 100: 524.

58. Kuit JA, Eppinga HG, Wallenburg HCS, Huikeshoven FJ. A randomized comparison of vacuum extraction delivery with a rigid and a pliable cup. Obstet Gynecol 1993; 82: 280–4.

59. Williams MC, Knuppel RA, O'Brien WF et al. A randomized comparison of assisted vaginal delivery by obstetric forceps delivery. Obstet Gynecol 1991; 78: 789–94.

60. Cohn M, Barclay C, Fraser R et al. A multicentre randomized trial comparing delivery with a silicone rubber cup and rigid metal vacuum extractor cups. Br J Obstet Gynaecol 1989; 96: 545–51.

61. Bird GC. The use of vacuum extractor. Clin Obstet Gynaecol 1982; 9: 641.

62. Mishell D, Kelly JV. The obstetrical forceps and the vacuum extractor: an assessment of their compressive forces. Obstet Gynecol 1962; 19: 204–6.

63. Gabbe SG, Niebyl JR, Simpson JL. Obstetrics: Normal and Problem Pregnancies, p. 387. Churchill Livingstone: New York, 1996.

64. Johanson RB, Menon BKV. Vacuum extraction versus forceps for assisted vaginal delivery. Cochrane Database of Syst Rev 2000; Issue 4.

65. Hofmeyr GJ, Gobetz L, Sonnendecker EWW et al. New design rigid and soft vacuum extractor cups: a preliminary comparison of traction forces. Br J Obstet Gynaecol 1990; 97: 681–5.

66. Johanson RB, Menon BKV. Soft versus rigid vacuum extractor cups for assisted vaginal delivery. Cochrane Database Syst Rev 2000; Issue 4.

67. Towner D, Castro MA, Eby-Wilkens E, Gilbert WM. Effect of mode of delivery in nulliparous women on neonatal intracranial injury. N Engl J Med 1999; 341: 1709–14.

68. Demissie K, Rhoads G, Smulian J et al. Operative vaginal delivery and neonatal and infant adverse outcomes: population based retrospective analysis. BMJ 2004; 329: 24–9.

69. Eason E, Labrecque M, Wells G et al. Preventing perineal trauma during childbirth: a systematic review. Obstet Gynecol 2000; 95: 464–71.

70. Bofill J, Rust OA, Devidas M et al. Neonatal cephalohematoma from vacuum extraction. J Reprod Med 1997; 42: 565–9.

71. Uchil D, Arulkumaran S. Neonatal subgaleal hemorrhage and its relationship to delivery by vacuum extraction. Obstet Gynecol Surv 2003; 58: 687–93.

72. Plauche WC. Subgaleal hematoma. A complication of instrumental delivery. JAMA 1980; 244: 1597–8.

73. Boo NY. Subaponeurotic haemorrhage in Malaysian neonates. Singapore Med J 1990; 31: 207–10.

74. Munsat TL, Neerhout R, Nyirjesy I. A comparative clinical study of the vacuum extractor and forceps. Am J Obstet Gynecol 1963; 85: 1083–90.

75. Zachau-Christiansen B, Villumsen A. Follow-up study of children delivered by vacuum extraction and by forceps. Acta Obstet Gynecol Scand 1964; 43 (Suppl 7): 31.

76. Center for Devices and Radiological Health. FDA Public Health Advisory: need for caution when using vacuum assisted delivery devices. 21 May 1998.

77. Blennow G, Svennignsen NW, Gustafson B et al. Neonatal and prospective follow-up study of infants delivered by vacuum extraction. Acta Obstet Gynecol Scand 1977; 56: 189–94.

78. Seidman DS, Laor A Gale R et al. Long-term effects of vacuum and forceps deliveries. Lancet 1991; 337: 1583–5.

25 Fetal malpresentations

Pierre F Lespinasse and Leslie Iffy

The labor process usually involves passage of the fetus through the birth canal in vertex presentation. In 2–3% of pregnancies, the presenting part is the breech.[1] In one out of 300, the fetus is in transverse lie or presents by the shoulder. Malpresentations are pathologic, since they make vaginal delivery difficult or impossible. They are also associated with an increased incidence of birth injuries.

Breech presentation

Breech presentation is common in early pregnancy, but its incidence decreases at term. The rate of breech presentation is still in the range of 7–10% among fetuses weighing less then 2500 g. Therefore, factors that cause preterm labor increase the incidence of breech delivery.

Breech presentations may be subdivided into three categories: frank breech, complete breech and footling breech, (Figure 25.1). The most common type is frank breech. Footling breech is seen relatively frequently in multiparas and in association with preterm labor.

The incidence of congenital malformations is about three-fold higher among fetuses in breech presentation than those in cephalic presentation.[2] Malformations frequently associated with breech presentation include anencephaly; hip dislocation; hydrocephaly; spina bifida; trisomies 13, 18, and 21; and meningomyelocele.

Breech presentation can be diagnosed with abdominal palpation or pelvic examination during the third trimester.[3] In all suspected cases, an ultrasound examination should be performed to confirm the presenting part, the attitude of the fetal head, and the type of breech. It will also help determine the location of the placenta, the estimated fetal weight and gestational age, the amount of amniotic fluid, and the presence or absence of pelvic masses that, by obstructing the birth canal, may have caused the abnormal fetal presentation.

In the days when virtually all breech presentations were managed by vaginal delivery,[4,5] the perinatal mortality rate for breech deliveries was 3–5 times higher than for vertex deliveries.[6,7] The main causes of fetal mortality and morbidity were prematurity, congenital malformations, intrapartum hypoxic insult, and birth trauma. Prolapse of the cord was, and remains

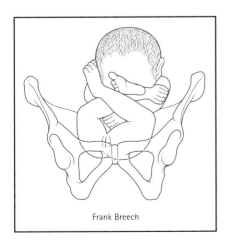
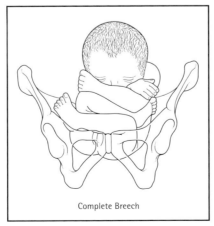
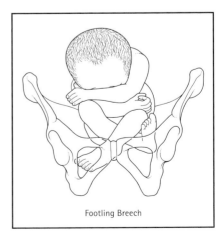

Frank Breech

Complete Breech

Footling Breech

Figure 25.1 Various types of breech presentation. (By permission of Drs Alvin Langer and Kay W. Kennedy, reproduced from Iffy L, Kaminetzky HA, eds. Principles and Practice of Obstetrics & Perinatology. New York: Wiley, 1981.)

a major problem in connection with breech presentation. Whereas the incidence of this complication is only 0.3% with cephalic presentation, it is in the range of 3–5% with breech presentation. This risk is particularly high in footling breech. In frank breech presentation, however, the incidence is close to that observed in cephalic presentation.

The gravest danger associated with breech delivery is arrest of the aftercoming head either by the pelvis or by the incompletely dilated cervix. The latter alternative is most threatening in premature deliveries, when the relatively small fetal body fails to dilate the cervix sufficiently for the passage of the head. It should be remembered that, whereas the progress of the head through the pelvis may take hours in cephalic presentation, the same must be accomplished within 2–3 minutes when the delivery of the head follows that of the body. The passage may be hindered further by deflexion of the head or by a nuchal arm or arms. The latter complication may occur as a result of either rapid descent of the fetal body in the birth canal or traction applied upon the lower extremities by the accoucheur.

Traumatic fetal injuries associated with vaginal breech delivery include spinal cord laceration and even transection; intraventricular hemorrhage; tentorial tear; fracture of the skull, vertebrae, ribs, or long bones; rupture of the spleen or the liver; and bleeding in the adrenals.[8,9] Injuries may also involve the muscles, the scrotum, and the testes. The latter may lead to testicular atrophy.

The relatively high perinatal mortality and morbidity rates[10] have resulted in the introduction of restrictions to elective breech vaginal delivery. The following factors have long been considered contraindications to attempted vaginal breech delivery:

(1) contracted pelvis[11]
(2) estimated fetal weight exceeding 3600 g
(3) poor obstetric history
(4) first pregnancy in a ≥35-year-old woman
(5) placenta previa
(6) dysfunctional labor
(7) prolapse of the umbilical cord
(8) prolonged premature rupture of the membranes
(9) footling breech
(10) less than 32 weeks' gestation
(11) hydrocephaly
(12) scarred uterus
(13) deflexed fetal head.

In recent decades, cesarean section has become the preferred method of delivery by most obstetricians. Some physicians and even medical organizations categorically reject the option of elective breech vaginal delivery currently and consider elective cesarean section the method of choice.[12,13] Others restrict elective breech deliveries to cases that fulfill certain specific criteria.[6,14–16]

Contemporary management

Since opinions differ with regard to the place of vaginal breech delivery in contemporary obstetric practice,[17–21] elective cesarean section for breech presentation is always an acceptable management choice. It is advisable to inform the patient about the differing opinions and involve her in the decision making. In order to give informed consent, the patient must be told that intrapartum complications may necessitate abandonment of a planned vaginal delivery.

Irrespective of the contemplated management, patients with breech presentation need close follow-up during the antepartum period. They should be advised about the risks of premature rupture of the membranes and preterm labor. When the breech presentation persists, the patient should undergo ultrasound examination to exclude conditions conducive to persistent malpresentation, such as pelvic tumors or fetal malformations. In the absence of such abnormalities, external version around 35–36 weeks is the recommended contemporary management.[22,23]

Patients selected for a trial of labor need to be hospitalized early. The presentation of the fetus and the absence of deflexion of the head should be confirmed by ultrasound at the time of admission. It is important to remember that any degree of pelvic contraction is an absolute contraindication to vaginal breech delivery. Computer tomography and magnetic resonance imaging can be used for pelvimetry, but their usefulness is disputed.[24] Before and after the procedure, the parturient must be monitored electronically. Rupture of the membranes must be avoided. Evidence of nonreassuring fetal heart rate or abnormal progress of labor is an indication for cesarean section.

Abdominal breech delivery can be performed under regional or general anesthesia. One should remember that extraction of the aftercoming head through a small incision can be as difficult as a complicated vaginal breech delivery. Fetal injuries, similar to those observed in connection with vaginal breech deliveries, can also occur with cesarean section. Complications such as extension of the uterine incision to the cervix or laterally to the uterine vessels may occur.

Breech delivery

Traditionally, the primary mode of delivering the breech fetus was through the vagina by a wide variety of techniques and maneuvers.[15] Maternal safety was the overwhelming concern, given the fact that modern antibiotics, blood banking, and safe anesthesia did not exist. In addition, techniques and facilities to sustain premature infants or those with congenital anomalies were not readily available.

To improve perinatal outcome, Hall and Kohl suggested, in 1956, the routine use of cesarean section for breech presentation.[25] Based on an analysis of 1456 breech-presenting fetuses, they concluded that cesarean section produced a lower perinatal mortality rate than vaginal delivery.[26] Since then, the rate of cesarean sections for breech presentation has risen from 5–10% up to 80–100%. On the ground of a large international study which involved a variety of obstetric centers with differing professional standards, Hannah et al. in 2000 concluded that elective vaginal breech delivery involved unacceptable fetal risks.[21,27] Their view was endorsed virtually immediately by British authorities.[28] Although the protocol on which the findings of the investigators rested incorporated management patterns that had been considered unacceptable in the USA for decades, the American College of Obstetricians and Gynecologists soon followed.

The turnaround did not go unchallenged. Several authorities have presented the view that Hannah et al's data excluded reference to the effect of cesarean sections upon subsequent pregnancies and, thus provided inadequate evidence for the support of their far-reaching conclusions.[6,14,15,29] The perinatal mortality rate associated with breech presentation has decreased since the widespread application of cesarean section; however, there has been a concomitant concern about the maternal risks of cesarean section, including infectious morbidity and the danger of rupture of the uterus in subsequent pregnancies. The latter complication along with a variety of others that occur with increased frequency after abdominal deliveries, such as placenta previa, placenta accreta, premature labor, and *in utero* fetal death, impose substantial risks upon future siblings of babies delivered by the abdominal route.

One alternative to abdominal delivery is external version.[23] Another alternative is selective trial of labor for breech fetuses. A randomized study which compared elective cesarean section with protocol-managed labor in frank breech fetuses at term found significant maternal morbidity when breech infants were delivered by cesarean section, with no dramatic improvement in the neonatal outcome.[30] Nonetheless, cesarean section is likely to remain the most frequent modality of delivery in breech presentation. When the opportunity arises for a selective trial of labor, the obstetrician must possess the skills necessary to conduct delivery vaginally. It is advisable to discuss the risks and benefits of the available options with the patient before any relevant decision making.

Although obviously less conducive to birth trauma than a vaginal breech delivery, abdominal extraction of the fetus presenting by the breech can involve considerable technical difficulties. Since the lower uterine segment is often uneffaced, it may be difficult to cut a long enough transverse incision for the delivery of the aftercoming head. Delay in completing the delivery process may cause fetal hypoxia, and undue force used during traction may result in traumatic injury.[31] In the same process, the incision may extend either laterally, involving the uterine blood vessels, or in the direction of the cervix, causing laceration difficult to repair. For this reason, careful inspection of contemplated incision site is important. When necessary, there should be no hesitation to apply a lower segment vertical incision in order to minimize the risks of these complications. If this opportunity has been forfeited, extension of the incision in an inverted 'T' fashion may resolve the problem at the expense of leaving behind a weak and vulnerable scar in case of future pregnancy. Development of Bandl's ring secondary to protracted labor may make the extraction of the fetus virtually impossible. Extension of the incision into a long classical cut may be the only solution in such instances. In cases of premature cesarean breech delivery, when the lower uterine segment is not developed, a lower segment transverse incision may be insufficient to deliver the head. In such cases, a vertical lower segment incision may be preferable.

The manipulative procedures to be described evolved decades and even centuries ago as a result of extensive application in everyday practice. With regard to elective breech delivery, one must remember the importance of certain precautionary measures[6]: (1) labor should not be induced; (2) oxytocin should not be used for uterine stimulation; (3) the second stage should not extend beyond 60 minutes; (4) the estimated fetal weight should not exceed 3600 g.

Vaginal breech delivery may occur spontaneously or may require partial or complete breech extraction. Personnel critical to a safe vaginal delivery in breech presentation include: (1) an obstetrician skilled in the relevant techniques; (2) an assistant to support the weight of the fetal body as the aftercoming head is delivered or, when needed, provide suprapubic pressure on the descending fetal head to maintain flexion; (3) a pediatrician to resuscitate the neonate if required; (4) an anesthesiologist to provide pain relief during the delivery; (5) appropriate nursing support; (6) operating room personnel scrubbed and gowned for instant cesarean section. Based solely on the mode of vaginal delivery, the best perinatal outcome has been found in association with spontaneous birth. The more complicated the procedure for vaginal breech delivery, the greater the perinatal morbidity and mortality risk.[4]

Spontaneous breech delivery

The only function of the obstetrician in spontaneous breech delivery is to support the body of the fetus, as the uterine contractions and the bearing-down efforts of the mother effect vaginal birth. The expulsion of the legs precedes the emergence of the buttocks in partial or complete breech presentations. As the fetal buttocks distend the perineum, episiotomy usually is required to prevent undue delay and maternal perineal lacerations. As the fetal body descends to the umbilicus, the physician supports, but does not place traction on, the fetal torso. With a few additional contractions, the fetal arms and shoulders are delivered. It is important to allow sufficient time for spontaneous delivery, bearing in mind, however, that once the body is expelled to the scapula, the umbilical cord becomes compressed between the head and the bony pelvis.

Assisted breech delivery

In the process of birth, the delivery of the fetal body occurs relatively quickly once the breech has emerged through the pelvic outlet and the trunk has begun its rotation. In the presence of adequate uterine contractions, reflected by the fact that the process of labor has followed Friedman's curve,[32] not more than one or two contractions are required for the delivery of the trunk up to the level of the scapula. The accomplishment of this process requires unimpeded uterine action and is facilitated by the parturient's abdominal and pelvic muscles. This important factor is bound to be lost or reduced if conduction or general anesthesia is used.[33]

When, prior to the delivery of the breech, cervical dilation and descent of the presenting part have been progressing at the normal rate, spontaneous delivery of the body up to the level of the shoulders occurs rather predictably without need for intervention on the part of those attending. Such a development provides the most favorable outlook. Interference prior to the delivery of the trunk, whether elective or indicated, increases the risks involved with the delivery of the head.[6,34] It is at the time of the birth of the fetus up to the shoulders that the greatest diameter of the head reaches the level of the pelvic inlet. In most instances, need exists for providing assistance with the delivery of the aftercoming head. The various maneuvers that facilitate this process will be discussed in some detail in the following sections.

Despite favorable cephalopelvic proportions, the premature fetus is liable to be stressed excessively or suffer birth injuries due to its fragile physical structure. Additional risks are introduced by the fact that the relative diameters of the breech, as compared to the head, are small, and the presenting part can pass through the cervix at a lesser degree of dilation than that required for the passage of the head. Thus, chances are high that the powerful musculature of the cervix will prevent delivery of the caput for a prolonged period of time. The delay is conductive to fetal hypoxia, and the physician's effort to overcome the resistance of the cervix to birth injuries.

On rare occasions, the normal rotation of the fetus is reversed and the chin instead of the occiput rotates toward the symphysis after the delivery of the body. In this situation, the chin interlocks with the symphysis; a collision which is bound to deflex the head. The end result is an almost insurmountable impasse.

Ideally, the malrotation should be prevented by facilitating the anterior rotation of the back before the full delivery of the trunk. Alternatively, an attempt should be made to correct the malrotation. This can be begun by an external maneuver; a fist over the symphysis displaces the chin toward one side. The effort is to be completed internally; a hand inserted into the vagina tries to rotate the occiput toward the desired direction. If this maneuver fails, as it often does, the 'reverse Prague maneuver' is the last resort. One hand grasps the fetal extremities and brings them, with gentle force, toward the abdomen of the mother. The other hand grasps the neck much in the same manner as in Mauriceau's maneuver, and traction is applied in an upward direction. If the effort succeeds, the fetus is born as if it turned a somersault. Since the use of some force is likely to be required under these exceedingly unfavorable circumstances, the maneuver involves considerable fetal risks. Therefore, it is

more of historical than clinical interest. In contemporary practice, 'abdominal rescue'[35] seems to be the preferable approach.

Partial breech extraction

Partial breech extraction involves the spontaneous delivery of the fetus to the umbilicus and the employment of obstetric maneuvers thereafter for delivery of the upper torso, shoulders, arms, and aftercoming head.[9,36] When spontaneous delivery of the fetus to the umbilicus is accomplished by the uterine contractions and maternal bearing-down efforts, the obstetrician places both hands around the fetal thighs with both thumbs over the sacrum and parallel to the fetal lumbar spine (Figure 25.2). The key to success is steady, gentle, sharp downward traction at the time of contraction at about a 60° angle with the back in the transverse diameter until the scapulae are outside the vulva. Care must be taken to avoid the birth injuries ascribed to this procedure. Although partial breech extraction may be necessary in some instances, the advisability of waiting until spontaneous delivery of the body up to the shoulder blades has been accomplished cannot be overemphasized.

Delivery of the shoulders and arms

Continuous traction upon the fetus is likely to entail unimpeded delivery of the shoulder girdle and arms, a mechanism traditionally attributed to Müller. An alternative, highly effective, and time-proven maneuver is somewhat more involved and requires careful observance of a series of steps.[9,34]

The classical method emphasizes the fact that there is more room in the space provided by the sacrum than under the symphysis. This approach stipulates that: (1) extraction of the

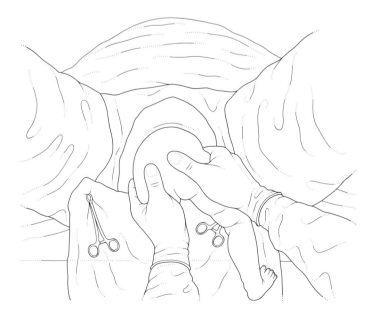

Figure 25.2 The initial step for partial breech extraction. (Reproduced from Burger. Operative Obstetrics, Franklin: Budapest, 1927.[52])

retained arm should be carried out in the space provided by the sacrum; (2) the right arm should be extracted with the right hand and the left arm with the left hand; (3) the arm should be brought out in front of the fetus and never behind the body; (4) any traction or pressure exerted upon the arm must be directed against a joint, usually at the elbow.

The procedure itself is carried out as follows. When the tendency of the rotation is such that the left shoulder is anterior and the right one is posterior, the legs of the fetus are grasped with the left hand, and, with a semicircular swing, they are lifted up to rest against the right inguinal area of the mother. The index and middle fingers of the right hand are inserted into the vagina over the perineum in such a manner that they follow the shoulder and upper arm and reach out for the elbow joint of the right arm. With pressure and traction upon the joint, the arm is swept out under the body in the space provided by the curve of the sacrum. The arm having been delivered, the limbs are grasped now with the right hand and brought with a broad 270° downward swing to the opposite inguinal area of the mother (Figure 25.3). Now the left hand is introduced into the vagina and the index and middle fingers sweep out the left arm in the same manner as described before. The delivery of the arms having been completed, that of the head follows. This procedure is highly useful for the prevention, as well as for the correction, of extension of the arm above the head. By the same token, rotation of the body in the wrong direction is likely to result in extension of the arm and difficulties with delivery of the head.[37]

Delivery of the head

Delivery of the head is a routine procedure required in most cases of breech delivery. It should be attempted without awaiting spontaneous birth. Thus, by definition, this is 'assisted breech delivery', part of the expected process when breech delivery is an elective procedure. Several excellent methods are available, probably equally satisfactory in experienced hands.

Mauriceau's maneuver. Interestingly, the maneuver was described, but not practiced, by Mauriceau. It was through the contributions of Levret, Smellie, and Veit that it achieved great popularity during the last three centuries. In the absence of spontaneous delivery up to and including the shoulders and the arms, the Mauriceau maneuver (as well as the other comparable techniques) follows the extraction of the arms immediately. The body of the fetus rests upon one arm as if the fetus were riding upon the forearm of the surgeon (Figure 25.4). The other arm holds the shoulders with the index and middle fingers surrounding the neck of the fetus. One finger (usually the index) of the supporting hand is inserted into the mouth of the fetus (Figure 25.5). The purpose of this hold is not traction (in fact, traction should be avoided very carefully), but flexion of the fetal head in order to permit the passage of the most favorable diameter of the vertex through the pelvis. Traction is exercised only by the upper hand and invariably in a downward direction, in the axis of the fetal spinal column, as depicted in Figure 25.4. With flexion of the fetal head carefully maintained throughout the traction, as the occiput is felt to clear the resistance offered

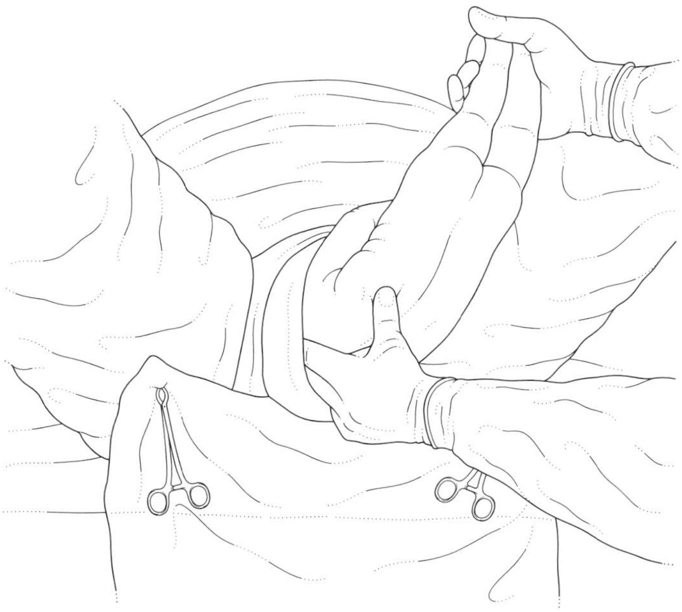

Figure 25.3 The classical method of extracting the arm during assisted breech delivery. (Reproduced from Burger. *Operative Obstetrics*, Franklin: Budapest, 1927.[52])

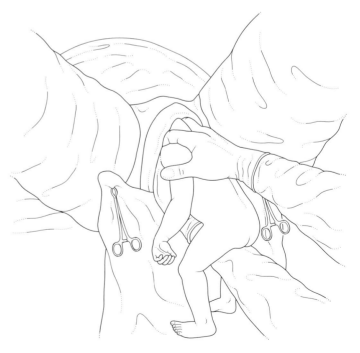

Figure 25.4 Extraction of the fetal head by the Mauriceau–Smellie–Veit maneuver. Note that the left hand simply supports the body of the fetus while the right one is used for traction. (Reproduced from Burger. *Operative Obstetrics*, Franklin: Budapest, 1927.[52])

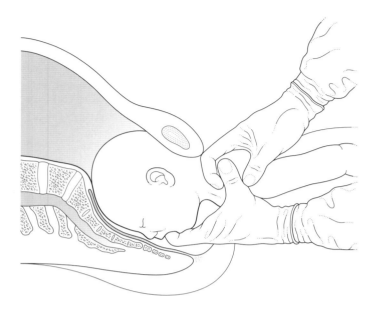

Figure 25.5 Lateral view of the extraction of the fetal head by the technique of Mauriceau. The index finger of the inside hand ensures flexion of the head and is not used for traction. (Reproduced from Burger. Operative Obstetrics, Franklin: Budapest, 1927.[52])

by the symphysis, the direction of the pull is changed gradually until, in the course of upward traction, the nose, forehead, and cranium are borne over the perineum.

The performance of episiotomy usually precedes the delivery of the breech. Alternatively, when the perineum does not offer resistance, it may precede the delivery of the head. Occasionally, in cases of multiparous women with lax perineal structures, breech delivery may be done without perineal incision. The considerations that are applicable to Mauriceau's maneuver are equally pertinent to other methods of breech delivery.

Bracht's maneuver. A simple and effective method for the delivery of the head is that recommended by Bracht. Even more than other procedures, this one mandates that the bladder be emptied immediately before the delivery. The technique requires the cooperation of two persons, one who handles the fetus and another who exercises pressure over the lower abdomen of the mother upon the fetal head. In Germany, where the technique enjoys particular popularity, the role of the person exercising pressure above the symphysis is perceived as the crucial one. Therefore, it is generally the attending physician who applies the pressure and the assistant, or assisting midwife, who holds and delivers the fetus. In general, the procedure is considered suitable for the completion of spontaneous birth, but not for one that requires partial or complete extraction. Accordingly, those attending should refrain from any action until the fetus is delivered up to the neck. If necessary, the arms are brought down with one of the earlier discussed methods. The assistant simply supports the body of the fetus in such a manner that with the birth of the upper body, the trunk is lifted up first to the level of and then above the symphysis. When the full delivery of the body is

accomplished, with two fists placed over the symphysis, the physician applies firm, continuous pressure against the head of the fetus. The latter is felt distinctly at this point immediately above the pubic bone. Under constant pressure and elevation of the body by the attending physician or the assistant, the fetus is delivered finally in a head-down position.[2] Undue pressure should be avoided, since it may result in 'cannonball'-type extrusion of the head from the pelvis, a high-risk situation for the sudden changes in intracranial pressure and their sequelae. In the practice of many European obstetricians, the Bracht maneuver is the first-line procedure. They resort to the Mauriceau maneuver on those rare occasions when the procedure fails.

Delivery by Piper's forceps. Instead of manual extraction, forceps may be applied to the aftercoming head. Piper's forceps[38] are used because of their wide shanks, fenestrations, cephalic curve, and reverse handle angle. Before the application of forceps to the aftercoming head, the fetus must be held by an assistant with some degree of extension at the neck. The feet are elevated upward above the plane of the abdomen and the arms are held by the assistant's other hand behind the back of the fetus. Some operators prefer to assume a kneeling position before introducing the left blade upward and diagonally across the introitus along the mentoocciptal line of the fetal head. A large episiotomy is essential so that during the introduction of the forceps blade, extension of the head is avoided. Before locking the forceps, it is important to be certain that the blades have been inserted with sufficient depth to have a good purchase on the fetal head. Traction is then made in a downward curve and in a continuous fashion until delivery is completed, with the forceps shanks not rising above the horizontal plane, as in the case of a reverse-curved Kielland's forceps delivery.

Piper's forceps were developed in 1924 for delivery of the aftercoming head. These forceps are designed to prevent injury to the fetal neck, to decrease compression of the fetal head, and to give the needed axis traction. Because of the absence of pelvic curve, one may encounter injury to the perineum.

Nuchal arms

Nuchal arms are a significant complication during breech delivery that may be prevented to a large degree. Rapid extraction of the fetal body should be avoided. It has been shown that umbilicus-to-mouth delivery times of up to 240 seconds (4 minutes) are usually associated with 5-minute Apgar scores of 7 or greater. If nuchal arms are present, the infant should be raised or lowered in the direction opposite to the nuchal arm and flexed over the opposite groin or buttocks of the mother. The operator's fingers should then be inserted along the humerus to the elbow, avoiding hooking the fetal arm, and, with the fingers as a splint, sweep the arm downward through the vulva. The trunk is then rotated so that the opposite nuchal arm is swept along the chest wall and the splinting maneuver repeated. The rule of delivering left arm with left hand and right arm with right hand must be remembered.

Total breech extraction

Total breech extraction is associated with a significant incidence of hypoxic and traumatic fetal injury. It should be performed only when the child is in jeopardy and cesarean delivery is not immediately available. During this procedure, no part of the fetal body other than the leg is delivered spontaneously. The operator places a hand in the birth canal, locates by palpation both or at least one of the fetal feet, and delivers the lower extremities by gentle traction. The fetal thighs are next grasped as in partial breech extraction and the fetal torso is delivered to the scapulae. The shoulder, arms, and aftercoming head are delivered as in partial breech extraction (Figure 25.2).

The anesthesiologist in the delivery room may be called upon to administer general anesthesia during total breech extraction in the absence of sufficient maternal pain relief. Hardly ever used in connection with elective delivery of singleton fetuses presenting by the breech, the technique is favored by some obstetricians for the delivery of the second twin, sometimes after the performance of an internal version.

Internal version

In contemporary obstetrics, the procedure of internal version is no longer an acceptable maneuver except for the delivery of the second twin. Although, even relatively recently, internal version and extraction have been used widely for the delivery of the second twin presenting as a vertex, such a stressful fetal manipulation is rarely justifiable. Spontaneous vertex delivery usually follows artificial rupture of the membranes; if not, delivery can be accomplished with the vacuum extractor. Thus, transverse lie of the second twin is probably the only good reason for internal version and extraction in modern obstetrics.[39]

The procedure requires general or conduction anesthesia. It consists of three steps: (1) introduction of the hands; (2) grasping the lower extremity or extremities; (3) version of the body.

Ideally, the membranes are intact until the hand is introduced to effect internal version of the body; then, they must be ruptured. The hand to be introduced is the one that corresponds with the side of the fetal legs – the left hand if the lower limbs are on the mother's right side, and the right hand if they are on the mother's left. If there is a choice, the upper foot is to be grasped when the fetal abdomen or chest is presenting, whereas the extraction of the lower limb is preferable when the presenting area is the fetal back. This promotes anterior rotation of the back and prevents anterior rotation of the chin and its earlier mentioned sequelae. In the absence of a choice, the leg that can be reached easiest is to be used for traction. Occasionally, it is possible to grasp both lower limbs, a circumstance that facilitates the procedure. While one hand is being introduced, the assisting hand holds the uterine fundus in order to prevent colporrhexis (Figure 25.6a).

The limb having been reached, traction is exerted upon it. The direction of the pull is toward the midline. Meanwhile, the external hand may divert the head from its lateral position toward the middle part of the fundus (Figure 25.6b).

The conclusion of internal version is identical with that of breech extraction as described earlier in this chapter. Internal uterine manipulations carry the risks of uterine rupture and cervical damage as well as that of colporrhexis. Therefore, exploration of the uterine cavity after the delivery of placenta and thorough inspection of the cervix and the vaginal vault are integral parts of the total operative procedure.

External version

External version can result in up to 70% reduction in the incidence of breech presentation at term.[40,41] Since many physicians favor the use of tocolysis, in order to facilitate the performance of this procedure, it should be remembered that major cardiac disorders and arrhythmia represent contraindications to the use of tocolytic agents.[21] Hibbard and Schulmann[42] effectively practiced prophylactic external version at week 34. Van Dorsten et al[43] conducted a randomized, controlled trial in which the external version was performed under terbutaline tocolysis at 37–39 weeks' gestation. It was successful in 68% of the cases, and all of these presented in labor subsequently with vertex presentations. Nulliparity, maternal obesity, engagement of the breech, and uterine anomaly tended to reduce the success rate of external version. In the control group, only 18% of the presenting breeches converted to vertex beyond week 37 of the pregnancy. Transient fetal heart rate decelerations were noted during version in 36% of the attempts (24% of successes and 63% of failures). These decelerations responded to cessation of manipulation. External cephalic version is less successful in cases of frank breech, where the splinting action of the extended fetal legs makes version difficult to perform.

Successful version is associated with an increased need for cesarean section on account of dystocia.[44] There is a relative contraindication in Rh-negative women because of the risk of accidents leading to fetomaternal transfusion. Other complications of external version include fetal distress; twisting, knotting, or laceration of the cord; placental separation; uterine rupture; premature labor; premature rupture of the membranes; and spinal cord transection *in utero*. For reasons mentioned above, Rh-negative mothers should be subjected to Kleinhauer–Betke's test after the procedure and should receive RhoGAM if evidence of fetomaternal transfusion is documented. Parity, sufficient amniotic fluid, and unengaged presenting part are conducive to a successful version. Previous cesarean or other penetrating uterine scar is a contraindication.

It is recommended that the external version procedure be carried out according to a prearranged protocol.[45,46] Although it can be attempted at any time before the occurrence of labor,[47] it is best to wait until the fetal lung has achieved maturity, yet the amount of the amniotic fluid has not decreased to such an extent as to hinder the manipulation of the fetus. This optimum time is probably the weeks 35–36 of gestation. It is necessary to

(a)   (b)

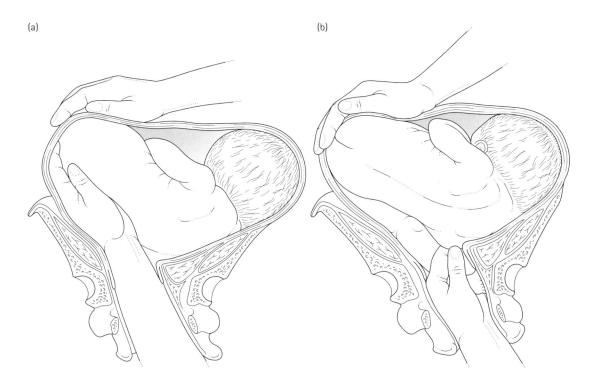

Figure 25.6 Internal version for the correction of transverse lie. (a) Introduction into the uterus of one hand while counterpressure is exerted by the assisting (outside) hand of the operator. (b) Traction applied toward the midline. (A classical nineteenth-century illustration by Halban-Seitz, reproduced from Iffy L, Kaminetzky HA, eds. Principles and Practice of Obstetrics & Perinatology. New York: Wiley, 1981.)

have facilities for electronic monitoring, ultrasound, and easy access to the operating room if circumstances require. The availability of at least one assistant for the performance of the procedure is considered essential.

For the performance of external version, the patient should take nothing by mouth for at least 6 hours before the procedure. The blood indices should be tested in anticipation of the procedure. The bladder must be empty. The placement of the patient into a head-down Trendelenburg position (about 15°) is conducive to the disengagement of the presenting breech from the pelvis. It is considered advantageous by some to spread fine talc powder over the abdomen in order to facilitate the maneuver. As mentioned earlier, the performance of a nonstress test at the end of the procedure is indicated in order to avoid overlooking fetal distress resulting from the version.

The exact position of the fetus having been established by ultrasound, the physician performing the procedure positions himself/herself in such a manner that he/she faces the fetus. The procedure itself begins with the operator lifting out the presenting breech from the pelvis and elevating it as high as possible without the use of undue force. Thereafter, the breech is displaced toward the direction of the fetal back, away from the pelvic inlet. At the same time, the other hand of the operator attempts to drive the head forward and downward as if encouraging the fetus to do a somersault. A useful alternative approach is to entrust the assistant with the elevation and displacement of

the breech in order to permit the operator to use both hands for driving the head through 180° into the pelvic inlet while the breech is moved gently upward in the opposite direction. It is to be remembered that the direction of version is counterclockwise in case of first breech presentation (fetal back turned to the mother's left side) and clockwise when the presentation is second breech (fetal back turned to the right side of the mother). It is axiomatic in good obstetric practice not to force the version in the absence of success with one or two attempts or when, after what appears to have been an accomplished external version, the fetus repeatedly returns to its original position. It is to be remembered, furthermore, that a breech presentation carries less risk than a transverse lie. Accordingly, care must be taken not to leave the fetus, initially presenting by the breech, lying in transverse or oblique position.

Contrary to what one might expect, external version in the case of transverse lie is more difficult than when the presentation is breech. Particularly, when permitted to prevail until the late third trimester, the shape of the uterus adjusts to the transverse lie of the fetus. Thus, when the axis of the body changes from transverse to longitudinal, it hinders the maintenance of the desired presentation. Whereas after a successful external version from breech presentation the fetus usually remains in vertex presentation, it tends to return to transverse hours or days after the procedure when version is attempted from a transverse lie.

If external version is employed, a number of rigid criteria must be met. The fetus must be judged normal, with no oligohydramnios or placenta previa demonstrated by standard sonography. External fetal monitoring should be utilized before and after the procedure. The breech should preferably be unengaged. It is performed at a gestation of 35–36 weeks so that, in the event of an accident requiring delivery, the fetal outcome will not be compromised by prematurity. The uterus must be nontender and not irritable. This is best ensured by a tocolytic agent,[48] such as 0.25 mg terbutaline administered 15–30 min before the attempt.

That difficulties arising during the labor process can be resolved by cesarean section is an old concept. On the other hand, it was accepted up to the last decades of the twentieth century that difficulties leading to the demise of the child may arise during the process of delivery in a variety of clinical situations. The latter include shoulder dystocia in the process of delivering a fetus presenting by the vertex, interlocking of the heads of twins (thus preventing the delivery of the first one), arrest of delivery of conjoined twins, and inability to deliver the aftercoming head in breech presentation. Fetal death or catastrophic injury deriving from these complications has generally been considered inevitable by obstetricians until recently.

The requirement of undertaking breech and twin deliveries under double-setup, along with the development of some new techniques discussed elsewhere in this volume, provides an opportunity for overcoming some difficulties during delivery that had inevitably led to fetal death or gross injury in the past. Relevant to breech presentation, 'abdominal rescue' represents a desperate, last-ditch effort to save fetal life in a situation when extraction of the aftercoming head or upper body appears impossible without potentially catastrophic fetal injury.[35,49] This maneuver requires the elevation of the body of the fetus by an assistant in order to improve circulation in the brain, and quick performance of a hysterotomy, typically by a vertical uterine incision, followed by extraction of the head, and the rest of the body abdominally. Under double setup, the same technique may be a practical solution whenever delivery of the aftercoming head becomes impossible for some unforeseen reason, such as deflexion of the fetal head during the process of delivery, resistance offered by an incompletely dilated cervix,[50] or interlocking of the heads of twins.

General considerations

It is widely believed that cesarean section offers improved outcome for the premature breech fetus weighing less than 1500–2000 g. It is thought that vaginal delivery of the premature breech fetus creates an increased risk of brain damage due to intracranial hemorrhage and birth trauma.[51] For fetuses above 2000 g, the benefit of cesarean section is less apparent.[30,53]

In case of a term fetus, a specific protocol must be implemented for selection of patients for vaginal breech delivery. This should include: (1) frank breech position; (2) immediate availability of cesarean section (including anesthesiologist and nursing staff); (3) estimated fetal weight 2000–3600 g; (4) adequate clinical pelvimetry, if necessary with radiographic confirmation; (5) absence of hyperextension of the fetal head; (6) absence of fetal distress; (7) absence of postmaturity; (8) normal progress of labor; (9), in case of second twin presenting by the breech, absence of a difference exceeding 3–4 mm between the biparietal diameters in favor of twin B.

It is an important principle that the membranes in breech labor must be left intact as long as possible. Since the small presenting parts permit the escape of much of the amniotic fluid after their rupture, breaking the membranes artificially is an invitation for cord-related complications.

The establishment of a plan with regard to the method of delivery by term (i.e., week 38) is of utmost importance. Labor frequently is preceded by rupture of the membranes, an event that carries the risk of prolapse of the cord and its dire sequelae. Since no tangible improvement in prenatal mortality and morbidity rates derives from continued fetal maturation beyond completed week 38, the risk/benefit ratio of procrastination beyond this time, in cases where vaginal delivery in contraindicated, is bound to be unfavorable. Accordingly, the recommended time for elective abdominal delivery is completed week 38 of gestation.

Transverse lie

When the long axis of the fetus is perpendicular to the axis of the mother, the technical term of transverse lie applies. The head or the breech occupies the iliac fossa. The shoulder presents and it is the point of designation. With regard to the definition of the position of the fetus, it needs to be determined whether the fetus is in a dorsoanterior or dorsoposterior position.

The incidence of transverse lie is about one out of 300 pregnancies. Those risk factors known to be conducive to breech presentation are also conducive to this entity.[54] Transverse lie can be easily detected by the Leopold maneuvers alone. On palpation, the corpus is wide and the fundal height is shortened. The head is palpated in one of the maternal flanks or iliac fossae. On pelvic examination, no presenting part is felt. A suspicion of transverse lie requires careful evaluation. The risks of early labor or rupture of membranes need to be brought to the attention of the patient. The exact presentation should be confirmed by ultrasound with the same considerations in mind that have been described for breech presentation.

It is advisable to attempt the external version maneuver earlier than in breech presentation since it becomes extremely difficult, if not impossible, by the last few weeks of gestation. By that time, the shape of the uterus has adjusted to the position of the fetus, and with the amount of amniotic fluid reduced, it can no longer accommodate the child in the longitudinal lie. For the same reason, versions that appear to be successful initially may often prove to be a failure a few days later.

Presumably on account of the loss of most of the amniotic fluid, fetuses in transverse lie fare poorly after the membranes have ruptured. For this reason, prolonged observation in connection with premature rupture of the membranes is not a viable option in transverse lie.

Because of the high risk of prolapse of the cord (10%), elective delivery at week 37 by cesarean section is recommended. If the fetal back is turned downward, a lower vertical or classical incision is needed. If the back is turned upward, the technique of abdominal delivery is essentially the same as in breech presentations.

References

1. Cruiskshank DP, White CA. Obstetric malpresentation: twenty years' experience. Am J Obstet Gynecol 1973; 116: 1097.
2. Braun FHT, Jones KL, Smith DW. Breech presentation as an indicator of fetal abnormality. J Pediatr 1975; 86: 419–21.
3. Thorp J, Jenkins T, Watson W. Utility of Leopold maneuvers in screening for malpresentation. Obstet Gynecol 1991; 78: 394–6.
4. Morgan ES, Kane SH. An analysis of 16,327 breech births. JAMA 1964; 187: 262–4.
5. Moore WT, Steptoe PP. The experience of the Johns Hopkins Hospital with breech presentation. An analysis of 1,444 cases. South Med J 1943; 36: 295.
6. Alarab M, Regan C, O'Connell MP et al. Singleton vaginal breech delivery at term: still a safe option. Obstet Gynecol 2004; 103: 407–12.
7. Eide MA, Oyen N, Skjaerven R et al. Breech delivery and intelligence: a population-based study of 8,738 breech infants. Obstet Gynecol 2005; 105: 4–11.
8. Brenner WE, Bruce RD, Hendricks CH. The characteristics and perils of breech presentation. Am J Obstet Gynecol 1974; 118: 700–12.
9. Weingold AB. The management of breech presentations. In: Iffy L, Charles D (eds), Operative Perinatology, p. 537 Macmillan: New York, 1984.
10. Ventura SJ, Martin JA, Curtin SC. Birth: final data for 1997. Nat Vital Stat Rep 1999; 47: 1–96.
11. Bhagwanani SG, Price HV, Laurence KM, Ginz B. Risks and prevention of cervical cord injury in the management of breech presentation with hyperextension of the fetal head. Am J Obstet Gynecol 1973; 115: 1159–61.
12. American Academy of Pediatrics and American College of Obstetricians and Gynecologists. Guideline for Perinatal Care, p. 109 (5th edition). Washington, DC, 2002.
13. Kotaska A. Inappropriate use of randomised trials to evaluate complex phenomena: case study of vaginal breech delivery. BMJ 2004; 329: 1039–42.
14. Apuzzio J, Iffy L, Weiss G. Mode of delivery in breech presentation. Acta Obstet Gynecol Scand 2002; 81: 1091.
15. Apuzzio J, Iffy L, Weiss G. Mode of term singleton breech delivery. Obstet Gynecol 2002; 99: 1131–3.
16. Van Roosmalen J, Rosendaal F. There is still room for disagreement about vaginal delivery of breech infants at term. Br J Obstet Gynaecol 2002; 109: 967–9.
17. Green PM, Walkinshaw S. Management of breech deliveries. Obstet Gynaecol 2002; 4: 87.
18. Gimovsky ML, Wallace RL, Schifrin BS, Paul RH. Randomized management of the non-frank breech presentations at term – a preliminary report. Am J Obstet Gynecol 1983; 146: 34–40.
19. Giuliani A, Scholl WM, Basver A Tamussino. Mode of delivery and outcome of 699 term singleton breech deliveries at a single center. Am J Obstet Gynecol 2002; 187: 1694–8.
20. Sibony O, Luton D, Oury JF, Blot P. Six hundred and ten breech versus 12,405 cephalic deliveries at term: is there any difference in the neonatal outcome? Eur J Obstet Gynecol Reprod Biol 2003; 107: 140–4.
21. Wong WM, Lao TT, Liu KL. Predicting the success of external cephalic version with a scoring system. A prospective, two-phase study. J Reprod Med 2000; 45: 201–6.
22. American College of Obstetricians and Gynecologists. External cephalic version. ACOG Practice Bulletin, No. 13, Feb 2004.
23. Hansen GF. Version of the fetus. In: Iffy L, Charles D (eds), Operative Perinatology, p. 471. Macmillan: New York, 1984.
24. Van Loon AJ, Mantingh A, Serlier EK et al. Randomized controlled trial of magnetic resonance pelvimetry in breech presentation at term. Lancet 1997; 350: 1799–804.
25. Hall JE, Kohl S. Breech presentation. Am J Obstet Gynecol 1956; 72: 977.
26. Hall JE, Kohl SG, O'Brien F et al. Breech presentation and perinatal mortality. Am J Obstet Gynecol 1965; 91: 655.
27. Hannah ME, Hannah WJ, Hewson SA et al. Planned caesarean section versus planned vaginal birth for breech presentation at term: a randomized multicenter trial. Lancet 2000; 356: 1375–83.
28. Lumley J. Any room left for disagreement about assisting breech birth at term? Lancet 2000; 356: 1369–70.
29. Hauth LT, Cuningham FG. Vaginal breech delivery is still justified. Obstet Gynecol 2002; 99: 1115–16.
30. Collea JV, Chein C, Quilligan EJ. The randomized management of frank breech presentation: a study of 208 cases. Am J Obstet Gynecol 1980; 137: 235–44.
31. Alexander J, Gregg JEM, Quinn MW. Femoral fractures at cesarean section. Case reports. Br J Obstet Gynaecol 1987; 94: 273.
32. Friedman EA. Labor: Clinical Evaluation and Management (2nd edition). Appleton-Century-Crofts: New York, 1978.
33. Whyte H, Hannah ME, Saigal S et al. Term Breech Trial Collaborative Group; outcomes of children at 2 years after planned cesarean birth versus planned vaginal birth for breech presentation at term: the International Randomized Term Breech Trial. Am J Obstet Gynecol 2004; 191: 864–71.
34. Iffy L, Toliver CW. Manual extraction procedures. In: Iffy L, Kaminetzky HA (eds), Principles and Practice of Obstetrics & Perinatology, p. 1521. John Wiley: New York, 1981.
35. Iffy L, Apuzzio JJ, Cohen-Addad N et al. Abdominal rescue after entrapment of the aftercoming head. Am J Obstet Gynecol 1986; 154: 623.

36. Martius G. Lehrbuch der Geburtshilfe, p. 299. (9th edition). Georg Thieme: Stuttgart, 1977.

37. Beischer NA. Pelvic contraction in breech presentations. J Obstet Gynaecol Br Commonw 1966; 73: 421–7.

38. Piper EB, Bachman C. The prevention of fetal injuries in breech delivery. JAMA 1929; 92: 217.

39. Winn HN, Cimino J, Powers J et al. Intrapartum management of nonvertex second-born twins: a critical analysis. Am J Obstet Gynecol 2001; 185: 1204–8.

40. Siddiqui D, Stiller RJ, Collins J, Laifer SA. Pregnancy outcome after successful external cephalic version. Am J Obstet Gynecol 1999; 181: 1092–5.

41. Zhang J, Bowes WA, Fortney JA. Efficacy of external cephalic version including safety cost benefits analysis and impact on the cesarean section rate. Obstet Gynecol 1993; 82: 306–12.

42. Hibbard LT, Schumann WR. Prophylactic external version in an obstetric practice. Am J Obstet Gynecol 1973; 116: 511–18.

43. Van Dorsten JP, Schifrin BS, Wallace RL. Randomized control trial of external cephalic version with tocolysis in late pregnancy. Am J Obstet Gynecol 1981; 141: 417–24.

44. Vezina Y, Bujold E, Varin J et al. Cesarean delivery after successful external cephalic version of breech presentation at term: a comparative study. Am J Obstet Gynecol 2004; 190: 763–8.

45. Hellstrom AC, Nilsson B, Stange L, Nylund L. When does external cephalic version succeed? Acta Obstet Gynecol Scand 1990; 69: 281–5.

46. Mancuso KM, Yancey MK, Murphy JA et al. Epidural analgesia for cephalic version: a randomized trial. Obstet Gynecol 2000; 95: 648–51.

47. Impey L, Lissoni D. Outcome of external cephalic version after 36 weeks' gestation without tocolysis. J Matern Fetal Med 1999; 8: 203–7.

48. Yanny H, Johanson R, Balwin KJ et al. Double-blind randomized controlled trial of glyceryl trinitrate spray for external cephalic version. Br J Obstet Gynaecol 2000; 107: 562–4.

49. Swartjes JM, Bleker OP, Schutte MF. The Zavanelli maneuver applied to locked twins. Am J Obstet Gynecol 1992; 166: 532.

50. Tchabo J, Tomai T. Selected external version of the second twin. Obstet Gynecol 1992; 79: 421–3.

51. Gravenhorst JB, Schreuder AM, Veen S et al. Breech delivery in very preterm and very-low-birth infants in the Netherlands. Br J Obstet Gynaecol 1993; 100: 411–15.

52. Burger K. Szülészeti Mütéttan, p. 117. Franklin Társulat: Budapest, 1927.

53. Collea JV. Malpresentations and cord accidents. In: Pernoll ML, Benson RC (eds), Current Obstetric and Gynecologic Diagnosis and Treatment, p. 23. Appleton & Lange: Norwalk, CT, 1987.

54. Hourihane MJ. Etiology and management of oblique lie. Obstet Gynecol 1968; 32: 512–19.

26 Delivery of twins and higher-order multiples

Isaac Blickstein and Louis G Keith

Changes in the epidemiology of multiple gestation influence the decision of how and when to deliver twins. The dramatic increase in the frequency of multiple birth has affected preterm deliveries.[1] The 2002 US vital statistics show that the twin birth rate reached a remarkable 3.1% of all live births; a 65% increase over the past two decades and a 38% increase since 1990.[2] In 2002, the incidence of triplets and higher-order multiples was 1.84 per 1000 live births compared to about 1:10 000 births after spontaneous conceptions.[2] The increased rates of multiple birth inevitably increase those of preterm deliveries because 12% of twins, 36% of triplets, and 60% of quadruplets are born before 32 weeks' gestation.[2] According to the US Centers for Disease Control, the main reason for the increase in preterm births is multiple gestation secondary to assisted reproductive technologies (ART), with 16% of all preterm deliveries in the USA (79 684 in 2002) being due to multiple births.[2]

Another important change is the increasing age of the mothers of multiples.[3] US data indicate that fewer mothers in the age group 15–29 years delivered their firstborn in 2002 than in 1990, whereas the first birth rate increased 25–30% in the age group 30–44.[2] In the past, pregnancies at older age were primarily unintended, and women usually delivered their last baby at an earlier age. At present, however, many women intentionally postpone childbirth until they achieve personal milestones. Because of the reduced fecundity associated with older age, there is a significant need for ART to achieve the desired pregnancy. Thus, social trends and available therapy act in concert to increase the risk of multiple births. Loos et al,[4] using data from the East Flanders Prospective Twin Survey, noted that in 1976 there was one induced twin maternity for every 32 spontaneous twins. In contrast, by 1996, this ratio was 1:1.02. With increasing frequencies of *iatrogenic* pregnancies, the proportion of previously infertile women delivering twins is increasing, leading to higher rates of 'premium pregnancies', for which any mode of delivery except a cesarean (justified or not) may be declined.[5]

The decision of how to deliver multiples may be further modified by recent publications demonstrating the reduced risk of elective cesarean, mainly in terms of maternal mortality, and describing the potential benefits of elective cesarean for both mothers and children in terms of reduced morbidity.[6] It could be inferred that if a cesarean section upon a woman's request is medically[6] and ethically[7] permissible, it would be logical to opt for a cesarean delivery of multiples, although the indication may seem subtle or unfounded by evidence.

The second consideration comes from a recent study documenting the advantage of a planned cesarean section for the term fetus in breech presentation without increasing the maternal complication rate compared to vaginal breech delivery.[8] As a result of this study based on singletons, many centers extrapolated its conclusions to twin births with any presentation other than vertex–vertex, and no longer undertake breech deliveries by the vaginal route irrespective of plurality. Consequently, many young residents presently lack the training, experience, and manual dexterity required for breech delivery. Indeed, a secondary analysis of the Term Breech Trial cited the presence of an experienced clinician at delivery among the significant factors that reduced the risk of adverse perinatal outcome among vaginal breech deliveries.[9] Because twin pairs include at least one breech or transverse lying twin in 50–60% of cases, assisted or operative deliveries are the rule rather than the exception. Indeed, a direct relationship exists between the cesarean section rate in twins and the combined delivery rate, suggesting that those who perform more abdominal deliveries in twins and are, thus, less experienced in vaginal deliveries of twins, are more likely to decide on a cesarean for the second twin.[10] In summary, because twin gestations frequently involve maternal and fetal complications, and are quite often considered 'premium' pregnancies, many clinicians prefer to deliver twins by the abdominal route for subtle reasons rather than clearcut indications.[5]

Cesarean section for all twins

The US cesarean delivery rate increased by 13% between 1989–91 and 1997–9 among twins delivered at ≥22 weeks and weighing ≥500 g.[11] This value represents average increases of 52%, 28% and 9%, among twin pregnancies delivered at 22–27, 28–33, and ≥34 weeks' gestation, respectively. Although the rates increased to a greater extent at earlier than at later gestational ages, the absolute number of cesareans was much higher at later gestational ages.[11] These rates are quite similar to the commonly cited rates of 50–60% abdominal births among twins and nearly 100% among triplets.[5] In the UK, the 2001 cesarean rate for twin deliveries was 59%.[12]

The clinician's problem is not reduction of the overall cesarean rate but avoiding unnecessary operations. In this respect, one addresses two important questions. First, are there specific maternal risks associated with abdominal delivery of twins?[13] Second, is there any solid evidence that cesarean section is safer for twins than vaginal delivery?

Regrettably, the first question has not been addressed in the literature adequately. On the other hand, the potential beneficial effect of cesarean section for twins has been studied extensively by case-control methodology. Hogle et al[14] recently reported their systematic review and meta-analysis aimed to determine whether a policy of planned cesarean section or vaginal delivery is favorable for twins. Their literature research ranging from 1980 through 2001 included studies that compared planned cesarean section to planned vaginal birth for babies weighing ≥1500 g or reaching at least 32 weeks' gestation. Only four studies with a total of 1932 infants were included in the analysis. A low, 5-minute Apgar score occurred less frequently in twins delivered by planned cesarean section (OR 0.5; 95% CI 0.3, 0.9) principally because of a reduction among pairs with twin A in breech presentation. Twins delivered by planned cesarean section spent longer time in the hospital, but, there were no significant differences in perinatal or neonatal mortality, neonatal morbidity, or maternal morbidity.

It follows that the decision for a cesarean in twins, intentionally or not, is based on qualitative variables. The quantitative variables suggest no advantage for abdominal delivery in the majority of cases.[5]

Vaginal delivery of twins

Malpresentation

Each twin may present as vertex or breech, or assume a transverse lie. To simplify the discussion, twins are vertex/nonvertex roughly 40% of the time; vertex/vertex 30% of the time; nonvertex/vertex 20% of the time; and nonvertex/nonvertex 10% of the time.[15] In many ways, decision making related to fetal presentation seems to be the easy way to deal with the optimal manner to deliver twins.

Vertex–vertex

Vertex–vertex pairs are generally considered *suitable* candidates for vaginal delivery albeit with a *few* exceptions related to size and/or gestational age. During the labor and delivery process of the first twin, the only sure thing to say is that twin B is likely to remain in the vertex presentation. This reservation emerges

from the observation that what appears to be vertex twin B is, in fact, more similar to an oblique presentation, because the position of twin A in the pelvis does not allow a true vertex presentation of twin B. Moreover, when twin B is surrounded by polyhydramnios, it might easily revert to a transverse lie after the delivery of its firstborn cotwin.

In the optimal setting, labor is allowed to progress under dual external monitoring of the twins. Most modern cardiotocographic machines can distinguish simultaneous signals from the two fetuses and record an adequate dual fetal heart rate tracing. However, this frequently necessitates the use of three belts on the maternal abdomen. Therefore, once the membranes of the presenting twin are ruptured, an internal (scalp) electrode is often used to replace one external Doppler electrode. The dual fetal heart rate tracing enables individual attention to the well-being of each fetus.

The preferred method of pain relief is regional anesthesia by epidural block.[16,17] Lumbar epidural anesthesia is recommended when vaginal delivery is anticipated. It also provides adequate anesthesia for interventions such as instrumental or cesarean delivery.

Once the first twin is delivered, the clamped umbilical cord should be marked in order to recognize it as belonging to twin A when the placenta is examined postpartum. Arguments favoring cord clamping in singletons suggest that this procedure enhances the separation of the placenta, an undesirable event before the delivery of twin B. To our knowledge, the practice of cord clamping for twin A has not been studied vis-à-vis the documented higher frequency of intrapartum placental abruption in twins.[18] A supporting argument of cord clamping of twin A refers to the possibility of blood loss from twin B via open vascular connections that are invariably found in monochorionic placentas. Cord clamping in this circumstance may avoid acute intrapartum twin-to-twin transfusion. For the same reason, umbilical cord-blood gases should be sampled from a segment of the cord distal to the clamp.

Immediately after the birth of twin A, the uterus often undergoes a strong, but brief, contraction. This is usually followed by a period of uterine quiescence, lasting a minute or two, before contractions resume for the delivery of twin B. This short period provides a window of opportunity for external manipulation of twin B, if necessary. In the case of vertex–vertex presentation, this may be used to perform external semiversion from oblique lie into longitudinal lie. To be able to do this, however, one needs three hands: one to perform a vaginal examination to establish the station of the presenting part, another to palpate the uterine fundus to determine the period of uterine relaxation, and a third one to hold a bedside ultrasound transducer to establish the correct presentation. Obviously, assistance is needed. When twin B is in the vertex position, a diluted solution of oxytocin should be administered via an infusion pump to ensure the resumption of uterine contractions. Amniotomy is expected to reduce the time interval between the deliveries of the twins. However, with a high station of the head, prolapse of the umbilical cord may occur if the membranes are ruptured intentionally or inadvertently. In one study, 26% of emergent cesareans for twin B, when both twins were in vertex presentation, resulted from cord prolapse of twin B.[19] It is therefore recommended that amniotomy be deferred until the head of twin B becomes engaged or a presenting umbilical cord is excluded.

At times, the head of twin B remains high above the pelvic inlet. This circumstance makes it clear that after the delivery of twin A, one is not dealing with an otherwise usual vertex delivery of a (remaining) singleton, but with the delivery of twin B. It is debatable whether the interdelivery interval should be more than the traditionally recommended 20 minutes. Leung et al[20] found that umbilical cord blood values of pH, P_{CO_2}, and base excess deteriorate with increasing twin-to-twin delivery interval. In their series, none of the second twins delivered within 15 minutes of the birth of twin A had a pH value under 7. However, 5.9% had such a value when delivered within 16–30 minutes, and 27% had this low pH value when delivered after an interval of over 30 minutes. Importantly, 73% of the twins with an interval of over 30 minutes had signs of fetal distress that required operative delivery. Erdemoglu and coworkers[21] found a linear relationship between the delivery interval and the 5-minute Apgar score. Pons et al[22] compared expectant to active management in the delivery of the second twin and found similar neonatal results. These data support the concept that prevailed before the 1980s, namely, that the time interval between the delivery of the twins should not exceed 20 minutes. Therefore, extension of this time limit to a maximum of 30 minutes should be subject to documentation of reassuring heart rate pattern of twin B by close electronic or ultrasonic surveillance.

Because twins are smaller than singletons, absolute cephalopelvic disproportion is rarely present. More commonly, relative disproportion is seen as a result of compound presentation. This is managed, as in the case of singleton birth, by gentle sweeping of the forelying extremity backward.

Delayed birth due to inadequate uterine contraction should be rare with the judicious use of oxytocin. Before delivery, the longitudinal lie of twin B should be reconfirmed. It has been found that 52% of cesarean sections performed for twin B in the 'safest' configuration (vertex A–vertex B) were done for change in presentation of twin B, with inability to perform version and extraction.[19]

Quite often, cervical dilation decreases after the delivery of twin A. This 'clamping down' of the cervix is attributed to the sudden decompression of the uterine cavity. However, the cervix in this case is different from a cervix with the same dilation in the active phase. Here, when 'clamping down' occurs, the time required to achieve again full dilation is short. With adequate uterine contractions, the cervix will usually regain its previous dilation within 5–15 minutes.

The uterine decompression following the birth of twin A is probably the main culprit in placental abruption.[18,19] It has been suggested that abruption occurs as a result of a sheering effect created by the different elasticity of the placenta and the uterine wall after decompression. Placental abruption needs emergency intervention.

Throughout the interval between births, the heart rate of twin B should be carefully monitored, and any sign of fetal distress should be effectively assessed. In the common scenario, the most relevant question is how soon the delivery of twin B is anticipated. When the cervix is fully dilated and the head is engaged, a vacuum extraction is a good option. Delivery of the second twin is the only circumstance where high-station vacuum extraction is permissible. However, this procedure should be reserved for special circumstances because the unengaged head of twin B has not undergone the necessary molding, and it may be difficult to place the vacuum cup on an unengaged head. Alternatively, internal podalic version (see below) and breech extraction can be performed. Thus, if prompt delivery of twin B is necessary, skillful instrumental delivery or internal version may be the first option, rather than abdominal delivery. If worst comes to worst, however, a combined twin delivery should be performed (see below).

Vertex–nonvertex

Vertex–nonvertex pairs are *possible* candidates for vaginal delivery, with *many* exceptions related to size and/or gestational age.[23] The ultimate goal is the safe delivery of twin B in breech presentation.[9] When twin B is in a transverse lie, it must first undergo version into the longitudinal lie (usually breech). Historically, this combination of presentations was subject to innumerable studies. Delivery of vertex–nonvertex twins is one of the highest challenges in manual dexterity (Figure 26.1).

When twin B presents by the breech, birth can be accomplished either by assisted breech delivery or by total breech extraction. In the former, amniotomy is delayed as much as possible to use the pressure effect of the amniotic sac on the cervix. Quite often, episiotomy is performed, and the breech is

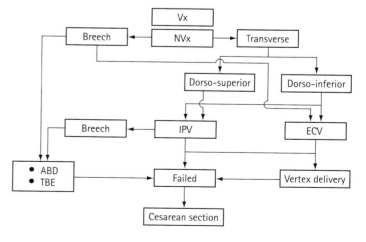

Figure 26.1 Options for vaginal birth of vertex–nonvertex twins (Vx–NVx). ECV = external cephalic version, IPV = internal podalic version, ABD = assisted breech delivery, TBE = total breech extraction.

delivered as in a singleton birth. Alternatively, the feet of twin B are grasped with intact membranes, and then the membranes are ruptured, and the fetus is delivered by total extraction. An alternative approach applies external version (EV) to the vertex. The pros and cons for each method are related to the size of twin B. Some authors recommend that the nonvertex second twin over 24 weeks' gestation and under 1700 g estimated fetal weight should undergo external cephalic version (ECV). If unsuccessful, a cesarean section should be performed. In contrast, in the nonvertex twin B over 1700 g, either EV or assisted breech extraction might be appropriate.[24] Others use a weight cutoff of 1500 g to select cases for vaginal birth.[25] It follows that breech delivery should not be performed on premature or growth-restricted twins with estimated weight under 1500 g.

When the nonvertex second twin is much larger than the firstborn twin, delivery in breech presentation may prove difficult. According to various sources, the uppermost tolerable difference ranges between 2 mm, as stated in the second edition of this volume, and 4 mm[26] in terms of bipariatal parameter.

Numerous case series have developed methods of delivery of the nonvertex twin B. While failing to reach a solid conclusion, the majority of authorities favor total breech extraction of the nonvertex second twin over external cephalic version.[27–30]

It is crucial to know the exact presentation of twin B immediately after the vaginal delivery of twin A. Bedside sonography can establish the relationship of the fetal back to the maternal pelvis. In addition, the position of the fetal head (right or left) should be known.

When twin B is in transverse lie, the fetus should be turned into a longitudinal lie. This may be performed either by EV or by internal podalic version. Both maneuvers are easiest accomplished under adequate anesthesia. This means that an anesthetist should be present in the delivery room for any emergency.

A transverse lie is either dorsoinferior or dorsosuperior when the back is directed downward toward the pelvis or upward, respectively. A dorsosuperior transverse lie requires a 90° version, a dorsoinferior lie may necessitate either a 270° somersault or a 90° version (backward somersault). Without ultrasound, neither maneuver is easy. Ideally, this procedure should be performed within the short period of uterine quiescence following the delivery of twin A. One may facilitate external or internal versions of the second twin by using intravenous nitroglycerin for uterine relaxation.[31] In one study, high-dose (0.1–0.2 mg/10 kg pregnant weight), intravenous nitroglycerin was used for internal podalic version of the second twin in transverse lie with intact membranes. Twenty of the 22 attempts were successful.[31]

If EV fails, one may revert to internal podalic version. This term refers to the introduction of the operator's hand into the birth canal in order to grasp the fetal legs after amniotomy and adequate episiotomy. In the past, this procedure was dependent on transabdominal palpation of the fetus. Currently, it is best performed under sonographic guidance. Once the legs are

grasped, the fetus is gently turned into the breech presentation, and delivered by total breech extraction. Like EV, internal podalic version is easier and less traumatic in the dorsosuperior lie. Uterine manipulation of the second twin does not increase the risk of postpartum metritis or neonatal sepsis, nor does the time interval between the deliveries of the twins. The rate of endometritis has been reported to be higher with twins delivered by cesarean section than in the general population of cesarean deliveries.[32,33]

Nonvertex first twin

Cesarean section is almost universally performed when the first twin presents as nonvertex.[34] A multicenter study of a large sample of breech-first twin pairs delivered in 13 European centers indicated that when the twins weighed under 1500 g, there was a 2.4-fold increased risk of depressed (<7) 5-minute Apgar scores and a 9.5-fold increased risk of neonatal mortality among pairs delivered vaginally compared with those delivered by cesarean section. However, when the breech-first twin weighed ≥1500 g, there was no difference in outcome.[35] As a rule of thumb, the criteria for singleton breech delivery could be applied to twin breech delivery also.

The potential complication of 'locked twins' (also known as 'entangled twins' or 'interlocking twins') is often cited as an argument against vaginal births. In this rare presentation, the chin of the breech-first twin is above the chin of the vertex-second twin. When the breech-first twin starts its descent, the chins become 'locked' and, with further descent, the heads become entrapped above or within the pelvis. Some ambiguity exists about which pairs are indeed 'locked'. For instance, twins that appear to be interlocking on imaging are not, in fact, locked but have the *potential to become* locked (Figure 26.2). The term 'locked twins' should be reserved for those cases where the breech of the first twin has been delivered halfway, and locking obstructs further descent of both twins. This devastating situation is rare, with an estimated prevalence of about 0.1%. It is not entirely clear whether the cited frequencies for cesarean births for 'locked twins' refer to twins that were actually 'locked', or whether imaging (probably radiography) led to an assumed 'dangerous' proximity between the chins. Because size matters in such an event, entrapment of the fetal heads is more likely in premature (and small) twins. Interestingly, no case of 'locked twins' was encountered in the large cohort compiled by Blickstein et al.[35] In Sweden, Rydhstrom and Cullberg[36] identified 29 cases in 26 428 (0.15%) twin pregnancies. Interlocking was attributed to growth restriction, birth weight under 2000 g, and antenatal fetal death. The intrapartum mortality was high: 38.9%. In order to facilitate unlocking, uterine relaxation may be achieved by beta-mimetic drugs[37] or nitroglycerin.[38] There is no generally accepted procedure to alleviate this obstetric emergency or that deriving from the accoucheur's inability to extract the aftercoming head arrested by entrapment by the cervix, deflexion of head, or absolute cephalopelvic disproportion. A modification of the Zavanelli

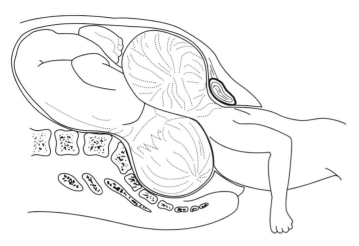

Figure 26.2 The mechanism of interlocking of fetal heads in breech–vertex combination in the course of attempted twin delivery.

maneuver employed in shoulder dystocia has been described to overcome this potentially catastrophic situation.[39] This involves pushing the partially delivered fetus back into the birth canal and then prompt classical cesarean section to effect emergent 'abdominal rescue' of the arrested first twin. Thereafter, the second twin is extracted in the usual manner. This new technique has gained some acceptance since its introduction almost two decades ago.[40]

Combined twin delivery

This term refers to cesarean section performed for twin B after the vaginal delivery of twin A. In its purest sense, combined twin delivery should thus be discussed under the subheading of cesarean delivery.[10] Jill Walton described this situation as 'the worst of both worlds – a tiring and often risky pregnancy, a tiring labour, a major abdominal operation, two lots of stitches and two new babies to care for' (*British Medical Journal*, 5 November 2002). It is safe to assume that no one intentionally plans a combined delivery. In a typical case, it occurs unexpectedly after the delivery of twin A, when an emergent situation is recognized, and the operator, in his/her best clinical judgment, considers an emergency cesarean for twin B as the safest option.

In the USA, the frequency of combined twin delivery is estimated to be 9.5%.[41] Interestingly, but not surprisingly, a direct, linear correlation was found between the frequency of cesarean section in twins and that of combined delivery.[10] When more cesareans are performed for both twins, less experience is gained in managing the often complicated delivery of twin B, and, thus, more combined twin deliveries are performed. Other investigators[42] demonstrated a statistically significant increase in combined vaginal cesarean and elective cesarean deliveries, with a decrease in the rate of vaginal deliveries.

Combined twin deliveries may occur in all combinations of presentation in which vaginal delivery is appropriate.[10] Using data from the large US multiple birth file, Wen et al[41] found that the cesarean rate for twin B increased when the mothers had medical or labor and delivery complications. Breech and other malpresentations were the most important predictors of emergent combined deliveries (population-attributable risk 33.2%). The need for emergent cesarean delivery of the second twin after vaginal delivery of the first twin was increased fourfold in such combinations. Operative vaginal delivery of the first twin was associated with a decreased rate of cesarean delivery for the second twin. In one study, the frequency of cesarean section for the second twin increased 7.6-fold if twin A was in vertex rather than breech presentation.[19]

It is important to remember that a prolonged interval between the vaginal delivery of twin A and the abdominal delivery of twin B may cause the uterus to contract around the malpresenting fetus, leading to difficult extraction during cesarean section. In this situation, nitroglycerin is the agent of choice in managing the 'entrapped' second twin.

In summary, it is not possible to avoid combined deliveries entirely unless cesarean section is performed in all twins. The operator must acknowledge the limits of his/her manual dexterity in what deserves to be included among the most formidable obstetric situations. If – for whatever reason – safe vaginal delivery of twin B cannot be expected, there is no need to test one's ability to handle cataclysmic situations. On account of this ever existing possibility, twin deliveries are invariably to be performed under double setup, in an operating room fully prepared for an abdominal operation on 1–2-minute notice. All personnel required for the operation must be scrubbed and gowned before the attempted vaginal twin delivery.

Vaginal birth after cesarean section (VBAC)

As a result of the currently high cesarean rates, there is a 1:3–1:6 chance that a given multipara carrying twins had a previous cesarean. The combination of a uterine scar with a multiple pregnancy and its associated uterine overdistention and fetal malpresentation constitutes a contraindication for a vaginal birth after cesarean (VBAC) in the opinion of most clinicians, even if the evidence does not entirely support this policy.[43–45] Therefore, when the patient is well motivated and is willing to accept the recognized risks of an attempted vaginal delivery,[25] and after the patient gives informed consent, VBAC can be accomplished in carefully selected cases. Both vertex–vertex and some vertex–nonvertex pairs may be candidates for vaginal delivery. However, when manipulations to deliver the second twin are anticipated, cesarean section is the appropriate choice. The frequency of combined deliveries is likely to be higher than in the general population. This fact should be included in the counseling process.

Special circumstances related to multiple births

Delivery of small twins

Currently, no prophylactic measure can reduce prematurity in multiple gestations. Generally, twins are delivered earlier and are smaller than singletons. Two-thirds of all twins are delivered before week 36 of gestation (14% under 33 weeks), and half of them weigh less than 2500 g (10% weighing under 1500 g).[2] Any planned mode of delivery should take these facts into consideration. One population-based study found that the overall chances of one or both twins weighing less than 1500 g were 10.8% and 5.9%, respectively. There was a significantly higher incidence among nulliparas than among multiparas (16.1% vs 7.5%).[46]

The presence of small twins, especially when they weigh under 1500 g and are before week 32, is a frequent argument against vaginal delivery. While ample data support the safety of vaginal deliveries of small singletons in the vertex presentation, few studies describe outcomes for small, vertex-presenting twins. Thus, decisions are frequently based on extrapolation from singleton series.

Recent population-based studies of very low-birth-weight (LBW) infants compared the outcomes of singletons, twins, and triplets[47] and those of twins A and B.[48] In this large Israeli database, the mode of delivery (vaginal vs abdominal) did not significantly influence the neonatal outcome. Importantly, the mode of delivery had no effect on the neurologic findings in the neonates.[47] In contrast, a French hospital-based study found a significantly higher incidence of periventricular leukomalacia among vaginally delivered twins weighing under 1500 g than among twins delivered by cesarean section.[49]

Delayed interval delivery

At times, one of the members of a multiple pregnancy is completely aborted or delivered remote from term. The uterus occasionally spontaneously ceases to contract after the birth of one or more grossly premature infant or infants. At this stage, one must decide whether to terminate the entire pregnancy or to perform the initial steps for a delayed interval delivery (also termed 'asynchronous delivery'). Such a procedure involves ligation of the umbilical cord as high as possible, preferably at the level of the external cervical os, and leaving the placenta of the aborted/delivered fetus *in situ*. The cervix then usually contracts while the pregnancy continues under close supervision.[50]

This heroic intervention is primarily used to salvage the remaining fetus(es) from the dismal outcome associated with extreme prematurity. The most serious concern is the fear of infection that may have caused the expulsion of the first fetus. Nevertheless, the literature is replete with cases and small series describing prolongation of the pregnancy after expulsion of the first fetus.

The following three points have been raised since the first reports on delayed interval delivery.

Firstly, in selected cases, the attempt to prolong the rest of the pregnancy may be justified,[51] since even modest prolongation at critical gestational ages can improve neonatal survival.[52] The selection criteria remain unclear. However, obviously, this daring intervention must be reserved for 'premium' pregnancies or for women with a history of infertility.[51]

Secondly, the prognosis is not bright. Although some studies show favorable outcome, this may reflect 'reporting bias', whereby failures remain unpublished.[53] Even if pregnancy is prolonged by several weeks, the outcome, in terms of risk of neurologic disability, is not favorable if the first twin was delivered at around 20 weeks. In other words, the time gained may save the retained fetus from mortality, but not from prematurity-related morbidity.[54,55] In a retrospective analysis of 80 multiple pregnancies with the birth of one child at a gestational age of 16–31 weeks, van Doorn et al[54] were able to postpone the delivery of the second (and third) infant in 10 out of 15 attempts, with a mean delay of 12 days, and a mean gestational age at the delivery of the remaining fetuses of 27 5/7 weeks. There was no difference in outcome between the first-born and the retained infant when the procedure was performed after 28 weeks. A recent US study found that asynchronous delivery occurred at a rate of 0.14 per 1000 births, mainly (86%) as a result of second-trimester rupture of membranes. The mean gestational age of the first delivered fetus was 21 ± 2.0 weeks and the median latency 2 days (range <1–70 days). Of the 19 retained fetuses, two died *in utero*, 10 died between birth and day 57 of life, and seven (37%) survived until hospital discharge. Six of the survivors had major prematurity-related sequelae, and only one (5%) was discharged without major consequences. More than half of the mothers suffered infectious morbidity, including one case of septic shock.[55]

Thirdly, the exact protocol for delayed deliveries has not been established. After the birth of the first infant, most practitioners keep the patient on bed rest until the pregnancy is completed, under close observation for signs of impending infection. Prophylactic antibiotics and tocolysis are the mainstay of therapy. There is dispute about the role of cervical cerclage. A survey of seven case series that previously identified all delayed interval deliveries found that despite routine prophylactic use of broad-spectrum antibiotics, intrauterine infection occurred after the first delivery in 36% of the cases. The incidence of maternal sepsis was 4.9%. The survey further indicated that cerclage was associated with a longer latency period than in cases without cerclage (median, 26 vs 9 days). The cerclage did not significantly increase the risk of intrauterine infection.[56] Interestingly, patients who already had a cerclage had shorter latency intervals.

In summary, the data indicate that delayed interval delivery is a feasible procedure and may prolong pregnancy beyond the limit of viability. Naturally, it should not be attempted without full disclosure to the patient of the serious maternal and fetal risks. These should be included in the patient's written informed consent in considerable detail.

Delivery of discordant twins

Significant intertwin size differences, per se, do not indicate cesarean section.[57] Nonetheless, as discussed elsewhere, discordance is an argument against vaginal delivery of vertex–nonvertex twins in whom twin B is significantly larger than twin A.

Delivery of monochorionic twins

Monochorionic (MC) twins deserve special consideration for three reasons. The first concerns the MC-diamniotic variety with or without the twin–twin transfusion syndrome (TTTS). To date, despite extensive research on antepartum management of TTTS, the preferential mode of delivery has not been determined. In the case of treated or untreated TTTS, it would seem that the burden of labor and delivery should not be imposed on these twins, who may be either seriously anemic (donors) or have decompensated cardiac function (recipient).

Another concern is the association of MC twinning with bizarre anomalies. One example is the delivery of the acardiac, acephalic twin (the so-called twin reversed arterial perfusion sequence (TRAP)) (Figure 26.3). The umbilical cord of the acardiac, acephalic twin is usually very short, and the diameters of this ovoid-shaped mass often are larger than the pelvic outlet or the 10–12-cm uterine incision performed at cesarean section. Accordingly, because extraction might prove traumatic and cause rupture of cord and exsanguination of the normal ('pump') twin, it seems reasonable to seek the welfare of the normal twin first. This may be accomplished only through cesarean section. Thus, after the uterine incision and the delivery of the normal twin, there is no rush to deliver the acardiac,

acephalic mass. Sometimes, despite the elastic nature of the mass, extraction through a narrow incision may be difficult. It is advisable to have a good grip on the mass in order to perform a controlled, slow delivery. Care must be taken to avoid lateral extension of the uterine incision toward the uterine arteries. One may use a 'corkscrew' device attached into the mass in order have a firm grasp and a safe extraction. The cutting of a 'smile' incision into the lower uterine segment is often warranted.

Another problem is the delivery of conjoined twins. In such rare circumstances, and particularly if the twins are to be spared a traumatic and destructive birth, cesarean section is preferred. Often, a classical incision is required for a safe dual delivery.

A matter of concern is the delivery of MC-monoamniotic twins (MA). Before the era of sonography, very few MA twins survived, because the diagnosis was not made in a timely manner. Cord entanglement is almost invariably present and may occur as early as week 12 of pregnancy. When such entanglement becomes sufficiently tight, one or both twins die (Figure 26.4). For many authorities, this 'ticking bomb' situation warrants delivery at 32 weeks, even without proving lung maturity. The wisdom of this protocol was questioned[52] by a series of 17 sets of MA twins delivered after 30 weeks with at least one twin still alive. The risks of early delivery in these pregnancies appear to outweigh the risk of fetal death. The argument used in defending this latter view is that twins of over 30 weeks' gestational age are too large to move around in the uterine cavity and are therefore unlikely to tighten the entangled cords. Most authors hold that the balance of the risks is in favor of delivery when pregnancy reaches 32 weeks.[58,59]

Labor induction and augmentation

About 20% of twin gestations may require induction of labor for fetal and/or maternal reasons. However, the overdistended

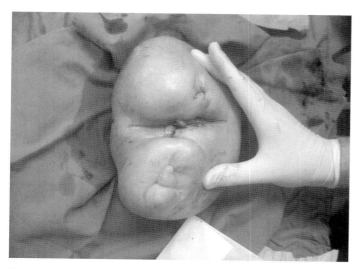

Figure 26.3 Acardiac, acephalic twin. The shortest diameter may be larger than the uterine incision, causing difficult extraction during cesarean section.

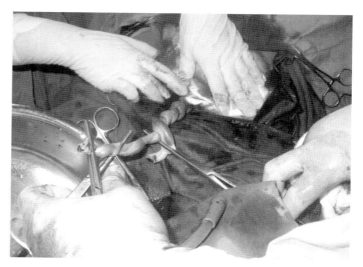

Figure 26.4 Cord entanglement in case of monoamniotic twins seen at cesarean section.

uterus is a relative contraindication for labor induction by means that may cause uterine hyperstimulation. Although pregnancy is often terminated by cesarean section, it seems that unfavorable cervical condition is no impediment for trial of labor in appropriate candidates. There is a report describing the effective use of an intrauterine balloon catheter for the induction of labor in carefully selected cases.[60]

The conflicting results in the older literature related to oxytocin induction or augmentation[61,62] were questioned in a recent study of 62 twin gestations matched with singleton controls.[63] Women with twin pregnancies and those with singletons responded similarly regarding maximum needed oxytocin dosage, time from oxytocin administration to delivery, and successful vaginal deliveries (90% in both groups).

Defining 'term' for twins

The discussion about the definition of 'term' in twins has been revitalized in the last few years. Since 'term' occurs earlier in twins than in singletons, one may argue that twins delivered later are exposed to risks associated with post-term pregnancy. This concept explains the increased risk of cerebral palsy observed in twins weighing more than 2500 g or delivered after 37 weeks.[64] The following lines of evidence suggest that 'term' occurs in twin pregnancies at 37–38 weeks:[64] (1) statistical deductions shows that the proportion of twins born after 38 weeks is similar to that of singletons born after 40 weeks; (2) growth curves of twins do not demonstrate a significant increase in size after 37 week (Figure 26.5); (3) fetal pulmonary and neurologic maturity is achieved by completed week 37; (4) perinatal mortality and morbidity rates decrease until 36 weeks but increase again thereafter.

In summary, ample circumstantial evidence supports the contention that twins should be delivered during week 38 of gestation.[65]

Delivery of triplets

Triplet delivery is more complex than that of twins. Therefore, the abdominal route is generally preferred.[45] However, it should be realized that in some centers the option of vaginal delivery of triplets has never been discarded.[66]

As the number of triplets increased worldwide due to the epidemic of multiple births,[1] and with the advent of sonography, fewer cases of triplets were misdiagnosed, and more centers gained experience with more triplets in a shorter time span[66-74] (Figure 26.6).

Delivery of triplets, by either route, is a logistic endeavor. As each of the infants deserves its own immediate postpartum care, there must be three neonatology teams. The obstetric team must include at least two operators, supported by an anesthesiologist. Including the midwives and nurses, a triplet delivery may require as many as 15–20 persons. The logistics involved in recruiting the necessary staff may be difficult. As the time of spontaneous birth cannot be predicted, a planned,

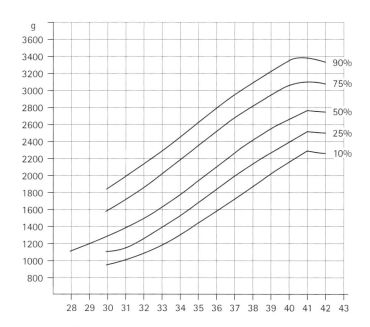

Figure 26.5 The average rate of growth of twins during the third trimester of gestation. Horizontal line: gestational age in weeks; vertical line: birth weight in grams. (Adapted from Bazsó J. et al. Ikermagzatok súlynövekedése a 28–42. terhességi hetekben. Magy Noorv Lapja 1969; 32: 248.)

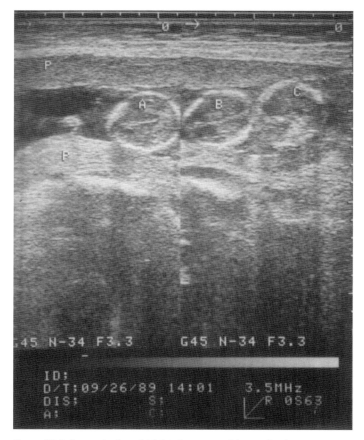

Figure 26.6 Demonstration of triplets by sonographic examination at 17 weeks' gestation.

daytime, elective cesarean section offers the simplest solution to the logistic problem.

Epilogue

And it came to pass in the time of her travail, that, behold, twins were in her womb. And it came to pass, when she travailed, that the one put out his hand: and the midwife took and bound upon his hand a scarlet thread, saying, This came out first. And it came to pass, as he drew back his hand, that, behold, his brother came out: and she said, How has thou broken forth? this breach be upon thee ... And afterward came out his brother, that had the scarlet thread upon his hand.' (Gen. 38:27–30)

The description of the delivery of Pharez and Zarah is a vivid documentation of the complexity of twin birth.[75] The midwife must have been experienced since she knew the diagnosis of twins intrapartum; otherwise, she could not have been ready to apply the scarlet thread to the firstborn. This biblical narrative summarizes the concept of the delivery of multiples: good clinical judgment and skills.

Generally speaking, cesarean section is the simplest and most efficient way to deliver multiples. This statement is especially true for a 'premium' pregnancy. In any particular case, the fact that vaginal delivery is *permissible* makes little sense if the operator is inexperienced in breech delivery. With training opportunities diminishing, the admission of lack of expertise should cause no embarrassment even for fully qualified obstetricians.

References

1. Blickstein I, Keith LG. The spectrum of iatrogenic multiple pregnancy. In: Blickstein I, Keith LG (eds), Iatrogenic Multiple Pregnancy: Clinical Implications, p. 1. Parthenon: New York, 2001.
2. Martin JA, Hamilton BE, Sutton PD et al. Births: final data for 2002. Natl Vital Stat Rep 2003; 52: 1.
3. Blickstein I. Motherhood at or beyond the edge of reproductive age. Int J Fertil Wom Med 2003; 48: 17.
4. Loos R, Derom C, Vlietinck R et al. The East Flanders Prospective Twin Survey (Belgium): a population-based register. Twin Res 1998; 1: 167.
5. Blickstein I. Cesarean section for all twins? J Perinat Med 2000; 28: 169.
6. Minkoff H, Chervenak F. Elective primary cesarean delivery. N Engl J Med 2003; 348: 946.
7. Minkoff H, Powderly KR, Chervenak F et al. Ethical dimensions of elective primary cesarean delivery. Obstet Gynecol 2004; 103: 387.
8. Hannah ME, Hannah WJ, Hewson SA et al. Planned caesarean section versus planned vaginal birth for breech presentation at term: a randomised multicentre trial. Term Breech Trial Collaborative Group. Lancet 2000; 356: 1375.
9. Su M, McLeod L, Ross S et al. Term Breech Trial Collaborative Group. Factors associated with adverse perinatal outcome in the Term Breech Trial. Am J Obstet Gynecol 2003; 189: 740.
10. Blickstein I, Zalel Y, Weissman A. Cesarean delivery of the second twin after the vaginal birth of the first twin – misfortune or mismanagement? Acta Genet Med Gemellol 1991; 40: 389.
11. Ananth CV, Joseph KS. Impact of obstetric intervention on trends in perinatal mortality. In: Blickstein I, Keith LG (eds), Multiple Pregnancy: Epidemiology, Gestation, and Perinatal Outcome. (2nd edition). Parthenon: London, 2004, pp 651–9.
12. The National Sentinel Caesarean Section Audit Report. Oct 2001. RCOG Clinical Effectiveness Support Unit.
13. Blickstein I. Maternal mortality in twin gestations. J Reprod Med 1997; 42: 680.
14. Hogle KL, Hutton EK, McBrien KA et al. Cesarean delivery for twins: a systematic review and meta-analysis. Am J Obstet Gynecol 2003; 188: 220.
15. Blickstein I, Smith-Levitin M. Twinning and twins. In: Chervenak FA, Kurjak A (eds), Current Perspectives on the Fetus as a Patient, p. 507. Parthenon: London, 1996.
16. Redick LF. Anesthesia for twin delivery. Clin Perinatol 1988; 15: 107.
17. Williams KP, Galerneau F. Intrapartum influences on cesarean delivery in multiple gestation. Acta Obstet Gynecol Scand 2003; 82: 241.
18. Ananth CV, Smulian JC, Demissie K et al. Placental abruption among singleton and twin births in the United States: risk factor profiles. Am J Epidemiol 2001; 153: 771.
19. Kurzel RB, Claridad L, Lampley EC. Cesarean section for the second twin. J Reprod Med 1997; 42: 767.
20. Leung TY, Tam WH, Leung TN et al. Effect of twin-to-twin delivery interval on umbilical cord blood gas in the second twin. Br J Obstetrics Gynaecol 2002; 109: 63.
21. Erdemoglu E, Mungan T, Tapisiz OL et al. Effect of inter-twin delivery time on Apgar scores of the second twin. Aust N Z J Obstet Gynaecol 2003; 43: 203.
22. Pons JC, Dommergues M, Ayoubi JM et al. Delivery of the second twin: comparison of two approaches. Eur J Obstet Gynecol Reprod Biol 2002; 104: 32.
23. Blickstein I, Schwartz Z, Lancet M et al. Vaginal delivery of the second twin in breech presentation. Obstet Gynecol 1987; 69: 774.
24. Houlihan C, Knuppel RA. Intrapartum management of multiple gestations. Clin Perinatol 1996; 23: 91.
25. Chervenak FA, Johnson RE, Berkowitz RL et al. Is routine cesarean section necessary for vertex-breech and vertex-transverse twin gestations? Am J Obstet Gynecol 1984; 148: 1.
26. Colon J, Apuzzio JJ, Evans H et al. Obstetric considerations of premium iatrogenic multiple pregnancy. In: Blickstein I, Keith LG (eds) Iatrogenic Multiple Pregnancy, p. 117. Parthenon: Cranford, 2000.
27. Fishman A, Grubb DK, Kovacs BW. Vaginal delivery of the nonvertex second twin. Am J Obstet Gynecol 1993; 168: 861.
28. Gocke SE, Nageotte MP, Garite T et al. Management of the nonvertex second twin: primary cesarean section, external

version, or primary breech extraction. Am J Obstet Gynecol 1989; 161: 111.

29. Hutton EK, Hannah ME, Barrett J. Use of external cephalic version for breech pregnancy and mode of delivery for breech and twin pregnancy: a survey of Canadian practitioners. J Obstet Gynaecol Can 2002; 24: 804.

30. Barrett J. Randomised controlled trial for twin delivery. BMJ 2003; 326: 448.

31. Dufour P, Vinatier D, Vanderstichele S et al. Intravenous nitroglycerin for internal podalic version of the second twin in transverse lie. Obstet Gynecol 1998; 92: 416.

32. Suonio S, Huttunen M. Puerperal endometritis after abdominal twin delivery. Acta Obstet Gynecol Scand 1994; 73: 313.

33. Alexander JM, Gilstrap LC 3rd, Cox SM et al. The relationship of infection to method of delivery in twin pregnancy. Am J Obstet Gynecol 1997; 177: 1063.

34. Blickstein I, Weissman A, Ben-Hur H et al. Vaginal delivery for breech-vertex twins. J Reprod Med 1993; 38: 879.

35. Blickstein I, Goldman RD, Kuperminc M. Delivery of breech-first twins: a multicenter retrospective study. Obstet Gynecol 2000; 95: 37.

36. Rydhstrom H, Cullberg G. Pregnancies with growth-retarded twins in breech-vertex presentation at increased risk for entanglement during delivery. J Perinat Med 1990; 18: 45.

37. Sevitz H, Merrell DA. The use of a beta-sympathomimetic drug in locked twins. Case report. Br J Obstet Gynaecol 1981; 88: 76.

38. Johansson BG, Helgadottir EA. A case of locked twins successfully treated with nitroglycerin sublingually before manual reposition and vaginal delivery. Acta Obstet Gynecol Scand 2001; 80: 275.

39. Iffy L, Apuzzio JJ, Cohen-Addad N et al. Abdominal rescue after entrapment of the aftercoming head. Am J Obstet Gynecol 1986: 154: 623.

40. Swartjes JM, Bleker OP, Schutte MF. The Zavanelli maneuver applied to locked twins. Am J Obstet Gynecol 1992; 166: 532.

41. Wen SW, Fung KF, Oppenheimer L et al. Occurrence and predictors of cesarean delivery for the second twin after vaginal delivery of the first twin. Obstet Gynecol 2004; 103: 413.

42. Persad VL, Baskett TF, O'Connell CM et al. Combined vaginal-cesarean delivery of twin pregnancies. Obstet Gynecol 2001; 98: 1032.

43. Sansergret A, Bujold E, Gaauthier RJ. Twin delivery after a caesarean: a twelve-year experience. J Obstet Gynecol Can 2003; 25: 294.

44. Delaney T, Young DC. Trial of labour compared to elective caesarean in twin gestations with a previous caesarean delivery. J Obstet Gynecol Can 2003; 25: 289.

45. ACOG Practice Bulletin. Vaginal birth after previous cesarean delivery. No. 54. Obstet Gynecol 2004; 104: 2003.

46. Blickstein I, Goldman RD, Mazkereth R. Risk for one or two very low birth weight twins: a population study. Obstet Gynecol 2000; 96: 400.

47. Shinwell ES, Blickstein I, Lusky A et al. Excess risk of mortality in very low birth weight triplets: a national, population based study. Arch Dis Child Fetal Neonatal Ed. 2003; 88: F36.

48. Shinwell ES, Blickstein I, Lusky A et al. Effect of birth order on neonatal morbidity and mortality among very low birth weight twins: a population based study. Arch Dis Child Fetal Neonatal Ed 2004; 89: F145.

49. Salomon LJ, Duyme M, Rousseau A et al. Periventricular leukomalacia and mode of delivery in twins under 1500 g. J Matern Fetal Neonatal Med 2003; 13: 224.

50. Platt JS, Rosa C. Delayed interval delivery in multiple gestations. Obstet Gynecol Surv 1999; 54: 343.

51. Tzafettas JM, Farmakides G, Delkos D et al. Asynchronous delivery of twins and triplets with an interval period ranging from 48 hours to 19 weeks. Clin Exp Obstet Gynecol 2004; 31: 53.

52. Farkouh LJ, Sabin ED, Heyborne KD et al. Delayed-interval delivery: extended series from a single maternal-fetal medicine practice. Am J Obstet Gynecol 2000; 183: 1499.

53. Fayad S, Bongain A, Holhfeld P et al. Delayed delivery of second twin: a multicentre study of 35 cases. Eur J Obstet Gynecol Reprod Biol 2003; 109: 16.

54. van Doorn HC, van Wezel-Meijler G, van Geijn HP et al. Delayed interval delivery in multiple pregnancies. Is optimism justified? Acta Obstet Gynecol Scand 1999; 78: 710.

55. Livingston JC, Livingston LW, Ramsey R et al. Second-trimester asynchronous multifetal delivery results in poor perinatal outcome. Obstet Gynecol 2004; 103: 77.

56. Zhang J, Johnson CD, Hoffman M. Cervical cerclage in delayed interval delivery in a multifetal pregnancy: a review of seven case series. Eur J Obstet Gynecol Reprod Biol 2003; 108: 126.

57. Blickstein I. The definition, diagnosis, and management of growth-discordant twins: an international census survey. Acta Genet Med Gemellol 1991; 40: 345.

58. Carr SR, Aronson MP, Coustan DR. Survival rates of monoamniotic twins do not decrease after 30 weeks' gestation. Am J Obstet Gynecol 1990; 163: 719.

59. Sau AK, Langford K, Elliott C et al. Monoamniotic twins: what should be the optimal antenatal management? Twin Res 2003; 6: 270.

60. Manor M, Blickstein I, Ben-Arie A et al. Case series of labor induction in twin gestations with an intrauterine balloon catheter. Gynecol Obstet Invest 1999; 47: 244.

61. Leroy F. Oxytocin treatment in twin pregnancy labour. Acta Genet Med Gemellol 1979; 28: 303.

62. Price JH, Marivate M. Induction of labour in twin pregnancy. S Afr Med J 1986; 70: 163.

63. Fausett MB, Barth WH Jr, Yoder BA et al. Oxytocin labor stimulation of twin gestations: effective and efficient. Obstet Gynecol 1997; 90: 202.

64. Blickstein I. Is it possible to reduce the incidence of neurolog-ical complications in multiple pregnancies? In: Carrera JM, Chervenak FA, Kurjak A (eds), Controversies in Perinatal Medicine. Studies on the Fetus as a Patient, p. 161. Parthenon: New York, 2003.

65. Dodd JM, Crowther CA. Elective delivery of women with a twin pregnancy from 37 weeks' gestation. Cochrane Database Syst Rev 2003; CD003582.

66. Pheiffer EL, Golan A. Triplet pregnancy. A 10-year review of cases at Baragwanath Hospital. S Afr Med J 1979; 55: 843.

67. Ron-El R, Caspi E, Schreyer P et al. Triplet and quadruplet pregnancies and management. Obstet Gynecol 1981; 57: 458.
68. Thiery M, Kermans G, Derom R. Triplet and higher-order births: what is the optimal delivery route? Acta Genet Med Gemellol 1988; 37: 89.
69. Feingold M, Cetrulo C, Peters M et al. Mode of delivery in multiple birth of higher order. Acta Genet Med Gemellol 1988; 37: 105.
70. Clarke JP, Roman JD. A review of 19 sets of triplets: the positive results of vaginal delivery. Aust N Z J Obstet Gynaecol 1994; 34: 50.
71. Wildschut HI, van Roosmalen J, van Leeuwen E et al. Planned abdominal compared with planned vaginal birth in triplet pregnancies. Br J Obstet Gynaecol 1995; 102: 292.
72. Bakos O. Birth in triplet pregnancies. Vaginal delivery – how often is it possible? Acta Obstet Gynecol Scand 1998; 77: 845.
73. Alamia V Jr, Royek AB, Jaekle RK et al. Preliminary experience with a prospective protocol for planned vaginal delivery of triplet gestations. Am J Obstet Gynecol 1998; 179: 1133.
74. Ziadeh SM. Perinatal outcome in 41 sets of triplets. Gynecol Obstet Invest 2000; 50: 162–5.
75. Blickstein I, Gurewitsch ED. Biblical twins. Obstet Gynecol 1998; 91: 632.

27 Birth injuries

Abraham Golan and Shimon Ginath

A substantial risk to the mother always existed at parturition. In the not-too-distant past, parturition was a very dangerous event in a woman's life, and many babies lost their mothers at birth. With the improvement of obstetric services, availability of blood transfusions, antibiotics, modern anesthetic methods, and the increasing popularity of hospital deliveries, maternal death has almost disappeared. There is a tendency today to abandon potentially traumatic vaginal deliveries and use cesarean sections whenever difficulties are expected, for the sake of both mother and fetus. However, maternal morbidity and injury during labor unfortunately still exist, especially in underdeveloped parts of the world where medical surveillance of deliveries is less effective than in the more developed countries. Iatrogenic or elective injury, such as episiotomy, may be still needed, sometimes in order to avoid more extensive birth trauma.

Elective procedures

Episiotomy

Although its popularity has been declining, episiotomy is still the most common obstetric operation.[1–17] Since it is described at length in another chapter, it is not discussed here any further.

Symphysiotomy

First used by Sigault in Paris in 1777, this operation consists of division of the symphysis pubis in order to increase the pelvic diameters and allow vaginal delivery in minor degrees of cephalopelvic disproportion.[18] The operation is performed with the patient in the lithotomy position, with both legs supported by an assistant on each side, limiting abduction and external rotation to avoid further accidental trauma to the pelvis. The bladder is emptied, and the catheter is left in place during the operation. After infiltration with 1% lidocaine solution, a short midline longitudinal incision of the skin over the symphysis is made, and the symphysis pubis is divided with a long, solid scalpel from behind forward and from above downward, introducing the knife behind the symphysis pubis at its upper border and keeping strictly to the midline. The surgeon uses a finger in the vagina to displace the urethra and the bladder neck laterally well to one side of the symphysis before cutting. The assistants continue to support the legs during the assisted delivery. A large episiotomy is performed. Traction is always directed away from the symphysis. A firm strapping or binding of the legs is applied for the support of the pelvis for 1 week.

In the majority of cases, proper healing takes place, and the pelvis regains its former stability. However, complications such as injury to the urethra, stress incontinence, infection, hemorrhage, and pelvic instability have been reported.

This operation probably has no place in developed countries nowadays when operating room facilities and personnel are readily available whenever necessary. However, it is still performed in rural areas in Africa and other underdeveloped regions. It has, in these cases, the advantages of avoiding a cesarean section for a moderately contracted pelvis and not weakening the uterus for future pregnancy. It also permanently increases the pelvic dimensions at all levels, allowing easier subsequent vaginal delivery.[19]

Injury to the perineum and vulva

Some degree of injury to the soft tissues of the external part of the birth canal is almost inevitable in primiparas and sometimes even in multiparas. The reasons for the injury of the perineum and vulva are, in general, quite similar:

(1) large fetal measurements, such as a large head or broad shoulders, occipitoposterior rotation, and face presentation
(2) precipitated labor and delivery, which do not allow gradual dilation of the tissues
(3) narrow bony passage due either to narrow subpubic angle or to a straight sacrum
(4) narrow soft-tissue passage, as in very young parturients, or extremely high perineum, whether primary or due to previous repair

(5) hasty or otherwise improper use of instrumentation or manual techniques

(6) insufficient control of the delivery due to an uncooperative patient or technical difficulties.

Injury to the vulva

The most frequent lacerations of the vulva are longitudinal on either side of the labium minor. They are usually shallow and bleed only slightly. Although many obstetricians leave them to heal spontaneously, poor wound approximation has been demonstrated in women who had not been sutured.[20] Therefore, it is preferable to close even a small superficial wound with a few stitches of rapidly absorbed polyglactin (Vicryl Rapide) 2-0, threaded on an atraumatic needle.

Periurethral lacerations are another variety of vulvar injury. These should always be sutured after inspection of the urethral orifice. In deeper lacerations, care has to be taken not to damage the urethra during repair. This can be done by the insertion of a catheter. Longitudinal laceration of the upper part of the vulva may include the clitoris or its preputium. Such a tear is often accompanied by bleeding. The ligation of all actively bleeding vessels is essential before the repair of the tear itself; otherwise, a hematoma will arise or continuous bleeding will require a secondary repair. Proper analgesia and use of very fine suture materials of Vicryl Rapide are important in this particular area due to its extensive vascularization and innervation.

Another site of vulvar lacerations is along the edge of the perineum in a transverse direction. These are not very common by themselves and sometimes represent a continuation of labial lacerations. More frequent is damage to this part of the vulva in combination with either a vaginal or a perineal tear. In most cases, its direction is longitudinal into the vagina, down to the perineum, or both.

Injury to the perineum

Tears of the perineum are longitudinal, extend from the vulva, and can reach the rectal canal.[17] It is of major importance to recognize the full extent of the damage, since the repair must be meticulous in order to avoid unnecessary complications. They are classified into four grades according to their extent:[21]

(1) *First-degree tear.* This is a short tear involving only the upper portion of the perineal body and the superficial tissues.
(2) *Second-degree tear.* This involves the whole length of the perineum and includes the perineal body. It reaches the sphincter ani, but does not involve it.
(3) *Third-degree tear.* This includes the anal sphincter, but does not extend into the anorectal canal.
(4) *Fourth-degree tear.* Sometimes called a complete perineal tear, this tear extends into the anorectal canal.

As this classification does not include the depth of external anal sphincter rupture or the involvement of the internal sphincter, it has been modified[22] as follows to allow differentiation between injuries to the external anal sphincter, the internal anal sphincter and the anal epithelium:

(1) *first:* injury to the skin only
(2) *second:* injury to the perineum involving perineal muscles but not the anal sphincter
(3) *third:* injury to perineum involving the anal sphincter complex
   (a) less than 50% of external anal sphincter thickness torn
   (b) more than 50% of external anal sphincter thickness torn
   (c) internal anal sphincter torn
(4) *fourth:* injury to perineum involving the anal sphincter complex and anal epithelium.

The following are principles of repair:[23]

- Suture as soon as possible after delivery to reduce bleeding and risk of infection.
- Check equipment and count swabs prior to commencing the procedure and count again after completion of the repair.
- Good lighting is essential to visualize and identify the structures involved.
- Ask for consultation if in doubt regarding the extent of trauma or structures involved.
- Difficult trauma should be repaired by an experienced operator under regional or general anaesthesia. Insert an indwelling catheter for 24 hours to prevent urinary retention.
- Ensure good anatomic alignment of the wound and give consideration to cosmetic results.
- Rectal examination after completing the repair will ensure that suture material has not been accidentally inserted through the rectal mucosa.
- After completion of the repair, inform the woman regarding the extent of trauma and discuss pain relief, diet, hygiene, and the importance of pelvic-floor exercises.

The repair of a first-degree tear is simple since the damage is superficial. After the wound is cleansed, hemostasis is ensured, and the edges of the wound are approximated with rapidly absorbed polyglactin (Vicryl Rapide) 2-0.

In second-degree tears, after hemostasis is secured, the torn perineal body exposes the edges of the two pillars of the pubococcygeal portion of the levator ani, and often the outer wall of the rectum becomes visible. The repair includes three or four interrupted sutures of rapidly absorbed polyglactin (Vicryl Rapide) 2-0, approximating the two separate portions of the levators. If the rectum is exposed, these sutures have to include its outer layer. Special care has to be taken not to enter the rectal cavity. After the tying of these sutures, the perineal body is approximated with interrupted sutures. Finally, the skin is closed with another layer of absorbable sutures (Vicryl Rapide 2-0). In patients with a thin subcutaneous layer, the two external layers, namely, the perineal body and fascia, and the skin may be sutured in one layer. The proper closure of the separated levators is important, since inadequate repair may be followed by rectocele at a later stage of the patient's life.

The repair of a third-degree tear includes the stages of a second-degree repair, preceded by the repair of the anal sphincter. In order to reunite the sphincter, its two edges have to be exposed. This is not always an easy task, since the torn edges usually retract. Nevertheless, they have to be pulled out from their retracted position on the sides of the anus in the direction of the retracted end, which is then elevated into view. It is essential to recognize the tissue and hold its whole thickness to achieve a good result. After both edges of the sphincter ani are exposed and identified, they are approximated, and the effect of this on anal closure is checked. Two or three interrupted, rapidly absorbed polyglactin (Vicryl Rapide) 2-0, sutures approximate the two edges of the sphincter, and another suture of rapidly absorbed polyglactin (Vicryl Rapide) 2-0, approximating the skin immediately above the anus, includes both edges of the sphincter. The repair of a third-degree perineal tear, according to the RCOG classification,[24] requires the following steps. The internal anal sphincter, which appears as a glistening, white, fibrous structure between the rectal mucosa and the external anal sphincter, is closed with continuous, rapidly absorbed polyglactin (Vicryl Rapide) 2-0. The external anal sphincter, which appears as a band of skeletal muscle with a fibrous capsule, can be sutured in an end-to-end manner, as described traditionally. Alternatively, it can be repaired by overlapping the edges of the torn sphincter, using larger surface area of tissue contact between the two torn ends.[25] Although colorectal surgeons prefer to use the overlapping method to repair the sphincter remote from delivery, the only two randomized, controlled studies showed similar outcomes in comparison of the primary overlap with approximation repair of third-degree obstetric tears.[26,27] It was recommended to use polydioxanone sulfate (PDS) 2-0 suture, a delayed absorbable monofilament suture, to allow the sphincter ends adequate time to scar together.[25] The repair of the sphincter is followed by that of the perineum, as described in the second-degree tear repair.

The first step in the repair of a fourth-degree tear is the suturing of the rectal mucosa. This is performed by approximating the torn edges of the rectum by external sutures through the submucosa. With this method, the needle does not enter the rectal lumen, and later contamination and disturbance of healing of the wound are minimal. Rapidly absorbed polyglactin (Vicryl Rapide) 4-0 is usually used. This layer of the rectal sutures is buried by the second layer of repair, the levators, and the procedure is accomplished by repair of the sphincter and the external layers of the perineum as described.

Many deliveries are performed under epidural anesthesia, and this is also efficient for perineal repair. Alternatively, local anesthesia can be used in first and second-degree tears, while general anesthesia is preferred in the more extensive variations. Postoperative care includes analgesics, prophylactic antibiotic therapy, sitz bath, and stool softeners, which are continued for about 2 weeks after the repair. Diet is normal, and no special local care is given except for the sitz bath. The patient is discharged when full anal control is ensured. Some stool softeners may be needed for a few weeks.

All women who have had a third- and fourth-degree tear repaired should be offered a follow-up examination at 6–12 months by a gynecologist or a colorectal surgeon. Endoanal sonography and anorectal manometry may prove useful as additional means for diagnosis and follow-up.[24]

Prevention of perineal tears

Many authors believe that the repair of an episiotomy, like that of any other surgical incision, is simpler than that of an uncontrolled tear. This classical belief has been challenged recently.[28] The preventive measures include allowance of gradual dilation of the tissues, controlled use of instruments, and, last but not least, assurance of good cooperation of the patient during delivery.

A variety of other preventive measures have been suggested by midwives in an attempt to protect against perineal trauma.[29] Kegel exercises, taking vitamins C and E to improve skin elasticity, avoiding the use of soap on the perineum during the last few weeks to avoid dryness of the skin's natural emollients, and prenatal perineal massage are all of questionable value. Although two randomized, controlled studies found some advantages for the use of antenatal perineal massage in reducing the incidence of second- or third-degree tear,[30,31] a third one concluded that perineal massage in the second stage of labor had no effect on the likelihood of an intact perineum, perineal trauma, pain, or subsequent sexual, urinary or fecal outcomes.[32]

Subsequent vaginal delivery may worsen anal incontinence. All women who had a third- and fourth-degree tear in their previous pregnancy should be counseled regarding the risk of developing anal incontinence or worsening symptoms with subsequent vaginal delivery.[24]

Vaginal lacerations

During labor and delivery, the vaginal tissues are under strain, as they are stretched and compressed at the same time or alternately. This is a natural occurrence, and if labor progress is normal, acute or permanent damage to the tissues is minimal. However, the following obstetric situations or interventions predispose to damage of the vagina:

(1) overt lacerations at different locations often combined with tears of other adjacent structures (cervix, perineum, and vulva)
(2) hematoma formation due to submucous tear of blood vessels.

Lacerations of the vagina occur more often with precipitated labor when gradual dilation of the tissue cannot occur, in cases of difficult vaginal delivery combined with a large fetus or pathologic presentations, in cases of instrumental delivery, and in prolonged labor when prolonged pressure on the tissues makes them edematous and brittle.

One of the rarest forms of vaginal laceration, namely, colporrhexis, or vault rupture, is a tear of the posterior cul-de-sac, with protrusion of intestines into the vagina. Colporrhexis necessitates careful repair under general anesthesia and excellent visualization. The intestine has to be carefully cleansed before replacing it into the peritoneal cavity, and the vaginal opening is then sutured with rapidly absorbed polyglactin (Vicryl Rapide) 2-0.

Longitudinal tears of the vagina are common. They follow the axis of the vagina, more frequently at the posterior wall. They can occur at normal spontaneous deliveries, but are more frequent in instrumental deliveries and prolonged and difficult labors. All detectable tears should be carefully visualized and sutured, care being taken for good hemostasis. The initial stitch must be taken well above the upper edge of the tear in order to include any retracted vessel that may bleed later if not closed. Vaginal tears combined with laceration of other structures may occur at both ends of the vagina.

Cervical tears may extend laterally and include the lateral fornix. This form may cause severe bleeding, since a branch of the uterine artery may be included. Repair of tears in this variety needs full operative conditions – anesthesia and perfect exposure by assistants and lights. Possible occult bleeding into the parametria has to be kept in mind. The vaginal tear is sutured from the side toward the cervix, followed by full repair of the cervical tear. Care must be taken not to damage the ureter, which can be in close proximity to an extensive tear.

Spontaneous vulvovaginal and combined perineovulvovaginal tears, and vaginal tear as an extension of episiotomy are another variety of vaginal lacerations. The same principles of treatment already described are applied.

Rarely, multiple vaginal abrasions and lacerations occur. Some of these can be sutured, but the mucosa can be so extensively damaged that suturing is impossible. In such cases, the best way to overcome the problem is tight tamponade of the vagina after inspection of the cervix and the fornices. The packing remains in place for up to 24 hours. Usually, good healing follows. A Foley catheter can be left in the uterine cavity to facilitate drainage.

Most vaginal lacerations heal quickly to full anatomic and functional integrity. One less noticed complication which can disturb the patient during the puerperium or later is granulation tissue formation. This tends to form at the edges of mucosal surfaces that have not been united. Its symptoms are spotting, contact bleeding, discharge, and, when sexual activity is resumed, dyspareunia. This minor complication can cause much discomfort. At the postnatal examination, small foci of granulation may be overlooked. Symptomatic patients are treated for vaginitis, bleedings are attributed to cervical erosion or uterine dysfunction, and the dyspareunia is often accepted as a 'normal' result of childbirth.

Careful search for granulation tissues must be a part of any postpuerperal examination. The vaginal parts of an episiotomy, sutured vaginal tears, and the complete surface of the vagina, even where no suturing was performed, must be examined. The treatment is simple; electrocautery as an office procedure, without the need of anesthesia, gives excellent results.

Hematoma formation

Hematomas may occur in the vulva, vagina, and, much less frequently, subperitoneally above the pelvic floor. Most hematomas become evident after delivery; however, rarely, the vaginal type may start during labor and disturb the progress of childbirth. If this is the case and correct diagnosis is made, incision and drainage of the hematoma may enable birth, but the lacerated vessels must be sutured immediately afterward.

As stated, hematomas usually become evident after delivery, but since their symptoms and signs develop slowly, most of them are discovered only hours later. The exception to this is the very rare instance of hematoma caused by laceration of a large vessel, often above the pelvic floor, which leads to blood volume decrease of significant degree, causing anemia and shock before giving any local signs or symptoms. The diagnosis of this situation is based mainly on the blood loss evident in progressive anemia and development of hypotension and shock, without any external loss through the birth canal. Sometimes some bulging of the fornix or parametria on the affected side may be detectable on vaginal palpation, accompanied by tenderness. Hematoma of this kind should be promptly treated, since the blood vessels must be tied. This can be best achieved by laparotomy by the retroperitoneal approach. In cases when the development of the hematoma is slow, it is sometimes self-limited and resolves spontaneously. This is often accompanied by fever due to resorption or infection; therefore, antibiotic treatment is indicated. Persistent fever during the puerperium in the presence of a parametrial mass is an indication for incision and drainage, which is preferentially performed abdominally. A parametrial hematoma may also evolve after cesarean section due to insufficient hemostasis and extravasation of the blood into the parametria.

Vulvar hematomas of smaller extent appear a short time after the completion of delivery. They usually result from incomplete hemostasis at suturing vulvar damage or from pricking of a vein during the procedure of repair. They are usually mild, cause little discomfort, and resolve spontaneously. Less frequently, vulvar hematoma results from a vaginal hematoma which dissects through the loose tissue into the vulvar region. These hematomas are usually unilateral and may reach considerable size if left untreated. They require surgical incision and drainage, and, most important, the torn vessels in the vagina have to be ligated.

The vaginal tissues, including the blood vessels, are under considerable strain during delivery. The tissues are stretched and compressed by the forces of labor and by the passage of the fetus. The congested blood vessels burst easily by pressure or tear in spontaneous delivery, but more often, at instrumental delivery. The hematoma formation usually starts during the second stage of labor, since, at this stage, the vessels are under maximal strain. However, even if ruptured, they are compressed, and blood effusion is slow or nil. After delivery, the intravaginal pressure decreases, and the open vessels, more often veins, start bleeding and cause hematoma formation. The extent of the hematoma and the rate of its growth depend on the location of the torn vessel and its size. Most hematomas remain undetected for a few hours after delivery, until the patient complains about intense pain and a tearing sensation in the vagina, about the rectum, and the perineal region. The pain increases, tenesmus can be felt, and, if the hematoma dissects its way under the bladder, difficulty in urination can be a symptom.

One must be attentive to the patient's complaints and be aware of the possibility of a hematoma formation at any stage of the puerperium. The diagnosis can then be made easily by vaginal and rectal palpation, and immediate treatment implemented. Surgical incision, under anesthesia with good exposure and illumination, facilitates clearing of the clots, after which the wound must be carefully searched for the bleeding vessels. All detectable bleeders must be ligated; however, this is sometimes a difficult task since the damage done by the hematoma itself causes secondary injury to capillaries, leading to diffuse oozing. Electrocoagulation can sometimes be used to overcome some of the difficulty. In some cases, tight vaginal packing for 24 hours may prove the only effective way to overcome the difficulties. Drainage of the wound is usually helpful.

Two additional types of vaginal hematomas must be kept in mind. First, a hematoma may develop in a repaired vaginal tear or episiotomy when hemostasis was inadequate. The open bleeding vessel can be anywhere in the wound, but the most probable site is a retracted vessel at its upper edge. Hence, it is most important to start any vaginal repair (tear or surgical incision) above the upper end of the wound. The usual pitfall causing delay in the diagnosis is that the pain arising from it is attributed to the sutured wound, and patients are given pain relievers and not examined sufficiently.

Second, a rather late form of hematoma formation is due to the delayed burst of a vessel, damaged by pressure necrosis during labor or delivery but bleeding only at a later stage. The symptoms are the same as in the other forms, but their onset is delayed. Thus, hematoma has to be thought of, even if previous vaginal and rectal examinations were normal.

The obstetrician is aware of the dangers of overt bleeding, searches for its cause, and applies treatment. Although occult bleeding is less frequent, the same awareness is necessary, since, if not discovered and treated, it may complicate an otherwise normal childbirth.

Attention is called to any complaint of pain in the vagina, rectum, or perineum, or pressure on the bladder – in cases of both a repaired wound and a woundless delivery – at any stage of the puerperium. Such pain must not be attributed to any cause before a thorough examination of the patient is performed.

Cervical tears

In normal labor, the cervix is gradually dilated, and the passage of the newborn causes only minimal damage that changes the appearance of the cervical os after involution. More severe tears occur when dilation is rapid or forceful, often accompanied by premature pushing of the newborn through an incompletely dilated cervix, as is sometimes the case in breech presentation or with an uncooperative patient. Manual displacement of the cervical edge during labor also causes cervical damage, as does an attempt at instrumental delivery before the cervix is completely dilated.

Scarring due to previous operations or cervical rigidity may also predispose to cervical tears. Special attention must be paid to parturients who had a cervical cerclage during pregnancy. It is customary to remove the McDonald-type cerclage at 37 weeks in order to enable healing of the cervix until labor starts. However, sometimes labor starts before the suture is removed, and the damage may become serious if the suture is not removed instantly. Many cervices are cicatrized or torn after cerclage, and the more worn off they are, the more they tend to tear. In such cases, abdominal delivery may be considered in order to prevent extension of a tear into the uterus or parametria.

Prolonged labor can weaken the cervical structure, and pressure necrosis occurs if a part of the cervix is compressed between the fetal head and the pelvic wall. In modern obstetrics, care is taken to prevent vaginal delivery in unfavorable conditions; thus, this type of injury is rare. Nonetheless, one must be acquainted with its symptoms and treatment.

In most cases, the injury is limited to the vaginal portion of the cervix; however, in some instances, the laceration may extend higher into the isthmic part of the uterus and thus form one of the variants of uterine rupture. Another possible extension is into the vaginal fornix.

The usual direction of a cervical laceration is longitudinal; however, a few cases of circular damage with complete ablation of the cervical ring have also been described. In such a case, if bleeding occurs, an attempt must be made to reconstruct the cervical lip along its entire circumference by approximating the endo- and exocervical mucosal lining, preferably with a continuous buttonhole stitch. However, although the damage is considerable since it usually results from prolonged compression, the lesion may not bleed at all and can be left to heal spontaneously.

Another unusual type of cervical damage can result from careless use of forceps, or of the vacuum cup when it is applied on an elongated part of the cervix and that portion is torn out at the delivery. The repair of such a lesion is a variation or a combination of the repairs of a circular ablation and a longitudinal tear; the tendency to one direction or the other depends on the extent of the absent tissue.

The most common cervical laceration is longitudinal, or radial; it can be single, or even multiple. The frequency of these lesions is higher than those diagnosed after delivery; since some do not bleed, their edges heal spontaneously and are discovered only later at a postnatal examination. The usual location of the radial cervical tear is lateral, although anterior or posterior locations are possible. These are usually connected with instrumental deliveries.

Cervical tear (and/or another lesion of the lower birth canal) should be suspected in any case of persistent bleeding in the presence of a well-contracted uterus. The vaginal canal and the whole circumference of the cervix must be visually explored. At least one but preferably two assistants should be available. In all delivery units, prepared sets containing the necessary instruments should be ready: four broad-bladed retractors at least 10 cm long, six ring forceps or sponge holders, two long needle holders, and two long, surgical tissue forceps.

The retractors are carefully inserted in the vagina and pushed up toward the fornices under visual control. The edge of the cervix is gripped by a ring forceps, and then another is applied about 60° in one direction and one more in the opposite one. The rest are applied successively in the same way; thus, the whole circumference of the cervix is held by the instruments. Any tear thus must become visualized between two forceps, and repaired immediately. The remaining forceps are taken off. The tear is well exposed by pulling the cervix to the opposite direction and toward the vaginal outlet. The suturing must start above the apex of the tear in order to include all retracted blood vessels and muscular tissue. We prefer one layer of interrupted, rapidly absorbed polyglactin (Vicryl Rapide) 2-0 sutures for this kind of repair. Interrupted suturing takes more time but enables good adaptation of tissues and prevents tension (Figure 27.1).

Continuous and especially buttonhole sutures are usually too tight and often cause necrosis, which interferes with unification of the wound edges, resulting in a residual defect that has to be repaired later.

Uterine rupture

Etiology, classification, and prophylaxis

Rupture of the uterus is one of the major catastrophes seen in obstetric practice (Figure 27.2). It carries a high rate of fetal and maternal mortality, of which it still is a major cause in developing countries. In a large series, the rate of uterine rupture was reported as 1:2900–1:4300 deliveries.[33–35] Rupture of an unscarred uterus is a rare event involving 1:17 000 deliveries.[36] In contrast, the reported rate of symptomatic uterine rupture of the scarred uterus in prospective cohort studies was 3.8 per 1000 trials of labor.[37] In a large series of ruptured uteri reported in 1980, there was a distinct difference in both fetal and maternal outcomes between the group with a previously scarred uterus, usually a previous cesarean section scar (approximately one-third of all uterine ruptures), and the group with no previous scarring[38] (Table 27.1).

The majority of reports of unscarred uterine ruptures come from rural areas in developing countries where poor antenatal care and obstetric facilities contribute to the occurrence of this grave complication. Common incriminating factors in previously unscarred uteri are cephalopelvic disproportion and grand multiparity (Table 27.2), but uncontrolled use of oxytocin is probably the leading etiologic factor these days. Special care should be exercised when oxytocin is used in the presence of any predisposing factor, such as grand multiparity, malpresentation, or a previous cesarean section scar, conditions that are relative contraindications to the use of oxytocin. Cephalopelvic disproportion is a major contraindication.

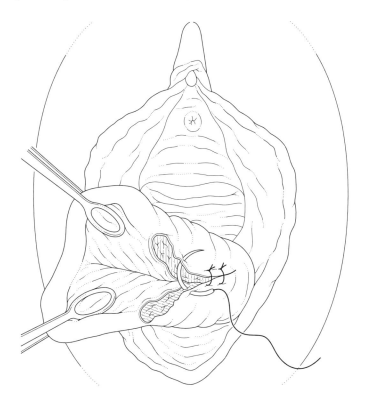

Figure 27.1 Repair of a cervical tear.

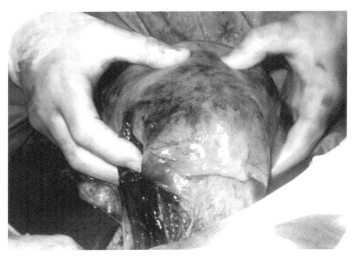

Figure 27.2 Ruptured uterus: unscarred, longitudinal tear.

Table 27.1 Clinical features of uterine rupture

Clinical features	Previously scarred uterus (n = 32)		Unscarred uterus (n = 60)		Total
Tachycardia only	1		4		5
Shock	3	(9%)	24	(40%)	27
Scar (or abdominal) tenderness or pain	9	(28%)	14	(23%)	23
Uterine bleeding	13	(40%)	40	(66%)	53
Hematuria	1		1		2
Cessation of contractions			4		4
Change in fetal position	2		6	(10%)	8
Disappearance of fetal heart sounds	3		17	(28%)	20
Routine examination of scar	9	(28%) } 47%			15
Operation for another reason	6	(19%)			

Reproduced from Golan A, Sandbank O, Rubin A. Rupture of the pregnant uterus. Obstet Gynecol 1980; 56: 549–54[38] with permission from Lippincott Williams & Wilkins.

Abruptio placentae and, in particular, Couvelaire uterus, with its extravasation of blood in the stretched and disrupted uterine wall, may predispose to uterine rupture. In our series, as many as 18% of the unscarred uterine ruptures were associated with abruptio placentae. The use of oxytocin in these patients may be particularly hazardous. One must realize that a patient with shock and tender abdomen, and without audible fetal heart sounds, diagnosed as having abruptio placentae, may have a ruptured uterus.

In our series, about one-third of uterine ruptures occurred after previous cesarean section.[38] A small number of these involved classical cesarean section scars. The incidence of rupture in these longitudinal, upper-segment scars was reported as 2.2–13% as compared to 0–0.5% in lower-segment scars.[39,40] The rupture of the latter usually takes place in labor, whereas a classic scar may rupture during pregnancy.

Uterine rupture after previous scarring due to hysterotomy or uterine perforation at operative hysteroscopy and dilation and curettage has been reported but is uncommon. The same is true of uterine rupture during difficult operative deliveries, malpresentations, and destructive operations, which are hardly seen these days.

Prophylaxis is the main way to fight this catastrophic obstetric complication. Improving medical facilities and antenatal care in rural areas and in developing countries, and implementation of family-planning programs will probably lower the incidence of rupture of the uterus. Great effort must be made in any obstetric unit in diagnosing even minor degrees of cephalopelvic disproportion or malpresentation, and in treating the grand multipara and all patients with suspected abruptio placentae as very high-risk patients. They should be attended and treated in a special high-risk intensive care zone in the labor ward by specially trained personnel. Difficult operative deliveries should be abandoned and replaced by cesarean sections. Vaginal birth after cesarean delivery (VBAC) should be attempted only on a patient who has had a previous transverse, lower-uterine-segment cesarean section for a nonrecurring condition, and after a careful assessment was favorable for delivery by the vaginal route. Previous postcesarean section sepsis can be an indicator of poor scar healing. Routine hysterosalpingograms in women who had cesarean sections demonstrate relatively often deficiencies of the uterine scars.[41] High correlation has been found between measurements of the lower uterine segment thickness by ultrasound preoperatively and by inspection intraoperatively.[42,43] However, such radiography or sonographies provides no absolute reassurance for the future resistance of the scar under the stress of labor; thus, each case should be assessed carefully and the management individualized. When vaginal delivery is decided upon, careful monitoring of labor is required along with adequate analgesia for an assisted second stage, if required.

A previous classical cesarean section should always be followed by a repeat section, and the same should be the case after repair of a uterine rupture.

Table 27.2 Etiologic factors involved in uterine rupture

Unscarred uterus	Cephalopelvic disproportion
	Oxytocin misuse
	Grand multiparity
	Abruptio placentae
	Malpresentations (face, brow, shoulder)
	Operative deliveries (forceps, internal version)
	Destructive operations
Previously scarred uterus	Cesarean section scar
	Hysterotomy scar
	Uterine perforation scar
	Myomectomy or metroplasty scar
	Previous repair of a ruptured uterus

Clinical presentation, diagnosis, and pathology

Vaginal bleeding, lower abdominal pain or tenderness, fetal distress, and shock are the most common clinical features. The rupture of a previously scarred uterus is a less dramatic event. Shock appears to be rare, vaginal bleeding and abdominal tenderness and pain being the main features. Obviously, less bleeding occurs from a separated uterine scar than from the fresh, torn edges of a primary uterine rupture. Other reported signs and symptoms include tachycardia, hematuria, cessation of contractions, change in fetal position, and disappearance of fetal heart sounds (Table 27.1).

The diagnosis of rupture of the uterus is usually a clinical one. Awareness of the risk of this condition is important in all high-risk patients. VBAC deserves special care and awareness. The clinical acumen of the obstetrician is of prime importance. Suspected rupture of the uterus is an indication for surgery.

The uterine tear may be complete, penetrating through the serosal layer of the uterus and communicating with the peritoneal cavity, or incomplete (dehiscence), leaving the serosa intact. It can be longitudinal, transverse, or compound. The most common type of tear in the unscarred uterus is the longitudinal one, which is usually complete. Rupture of the previously scarred uterus is usually transverse and incomplete, as most ruptures are in fact dehiscent scars.[38] In 12–22% of the cases, bladder lacerations accompany ruptures. These are almost always related to a previous cesarean section scar. The main symptoms are hematuria or meconium-stained urine.[44]

Treatment and outcome

The basic treatment of a patient with a ruptured uterus is immediate resuscitation and surgery. Most publications advise hysterectomy. However, especially in young women, there may be good reasons for preserving the uterus. In general, the surgical procedure employed must be individualized, and it is dependent upon the type, location, and extent of the laceration. The decision to perform a total or a subtotal hysterectomy should depend on whether the cervix or vagina is involved and on the patient's condition. When the dehiscence of a previous cesarean section scar is repaired, the edges should be excised prior to the repair. The repair is performed with polyglactin (Vicryl) 2-0 sutures, two continuous layers for a lower-segment rupture repair and three continuous layers for an upper-segment rupture repair. Special care must be taken to secure hemostasis at the apexes of the tear. Repair of a ruptured uterus is mainly considered when future fertility is desired. When there is only slight dehiscence of a uterine scar, or when a tear is linear and easily reparable in a young patient of low parity, further pregnancies may be allowed after adequate repair.

Careful postoperative attention and support are needed, as, even after surgery is completed, the patient is still at risk of complications of hemorrhage, sepsis, and thromboembolic phenomena. In case of damage to the bladder, drainage with an indwelling catheter is needed for 5–7 days. It is an important means of preventing fistula formation.

Rupture of the uterus is still an important cause of maternal death in obstetric practice. In a recent publication describing the trends in pregnancy-related mortality and risk factors for pregnancy-related deaths in the USA for the years 1991–7, uterine rupture accounted for 1.7% of all maternal deaths.[2] In the UK, it accounted for 1.9% of all maternal deaths for the years 1994–6.[45] It is worth noting that there are considerably fewer maternal deaths among ruptured scarred uteri than among ruptured unscarred uteri. No maternal deaths were reported in the former group. In the unscarred group, the maternal mortality was 6.5–10% in various large series.[38,46] The fetal mortality rate was high as a result of separation of the placenta; in the unscarred group, it was 46–74%, but only 22–28% in the scarred group.[38]

Early miscellaneous injury

Symphysiolysis

Peripartum pubic symphysis separation is a recognized complication of pregnancy, estimates of its incidence ranging from 1:300–1:30 000.[47] Some degree of relaxation of the pelvic joints is present in all pregnant women. It is regarded as a preparatory process for delivery. The peptide hormone relaxin, structurally related to insulin and insulin-like growth factor, and primarily secreted by the corpus luteum and the placenta during pregnancy, is involved in a variety of functions.[48] It was isolated and studied as a substance that dissolved the anterior pelvis in guinea pigs late in pregnancy.[49] Although there is no proof for this role of relaxin in human subjects, the genetic machinery for production of relaxin does exist in humans, and may explain this phenomenon.[50]

The amount of relaxation of the pelvic joints during pregnancy may be quite considerable. The two pubic bones may become separated by a few centimeters without any symptom, complaint, or other difficulty for the pregnant woman. However, in other cases, a much smaller separation may be very painful and severely debilitating. This sometimes occurs during the later part of pregnancy and probably is combined with relaxation of the two sacroiliac joints.

Symphysiolysis is an infrequent affliction of the pelvic joint. It is characterized by loosening of the ligamentous support of the joint, and hence, a free sliding movement of the bones, mainly in the direction of the body axis. This comes into effect most prominently during gait and is accompanied by severe pain, which often interferes with mobilization. During walking, the body weight is alternately shifted from one leg to the other, this shift being transferred through the pelvic girdle. In the case of a loose symphysis pubis, at each step the pelvic bone is elevated in relation to the opposite side. This can be demonstrated by radiography if exposures are taken as the patient stands on each of her legs (Figure 27.3). The source of the pain can be of dual origin, due to friction of the bones or to excessive stretching of the joint ligaments.

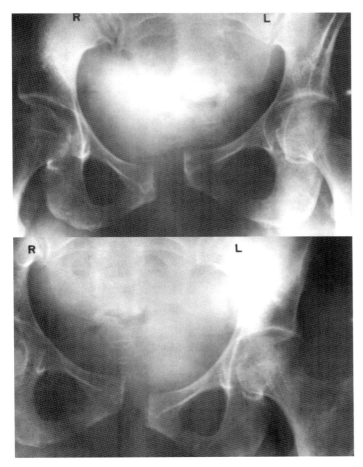

Figure 27.3 Radiographs of patient with symphysiolysis, standing alternately on each leg. Note change of joint as body weight shifts (antero-posterior plane).

The most prominent symptom of symphysiolysis is pain in the joint at any movement involving the pelvis. Gait is most severely inhibited, and even movements in bed often cause severe discomfort. Pressure on the joint usually elicits pain. Another diagnostic measure is to adduct and abduct the thighs against external counterpressure exerted by the examiner. In normal condition, this is painless; if the joint is affected, the procedure is painful. As already stated, radiologic proof can be documented by special techniques.

Symphysiolysis often occurs after difficult delivery, either spontaneous or instrumental. It is possible that in some cases the ligaments supporting the joint are ruptured during a traumatic or forceful delivery. Recovery from symphysiolysis usually occurs within 6–8 weeks.

The treatment of pelvic relaxation is mainly symptomatic, both during pregnancy and after delivery. Tight binding of the pelvis usually permits free movement, although sometimes it is accompanied by discomfort. The puerpera should be encouraged to move in order to prevent other complications. Non-steroidal anti-inflammatory drugs (NSAIDs) are in common use. Injection of corticosteroids into the joint has been tried, but the results are controversial. Local injection of anesthetics is of help in difficult cases and may promote mobilization. Orthopedic repair of the joint is very rarely needed.

Damage of the coccyx

During delivery, the coccyx is pushed backward in order to enlarge the pelvic outlet. This physiologic movement, if exaggerated, can cause tearing of the sacrococcygeal joint or, in some cases, fracture of the coccyx. This is most likely to occur in cases of difficult deliveries of large infants, occipitoposterior positions, and instrumentation, or if the coccyx points sharply forward. Damage to the joint or the bone itself is usually painful. It disturbs the patient mainly in the sitting position, but also when she lies in bed or defecates.

Diagnosis is by combined rectal and external examination. This procedure discloses tenderness and sometimes swelling of the surrounding tissues. A lateral radiograph of the sacroiliac joint can be helpful. Spontaneous healing is the rule in most cases; however, sometimes healing is by ankylosis, often with a coccyx directed anteriorly, a result which can obstruct the next labor. In some cases, pain continues for prolonged periods. It can be treated by injection of local anesthetics, but surgery may be indicated in severe cases.

Peroneal palsy

Peroneal palsy is a rare complication attributable to improper and prolonged strapping of the legs during delivery. If the legs are strapped too tightly and externally to the supportive poles, pressure on the peroneal nerve may cause palsy, with foot-drop resulting. Today, when strapping is no longer popular and supportive poles are used infrequently, this complication is hardly seen. Usually, no permanent damage is left; however, this preventable complication unnecessarily prolongs puerperal convalescence. Treatment is by physiotherapy combined with foot support to facilitate free movement. Even if wide abduction is needed for delivery, the legs can be freed for the third stage and, if necessary, strapped again for any further procedure.

Miscellaneous cervical damage

In most instances, obstetric trauma of the cervix is disclosed soon after delivery or in the early puerperium. In these detected cases, the lesion should be repaired upon diagnosis. Unfortunately, in some cases, cervical damage is unsuspected and spontaneous healing takes place, resulting, albeit infrequently, in permanent damage to the structural and functional integrity of the cervix.

The factors contributing to such cervical damage include mainly those also causing cervical incompetence. Previous cervical surgery predisposes to damage during labor and delivery. Cervical cerclage is a quite frequent cause of inconspicuous cervical tears, fenestration, and fibrosis.

Most of the injuries, mainly lateral tears, partial muscular retractions, and eversion of endocervical mucosa, are detected at postpartum examination. They should be corrected at the earliest occasion, since further involvement may be expected at a future delivery. Infrequently, cervical damage is undetectable at first examination, and its existence becomes obvious only at some later stage. Cervical scarring and fibrosis may result in cervical dystocia due to rigidity and failure to dilate. If neglected, new tears, often severe, or even annular detachment of the cervix may occur. Cervical damage may cause problems of infertility due to chronic cervicitis or extensive damage to the endocervical glands.

Urinary fistula

Urinary incontinence after childbirth may herald the formation of a urinary fistula. In his monograph on vesicovaginal fistula, Chassar-Moir,[51] reported that almost one-third of the fistulas he operated on were of obstetric origin. Mahfouz,[52] reporting on 758 cases in Egypt, found that obstetric trauma was the most common cause of urinary fistulas. These were also the findings in two large series reported from South Africa.[53,54] The main causes of urinary fistulas were protracted labors, difficult forceps deliveries, cesarean sections, ruptured uterus, and symphysiotomy. However, it seems that with the improvement of obstetric services, obstetric trauma as the predisposing factor for urinary fistulas is becoming rare.

Two types of fistulas occur. The most common type is caused by pressure necrosis. In prolonged labor with cephalopelvic disproportion, the bladder neck and urethra are compressed between the fetal head and the symphysis pubis. When this compression is prolonged, these tissues become ischemic and undergo necrosis. This leads to urinary incontinence, usually appearing 7–10 days later when the necrotic tissue sloughs out, forming a hole in the bladder base communicating with the vagina. It is usually located between the cervix and the external urethral meatus, involving the bladder neck and the anterior vaginal wall. Such fistulas vary in size, from some that hardly admit a probe to large ones easily recognized on vaginal inspection.

The second type is the traumatic fistula caused by direct injury to the bladder at difficult forceps delivery, craniotomy, or whenever a uterine or large anterior cervical tear involving the bladder is overlooked. Such circumstances are rare today. At cesarean section, especially at a repeat operation, damage can be done to the bladder during its downward displacement and, also on opening the uterus or its subsequent suturing. Blood-stained urine is a warning sign.

Immediate effective continuous drainage of the bladder is mandatory. Small obstetric vesicovaginal fistulas may heal spontaneously if the bladder is effectively drained by an indwelling catheter. If no healing occurs within 3 months, surgical repair is necessary. It was always considered unwise to attempt surgical repair too soon after the causative trauma. Apart from achieving reduction in size by spontaneous healing, in time the local blood supply improves, the slough separates, and the inflammation subsides, providing better conditions for surgery.

Sometimes ureterovaginal fistula may occur. Injury to a ureter during cesarean section or a repair of a ruptured uterus may result in ureterovaginal or ureterocervical fistula. Corrective surgery is usually the treatment. The urologist should be involved in the management of such fistulas.

Rectovaginal fistula

Although less common than the vesicovaginal fistula, the rectovaginal fistula is a very distressing consequence of birth trauma. Fortunately, this complication has become extremely rare. Three main situations are considered to cause rectovaginal fistula. The first is prolonged and firm compression of the posterior vaginal wall by the presenting part toward the bony birth canal. This continuous compression causes impairment of the circulation, edema, and necrosis of the tissues, leading finally to a fistula formation. Such a fistula may appear any time during the puerperium. The second causative factor is faulty repair or healing process of a fourth-degree perineal tear. The third is unnoticed damage of the rectum during repair of a third-degree tear, an episiotomy, or a deep vaginal tear. Gynecologic or colorectal surgeons should be involved in the management of such fistulas.

Genital prolapse

Pelvic organ prolapse is a major health issue for women. Women with normal life expectancy have an 11% chance of undergoing at least one operation for pelvic organ prolapse or urinary incontinence during their lifetime.[44] The causal basis of genital prolapse is multifactorial. Birth trauma to the pelvic floor and other surrounding tissues supporting the uterus and adjoining structures is of basic and major importance.[55,56]

Genital prolapse also occurs in other mammals, but is much less frequent in quadrupeds. The erect posture of the human female exerts a dual influence on the pathogenesis of genital prolapse. First, the evolutionary process of the erect posture of the human species caused an adaptational strengthening of the pelvic girdle. This structure has to carry the weight of the body, transferred to the legs; therefore, the bones became stronger and thicker, resulting in the narrowing of the internal measures of the bony birth canal. The relatively large human fetus, as compared to other species, further increases the problem of passage through the tightly fitting birth canal. The birth process in most species is much easier and less traumatic due to larger space and smaller fetal size, thus resulting in less damage to the pelvic musculature and fascia.

Second, the fascial and muscular support of the human pelvic floor is under continuous strain from intra-abdominal pressure, which in the erect posture is also influenced by the forces of gravity. In order to resist this continuous strain, the pelvic floor has to be strong and undamaged; otherwise, its supportive function of the pelvic organs fails. Some amount of damage to the floor is almost inevitable in childbirth, and the additional pressure due to the erect posture exacerbates the condition.

Genital prolapse may occur shortly after childbirth if the damage is extensive, but it is far more frequent with advancing age when additional contributing factors come into effect. These include general weakening of connective and estrogen-dependent tissues in the pelvis, often aggravated by recurrent or chronic abdominal pressure due to constipation, chronic cough, or obesity.

DeLee[57] explained the principles of pelvic floor damage as follows:

(1) The head advancing through the hiatus genitalis stretches the vagina radially and longitudinally – sometimes it also wipes the vagina off its fascial anchorings, sliding it downward and outward.

(2) The head stretches the pelvic fascia over the levator ani and, between the rectum and the vagina and the layer behind the rectum, also radially and longitudinally, and this also permits the rectum to be wiped downward and slide off its fascial attachments to the levator ani.

(3) The head often tears or overstretches the fascia over the levator ani, especially those bundles which hold the pillars of the muscle in position at the sides of the rectum, spanning the hiatus genitalis, and this permits the pillars to separate, diastasis of the levator pillars resulting – the disorder is similar to that of diastasis recti abdominalis. This diastasis of the levator pillars and the wiping or sliding of the rectum and vagina downward and outward are the essential features of most pelvic floor injuries, and have been, we think, the least noticed by current writers.

(4) The tears in the levator ani muscle are usually due to improper treatment, and they occur, least commonly, near the insertion of the muscle on the pubic ramus (usually due to cutting by the forceps) and more commonly at the sides of the rectum, behind, near the raphe.

(5) Labor always ruptures the urogenital septum, tearing it in all directions, and also from its ramifications with the endopelvic fascia, both above and below the levator ani.

(6) The fascia between the rectum and the bladder is also stretched or torn, also radially and in a downward direction, tearing the vagina and bladder off its anchoring to the upper surface of the endopelvic fascia over the levator ani and the posterior surface of the pubis.

It is thus evident that most of the damage resulting from labor is due to injury, rupture, distraction, and displacement of the fascia, and less to tearing of the muscles. The more difficult childbirth is, the more damage is to be expected. Macrosomia, constitutional or as seen with postmaturity or diabetes, is an important factor. Too conservative obstetric practice and prolonged trials of labor could be involved. Occipitoposterior and difficult breech deliveries, shoulder dystocia, and hastily managed instrumentation due to emergency situations all contribute to pelvic floor damage.

The site of the late disorder depends on the site of the initial injury. The most common lesion is the diastasis of the levator ani pillars, which destroys the posterior and lateral support of the vagina, resulting in a relaxed and atonic vaginal inlet with a tendency to rectocele formation. The atonic vagina itself may cause, at any stage, sexual insufficiency and, in combination with a sagging perineum, recurrent vaginal infections.

This form of injury to the pelvic floor is usually due to large fetal parts, but its extent depends on the preventive measures taken. The performance of episiotomy and good repair may be of importance, and so may judicious management of the second stage of labor, allowing gradual relaxation of the pelvic and perineal structures.

An even deeper tear affects the muscular bundles of the pubococcygeus, which, in combination with detachment of the rectum from its superior anchorage to the pelvic fascia, leads to the formation of a high rectocele as the vaginal wall slides along with the loosened rectum.

Damage to the posterior part of the pelvic support arises more commonly in cases of continuous pressure and tension at this region. Undetected and prolonged anterior asynclitism may be of importance.

Affliction of the fascia supporting the bladder and the urethra causes, at a later stage, anterior vaginal wall prolapse, combined with cystocele, urethrocele, or both. In some instances, this leads to functional disturbances of the bladder and its control, resulting in stress incontinence.

Untimely pushing or pulling of the fetus through an insufficiently prepared birth canal often damages the uterine anchorage and the ligamentous support of the uterus. This predisposes to uterine prolapse at a later stage. Solitary damage to the ligaments is less common and leads to cervical elongation or uterine prolapse. More commonly, it is combined with additional damage to the pelvic floor, resulting later in prolapse, combined with other forms of vaginal relaxation.

Although many of these injuries can be prevented by proper obstetric management, some will occur due to the large size of the fetus. As only a small part of this damage can be detected immediately after delivery, the rest will remain obscure until a later stage, when additional strain is exerted on the pelvic support.

Urinary incontinence

Urinary incontinence can occur at any age; however, it is much more common in parous women late in their reproductive years. Obstetric injury to the urethrovesical support is the most common factor predisposing to the development of stress incontinence, although many years may intervene between childbirth and the onset of symptoms. Vaginal birth may increase the risk of stress and mixed urinary incontinence, but not of urge urinary incontinence and overactive bladder.[58,59] However, in the EPINCONT study,[60] the risk of urinary incontinence was higher after vaginal delivery than cesarean section (21% vs 15.9%). It was even higher after cesarean section than in nulliparous women (15.9% vs 10.1%) As compared with nulliparous women, women who had cesarean section had an adjusted odds ratio for any incontinence of 1.5 (95% CI,

1.2–1.9), and women who had vaginal delivery had an adjusted odds ratio for any incontinence of 2.3 (95% CI, 2.0–2.6). The adjusted odds ratio for any incontinence associated with vaginal delivery as compared with cesarean section was 1.7 (95% CI, 1.3–2.1). The authors recommend that these findings not be used to justify an increase in the use of cesarean section.

In a difficult labor, the bladder is compressed between the advancing fetal head and the symphysis pubis, and its fascial supports may be weakened. Some degree of stress incontinence may also appear during pregnancy, but this is only temporary and usually disappears after delivery.[61]

Dyspareunia

Dyspareunia resulting from childbirth can occur either shortly after resuming sexual activity or at any later stage of the woman's life. At the later stage, additional components usually play an important role, such as hormonal deficiency and aging of the tissues. In its milder forms, dyspareunia is probably quite common; however, women tend to accept it as a result of childbirth. They do not complain, and many times its pathologic meaning is brought to their attention only by the physician.

Damage to the birth canal and its repair accounts for these cases of dyspareunia. Too tight a repair of a vaginal tear or of an episiotomy can make coitus difficult and uncomfortable, a too tightly repaired perineum can make sexual relations almost impossible, and, if insisted on, very painful. One must be careful in repair of multiple lacerations, since here lies the danger of a too perfect repair and multifocal fibrosis.

A frequent, but often overlooked, cause of coital discomfort soon after the puerperium is formation of granulation tissue in the vagina. Causes of deep dyspareunia resulting from childbirth include organized hematomas and scars in the parametria or the vaginal vault.

In many instances, no interference with sexual activity appears during the fertile age; however, when additional factors resulting from aging appear, mainly atrophy and tightening due to hormonal deprivation, dyspareunia becomes evident.

Allen–Masters syndrome

In 1955, Allen and Masters[62] described the syndrome, named after them, of a tear in the posterior leaf of the broad ligament, extreme retroversion of the uterus, and a freely movable cervix termed a 'universal joint cervix'. They established an anatomic basis for the pelvic congestion syndrome described earlier by Taylor,[63] showing that the anatomic defect is a tear at the base of the broad ligament, on one or both sides, which can also include the sacrouterine ligaments. They assumed that the loss of support of the blood vessels leads to kinking and subsequently venous congestion. In the majority of cases, a conglomerate of congested veins is visible through the defect in the broad ligament, and almost invariably some amount of serous fluid is found in the pouch of Douglas. The venous congestion produces softness of the lower part of the uterus, which further weakens the uterine support, resulting in the 'universal joint cervix', with hypermobility of the cervix in relation to the uterus.

The clinical features of the syndrome include dysmenorrhea, menorrhagia, dyspareunia, continuous pelvic pain and discomfort, pain on defecation, general weakness, emotional instability, and headaches. The syndrome is not difficult to diagnose on a clinical basis; however, laparoscopy can be a helpful diagnostic aid. Endometriosis might be an alternative in the differential diagnosis.

A traumatic obstetric event has been suggested as the etiologic factor involved in the majority of these cases. Compromise of the uterine support usually follows some traumatic obstetric incident such as a difficult instrumental delivery, breech extraction, prolonged labor, manual removal of placenta, and puerperal curettage. As most of the complaints of this syndrome are nonspecific, the gynecologist must be aware of its existence.

* * *

Birth trauma may have an impact on a woman's health far beyond its immediate influence. It is imperative that such trauma be promptly and properly diagnosed and treated in order to avoid further complications and modifications of the woman's health, sexual life, and social well-being.

References

1. Angioli R, Gomez-Marin O, Cantuaria G, O'Sullivan MJ. Severe perineal lacerations during vaginal delivery: the University of Miami experience. Am J Obstet Gynecol 2000; 182: 1083–5.
2. Berg CJ, Chang J, Callaghan WM, Whitehead SJ. Pregnancy-related mortality in the United States, 1991–1997. Obstet Gynecol 2003; 101: 289–96.
3. Carroli G, Belizan J, Stamp G. Episiotomy for vaginal birth. Birth 1999; 26: 263.
4. Coats PM. Chan KK, Wilkins M, Beard RJ. A comparison between midline and mediolateral episiotomies. Br J Obstet Gynaecol 1980; 87: 408–12.
5. David MP, Boiman O, Avni A. Anti-inflammatory effect of oxyphenbutazone on episiotomy healing. Int Surg 1976; 61: 555–6.
6. Droegemuller W. Cold sitz baths for relief of postpartum perineal pain. Clin Obstet Gynecol 1980; 23: 1039–43.
7. Goldberg J, Holtz D, Hyslop T, Tolosa JF. Has the use of routine episiotomy decreased? Examination of episiotomy rates from 1983 to 2000. Obstet Gynecol 2002; 99: 395–400.
8. Hausler G, Hanzal E, Dadale C, Gruber W. Necrotizing fasciitis arising from episiotomy. Arch Gynecol Obstet 1994; 255: 153–5.
9. Kettle C, Hills RK, Jones P. Continuous versus interrupted perineal repair with standard or rapidly absorbed sutures after spontaneous vaginal birth: a randomised controlled trial. Lancet 2002; 359: 2217–23.

10. Kettle C, Johanson RB. Absorbable synthetic versus catgut suture material for perineal repair. Cochrane Database Syst Rev 2000; 2: CD000006.

11. Macdonald R, Smith PJ. Extradural morphine and pain relief following episiotomy. Br J Anaesth 1984; 56: 1201–5.

12. Niv D, Wolman I, Yashar T et al. Epidural morphine pretreatment for postepisiotomy pain. Clin J Pain 1994; 10: 319–23.

13. Ould F. Treatise of Midwifery. Nelson and Conner: Dublin, 1742.

14. Ramler D, Roberts J. A comparison of cold and warm sitz baths for relief of postpartum perineal pain. J Obstet Gynecol Neonatal Nurs 1986; 15: 471–4.

15. Shiono P, Klebanoff MA, Carey JC. Midline episiotomies: more harm than good? Obstet Gynecol 1990; 75: 765–70.

16. Shy KK, Eschenbach DA. Fatal perineal cellulitis from an episiotomy site. Obstet Gynecol 1979; 54: 292–8.

17. Signorello LB, Harlow BL, Chekos AK, Repke JT. Midline episiotomy and anal incontinence: retrospective cohort study. BMJ 2000; 320: 86–90.

18. Dumont M. [The long and difficult birth of symphysiotomy, or from Severin Pineau to Jean-Rene Sigault]. J Gynecol Obstet Biol Reprod (Paris) 1989; 18: 11–21.

19. Bjorklund K. Minimally invasive surgery for obstructed labour: a review of symphysiotomy during the twentieth century (including 5000 cases). Br J Obstet Gynaecol 2002; 109: 236–48.

20. Fleming VEM, Hagen S, Niven C. Does perineal suturing make a difference? The SUNS trial. Br J Obstet Gynaecol 2003; 110: 684–9.

21. Cunningham FG, Gant FN et al. Williams' Obstetrics. McGraw-Hill: New York, 2001.

22. Sultan AH. Obstetrical perineal injury and anal incontinence. Clin Risk 1999; 5: 193–6.

23. Royal College of Obstetricians and Gynaecologists. Methods and Materials used in Perineal Repair. Guideline No. 23. RCOG Press: London, 2004.

24. Royal College of Obstetricians and Gynaecologists. Management of Third and Fourth-Degree Perineal Tears Following Vaginal Delivery. Guideline No. 29. RCOG Press: London, 2001.

25. Leeman L, Spearman M, Rogers R. Repair of obstetric perineal lacerations. Am Fam Physician 2003; 68: 1585–90.

26. Fitzpatrick M, Behan M, O'Connell PR, O'Herlihy C. A randomized clinical trial comparing primary overlap with approximation repair of third-degree obstetric tears. Am J Obstet Gynecol 2000; 183: 1220–4.

27. Tjandra JJ, Han WR, Goh J et al. Direct repair vs. overlapping sphincter repair: a randomized, controlled trial. Dis Colon Rectum 2003; 46: 937–42; discussion 942–3.

28. Carroli G, Belizan J. Episiotomy for vaginal birth. Cochrane Database Syst Rev 2000; 2: CD000081.

29. Bruce E. Everything you need to know to prevent perineal tearing. Midwifery Today Int Midwife 2003; 10–13.

30. Labrecque M, Eason E, Marcoux S et al. Randomized controlled trial of prevention of perineal trauma by perineal massage during pregnancy. Am J Obstet Gynecol 1999; 180: 593–600.

31. Shipman MK, Boniface DR, Tefft ME, McCloghry F. Antenatal perineal massage and subsequent perineal outcomes: a randomised controlled trial. Br J Obstet Gynaecol 1997; 104: 787–91.

32. Stamp G, Kruzins G, Crowther C. Perineal massage in labour and prevention of perineal trauma: randomised controlled trial. BMJ 2001; 322: 1277–80.

33. Gardeil F, Daly S, Turner MJ. Uterine rupture in pregnancy reviewed. Eur J Obstet Gynecol Reprod Biol 1994; 56: 107–10.

34. Ofir K, Sheiner E, Levy A et al. Uterine rupture: risk factors and pregnancy outcome. Am J Obstet Gynecol 2003; 189: 1042–6.

35. Waterstone M, Bewley S, Wolfe C. Incidence and predictors of severe obstetric morbidity: case-control study. BMJ 2001; 322: 1089–93.

36. Miller DA, Goodwin TM, Gherman RB, Paul RH. Intrapartum rupture of the unscarred uterus. Obstet Gynecol 1997; 89: 671–3.

37. Guise JM, McDonagh MS, Osterweil P, et al. Systematic review of the incidence and consequences of uterine rupture in women with previous caesarean section. BMJ 2004; 329: 19–25.

38. Golan A, Sandbank O, Rubin A. Rupture of the pregnant uterus. Obstet Gynecol 1980; 56: 549–54.

39. Dewhurst CJ. The ruptured caesarean section scar. J Obstet Gynaecol Br Emp 1957; 64: 113–18.

40. Halperin ME, Moore DC et al. Classical versus low-segment transverse incision for preterm caesarean section: maternal complications and outcome of subsequent pregnancies. Br J Obstet Gynaecol 1988; 95: 990–6.

41. Poidevin LO, Bockner VY. A hysterographic study of uteri after caesarean section. J Obstet Gynaecol Br Emp 1958; 65: 278–83.

42. Rozenberg P, Goffinet F, Phillippe HJ, Nisand I. Ultrasonographic measurement of lower uterine segment to assess risk of defects of scarred uterus. Lancet 1996; 347: 281–4.

43. Tanik A, Ustun C, Cil E, Arslan A. Sonographic evaluation of the wall thickness of the lower uterine segment in patients with previous cesarean section. J Clin Ultrasound 1996; 24: 355–7.

44. Olsen AL, Smith VJ, Bogstrom JO et al. Epidemiology of surgically managed pelvic organ prolapse and urinary incontinence. Obstet Gynecol 1997; 89: 501–6.

45. Why Mothers Die. Report on Confidential Inquiries into Maternal Deaths in the United Kingdom 1994–1996. RCOG Press: London, 1998.

46. Schrinsky DC, Benson RC. Rupture of the pregnant uterus: a review. Obstet Gynecol Surv 1978; 33: 217–32.

47. Snow RE, Neubert AG. Peripartum pubic symphysis separation: a case series and review of the literature. Obstet Gynecol Surv 1997; 52: 438–43.

48. Baccari MC, Calamai F. Relaxin: new functions for an old peptide. Curr Protein Pept Sci 2004; 5: 9–18.

49 Hisaw FL. Experimental relaxation of the pubic ligament of the guinea pig. Proc Soc Exp Biol Med 1926; 23: 661–3.

50. Ziel HK. A guest editorial: dialog between basic and clinical science: relaxin as a possible cause of symphyseal separation. Obstet Gynecol Surv 2001; 56: 447–8.

51. Chassar-Moir J. The Vesico-Vaginal Fistula. Baillière Tindall and Cassell: London, 1967.

52. Mahfouz N. Urinary fistulae in women. J Obstet Gynaecol Br Emp 1957; 64: 23–34.

53. Coetzee T, Lithgow DM. Obstetric fistulae of the urinary tract. J Obstet Gynaecol Br Commonw 1966; 73: 837–44.

54. Lavery DW. Vesico-vaginal fistulae; a report on the vaginal repair of 160 cases. J Obstet Gynaecol Br Emp 1955; 62: 530–9.

55. Dannecker C, Anthuber C. The effects of childbirth on the pelvic floor. J Perinat Med 2000; 28: 175–84.

56. Sze EH, Sherard GB 3rd, Dolezal JM. Pregnancy, labor, delivery, and pelvic organ prolapse. Obstet Gynecol 2002; 100: 981–6.

57. Gabbe SJ, DeLee JB. The prophylactic forceps operation. Am J Obstet Gynecol 1920; 1: 34–44.

58. Burgio KL, Zyczynski H, Locher JL et al. Urinary incontinence in the 12-month postpartum period. Obstet Gynecol 2003; 102: 1291–8.

59. Parazzini F, Chiaffarino F, Lavezzari M et al. Risk factors for stress, urge or mixed urinary incontinence in Italy. Br J Obstet Gynaecol 2003; 110: 927–33.

60. Rortveit G, Daltveit AK, Hannestead YS et al. Urinary incontinence after vaginal delivery or cesarean section. N Engl J Med 2003; 348: 900–7.

61. Viktrup L, Lose G, Rollf M, Barfoed K. The symptom of stress incontinence caused by pregnancy or delivery in primiparas. Obstet Gynecol 1992; 79: 945–9.

62. Allen WM, Masters WH. Traumatic laceration of uterine support; the clinical syndrome and the operative treatment. Am J Obstet Gynecol 1955; 70: 500–13.

63. Taylor HC Jr. Life situations, emotions and gynecologic pain associated with congestion. Res Publ Assoc Res Nerv Ment Dis 1949; 29: 1051–6.

28 Puerperal inversion of the uterus

Watson A Bowes, Jr. and Peter T Watson

References to uterine inversion can be found in Hindu ayurvedic literature (2500–600 BC), but Hippocrates is said to be the first to give an accurate description of the problem and offer a treatment regimen.[1] In the first half of the twentieth century, puerperal inversion of the uterus was associated with high mortality (12–40%) because of delay in diagnosis, lack of anesthesia, and inadequate management of hemorrhage, shock and infection.[2–6] Since 1960, the outcome for puerperal uterine inversion has improved remarkably as a result of early diagnosis, adequate treatment of shock, and prompt manual reinversion of the uterus.[6–14]

Classification

The following classification is based on the time of diagnosis[15] and the relationship of the inverted uterine fundus to the cervix and the perineum:

(1) *Acute puerperal inversion.* The inversion is noted shortly after delivery and before there is significant contraction of the cervix (usually within a few hours of delivery).
(2) *Subacute puerperal inversion.* The inversion is noted within 4 weeks after delivery and after contraction of the cervix has occurred.
(3) *Chronic inversion.* More than 4 weeks have elapsed since the inversion and cervical contraction occurred.
(4) *Incomplete inversion.* No part of the corpus of the uterus extends past the cervix.
(5) *Complete inversion.* The inverted corpus extends beyond the cervix.
(6) *Prolapsed inversion.* The inverted uterus extends beyond the introitus.

This chapter will be devoted to the diagnosis and management of acute or subacute puerperal uterine in version.

Incidence

In nine studies of pregnancies in North America complicated by puerperal inversion of the uterus that have occurred since 1960 (Table 28.1), the incidence of the complication varied from one in 1739 to one in 6407 deliveries (average 1/2870).[6–14] The problem, therefore, remains sufficiently uncommon that any single practitioner may encounter only one or two such complications in a professional lifetime, and no obstetric service or individual gains enough experience to test management protocols in any reasonable prospective study. Consequently, the assessment of this problem depends upon the retrospective review of case reports and series with small numbers of patients.

Epidemiology

There is no consistent epidemiologic characteristic of puerperal inversion of the uterus, with the possible exception of parity. In several studies, the proportion of nulliparous patients has been higher in cases of uterine inversion than in the total birthing population.[2,9,11,16] Other series have not confirmed the association of acute puerperal inversion with primiparity.[6–8]

Etiology

The etiology of acute puerperal uterine inversion is not known with certainty. The following conditions have been suggested as predisposing or causal factors: manual removal of the placenta, improper fundal pressure, excessive cord contraction, injudicious use of oxytocics, short umbilical cord, abnormally adherent placenta, and fundal implantation of the placenta. In almost all cases of uterine inversion in which the site of implantation of the placenta was recorded, it was noted to be in the fundus of the uterus.[3,4,7,11] Fundal implantation of the placenta occurs in only approximately 10% of pregnancies. The uterine wall (myometrium) beneath the placental implantation site is thin in comparison to the remainder of the uterus. It is presumed that when this thin area of endometrium is in the fundus

Table 28.1 Acute inversion of the uterus

Author and site	Years of study	Number of patients and incidence	Method of reinversion	Placental management (removal or leave intact)	Tocolytics
Kitchen et al, U. of Virginia[6]	1960–74	11 1/2284	All replaced vaginally	No data. Discussion advises removal if replacement difficult without doing so	Tocolytics not used
Watson et al, U. of Colorado[7]	1969–78	18 1/1739	All replaced vaginally	All replacements occurred after placenta had been separated from uterine wall	Tocolytics not used
Cumming & Taylor, U. of Calgary[8]	1966–77	9 1/2176	7 replaced vaginally 1 laparotomy, 1 hysterectomy	8 removed before replacement 1 no information given	Tocolytics not used
Platt & Druzin U. of Southern California[9]	1972–77	28 1/2148	27 replaced vaginally 1 laparotomy	No data or discussion of management of the placenta	$MgSO_4$ recommended but no data given
Brar et al, U. of Southern California[10]	1977–86	54 1/2495	52 acute inversions replaced vaginally 2 subacute inversions replaced with laparotomy	No data. Statement that less blood loss noted if placenta left intact	18 treated with tocolytics (terbutaline or $MgSO_4$)
Shah-Hosseini & Evrard, Women and Infants Hospital of Rhode Island[11]	1978–88	11 1/6407	9 replaced vaginally 1 Huntington procedure, 1 hysterectomy	No data. Discussion mentioned the oft-repeated notion that blood-loss is less if uterus replaced before the placenta is removed	No data or discussion about use of tocolytics
Catazarite et al, U. of New Mexico[12]	1983–84	6 1/1200	All replaced vaginally	No data or discussion of management of placenta	2 treated with terbutaline 2 treated with $MgSO_4$
Abouleish et al, U. of Texas, Houston[13]	1987–93	18 1/3643	All replaced vaginally	No data or discussion of management of placenta	5 received terbutaline
Baskett, Dalhousie U. of Halifax, NS[14]	1977–2000	40 1/3737	27 cases of acute inversion after vaginal delivery, all replaced vaginally 13 cases of acute inversion with cesarean delivery	No data or discussion of management of placenta	No data

of the uterus, a slight inward dimpling of the uterus may occur as the placenta begins to separate. Thereafter, a progressive inversion ensues, with each contraction extending the inversion as the uterus virtually delivers itself inside out. Such maneuvers as fundal pressure or traction on the umbilical cord may enhance the inversion tendency, but they are probably not independent causal factors. A substantial proportion of uterine inversions occur spontaneously where there has been no uterine or cord manipulation.[2,3]

There are several reports of uterine inversion occurring at the time of cesarean delivery.[14,17–19] Among the 40 cases of uterine inversion reported by Baskett, 13 occurred at the time of cesarean delivery.[14] The author noted that inversion of the

uterus at the time cesarean occurred in each case immediately after manual removal of the placenta. Although this may be evidence that manual removal of the placenta is a cause of puerperal uterine inversion, there was no control group of cesarean deliveries performed with spontaneous delivery of the placenta.

Pathophysiology

Acute puerperal inversion of the uterus is almost always associated with uterine hemorrhage and shock. Some authorities have suggested that the degree of cardiovascular collapse is out of proportion to the hypovolemia resulting from blood loss;[2,5] however, it is probable that blood loss does account for the hypotension and tachycardia experienced by many of these patients.[7] The placenta is frequently attached to the inverted fundus, suggesting that the inversion process begins before separation of the placenta has occurred by cleavage along the decidua basalis.

If a complete inversion occurs, the cervix forms a ring or collar around the inverted fundus. This results in edema and vascular congestion, promoting additional blood loss and further edema, which, in turn, aggravates the cervical constriction. Prolonged inversion may result in tissue necrosis and infection, but, with prompt recognition and treatment, these complications are seen only rarely in modern obstetric services.

Mortality

Reviews of the literature that included predominantly cases reported prior to 1940 record maternal mortality rates of 13–70%.[1,3,4] Kitchin et al quoted one report from the Committee on Maternal Health of the Ohio Medical Association in 1963 listing six maternal deaths from uterine inversion.[6] The obstetric population in which these six deaths occurred is not known; therefore, the maternal mortality rate represented by these cases cannot be determined.

Selected series of cases suggest there was no improvement in the mortality rate of puerperal uterine inversion until 1960. McCullagh summarized 233 cases from 1911 to 1924 and found a mortality rate of 16%.[4] Bell et al reported 76 cases from the literature from 1940 to 1952 and found 13 (17%) deaths.[2] Burke and Hofmeister reviewed 22 cases published in the literature from 1957 to 1962 and added 19 cases from nine Milwaukee hospitals with an accumulated death rate of 23%.[20] However, in nine recent series from obstetric services in North America including 195 cases of puerperal inversion of the uterus since 1960, no deaths were reported (Table 28.1).[6–14]

Prevention

Measures to prevent uterine inversion include recognizing those patients who are at high risk of the complication and avoiding any of the precipitating factors in their management. Fundal implantation of the placenta is the single most common prerequisite of uterine inversion. With the use of ultrasound, which is now common in the third trimester of pregnancy, those patients with fundal implantation, in many cases, will be identified prior to labor. In such patients, there should be no more than minimal traction on the umbilical cord and only very gentle pressure on the uterine fundus during the third stage of labor. These patients must also be observed carefully for signs of spontaneous inversion during and after the third stage of labor.

There is debate among experts on the role of oxytocin in either precipitating[5,6,21] or preventing uterine inversion.[14]

Active management of the third stage of labor, which involves giving intravenous oxytocin after delivery of the infant's shoulder, has been shown to reduce blood loss, postpartum hemorrhage, and the need for blood transfusion.[22] Baskett studied a series of 40 pregnancies complicated by acute postdelivery inversion of the uterus at a regional tertiary-level maternity hospital in Nova Scotia (1977–2000).[14] When the period 1989–2000 was compared to the period 1977–89, there was a fourfold decrease in the incidence of acute inversion of the uterus after vaginal delivery. This decrease followed the introduction of active management of the third stage of labor. In one large series of 10 082 patients in which oxytocin was given prior to delivery of the placenta, there were no uterine inversions.[23] These studies suggest that giving oxytocin after delivery of the infant's shoulders is a useful measure to reduce the risk of uterine inversion.

Diagnosis

Successful management of puerperal inversion of the uterus depends upon early recognition and diagnosis, prompt and efficient treatment of hemorrhage and shock, and reinversion of the uterus at the earliest opportunity.

Diagnosis is straightforward if an acute, total inversion occurs in the third stage of labor. The dramatic appearance of the placenta adherent to the inverted uterine corpus protruding through the introitus is an unforgettable sight. Even in cases where the placenta separates immediately before the inversion occurs, the beefy red tumor, the size of an infant's head, protruding through the introitus is recognized as an inverted uterus. More difficult is the diagnosis of a nonprolapsed or incomplete inversion which occurs after the third stage of labor.[24] Routine visual examination of the cervix after delivery of the placenta will result in the early detection of some cases of incomplete inversion. Lewin and Bryan[25] reported a case of puerperal inversion of the uterus in which magnetic resonance imaging was used to confirm the diagnosis when physical examination and sonograms were equivocal. Some authors have also advocated manual exploration of the uterus immediately after delivery of the placenta as a means of making the earliest possible diagnosis of uterine inversion.[6]

The only symptoms may be hemorrhage and shock. In all cases of puerperal hemorrhage, uterine inversion must be kept in mind if subtle cases are not to be misdiagnosed. Palpation of the abdomen may reveal a suspicious absence of the uterine fundus, a sign which should always alert one to uterine inversion. Thereafter, a careful inspection of the vagina, both visually and manually, will discover the cause of the hemorrhage in cases of inversion of the uterus. Occasionally, physicians have been misled by assuming that the prolapsed fundus is a large leiomyomata or cervical polyp.[4] Whenever a mass is visualized or palpated in the cervix or vagina in the immediate postpartum period, especially when there is unexplained blood loss or hypotension, the diagnosis of uterine inversion should be suspected. Delay in recognizing this complication increases the difficulty of reinverting the corpus because of cervical contraction and edema, which may enhance blood loss and shock and increase the chance of infection and tissue necrosis.

Treatment

A major reason for the high mortality reported in earlier series of uterine inversion was inadequate therapy for blood loss and shock. Modern use of prompt replacement of blood volume, using crystalloid or colloid solutions and blood products, can usually be accomplished before the serious side effects of prolonged hypotension occur. Immediately upon making the diagnosis of inverted uterus, or in cases of acute postpartum hemorrhage, one or more large-bore, intravenous infusion lines should be established. An infusion of a crystalloid solution, such as 5% dextrose/lactated Ringer's, is begun, while whole blood and packed red cells are obtained. Vital signs, including pulse and blood pressure, should be monitored frequently, as should urine output. As soon as blood volume is being restored, efforts should be made to replace the uterus in its normal anatomic position.

Restoration of the uterus to its normal position will frequently require general anesthesia. As soon as the diagnosis of an acute puerperal uterine inversion occurs, and while adequate intravenous infusions of crystalloid solutions are being established and blood products ordered, an anesthesiologist should be summoned.

Before administering inhalation anesthesia, a tocolytic drug can be administered; this will often allow manual reinversion of the uterus.[9,10,12,13,26] As noted in the series listed in the Table 28.1, tocolytic drugs commonly used for preterm labor inhibition, such as magnesium sulfate (4 g, IV) or terbutaline (0.25 mg, IM), have been used for treatment of acute puerperal uterine inversion. There is also enthusiasm for the use of nitroglycerine, which has been used in a variety of clinical situations requiring acute emergency uterine relaxation.[27] Although there are a number of case reports demonstrating that nitroglycerin (100 μg, IV) is effective in providing transient uterine relaxation during manual replacement of the inverted uterus,[28–30] there are insufficient data to establish one or another tocolytic drug as being superior in either effectiveness or safety for treatment of the inverted uterus. Moreover, tocolytic therapy is not successful in all cases, and inhalation anesthesia may be necessary in refractory situations. Once the uterus is manually reinverted, prompt administration of a uterotonic medication is necessary to avoid reinversion.[12,31]

The method most widely used and most likely to be successful for manually replacing the uterus was first described by Johnson in 1949.[32] He described nine cases of puerperal inversion of the uterus and the technique of replacement (Figure 28.1).

To replace the inverted uterus the entire hand is placed in the vagina with the tips of the fingers at the uterocervical junction and the fundus uteri in the palm of the hand. The entire uterus is then lifted out of the pelvis and forcefully held in the abdominal cavity above the level of the umbilicus. It is necessary to hold the uterus in this position for a period of three to five minutes, at which time the fundus recedes from the palm of the hand.... It is emphasized that in order to accomplish this procedure the entire hand and two-thirds of the length of the forearm must be placed in the vagina; otherwise the pull and tension of the ligaments are not sufficient to correct the condition.

Johnson explained that the mechanism of fundal replacement by this method depends upon traction, which occurs on the uterine ligaments when the uterus is elevated into the abdomen. Among the nine patients treated by Johnson, there were two chronic inversions, one subacute inversion, and six acute inversions. All patients survived. Recent series have confirmed the effectiveness of this technique (Table 28.1).

A hydrostatic method of inducing replacement of the inverted uterus was first described by O'Sullivan in 1945.[33] This method involves infusion of 1000–2000 ml warm saline into the vagina with the patient in the lithotomy position. Fluid is prevented from escaping from the vagina by blocking the introitus with the operator's hand. Momani and Hassan reported five consecutive cases of acute puerperal uterine inversion that were successfully reduced within 5–10 minutes by this method.[34] Although reported as being used with success in the UK, Australia, and the Middle East, the hydrostatic method has not been reported in recent series from North America.

Whether to remove an adherent placenta from the uterine fundus before attempting manual replacement is controversial. There is no consensus in the medical literature: several authors strongly advise against removing the placenta prior to manual replacement,[17,35] while others suggest that its removal is not dangerous,[8] and still others claim that removal of the placenta will actually facilitate replacement of the inverted fundus.[6] As noted in the series summarized in Table 28.1, there are remarkably little data about management of the placenta upon which to establish an evidence-based opinion. In the absence of such data, perhaps the most practical advice is to remove the placenta if that can be accomplished easily and with minimal trauma and blood loss. But if the placenta seems unusually adherent, or if its removal will cause an appreciable delay, manual elevation of the uterus should be accomplished with the placenta intact. The placenta can then be removed manually when the fundus is repositioned.

All physicians, nurse midwives, and nurses entrusted with the care of women in labor should be familiar with the diagnosis and management of acute inversion of the uterus, because its infrequent occurrence precludes the supervised training of each individual in the technique of manual replacement. Since prompt therapy is the key to successful replacement and low morbidity, treatment will often have to be initiated by the

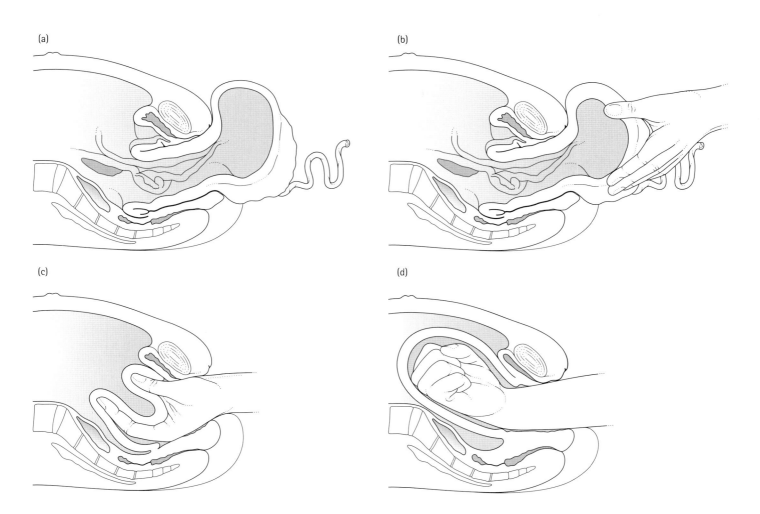

Figure 28.1 Manual replacement of the inverted uterus. (a) Complete acute inversion of the uterus with the placenta attached to the uterine fundus. (b) The inverted fundus is grasped in the palm of the hand with the fingers directed toward the posterior fornix. (c) The uterus is lifted out of the pelvis and directed with steady pressure toward the umbilicus. (d) The fundus is held in position for 3 min. (Reproduced from Watson P, Besch N, Bowes WA Jr et al. Management of acute and subacute puerperal inversion of the uterus. Obstet Gynecol 1980; 55: 12–16[7] with permission from Lippincott Williams & Wilkins.)

practitioner at hand, who may have never personally managed such a case.

On rare occasions, manual replacement fails. In these situations, the procedure described by Huntington[36] will usually suffice. Huntington et al[37] reported the successful treatment of five cases of acute puerperal inversion with this procedure. The operation is accomplished by performing a laparotomy incision in the lower abdomen. The inverted fundus will be apparent (Figure 28.2), with the round ligaments disappearing into the inverted crater. The uterus is grasped in two places with clamps 1 inch (2.54 cm) within the crater, and gentle traction is exerted. A second set of clamps is then placed an inch beyond the first clamps, and so on, until the fundus is repositioned. Occasionally, pressure on the inverted fundus from an assistant's hand in the vagina will aid in the repositioning procedure. Tews et al described a modification of the transabdominal approach in which the bladder is dissected away from the cervix and a longitudinal incision is made into the vagina below the con-

traction ring. Two fingers inserted through this incision assist in applying upward pressure on the invaginated uterus.[38]

If the traction method described by Huntington[36] does not succeed in repositioning the fundus because the cervix is too tightly contracted, as may occur with subacute uterine inversion, a vertical incision is made through the posterior wall of the uterus where the inversion disappears from the abdomen. The inversion is then corrected by upward pressure from within the vagina by an assistant, a procedure described by Haultain[39] (Figure 28.3). Modifications of this procedure have been described in which an anterior incision is made in the uterus.[24] In addition, the Spinelli procedure (transvaginal incision in the anterior wall of the inverted and prolapsed uterus) has been reported for replacement of the uterine fundus in some cases of refractory inversion.[2]

Bell et al[2] collected 76 cases of puerperal inversion of the uterus reported in the US and UK literature from 1940 to 1952. Fifteen (20%) of these cases were treated surgically, five with

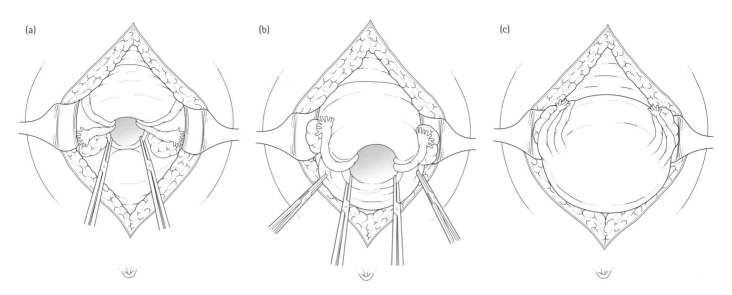

Figure 28.2 Huntington procedure for correction of uterine inversion. (a) The surface of the uterus is grasped with two Allis or Ochsner clamps approximately 1 inch (2.54 cm) within the crater, and gentle traction is applied. Pressure on the inverted fundus through the vagina by an assistant may facilitate the procedure. (b) As the uterine corpus is drawn out of the crater, an additional set of clamps is used to grasp the round ligaments 1 inch beyond the first set of clamps. (c) The uterine corpus after resolution of the inversion. (Figures 28.2 and 28.3 are original drawings based upon Figures 18–21 in Douglas RG, Stromme WB. Operative Obstetrics, (3rd edition). Appleton-Century-Crofts: New York, 1976.)

the Huntington procedure, one with the Haultain method, three with the Spinelli procedure, and six with hysterectomy. Among 182 cases of puerperal inversion of the uterus after vaginal delivery reported since 1960 (Table 28.1), surgical therapy was required in only seven (4%).[6–14] It is likely that earlier recognition, tocolytic drugs, improved anesthesia, and prompt use of the manual procedure to reposition the uterus have reduced the need for surgical intervention. It is reasonable to

administer a course of antibiotics after either manual or surgical treatment of uterine inversion. Blood loss, contamination of the endometrium, and tissue trauma all predispose the patient to puerperal infection.

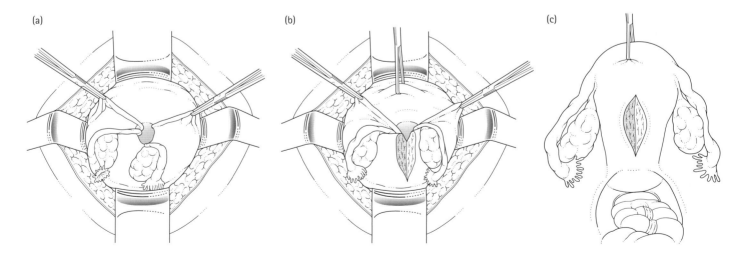

Figure 28.3 Haultain procedure for correction of uterine inversion. (a) A longitudinal incision is made posteriorly through the uterine wall to include the constriction ring. The corpus is then repositioned by pressure on the inverted fundus through the vagina by an assistant. (b) Once the corpus is repositioned, the incision on the posterior surface of the uterus must be sutured closed in a manner similar to that of closing the incision after classic cesarean delivery. (c) The reconstructed uterus.

Recurrence

The precise risk of recurrence of puerperal uterine inversion is not known. There are isolated reports of recurrent uterine inversion after manual repositioning. Some of these occurred in the postpartum period of the same pregnancy,[2,40] and others occurred in subsequent pregnancies.[16,21] Miller[41] reported the incidence of recurrence of inversion in subsequent pregnancies to be 26% and found the recurrence risk was higher when the inversion had been corrected manually (40%) than when it had been treated surgically (0%). However, recurrence of uterine inversion after surgical repair has been reported.[42] Even if future studies demonstrate a lower risk of recurrence than that given by Miller,[41] a patient with a history of uterine inversion must be considered at greater risk of recurrence in subsequent pregnancies. Such a past history would justify an ultrasound examination to determine the location of placental implantation. If fundal implantation is identified, intrapartum management of this patient should include use of oxytocin after delivery of the shoulders of the infant, and minimal cord traction or fundal pressure in delivery of the placenta.

Acknowledgements

Inasmuch as there are no randomized, controlled trials and no well-designed cohort or case-control analytic studies about puerperal inversion of the uterus, statements regarding etiology, pathophysiology, diagnosis, and management in this chapter are based upon level II-3 and level III evidence, that is, evidence obtained from multiple time series and opinions of respected authorities, based on clinical experience and descriptive studies. Recommendation for management should be regarded as level B, that is, based on limited or inconsistent scientific evidence.[43]

References

1. Fenton AN, Singh BP. Acute puerperal inversion of the uterus. Obstet Gynecol Surv 1950; 5: 781–95.
2. Bell JE Jr, Wilson F, Wilson L. Puerperal inversion of the uterus. Am J Obstet Gynecol 1953; 66: 767–80.
3. Das P. Inversion of the uterine. Br J Obstet Gynaecol 1940; 47: 525–48.
4. McCullagh WMH. Inversion of the uterus. A report on three cases and an analysis of 223 recently recorded cases. J Obstet Gynaecol Br Emp 1925; 32: 280–5.
5. Schaeffer G, Veprovsky EC. Inversion of the uterus. Surg Clin North Am 1949; 29: 599–610.
6. Kitchin JD III, Thiagarajah S, May HV, Thornton WN. Puerperal inversion of the uterus. Am J Obstet Gynecol 1975; 123; 51–8.
7. Watson P, Besch N, Bowes WA Jr. Management of acute and subacute puerperal inversion of the uterus. Obstet Gynecol 1980; 55: 12–16.
8. Cumming DC, Taylor JT. Puerperal uterine inversion: report of nine cases. Can Med Assoc J 1978; 118: 1268–70.
9. Platt LD, Druzin MKL. Acute puerperal inversion of the uterus. Am J Obstet Gynecol 1981; 141: 187–90.
10. Brar HS, Greenspoon JS, Platt LD et al. Acute puerperal uterine inversion: new approaches to management. J Reprod Med 1989; 34: 173–7.
11. Shah-Hosseini R, Evrard JR. Puerperal uterine inversion. Obstet Gynecol 1989; 73: 567–70.
12. Catanzarite VA, Moffit KD, Baker ML, et al. New approaches to the management of acute puerperal uterine inversion. Obstet Gynecol 1989; 68: 7S-10S.
13. Abouleish E, Ali V, Joumaa B et al. Anaesthetic management of acute puerperal uterine inversion. Br J Anaesth 1995; 75: 486–7.
14. Baskett TF. Acute uterine inversion: a review of 40 cases. J Obstet Gynaecol Canada 2002; 24: 953–6.
15. Kellogg FS. Puerperal inversion of the uterus. Classification for treatment. Am J Obstet Gynecol 1929; 18: 815–17.
16. Henderson H, Alles RW. Puerperal inversion of the uterus. Am J Obstet Gynecol 1948; 56: 133–42.
17. Kriplani A, Relan S, Kumar RK et al. Complete inversion of the uterus during caesarean section: a case report. Aust N Z J Obstet Gynaecol 1996; 36: 17–19.
18. Rudloff U, Joels LA, Marshall N. Inversion of the uterus at ceasarean section. Arch Gynecol Obstet 2003; 3: 224–6.
19. Banerjee N, Deka D, Roy KK et al. Inversion of uterus during cesarean section. Eur J Obstet Gynecol Reprod Biol 2000; 91: 75–7.
20. Burke JW, Hofmeister FJ. Uterine inversion obstetrical entity or oddity. Am J Obstet Gynecol 1965; 91: 934–40.
21. Heyl PS, Stubblefield PG, Phillippe M. Recurrent inversion of the puerperal uterus managed with 15(s)-15-methyl prostaglandin $F_{2\alpha}$ and uterine packing. Obstet Gynecol 1984; 63: 263–4.
22. Penderville W, Elbourne D, Chalmers I. The effects of routine oxytocic administration in the management of the third stage of labour: an overview from controlled trials. Br J Obstet Gynaecol 1988; 95: 3–16.
23. Fleigner JR, Hibbart BM. Active management of the third stage of labour. BMJ 1966; 2: 622–3.
24. Romo MS, Grimes DA, Strassle PO. Infarction of the uterus from subacute incomplete inversion. Am J Obstet Gynecol 1992; 166: 878–9.
25. Lewin JS, Bryan PJ. MR imaging of uterine inversion. J Comput Assist Tomogr 1989; 13: 357–9.
26. De Villiers VP. Intravenous hexoprenaline in the reduction of acute puerperal inversion of the uterus. S Afr Med J 1977; 51: 664–5.
27. Smith GN, Brien JF. Use of nitroglycerin for uterine relaxation. Obstet Gynecol Surv 1998; 53: 559–65.
28. Altabef KM, Spencer JT, Zinberg S. Intravenous nitroglycerin for uterine relaxation of an inverted uterus. Am J Obstet Gynecol 1992; 16: 1237–8.
29. Dayan SS, Schwalbe SS. The use of small-dose intravenous nitroglycerin in a case of uterine inversion. Anesth Analg 1996; 82: 1091–3.

30. Bayhi DA, Sherwood CDA, Campbell CE. Intravenous nitroglycerin for uterine inversion. J Clin Anesth 1992; 4: 487–8.

31. Thiery M, Delbeke L. Acute puerperal uterine inversion: two-step management with a B-mimetic and a prostaglandin. Am J Obstet Gynecol 1985; 153: 891–2.

32. Johnson AB. A new concept in the replacement of the inverted uterus and a report of nine cases. Am J Obstet Gynecol 1949; 57: 557–62.

33. O'Sullivan JV. Acute inversion of the uterus. BMJ 1945; 2: 282–3.

34. Momani A, Hassan A. Treatment of puerperal uterine inversion by the hydrostatic method; reports of five cases. Eur J Obstet Gynecol Reprod Biol 1989; 32: 281–5.

35. Campbell J, Pash J, Walters WAW. Acute inversion of the uterus and its management. Med J Aust 1972; 2: 475–6.

36. Huntington JL. Acute inversion of the uterus. Boston Med Surg J 1921; 15: 376.

37. Huntington JL, Irving FC, Kellogg FS. Abdominal reposition in acute inversion of the puerperal uterus. Am J Obstet Gynecol 1928; 15: 34.

38. Tews G, Ebner T, Yaman C et al. Acute puerperal inversion of the uterus – treatment by a new abdominal uterus preserving approach. Acta Obstet Gynecol Scand 2001; 80: 1039–40.

39. Haultain FWN. The treatment of chronic uterine inversion by abdominal hysterectomy with a successful care. BMJ 1901; 2: 974.

40. Silver DF, Heyl PS, Linfert JB. Delayed uterine re-inversion: a unique symptom complex. Am J Obstet Gynecol 2004; 191; 378–9.

41. Miller NF. Pregnancy following inversion of the uterus. Am J Obstet Gynecol 1927; 13: 307–22.

42. Steffen E. Puerperal inversion of the uterus occurring in consecutive pregnancies in the same patient. Am J Obstet Gynecol 1957; 74: 655–7.

43. American College of Obstetricians and Gynecologists. Reading the medical literature: applying evidence to practice. Compendium of Selected Publications, pp. 259–70. Washington, DC, 2004.

29 Wound healing, sutures, knots, needles, drains, and instruments

Jesús R Alvarez and Vijaya Ganesh

It is imperative for a surgeon to have a basic understanding of the mechanisms that control wound healing. Due to the increased knowledge acquired in the biomechanics of wound healing, a modern surgeon now practices and develops new surgical skills with a better understanding of what to use, for how long, and when.

Surgical wound healing

Tissue loss or damage causes either regeneration or repair by scar tissue, or a combination of both. Human tissue heals by scarring with the exception of the epidermis, bone, liver, and the mucosa of the intestinal tract, which heal by regeneration.

Wound healing is classified as healing by first, second, or tertiary (delayed primary) intention (Figure 29.1).

Primary or first intention healing occurs when the edges of a wound are approximated, such as a surgical skin incision closed with sutures. The apposition of the tissue layers permits a rapid re-epithelialization sealing of the incisional defect with minimal scarring.

Secondary intention type of healing occurs when the wound edges are not approximated and are left open to granulate and heal. This is seen in burns, in punch biopsies, or in cases of infected wounds or incisions left open to allow closure spontaneously. With a combination of contraction and granulation, the wound eventually epithelializes. This healing process can be slow and may produce extensive scarring.

Delayed primary closure, or healing by tertiary intention, occurs when an open wound is closed several days after the injury. This method is used for wounds with gross contamina-tion. This type of wound management may be used when a ruptured tuboovarian abscess is encountered during a laparotomy. After the closure of the peritoneum and the fascia, the subcutaneous layer and the skin are packed with sterile wet dressings, and the wound is left open for several days. The wound is then closed several days later after the contamination has been diminished. Successful closure depends on the condition of the wound edges and the absence of significant bacterial colonization. The best timing for such closure is 3–4 days. Delayed closures after 1 week do not heal well due to an increase of collagen deposition.[1]

The biologic events involved in wound healing are conceptually defined as *inflammation*, *epithelialization*, *granulation*, *fibroplasia*, and *contraction*. These steps occur simultaneously and should not be seen as separate processes. These are nonspecific mechanisms activated by the tissue injury.

An inflammatory response is the initial stage of wound healing. When tissue injury occurs, vasoconstriction traps platelets at the wound site. The coagulation cascade is stimulated, forming a stable clot at the site of injury. This vasoconstriction lasts approximately 10 minutes and is followed by vasodilation, which causes edema. The platelets degranulate, and biologically active products are generated, stimulating the converting fibroblasts and endothelial cells into reparative entities.

Monocytes and leukocytes are stimulated to migrate into the site of injury secondary to chemoatractant products released in this inflammatory phase. Their function is to remove debris and bacteria by active phagocytosis and complement-induced lysis. Monocytes then differentiate into macrophages, which are crucial to wound healing. Macrophages continue to consume

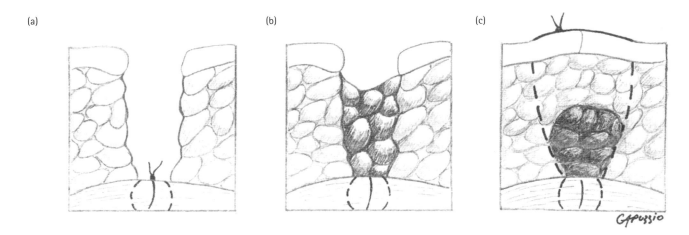

Figure 29.1 Wound healing by primary (a), secondary (b), and tertiary (c) intention.

tissue and bacterial debris but, more importantly, also secrete a plethora of growth factors.[2] These further stimulate fibroblasts and epithelial cells to initiate granulation tissue formation.

During the granulation phase, fibroblast proliferation (fibroplasia), endothelial cell division, and angiogenesis occur. This process produces a new, loose, extracellular matrix composed of collagen (mostly types I and III), fibronectin, hyaluronic acid, and adhesion glycoproteins that maintain the matrix together.

Epithelialization occurs by migration of marginal basal cells. These cells are derived from the fixed basal layer zone adjacent to the tissue injury site. The daughter cells migrate over the new wound matrix in an immature form. They release type IV collagen and mature, epithelial cells that move under the scab. Glycoproteins in the matrix and hemidesmosomes maintain the integrity of these cells, and a watertight seal is produced 24 hours after tissue injury. Keratin will then form as these epithelial cells eventually mature.

Fibroplasia is the step in wound healing that ultimately forms a fibrous scar secondary to collagen deposition. It also determines the strength of the scar produced. The tensile strength of a wound varies depending on the type of tissue and the time since the injury. The tensile strength of a skin wound increases in the course of 6 weeks.[3] Fibroblasts migrate to the site of tissue injury secondary to the chemoattractants released by macrophages. These fibroblasts deposit collagen on the fibrin and fibronectin sheets after the clot forms. New collagen fibers can be appreciated 3 days after injury. Fibroblasts also release mucopolysaccharides and glycoproteins. They are the major contributors to the new extracellular matrix formed.

Wound contraction occurs in an open wound when the surrounding uninjured skin edges are brought together. This process occurs simultaneously with the fibroplasia phase of healing. The cell responsible for the process of wound contraction is the myofibroblast. Wound contraction is an active process produced by contractile proteins within the cells. Myofibroblast cells have gap junctions and cell to matrix links. These are

beneficial because they reduce the area of scar tissue covering the injury. The tissue between the edges of the skin is a scar, lacking normal skin appendages and incorporating disorganized collagen fibers.

Suture material

The Edwin Smith papyrus from 3000 BC describes the use of linen strips and animal sinews for simple wound closure. Celsus, the Roman physician, advocated ligation of blood vessels. Although sutures have been used for many centuries, it was only in the second half of the nineteenth century that suturing became practical and safe, after the introduction of asepsis by Semmelweis and Pasteur.[4]

The suture is characterized by the type of material and the gauge of the suture, according to the US Pharmacopeia (USP) system. This characterization is based on the rate of absorption. If the tensile strength is lost within 60 days, the suture is categorized as 'absorbable'. This term implies that eventually the suture will disappear from the tissue implantation site. *Nonabsorbable sutures* are those which maintain their tensile strength for more than 60 days.

A surgeon has a wide choice of suture materials available today. The decision of which type of suture to be used should be based on the knowledge of the physical and biologic properties of the suture material, and the healing ability of the sutured tissue.

Absorbable sutures

Absorbable material may be either organic (catgut) or synthetic. The organic sutures are lysed by body enzymes.[5,6] In the first stage, the strength of the material is lost, and later the suture is totally absorbed.

The *organic absorbable sutures* used in operative obstetrics are chromic catgut or plain sutures. Catgut may be chromicized ('chromic catgut') or plain. The difference is in the strength of the suture material and the time needed for absorption. The manufacturers used to mark catgut with the number of days it was supposed to take until it was completely absorbed. The strength of the knot of both types of catgut is lessened by 50% after 1 week. Plain material is absorbed within 12 days, while the chromic suture keeps for about 28 days. Catgut suture absorption is caused by a proteolytic enzymatic reaction. This causes a marked inflammatory response in the tissue that is approximated with this suture.

Although a number of papers have claimed to show the superiority of synthetic absorbable sutures over natural ones,[7,8] the majority of US obstetric and gynecologic surgeons still prefer chromic catgut to any other material.[5]

Chromic suture

This suture is used when performing bilateral uterine artery ligation, closure of the uterine incision, approximation of the peritoneal surfaces, tubal ligation, and closure of episiotomies and lacerations after vaginal delivery. It is customary to use no. 1.0 chromic suture for a nonpermanent hypogastric artery ligation, because it is unlikely to lacerate the tissue, and is quickly absorbed in the body.

Plain gut

This gut suture is used in obstetrics for tubal ligation and for approximation of the subcutaneous tissue. It is the ideal material (2.0 plain gut) for a modified Pomeroy tubal ligation because of its quick absorption.[9]

The *synthetic absorbable suture* material is absorbed by hydrolysis, and not by enzymatic reaction.[5,6] Because of this, synthetic sutures provoke less tissue reaction, have great tensile strength, and are absorbed less rapidly (Table 29.1). These synthetic absorbable sutures can be categorized further into braided and monofilament sutures.

Since the 1970s, two types of braided absorbable sutures have been used. Braided sutures have great tensile strength but may induce bacterial infection.

Polyglycolic acid (Dexon)

This is a braided, absorbable, synthetic suture material with greater tensile strength than catgut. Dexon causes minimal tissue reaction, retains 50–60% of its tensile strength for 14 days, and is reabsorbed by hydrolysis after 60–90 days. Dexon is useful for the closure of fascia, tendons, muscle, and capsules.

Polyglactic acid (Vicryl)

This is a braided, absorbable, synthetic suture material similar to Dexon. Breakdown is by hydrolysis, causing minimal inflammatory reaction. After 14 days, Vicryl has a tensile strength of 50%. It is usually absorbed after 60–90 days. Since braided sutures induce bacterial infection, an antibiotic-coated Vicryl suture was developed, but it failed to decrease infection rates.

Polyglactin 910 (Vicryl Rapide)

This braided suture was first used in Europe and is available now in the USA. It is chemically similar to Vicryl, but has lower molecular weight. Its absorption is by hydrolysis. It has a tensile strength of 1 week, similar to that of catgut. Vicryl Rapide is mostly used in for episiotomies and in skin closure.

Poliglecaprone 25 (Monocryl)

This is a monofilament suture similar in absorption time to chromic catgut. The tensile strength of this suture is 50–60% in 7 days. It is absorbed by hydrolysis, causing minimal inflammatory response. After 21 days, it has lost all its tensile strength, so it is not recommended for fascial closure.

Polyglyconate (Maxon) and polydioxanone (PDS)

These sutures have similar characteristics and biologic properties. They are monofilament polymers with a slow absorption rate. Both have a tensile strength of 80% by 2 weeks and of 50% by 4 weeks. Since they are monofilament and not braided, bacterial infection secondary to the suture material is not common. It is rare for an inflammatory response to this suture material to occur even though its complete absorption may take months.

Synthetic absorbable sutures are frequently used in modern operative obstetrics. Vicryl suture is the one most frequently used for uterine incision closure, hysterectomy, ligament and vessel suture ligation, skin closure, and episiotomy repair. Because it causes minimal inflammatory reaction, episiotomy repair with Vicryl is less likely to cause short-term perineal pain than chromic catgut. Nevertheless, the length of time taken for the synthetic material to be absorbed is of concern.[10] Vicryl Rapide and Monocryl are probably the best sutures for episiotomy closure, since they have minimal inflammatory response and have the same properties as chromic catgut.

Monocryl suture is now widely used for closure of uterine incisions, myomectomies, reapproximation of peritoneal surfaces and the subcutaneous layer, episiotomies, and skin closure. Because of its short tensile strength, it should never be used in fascial closure. It creates minimal inflammatory tissue response, making it ideal for myomectomy (decreasing the risk of adhesions) and episiotomy repair. It is the best suture for skin subcuticular closure. Due to its short reabsorption time, it is not necessary to remove these sutures, thus lessening the patient's discomfort and anxiety.[11] Because this is a monofilament suture, the risk of bacterial infection is minimal.

PDS is a synthetic polymer monofilament suture material. It has high tensile strength and long duration, making it ideal

Table 29.1 Comparison of the biomechanical properties of absorbable suture materials

Absorbable suture	50% Tensile strength	Complete absorption
Plain	3 days	10 days
Chromic	7 days	21 days
Monocryl	7 days	21 days
Vicryl	14 days	60–90 days
PDS	>42 days	>6 months

for fascial closure. PDS maintains its integrity even in the presence of a bacterial infection. Its disadvantages are that it is stiff, is difficult to handle, and has poor knot security.

Nonabsorbable sutures

Nonabsorbable sutures maintain their tensile strength for over 60 days and are absorbed only after a long period of time.

Polypropylene (Prolene)

This is a monofilament linear polymer suture. Prolene causes the least immune reaction of any suture materials. This suture has been retrieved after 2–6 years and still maintained its tensile strength.[12]

Nylon

Nylon suture is available as a monofilament (Ethilon, Dermalon) or a multifilament (Neurolon, Surgilon). Neither form causes tissue reaction and may be used in the presence of bacteria since nylon is inert. Nylon is usually absorbed after 2 years. Its disadvantage is knot slippage, so careful attention should be used when tying it.

Polyester

These types of sutures have great strength and durability, but since they are braided, they are not recommended in the presence of bacteria. Mersilene is an uncoated type of suture. It is frequently used for cervical cerclage. The advantage of this suture is that it possesses great knot security.

Silk

This is a protein filament obtained from silkworm larvae. It is braided, has great tensile strength, and is easy to handle. The major advantage of this suture is its knot security. However, silk acts as a source of infection, and therefore its popularity has diminished.

Staples

Skin staples are frequently used in obstetrics for closure, especially in a vertical skin incision. The only benefit of staples over subcuticular stitches is speed. However, skin staples may cause more pain and a less favorable cosmetic result.[13–15] Internal stapling devices are rarely used in obstetrics.

Nonabsorbable sutures such as Prolene and Mersilene are both used for cervical cerclage.

For fascial closure, the suture must be chosen by its tensile strength, the type of laparotomy incision made, and the quality of the fascial layer to be approximated. When performing a fascial closure, one should not lock the suture, since this causes necrosis and weakens the fascia. If a vertical incision is performed, the fascia should always be reapproximated either with PDS, or with a nonabsorbable suture, such as nylon. Neither Vicryl nor Dexon should be used for a vertical fascial closure. The best fascial closure for a vertical incision is a continuous, running mass closure because it has a significantly greater wound strength, and decreases closure time when compared to

the interrupted technique.[16] If a transverse incision is performed and the patient has no medical problems, the fascial closure can be performed with Vicryl or Dexon. If the patient has diabetes, is morbidly obese, or had previous surgery, closure of the fascia should be done with PDS.

Knots

Surgery is both a science and an art. Dexterity and speed in tying knots constitute an art which only practice can make perfect.[17]

The surgical knots used in operative obstetrics can be divided into two categories: sliding knots (identical or non-identical) and flat knots (square and surgeon's). A sliding knot is formed when two half-hitches are tied, applying greater tension on one segment of the suture. A flat knot is formed when two half-hitches are tied applying the same tension to both segments of the suture.

Sliding knots have a tendency to slip and are less secure. However, they are easy to make and are frequently used in operative obstetrics.[18] It is better to use a sliding knot in certain situations, as when tying deep in the pelvis. The addition of several throws to a sliding knot improves the knot's security.[19]

Flat knots are the most secure of the surgical knots if the number of throws is adequate.[20] When unnecessary throws are used, the risk of infection increases. Studies have shown that a minimum of four throws should be used to achieve optimum knot-holding capacity when using a flat knot on a nonmonofilament absorbable suture.[21]

Investigations to determine the security of knots tied with one looped end and one free end versus knots with two free ends have been done. It has been demonstrated that knots with one looped and one free end are weaker than those tied with two free ends.[22] Therefore, a continuous suture line is best tied with a knot having two free ends (Figure 29.2).

Needles

Currently, the needle is attached to the suture material by the manufacturer and is atraumatic; therefore, the type of eye of the needle meticulously described in former textbooks is no longer relevant.

Curved needles are usually used for sutures. The diameter of the curve depends on the bulk of the material to be sutured. The profile of the needle (transverse section) is of two main types: round and cutting. Cutting needles may be of different shapes, such as reverse cutting with the point away from the curve, tapering in the form of a spatula, and so forth. Needles may be of various lengths, usually in the range 13–50 mm. Several sutures have needles attached to each end. Soft and friable tissue should be sutured with round needles, and thick or hard tissue with a cutting needle. Therefore, the uterus and the peritoneum are transfixed with round needles, while the use of

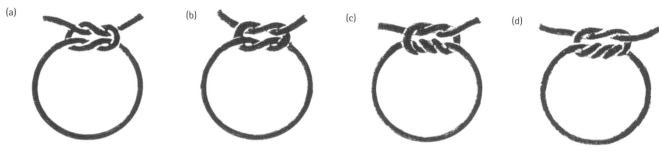

Figure 29.2 (a) Square knot; (b) granny knot; (c) surgeon's square knot; (d) surgeon's granny knot. (Drawing by Julian Gaspar.)

cutting ones is recommended for the fascia and the skin. The use of different types of cutting needles and straight needles will depend on the preference of the surgeon. Hand needles, which require no needle holder, shorten operation time and are therefore popular in the UK. They have gained little acceptance, however, in the USA.

Drains

The earliest documented use of a drainage system was by Celsus in the first century AD. He placed lead and bronze tubes into the abdominal cavity as gravity drains. In contemporary surgery, the use of prophylactic drains for peritoneal contamination has been abandoned because they are quickly surrounded by bowel and omentum.[23]

Currently, there are four type of drains used: (1) the Penrose drain; (2) the closed-suction drain; (3) the sump drain; (4) the closed-suction Penrose drain. In obstetrics, the Penrose drain and the closed-suction drain are most frequently used. These drains are brought through a separate stab wound, not through the surgical incision, to prevent infection in the suture line, weakness of the fascia, and subsequent hernia.

Penrose drain

This is a very efficient drain; however, it increases the risk of secondary infection.[24] It is a latex drain which varies in size and diameter. It is used for drainage of blood, pus, or serosanguineous fluid from a cavity.

Closed-suction drain (Jackson Pratt)

Closed-suction drains of silicone are minimally irritating to tissues. These drains have a low incidence of secondary infection, but tend to clog and cease functioning earlier than the Penrose drain.[24]

To drain or not to drain is still an area of controversy. Some studies in surgery have shown no benefit from intra-abdominal drains. Besides, intra-abdominal drains can cause adhesions and ultimately bowel obstruction. However, it is advisable to place an intra-abdominal drain whenever hemostatic control is not optimal during a cesarean section. This may occur in cases of

ruptured uterus, severe preeclampsia, and superimposed HELLP syndrome, and in patients on anticoagulation therapy.

Some studies have suggested that the use of drains in the subcutaneous space may reduce the incidence of postoperative complications in obese women who have at least 2 cm of subcutaneous tissue.[25] Nevertheless, suture closure of the subcutaneous fat during a cesarean section is probably better than placement of a subcutaneous drain.[26]

Instruments for operative obstetrics

The instrument table should include the proper armamentarium and drapes for operative obstetrics. The following list of instruments includes the equipment necessary to perform a cervical cerclage, dilation and curettage, cesarean section, and hysterectomy. Other surgeons may use different instruments, according to their own preferences and experience.

Cerclage set

Item description	Quantity
Ring forceps	4
Long Heaney needle holder	1
Long Heaney needle	1
Kelly's	2
Scissors (long straight Mayo)	1
Retractors – lateral (Sims)	2
Heavy weighted speculum	1
Forceps plain	1
Forceps w/teeth	1
Russian forceps	1
Sound	1
Aneurysm – L-hand	1
Aneurysm – R-hand	1
Disposable scalpel Size 10	1
Disposable scalpel Size 12	1
Disposable scalpel Size 15	1

Cesarean section tray

Item description	Quantity
Knife handle	2
Sponge sticks	5
Retractors	
Balfour blade	1
Richardson (large)	2
Richardson (small)	2
Army/Navy	2
Forceps	
Mouse tooth	2
Plain	2
Plain (large)	1
Mouse tooth (large)	1
De Bakey vascular	1
Needle holders	
Large	1
Small	1
Clamps	
Towel	6
Mosquito	14
Kelly	7
Babcock	4
Kocher	6
Allis	4
T-clamp	10
Scissors	
Metzenbaum	2
Straight Mayo	2
Curved Mayo	2
Bandage	1
Kidney basin	1
Light handles	2
Stat pack (wrapped separately in a surgical towel)	
Mosquito	6
Kelly	4
Kocher	2
T-clamps	5
Knife handles	2
Suture scissors	1
Curved Mayo	1
Bandage scissors	1
Metzenbaum scissors	1
Allis clamp	2
Needle holder	2
Forceps (plain and toothed)	2

Hysterectomy tray

Item description	Quantity
Knife handle	2
Knife handle long	1
Balfour retractor and blade	1
Ribbon retractor small	1
Ribbon retractor medium	1
Ribbon retractor large	1
Army-Navy retractor	2
O'Connor–Sullivan w/blade	1
Richardson retractor small	2
Richardson retractor medium	2
Richardson retractor large	2
Deaver retractor small	2
Deaver retractor medium	2
Deaver retractor large	2
Cystic duct forceps	1
Needle holder 8 inch	2
Needle holder 6 inch	2
Tissue forceps w/teeth 8 inch	2
Dressing forceps plain 8 inch	2
Adson forceps w/teeth	2
Babcock clamps 8 inch	4
Kocher clamps	6
Allis clamps	8
Halstead clamps	4
Right angle clamps	4
Tonsil clamps	6

D & C tray

Item description	Quantity
Lateral retractor, L-shaped blades	1
Heavy weighted speculum	1
Leaves speculum (medium or large)	1
Hank dilators	
Set no. 1	
9/10	1
11/12	1
13/14	1
15/16	1
17/18	1
19/20	1
Set no. 2	
17/18	1
19/20	1
21/22	1
23/24	1
25/26	1
27/28	1
Uterine curette sharp no. 1	1
Uterine curette sharp no. 2	1
Uterine curette sharp no. 3	1
Uterine curette sharp no. 4	1
Uterine curette sharp no. 5	1
Curette, Heaney endometrial (serrated cup)	1
Curette, endocervical (tip end is square)	1
Uterine sound (tip end has a ball tip)	1
Thumb tissue forceps	1
Thumb dressing forceps	1
Baum's tenaculums	2
Allis tissue clamps	2
Polyp forceps	1
Mayo Hager needle holder	1
Mayo dissecting scissors	1
Forrester sponge forceps straight	4
Curved Allis	1

References

1. Edlich RF, Rogers W, Kasper G et al. Studies on the management of the contaminated wound. I. Optimal time for closure of contaminated open wounds. Am J Surg 1969; 117: 323–9.
2. Rappolee DA, Mark D, Banda MJ et al. Wound macrophages express TGF-alpha and other growth factors *in vivo*: analysis by mRNA phenotyping. Science 1989; 241: 708–12.
3. Madden JW, Peacock EE Jr. Studies on the biology of collagen during healing. III. Dynamic metabolism of scar collagen and remodeling in dermal wounds. Ann Surg 1971; 174: 511–20.
4. Stroumtsos A. Perspectives on Sutures. David and Geek, American Cyanamid Company, 1978.
5. Hartko WJ, Ghanekar G, Kemmann E. Suture materials currently used in obstetric-gynecologic surgery in the United States. Obstet Gynecol 1982; 9: 241.
6. Holmlund D, Tera H, Wiberg Y et al. Sutures and Techniques for Wound Closure. Medical and Surgical Publications, Naimark and Barba: New York, 1978.
7. Gallitano AL, Kondi ES. The superiority of polyglycolic acid sutures for closure of abdominal incision. Surg Gynecol Obstet 1973; 37: 794–6.
8. Kronborg O. Polyglycolic acid (Dexon) versus silk for fascial closure of abdominal incision. Acta Chir Scand 1976; 142: 9–12.
9. Bishop E, Nelms WF. A simple method of tubal sterilization. N Y State J Med 1930; 30: 214.
10. Kettle C, Johanson RB. Absorbable synthetic versus catgut suture material for perineal repair. Cochrane Database Syst Rev 2000; (2): CD000006.
11. Parell GJ, Becker GD. Comparison of absorbable with nonabsorbable sutures in closure of facial skin wounds. Arch Facial Plast Surg 2003; 5: 488–90.
12. Edgerton MT. The Art of Surgical Technique. Williams & Wilkins: Baltimore, MD, 1988.
13. Eldrup J, Wied U, Andersen B. Randomised trial comparing Proximate stapler with conventional skin closure. Acta Chir Scand 1981; 147: 501–2.
14. Ranaboldo CJ, Rowe-Jones DC. Closure of laparotomy wounds: skin staples versus sutures. Br J Surg 1992; 79: 1172–3.
15. Frishman GN, Schwartz T, Hogan JW. Closure of Pfannenstiel skin incisions. Staples vs. subcuticular suture. J Reprod Med 1997; 42: 627–30.
16. Seid MH, McDaniel-Owens LM, Poole GV Jr, Meeks GR. A randomized trial of abdominal incision suture technique and wound strength in rats. Arch Surg 1995; 130: 394–7.
17. Bashir Zikria, Ethicon Knot Tying Manual, 1996.
18. Trimbos JB. Security of various knots commonly used in surgical practice. Obstet Gynecol 1984; 64: 274–80.
19. Ivy JJ, Unger JB, Mukherjee D. Knot integrity with nonidentical and parallel sliding knots. Am J Obstet Gynecol 2004; 190: 83–6.
20. Brouwers JE, Oosting H, Haas D, Kloppers PJ Dynamic loading of surgical knots. Surg Gynecol Obstet 1991; 173: 443–8.
21. Brown RP. Knotting technique and suture materials. Br J Surg 1992; 79: 399–400.

22. Annunziata CC, Drake DB, Woods JA et al. Technical considerations in knot construction. I. Continuous percutaneous and dermal suture closure. J Emerg Med 1997; 15: 351–6.

23. Stylianos S, Martin, EC, Starker PM et al. Percutaneous drainage of intra-abdominal abcesses following abdominal trauma. J Trauma 1989; 29: 584–8.

24. Berlin RB, Javna SL. Closed suction wide area drainage. Surg Gynecol Obstet 1992; 174: 421.

25. Allaire AD, Fisch J, McMahon MJ. Subcutaneous drain vs. suture in obese women undergoing cesarean delivery. A prospective, randomized trial. J Reprod Med 2000; 45: 327–31.

26. Chelmow D, Rodriguez EJ, Sabatini MM. Suture closure of subcutaneous fat and wound disruption after cesarean delivery: a meta-analysis. Obstet Gynecol 2004; 103: 974–80.

30 Cesarean section

Joseph J Apuzzio and Charbel G Salamon

Cesarean section has had a tumultuous and controversial history. The operation was seldom used before the end of the nineteenth century because of its prohibitive maternal mortality; it was utilized at a rate of less than 5% of births until 1960.[1,2] A dramatic rise in abdominal deliveries has occurred over the past three decades. The cesarean delivery rate in the USA in 1970 was 5.5%, compared to 26.1% in 2002.[3] Approximately one in ten women in spontaneous labor delivers by cesarean. Several factors have contributed to this change:[4,5]

- Women are delaying childbearing, leading to more births among women of older age. This group has a high rate of cesarean deliveries.
- A higher proportion of births are occurring in nulliparous women, who are also at higher risk of cesarean delivery.
- Continuous fetal monitoring has increased the cesarean delivery rate for nonreassuring fetal status.
- There are concerns about legal action in the event of an adverse outcome.
- A diagnosis of dystocia is made more frequently and managed by cesarean delivery.
- Term vaginal breech delivery is discouraged.
- There is routine repeat cesarean birth. In 2001, 39% of all cesarean deliveries were repeat cesarean births,[3] making this one of the leading indications for abdominal delivery.
- There is cesarean section on 'demand'.

The final goal of any operative indication is that the necessity of performing the operation would appear as valid in retrospect as it does in prospect. Although this goal may never be achieved in all cases, it should be sought.

Historical review

Prior to the end of the nineteenth century, cesarean section was one of the most fatal of surgical operations. In 1885, the mortality rate in Great Britain and Ireland was 85%.[6] The rate was 92% in New York City in 1887. Not one woman survived cesarean section from 1786 to 1876 in greater Paris. Paradoxically, the mortality rate was less than half (40%) of the usual rates when women in desperation did sections on themselves or delivered abdominally after having been gored by the horns of cattle. Many factors contributed to the risks of cesarean section. Several reports underscored the necessity of performing it during early labor.[7–9] When the operation was done as a last resort, the maternal mortality rate was 92% in New York and 75% in Louisiana.

In 1882, Sanger's[10] epic monograph provided the basis for a revolution in obstetrics. Contending that the treatment of the uterine wound was crucial, he urged that buried sutures should be used to close it. The new technique converted a fatal operation into a relatively safe procedure.

In 1930, Williams showed that the 'timely operation' was still crucial, since the maternal mortality rate was less than 2% when section was done during the early stages of labor, 10% when it was done during advanced labor, 15% following induction of labor, and 27% after failed forceps maneuvers.[11] Many of the current indications for cesarean section fall into the last three categories; hence, they would be associated with a prohibitive maternal mortality if progress had not been made.

Maternal mortality rates decreased steadily with the introduction of safe blood transfusion, antibiotics, and safe anesthesia. Before this time, hemorrhage and infection had been leading causes of maternal death. Transfusions treated hemorrhage by direct blood replacement to prevent shock, and infection by preventing anemia and low resistance to sepsis. Infection was treated directly with antibiotics, often preventing death in previously lethal situations. Progress with anesthesia enabled cesarean section to be used safely in emergency situations.

Before 1960, there were no means to determine fetal well-being in the uterus or the chances of newborn survival outside the uterus. The pregnant uterus was an emotional, as well as physiologic, barrier to investigation. Some early discoveries with therapeutic promise provided cogent reason to invade the uterus on a therapeutic rather than on a purely investigative basis.[12] Thus, the emotional restraint was broken, and the new field of fetal medicine emerged. Fetal well-being was determined by measuring excreted metabolic products, such as urinary estriol, and the fetal response to the stress of uterine contraction or correlated fetal movement and heart rate.

Ultrasound provided an accurate means of determining fetal size and growth. Sampling fetal blood during labor was possible for direct biochemical analysis. The maturity of fetal lungs before birth was measurable, so that the chances for fetal survival could be predicted. Intrauterine transfusion became possible.

New knowledge of fetal medicine combined with increasing concern for maternal safety necessitated a reconsideration of classic indications and provided evidence that the operation could be utilized as an alternative to difficult vaginal operations. The focus of attention shifted from the mother to the fetus, and expectations for reduced perinatal morbidity and mortality rates increased. *Perfect fetal results* became the primary goal. Cesarean section provided the means for fulfilling these expectations. However, two points were overlooked in this transition: (1) some of the sections were not necessarily based on valid, evidence-based medicine; (2) cesarean section was not a perfectly safe procedure for the mother. In retrospect, traditional indications have changed so markedly that there are only limited guidelines for the use of the operation in obstetrics.[13]

Indications for cesarean section

Sections may be performed for maternal, fetal, or combined indications. Maternal indications include those done in the mother's interest when vaginal birth is dangerous or impossible. A section would be done for fetal indication when the fetal risk is less with abdominal than with vaginal birth. When it is in the interest of both mother and fetus to have a cesarean delivery, we have a combined indication.

The four most common indications for cesarean section account for approximately 70% of these deliveries:

(1) failure to progress in labor
(2) nonreassuring fetal status (nonreassuring antepartum fetal testing by nonstress test, biophysical profile, fetal blood sampling, Doppler assessment, contraction stress test, fetal heart rate monitoring, etc.)
(3) previous cesarean delivery or hysterotomy (secondary to myomectomy or uterine surgery, etc.)
(4) fetal malpresentation (breech, transverse lie, etc.).

The interests of the mother and fetus do not always coincide. The decision making requires experience, clinical judgment, logic, and consideration of the wishes of the parents. The right decision results from understanding all factors, rather than relying on a tabulated list of indications. Decisions should take into account any conflict between the interests of the mother and the fetus.

Maternal indications

From the maternal perspective, the crucial questions are as follows:

- How soon must the process be terminated by delivery?
- How soon can vaginal birth be accomplished?
- What are the chances of severe complications arising as a result of any delay in delivery?
- To what extent will a major operation (cesarean section) be dangerous for the mother?

Absolute indications

(1) Patients with total placenta previa must always be delivered by section, even if the fetus is dead. Low-lying placenta previa is considered by many as an indication for section, although, as a maternal indication, the imperativeness of the indication varies somewhat with the degree of the previa.
(2) Abruptio placentae is an absolute indication for section if the hemorrhage is severe and the fetus is not immediately deliverable. In this situation, section may be indicated even in the presence of fetal death. However, if the fetus is immediately deliverable, vaginal birth may be preferable for the mother's sake. Marginal abruption ('marginal sinus rupture'), on the other hand, is not a maternal indication for section because complications such as severe hemorrhage, clotting disorders, and renal failure, sometimes associated with central abruption, do not arise.
(3) Most neurologists feel that section should be performed if the patient has had cerebral hemorrhage or has an aneurysm because any second-stage bearing-down effort is usually contraindicated.
(4) Mechanical obstruction to vaginal birth (such as large leiomyoma or condyloma acuminata, severely displaced pelvic fracture, cervical myoma, or pedunculated ovarian tumor). All myomas do not require section, however, some will be drawn upward as the lower uterine segment develops.
(5) Virtually everyone agrees that the cervix should not be dilated with invasive carcinoma of the cervix. Pregnant women with carcinoma *in situ* or microinvasive disease (up to 3 mm in depth, having undergone full evaluation during pregnancy with a conization showing negative margins) may be followed to term and delivered vaginally, with re-evaluation and treatment at 6 weeks postpartum.[14] Recurrences have been reported at the episiotomy site in women who delivered vaginally; this area should be inspected and palpated during post-treatment surveillance.[14] Delivery in women with larger-volume, invasive cervical cancer should be by classical cesarean delivery to avoid potential cervical hemorrhage and possible dissemination of tumor cells during labor and vaginal birth, although the latter risk is controversial.[15,16] A classical cesarean and radical hysterectomy with therapeutic lymphadenectomy is the treatment of choice for early lesions, after fetal pulmonary maturity is established.

(6) Repaired and healed vesicovaginal fistulas are generally considered absolute indications, since the stretching of the vagina during birth may reopen the fistula. The exceptions are repairs close to the introitus, which may be protected by episiotomy.

(7) Some abnormal fetal presentations and positions constitute strong maternal indications for section. A transverse presentation is one example because of the danger of uterine rupture. A face presentation with a persistent mentum posterior position is also an indication, because the fetus is undeliverable. Face presentations in other positions, mentum anterior, do not necessarily imply that a section should be performed. During early labor, a brow presentation does not indicate immediate operative birth because there is often spontaneous conversion to an occiput or face presentation, but it is an indication if the brow presentation persists.

(8) Cephalopelvic disproportion so pronounced that vaginal birth would be impossible is rare. This indication for section is more fetal than maternal. The key question is whether or not the mother would be injured by waiting longer, stimulating the labor with oxytocics, or attempting vaginal birth.

Relative indications

(1) Gestational hypertensive diseases, preeclampsia, and eclampsia are relative maternal indication for section, depending upon severity of the disease and how soon delivery must occur. Most clinicians would choose induction of labor if there was time, but if the condition is rapidly progressing, section is a means of immediate delivery.

(2) Maternal cardiac disease is not an absolute indication for cesarean section. The stress of major surgery should not be superimposed upon a failing or potentially failing heart. The goal for these patients is a short second stage, with minimal bearing down. The mother should give birth with the least possible stress. Obviously, if there is indication for section, such as disproportion, the operation need not be avoided.

(3) Patient choice for cesarean delivery is rising, reaching 1.87% of births in the USA in 2001. These deliveries accounted for 22% of primary preplanned cesarean births.

Finally, maternal pelvic infection is a relative contraindication. The classic prohibition against section in a patient with sepsis is still valid. The gravida should be delivered before she becomes seriously infected. Cesarean section remains a particularly dangerous operation when clinical infection is present. When the uterus is infected and there is strong maternal or fetal indication for abdominal delivery, consideration should be given to cesarean hysterectomy when the family is complete.

Fetal indications

When the fetus is jeopardized by an attempt at vaginal birth, there is a *fetal* indication for cesarean section. An example of a strong fetal indication without a maternal component is a prolapsed umbilical cord. The fetus is seriously threatened, but the mother's life or health is not. Section is strongly indicated unless the patient is immediately deliverable vaginally or the fetus is dead.

Fetal indications can be grouped into several categories. Some indications are mandatory, such as a nonreassuring fetal heart tracing that does not respond to fetal stimulation in labor. Sometimes there is a fetal indication when the pregnancy is complicated by diabetes mellitus, pregnancy-induced hypertension, or renal disease and tests for fetal well-being become ominous. In this situation, a hostile intrauterine environment may warrant delivery without delay.

Other signs of hostile intrauterine environment include oligohydramnios, thick, pea-soup amniotic fluid (not merely stained fluid), and evidence of fetal bleeding during labor. Most clinicians would consider these conditions as fetal indications for cesarean section.

Other recognized indications include evidence of intrauterine infection and threat of birth trauma. Cephalopelvic disproportion and failure to progress often are used as a wastebasket diagnosis. This group may include patients who have labored in the second stage with ruptured membranes for several hours without descent of the head.[17] At the other extreme are patients with dysfunctional contractions in the latent stage who in retrospect were not even in labor.

Most fetuses in the breech presentation are delivered by cesarean section.

Currently, cesarean section often is utilized for twins mainly to provide the second twin with maximum safety at birth. Mortality and morbidity rates usually are higher for the second twin than for the first twin. This is not because all second-twin vaginal births are traumatic, but because there are few good solutions when trouble arises.

When a nonreassuring fetal heart tracing is encountered, the clinician must choose between vaginal birth or emergency section for the second twin. Vaginal birth is the desirable choice only when there is good chance of success without trauma, and emergency section is impossible. This is a difficult choice and depends upon specific circumstances at the time. If a cesarean section for the second twin is necessary after vaginal delivery of the first twin, one should not forget to repair the episiotomy if it was performed.

Cesarean section is almost always utilized for triplet and quadruplet births in the interest of fetal survival if pregnancy has progressed to the point of fetal viability.

In certain circumstances, abruptio placentae offers a strong fetal indication. When part of the placenta is separated, immediate fetal death results if the remaining functioning placenta is insufficient to support life. In some cases, a portion of placenta remains functional and will sustain life only for a short time. For these, early section can be lifesaving for the fetus. In other cases, the abruption is so small that the fetomaternal exchange is not really compromised. Since there is no accurate way to determine placental reserve, section is often the best method to ensure the birth of a live fetus.

In cases of placenta previa, fetal survival is unlikely with vaginal birth. In addition, the methods used for vaginal birth with placenta previa were often directly traumatic to the fetus.

Certain presentations can expose the fetus to birth trauma. Even in early labor, transverse presentations are extremely dangerous to the fetus because of the risk of prolapsed cord. The potential trauma of version and extraction thus provide an absolute fetal indication.

Maternal infection may be a fetal indication. Currently, section is recommended for the fetus if there is an active herpetic lesion present in the maternal genital tract.

The American College of Obstetrics and Gynecology (ACOG) issued an opinion that elective cesarean delivery should be discussed and recommended for all human immunodeficiency virus (HIV)-infected pregnant women with viral loads above 1000 copies/ml.[18] If the decision is made to perform an elective cesarean delivery, the ACOG recommends it be done at 38 weeks' gestation, due to the potential risk of labor and membrane rupture before the woman reaches 39 weeks' gestation, which is the standard recommended time for operative deliveries in women without HIV infection.

Zidovidine (ZDV) prophylaxis should be provided regardless of the mode of delivery, as the available data indicate that ZDV provides an additional protective effect in women undergoing elective operative delivery. Intravenous ZDV should begin 3 hours prior to surgery. Because of the potential for increased postoperative maternal morbidity in HIV-infected women undergoing operative delivery, clinicians may opt to administer perioperative antibiotic prophylaxis.

In women at very low risk of transmission, such as those with low or undetectable viral load, the additional benefit provided by elective cesarean section may be marginal. The potential benefit of elective cesarean section should be discussed with all HIV-infected pregnant women, and the decisions regarding operative delivery will need to be individualized according to the woman's clinical, immunologic, and virologic status.

The influence of the mode of delivery on perinatal transmission of hepatitis C virus (HCV) is incompletely understood. Cesarean section is associated with a reduced risk of HCV transmission in women who are HCV/HIV coinfected.[19,20]

A difficult clinical situation arises when there is an indication for delivery and several days of induction have been unsuccessful. Whether or not a section is indicated depends upon the strength of the indication for delivery – not upon the fact that there is failed induction. One should not induce patients without a good indication for delivery, expecting that an easy induction will ensue.

Some data indicate that grossly premature fetuses do not withstand the stress of labor well. Accordingly, obstetricians tend to use relatively liberal criteria for cesarean section when the gestation is long before term, but the fetus is considered viable, particularly when tracings of the fetal heart-rate monitoring indicate significant and recurrent cord compression, a circumstance predisposing to intracerebral hemorrhage.

If the fetus is dead, the mother should be delivered vaginally unless there is a maternal indication for cesarean section. Similarly, if the fetus is clearly so small as to be nonviable, a section should not be performed for fetal indication. When there is no reasonable chance for fetal survival, the mother should not be exposed to the risk of an operation.

Combined indications for cesarean delivery

There are combined indications for cesarean section with maternal and fetal components that can be additive. Abruptio placentae and pregnancy-induced hypertension are such examples.

Years ago, there were few sections for fetal indications because the operation was dangerous for the mother. Her interests always superseded those of the fetus. Now, section is safe enough; nonetheless, it endangers the mother in the interests of the fetus. This being the case, what should be done when the fetus has little chance of survival no matter how delivered? Many weeks before term, there may be strong fetal indication for cesarean section with relatively little chance of survival, and in some cases, increased maternal danger.

There is no easy answer, but the clinician's dilemma brings up the third consideration: legal liability for results. Legal liability has increased in all areas of medicine, but obstetrics is considered one of the most serious areas for several reasons. There is a certain irreducible fetal morbidity, yet society is coming to expect perfect results. In recent years, performing a cesarean section has been safer from a legal point of view than persisting with a vaginal birth. The impression has developed that if a section was performed, everything possible was done and that any untoward results with vaginal birth could not be defended. Whether or not true from a legal point of view, this impression has had a great impact clinically.

The recent increase in the number of cesarean sections for dystocia, fetal distress, and breech presentation probably reflects an increased concern for the fetus and an effort to reduce perinatal mortality and morbidity. Since cesarean section increases the danger to the mother, there is crucial need to ensure that every operation performed is necessary for one or both of the patients. Critical understanding of the indications and a logical decision-making process should help clinicians to attain this goal.

Repeat cesarean section

The dictum 'once a cesarean always a cesarean' was stated in 1916 because the risk of uterine rupture after a previous section was considered unduly high.[18] It took more than half a century before the concept was almost totally accepted.[19] In the ensuing decade, clinicians have decided that the dictum is not true and that most patients with previous sections can be delivered vaginally safely.

The US national enthusiasm for vaginal birth after cesarean delivery (VBAC) led to a decrease in the cesarean delivery rate, which reached 20.7% in 1996. During the same period (1989–1996), the VBAC rate increased from less than 18.9% to 28.3%. Some third-party payers and managed-care organizations even mandated that all women who had previous cesarean deliveries undergo trials of labor. Many physicians were pressured into offering VBAC to unsuitable candidates or to women who wanted to have a repeat cesarean delivery. As the VBAC rate increased, so did the number of well-publicized reports of uterine rupture and other complications during trials of labor after previous cesarean deliveries. As a result, many physicians and hospitals have discontinued the practice altogether. This abrupt change in practice has contributed to the cesarean delivery rate in the USA increasing again, reaching an all-time high of 26.1% in 2002, while the VBAC rate decreased by 55% to 12.6%.

Currently, the debated topic is whether or not patients with a previous section and no contraindication to vaginal birth should be subjected to a repeat section without trial of labor.

Candidates for VBAC

The American College of Obstetricians and Gynecologists' (ACOG) guidelines for identifying women who are potential candidates for VBAC include the following criteria:[21]

- no traditional contraindications to labor or vaginal birth.
- only one or two previous low transverse uterine incisions (However, an ACOG Task Force on Evaluation of Cesarean Delivery recommended restricting VBAC attempts to women with only one previous low transverse incision.[22])
- no other uterine scars
- no history of previous uterine rupture
- a clinically adequate pelvis
- a physician immediately available throughout active labor who is capable of making the decision for and performing an emergency cesarean delivery
- availability of anesthesia and nursing personnel for emergency cesarean delivery with delivery within 30 minutes of the decision to operate
- pregnancy of 37–40 weeks' gestation.[22]

More data are required before recommendations can be made for women with two or more previous cesarean deliveries, unknown uterine scar,[23] multiple gestation,[24] postterm[25] or preterm[22] pregnancy, low vertical incision,[26] induction,[27] or suspected macrosomia.[28]

Contraindications

VBAC should not be attempted in women at high risk of uterine rupture or with contraindications to labor or vaginal birth. Contraindications for VBAC include:[21]

- prior classical or inverted T-shaped uterine incision or other transfundal uterine surgery (such as myomectomy)
- previous uterine rupture
- medical or obstetric complication that precludes vaginal birth (such as placenta previa)
- inability to perform emergency cesarean delivery due to factors related to the facility, surgeon, anesthesia, or nursing staff
- two prior uterine scars and no vaginal deliveries.

Most unknown scars are the result of low transverse incisions. Women with an unknown scar in the setting of risk factors for a previous classical or T incision (preterm breech birth before 28 weeks of gestation and transverse lie) should be considered at higher risk of uterine rupture with a trial of labor.

If VBAC is offered, experience shows that about 50–70% of the attempts will be successful.[29]

Types of cesarean operations

Each type of cesarean operation has advantages and disadvantages. Obstetricians should be experienced with the different types of operations and cesarean hysterectomy. Both of the lower-segment techniques to be discussed are useful, depending on the stage of gestation and the clinical situation.

Skin incisions

Both transverse and vertical skin incisions are used for cesarean sections. Vertical incisions have the advantage of providing rapid entry into the peritoneal cavity and good exposure. The midline incision is commonly used, as it is easy to effect and to close. This results in minimal dissection of cleavage planes between muscle and fascia helps prevent wound infections.

All vertical skin incisions place stress on the suture line, making postoperative hernia formation more common than with the transverse incision. However, this does not appear to be an important practical factor, since patients with cesarean section are usually young and have a good musculature.

Transverse incisions have become increasingly popular for section. For cosmetic purposes, the Pfannenstiel incision is often used. This incision, which can often be made within the pubic hairline, is barely visible postoperatively. One problem with this incision may be exposure. Because anterior rectus fascia must be dissected from the muscle, there is opportunity for wound infection. If exposure is inadequate with a classic Pfannenstiel, the Cherney modification (rectus tendons divided at pubis) will provide generous exposure. Excellent exposure is obtained with the Maylard incision, a transverse incision through all layers, but this necessitates cutting through the rectus muscles and ligating the inferior epigastric vessels.

Sometimes, with a Pfannenstiel incision, the intact rectus muscles hinders the delivery of the head. In this case, the medial two-thirds of each rectus can be cut without worrying about the inferior epigastric vessels. If this is done, one should resuture the rectus muscles so that they heal in an intact manner.

The choice of incision seems to depend primarily upon how the clinician was trained and what the custom is in the area of practice. Individuals trained to utilize Pfannenstiel incisions often use this incision almost exclusively. Irrespective of the original incision, the peritoneum usually is opened vertically.

Lower-segment transverse section

Lower-segment transverse section is the standard routine procedure, which is easy to perform, as the incised area is less vascular and the uterus is easy to suture. However, there are potential problems. The length of the incision is limited by the width of the anterior lower uterine segment between the round ligaments. Any lateral extension might result in tearing of the uterine arteries and veins, resulting in hemorrhage and/or hematoma. Therefore, the incision may be difficult to use for premature birth where the lower uterine segment is underdeveloped and narrow. In these cases, a lower-segment vertical incision may be preferable. If, at operation, there is insufficient space for a transverse incision, a vertical incision can be made in the middle of the superior flap to form an inverted 'T'. The junction joint of both incisions is difficult to close and probably is always weak, so a T incision should be used only as a last resort to deliver the fetus.

If either or both of the ascending uterine arteries at the lateral angles of the incision are torn, they can easily be repaired. The vessels (both artery and veins may be injured) should be temporarily clamped to prevent bleeding, and ligated superior and inferior to the incision with an encircling mattress suture. Removal of the clamps should result in no bleeding. Then the hysterotomy incision can be closed in the usual manner. This technique provides far better hemostasis for major vessels than merely trying to stop bleeding by the usual closure of the incision. With upward traction on the uterus, the ureters are far away from the torn vessels so need not be a concern.

In summary, the lower-segment transverse incision is ideal for most patients (Table 30.1).

Operative technique

After the abdomen is opened, the peritoneal reflection between the bladder and uterus is identified. A bladder flap is developed to mobilize the loose visceral peritoneum between the bladder and uterus; the peritoneum is picked up about 1 cm below its firm attachment to the uterus and incised laterally toward the round ligaments (Figure 30.1). This step should be carried out under direct vision with a bladder retractor inferiorly and Richardson retractors laterally so that the round ligaments can be seen. Note of any uterine rotation is made to assist in later extension of the uterine incision.

With the bladder peritoneum grasped with thumb forceps and stretched away from the uterus, blunt finger dissection with the finger tip against the uterine surface is used to separate the

Table 30.1 Advantages, problems, and dangers of lower-segment transverse section

Advantages
  Incision lies entirely in lower segment
  Incisional area less vascular than upper segment
  Lower segment easier to suture than upper
  Easy to cover incision with bladder peritoneum
Technical problems
  Incision length limited by lateral margins of uterus
    Problem with premature birth
    Problem with abnormal presentation
  Angles may be difficult to suture
Specific dangers
  Injury to vessels at lateral margins of uterus
  Hemorrhage and hematoma at angles

posterior surface of the bladder from the anterior surface of the lower uterine segment (Figure 30.2). Sharp dissection may be necessary if the patient has had a previous section; otherwise, blunt finger dissection will usually cause less bleeding.

At this point, any rotation of the uterus is noted, and a transverse incision is made in the midline of the uterus. Extension of the incision may be made with bandage scissors or by placing one and then two fingers into the incision and extending it laterally by 'tearing' the muscles, since the muscle bundles separate easily (Figure 30.3).

Each method has pros and cons. Cutting the lower uterine segment with bandage scissors allows a precise termination of the lateral margin of the incision, so there is no injury to major

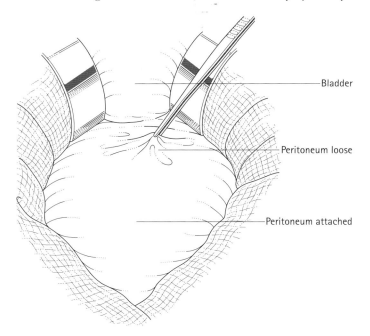

Figure 30.1 Mobilization of bladder flap; peritoneum on the anterior surface of the uterus is picked up just below (caudad) its firm attachment and incised laterally from the midline to each round ligament.

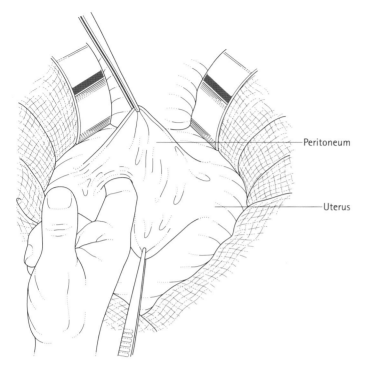

Figure 30.2 Mobilization of bladder flap; the inferior edge of peritoneum is elevated with forceps and put on stretch. Blunt finger dissection separates the peritoneum and bladder from the lower uterine segment.

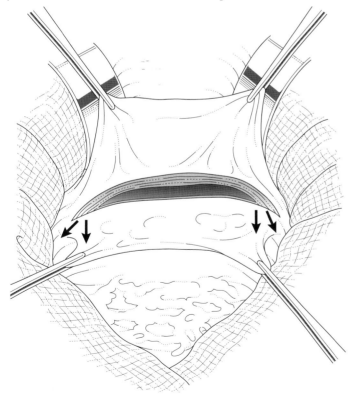

Figure 30.3 Transverse incision into the uterus; after the uterus is opened in the midline by means of a small incision, the opening is enlarged laterally by 'tearing' with fingers in a lateral and cephalad direction (arrows).

vessels. A problem is that several arcuate arteries may run transversely across the uterus, resulting in increased blood loss. Enlarging the initial incision by tearing usually avoids injury to the arcuate arteries. Experience is necessary to enlarge the initial incision symmetrically and yet not tear into the ascending uterine artery and vein. When tearing, it is important to pull toward the fundus of the uterus (cephalad), as well as laterally. This will ensure that the lateral ends of the resulting incision curve upward where the lower uterine segment between the round ligaments is wider. How well the incision has been made is easily determined by observation after delivery.

With either method, it is important that the original incision be made through the entire uterine wall. There is a plexus of arteries and veins about one-third of the way through the uterine wall which, if the incision is inadvertently enlarged by either blunt or sharp dissection in this plane, can cause severe hemorrhage. Sometimes, there is concern about injuring the fetus by cutting too deeply. In this case, the lateral margins of the short (2 cm) transverse incision can be picked up with Allis clamps after the incision is started to hold the uterine tissue away from the fetal head.

Another method is routinely used by some obstetricians to avoid fetal injury. The central, small, transverse uterine incision is made through almost the entire thickness of the uterine wall. Then a hemostat is used to tease through the remaining few millimeters of uterine wall. When amniotic fluid appears, the incision can be enlarged by either of the previously mentioned techniques.

It is crucial with any section that the uterine incision be large enough for atraumatic delivery. When the section is performed to prevent the stress of labor with a fragile premature fetus, it would be absurd to have a traumatic birth because the incision was too small. The incision must not be extended so far laterally as to injure arteries and veins, but if it seems too small for atraumatic birth, the incision can be enlarged by incising vertically in the center of the superior flap to create an inverted T.

Immediately after delivery, until the placenta separates, the operative field is usually bloodless for a few minutes. During this time, operative bleeding can be reduced by mobilizing the uterine incision with T and Allis clamps and beginning the closure. T clamps can be placed at the angles of the incision and at other areas where bleeding is active. Traditionally, the placenta is removed first and then suturing begins. Alternatively several sutures could be placed beginning immediately from the angle before the placenta separates and the field becomes covered with blood (Figure 30.4). After the removal of the placenta, the suturing of the incision can be continued rapidly.

Some surgeons exteriorize the uterus, which facilitates exposure and may result in a quicker repair. However, there is some evidence that exteriorization increases maternal discomfort and nausea, but does not increase the risk of infection.[30] This point is controversial.

The uterus can be closed in a single layer, a method which decreases operating time.[31] However, it is not clear whether

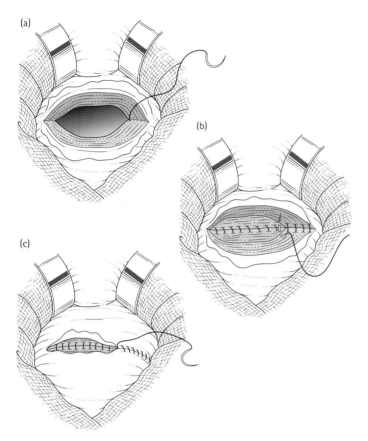

Figure 30.4 Closing the uterus; a low-segment transverse incision is usually closed in two layers. Care is taken to place angle sutures lateral to the apex of the incision and approximate myometrium (a). The second layer should cover the first suture line (b). The peritoneum is closed so that the lower flap covers the incision (c).

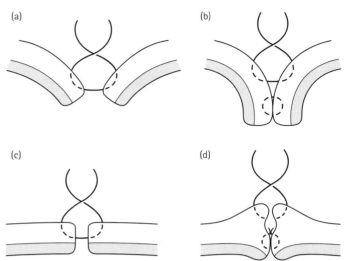

Figure 30.5 Suturing the uterus; the uterus should be sutured so that the myometrium, rather than the endometrium, is approximated and that the second suture line covers the first. The uterine tissue, therefore, should be inverted – panels (a) and (b) show how this can be accomplished even when the uterine wall is thin; (c) and (d) show the technique when the two edges are thicker.

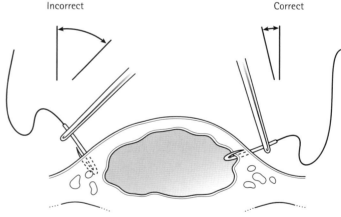

Figure 30.6 Suturing the angles; the lower uterine segment is convex after birth, although the peritoneum on the anterior surface of the broad ligament makes it appear flat. Care must be taken, therefore, to place angle sutures into the uterine muscle rather than into the peritoneum and vessels at the lateral margins.

patients who have a single-layer closure are at increased risk of complications during the next pregnancy compared to those who undergo a two-layer closure.

To close the uterus in two layers, a continuous running suture is used. Care must be taken to avoid the endometrium and to invert the two flaps so that myometrium is opposed to myometrium (Figure 30.5). After one again inverts the tissue, a second line of continuous running sutures is placed to cover the first one. When suture lines have been placed properly, the first is covered by the second, and the only sutures visible are the ties at each angle for the second layer. Some operators utilize a Lembert suture rather than a continuous running suture for the second layer.

Care must be given to suturing the angles properly. The most common mistake is to neglect the uterine curvature and thus not suture perpendicular to the uterine wall (Figure 30.6). This results in vessel injury and sutures with very little purchase on the myometrium. It is easy to avoid this mistake if each angle suture is placed by the operator on the opposite side of the table, and the incision is closed by suturing to the midline.

Any suture line will become loose in a few days because of uterine involution. The aspect of healing in the face of tissue catabolism and involution is normally present only under one circumstance in the entire field of surgery – the uterine incision of cesarean section! This raises the point of continuous compared to interrupted sutures for uterine closure. Poidevin's work in the 1960s[32] seemed to show that there is less chance of a uterine scar defect if interrupted sutures are used. This would seem logical, yet, few operators ever use interrupted sutures. With the new emphasis on vaginal birth after a previous section, this entire area of investigation should be renewed.

Factors that may affect the strength of the closure need to be studied. These include choice of suture material, closure technique, and presence of postoperative infection. In women contemplating subsequent pregnancies, the surgeon should consider using a polyglactin suture and/or a double layer closure.

Since vascular muscle tissue is easily torn, suturing the uterus is difficult. A fairly heavy suture with a large diameter is best (no. 1-0 or 0), because it will not cut through the muscle even though it is tied snugly. The diameter of the heavy suture, rather than its strength, is the critical factor. To avoid tearing apart or cutting through the myometrial fibers, each bite should be big enough so that the suture gets a good purchase on the tissue. When bleeding points remain after the second row of sutures, they can best be controlled by figure-of-8 stitches over the site tied snugly but not tightly. The sutures should be placed away from, but still around, the bleeding site and tied to compress the tissue.

Closure of the peritoneal bladder flap or the parietal peritoneum is not generally performed, as there is no conclusive evidence that such closure has benefits (such as reduction in infectious morbidity, analgesia requirements, or bowel function).[33] The effect on adhesion formation is unclear. Discordant results have been reported;[34,35] thus, if the peritoneum is closed to prevent adhesions, it should be done by a fine 3:0 suture. Intra-abdominal irrigation does not reduce maternal morbidity beyond the reduction achieved with prophylactic antibiotics alone.[36]

The fascia is typically closed with a delayed-absorbable suture using a continuous stitch. Difficulty with hemostasis is usually not a major issue; however, care should be taken to avoid too much tension when closing the fascia: approximation, not strangulation, is the appropriate goal. A delayed-absorbable monofilament (such as polydiaxanone (PDS) or polyglyconate) or permanent monofilament suture (such as polypropylene or polybutester) is recommended for patients at high risk of fascial dehiscence, especially with a vertical incision. These patients include those who are obese, diabetic, immunosuppressed, or undernourished, as well as women with a history of prior fascial herniation. A running Smead-Jones closure can be considered in such cases to enhance the tensile strength of the incision.[37]

Appropriate antibiotic use, careful handling of tissue,[38] and judicious use of electrical cautery appear to decrease the risk of seroma formation and infection. Closure of the subcutaneous adipose layer with plain catgut suture is also helpful and is recommended if the layer is deep. This was illustrated by a meta-analysis showing that suture closure of the subcutaneous adipose layer at cesarean delivery decreased the risk of subsequent wound disruption by one-third in women with subcutaneous tissue depth greater than 2 cm but not ≤2 cm.[36] Closure of the dead space seems to inhibit accumulation of serum and blood, which can lead to a wound seroma and subsequent wound breakdown.[39] This occurrence is a major cause of morbidity, can be costly, and lengthens the recovery time for the patient.

Finally, reapproximation of the skin may be performed with staples or suture.[40] If the skin incision was transverse, the staples may be removed in about 3 days. If a vertical incision was performed, the staples are left in place for at least 5–7 days, and longer in a patient at high risk of wound complications, since there is more tension on the skin edges of a vertical incision.

Vascular anatomy and uterine hemorrhage control

A major contributing factor in uterine hemorrhage control is confusion about the vascular anatomy. Several factors are important to keep in mind. The uterus is supplied by four major arteries – two uterine and two ovarian. To shut off all blood flow, one would need to ligate all four arteries, as well as the two ascending vaginal branches of the pudendal arteries. In addition, arterial anastomoses are such that the uterus should be considered as one system in equilibrium. Blood freely flows from one area or one vessel to any other vessel. Arcuate arteries originate from the uterine arteries at the lateral margins and course around the uterus (back and front) with multiple anastomoses in the midline.

From an operative point of view, this means that a bleeding point is best controlled by placing fairly deep mattress sutures around the site of hemorrhage, since ligation of a specific vessel is impossible. These sutures should be placed about 1 cm away from the bleeding site.

If there is inadvertent injury to the uterine arteries or veins along the lateral margin of the uterus, all the vessels in the area can be safely ligated.

To control bleeding, a horizontal mattress suture is placed that passes through the uterine muscle and around the vessels. A large suture (no. 1-0) should be used so that it can be tied snugly and still not cut through the muscle. A suture is placed above and below the injury, and these two sutures should control all bleeding in the ascending vessels. Any attempt to dissect and ligate vessels individually will produce more tissue injury and hemorrhage.

The risk of extensive uterine injury or extension of the incision into the uterine vessels is usually low; only 1–2% of all patients having cesarean deliveries require blood transfusion.[41] Hemorrhage may be due to uterine atony, placenta accreta, or lacerated vessels. Lacerations extending into the lateral vagina and broad ligament should be evaluated carefully and repaired with meticulous attention to the position of the ureter.

Lower-segment vertical section

A vertical incision is still sometimes utilized for cesarean sections and in some instances has clear advantages over the transverse incision (Table 30.2). The vertical incision can be enlarged easily, since its length is not limited by vital structures (major vessels on the lateral margin of the uterus). It is useful for the delivery of premature infants because it is not limited by the size of the lower uterine segment. With abnormal presentations, such as breech or transverse, these advantages are significant.

Table 30.2 Advantages, problems, and dangers of the lower-segment vertical section

Advantages
    Lower-segment incision
    Incision easy to outline
    Incision length not limited
Technical problems
    Extensive bladder dissection
    Upper-segment extension
    Upper segment difficult to suture
Specific dangers
    Bladder injury from extension
    Poor scar in upper-segment extension

There are also some disadvantages. The lower-uterine segment is short, unless the patient has been in labor, and, without due care, the bladder may be injured in making the incision or from extension during birth. Moreover, with a short lower segment, it may be necessary to continue the incision into the upper segment. Because muscle must be incised rather than separated, the vertical incision may be more vascular than the transverse one.

Operative technique

The procedure is started the same way as the lower-segment transverse procedure. The peritoneum between uterus and bladder is picked up just below its firm attachment to the uterus and incised transversely toward the round ligaments. Blunt dissection is used to separate the bladder from the uterus. A small incision is made through the uterine wall in the midline after noting any rotation of the uterus. Large bandage scissors are used to extend this incision. First, the incision is extended downward to a point 1 or 2 cm above the bladder reflection (Figure 30.7). This is a critical distance because, if the incision is carried to the reflection, the bladder may be injured when the baby is born. Then, with bandage scissors, the incision is extended upward to a length sufficient for delivery.

If only the lower segment is involved, closure is done with two layers of running sutures.

Classical cesarean section

There are few indications for the classical operation in contemporary obstetrics. In this operation, the entire uterine incision is placed in the upper segment, so structures over the bladder should not be disturbed (Table 30.3).

Pregnant women with invasive carcinoma of the cervix should have a classical section in order to avoid areas involved with tumor. Other indications may be a major degree of placenta previa, when the operator wishes to avoid cutting through the placenta attached to the lower segment or neglected transverse lie, or possibly one with the back turned downward. A classical section might be desirable after previous vesicovaginal fistula repair when there are extensive bladder

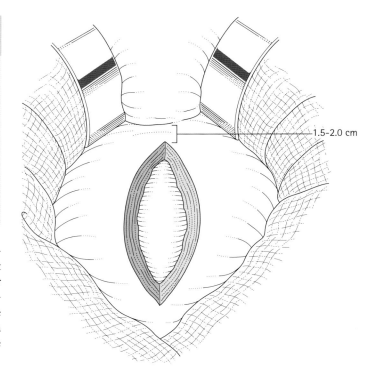

Figure 30.7 Uterine incision with lower-segment vertical section; the uterus is opened by making a small incision in the midline. This incision is extended downward to a point 1–2 cm above the bladder reflection. This will help ensure that the bladder is not injured as the fetus is delivered.

adhesions to the uterus, and in some cases of uterine sacculation. The advantage to the procedure is that the operative field avoids the bladder and the lower segment. Since the lower-segment vertical incision can always be extended superiorly for exposure, there is little indication for a classical cesarean section unless there is cogent need to exclude the entire lower segment from the operative site.

The classical cesarean operation has several disadvantages. An incision in the upper part of the uterus is more likely to rupture in a subsequent pregnancy than one in the lower segment, and such ruptures tend to occur prior to the onset of labor.

Table 30.3 Advantages, problems, and dangers of classical cesarean section

Advantages
    Cervix and bladder not dissected (carcinoma of the cervix, fistulas)
    No limitation in uterine incision length
Technical problems
    Closing incision difficult
    Vascular incision hemorrhage
Specific dangers
    Poor uterine closure
    Subsequent uterine rupture
    Adhesion of bowel to incision wound, postoperative ileus

Operative technique

Technically, opening the uterus is less difficult than a low vertical section. The uterus is incised through its full thickness in the midline with a knife. Bandage scissors are used to extend the incision vertically, starting from an inferior point just above the firm attachment of the bladder peritoneum and extending as far as necessary to provide exposure for birth.

The uterine incision must be carefully closed with several layers of interrupted or running sutures.

Extraperitoneal approaches to the uterus

Physick first described extraperitoneal cesarean section more than 150 years ago in an attempt to reduce mortality.[42] Mainly used to decrease infectious morbidity, this approach has fallen into disfavor because of its technical difficulty, longer operating time, and lack of advantage in the antibiotic era, and thus it will not be discussed in this chapter. Those who are interested in this topic should see the second edition of this book.

Technical complications associated with cesarean section

Adherent bladder

Unless the patient has had a previous operation, there is usually an excellent cleavage plane between the uterus and bladder, and bladder mobilization is easy. However, bladder dissection may be a problem if there is scarring from a previous section or if there are varicosities on the surface of the uterus or bladder. If blunt dissection is used to mobilize the bladder, these veins, which are friable, often rupture. An avascular cleavage plane exists between the two structures, but sharp dissection must be employed for this mobilization (Figure 30.8). This is not difficult technically, if the bladder is picked up with a tissue forceps and placed on stretch away from the uterus to expose the vesicouterine plane.

Since sharp dissection is not difficult for one with experience, every pelvic surgeon should be competent in the technique so that it can be utilized when blunt dissection would be impossible.

One last resort would be an intentional bladder dome cystotomy to help delineate the bladder and therefore perform a clean, sharp dissection. This approach would prevent multiple, small serosal or muscularis, or full-thickness injuries during extremely difficult dissection and thus decrease the risk of fistula formation.

Placental obstruction at section

Sometimes the placenta is encountered upon opening the uterus. This occurs in the following two situations: (1) with a classical section, when the placenta is on the anterior wall of

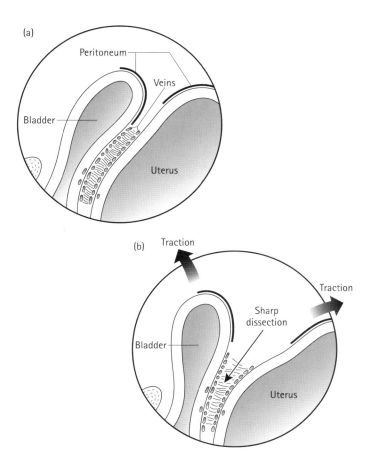

Figure 30.8 Sharp dissection of adherent bladder; there is an avascular, fascial cleavage plane between bladder and uterus that can be identified if the bladder and uterus are separated by traction on both at a 60° angle. The plane for sharp dissection lies halfway between the two organs.

the uterus; (2) with a low cervical section done for placenta previa.

The management of this problem is controversial. Many operators cut through the placenta, but this opens the fetal circulation, and even a small amount of fetal bleeding may be dangerous. The umbilical cord should be clamped immediately if the placenta is incised. Probably a safer procedure is to push the placenta to the side or actually remove it first. There is more maternal bleeding, but it is less dangerous to the infant than fetal hemorrhage.

Difficulties in delivering the fetus

There is difficulty in delivering the fetal head if it has become tightly wedged into the pelvis after prolonged labor. In this situation, someone in the operating theater can provide upward pressure on the head by inserting two fingers from a sterile gloved hand in the vagina. If this difficulty is expected, preparation for this maneuver should be made in advance. In addition, the operator can push his or her hand down into the pelvis between the fetal head and the symphysis, elevate the head and deliver it from the uterus. Some obstetricians use forceps or a vacuum extractor to deliver the head. Difficulties also can arise with breech or transverse presentations. It is helpful to remember that the inferior pole of the fetus must be delivered first through any lower-segment incision, but the superior pole may come first through a classical incision.

Incision into the vagina

One important question for the surgeon at cesarean section is where to make the transverse incision in the uterus. If it is too high, it may be near the thicker upper uterine segment. An incision that is too low is not usually a problem. However, incisions have actually been made into the vagina rather than the uterus.[43] In such cases, the patients had been in the second stage of labor for several hours, and the section was done for disproportion. The lower uterine segment was thin and the bladder was easily mobilized. Once the anatomy is recognized, the repair is usually easy and patients have uneventful recovery.

A somewhat similar situation may arise in the event of sacculation of the uterus. In this case, both the vagina and the bladder may be drawn up as high as the level of the navel. The incision under such circumstances is likely to involve both the bladder and the vagina. This complication is to be suspected when the cervix is high in the vaginal canal and cannot be reached by the examining finger during pelvic examination. When diagnosed in advance, inadvertent placement of the incision and thus injury of the bladder and vagina can be avoided by utilizing a high midline skin incision in anticipation of a uterine entry at or above the level of the umbilicus.

Fetal monitoring at cesarean section

Electronic fetal monitoring is commonplace in labor and is particularly necessary in high-risk pregnancies or at times when there is a nonreasurring fetal heart-rate tracing. The most effective way to monitor during cesarean section is a subject of much concern and discussion. Often there is a hiatus in fetal monitoring from the time when the electrode is removed until the time when the baby is born. This time interval should be minimized, but time may be lost in preparing and draping the patient. Sometimes, after draping, a regional anesthetic will not be satisfactory and the anesthesiologist will recommend waiting for a few more minutes. The result is that the fetus is not monitored at a potentially crucial time.

Certain procedures may prevent this problem:

- If an internal scalp electrode is applied, it is left on until the head is delivered at section; then the wire is cut and pulled out vaginally.
- Regional anesthesia is checked while the external monitor is applied before draping.
- A clock is started when the external or internal electrode is removed, and the obstetrician is notified about time.

Obstetric conditions affecting cesarean section

Certain obstetric conditions affect cesarean section from a technical point of view; the clinician should understand the pathophysiology and be prepared. In addition to being an indicator for section, placenta previa may complicate the procedure. There is less myometrium in the thinned-out lower segment, and since muscular contraction is the basis of uterine hemostasis postpartum, there may be severe uncontrolled hemorrhage with placenta previa. Sometimes one can visualize large vessels that may be covered only with peritoneum and endometrium. If seen, vessels can be ligated with sutures running through the entire thickness of the uterine wall. There is such an abundance of the uterine blood supply that a small area of the wall can be isolated to control hemorrhage without fear. If the placental site is denuded of myometrium and mattress sutures will not stop bleeding, internal iliac ligation or even hysterectomy may be necessary.

There is controversy about the management of abruptio placentae at cesarean section. Traditionally, it was said that hysterectomy was necessary when there was bleeding into the myometrium (Couvelaire uterus). It is now known that most of the time the Couvelaire uterus contracts well and that removal is rarely necessary. This is common sense, because Couvelaire uterus is diagnosed only at section, although it must occur and remain undiagnosed in patients who give birth vaginally. The critical point with abruption is whether or not the uterus contracts sufficiently to provide hemostasis.

This raises another point of uterine physiology: a uterus may contract well after it is sutured and yet remain flaccid as long as the incision is open. With uterine atony, a further operation would be valid only after oxytocics medication had been utilized and the uterus had been closed. This physiologic fact is the counterpart of the observation that when section is performed for tetanic contraction, the uterus often relaxes as soon as the incision is made.

Finally, placental adherence such as placenta accreta may complicate cesarean section. In this situation, there is no cleavage plane between placenta and uterus. As a result, the placenta cannot be removed without injury to the myometrium with resulting hemorrhage. When the condition involves more than a minor area of attachment, hysterectomy is indicated. In selected patients who feel that another pregnancy is important, one might consider leaving the placenta in place, suturing bleeding sites with mattress sutures, and using drugs such as methotrexate to promote early placental death. However, the risks of this approach are considerable and unacceptable to most patients.

Cesarean section in the obese patient

Obese women are at increased risk of needing a cesarean delivery. This may be related to a higher incidence of pregnancy complications necessitating induction of labor or soft tissue dystocia in the maternal pelvis.[44] In one large, prospective study, the cesarean delivery rates in primigravid women with first-trimester body-mass index of <30 (controls), 30–34.9 (obese group), and ≥35 (morbidly obese group) were 21%, 34%, and 47%, respectively.[45]

The optimal surgical approach for the massively obese patient is not clear. A high (supraumbilical) transverse incision is one option, as it has the strength of the transverse repair, avoids burying the incision under a large panniculus, and affords excellent exposure. However, is not safer than a low transverse incision.[46] The supraumbilical incision is often anatomically directly over the lower uterine segment because the large pannus draws the umbilicus caudally.

Although the Pfannenstiel incision is unsatisfactory because it provides limited exposure even in the thin patient, Cherney's modification provides excellent exposure. If any of the transverse incisions are chosen, the upper flap can be turned back upon itself and suspended with skin clips so that it is held entirely out of the operative field.

Another contributing factor to wound infections is subcutaneous bleeding or serous oozing. Closure of the subcutaneous fat tissue with (3:0 plain catgut) has been shown to decrease seroma formation by one third.

For the prevention of thromoembolic complications in obese patients, the prophylactic use of heparin perioperatively is usually indicated.

Remote effects of cesarean section

There are some short- and long-term sequelae to cesarean section. An enormous physical effort is required to care for a newborn during the first few months of life. When a woman is also recovering from a major operation, the difficulty is compounded. A protracted convalescence is expected after a major operation. The woman delivered by section also must take care of a baby. In the presence of a chronic illness, she is under tremendous stress during the postpartum period. Some patients with chronic cardiac disease remain compensated with protected care during pregnancy but promptly go into circulatory failure after returning home with the baby.

The average blood loss is about twice as great with section as with a vaginal birth and there is a higher incidence of transfusion and hence of transfusion-related complications.

One long-term consequence of cesarean section is a high likelihood of future operations and the fact that these operations may be increasingly difficult. Once delivered abdominally, many women will have repeat operations for subsequent pregnancies. After cesarean section, there is an increased chance of uterine rupture, which may result in fetal death and frequently requires hysterectomy. Cesarean section, therefore, can compromise long-term childbearing ability.

Certain complications of cesarean section can lead to other operations. Adhesions and pelvic pain may necessitate exploratory celiotomy. An incisional hernia can require a second operation years after the first one.

Cesarean section can make a subsequent operation more problematic. There may be difficulty in dissection of the bladder from the cervix, and there is an increased possibility of bladder injury. In the presence of a weak scar, the risk of uterine perforation during dilation and curettage, or other methods of induced abortion, increases. The risk of placenta implantation abnormalities, such as accrete, increta, and percreta, is also increased with each cesarean delivery.

Because cesarean section can have deleterious long-term consequences, it should be performed only when there is a valid indication.

Postoperative infection

The most common infections after cesarean delivery are endometritis, urinary tract infection, respiratory tract infection, wound infection, and septic pelvic thrombophlebitis; occasionally, there is pelvic abscess.

The most frequent postoperative infection after cesarean delivery is endometritis. The mean risk of postoperative endomyometritis after cesarean delivery is 35–40% in the absence of prophylactic antibiotics.[47] This rate is as low as 4–5% after scheduled cesarean delivery with intact membranes and as high as 85% after an extended labor with ruptured membranes.[48] Prophylactic antibiotics reduce the overall rate of infection by approximately 60%.[45]

The classical definition of febrile morbidity is an elevated oral temperature of 100.4 °F (38 °C) or more on two occasions at least 6 hours apart from day 2 to day 10 postpartum. However, it is recognized that postpartum day 1 should not be excluded from this definition, since some organisms, such as group B β-hemolytic streptococcus, tend to cause temperature elevation within 12–24 hours of cesarean delivery.

The patient who satisfies the definition of febrile morbidity after cesarean section must be examined completely for any other focus of infection or atelectasis. Typical findings of endometritis include uterine and abdominal tenderness; but these are 'soft' signs of infection, since a recent, normal postcesarean patient would also be expected to have a tender uterus and abdomen. The most important aspect of the diagnosis of endometritis is that it is a diagnosis by exclusion of other causes of febrile morbidity.

Risk factors for endometritis are listed in Table 30.4. However, the most important risk factor is the mode of delivery. Patients delivered by cesarean section are 10–20 times more likely to develop infection than those delivered vaginally.

Table 30.4　Risk factors for endometritis

Cesarean delivery
Prolonged duration of labor
Prolonged duration of rupture of membranes
Frequent pelvic examination intrapartum
Obesity
Internal uterine monitoring

The standard laboratory workup for endometritis includes a complete blood count with differential, blood, urine, and endocervical specimens for culture; and blood urea nitrogen and serum creatinine.

The causative organisms of endometritis are multiple and the infection is considered polymicrobial. The more common pathogens include peptococcus and peptostreptococci, group B β-hemolytic streptococcus, *Escherichia coli*, and the *Bacteroides* group of organisms. Approximately 10–14% of patients with endometritis after cesarean delivery also have associated bacteremia. If the group B β-hemolytic streptococcus is determined to be the causative organism, the pediatrician should be notified, since this organism may cause devastating, fulminant neonatal sepsis.

Antimicrobial therapy for endometritis after cesarean section should include a broad-spectrum antibiotic appropriate for a polymicrobial infection. Standard therapy is clindamycin and gentamicin, but other antibiotics are also effective as a single-agent therapy. A suggested scheme is seen in Table 30.5.

Patients treated for endometritis with appropriate antibiotics should show improvement within 48 hours. A worsening of the clinical condition as determined by clinical examination, increasing white blood cell count, etc., requires a re-evaluation of the mother. If available, the bacteriology reports from previously obtained culture specimens should guide further antibiotic therapy. If the initial antibiotic regimen included clindamycin and gentamicin, the addition of ampicillin for enterococcal coverage is prescribed. If the initial antibiotic coverage was an extended-spectrum penicillin, such as Timentin, Unasyn, Zosyn, or a cephalosporin, the addition of an amino-

Table 30.5　Atimicrobial therapy for postcesarean endometritis

- Clindamycin 900 µg every 8 hours and gentamicin 3–5 µg/kg body weight per day IV or IM divided every 8 hours *or* gentamicin 5–7 µg/kg body weight IV every 24 hours
- Cefoxitin 1–2 g IV or IM every 6 hours (or equivalent cephalosporin)
- Ticarcillin and clavulanate (Timentin®) 3.1 g IV every 4–6 hours
- Ampicillin plus sulbactam (Unasyn®) 1.5–3 g IV or IM every 6 hours
- Piperacillin plus Tazobactam (Zosyn®) 3.375–4.5 g IV every 6 hours
- Ertapenem (Invanz®) 1 g IV or IM every 24 hours

glycoside is appropriate. It is advisable to obtain peak and trough serum values to guide aminoglycoside dosage if gentamicin is prescribed every 8 hours. Alternatively, gentamicin may be prescribed once a day at a dose of 5 mg/kg body weight per day with no need to obtain peak and trough serum levels.

A small percentage of patients with endometritis will fail to respond to the adjusted antibiotic therapy. This group of patients should be evaluated for septic pelvic thrombophlebitis and/or a pelvic abscess. A heparin challenge test may be prescribed in these cases along with the triple antibiotic regimen of clindamycin, gentamicin, and ampicillin. If septic pelvic thrombophlebitis is present, the patient usually responds rather rapidly to heparin. The dose of heparin should be adjusted so that the partial thromboplastin time (PTT) is approximately 1.5–2 times normal. If the patient fails to respond to triple antibiotics and heparin, one should search for other causes such as pelvic abscess. Re-examination of the patient and appropriate diagnostic tests, including pelvic sonography and computed tomography (CT), should be ordered if appropriate. Should an abscess or wound infection be present, drainage is usually required.

Cesarean hysterectomy

Absolute indications for cesarean hysterectomy are relatively rare. The most common indication is intractable uterine bleeding that cannot be controlled by other, more conventional means.

Severe forms of placenta previa sometimes necessitate hysterectomy. When the placenta is implanted upon the thin lower segment, there may be too little muscle to provide uterine hemostasis after birth. In these cases, the operation is particularly difficult because the tissues around the cervix are even more vascular than they are with a normal pregnancy. Placenta accreta (increta, percreta) may also coexist with placenta previa, necessitating hysterectomy. This complication should always be kept in mind when the placenta fails to separate easily or in patients who are having repeat cesarean delivery with an anterior low placenta.

Another indication for cesarean hysterectomy is rupture of the uterus. However, the uterus may be saved if the patient is anxious to have more children, and conservative surgery is possible technically, since the uterus can function even after major operations. Some conditions provide valid indications for hysterectomy but do not occur commonly. Large uterine myomas are one example. There may be an indication for cesarean hysterectomy in cases of severe infection.

For the purpose of sterilization, cesarean hysterectomy is a more extensive and potentially morbid procedure than section and tubal ligation. Thus, only in association with other indications for removal of the uterus can cesarean hysterectomy be considered as the procedure of choice.

Technically, the operation proceeds as any other cesarean section until after the baby is born. Thereafter, the same principles of abdominal hysterectomy apply with certain particularities that emerge from the gravid uterus and the emergent situation. Usually, the uterus is closed quickly in one layer to attempt to decrease blood loss or one could move on with the hysterectomy.

The pelvic tissues are edematous, and rough application of clamps will cause tearing. The uterus is usually exteriorized and placed under tension. Then the round ligaments are divided first, followed by the cornual region of the fallopian tubes and the utero-ovarian ligaments. Next, the uterine vessels are skeletonized and the bladder is dissected off the lower uterine segment and the cervix, utilizing sharp or blunt dissection as appropriate.

As the uterus enlarges during pregnancy, it stretches the broad ligaments, so that there is considerable slack immediately postpartum. This change in anatomic configuration makes it easy to clamp the broad ligament more laterally than usual during cesarean hysterectomy and thus to endanger the ureter (Figures 30.4 and 30.9).

Supracervical hysterectomy is preferred whenever possible in this setting due to its decreased morbidity in a patient population that is already hemodynamically compromised and unstable. In this case, the uterosacral ligaments are identified and the uterus amputated above their level.

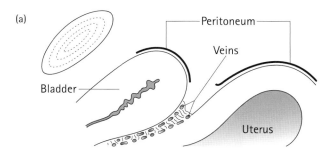

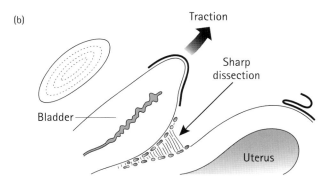

Figure 30.10 With bladder and uterine varicosities (a), sharp dissection (b) is mandatory to separate the structures without bleeding.

If total hysterectomy is needed (placenta previa, placenta accreta, cervical lesions, bleeding from the cervix, etc.), the next problem is identifying the boundary between cervix and vagina and attaining vaginal hemostasis (Figure 13.10). Cervical boundaries are difficult to determine after advanced labor when the cervix is very thin. However, they can be identified by pinching the upper vagina between thumb and forefinger, moving the hand superiorly, and determining where the cervix extends into the vagina. Another method involves palpating the inside of the vagina to identify the cervical lip. The vagina is entered after the cervix is identified and incised with scissors. A last resort would be empirically to transect the tissue 0.5–1 cm below the lower edge of the uterosacral ligaments insertion.

The postpartum vagina is always vascular and heavy bleeding may ensue. Usually, this can be controlled by temporary application of ring forceps. If not, figure-of-8 sutures can be placed in the vaginal cuff as it is incised. Care must be taken to identify both ureters if total hysterectomy is undertaken.

Operative complications

Injury to the urinary tract

Urinary tract injuries are uncommon with cesarean section, occurring in approximately 1% of cesarean deliveries. When recognized during the operation, most are easily repaired and the 'cure rate' is excellent.

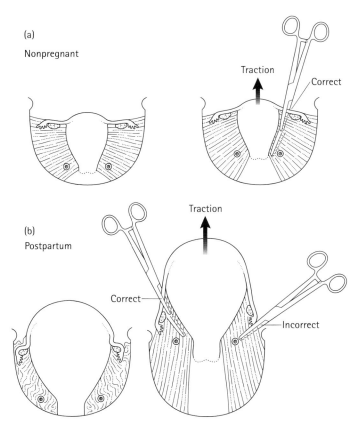

Figure 30.9 Instead of being taut (a), the broad ligaments are slack (b), allowing inadvertent placement of clamps to endanger vital structures.

Bladder injuries

Bladder injuries are at times almost inevitable. Risk factors include previous pelvic surgery such as previous cesarean section and cesarean hysterectomy. Another problem is that there may be marked engorgement of the veins on both the bladder and the uterus. These veins rupture easily, requiring the operator to dissect in a bloody field. When these anatomic variations are combined with the necessity for haste in delivering a potentially compromised fetus, it is apparent that an unavoidable laceration of the bladder is more probable.

It is important to make a firm diagnosis and to outline the extent of the injury. A finger inserted through the laceration can do this. It is a mistake to begin suturing the rent before its extent has been assessed. When there is any doubt about bladder injury, methylene blue dye in normal saline or sterile milk can be instilled into the bladder through the indwelling Foley catheter. Either of the two will quickly identify the point of leakage, but milk has the added advantage that it can be used repeatedly, so the bladder can be tested again after the repair.

Sometimes only the muscularis layer of the bladder is injured and the mucosa is intact. These injuries may not be identified unless the bladder is filled with fluid (100–200 μl). Identification is important, as fistulas may ensue if the muscularis is not oversewn and if the bladder is not immobilized postoperatively. This type of injury is easily repaired with a fine suture such as 2:0 or 3:0 Vicryl, or 2:0 or 3:0 chromic suture.

Basically, repair of bladder injuries involves inverting the tissue with two layers of sutures and immobilizing the bladder postoperatively. The suture lines should be free from tension. When fistulas develop after primary injuries that have been diagnosed and repaired it is almost always because the sutures have been placed under tension (Figure 30.11). Before suturing, the bladder should be mobilized for 1.5–2.0 cm all around the injury so that there is sufficient tissue to invert (Figure 30.11). Two layers of continuous running suture, such as 2:0 Vicryl or 2:0 chromic suture, are used to close the defect. The bladder should be immobilized for 7–10 days with catheter drainage. If the laceration is well sutured without tension and the bladder is immobilized, there is little risk of fistula formation.

Usually, abdominal drains are not needed, but if they are present, there is no problem if some urine leaks through the repair. The problem occurs when there is leakage and no drain. If the operator is not absolutely sure that there is no leakage, it is safer to use drains.

Ureteral injuries

Ureteral injuries are uncommon with cesarean section but may occur with cesarean hysterectomy, particularly if there is bleeding deep in the pelvis. One helpful suggestion is to use sponge forceps to clamp when there is sudden hemorrhage and the anatomic landmarks are not identifiable. Any pelvic structure, including the ureter, can be caught within sponge forceps without inflicting injury. Once hemostasis has been achieved and the field is dry, the forceps can be removed and other clamps applied.

Ureters can be injured in several ways: severed either partly or completely or ligated by a suture. Ureteral injury is seldom evident at operation and must be suspected in the postoperative period to be diagnosed. There should be a high index of suspicion of ureter injury when the operation has not progressed in a routine manner as expected, especially if both ureters have not been identified in performing a total hysterectomy.

There are several ways to survey the ureter for possible damage. Palpation is the easiest but direct visualization is preferred.

In dissecting the ureter to identify injury, the operator separates the tissue anterior to the ureter so that the structure can be visualized in its bed from pelvic brim to bladder (Figure 30.12). This provides visual proof that the ureter has not been severed, ligated, or sutured. As noted in the section on iliac ligation, the ureter remains on the medial leaf of the peritoneum in the area between the pelvic brim and the broad ligament. It enters the broad ligament through the so-called tunnel, passes inferiorly, and comes medially toward the midline as it enters the bladder. To unroof the ureter, tissue on the medial leaf of the peritoneum just anterior to the ureter is opened so that the ureter itself is exposed. Right-angle clamps can be used to mobilize a free space anterior to the ureter before the tissue is incised. The same technique is used in the broad ligament, except that the uterine vessels pass over the ureter, so the tissue must be clamped as well as incised (Figure 30.13). Since the broad ligament is anterior to the uterus and is vascular, this technique of opening a tunnel, clamping, and incising is used repeatedly in the dissection from the broad ligament tunnel to the bladder (Figure 30.13).

If one were to image the ureter on end and look from the pelvic brim toward the bladder, the ureter would be mobilized anterolaterally in the pelvic portion, anteriorly in the broad ligament area, and anteromedially near the bladder (Figure 30.12).

To check the integrity of the ureter, one may pass ureteral catheters from the bladder into each ureter through a cystoscope. If this can be accomplished successfully, the ureter has

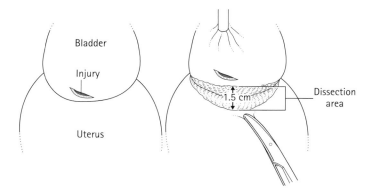

Figure 30.11 Before repair of the bladder, tissue around an injury is dissected in such a manner that the rent can be closed without tension on the sutures.

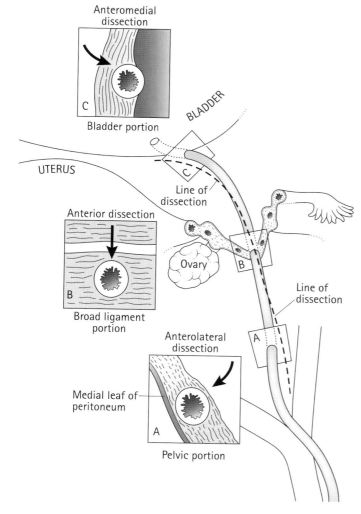

Figure 30.12 The broad ligament is split open and the vessels are clamped. This permits visualization of the ureter. The tissues in different areas (A, B, and C) are mobilized to visualize the ureter at different levels of the pelvis.

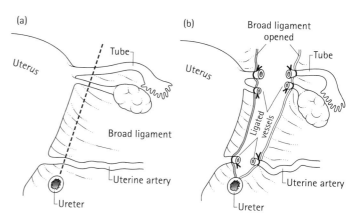

Figure 30.13 The uterine and ovarian vessels must be clamped (a) and ligated in order to open the broad ligament (b) and 'unroof' the ureter.

inserted from above if the ureter has been severed or from below by cystoscopy.

In end-to-end anastomosis, the ureter should be repaired without tension by placing four or five 3:0 Vicryl catgut sutures in the ureter. The anastomosis need not be watertight. The point is to approximate the epithelium ends. When injury has occurred near the bladder, there are two ways to insert the ureter into the bladder.

The traditional method used by gynecologists is a blind insertion. The end of the ureter is split for about 1 cm, making two flaps. A small stab incision is made into the bladder. Then a mattress suture is placed in each flap so that the loop is inside the ureter. With atraumatic French eye needles, these sutures are carried into the bladder through the incision and brought out through the bladder wall (Figure 30.14). When the sutures are pulled up, the ureter is drawn into the bladder with the flaps

not been severed or ligated. Unfortunately, the fact that the catheter cannot be passed does not always prove that the ureter has been injured.

In the case of ureteral injuries, the ureter is usually splinted with a catheter, and the site of the repair is drained. If the ureter is ligated or sutured, the suture simply needs to be removed, and a stent should be placed and should remain in place for about 2 weeks. If the ureter has been severed, the choice of procedure depends upon how close to the bladder the injury occurred. Stricture is a fairly common complication with end-to-end anastomosis; thus, implantation into the bladder is often preferable.

A ureteral catheter or plain polyethylene tubing can be used as a splint. The catheter has an advantage in that one can determine exactly where the catheter tip is in relation to the kidney by the measuring bands. Some feel that polyethylene causes less tissue reaction. The splinting catheter can be

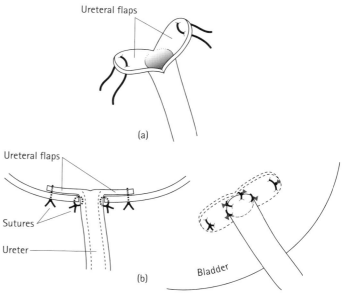

Figure 30.14 Blind ureteral implantation with utilization of flaps.

spread against the bladder wall (Figure 30.14). Two or three fine sutures are used to tack the adventitia of the ureter to the outside of the bladder. This repair does not prevent reflux; nevertheless, it has been used successfully in the past.

The other method of transplantation is more complex. The bladder is opened so that both its outside and inside are visible. A tunnel is made through the muscularis and the ureter is brought into the bladder. Mucosa is tacked to mucosa under direct vision, and the ureter is also tacked to bladder muscularis on the outside of the bladder. There is usually no reflux from the natural ureteral orifice in the trigone after ureteral implantation at another site, but if the distal end of the ureter is identifiable at the bladder, it should be ligated.

Surgical repair of ureteral injuries that require other structures as ureteral substitutes may be necessary when part of the ureter has been removed.

If a ureteral catheter has been placed abdominally and cystoscopy is not available, the catheter can easily be brought out of the bladder. The operator should have someone to place a uterine dressing forceps into the urethra. The operator then takes the handle of the forceps in one hand and uses the other hand in the abdomen, but outside the bladder, to guide the tip of the catheter into the mouth of the forceps. (Of course, the one hand holding the forceps in the urethra is contaminated.) This approach works because human beings can touch fingers of opposite hands together blindly and can bring one finger to the tip of an instrument held in the other hand. Surgeons have often waited for hours until the patient could be cystoscoped to bring the tip of a ureteral catheter out of the bladder, simply because they did not know of this simple technique. The bladder should be catheterized and the ureteral catheter tied to the Foley catheter so that it is not expelled by ureteral peristalsis. It remains in place to splint the ureter for about 1 week.

Intestinal injuries

Injuries to the large and small bowel are uncommon with cesarean section. Most patients are young and have had few previous operations, and the adhesions from previous sections are anterior to the uterus. Bowel is uncommonly involved in these adhesions. Even with cesarean hysterectomy, when the cul-de-sac is included in the operative field, adhesions are rare. The chance that bowel will be injured is much less with section than with hysterectomy for the usual gynecologic indications.

However, with operative bowel injury, the diagnosis is crucial. An undiagnosed injury will result in serious postoperative complication and peritonitis. Diagnosis is made by inspection of the area of possible trauma. Unless there is a cogent reason to proceed with the operation, it is usually wise to stop and examine the bowel at the time of the suspected injury. If this cannot be done (as when the section must proceed to deliver a fetus in distress), the injured loop of bowel should be marked in some way. It is easy to 'lose' a traumatized area and have great difficulty finding it subsequently.

Another method that can be used to survey the bowel (both large and small) in the true pelvis for even the smallest perforation is as follows: the pelvis is filled with physiologic saline (approximately 100 ml may be required) and the bowels submerged. After a few moments, air from the rent will rise to the surface, and if the bowel is 'milked', gas coming from any injury through the bowel wall will be evident. This method will help to pinpoint the site of the perforation more precisely than simple inspection.

The principles of the repair of surgical injuries to the bowel are quite different from those employed in gynecologic surgery. First, the closure must be done precisely and meticulously so that it is absolutely watertight. Repair of the bowel is always based on the inversion of the tissue, so that serosa is approximated with serosa. This is important, since there is little margin for error in suturing. A mistake cannot be 'oversewn'. The sutures must be placed precisely as to depth. A suture in the external layer must not penetrate through the bowel wall, since that would make a potential tract for microbial contamination with bowel flora.

It is important to preserve an adequate bowel lumen. This is a greater problem with small than with large bowel. One technique for this is to close all injuries transversely if at all possible. Thus, consideration should be given to closing a longitudinal injury transversely if it is not too long. Suture bites must be small so that an unnecessarily large amount of bowel wall is not to be used in the repair.

During the course of the repair of both large and small bowels, the contaminated operative field should be packed off with laparotomy pads, and atraumatic rubber-shod clamps should be placed on each side of the injury to prevent continuous contamination during the procedure. Stay sutures used as guides and also for traction are placed beyond the ends of the rent. These sutures of no. 3:0 Vicryl will subsequently be the angle sutures of the inside layer (Figure 30.15). Fine atraumatic bowel suture,

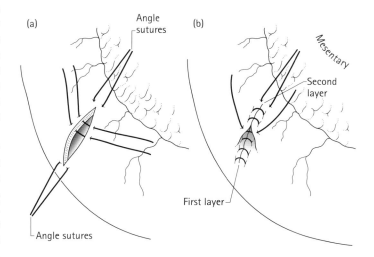

Figure 30.15 Bowel injuries are closed in two layers (a and b) by carefully inverting the bowel wall.

such as 4:0 Vicryl, is used for the inner layer of continuous running sutures. Stitches are taken in such a manner that the edges are inverted, with no suture material between the two serosal edges. A running Lembert suture is useful for this. Care is to be taken to ensure that the edges are not everted when the suture is tied at the end.

The inner suture line is reinforced with a second row of Lembert sutures (3:0 silk or 3:0 Vicryl) (Figure 30.15), which must not pass through the entire wall but only into the muscularis layer. After this part of the operation is complete, a thumb and forefinger are used to feel that the lumen is open. They should touch freely without surrounding constriction. As soon as the injury is repaired, the potentially contaminated packs around the field should be removed, and the operator and assistants should change gloves, since they may have been contaminated with bowel flora. The upper abdomen should not be explored after bowel surgery unless there is a compelling reason.

Bowel injuries requiring resection and anastomosis are beyond the scope of this discussion. The operator who is not experienced in these surgical techniques should have a general surgical consultant when necessary.

Incidental pelvic pathology

It is unusual to find significant pathology at cesarean section, since most patients are young and healthy. In general, a decision and plan of management are based upon the pathology encountered, the indication for section, and the condition of the patient. The last is usually no deterrent to treatment unless it is an emergency section for maternal reasons with a hemodynamically unstable patient. The serious potential for infection with section is an important consideration in additional operations.

Ovarian tumors are the most common pathologic lesions encountered at the time of cesarean section. For the most part, they should be treated as they would be at any other abdominal operation. Cystectomy or oophorectomy is certainly not contraindicated, but many feel that myomectomy is, because of its predilection for morbidity. Small pedunculated myomas or those actually involved in the incision should be removed.

There has been controversy about elective appendectomy at cesarean section. Theoretically, the operation would seem to be contraindicated because of potential contamination by bowel contents. On the other hand, there are large reported series indicating that appendectomy can be done safely at the time of routine section.

Postoperative course and management

Patients who deliver by cesarean section are not generally ill before the operation, and they recover quickly afterwards. They should be ambulated on the day of the operation if possible to decrease the risk of postoperative morbidity such as deep vein thrombosis. The next day, they can have a diet as tolerated.

The Foley catheter can be removed immediately after the operation or the next day. Physiologically, a urinary catheter is probably unnecessary during the postoperative period. An important aspect of postoperative care is deep breathing and coughing, particularly after general anesthesia. Thus, prophylactic incentive spirometry is important to prevent pulmonary complications.

Vaginal bleeding should be observed, and if it is excessive, evaluation and treatment can be given.

Postoperative complications

With the exception of infection, severe postoperative complications after cesarean section are uncommon. Atelectasis especially after general anesthesia is one of the most common problems and should be suspected when there is a fever spike within the first 24 hours after delivery. Diagnosis is made by auscultation of the chest and radiologic examination. Treatment consists of incentive spirometry and deep breathing every couple of hours, coughing, and sometimes intermittent positive-pressure breathing four times a day for 15 minutes.

Urinary tract infections are also common postpartum. Bacteriuria and urinary tract infection are common during pregnancy, and they can be treated effectively postpartum if not treated prior to delivery.

Ileus and obstruction

Ileus does not usually develop after pelvic surgery unless the bowel has been handled extensively or there is infection. In order to prevent the occurrence of the latter, the abdomen should probably not be explored at the time of cesarean section unless there is a specific indication. The upper abdomen should not be explored in an infected patient without a compelling reason. The upper abdomen is difficult to explore before the fetus is removed from the uterus, and the potential danger of spreading infection after the section is completed contraindicates routine exploration.

Postoperative ileus can be diagnosed when the abdomen is quiet on auscultation and becomes distended. Any oral intake should be stopped when ileus is suspected and nasogastric suction initiated if the patient is vomiting. If the condition is secondary to peritonitis, the primary infection needs to be treated with appropriate antibiotics. When bowel sounds return and the patient is passing gas, the tube can be clamped and then removed, and the patient can take sips of clear fluid.

Bowel obstruction after cesarean section is an unusual but serious complication. It can be differentiated from paralytic ileus, because at the onset there will be bowel sounds present and often the peristaltic sounds will coinside with crampy abdominal pain. The radiologic examination (CT scan with contrast) is usually diagnostic. Patients with a suspected bowel obstruction should have bowel rest and nasogastric tube suction. General surgery consultation may be needed when a surgical intervention is contemplated.

Pulmonary embolism

Pulmonary embolism is a serious complication of deep venous thrombosis in which a thrombus becomes dislodged and passes through the vena cava and the right heart into the pulmonary arterial tree. The clinical picture will depend upon the size of the clot. A small clot will pass to the periphery of the lung and produce a small wedge-shaped infarct. There may be a few symptoms or mild chest pain. Often there is tachycardia, chest pain, cyanosis, and dyspnea. Subsequently, there will be a transient pleural friction rub, bloodstained sputum, and, finally, pleural effusion. A radiologic examination 12 hours after the initial symptoms will usually demonstrate the lesion. Even small infarcts are likely to be followed by others; thus, they are serious.

Diagnosis is made by spiral CT, pulmonary arteriography, ventilation perfusion scan, and, rarely, pulmonary angiography. Venous Doppler studies of the lower extremities are noninvasive and may be helpful. Arterial blood gases are also mandatory to quantify the degree of hypoxia and direct the resuscitation effort.

If a large clot blocks the pulmonary arterial tree, the signs and symptoms are more dramatic. Chest pain, acute cyanosis, dyspnea, and shock may be apparent. The patient may not be stable enough for CT scan or ventilation perfusion scans. An ECG and a bedside echocardiogram will demonstrate the acute, right-sided heart strain or failure. The clot could be so large that it obstructs the bifurcation of the pulmonary artery, and the embolism may be immediately fatal. The clot produces intense arteriospasm and vagal stimulation. The administration of oxygen, heparin, morphine, and intermittent positive pressure are indicated as emergency measures. Today, in many hospitals, embolectomy is a feasible procedure for massive embolism if the patient does not succumb immediately. Alternatively, thrombolysis, either systemic or through a pulmonary arterial angiography catheter, can be lifesaving.

Heparin or low-molecular-weight heparin anticoagulation is the treatment for hemodynamically stable patients with postoperative thromboembolic complications as soon as the diagnosis is entertained. Diagnostic studies can then be performed.

Wound disruption

Wound disruption is another rare but frightening complication of abdominal surgery. It may occur without any warning. Slight abdominal pain and a serous or serosanguineous discharge from the wound are ominous signs. The skin may open up so that the bowel can be palpated upon exploration or the abdomen may break open during a cough. Whenever wound disruption is suspected, the incision should be explored in the operating room under anesthesia.

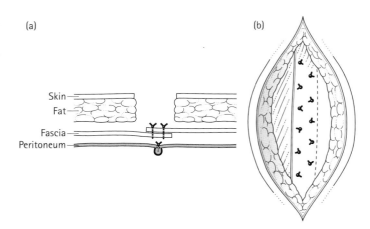

Figure 30.16 The fascia is imbricated in order to provide double thickness at the suture line.

Closure is a debatable question. In general, surgeons use a permanent suture, and most prefer monofilament material such as Prolene. Some close with through-and-through sutures either including or excluding the peritoneum. Others employ a layer closure with meticulous suturing of peritoneum, fascia, subcutaneous tissue, and skin. A few imbricate the fascia so that there is a larger area for adhesion.

For imbrication, the fascial flaps are freed of subcutaneous fat for 1 to 2 cm. The flaps are overlapped by about 1 cm for suturing (Figure 30.16a). The fascia is closed with two rows of mattress sutures, making a double layer of fascia at the suture line (Figure 30.16b).

Acknowledgment

We particularly thank R. Clay Burchell, MD, for his assistance with the previous edition of this chapter.

References

1. Bottoms SF, Rosen MG, Sokol RJ. The increase of cesarean birth rate. N Engl J Med 1980; 302: 559–63.
2. Petitti D, Olson RO, Williams RL. Cesarean section in California: 1960 through 1975. Am J Obstet Gynecol 1979; 133: 391–7.
3. www.cdc.gov.
4. Cunningham FG, McDonald PC, Gant NF, et al. Williams' Obstetrics (21st edition). McGraw-Hill: New York, 2001.
5. http://odp.od.nih.gov/consensus/cons/027/027_statement.htm#1.
6. Budin in Tarnier et Budin: Traité de l'art des accouchements, Vol. 4., p. 495, 1901.
7. Eastman NJ. The role of frontier America in the development of cesarean section. Am J Obstet Gynecol 1932; 24: 919.
8. Harris RP. Cattle-horn lacerations of the abdomen and uterus in pregnant women. Am J Obstet 1887; 20: 673.
9. Lungren SS. A case of cesarean section twice successfully performed on the same patient. Am J Obstet 1881; 14: 78.

10. Sanger J. Der Kaiserschmitt bei Uterusfibromen nebst Vergleichender Methodik der Sectio caesarea und der Porro Operation. W. Engelmann: Leipzig, 1882.

11. Williams JW. Obstetrics: A Textbook for the Use of Students and Practitioners (6th edition). D Appleton & Co: New York, 1930.

12. Liley AW. Liquor amnii analysis in the management of the pregnancy complicated by rhesus sensitization. Am J Obstet Gynecol 1961; 82: 1359–70.

13. O'Driscoll KO, Foley M. Correlation of decrease in perinatal mortality and increase in cesarean section rates. Obstet Gynecol 1983; 61: 1–5.

14. Committee on Practice Bulletins – Gynecology. Diagnosis and treatment of cervical carcinomas, no. 35, May 2002. Obstet Gynecol 2002; 99: 855.

15. Van der Vange N, Weverling GJ, Ketting, BW et al. The prognosis of cervical cancer associated with pregnancy: a matched cohort study. Obstet Gynecol 1995; 85: 1022–6.

16. Sood AK, Sorosky JI, Mayr N et al. Cervical cancer diagnosed shortly after pregnancy: prognostic variables and delivery routes. Obstet Gynecol 2000; 95: 832–8.

17. Roemer F, Rowland D, Nuamah I. Retrospective study of fetal effects of prolonged labor before cesarean delivery. Obstet Gynecol 1991; 77: 653–8.

18. ACOG Committee Opinion Number 234. Scheduled cesarean delivery and the prevention of vertical transmission of HIV infection. Obstet Gynecol 2000; 95: 1.

19. Thomas SL, Newell ML, Peckham CS et al. A review of hepatitis C virus (HCV) vertical transmission: risks of transmission to infants born to mothers with and without HCV viraemia or human immunodeficiency virus infection. Int J Epidemiol 1998; 27: 108–17.

20. ACOG Committee Opinion Number 220, August 1999. Breast feeding and the risk of hepatitis C virus transmission. Committee on Obstetric Practice. American College of Obstetricians and Gynecologists. Int J Gynaecol Obstet 1999; 66: 307.

21. American College of Obstetricians and Gynecologists. Vaginal birth after previous cesarean delivery. ACOG Practice Bulletin no. 54. Washington, DC, 2004.

22. American College of Obstetricians and Gynecologists' Task Force on Cesarean Delivery Rates: Evaluation of Cesarean Delivery. American College of Obstetricians and Gynecologists: Washington, DC, 2000.

23. Miller DA, Diaz FG, Paul, RH. Vaginal birth after cesarean: a 10-year experience. Obstet Gynecol 1994; 84: 255–8.

24. Miller DA, Mullin P, Hou D, Paul RH. Vaginal birth after cesarean section in twin gestation. Am J Obstet Gynecol 1996; 175: 194–8.

25. Yeh S, Huang X, Phelan JP. Postterm pregnancy after previous cesarean section. J Reprod Med 1984; 29: 41–4.

26. Shipp TD, Zelop CM, Repke JT et al. Intrapartum uterine rupture and dehiscence in patients with prior lower uterine segment vertical and transverse incisions. Obstet Gynecol 1999; 94: 735–40.

27. American College of Obstetricians and Gynecologists. Induction of labor. ACOG Practice Bulletin 10. ACOG: Washington, DC, 1999.

28. Elkousy MA, Sammel M, Stevens E, Peipert JF. The effect of birth weight on vaginal birth after cesarean delivery success rates. Am J Obstet Gynecol 2003; 188: 824–30.

29. Phelan JP, Clark SL, Diaz F et al. Vaginal birth after cesarean. Am J Obstet Gynecol 1987; 157: 1510–15.

30. Wilkinson C, Enkin MW. Uterine exteriorization versus intraperitoneal repair at caesarean section. Cochrane Database Syst Rev 2000; CD000085.

31. Bujold E, Bujold C, Hamilton EF et al. The impact of a single-layer or double-layer closure on uterine rupture. Am J Obstet Gynecol 2002; 186: 1326–30.

32. Poidevin LOS. The value of hysterography in the prediction of cesarean section wound defects. Am J Obstet Gynecol 1961; 81: 67–71.

33. Wilkinson CS, Enkin MW. Peritoneal non-closure at caesarean section. Cochrane Database Syst Rev 2000; CD000163.

34. Cheong YC, Bajekal N, Li TC. Peritoneal closure to close or not to close. Human Reprod 2001; 16: 1548–52.

35. Lyell D, Caughey A, Hu E, Daniels K. Peritoneal closure at primary cesarean section decreases adhesion formation. Am J Obstet Gynecol 2004; 189: S61.

36. Harrigill KM, Miller HS, Haynes DE. The effect of intraabdominal irrigation at cesarean delivery on maternal morbidity: a randomized trial. Obstet Gynecol 2003; 101: 80–5.

37. Wallace D, Hernandez W, Schlaerth JB et al. Prevention of abdominal wound disruption utilizing the Smead-Jones closure technique. Obstet Gynecol 1980; 56: 226–30.

38. Lyon JB, Richardson AC. Careful surgical technique can reduce infectious morbidity after cesarean section. Am J Obstet Gynecol 1987; 157: 557–62.

39. Chelmow D, Rodriguez EJ, Sabatini MM. Suture closure of subcutaneous fat and wound disruption after cesarean delivery: a meta-analysis. Obstet Gynecol 2004; 103: 974–80.

40. Alderdice F, McKenna D, Dornan J. Techniques and materials for skin closure in caesarean section. Cochrane Database Syst Rev 2003; CD003577.

41. Petitti DB. Maternal mortality and morbidity in cesarean section. Clin Obstet Gynecol 1985; 28: 763–9.

42. Physick P. In Dewees WP (ed.), A Compendious System of Midwifery, p.580. HC Carey & I Lea: Philadelphia, 1824.

43. Goodlin RC, Scott JC, Woods RE, Anderson JC. Laparoelytrotomy or abdominal delivery without uterine incision. Am J Obstet Gynecol 1982; 144: 990–1.

44. Kaiser PS, Kirby RS. Obesity as a risk factor for cesarean in a low-risk population. Obstet Gynecol 2001: 97; 39–43.

45. Weiss JL, Malone FD, Emig D, et al. Obesity, obstetric complications and cesarean delivery rate – a population-based screening study. Am J Obstet Gynecol 2004; 190: 1091–7.

46. Houston MC, Raynor BD. Postoperative morbidity in the morbidly obese parturient woman: supraumbilical and low transverse abdominal approaches. Am J Obstet Gynecol 2000; 182: 1033–5.

47. Duff P. Pathophysiology and management of postcesarean endomyometritis. Obstet Gynecol 1986; 67: 269–76.

48. Hopkins L, Smaill F. Antibiotic prophylaxis regimens and drugs for cesarean section. Cochrane Database Syst Rev 2000; CD001136.

31 Prevention of surgical site infection

Joseph J Apuzzio and Javier Garcia

Postoperative surgical site infections remain a major source of illness and result in longer hospitalization and higher costs to the health-care system. These infections number approximately 500 000 per year, among an estimated 27 million surgical procedures,[1] and account for 24% of the estimated 2 million nosocomial infections in the USA each year (second only to urinary tract infections).[2] Therefore, it is important to reduce surgical site infection by a comprehensive approach. While principles of infection control remain unchanged, new technologies, materials, equipment, and data require continual evaluation. Infection-control practices currently include traditional methods of infection prevention and appropriate preoperative antibiotic prophylaxis. In this chapter, we will review the various practices associated with surgical site infection prevention.

Surgical attire

Surgical mask, shoe covers, and surgical caps

Conventionally, a surgical mask is worn during the operation to avoid microbial contamination of the incision. Surgical mask and eye protection with solid side shields or a face shield additionally protect mucous membranes of the eyes, nose, and mouth during procedures likely to generate splashing or spattering of blood or other body fluids. Masks should be changed between surgical cases, if the outer surface becomes contaminated with either secretions, or from touching the mask with contaminated fingers. When airborne infection isolation precautions are necessary (as for TB patients), a National Institute for Occupational Safety and Health (NIOSH)-certified particulate-filter respirator (such as N95, N99, or N100) should be used.[3]

Shoe covers are also routinely used during surgery, offering protection from blood and other body fluids. Shoe covers have failed to demonstrate a decrease in surgical site infection.[4,5] In addition, Humphreys et al[5] did not demonstrate a reduction of bacterial counts on the operating room floor when shoe covers were used.

A few reports have identified surgical incision contamination by organisms shed from the hair and scalp of the surgical team. The Centers for Disease Control and Prevention (CDC) recommend wearing a surgical cap or hood to cover fully hair on the head and face when entering the operating room.[6]

Scrub suits

Protective clothing (scrub suits) should be worn to prevent contamination from street clothing and to protect the skin of health-care personnel from exposure to blood and body secretions. Guidelines and regulations for laundry practices and restrictions regarding wearing scrub uniform outside the surgical area vary extensively from institution to institution. Data are lacking on the repercussions of these factors in surgical site infection.

All protective clothing should be changed when it becomes visibly soiled and as soon as feasible if penetrated by blood or other potentially infectious fluids. Scrub suits should also be removed before leaving the hospital.[6–8]

Sterile gowns and drapes

These items are used to separate and protect the surgical field from contaminants. Surgical gowns are worn by every member of the surgical team participating in the procedure. Sterile drapes are used to cover the patient. There is great heterogeneity regarding the characteristics of available products. Gowns and drapes can be disposable or made of reusable fabric. The CDC recommends that regardless of the material utilized, both should be impermeable to liquids and viruses[6] (Figure 31.1).

Gloves

Health-care professionals wear gloves to prevent contamination of their hands when touching mucous membranes, blood, or secretions, and also to reduce the likelihood that microorganisms on their hands will be transmitted to patients during surgical or other procedures. Medical gloves, both patient examination and surgeon's gloves, are manufactured as single-

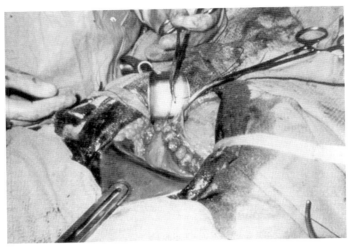

Figure 31.1 Isolation of the skin during cesarean delivery. The skin towels are soaked with blood. It is advisable to replace them with dry towels as soon as circumstances permit.

use, disposable items that should be used for only one patient and discarded. Gloves should also be replaced and discarded when torn or punctured.

Sterile surgeon's gloves must meet standards for sterility assurance established by the US Food and Drug Administration (FDA) and are less likely than patient examination gloves to harbor pathogens that could contaminate an operative wound.[9] Sterile gloves are put on after donning sterile gowns. Appropriate sizes should be readily accessible. The FDA regulates the medical glove industry and sets quality levels, but even intact gloves eventually can fail with exposure to mechanical (e.g., puncture) and chemical hazards. Data obtained from dental health literature reports a slight increase in formation of micropunctures after a hand rub with alcohol.[10] Hence, hands should be thoroughly dried before gloving. Although the effectiveness of wearing two pairs of gloves in preventing disease transmission has not been demonstrated, the majority of studies have shown a lower frequency of inner glove perforation and visible blood on the surgeon's hands when double gloves are worn.[11,12] Wearing double gloves has minimal impact in manual dexterity and tactile sensitivity during surgery.[13,14] Additional

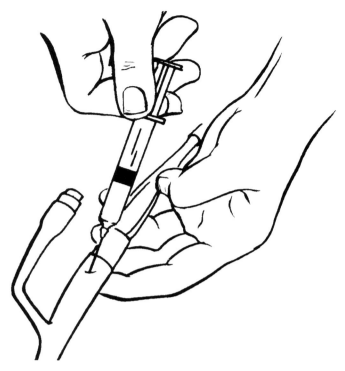

Figure 31.2 Aseptic technique for obtaining a urine specimen for culture

protection might also be provided by utilization of specialty products (such as orthopedic surgical gloves) (Figure 31.2).

Gloves should be replaced during surgery when punctured or contaminated by microorganisms. For example, gloves should be replaced after delivering the fetus when the hand reaches into the birth canal during cesarean delivery to delivery the fetal head from a gravida whose cervix is dilated and has arrest of labor. The cervix contains many bacteria which are opportunistic and may cause postpartum infection (Table 31.1).

Perioperative interventions

Hand wash

For the last century, hand hygiene has been accepted as a primary mechanism of infection control. Current guidelines recommend plain soap for hand washing unless patient care involves invasive procedures or when hands are visibly dirty or contaminated with blood or other potentially infectious substances. There is evidence that infection rates in adult or neonatal intensive care units or surgery may be further reduced when antiseptic products are used.[15,16] If hands are not visibly soiled, an alcohol-based hand rub can also be used. Alcohol-based formulations are superior to antiseptic detergents for rapid microbial killing on skin and, with the addition of appropriate moisturizers, are probably milder and better tolerated by health-care personnel, since acceptance is a major factor for compliance with recommended hand hygiene protocols (Table 31.2).

Table 31.1 Partial list of microorganisms isolated from the normal cervix

Aerobes	Anaerobes
Lactobacillus	Bacteroides sp.
Escherichia coli	Peptococcus
Staphylococcus epidermidis	Peptostreptococcus
Proteus mirabilis	Clostridial sp.
Candida sp.	Bifidiobacterium
	Eubacterium
	Veillonella
	Bacteroides fragilis

Table 31.2 Agents for cleaning hands before surgical and other invasive procedures*

Procedure	Hand washing	Gloves	Preparation of patient's skin
Catheterization of the bladder	Soap and water	Sterile recommended	Prepare urethral meatus with antiseptic solution
Insertion of intravenous or arterial cannula	Soap and water or antiseptic	Optional	Fast-acting antiseptic is desirable, preferably tincture of iodine
Insertion of central catheter	Antiseptic	Sterile	Fast-acting antiseptic, preferably tincture of iodine
Abdominal paracentesis	Soap and water or antiseptic	Sterile	Fast-acting antiseptic, preferably tincture of iodine
Laparoscopy or insertion of peritoneal catheter	Antiseptic	Sterile recommended	Antiseptic solution; hair to be clipped with scissors immediately before the procedure
Major operations (cesarean section)	Antiseptic solution	Sterile – to be changed after contact with contaminated amniotic fluid or lower segment of the uterus after rupture of the membranes	Skin to be scrubbed with detergent. Shaving should precede surgery by a short interval. Skin should be isolated from the field of the operation by sterile towels

*Adapted from Simmons BP. Guidelines for Hospital Environmental Control. National Technical Information Service, US Department of Commerce, Springfield, VA, 1981.

Irritant contact dermatitis, which is associated with frequent hand washing, has a prevalence as high as 10–45%. Use of hand lotions to prevent skin dryness associated with hand washing is recommended. However, moisturizing products should be assessed for compatibility with any topical antimicrobial being used.[16] Soap and antiseptic products should be appropriately stored and maintained; attention must be given to manufacturers' directions since liquid products can become contaminated or support the growth of microorganisms.[16,17]

Surgical scrub

Participating members of the surgical team that will have contact with the sterile field should wash their hands and forearms by performing surgical scrub immediately before gowns and gloves are fitted.[6] Povidone-iodine and chlorhexidine are the agents most frequently used by surgical teams. The introduction of alcohol-based products (alcoholic chlorhexidine and propanol-containing solutions) has been received with great acceptance. This new product was also found to have less residual antimicrobial activity than 7.5% povidone-iodine or 4% chlorhexidine gluconate.[18] Hand cleansing utilizing an aqueous alcoholic solution should be preceded by a 1-minute nonantiseptic hand wash before the first procedure of the day.[19] The duration of a surgical scrub traditionally was established to be 10 minutes, but recent studies suggest that scrubbing for at least 2 minutes is as effective. The CDC guidelines for prevention of surgical site infection published in 1999 recommend performing hand and forearm scrub for 2–5 minutes.[6,20–22]

Nails and rings

Although the relationship between fingernail length and wound infection is unknown, keeping nails short is considered essential because the majority of flora on the hands are found under and around the fingernails. Sharp nail edges or broken nails are also likely to increase glove failure by puncture. Hand carriage of Gram-negative organisms has been determined to be greater among wearers of artificial nails. In addition, artificial fingernails have been implicated in multiple outbreaks in hospital intensive-care units and operating rooms.[23–26]

Jewelry should not interfere with glove use or alter glove integrity. Skin underneath rings is heavily colonized with microorganisms. A study of the skin flora of nurses who work in intensive-care units determined that rings were the only substantial risk factor for carriage of Gram-negative bacilli and *Staphylococcus aureus*. However, other studies have demonstrated that mean bacterial colony counts on hands after handwashing were similar among persons wearing rings and those not wearing rings.[27]

Preoperative hair removal from surgical incision site

Microscopic skin cuts after shaving become foci of bacterial proliferation, causing an increase in operative site infections. Some evidence suggests that hair removal by any means is associated with increased risk of wound infection.[28,29] Shaving immediately prior to the operation proved to be associated with a decreased rate of surgical site infection when compared to shaving within 24 hours or more that 24 hours before surgery.[30]

Clipping hair rather than shaving immediately before surgery also was associated with lower risk of infection than clipping or shaving the night before an operation.[31–38] Depilatory agents have been associated with greater decreases in infection rates than the other techniques for hair removal.[30,39] Local hypersensitivity reactions can occur occasionally. The CDC recommends removing hair at or around the incision site only if it interferes with the operation. Hair should be removed immediately before the operation, preferably by clippers.[6]

Skin preparation in the operating room

Several agents are available for preoperative skin preparation (Table 31.2). Most centers utilize povidone-iodine or chlorhexidine gluconate, both of which have a broad antimicrobial spectrum. Studies comparing the use of these agents for hand scrub have determined that chlorhexidine has a superior reduction in skin flora with greater residual activity and furthermore is not inactivated by blood.[40,41] Chlorhexidine is also the agent of choice when patients are allergic to iodine products.

Preparation of the surgical skin site begins after removing all gross contamination that could interfere with application of the antiseptic solution. The skin is prepared in concentric circles, beginning at the area of the proposed incision and moving outward. Certain modifications to the traditional preoperative skin preparation have been described, including removal or wiping of the antiseptic solution applied and utilization of antiseptic impregnated adhesive drapes among others. However, none of these variations have been shown to represent an advantage.[6] However, the antiseptic solution should remain on the surgical site for at least several seconds, and some surgeons allow it almost to dry on the skin before the incision is made.

Asepsis and surgical technique

Asepsis is an extension of the concept of hygiene, based on the awareness of the various routes by which infection can spread. This notion includes many different methods to prevent transmission of pathogenic organisms. Rigorous adherence to the principles of asepsis by all scrubbed personnel is the foundation of surgical site infection prevention.[6] Traffic patterns and personnel moving in and around the operating room should be at a minimum, since an association between the number of people moving and levels of microbial counts in the air exists.[42] Optimal surgical technique and experience of the surgeon reduces the risk of infection in obstetric and general surgery.[43,44] Minimizing blood loss and tissue trauma during surgery, removing necrotic tissue, avoiding injury to neighboring structures, and hypothermia represent basic principles of surgical technique directly associated with surgical site infection prevention. Foreign bodies, including suture material, may promote an inflammatory reaction and a subsequent infection. In general, monofilament sutures appear to have the lowest infection-promoting effect.

Postoperative care

Most incisions after obstetric surgery are closed primarily. The incision usually is covered with a sterile dressing for several days. Immobilization provided by the sterile dressing contributes to the healing process. Data are lacking to assess the value of covering the incision after that period of time. It is also undetermined whether showering or bathing is detrimental to wound healing.[6] The incision should be assessed on a daily basis and surgical staples are removed usually on the fourth day after surgery. Ambulation is encouraged by the first 24 hours postoperatively; the patient should get out of bed briefly with assistance, and by the second day, walking is expected. Bladder catheters are usually removed the next morning after the surgery after verification of adequate urinary output. Early discharge is advised; however, adequate discharge planning requires individualization of care. Many patients return home before surgical incisions are fully healed; therefore, instruction on signs and symptoms of infection or other complications must be stressed.

Operative room environment

Ventilation systems

Operating room air may contain microbial-laden dust, respiratory droplets, skin particles, and other microscopic contaminants. Levels of microorganisms in the air are associated with the number of health-care personnel in the operating room.[45] Operating rooms should be maintained at positive pressure with respect to adjacent areas. All ventilation or air-conditioning systems should have two filter beds in series, with the efficiency of the first filter bed being over 30% and that of the second being over 90%. Air should be introduced from the ceiling and exhausted near the floor. A minimum of 15 air changes of filtered air per hour should be produced, of which 20% should be fresh air. Recommended relative humidity ranges are 30–60%, with room temperatures between 68–73°F (depending on normal ambient temperatures). A more comprehensive review on ventilation parameters in the operating room is available from the American Institute of Architects in collaboration with the US Department of Health and Human Services.[46]

Laminar airflow is designed to mobilize ultraclean air at a constant velocity, producing a sweeping action over microscopic particles. Recirculated air is passed through a high-efficiency particulate air filter, which can remove particles larger than 0.3 μm in diameter with efficiency superior to 99%. While this measure has been demonstrated to reduce infections in orthopedic surgery marginally,[47] there are no data regarding laminar airflow and obstetric surgery. Other interventions, such as intraoperative ultraviolet (UV) radiation, have not been shown to decrease infection rates.[48]

Housekeeping

Cleaning is a form of decontamination that renders the environmental surface safe by removing organic matter, salts, and visible soils, all of which interfere with microbial inactivation. The physical action of scrubbing with detergents and surfactants, and rinsing with water removes substantial numbers of microorganisms. Evidence does not support the notion that housekeeping surfaces (e.g., floors, tables, walls, lights) pose a risk of disease transmission.[6] The majority of housekeeping surfaces need to be cleaned only with detergent and water or an Environmental Protection Agency (EPA)-registered hospital disinfectant/detergent, depending on the nature of the surface and the type and degree of contamination. There are no data to support routine disinfecting of environmental surfaces and equipment.[6] Schedules and methods vary according to institutional guidelines. When visible soiling occurs during surgery, an EPA-approved hospital disinfectant effective against hepatitis B virus (HBV) and human immunodeficiency virus (HIV) or an EPA-registered hospital disinfectant with a tuberculocidal claim (i.e., intermediate-level disinfectant) should be used before the next operation as part of the Occupational Safety and Health Administration (OSHA) requirements. In settings where resources are limited, a 1:100 dilution of sodium hypochlorite (approximately ¼ cup of 5.25% household chlorine bleach to 1 gallon of water) is an inexpensive and effective alternative. There is no evidence to recommend special cleaning procedures or closing of an operating room after a contaminated operation has occurred.[6]

Universal precautions

In 1983, the CDC published a document entitled 'Guideline for Isolation Precautions in Hospitals' that contained a section entitled 'Blood and Body Fluid Precautions'. The recommendations in this section called for blood and body fluid precautions when a patient was known or suspected to be infected with bloodborne pathogens. In August 1987, the CDC published a document entitled 'Recommendations for Prevention of HIV Transmission in Health-Care Settings'.[49] In contrast to the 1983 document, the 1987 document recommended that blood and body fluid precautions be consistently used for all patients regardless of their bloodborne infection status. This extension of blood and body fluid precautions to all patients is referred to as 'universal blood and body fluid precautions' or 'universal precautions'. Under these universal precautions, blood and certain other body fluids of all patients are considered potentially infectious for HIV, HBV, and other bloodborne pathogens. Universal precautions are intended to prevent parenteral, mucous membrane, and nonintact skin exposures of health-care workers to bloodborne pathogens. In addition, immunization with HBV vaccine is recommended as an important adjunct to universal precautions for health-care workers exposed to blood.

Table 31.3 Wound care in contaminated patients

(1) Wash hands and put on sterile gloves.
(2) Remove soiled dressing and place in disposable plastic bag.
(3) Remove soiled gloves and rewash hands, if necessary.
(4) Put on sterile gloves and clean wound with sterile materials (gauze pads, Q-tips, etc.) from the center outward, being careful not to recontaminate an area already cleaned.
(5) Apply sterile dressing to the wound.
(6) Discard gloves and all waste material in a sealed plastic bag.
(7) Wash hands before examining the next patient.

Blood is the single most important source of HIV, HBV, and other bloodborne pathogens in the occupational setting. Universal precautions apply to vaginal secretions as well. Since the obstetric practice is often faced, during emergencies or at the time of delivery, with potential risk of exposure to hazardous secretions, strict adherence to universal precaution practices must be followed on all cases. Consistent utilization of protective barriers such as gloves, masks, and protective eye wear or face shields should be used to reduce the risk of exposure of the health-care worker's skin or mucous membranes to potentially infective materials (Table 31.3).

Prophylactic antibiotics for cesarean delivery

Postoperative infectious complications after cesarean section include febrile morbidity, endometritis, wound infection, urinary tract infection, and other serious infectious complications such as bacteremia, pelvic abscess, necrotizing fasciitis, septic pelvic thrombophlebitis, and septic shock. These complications represent a substantial cause of maternal morbidity and are associated with a significant increase in length of hospital stay.[50] The objective of prophylactic antibiotics is to attain therapeutic levels when surgical manipulation and possible bacterial contamination occur.[51] Nevertheless, antibiotic prophylaxis should not replace proper pre- and intraoperative asepsis, correct surgical technique, and meticulous hemostasis. The antimicrobial agent selected should have adequate pharmacokinetics during the pregnant state, achieving satisfactory concentration in maternal circulation and fetal compartments rapidly, since only short courses are used; agents also must have a good safety profile and be inexpensive.[35–37]

The single most important risk factor for postpartum maternal infection is cesarean delivery.[38] Other conditions that have been associated with an increased risk of infection after cesarean section include duration of labor, duration of rupture of membranes, increased number of vaginal examinations during labor, internal fetal monitoring, urinary infection, emergent cesarean section, operative blood loss, general anesthesia, experience of the surgeon, anemia, diabetes, bacterial vaginosis, socioeconomic status of the patient, and number of prenatal visits.[52–57] The Cochrane Library review included a total of 81 randomized case-control trials with nearly 12 000 women enrolled. Results obtained from those studies were remarkably consistent, demonstrating that prophylactic antibiotics are efficacious in decreasing rates of postpartum endometritis, wound infection, urinary infection (positive urine culture), febrile morbidity overall, and serious infection. Postpartum endometritis was reduced drastically by two-thirds to three-quarters.[52]

Antibiotic prophylaxis for an elective procedure had been controversial, with a number of randomized trials finding no evidence of decreased postoperative morbidity.[58–60] Smaill and Hofmeyr in their review for the Cochrane Library concluded that the reduction of postcesarean endometritis was equivalent whether the procedure was performed on an elective or nonelective basis.[52] These data were corroborated by a meta-analysis[61] that included seven randomized trials of non-laboring women with intact membranes and demonstrated reduction of postpartum fever and endometritis after antibiotic prophylaxis. As for the outcome wound infection after elective abdominal delivery, the reduction was determined to be merely significant. Only 15 trials included in the same literature review addressed the duration of hospital stay. Patients who received prophylaxis reduced the duration of hospitalization stay by approximately 0.5 days.[62]

Hopkins and Smaill[63] reviewed 51 randomized trials comparing antibiotic regimens and concluded that ampicillin and first-generation cephalosporins, such as cefazolin, have equivalent efficacy in the reduction of febrile morbidity, endometritis, and other postoperative infectious complications. Antimicrobials with a wider spectrum, such as second- or third-generation cephalosporins, carbapenems, or extended-spectrum penicillins, failed to demonstrate an additional benefit. Furthermore, multiple-dose regimens or multiple-agent combinations offer no advantage over a single dose and are likely to increase cost and antimicrobial resistance.

In many centers, a single 2-g dose of cefazolin is the preferred agent. Clindamycin may be an appropriate choice for penicillin-allergic patients; however, distribution in the umbilical cord and amniotic fluid is less predictable.[36,64] Optimal timing for antibiotic prophylaxis is not well defined and needs to be addressed in an appropriately designed trial. Gordon and collaborators[65] reported that administration of ampicillin immediately after the cord is clamped was comparable to preoperative administration. Since then, most obstetricians have adopted that practice.

Several potential concerns regarding the prophylactic utilization of antibiotics have emerged. Changes in pathogenic organisms believed to be caused by selection of resistant endogenous flora, as well as infection with nosocomial strains, embody fundamental mechanisms accountable for the rise in antimicrobial resistance. Allergic reactions and anaphylaxis represent another potential complication of antibiotic prophylaxis. Cephalosporins have a low cross-allergenicity with penicillin (2–7%).[48] Urticaria or other mild reactions

occur in 1–3%. Anaphylaxis with these antibiotics is a rare event (0.001–0.1%).[51,66] Only a minority of trials describe adverse reactions to prophylaxis, making any determination of its incidence difficult. Overall, the most common side effects reported include skin rash and phlebitis at the intravenous site (1.5%).[36]

Antibiotic prophylaxis for other obstetric procedures

Subclinical or clinically evident chorioamnionitis after prophylactic cervical cerclage occurs at rates of 1–16%.[67] In women with cervical dilation, effacement, and shortening (which represent candidates for emergency cerclage), rates of postoperative infections have been reported to be 9–33%.[62,68] Additionally, the increased risk of rupture of membranes after an urgent procedure makes the administration of prophylactic antibiotics an appealing intervention. However, no randomized trial has presented clear data to support antibiotic prophylaxis in either of these procedures. Manual extraction of the placenta is associated with an increase in postcesarean section endometritis, even in the presence of antibiotic prophylaxis.[69–71]

There are no published studies to support antibiotic prophylaxis after a vaginal birth where manual removal of the placenta has been required; however, in some centers, administration of antimicrobials is common and may represent a reasonable practice.

References

1. Centers for Disease Control and Prevention, National Center for Health Statistics Vital and Health Statistics. Detailed Diagnoses and Procedures, National Hospital Discharge Survey 1994, vol. 127. Hyattsville, MD: Department of Health and Human Services, 1997.
2. Haley RW, Culver DH, White JW, Morgan WM, Emori TG. The nationwide nosocomial infection rate: a new need for vital statistics. Am J Epidemiol 1985; 121: 159–67.
3. CDC. Guidelines for preventing the transmission of Mycobacterium tuberculosis in health-care facilities, 1994. MMWR 1994; 43(no. RR-13).
4. Weightman NC, Banfield KR. Protective over-shoes are unnecessary in a day surgery unit. J Hosp Infect 1994; 28: 1–3.
5. Humphreys H, Marshall RJ, Ricketts VE, Russell AJ, Reeves DS. Theatre over-shoes do not reduce operating theatre floor bacterial counts. J Hosp Infect 1991; 17: 117–23.
6. Mangram AJ, Horan TC, Pearson ML, Silver LC, Jarvis WR. Guideline for Prevention of Surgical Site Infection, 1999. Centers for Disease Control and Prevention (CDC) Hospital Infection Control Practices Advisory Committee. Am J Infect Control 1999; 27: 97–132.

7. US Department of Labor, Occupational Safety, and Health Administration. 29 CFR Part 1910.1030. Occupational exposure to bloodborne pathogens; needlesticks and other sharps injuries; final rule. Fed Regist 2001; 66: 5317–25. As amended from and includes 29 CFR Part 1910.1030. Occupational exposure to bloodborne pathogens; final rule. Fed Regist 1991; 56: 64174–82.

8. US Department of Labor, Occupational Safety, and Health Administration. OSHA instruction: enforcement procedures for the occupational exposure to bloodborne pathogens. Washington, DC: US Department of Labor, Occupational Safety, and Health Administration, 2001; directive no. CPL 2–2.69.

9. Food and Drug Administration. Glove powder report. Rockville, MD: US Department of Health and Human Services, Food and Drug Administration, 1997.

10. Pitten FA, Herdemann G, Kramer A. The integrity of latex gloves in clinical dental practice. Infection 2000; 28: 388–92.

11. Punyatanasakchai P, Chittacharoen A, Ayudhya NI. Randomized controlled trial of glove perforation in single- and double-gloving in episiotomy repair after vaginal delivery. J Obstet Gynaecol Res 2004; 30: 354–7.

12. Malhotra M, Sharma JB, Wadhwa L, Arora R. Prospective study of glove perforation in obstetrical and gynecological operations: are we safe enough? J Obstet Gynaecol Res 2004; 30: 319–22.

13. Watts D, Tassler PL, Dellon AL. The effect of double gloving on cutaneous sensibility, skin compliance and suture identification. Contemp Surg 1994; 44: 289–92.

14. Wilson SJ, Sellu D, Uy A, Jaffer MA. Subjective effects of double gloves on surgical performance. Ann R Coll Surg Engl 1996; 78: 20–2.

15. Hospital Infection Control Practices Advisory Committee Guideline for Isolation Precautions in Hospitals. Am J Infect Control 1996; 24: 24–52.

16. Larson E and the 1992, 1993, and 1994 APIC Guideline Committees. APIC Guideline for Handwashing and Hand Antisepsis in Health Care Settings. Am J Infect Control 1995; 23: 251–69.

17. Archibald LK, Corl A, Shah B et al. Serratia marcescens outbreak associated with extrinsic contamination of 1% chlorxylenol soap. Infect Control Hosp Epidemiol 1997; 18: 704–9.

18. Wade JJ, Casewell MW. The evaluation of residual antimicrobial activity on hands and its clinical relevance. J Hosp Infect 1991; 18 (Suppl B): 23–8.

19. Parienti JJ, Thibon P, Heller R et al. Antisepsie chirurgicale des mains Study Group. Hand-rubbing with an aqueous alcoholic solution vs traditional surgical hand-scrubbing and 30-day surgical site infection rates: a randomized equivalence study. JAMA 2002; 288: 722–7.

20. Hingst V, Juditzki I, Heeg P, Sonntag HG. Evaluation of the efficacy of surgical hand disinfection following a reduced application time of 3 instead of 5 min. J Hosp Infect 1992; 20: 79–86.

21. Wheelock SM, Lookinland S. Effect of surgical hand scrub time on subsequent bacterial growth. AORN J 1997; 65: 1087–92; 1094–8.

22. Deshmukh N, Kramer JW, Kjellberg SI. A comparison of 5-minute povidone-iodine scrub and 1-minute povidone-iodine scrub followed by alcohol foam. Mil Med 1998; 163: 145–7.

23. McNeil SA, Foster CL, Hedderwick SA, Kauffman CA. Effect of hand cleansing with antimicrobial soap or alcohol-based gel on microbial colonization of artificial fingernails worn by health care workers. Clin Infect Dis 2001; 32: 367–72.

24. Hedderwick SA, McNeil SA, Lyons MJ, Kauffman CA. Pathogenic organisms associated with artificial fingernails worn by healthcare workers. Infect Control Hosp Epidemiol 2000; 21: 505–9.

25. Passaro DJ, Waring L, Armstrong R et al. Postoperative Serratia marcescens wound infections traced to an out-of-hospital source. J Infect Dis 1997; 175: 992–5.

26. Parry MF, Grant B, Yukna M et al. Candida osteomyelitis and diskitis after spinal surgery: an outbreak that implicates artificial nail use. Clin Infect Dis 2001; 32: 352–7.

27. Salisbury DM, Hutfilz P, Treen LM, Bollin GE, Gautam S. The effect of rings on microbial load of health care workers' hands. Am J Infect Control 1997; 25: 24–7.

28. Mishri SF, Law DJ, Jeffery PJ. Factors affecting the incidence of post-operative wound infection. J Hosp Infect 1990; 16: 223–30.

29. Moro ML, Carrieri MP, Tozzi AE, Lana S, Greco D. Risk factors for surgical wound infection in clean surgery: a multicenter study. Italian PRINOS study group. Ann Ital Chir 1996; 67: 13–19.

30. Seropian R, Reynolds BM, Wound infections after preoperative depilatory versus razor preparation. Am J Surg 1971; 121: 251–4.

31. Alexander JW, Fischer JE, Boyajian M, Palmquist J, Morris MJ. The influence of hair-removal methods on wound infections. Arch Surg 1983; 118: 347–52.

32. Masterson TM, Rodeheaver GT, Morgan RF, Edlich RF. Bacteriologic evaluation of electric clippers for surgical hair removal. Am J Surg 1984; 148: 301–2.

33. Sellick JA Jr, Stelmach M, Mylotte JM. Surveillance of surgical wound infections following open heart surgery. Infect Control Hosp Epidemiol 1991; 12: 591–6.

34. Ko W, Lazenby WD, Zelano JA, Isom OW, Krieger KH. Effects of shaving methods and intraoperative irrigation on suppurative mediastinitis after bypass operations. Ann Thorac Surg 1992; 53: 301–5.

35. ACOG. Prophylactic antibiotic in labor and delivery. Int J Gynaecol Obstet 2004; 84: 300–7.

36. Fiore Mitchell T, Pearlman MD, Chapman RL, Bhatt-Mehta V, Faix RG. Maternal and transplacental pharmacokinetics of cefazolin. Obstet Gynecol 2001; 98: 1075–9.

37. Chamberlain A, White S, Bawdon R, Thomas S, Larsen B. Pharmacokinetics of ampicillin and sulbactam in pregnancy. Am J Obstet Gynecol 1993; 168: 667–73.

38. Gibbs RS. Infections following classical cesarean section. Obstet Gynecol 1980; 55: 167–9.

39. Hamilton HW, Hamilton KR, Lone FJ. Preoperative hair removal. Can J Surg 1977; 20: 269–71; 274–5.

40. Brown TR, Ehrlich CE, Stehman FB, Golichowski AM, Madura JA, Eitzen HE. A clinical evaluation of chlorhexidine gluconate spray as compared with iodophor scrub for preoperative skin preparation. Surg Gynecol Obstet 1984; 158: 363–6.

41. Lowbury EJ, Lilly HA. The effect of blood on disinfection of surgeons' hands. Br J Surg 1974; 61: 19–21.

42. Ayliffe GA. The role of ventilation systems in the prevention of hospital infection. Health Estate J 1994; 48: 6–8.

43. Miller PJ, Searcy MA, Kaiser DL, Wenzel RP. The relationship between surgeon experience and endometritis after cesarean section. Surg Gynecol Obstet 1987; 165: 535–9.

44. Chia JY, Tan KW, Tay L. A survey of postoperative wound infections in obstetrics and gynaecology – the Kandang Kerbau Hospital experience. Singapore Med J 1993; 34: 221–4.

45. Ayliffe GA. Role of the environment of the operating suite in surgical wound infection. Rev Infect Dis 1991; 13 (Suppl 10): S800–4.

46. Sehulster L, Chinn RY; CDC; HICPAC. Guidelines for environmental infection control in health-care facilities. Recommendations of CDC and the Healthcare Infection Control Practices Advisory Committee (HICPAC). MMWR Recomm Rep 2003; 52(RR-10): 1–42.

47. Lidwell OM, Elson RA, Lowbury EJ et al. Ultraclean air and antibiotics for prevention of postoperative infection. A multicenter study of 8,052 joint replacement operations. Acta Orthop Scand 1987; 58: 4–13.

48. Taylor GJ, Leeming JP, Bannister GC. Wound disinfection with ultraviolet radiation. J Hosp Infect 1995; 30: 85–93.

49. Update: universal precautions for prevention of transmission of human immunodeficiency virus, hepatitis B virus, and other bloodborne pathogens in health-care settings. MMWR Morb Mortal Wkly Rep 1988; 37: 377–82; 387–8.

50. Henderson E, Love EJ. Incidence of hospital-acquired infections associated with caesarean section. J Hosp Infect 1995; 29: 245–55.

51. Kelkar PS, Li JT. Cephalosporin allergy. N Engl J Med 2001; 345: 804–9.

52. Smaill F, Hofmeyr GJ. Antibiotic prophylaxis for cesarean section. Cochrane Database Syst Rev 2002; 3: CD000933.

53. Webster J. Post-caesarean wound infection: a review of the risk factors. Aust N Z J Obstet Gynaecol 1988; 28: 201–7.

54. Magann EF, Washburne JF, Harris RL, Bass JD, Duff WP, Morrison JC. Infectious morbidity, operative blood loss, and length of the operative procedure after cesarean delivery by method of placental removal and site of uterine repair. J Am Coll Surg 1995; 181: 517–20.

55. Desjardins C, Diallo HO, Audet-Lapointe P, Harel F. Retrospective study of post-cesarean endometritis 1992–1993, Notre Dame Hospital, Montreal, Canada. J Gynecol Obstet Biol Reprod (Paris) 1996; 25: 419–23.

56. Killian CA, Graffunder EM, Vinciguerra TJ, Venezia RA. Risk factors for surgical-site infection following cesarean section. Infect Control Hosp Epidemiol 2001; 22: 613–17.

57. Watts DH, Krohn MA, Hillier SL, Eschenbach DA. Bacterial vaginosis as a risk factor for post-cesarean endometritis. Obstet Gynecol 1990; 75: 52–8.

58. Bagratee JS, Moodley J, Kleinschmidt I, Zawilski W. A randomised controlled trial of antibiotic prophylaxis in elective caesarean delivery. Br J Obstet Gynaecol 2001; 108: 143–8.

59. Yip SK, Lau TK, Rogers MS. A study on prophylactic antibiotics in cesarean sections – is it worthwhile? Acta Obstet Gynecol Scand 1997; 76: 547–9.

60. Rizk DE, Nsanze H, Mabrouk MH, Mustafa N, Thomas L, Kumar M. Systemic antibiotic prophylaxis in elective cesarean delivery. J Gynaecol Obstet 1998; 61: 245–51.

61. Chelmow D, Ruehli MS, Huang E. Prophylactic use of antibiotics for nonlaboring patients undergoing cesarean delivery with intact membranes: a meta-analysis. Am J Obstet Gynecol 2001; 184: 656–61.

62. Kurup M, Goldkrand JW. Cervical incompetence: elective, emergent, or urgent cerclage. Am J Obstet Gynecol 1999; 181: 240–6.

63. Hopkins L, Smaill F. Antibiotic prophylaxis regimens and drugs for cesarean section. Cochrane Database Syst Rev 2000; 2: CD001136.

64. Heikkinen T, Laine K, Neuvonen PJ, Ekblad U. The transplacental transfer of the macrolide antibiotics erythromycin, roxithromycin and azithromycin. Br J Obstet Gynaecol 2000; 107: 770–5.

65. Gordon HR, Phelps D, Blanchard K. Prophylactic cesarean section antibiotics: maternal and neonatal morbidity before or after cord clamping. Obstet Gynecol 1979; 53: 151–6.

66. Shephard GM. Allergy to beta-lactam antibiotics. Immunol Allergy Clin North Am 1991; 11: 611–33.

67. Harger JH. Cerclage and cervical insufficiency: an evidence-based analysis (review). Obstet Gynecol 2002; 100: 1313–27; erratum in: 2003; 101: 205.

68. Shellhaas CS, Iams JD. Ambulatory management of preterm labor (review). Clin Obstet Gynecol 1998; 41: 491–502.

69. Atkinson MW, Owen J, Wren A, Hauth JC. The effect of manual removal of the placenta on post-cesarean endometritis. Obstet Gynecol 1996; 87: 99–102.

70. Lasley DS, Eblen A, Yancey MK, Duff P. The effect of placental removal method on the incidence of postcesarean infections. Am J Obstet Gynecol 1997; 176: 1250–4.

71. Magann EF, Washburne JF, Harris RL, Bass JD, Duff WP, Morrison JC. Infectious morbidity, operative blood loss, and length of the operative procedure after cesarean delivery by method of placental removal and site of uterine repair. J Am Coll Surg. 1995; 181: 517–20.

32 Anesthetic procedures in obstetrics

Joel Mann Yarmush and Jonathan David Weinberg

Obstetric anesthesia is a subspecialty with many unique features not found in other areas of anesthetic practice. The altered physiology of pregnancy increases the risk of anesthetic morbidity in otherwise healthy patients. In addition, the obstetric population increasingly includes older and sicker patients, further complicating their anesthetic management.

Often, labor management decisions directly affect anesthesia requirements and vice versa. Each patient's labor course may suddenly require emergency surgical intervention with accompanying anesthetic considerations. Obstetricians and anesthesiologists must coordinate plans for management in order to facilitate delivery, while minimizing the risk to the mother. It behooves every obstetrician to become aware of the benefits, alternatives, and risks of obstetric anesthesia procedures.

Analgesia for labor and delivery

Pain pathways

Pain of the pelvic viscera is carried via autonomic (sympathetic and parasympathetic) nerve pathways (Figure 32.1) to the dorsal horn of the spinal cord (Figure 32.2).[1] These fibers are thin and unmyelinated, and transmission is easily blocked with dilute local anesthetic solutions at the appropriate level.

In the first stage of labor, pain is caused by uterine contractions, cervical dilation, and stretching of the lower uterine segment. Impulses of these painful stimuli travel via sympathetic fibers at the T10–L1 dermatomes. A bilateral selective sympathetic block of these dermatomes would provide analgesia for this stage but is generally impractical.[2] A paracervical block could also provide analgesia for this stage, but it has its drawbacks (discussed later). A lumbar epidural block, hereafter known simply as epidural block, typically is administered at the L3–L4 level and can easily be adjusted to provide analgesia to the T10–L1 dermatomal level.

In the second stage of labor, pain is caused partially by the above factors, but principally by distention of the vagina and perineum as the fetus descends. These additional pain impulses travel via S2–S4 parasympathetic fibers. A pudendal block could provide analgesia for most of the pain during this stage. An epidural block may have to be extended to reach these lower levels, but can provide complete analgesia for this stage. A caudal block, which is a sacral epidural block, can also be used for the second stage of labor. These blocks will be discussed later.

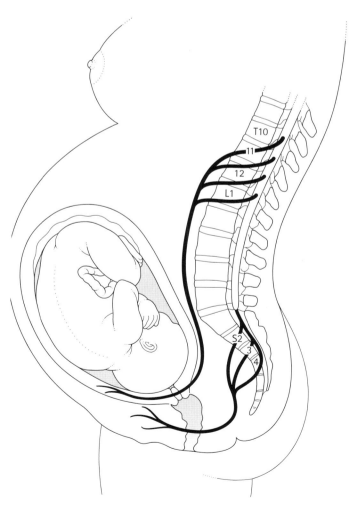

Figure 32.1 Autonomous nerve pathways for noxious stimuli.

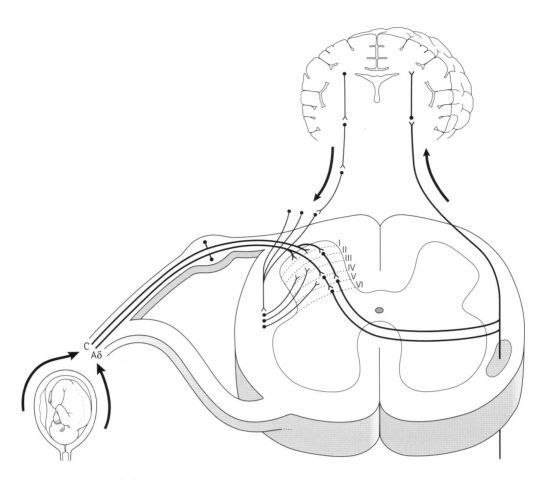

Figure 32.2 The dorsal horn of the spinal cord where nerves synapse.

Sometimes the pain is not successfully treated as above despite adequate coverage of the corresponding autonomic plane. This may be due to irritation of the body wall adjacent to the visceral structures. Impulses of painful stimuli from these somatic structures are conveyed to the spinal cord via somatic sensory fibers. These are thicker, myelinated fibers, which are less easily blocked and require a more concentrated local anesthetic at the appropriate level. Similarly, pain from manipulation of the uterus may originate from higher segmental levels innervating the peritoneum (T6–T10).

From the dorsal horn, the nerve impulse proceeds along ascending pathways to higher centers in the brain where pain is ultimately perceived. These impulses may be altered, usually resulting in attenuation, via descending pathways from the brain.

Different medications and techniques can affect the pathway at various points to modify the perception of pain.[3] Systemic opioids (endogenous or exogenous) decrease painful stimuli indirectly by activating the descending pathways. Nonpharmacologic modes, such as the psychoprophylactic method of Lamaze, also decrease painful stimuli via descending modulation. Conversely, anxiety and emotional distress may block this modulation, thereby increasing the perception of pain.

Neuraxial (i.e., spinal or epidural) opioids act at opioid receptors located in the dorsal horn itself to inhibit transmission of painful stimuli. Alpha-2 agonists, such as clonidine and epinephrine, also modulate painful stimuli via receptors in the dorsal horn.

Inhalational agents act by disrupting transmission of stimuli to the spinal cord and between the spinal cord and the brain, and by interfering with awareness of the pain at the cerebral cortex.

Systemic medications

It is widely accepted that neuraxial analgesia with local anesthetics and/or opioids is usually the best technique for relieving discomfort during labor and delivery.[4,5] Medical contraindications, patient desire for alternative methods, and lack of trained personnel may make neuraxial blockade unfeasible. Systemic medications are a popular alternative.

Systemic opioids

Opioids are the most commonly used systemic medications for labor analgesia.[6] Pure agonists, such as morphine and meperidine, are effective at opioid receptors in the spinal cord and in the brain without any intrinsic limit to their effect. Sedation and respiratory depression are the side effects of greatest concern in the labor suite, although pruritus, nausea, and ileus can also be troublesome. Diffusion across the placenta is a potential problem, particularly with the more lipophilic agents (e.g., fentanyl, sufentanil), possibly resulting in hypoventilation of the newborn, and in diminished variability of the fetal heart rate. Partial agonists, such as buprenorphine, are said to have a ceiling effect due to their reduced intrinsic activity at opioid receptors. Opioid agonist-antagonists, such as butorphanol and nalbuphine, exhibit both agonist and antagonist properties. Consequently, both their desirable and undesirable effects are somewhat limited. They have become relatively popular for parturients as the potential for harm to the fetus, while not eliminated, is reduced relative to the pure agonists. Agonist-antagonists can also trigger withdrawal in opioid-tolerant patients.

Regional and neuraxial analgesia

Table 32.1 outlines regional and neuraxial techniques and indications used in the parturient. These include epidural, caudal, spinal, combined epidural/spinal, paracervical, and pudendal blocks. It should be emphasized that the goal of these techniques is analgesia, the relief of pain, rather than anesthesia, the complete absence of sensation.

Lumbar epidural analgesia

In obstetrics, epidural analgesia has gained widespread popularity, and is the most common anesthetic intervention in many centers. A slender catheter can be placed through a blunt needle positioned just outside the dural sac. Medications can then be injected via the catheter, to effect analgesia either at the

Table 32.1 Regional anesthetic techniques for parturients

Procedure	Common usage
Local infiltration	Episiotomy
Paracervical block	First-stage labor
Lumbar sympathetic block	First-stage labor
Pudendal block	Second-stage labor
Lumbar epidural block	Labor, delivery, cesarean section, uterine manipulation
High caudal	Labor, delivery
Low caudal	Second-stage labor, delivery
Subarachnoid block	Cesarean section, uterine manipulation
Saddle block	Second-stage labor, delivery, episiotomy

nerve roots in the epidural space or at the spinal cord by diffusion into the subarachnoid space. The technique offers the advantages of continuous use and safe, reliable analgesia. It also allows for the rapid conversion to a more dense or extensive analgesic, or to a surgical anesthetic if needed for abdominal or instrumental delivery, manual placental extraction, repair of perineal laceration, and other obstetric procedures.

Controversy exists as to the relationship between epidural analgesia and the progress of labor.[5,7–9] Some studies have shown that the second stage of labor can be prolonged, with an increased incidence of forceps delivery, when epidural analgesia is employed. This has been attributed to decreased maternal pushing associated with blunted oxytocin release (Ferguson's reflex), or excessive motor blockade and diminished sensation. Other studies dispute these findings.[10] Moreover, only a few retrospective or nonrandomized studies have shown a relationship between epidural analgesia and cesarean section for dystocia.[11–14] Many believe that dystocia makes parturients likely to choose epidural analgesia, and not vice versa.[15–17]

Labor epidural analgesia, when originally introduced, consisted entirely of repeated boluses of local anesthetic. In order to be effective and sufficiently long-lived, high concentrations were often used. The consequence of this was that patients experienced weakness and numbness of their legs. If there is a causal relationship between epidural analgesia and prolongation of the second stage of labor and dystocia, it is most likely associated with this type of epidural technique.[18]

Over time, other agents such as opioids and alpha-2 agonists were found to have analgesic properties when administered neuraxially. These agents were added to the epidural injectate to allow a decrease of the concentration of local anesthetic while maintaining adequate analgesia. The current trend has been to reduce the concentration of each of the agents as much as possible.[19,20] These epidural solutions, called 'ultralight' or 'mobile' in the anesthesiology literature, produce so little motor block that patients can often ambulate while under their effect, hence the moniker 'walking epidural'. Although few patients actually ambulate while laboring with a 'walking epidural', the benefits of avoiding the untoward effects of local anesthetics are evident.

Contraindications for epidural (and most other regional) blocks include patient refusal, local or widespread infection, coagulopathy, and hypovolemia. If a bleeding tendency is suspected, laboratory studies should be obtained before placing the block. If no potential bleeding tendency is suspected, no special laboratory studies need be obtained.[21]

Intravenous access should be established prior to epidural placement.[22] During the onset of an epidural anesthetic, sympathetic blockade and resultant vasodilation and hypotension may occur quickly if the patient is hypovolemic. Since uterine blood flow is not autoregulated, a decrease in systemic blood pressure will cause a decrease in uterine blood flow. If large decreases occur, uteroplacental insufficiency may ensue. This should be treated promptly with vasopressors. Hydration with 0.5–2 l iso-osmolar crystalloid without dextrose is suggested before and during the initial dose(s) of epidural local anesthetics to blunt the hypotensive effects from vasodilation. An ultralight labor epidural produces less vasodilation and hypotension. Preloading may be unnecessary if the local anesthetic concentration is sufficiently low. This would also avoid any potential inhibition of labor that may be seen with rapid infusion of intravenous fluids.[23]

The insertion of an epidural catheter requires sterile technique, with appropriate skin preparation and draping. The patient may be placed in the lateral or sitting position with the back maximally flexed. Placing the needle below the L2 level (usually L3–L4) minimizes the risk of trauma to the spinal cord, which terminates at the level of the L1–L2 intervertebral disk in most adults. There are several methods for identifying the epidural space, but the most commonly employed is the 'loss of resistance' technique. In this technique, a syringe is attached to the epidural needle and pressed to assess the resistance to injection between needle advances. As the needle passes from the ligamentum flavum into the epidural space, there is a marked reduction in the resistance to injection.

After localization of the epidural space and placement of the catheter, a test dose containing local anesthetic and epinephrine should be given to rule out incorrect placement. The test dose is designed so that intravenous injection will cause a brief, inconsequential increase in maternal heart rate, and subarachnoid injection will yield a manageable (low-level) spinal anesthetic. The test dose should not be given during a contraction, lest there be confusion as to the cause of any increase in maternal heart rate or interference with the patient's reporting of symptoms.

Significant complications of epidural analgesia other than hypotension are rare, especially with the use of a test dose and careful aspiration before injection. They include local anesthetic toxicity and high spinal anesthesia. Any discussion of the risk associated with epidural analgesia must also take into consideration the reduction in risk from the avoidance of general anesthesia (discussed below) and systemic analgesics, and the greater freedom it affords the obstetrician to choose the most appropriate management without concern for the discomfort of the patient. If systemic toxicity does occur, it is usually manifest as self-limiting bouts of tingling or dizziness. Seizures resulting from toxicity are extremely rare but may require ventilatory support and treatment with benzodiazepines or barbiturates. High spinal anesthesia can occur if too large a volume of local anesthetic is injected into the subarachnoid space. Spread of neural blockade may then extend upward to the cranial nerves, whereupon ventilatory and cardiovascular support is indicated.

The incidence of inadvertent dural puncture is less than 0.5% in trained hands. The incidence in training centers may be as high as 1–2%.[24] As the epidural needle is relatively large bore (i.e., no. 17 gauge), the incidence of a postdural puncture headache is greater than 50% when the dura has been punctured with an epidural needle. The headache can be severe but characteristically improves when the patient is recumbent. An epidural blood patch may then be warranted.[25] This involves

locating the epidural space near the dural puncture and injecting 12–20 ml of the patient's own aseptically obtained blood. Relief is usually rapid and complete, although the headache can occasionally recur. The risks of epidural blood patch include making a second dural puncture and infection.

Caudal analgesia

Caudal analgesia is epidural analgesia obtained by placing medication in the caudal canal, which is contiguous with the epidural space. Either a single-shot injection or a continuous infusion can be used. The patient should be hydrated, as with a lumbar epidural, and sterile technique must be observed. The patient is usually placed in the lateral position and the needle inserted through the sacral hiatus. The *dura* normally ends at about the S1 or S2 level, and therefore subarachnoid injection is infrequent. However, one should always aspirate before any injection to check for blood or cerebrospinal fluid (CSF).

Other risks and contraindications of caudal anesthesia are similar to those for lumbar epidural. The risk of infection is somewhat higher than that of lumbar epidural, particularly if a catheter is left in place for an extended period of time. Great care must be taken to avoid injecting the presenting part of the fetus. To assess this possibility, we recommend a rectal examination before injection or catheter placement.[26]

Spinal analgesia

Spinal analgesia for labor is produced by the subarachnoid administration of opioids with or without very small amounts of local anesthetics.[27,28] A special type of spinal block, namely, the saddle block, usually uses local anesthetics alone.[29] The blocks are administered in a manner similar to that for lumbar epidural analgesia above. The same positioning, sterile technique, and hydration are needed. Proper needle placement is easier, since a direct indicator (CSF) is present. The needle is placed beyond the epidural space, through the *dura*, and into the subarachnoid space, where CSF is located.

Spinal analgesia can be provided with opioids alone, without the hemodynamic alterations seen when local anesthetics are used. If hydrophilic morphine is used, onset is slow (15–30 min), but the duration of action is long (12–24 h). If lipophilic opioids are used (e.g., fentanyl and sufentanil), onset is rapid (5–15 minutes), but the duration is shorter (2–6 h). This type of analgesia is not without side effects. Systemic absorption of spinal opioids may lead to mild respiratory depression, nausea, vomiting, urinary retention, and pruritus. Additionally, long-acting morphine can remain suspended in the CSF, where rostral migration to the medulla can cause delayed respiratory depression, appearing some 12–16 hours after administration. Despite these side effects, spinal opioids have little apparent effect on the progress of labor. They can be used alone for the first stage of labor. However, they provide inadequate analgesia for the second stage.

Spinal analgesia as a saddle block has minimal risks. By injecting a solution with a specific gravity greater than CSF, and leaving the patient in the sitting position until the anesthetic has 'set' (usually about 10–15 minutes), a block of only the sacral fibers can be obtained, obviating potential high spinal anesthesia. The incidence of hypotension is reduced if the block is limited to the sacral fibers, and local anesthetic toxicity is seldom (if ever) seen due to the small dose involved. The resulting block is not useful for the first stage of labor but is excellent for both delivery and repair of the episiotomy.

The incidence of postdural puncture headache after spinal analgesia is related to the size and shape of the needle used. Use of a 25- or 26-gauge, cutting-type spinal needle (e.g., Quincke) is associated with an incidence of less than 2%. However, in parturients, the incidence may be higher. Use of a 25- or 26-gauge, pencil-point-type spinal needle (e.g., Whitaker, Sprotte, and Gertie Marx) is usually associated with a much lower incidence of postdural puncture headache than seen with a cutting-type needle (less than 1%).[30]

Combined epidural/spinal analgesia

Combining spinal opioids with an epidural analgesic offers some advantages over each treatment administered separately.[31,32] Once an epidural needle is properly positioned, a very small spinal needle (e.g., 27-gauge, pencil-point needle) can be placed through it, puncturing the *dura*. After medication is introduced into the subarachnoid space, the spinal needle is withdrawn, and a catheter is advanced via the epidural needle into the epidural space. This technique can be used to administer subarachnoid (spinal) lipophilic opioids, resulting in the rapid development of analgesia, which can then be followed by epidural medications as needed.

Paracervical block

Paracervical block is an easily performed technique for the first stage of labor.[33,34] With the patient in the lithotomy position, a needle is placed lateral to the cervix into the submucosa at the 3 o'clock position. A dose of 5–10 ml of local anesthetics is administered after aspiration, and then repeated at the 9 o'clock position. This blocks all sensory fibers of the uterus, cervix, and upper vagina. Unfortunately, severe fetal bradycardia is a common side effect of this procedure. If this technique is to be used, minimizing drug dosages and injecting only superficially after careful aspiration can help prevent fetal bradycardia. Continuous fetal heart-rate monitoring is essential. Uteroplacental insufficiency and pre-existing fetal distress are contraindications. Possible etiologies for fetal bradycardia include spasm of the uterine artery and direct transfer of local anesthetic to the fetus. In addition, once cervical dilation has progressed, direct injection into the presenting part is possible. Thus, the placement of the needle requires great care.

Pudendal block

The pudendal block is an easily performed technique for the second stage of labor.[34] The transvaginal approach is generally used. After palpating the ischial spine, a needle guide, or Iowa trumpet, is placed under the spine and the needle advanced approximately 1 cm into the sacrospinous ligament. A 10-ml dose of local anesthetic is then administered and the technique is repeated on the contralateral side. With proper aspiration and use of dilute local anesthetics, the risk of toxicity is minimal.

Inhalational analgesia

This method involves giving subanesthetic doses of inhalational anesthetic agents for analgesia. It can provide excellent first-stage labor analgesia and fair or good second-stage labor analgesia. The technique is easily administered. It is, in fact, too easily administered and can result in loss of consciousness and loss of protective airway reflexes, with resultant aspiration. Patients need to be monitored continuously and verbal contact must be maintained while administering the anesthetic. Therefore, this technique has fallen into disfavor.

Anesthesia for cesarean section

Induction or administration of general anesthesia

While regional anesthetic techniques have gained wide popularity for cesarean section, there are still times that a general anesthetic (GA) is needed.[35]

Obstetric patients should be interviewed and examined by anesthesia personnel. This will ensure adequate history and physical examination, even if the patient is hurriedly rushed into the operating suite for emergency surgery. When available, laboratory values should be checked and the chart reviewed with the obstetrician. Particular attention should be paid to prior anesthetic history, medical problems, current medications, allergies, and social history. Physical examination should focus on the patient's cardiopulmonary status and airway. A large-bore IV line should be present. A nonparticulate antacid should be administered orally to minimize the risk of aspiration.

The operating room (OR) should have a fully equipped anesthesia machine, with appropriate alarms, that has been thoroughly checked. Suction apparatus and prepared airway equipment should be present. Monitoring for blood pressure, heart function, arterial oxygen saturation, temperature, end-tidal carbon dioxide, inspired oxygen concentration, and neuromuscular blockade should be at hand.[36] In addition, all routine and emergency drugs should be prepared in advance or be immediately available.

Once in the OR, the patient should be positioned supine, with the uterus displaced leftward. The IV should be checked and flushed if necessary, and monitors applied. The patient should be given 100% oxygen to breathe for 3–5 minutes, or alternatively told to take four to eight deep breaths of 100% oxygen. This serves to load the alveoli with oxygen, thus minimizing the incidence of hypoxia while she is apneic during induction.[37]

Anesthesia should not be induced until the surgeons are ready to make an incision. This minimizes exposure of the fetus to the anesthetics. If a separate neonatal resuscitation team is to be present, and time permits, the induction of anesthesia should wait until the resuscitation team is ready.

Since parturients have increased gastric pressure and delayed gastric emptying, all obstetric patients are at an increased risk of aspiration and are considered to have a 'full stomach'. This 'full stomach' and a reduced esophageal sphincter tone necessitate a 'rapid-sequence' induction of anesthesia. Pressure on the cricoid cartilage, sufficient to occlude the underlying esophagus, is maintained by an assistant during this induction from the time consciousness is lost until after tracheal intubation is confirmed. An induction agent and a muscle relaxant are given together, and the patient is not ventilated until after the endotracheal tube is placed. This technique minimizes passage of air into the stomach, reducing the chance of vomiting and aspiration. However, it depends on a successful intubation before the alveolar oxygen is consumed, which can be a distressingly short period of time in the parturient.

The patient is intubated once adequate muscle relaxation is achieved (60–90 seconds). A 7.0-mm internal diameter endotracheal tube is usually used, but smaller tubes also should be available. Obstetric patients frequently have edematous pharyngeal mucosa, which makes the passage of a tube that would easily fit in a nonpregnant woman's trachea difficult.

Inability to intubate is a life-threatening emergency that is more common among parturients than among nonpregnant women. For patients with a suspected difficult airway, awake intubation should be considered using oral, nasal, or fiber-optic techniques. If intubation is not possible after rapid-sequence induction, the choices for subsequent action include continuing with GA with a laryngeal mask airway or a face mask, waking up the patient and trying an awake intubation, or performing a cricothyroidotomy. If there is no fetal distress, waking up the patient may be the safest alternative. At that point, regional anesthesia should be considered.[38]

Maintenance of anesthesia typically requires no more than 50% nitrous oxide and a reduced concentration of potent inhalational agent (e.g., 1% sevoflurane or 3% desflurane). Limiting concentrations to these amounts of gaseous anesthetics minimizes the deleterious effects on the fetus and parturient.

High concentrations of potent inhalation agents decrease uterine tone, causing increased blood loss. For uterine tetany or for procedures where profound uterine relaxation is needed, higher concentrations of potent inhalational agents may, nevertheless, be needed.

After delivery of the fetus, narcotics and other ancillary drugs may be given.

At the end of the procedure, any nondepolarizing muscle relaxant effects are pharmacologically reversed and the stomach is suctioned. The patient is extubated only after regaining full motor strength and all protective airway reflexes. The patient is transferred to the recovery room where supplemental oxygen is given. Circulatory status, arterial oxygen saturation, and any other necessary vital signs are monitored until recovery is complete.

GA has been associated with lower 1-minute Apgar scores than regional anesthesia, especially when high doses of inhalational anesthetic are used.[39] This effect is more pronounced as the time from induction of GA to delivery increases. Proper neonatal management in nonemergent cases results in comparable 5-minute Apgar scores. Neurobehavioral scores have been shown to be transiently decreased in neonates delivered under GA.[40]

Major complications of GA for cesarean section include asphyxia due to difficulty in maintaining a patent airway and pneumonia due to aspiration of gastric contents. Over the last quarter of a century, while the incidence of cesarean section has increased dramatically, the rates of maternal and fetal mortality have decreased. Certainly, improved anesthetic management has contributed to this result. The institution of better protection against aspiration, more sophisticated monitoring, and the decreased use of GA are examples of this.[35,41] Still, one of the greatest risks for the parturient undergoing cesarean section is anesthesia.

Major regional anesthesia

Regional anesthesia is the generally preferred technique for cesarean section because it obviates the hazards associated with GA in the obstetric patient.[42] It allows the mother to interact immediately with her baby and offers the opportunity for better operating conditions. As the time from skin incision to uterine incision has little effect on Apgar scores under regional anesthesia,[43] there is ample time to obtain hemostasis. Better hemostasis and maintenance of normal uterine tone may explain the decreased blood loss seen with regional as compared to GA for cesarean section.

Regional techniques must supply neural blockade from the upper thoracic (T4–T6) to the fifth sacral dermatomes for cesarean section. Lumbar epidural anesthesia offers several advantages over spinal anesthesia. Since a catheter can be inserted for continuous or intermittent infusion, greater intraoperative control of duration and level of neural blockade is possible. In addition, postoperative analgesia is easily titrated and maintained as well. Conversely, spinal anesthesia has several advantages over epidural anesthesia in that it is easier and quicker to administer, has a lower failure rate, is less often patchy or unilateral, and usually results in a denser anesthetic with less residual sensation. As is the case for labor analgesia, a combined epidural-spinal technique can be employed to harness the advantages of each technique. Caudal anesthesia would require a very large volume of local anesthetic agent and is, therefore, seldom chosen.

Anesthetic alternatives in obstetrics

Preterm labor

Preterm neonates have an increased incidence of morbidity and mortality as compared to full-term babies. Respiratory complications are prevalent. Therefore, depressant drugs, such as systemic narcotics and inhalational agents, should be avoided if possible. Epidural analgesia is the technique of choice for premature labor and subsequent delivery.[44] Spinal or epidural anesthesia can be used for cesarean section.

Abnormal position or presentation

Patients with an abnormally positioned or presented fetus typically experience more pain, and request analgesia earlier in labor than their counterparts. Consequently, an association has been noted between epidural analgesia, particularly if administered early in labor, and fetal malpresentation. The weight of the evidence points to the malpresentations causing the request for epidural analgesia, rather than the other way around.[15-17] Surely, if the local anesthetic concentration is kept low enough to maintain pelvic muscle tone, it is unlikely that labor epidural analgesia will cause fetal malpresentation.

Abnormal position or presentation of the fetus increases the morbidity and mortality associated with delivery. Anesthetic intervention may not always be required, but must always be considered. Urgent intervention to relax the uterus requires rapid administration of medications, which may include general anesthetics. Anesthesia personnel should be readily available for every delivery of this type.

Spontaneous internal rotation during labor is facilitated by intact perineal muscle tone. The concentration of epidurally administered anesthetics should be kept low so as not to relax the perineal musculature.

Low-forceps delivery can be accomplished with local perineal infiltration or pudendal nerve block. Midforceps delivery requires a more complete anesthetic. External or internal version is usually best performed with abdominal wall muscle relaxation provided by neuraxial anesthesia.[45,46] Vacuum extraction can be performed with minimal or no anesthesia.

Breech presentation often proceeds to cesarean section and may, therefore, benefit from pre-emptive epidural anesthesia.[46]

Multiple gestation

Multiple gestation is often associated with prematurity and breech presentation. Epidural anesthesia is considered by many to be the anesthetic of choice for labor and subsequent delivery.[46] Internal or external version or breech extraction of the second baby may be needed and may necessitate anesthetic intervention. Uterine hypertonus after the first twin's delivery may require GA or other uterine relaxants. Anesthesia personnel should be in attendance during delivery.

Antepartum and postpartum hemorrhage

Antepartum hemorrhage is usually caused by placenta previa or abruptio placentae. Cardiovascular support and GA for cesarean section are often indicated.

Postpartum hemorrhage after vaginal delivery is usually caused by retained placenta, uterine atony, or vaginal lacerations. Manual exploration of the uterus is necessary for management of the retained placenta. Uterine relaxation may be required and can be achieved with an existing regional block for analgesia accompanied by intravenous infusion of a beta agonist or nitroglycerin for smooth muscle relaxation.[47,48] Alternatively, GA with rapid sequence induction and endotracheal intubation may be utilized.

Uterine atony may result in severe blood loss; therefore, an increase in uterine tone is imperative. Potent inhalational agents should be discontinued. Intravenous oxytocin and directly administered prostaglandin F_2 can also be given. If bleeding continues, emergency surgical intervention may be required.

Preeclampsia–eclampsia

In preeclampsia, anesthesia personnel are confronted with a hypertensive, intravascularly depleted patient who is very sensitive to cardiovascular insult and who teeters between hypovolemia and congestive heart failure. Painful uterine contractions cause an increase in catecholamines and a decrease in uteroplacental perfusion. This can be magnified in the already tenuous preeclamptic patient. For this and other previously stated reasons, lumbar epidural analgesia is indicated.[49] All preeclamptic patients with normal bleeding and coagulation times should benefit from epidural analgesia for labor and delivery, or anesthesia for cesarean section, unless otherwise contraindicated.

Anesthesia personnel must maintain a low threshold for placement of invasive monitoring in the severe preeclamptic. Usually, arterial and central venous catheters are sufficient. Placement of a pulmonary artery catheter may be needed, but is associated with increased morbidity. The benefits of such a procedure must be weighed against its associated risks.

Hypertensive patients are often taking antihypertensive medications such as hydralazine or alpha-methyldopa. If induction of GA is planned, short-acting IV antihypertensive drugs may be necessary to prevent excessive increases in blood pressure. Sodium nitroprusside, nitroglycerine, labetalol, or esmolol limited to very short periods of time should have little adverse neonatal effects.

Magnesium sulfate is the anticonvulsant of choice in the USA for seizure prophylaxis in the preeclamptic patient.[50] Of particular note are its neuromuscular and cardiac effects at high doses. It can cause muscle weakness and even paralysis. Cardiac bradyarrhythmia and depression are rare, but are occasionally seen with high serum magnesium levels. Discontinuation of the magnesium, intubation, and ventilatory support are usually all that are needed; but calcium may be required to antagonize the magnesium. Magnesium also crosses the placenta and with high serum levels can cause depression in the neonate.

Diazepam, as an anticonvulsant, is commonly used throughout the world in preeclamptic patients. However, it may be associated with neonatal depression.

Coexisting conditions

Diabetes mellitus
Diabetes mellitus is the most common coexisting medical illness seen in parturients. There is slightly increased maternal and neonatal morbidity and mortality in this population. The usual problems are maternal hyperglycemia and compromised uteroplacental flow. Epidural analgesia decreases catecholamine release and may improve uteroplacental flow in the diabetic mother.[51] Concomitant cardiovascular, renal, and neurologic disease may further influence anesthetic management.

Bronchial asthma
Most patients with asthma find that their disease is relatively quiescent during pregnancy.[52] However, these patients are at risk of exacerbation of their asthma in the setting of a trigger. Unfortunately, much about GA – including the foreign body in the airway and the cold, dry inhaled gasses – can trigger bronchospasm in susceptible individuals. In elective situations, a regional analgesic or anesthetic is the optimal choice. The poorly controlled asthmatic who requires an emergency cesarean section and who does not have an epidural catheter presents an ethical dilemma, requiring physicians to choose between the safety of the fetus and that of the mother. The early placement of an epidural catheter is the easiest way around this dilemma.

Cardiac disease
The hyperdynamic parturient with coexisting cardiac disease has an increased risk of morbidity and mortality.[53] Cardiovascular stressors such as painful uterine contractions should be avoided if possible. Epidural analgesia is usually considered the anesthetic of choice, especially for patients with left-to-right cardiac shunts or valvular regurgitation, as the reduction in systemic vascular resistance promotes forward ejection by the left ventricle. However, in patients with right-to-left cardiac shunts or valvular stenosis, epidural analgesia must be performed with extreme caution. Peripheral vasodilation and hypotension may be particularly detrimental in these patients, causing hypoxia and uteroplacental insufficiency.

Patients with cardiac disease in which the cardiovascular effects of regional anesthesia are undesirable may benefit from neuraxial opioids alone. Alternatively, an epidural technique which uses a very low concentration of local anesthetics, so as not to interfere with sympathetic nervous system outflow, may be acceptable.

Intensive hemodynamic monitoring may be indicated, and early and close coordination between anesthesiologist and obstetrician is essential.

Multiple sclerosis
Controversy exists regarding the patient with multiple sclerosis. Spinal anesthesia has been reported to increase the relapse rate, but definitive studies have not been performed. Epidural anesthesia has been used successfully.

Sickle cell anemia
In sickle cell anemia, epidural or spinal anesthesia must be performed with caution. The patient must be well hydrated with hypo-osmolar fluids (e.g., 50% normal saline) and hypotension prevented. Hypoxia may be obviated with supplemental oxygen, but stasis, especially in the lower extremities, may still precipitate a sickle cell crisis.

Acquired immunodeficiency syndrome
Acquired immunodeficiency syndrome (AIDS) is becoming more prevalent in the obstetric population. There are no known medical contraindications to any form of anesthesia in this group.[54] Aseptic technique and universal precautions should be maintained in this and all other parturients.

One must weigh the effects of major regional blockade in patients prone to develop peripheral neuropathy against its benefits.

Recreational drugs
The use of recreational drugs by pregnant women is prevalent in the USA.[55] Alcohol is commonly abused. Anesthetic considerations include withdrawal and organ (especially liver) dysfunction. Regional anesthesia is preferred, if no contraindications exist. An altered response to anesthetics may be present and dosages must be tailored accordingly.

Cocaine, or 'crack', is another abused drug. It is an ester local anesthetic with vasoactive effects. It enhances sympathetic nervous activity by blocking presynaptic reuptake of norepinephrine, and causes hemodynamic lability. In obstetrics, it is associated with spontaneous abortion, abruptio placentae, and congenital malformations. Anesthetic considerations include potential adverse interaction with other medications.[56] Concerns about systemic local anesthetic toxicity may theoretically prevent routine use of epidural anesthesia. Spinal anesthesia or saddle block uses small amounts of local anesthetic and may be preferable. GA with appropriate invasive monitoring is still commonly used for cesarean section.[57] Acutely intoxicated patients may be relatively resistant to the effects of anesthetic agents, while chronic users who are not acutely intoxicated may be abnormally sensitive. Ephedrine, which is often used to increase the blood pressure by promoting the presynaptic release of norepinephrine, may have an exaggerated effect in the acutely intoxicated patient, and a blunted effect in the chronic user. Additionally, chronic users often develop cardiomyopathy, which can become more symptomatic in the cardiovascular milieu of pregnancy.

Summary

The obstetric patient population has become older and more medically complicated over the past several decades. Despite this, maternal morbidity and mortality attributable to obstetric anesthesia have declined, even as more patients require or request anesthetic interventions.[58] This may be attributable to many factors, including a greater understanding of the causes of morbidity, improved monitoring, better medications, a reduction in the use of relatively risky techniques such as GA, and enhancement of the safety and efficacy of epidural analgesia.

Changing attitudes may also have contributed to enhanced patient safety in the labor and delivery suite. As obstetricians and anesthesiologists developed appreciation of, understanding of, and respect for one another's concerns, they have become more effective partners in delivering optimal care for the patients they serve.

References

1. Lowe NK. The nature of labor pain. Am J Obstet Gynecol 2002; 186: S16–24.

2. Meguiar RV, Wheeler AS. Lumbar sympathetic block with bupivacaine: analgesia for labor. Anesth Analg 1978; 57: 486–92.

3. Sawynok J. The 1988 Merck Frosst Award. The role of ascending and descending noradrenergic and serotonergic pathways in opioid and non-opioid antinociception as revealed by lesion studies. Can J Physiol Pharmacol 1989; 67: 975–88.

4. Task Force on Obstetric Anesthesia. Practice Guidelines for Obstetrical Anesthesia. A Report by the American Society of Anesthesiologists, pp. 8–13. American Society of Anesthesiologists: Park Ridge, IL, 1999.

5. Canton D, Frölich MA, Euliano TY. Anesthesia for childbirth: controversy and change. Am J Obstet Gynecol 2002; 186: S25–30.

6. Bricker L, Lavender T. Parenteral opioids for labor pain relief: a systematic review. Am J Obstet Gynecol 2002; 186: S94–109.

7. Leighton BL, Halpern SH. The effects of epidural analgesia on labor, maternal, and neonatal outcomes: a systematic review. Am J Obstet Gynecol 2002; 186: S69–77.

8. Lieberman E, O'Donoghue C. Unintended effects of epidural analgesia during labor: a systematic review. Am J Obstet Gynecol 2002; 186: S31–68.

9. Thacker SB, Stroup DF. Methods and interpretation in systematic reviews: commentary on two parallel reviews of epidural analgesia during labor. Am J Obstet Gynecol 2002; 186: S78–80.

10. Sharma SK, McIntire DD, Wiley J et al. An individual patient meta-analysis of nulliparous women. Anesthesiology 2004; 100: 42–8.

11. Lieberman E, Lang JM, Cohen A et al. Association of epidural analgesia with cesarean delivery in nulliparas. Obstet Gynecol 1996; 88: 93–100.

12. Newton ER, Schroeder BC, Knape KG et al. Epidural analgesia and uterine function. Obstet Gynecol 1995; 85: 749–55.

13. Thorp JA, Parisi VM, Boylan PC et al. The effect of continuous epidural analgesia on cesarean section for dystocia in nulliparous women. Am J Obstet Gynecol 1989; 161: 670–5.

14. Zhang J, Klebanoff MA, DerSimonian R. Epidural analgesia in association with duration of labor and mode of delivery: a quantitative review. Am J Obstet Gynecol 1999; 180: 970–7.

15. Chestnut DH. Does epidural analgesia during labor affect the incidence of cesarean delivery? Reg Anesth 1997; 22: 495–9.

16. Panni MK, Segal S. Local anesthetic requirements are greater in dystocia than in normal labor. Anesthesiology 2003; 98: 957–63.

17. Thompson TT, Thorp JM Jr, Mayer D et al. Does epidural analgesia cause dystocia? J Clin Anesth 1998; 10: 58–65.

18. Littleford J. Effects on the fetus and newborn of maternal analgesia and anesthesia: a review. Can J Anesth 2004; 51: 586–609.

19. Breen TW, Shapiro T, Glass B et al. Epidural anesthesia for labor in an ambulatory patient. Anesth Analg 1993; 77: 919–24.

20. Comparative Obstetric Mobile Epidural Trial (COMET) Study Group UK. Randomized controlled trial comparing traditional with two 'mobile' epidural techniques. Anesthesiology 2002; 97: 1567–75.

21. Simon L, Santi TM, Sacquin P et al. Pre-anaesthetic assessment of coagulation abnormalities in obstetric patients: usefulness, timing and clinical implications. Br J Anaesth 1997; 78: 678–83.

22. Kinsella SM, Pirlet M, Mills MS et al. Randomized study of intravenous fluid preload before epidural analgesia during labour. Br J Anaesth 2000; 85: 311–13.

23. Cheek TG, Samuels P, Miller F et al. Normal saline i.v. fluid load decreases uterine activity in active labour. Br J Anaesth 1996; 77: 632–5.

24. Choi PT, Galinski SE, Takeuchi L et al. PDPH is a common complication of neuraxial blockade in parturients: a meta-analysis of obstetrical studies. Can J Anesth 2003; 50: 460–9.

25. Safa-Tisseront V, Thormann F, Malassiné P et al. Effectiveness of epidural blood patch in the management of post-dural puncture headache. Anesthesiology 2002; 97: 1567–75.

26. Finster, Poppers PJ, Sinclair JC et al. Accidental intoxication of the fetus with local anesthetic during caudal anesthesia. Am J Obstet Gynecol 1965; 92: 922–4.

27. Brill S, Gurman GM, Fisher A. A history of neuraxial administration of local analgesics and opioids. Eur J Anaesthesiol 2003; 20: 682–9.

28. Stephens MB, Ford RE. Intrathecal narcotics for labor analgesia. Am Fam Physician 1997; 56: 463–70.

29. Egerton CD. Saddle block anesthesia in obstetrics. Am J Obstet Gynecol 1954; 68: 1098–1104.

30. Vallejo MC, Mandell GL, Sabo DP et al. Postdural puncture headache: a randomized comparison of five spinal needles in obstetric patients. Anesth Analg 2000; 91: 916–20.

31. Hepner DL, Gaiser RR, Cheek TG et al. Comparison of combined spinal-epidural and low dose epidural for labour analgesia. Can J Anesth 2000; 47: 232–6.

32. Norris MC, Fogel ST, Conway-Long C. Combined spinal-epidural versus epidural labor analgesia. Anesthesiology 2001; 95: 913–20.

33. Rosen MA. Paracervical block for labor analgesia: a brief historic review. Am J Obstet Gynecol 2002; 186: S127–30.

34. King JC, Sherline DM. Paracervical and pudendal block. Clin Obstet Gynecol 1981; 24: 587–95.

35. Dresner MR, Freeman JM. Anaesthesia for caesarean section. Best Pract Res Clin Obstet Gynaecol 2001; 15: 127–43.

36. American Society of Anesthesiology House of Delegates. Standards for Basic Anesthesia Monitoring. American Society of Anesthesiologists: Park Ridge, IL, approved 21 October 1986 and affirmed 15 October 2003.

37. Pandit JJ, Duncan T, Robbins PA. Total oxygen uptake with two maximal breathing techniques and the tidal volume breathing technique: a physiologic study of preoxygenation. Anesthesiology 2003; 99: 841–6.

38. Kuczkowski KM, Reisner LS, Benumof JL. Airway problems and new solutions for the obstetric patient. J Clin Anesth 2003; 15: 552–63.

39. Sener EB, Guldogus F, Karakaya D, et al. Comparison of neonatal effects of epidural and general anesthesia for cesarean section. Gynecol Obstet Invest 2003; 55: 41–5.

40. Dick WF. Anaesthesia for caesarean section (epidural and general): effects on the neonate. Eur J Obstet Gynecol Reprod Biol 1995; 59: S61–7.

41. Hawkins JL, Koonin LM, Palmer SK et al. Anesthesia-related deaths during obstetric delivery in the United States, 1979–1990. Anesthesiology 1997; 86: 277–84.

42. Hager RM, Daltveit AK, Hofoss D et al. Complications of cesarean deliveries: rates and risk factors. Am J Obstet Gynecol 2004; 190: 428–34.

43. Datta S, Ostheimer GW, Weiss JB et al. Neonatal effect of prolonged anesthetic induction for cesarean section. Obstet Gynecol 1981; 58: 331–5.

44. Gutsche BB, Samuels P. Anesthetic considerations in premature birth. Int Anesthesiol Clin 1990; 28: 33–43.

45. Mancuso KM, Yancey MK, Murphy JA et al. Epidural analgesia for cephalic version: a randomized trial. Obstet Gynecol 2000; 95: 648–51.

46. Pratt SD. Anesthesia for breech presentation and multiple gestation. Clin Obstet Gynecol 2003; 46: 711–29.

47. Morgan PJ, Kung R, Tarshis J. Nitroglycerin as a uterine relaxant: a systematic review. J Obstet Gynaecol Can 2002; 24: 403–9.

48. David M, Hamann C, Chen FC et al. Comparison of the relaxation effect in vitro of nitroglycerin vs. fenoterol on human myometrial strips. J Perinat Med 2000; 28: 232–42.

49. Mandal NG, Surapaneni S. Regional anaesthesia in pre-eclampsia: advantages and disadvantages. Drugs 2004; 64: 223–36.

50. Duley L. Pre-eclampsia and the hypertensive disorders of pregnancy. Br Med Bull 2003; 67: 161–76.

51. Datta S, Brown WU Jr, Ostheimer GW et al. Epidural anesthesia for cesarean section in diabetic parturients: maternal and neonatal acid-base status and bupivacaine concentration. Anesth Analg 1981; 60: 574–8.

52. Kwon HL, Belanger K, Bracken MB. Effect of pregnancy and stage of pregnancy on asthma severity: a systematic review. Am J Obstet Gynecol 2004; 190: 1201–10.

53. Sullivan JM, Ramanathan KB. Management of medical problems in pregnancy – severe cardiac disease. N Engl J Med 1985; 313: 304–9.

54. Avidan MS, Groves P, Eliot M et al. Low complication rate associated with cesarean section under anesthesia for HIV-1-infected women on antiretroviral therapy. Anesthesiology 2002; 92: 320–4.

55. Birnbach DJ. Anesthetic management of the drug-abusing parturient: are you ready? J Clin Anesth 2003; 15: 325–7.

56. Krzysztof M, Kuczkowski MD. The cocaine abusing parturient: a review of anesthetic considerations. Can J Anesth 2004; 51: 145–54.

57. Yarmush JM, Carlson RM. Obstetric anesthesia. In: Iffy L, Apuzzio JJ, Vintzileos AM (eds), Operative Obstetrics, pp. 262–80 (2nd edition). McGraw-Hill: New York, 1992.

58. Grant GJ, Halpern S. Obstetric anesthesia: update 2004. Contemp Ob Gyn 2004: 49: 45–57.

33 Invasive cardiovascular monitoring

Joanie Hare-Morris and Brian Kirshon

Pulmonary artery catheter

Swan and associates originally described the pulmonary artery catheter in the early 1970s as cardiologists and anesthesiologists initially utilized it as a management tool in the critically ill patient allowing invasive serial hemodynamic monitoring.[1] The first publication on the use of the pulmonary artery catheter in obstetrics appeared in 1980, and in the last 20 years, it has become part of the armamentarium of the obstetrician-gynecologist.[2-4] Numerous clinical reports utilizing pulmonary artery catheterization have helped described the pathophysiology of various obstetric emergencies.[4-10] This chapter deals with invasive hemodynamic monitoring of critically ill patients, and will enable the clinician to recognize serious problems early and select appropriate diagnostic and therapeutic measures in a timely fashion.

Pulmonary artery catheter placement

Pulmonary artery catheters are prepackaged in several commercial trays containing the necessary equipment. This procedure is performed by a sterile method using continuous electrocardiographic monitoring. An experienced obstetrician, cardiologist, or anesthesiologist who performs this procedure on a regular basis should perform the placement. The procedure for pulmonary artery catheter placement involves two phases. The initial phase is establishment of central venous access with a large-bore sheath, and the second phase is placement of the pulmonary catheter. The internal or external jugular, subclavian, femoral, and antecubital veins have all been described as entry sites. The subclavian vein approach has a higher incidence of complications, including pneumothorax, hemothorax, and puncturing the subclavian artery.[11,12] The femoral vein is associated with infection and thrombosis, and requires fluoroscopy for catheter placement. The antecubital vein may be utilized when the neck or thoracic access is difficult, or in the presence of coagulopathy. This vein is associated with greater technical difficulty in placement; however, the patient with impaired coagulation is an ideal candidate for the antecubital approach to avoid a potential intrathoracic bleed. The right internal jugular vein is the preferred site of central venous access due to its direct flow to the heart, and thus direct accessibility of the right ventricle. The right internal jugular vein also has less risk of pneumothorax.[13-15]

The gowned and gloved operator uses a sterile method to place the pulmonary artery catheter. The patient is supine, placed in Trendelenburg's position, and the head is turned to the left. The skin is initially punctured with a 21-gauge needle, and local anesthetic is infiltrated into the junction of the sternocleidomastoid muscles, with constant aspiration of the syringe. The internal jugular vein is identified by directing the needle at a 30° angle superior to the plane of the skin and aiming toward the ipsilateral nipple. The internal jugular vein is identified by the presence of free-flowing venous blood. Next, the smaller needle is removed, and a large, 16- or 18-gauge needle and syringe are directly placed into internal jugular vein. The syringe is removed and the guide wire is placed through the needle into the internal jugular vein.

Once the guide wire is successfully advanced without resistance, the needle is removed, a scalpel is used to widen the skin, and the introducer sheath-vein dilator is passed over the guide wire. The proximal tip of the guide wire must at all times be visible while placing the introducer sheath-vein dilator in view of the potential loss of the guidewire in the internal jugular vein. Once the introducer sheath-vein dilator has been placed, the guide wire is removed while the patient is asked to hold her breath to prevent air embolism. Current introducer systems contain an accessory port attached to the proximal end of the introducer sheath that includes a one-way valve that prevents air introduction into the central venous system. Heparin flush is infused to keep the lines open through the accessory port of the introducer sheath.

Phase two involves the actual placement of the pulmonary artery catheter (Figure 33.1). Continuous electrocardiographic monitoring is required during placement of the catheter to detect ventricular ectopy and arrhythmia. Intravenous lidocaine (100 mg) should be readily available for any significant ventricular arrhythmia that may occur. The typical catheter for hemodynamic monitoring is radiopaque, 110 cm long, and

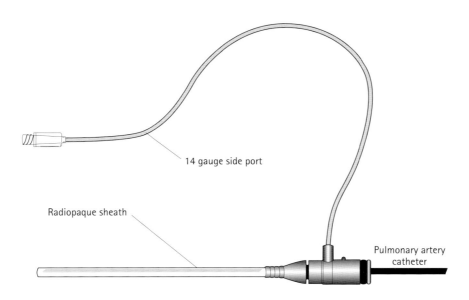

Figure 33.1 Introducer sheath for the pulmonary artery catheter.

marked at 10-cm intervals from the catheter tip. The catheter is attached to the physiologic monitor. The catheter tip is introduced through the sheath and advanced without force. All of the lumens of the catheter are flushed with heparin, and the balloon is tested with 1 ml air. The pulmonary artery catheter is advanced approximately 20 cm, using the markings which allow one to advance the catheter without fluoroscopy. At this point, the balloon is inflated and the catheter is advanced further into the central venous system by the blood flow. The catheter has been attached to a pressure transducer, and minute catheter tip movements will produce characteristic waveforms and pressure on the monitors.[16]

The standard flow-directed thermodilution pulmonary artery catheter includes a distal lumen at the catheter tip, a proximal lumen 30 cm from the catheter tip, a balloon lumen, and a thermistor. The pulmonary artery catheter generates vital measurements. The distal lumen measures pulmonary capillary wedge pressure when the balloon is inflated and pulmonary artery pressure when the balloon is deflated. The proximal port terminates in the right atrium or superior vena cava; it measures central venous pressure and can administer fluids and drugs. Cardiac output and core body temperature are measured in conjunction with a thermodilution computer. Cardiac output can be calculated by injecting fluid of known temperature through the proximal port. The rapidity of temperature change at the distal thermistor allows calculation of cardiac output.[4]

Waveforms

As the balloon-tipped catheter is advanced into the chest cavity, inspiration is marked by a decline in pressure, while expira-

tion produces a pressure rise. Entrance into the right ventricle is noted by a high spiking waveform with diastolic pressures of 0–5 mmHg. Complications may arise when the catheter impinges on the intraventricular septum, and arrhythmia may occur. This potential warrants rapid advancement of the catheter through the right ventricle into the pulmonary artery. Premature ventricular contractions may also occur during this process. If a delay in advancing the balloon into the right ventricle and pulmonary artery occurs then, balloon deflation and catheter withdrawal into the right atrium should be rapidly accomplished. When ventricular ectopy persists, a bolus of 50–100 mg lidocaine intravenously is indicated.

Entrance into the pulmonary artery usually occurs at 40–50 cm of catheter length and is characterized by a rise in the diastolic pressure above 5 mmHg. Secondly, a dicrotic notch of the peak systolic waveform is often seen, representing pulmonic valve closure. It should be emphasized that a dicrotic notch may occasionally be seen with right ventricular waveforms as well. With further advancement of the catheter into the pulmonary artery, a damped tracing with respiratory variation marks the pulmonary capillary wedge pressure. The pulmonary capillary wedge pressure is so called because the balloon is 'wedged' into the distal pulmonary artery, allowing the tip to equilibrate with the pressure of the pulmonary capillary bed. If the balloon is deflated, a pulmonary artery tracing reappears. The diastolic pulmonary artery pressure should exceed the pulmonary capillary wedge pressure. A catheter sheath is recommended to maintain sterility during advancement, withdrawal, and catheter manipulation. The waveforms in relation to the catheter position are illustrated in Figure 33.2.

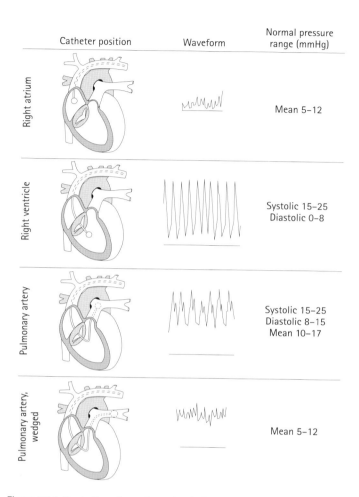

Figure 33.2 Illustration of waveforms in relation to catheter position.

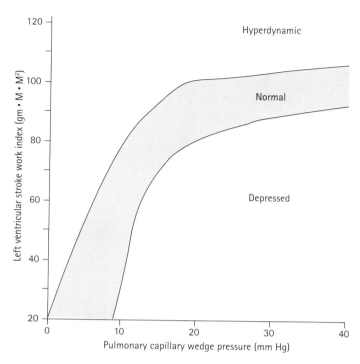

Figure 33.3 Starling curve of left ventricular stroke work index as a function of pulmonary capillary wedge pressure.

Measurements provided by pulmonary artery catheterization

Central venous pressure

Prior to the introduction of pulmonary artery catheterization, the central venous pressure (CVP) was utilized as the sole central parameter assessing cardiac function and volume status. The right-ventricular, end-diastolic filling pressure is assessed from CVP measurement, and the pulmonary capillary wedge pressure assesses the left-ventricular, end-diastolic filling pressure. The normal CVP in healthy, nonpregnant subjects is 1–8 mmHg, and in pregnant subjects this reading is usually unchanged. Preload is determined by intraventricular pressure and volume, thus setting the initial myocardial fiber length. A Starling ventricular function curve plotting cardiac output against CVP for right-heart function, or against pulmonary capillary wedge pressure for left-heart function, can delineate when a failing heart requires a higher preload of filling pressure to achieve the same cardiac output as a normally functioning heart (Figure 33.3). Therapeutic manipulation of ventricular filling pressures and simultaneous measurement of cardiac output allows calculation of optimal preload. Preload can be increased by the administration of crystalloid, colloid, or blood, and decreased by the use of diuretics or vasodilator. A high CVP reading is suggestive of fluid overload and/or ventricular dysfunction, while a low CVP reflects a low intravascular fluid volume relative to the intravascular capacity. The CVP measures preload of the right ventricle. The inaccuracy and fallacy of extrapolating the CVP to left-heart function will be discussed later.[9,17,18]

Pulmonary capillary wedge pressure

One of the major advantages of the pulmonary artery catheter over a simple central venous catheter is the ability to measure the pulmonary capillary wedge pressure (PCWP). The left-ventricular, end-diastolic pressure of the left-atrial pressure represents the left heart preload. This is the equivalent of the left-atrial pressure in diastole with a normal open mitral valve. Without catheterizing the left heart, this can be obtained from the pulmonary capillary bed pressure. By inflating the catheter tip balloon, the resultant PCWP estimates left-ventricular, end-diastolic filling pressure or PCWP.[19] Pulmonary artery diastolic pressure accurately correlates with the PCWP in the absence of intrinsic pulmonary disease in many cases and, if confirmed in a given patient, may be substituted for the PCWP if wedging becomes technically difficult.[20]

The PCWP serves as an index of left-ventricular filling pressure and helps guide maneuvers to optimize cardiac output. Furthermore, the PCWP can be monitored to prevent the development of hydrostatic pulmonary edema, and to help define the etiology and monitor treatment of pre-existing pulmonary edema. The normal nonpregnant PCWP is 6–12 mmHg. Bader et al found a mean PCWP of 5.4 mmHg (range: 1–9 mmHg) in 16 normal, resting pregnant patients at 28–40 weeks' gestation.[21] Groenendijk et al reported a mean PCWP of 9 mmHg (range: 6–12 mmHg) in four normal, pregnant patients at 28–34 weeks' gestation.[22] Clark et al catheterized 10 normal, pregnant subjects at 35–38 weeks' gestation and found a mean PCWP of 8 ± 2 mmHg.[23]

As central venous cannulation may be safer than pulmonary artery catheterization, CVP has been used to gauge intravascular volume, as an indirect measure of left-sided filling pressure. This may be misleading in seriously ill patients, as asymmetries of ventricular function are common.[24,25] When right-heart failure occurs secondary to left-heart failure, CVP will reflect left-heart conditions. However, this rise in CVP due to failure or overload of the left heart is a relatively late event. A marked discrepancy between the CVP and the PCWP is seen in disease states affecting the systemic but not the pulmonary circulation (such as pregnancy-induced hypertension).

Cardiac output

Cardiac output (CO), the amount of blood that is pumped by the heart per unit of time, is measured in l/minute. Cardiac output is determined by the heart rate and stroke volume. Dilutional techniques are the usual methods employed to calculate cardiac output with the pulmonary artery catheter. Thermodilution is a rapid and highly reproducible measurement of cardiac output.[12] Oxygen is the indicator in the Fick method. Oxygen consumption is measured in the steady state by analyzing inhaled and exhaled gases. Mixed central venous blood and arterial blood are used to calculate the change in oxygen content (arterial O_2 content – venous O_2 content). Cardiac output is calculated by the following formula:

$$\frac{\text{Cardiac output (CO)}}{\text{(l/minute)}} = \frac{O_2 \text{ consumption ml/minute} \times 100}{\text{arterial } O_2 \text{ content} - \text{venous } O_2 \text{ content}}$$

The cardiac index is obtained by dividing cardiac output by square meters of body surface area, as in the following formula:

$$\text{Cardiac index (CI)} = \frac{\text{cardiac output}}{\text{body surface area (m}^2)}$$

If oxygen consumption and arterial oxygen content are constant, cardiac output is proportional to mixed venous oxygen content.

Dye dilution techniques, which can be cumbersome, are conceptually similar to the Fick technique, except that steady state is not achieved. Thermodilution techniques with cold fluid can be used, although fluid at room temperature may elim-inate errors due to inaccurate measurement of injected fluid and warming of fluid within the catheter.[23,26,27]

Potential sources of error with thermodilution estimation of cardiac output included inaccurate measurement of solution temperature prior to injection and uneven or slow injection. In addition, if the catheter tip is against the vessel wall or out of the main flow, inaccuracies may occur. The accuracy of measurements may be evaluated by examining the thermodilution curve (Figure 33.4).

Systemic vascular resistance

The systemic vascular resistance (SVR) represents the resistance to blood flow through the body's vascular tree. The systolic and diastolic blood pressure, combined with measurements of cardiac output and CVP, is used to calculate the SVR and the mean arterial pressure (MAP) as follows:

$$\text{SVR (dyn/s per cm}^{-5}) = \frac{(\text{MAP} - \text{CVP}) \times 80}{\text{cardiac output}}$$

$$\text{MAP} = \text{diastolic} + \varrho e \ (\text{systolic} - \text{diastolic})$$

Conversion factor: 1 mmHg 1l per minute = 80 dyn/s per cm^{-5}

The normal SVR is 900–1200 dyn/cm^{-5}. During pregnancy, the SVR may be as low as 800 dyn/cm^{-5}. Clark et al found the mean SVR in pregnancy to be 1333 ± 33 mmHg.[28] The SVR may be decreased in patients with anemia, thyrotoxicosis, arteriove-

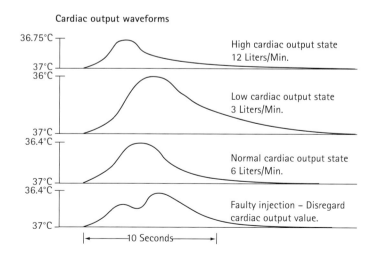

Cardiac output waveforms

36.75°C ⌐
37°C ⌐   High cardiac output state
          12 Liters/Min.
36°C ⌐
          Low cardiac output state
          3 Liters/Min.
37°C
36.4°C ⌐
          Normal cardiac output state
          6 Liters/Min.
37°C
36.4°C ⌐
          Faulty injection – Disregard
          cardiac output value.
37°C
|⟵——10 Seconds——⟶|

Figure 33.4 Thermodilution curves for estimating cardiac output.

nous fistula, septic shock, and liver cirrhosis.[29-31] The SVR may be increased in patient heart failure, cardiogenic shock, and hypertension.[17,22,32,33] Arterial dilators, such as hydralazine, nifedipine, and nitroprusside, may cause a decrease in SVR. Arterial constrictors such as dopamine or norepinephrine may be used to increase the SVR.[8,33,34]

Mixed venous oxygen saturation

The mixed venous oxygen saturation (SV_{O_2}) reflects the balance between oxygen delivery and oxygen utilization. It reflects tissue perfusion, the variation in oxygen requirements of different organs, and the affinity of hemoglobin for acceptance and subsequent release of oxygen. The clinically acceptable range for SV_{O_2} is 68-77%. A 10% decrease from initial baseline values is clinically significant. The mixed venous oxygen saturation reflects peripheral oxygen availability.[12] Any of the following factors may be responsible for a decline of the SV_{O_2}:

(1) acute decrease in cardiac output
(2) hemoglobin concentration
(3) arterial oxygen saturation
(4) tissue oxygen consumption.

Continuous SV_{O_2} monitoring can serve as an early marker of hemodynamic malfunction.[35] The SV_{O_2} can be used to evaluate rapidly any clinical manipulation. For example, increasing the positive end-expiratory pressure (PEEP) to improve oxygenation may result in a decline in SV_{O_2} due to decline in cardiac output. Continuous SV_{O_2} may also be used when titrating vasoactive or inotropic drugs. The SV_{O_2} will frequently fall before any other evidence of hemodynamic instability is manifested, making it very useful as an early warning system.[20,36] Likewise, a rise in SV_{O_2} with a stable cardiac output is a good prognostic sign associated with clinical improvement.

The average mixed venous oxygen tension (PV_{O_2}) is 40 mmHg. In humans, unconsciousness accompanies a PV_{O_2} of less than 20 mmHg, and irreversible brain damage occurs below 12 mmHg.[37,38] During pregnancy, an increase in cardiac output in excess of oxygen utilization causes the PV_{O_2} and SV_{O_2} to increase.[39] Labor alters these parameters by lowering the PV_{O_2} and SV_{O_2} during contractions, and elevating them to nonlaboring levels between contractions.[40] Table 33.1 depicts the hemodynamic and ventilatory parameters in pregnant and nonpregnant patients.

Indications for pulmonary artery catheterization in obstetric patients

▪ Hypovolemic shock, resulting from massive blood loss with large transfusion requirements, particularly in the face of oliguria or pulmonary edema
▪ Septic shock, especially when accompanied by hypotension or oliguria and when vasopressor therapy is needed
▪ Severe pregnancy-induced hypertension complicated by pulmonary edema and oliguria unresponsive to initial fluid challenge

Table 33.1 Normal central hemodynamic parameters in healthy nonpregnant and pregnant patients

	Nonpregnant	Pregnant
Cardiac output (l/min)	4.3 ± 0.9	6.2 ± 1.0
Heart rate (beats/min)	71 ± 10	83 ± 10
Systemic vascular resistance (dyne × cm × sec^{-5})	1530 ± 520	1210 ± 266
Pulmonary vascular resistance (dyne × cm × sec^{-5})	119 ± 47	78 ± 22
Colloid oncotic pressure (mmHg)	20.8 ± 1.0	18.0 ± 1.5
Colloid oncotic pressure – Pulmonary capillary wedge pressure (mmHg)	14.5 ± 2.5	10.5 ± 2.7
Mean arterial pressure (mmHg)	86.4 ± 7.5	90.3 ± 5.8
Pulmonary capillary wedge pressure (mmHg)	6.3 ± 2.1	7.5 ± 1.8
Central venous pressure (mmHg)	3.7 ± 2.6	3.6 ± 2.5

Reproduced from Clark SL, Cotton DB, Lee W et al. Central hemodynamic assessment of normal term pregnancy. Am J Obstet Gynecol 1989; 161: 1439.[23]

- Ineffective intravenous antihypertensive therapy
- Adult respiratory distress syndrome requiring ventilatory support
- New York Heart Association functional classes III and IV patients in labor or during surgery
- Pulmonary edema, from any etiology, unresponsive to initial therapy
- Amniotic fluid embolism
- Pulmonary hypertension in labor or surgery[16,41]

Specific indications for hemodynamic monitoring

Hypovolemic shock

The term 'shock' refers to a morbid condition in which the patient's functional intravascular blood volume is below that of the capacity of the body's vascular bed. This results in a lowering of blood pressure and decreased tissue perfusion. Without treatment, this leads to cellular acidosis, hypoxia, end-organ tissue dysfunction, and death.[29] Two other causes of shock should be mentioned; namely, cardiogenic shock due to cardiac failure (high PCWP) or pump failure, and neurogenic shock due to loss of sympathetic control of vascular resistance (low SVR), such as that seen with a high spinal block.[42]

Clinicians frequently underestimate puerperal blood loss by as much as 50%. Normal vital signs do not preclude imminently dangerous hypovolemia, since relative bradycardia has been described with intraperitoneal bleeding.[43] The patient in shock from hypovolemia will have low CVP and PCWP, accompanied by a low cardiac output and high SVR. Conversely, the patient in septic shock will have low CVP, PCWP, and SVR accompanied in the early stage of the process by elevated cardiac output. The cardiac output will subsequently decline if shock continues. The patient with protracted hemorrhagic shock develops secondary changes in the microcirculation, that affect circulating blood volume. In early hypovolemic shock, there is a tendency to draw fluid from the interstitial space into the capillary bed. However, later in the shock state, damage to the capillary endothelium can lead to further loss of intravascular volume. The clinical implication is that a disproportionately large volume of fluid is necessary to resuscitate patients in severe shock. Prolonged shock may alter active transport of electrolytes, with fluid movement into cells and a further decline in interstitial fluid that results in a further decline in intravascular volume. Acute blood loss should first be managed by restoration of intracellular volume. The patient should not be transfused if volume expansion alone restores or maintains normal vital signs.[24] Crystalloid administration as well as colloid administration is recommended to assist in the restoration of the circulation blood volume.[44]

Large volumes of crystalloid can diminish the colloid osmotic pressure (COP), and, for a given volume, expand the plasma less and for a shorter period of time than colloids. A randomized, prospective clinical trail comparing 5% albumin, 6% hetastarch, and 0.9% saline for resuscitation of patients in hypovolemic or septic shock found that two to four times the volume of saline compared to albumin and hetastarch was required to reach the same hemodynamic endpoint. Saline decreased the COP (34%), whereas albumin and hetastarch significantly increased the COP compared with initial values throughout the study period.[44]

Enormous volumes of crystalloids necessary to resuscitate the profoundly shocked patient will reduce the COP to PCWP gradient and predispose to pulmonary edema.[45,46] Although it remains controversial as to whether crystalloids to replenish extracellular water or colloids to correct intravascular hypovolemia should be administered, either or both are required for rapid restoration of intravascular volume and hemodynamic stability in the obstetric patient.[47] During the antepartum period, correction of maternal hypovolemia with volume is preferable to inotropic support, as inotropic drugs, such as dopamine, decrease uterine blood flow in healthy and hypotensive pregnant sheep.[48,49]

Current blood banking policies call for initial resuscitation to require administration of packed red blood cell component therapy, with volume expansion provided by crystalloids or colloids, to be administered to improve oxygen delivery in patients with decreased red cell mass due to hemorrhage.[50,51] With massive hemorrhage, a coagulation disorder does not exclusively produce dilution of clotting factors. Stress, tissue injury, bacteremia, and shock individually and collectively contribute to depletion of coagulation factors. Physiologic changes that accompany blood loss, such as metabolic acidosis, hypothermia, hypocalcemia, and hypokalemia, may also inhibit coagulation. However, during massive blood replacement, correction of specific coagulation defects with fresh frozen plasma, cryoprecipitate, and platelets will minimize further transfusion requirements.[50–52]

Hypofibrinogenemia, coupled with fluid depletion, is best managed with fresh frozen plasma, which contains all coagulation factors. A unit of fresh frozen plasma has a volume of approximately 200–250 ml. Cryoprecipitate can be used when volume depletion is absent. A unit of cryoprecipitate has a volume of 10–15 ml. A fibrinogen concentration of less than 100 mg/dl in the face of active bleeding should be corrected. Ten units of cryoprecipitate should raise the fibrinogen by 100 mg/dl. Thrombocytopenia below 50 000/mm^3 with anticipated surgery, or in the presence of bleeding should be corrected with platelet concentrate transfusion. Each unit of platelet concentration will raise the platelet count by 5000 to 10 000/mm^3 and has a volume of approximately 50 ml. The usual dose for platelet transfusion in massive hemorrhage is 6–10 units.[50,52]

Septic shock

Although bacteremia, the presence of viable bacteria in the blood, is not an uncommon event in the obstetric patient, less than 5% of bacteremic patients develop septic shock.[53] Sepsis is defined as a systemic response to infection, whereas septic shock is sepsis-induced hypotension and inadequate tissue perfusion.[30] The most common causes of septic shock in the obstetric patient are pyelonephritis, postpartum endometritis, chorioamnionitis, and necrotizing fasciitis. Despite a lower mortality with septic shock in the pregnant patient than the nonpregnant patient, sepsis still remains a major cause of maternal death.[46,54–57] The cornerstone of therapy for septic shock centers on aggressive volume expansion to correct either an absolute or relative hypovolemia and inotropes to treat hypotension.[30,56,58,59] Contemporary management emphasizes oxygen delivery and organ perfusion. Considerable quantities of fluid are often needed, favoring the use of the flow-directed pulmonary artery catheter to guide fluid administration.[60]

In addition, vasoactive agents should be used if fluid resuscitation proves inadequate in restoring optimal cardiovascular function. The initial agent, dopamine hydrochloride, a drug with dose-dependent alpha- and beta-adrenergic effects, is used if hypotension persists after volume administration.[61] A selective increase in mesenteric and renal blood flow occurs with low-dose dopamine therapy below 5 μg/kg per minute. At this dosage, the predominant effects are an increase in myocardial contractility and cardiac output, and an increase in renal perfusion without increasing myocardial oxygen consumption. A simple way to deliver dopamine is to use the following formula:

1.5 × weight (kg) = amount in mg added to 250 ml 5% dextrose in water

At 10 ml/hour, this concentration delivers 1 μg/kg per minute. With increasing doses of dopamine, alpha effects predominate with marked vasoconstriction and a further adverse reduction in tissue perfusion. Most of the other pressor agents available produce an increase in blood pressure at the expense of rather significant vasoconstriction. Since these effects are undesirable, their indications in septic shock are limited to the patient in whom dopamine cannot support blood pressure.

In shock unresponsive to dopamine (that is, cannot support blood pressure to at least a systolic blood pressure of 80 mmHg accompanied by a low SVR), one should consider phenylephrine (Neosynephrine), and, if the patient is unresponsive, norepinephrine (Levophed). Phenylephrine is a postsynaptic alpha receptor stimulator with little effect on beta receptors in the heart. It is used primarily to increase SVR to above 600 dyn/s per cm^{-5} (dose = 0.5–5.0 μg/kg per minute). Norepinephrine is a powerful stimulator of both the alpha and beta receptors. It causes both vasoconstriction and inotropic stimulation of the heart (dose = 1–5 μg/minute). If cardiac output cannot be supported above 4 l/minute despite maintaining SVR, isoproterenol (Isuprel) may be added. Isoproterenol is a potent stimulator of beta receptors and causes increases in cardiac contractility and heart rate (dose = 1–20 μg/minute). However, these drugs are used only as the last resort (Table 33.2)

Table 33.2 Inotropic drugs for management of shock

Agent	Dose	Hemodynamic effect
Dopamine: low dose	< 5 μg/kg/min	↑CO, vasodilation of renal arteries
Dopamine: high dose	10–20 μg/kg/min	↑CO, ↑SVR
Dobutamine	2.5–15 μg/kg/min	↑CO, ↓SVR or ↑SVR
Phenylephrine (Neosynephrine)	40–180 μg/kg/min	↑SVR
Norepinephrine (Levophed)	2–12 μg/kg/min	↑CO, ↑SVR
Isoproterenol (Isuprel)	0.5–5 μg/kg/min	↓CO, ↑SVR

Reproduced from Counts. Ann Surg 1979; 190: 91–9[49] with permission from Lippincott Williams & Wilkins.

Needless to say, antimicrobial therapy, electrolyte and coagulation correction, and surgical therapy, if indicated, are mandatory in the treatment of septic shock. The response to therapy should be reflected in the continuous SV$_{O_2}$, cardiac output, and PCWP. The patient in septic shock will have a low CVP, PCWP, and SVR accompanied in the early stage of the process by elevated cardiac output, but, as the process continues, the cardiac output and the SV$_{O_2}$ decline. The earliest sign of either deterioration or improvement of the shock state may be either a fall or a rise in the mixed venous oxygen saturation, respectively.

Pulmonary edema

The greatest utility of invasive hemodynamic monitoring in obstetrics may lie in differentiation of hydrostatic pulmonary edema due to heart failure (high PCWP) from permeability pulmonary edema due to lung failure (low PCWP).[62] Reduction of COP, alteration of capillary membrane permeability, and elevated pulmonary vascular hydrostatic pressures all lead to extravasation of fluids into the interstitial and alveolar spaces, resulting in pulmonary edema.[57] Pregnancy is known to lower COP, and COP is lower in preeclamptic than in normal, pregnant patients. COP decreases further postpartum, secondary to supine positioning, bleeding at delivery, and intrapartum infusion of crystalloid solutions. One may see the development of hydrostatic pulmonary edema at lower pressures in pregnancy because of the lower COP.[23,44,60]

McHugh et al have correlated radiographic findings of pulmonary edema with absolute PCWP in patients with myocardial infarction.[63] Pulmonary congestion was apparent at a PCWP of 18 mmHg, was mild to moderate at 18–25 mmHg, and was moderated to severe at 20–30 mmHg. Frank pulmonary edema developed at PCWP above 30 mmHg. This model represents pure hydrostatic pulmonary edema secondary to the left-ventricular or acute volume overload. Thus, the treatment of pulmonary edema in this model should be directed at improving myocardial contractility and reducing the preload.

Pulmonary edema also can result from damage to the pulmonary alveolar capillary membrane by any of a host of insults, including sepsis (most common), pneumonia, and hypersensitivity reactions mediated by non-HLA leukoagglutinins at the time of blood transfusion.[2,24,38,64,65] A disturbance of membrane permeability results in influx of both protein and water into the pulmonary interstitium and the alveolus, despite normal cardiac function and filling pressures. This process may result in adult respiratory distress syndrome (ARDS) if the source of the injury is not eradicated. The diagnosis of ARDS is made on the basis of progressive hypoxemia, low or normal PCWP, diffuse infiltrates on chest radiograph, and decreased pulmonary compliance.[31] The therapeutic goals in pulmonary edema due to permeability defects are to maintain filling pressures in the low-normal range and minimize transudation of protein and fluid into the lungs while eradicating the source of injury.

Hypoxemia requires ventilatory support to maintain adequate gas exchange at nontoxic levels of inspired oxygen (FIO_2 < 60%). Positive end-expiratory pressure (PEEP) is usually necessary to accomplish this goal, and serial monitoring of arterial blood gases is essential. In interpreting hemodynamic values, consideration must be given to the artificial increase on PCWP from PEEP. Hydrostatic forces continue to play a major role in the degree of pulmonary edema experienced by patients with damaged membranes. By lowering filling pressures from high-normal and normal levels to low-normal levels, transudation of proteins may be lessened.

The normal fetus will tolerate a maternal Pa_{O_2} greater than 60 mmHg with oxygen saturation greater than 90%. However, lower saturations or marginally decreased saturations associated with a fetus experiencing labor or already compromised by placental insufficiency may be tolerated poorly.

Severe preeclampsia

Most patients with severe preeclampsia can be quite adequately managed without central monitoring. Controversy exists regarding the routine use of invasive hemodynamic monitoring in severe preeclampsia. Benedetti et al have recommended invasive monitoring in severe preeclampsia because of the associated hypovolemia.[2] The routine use of invasive monitoring in uncomplicated severe preeclampsia is not recommended. The potential morbidity of pulmonary artery catherization is not justified.[2,66,67] The indications for pulmonary artery catheterization in severe preeclampsia include[41]:

(1) complications related to central volume status
(2) pulmonary edema of uncertain etiology
(3) pulmonary edema unresponsive to conventional therapy
(4) persistent oliguria despite aggressive volume expansion
(5) induction of conduction anesthesia in hemodynamically unstable patients
(6) medical complications that would otherwise require invasive monitoring.

The development of antepartum pulmonary edema in patients with severe preeclampsia usually reflects left-ventricular dysfunction or iatrogenic fluid overload.[68] It is extremely uncommon to develop pulmonary edema in severe pregnancy-induced hypertension in the absence of iatrogenic fluid administration. Invasive hemodynamic monitoring in this setting may also identify the relatively uncommon case of noncardiogenic pulmonary edema. In addition, the pulmonary artery catheter permits more rapid and precise optimization of hemodynamic parameters.

Volume expansion in hypovolemic preeclampsia results in a decrease in SVR and an increase in cardiac output.[17,36,69–72] Mean arterial pressure usually is unaffected by the fluid administration or may actually fall.[22,71,73] The need for volume expansion in preeclamptic patients undergoing vasodilator therapy remains controversial.[74] The abrupt reduction in blood pressure in the hypovolemic, hypertensive patient can result in circulatory collapse, and cerebral ischemic damage has been described.[75,76] The correction of hypovolemia prior to nitroprusside or nitroglycerin administration in a case that fails to respond to hydralazine is essential, since sudden and profound drops in blood pressure occur with these drugs when intravascular volume is depleted. The need for volume expansion prior to vasodilator therapy is necessary in preparation for epidural placement.[9,45]

Oliguria

The pathophysiologic basis of persistent oliguria in the setting of severe preeclampsia is still not well understood. Oliguria is defined as urine output less than 30 ml/hour over 2 consecutive hours. This may also be related to a rise in serum creatinine. A common therapeutic approach is to employ a limited fluid challenge to restore adequate urine output.[5] The 'fluid challenge' may be administered in the following fashion:

(1) administer 5–20 ml/minute of intravenous fluid over 10 minutes with observation of the PCWP. If the pressure increases by more than 7 mmHg, the next fluid bolus is withheld.
(2) if the PCWP does not exceed 3 mmHg, a repeat challenge is administered. The optimal range for the PCWP in these patients is 10–12 mmHg. Another fluid infusion is repeated until the desired wedge pressure is reached.
(3) a fluid challenge of 500–1000 ml normal saline or lactated Ringer's solution may be administered over 30 minutes. If there is no response, one should consider repeating the fluid challenge or cardiac catheterization.

Clark et al described three different hemodynamic subsets of preeclamptic patients with oliguria, based on invasive monitoring parameters of patients with oliguria.[5] The first group had low capillary wedge pressures, hyperdynamic left-ventricular function, mild to moderate elevation of SVR, and renal artery vasospasm. These patients responded to volume expansion to resolve their oliguria because of intravascular volume depletion.

The second group of oliguric patients had normal or elevated PCWP, normal cardiac output, and normal SVR. The pathophysiology of oliguria in this set of patients was renal artery vasospasm, and it responded to vasodilator therapy. Kirshon et al demonstrated a significant increase in urine output and free water clearance while treating six oliguric, euvolemic, severe preeclamptic patients with low-dose dopamine (1–5 μg/kg per minute).[77]

The third group of oliguric patients had elevated PCWP and SVR with depressed ventricular function accompanied by pulmonary edema. These patients respond to volume restriction and afterload reduction.[5] Finally, PCWP generally rises postpartum, at which time a pulmonary artery catheter is useful in detecting incipient pulmonary edema in complicated cases.[9,45]

Complications of pulmonary artery catheterization

The major potential problem with pulmonary artery catheterization lies in obtaining central venous access rather than floating the pulmonary artery catheter. Mitchell and Clark reported complication rates with invasive hemodynamic monitoring of 0.4–9.0%, with an inability to pass the catheter in 5–10% of cases.[14] Potential complications of pulmonary artery catheterization include air embolism, thromboembolism, pulmonary infarction, catheter-related sepsis, direct trauma to the heart or pulmonary artery, postganglionic Horner's syndrome, and catheter entrapment (Table 33.3). The complication of immediate significance is that of pneumothorax and insertion site infection, which occurs in 0.3–5% of patients undergoing this procedure.[11,15] Traumatic injury to any structure in the neck or chest, such as hemothorax, may occur when one attempts percutaneous access. Damage to the subclavian, carotid, and internal mammary arteries can occur; and damage to the thoracic duct, phrenic nerve, brachial plexus, vagus nerve, and recurrent laryngeal nerve has been reported.[14] Pulmonary infarction and/or hemorrhage resulting from the pulmonary artery catheter balloon occur rarely. Catheter migration into the pericardial or pleural space, with resultant tamponade or hydrothorax, respectively, has been described. Infection can occur, but is minimized by proper technique.

Controversy exists as to the site of central venous access. Eisenhauer et al reported a 4.2% complication rate with subclavian catheterization and a 0.4% complication rate for the internal jugular approach.[78] However, Kaiser et al reported no complications in 100 consecutive patients randomized to sub-

Table 33.3 Pulmonary artery catheter complications

At insertion	After placement
Pneumothorax	Pulmonary infarction
Thrombosis	Pulmonary artery rupture
Arterial puncture	Infection
Air embolization	Balloon rupture
Catheter knotting	Endocardial/valvular damage
Cardiac arrythmias	

clavian versus the internal jugular approach.[13] In this group of patients, the subclavian route was successful 98% of the time compared to an 84% success rate with the internal jugular approach. The left-sided approach is more likely to result in vascular injuries due to adjacent vessels and difficult manipulation required when placing the sheath or catheter. The right internal jugular vein is preferred because it enters the superior vena cava in a relatively direct fashion, without the abrupt bends encountered on the left side.[11] The technique is probably best left to the judgment and skill of the operator. A chest radiograph taken after insertion will help exclude a pneumothorax and can determine the position of the pulmonary artery catheter.

Noninvasive hemodynamic monitoring

The risk of pulmonary artery catheterization is minimal in experienced hands; however, the development of noninvasive hemodynamic assessment has dramatically changed the need for invasive monitoring. Two-dimensional and Doppler echocardiography provides an extremely useful and noninvasive method for assessing cardiovascular function. Echocardiography using Doppler, pulse wave, and M-Mode can calculate stroke volume, cardiac output, cardiac index, left- and right-ventricular filling pressure, pulmonary artery systolic pressure, left-ventricular stroke volume, and right-atrial pressure.[79–83] Information has been formulated from the use of echocardiography in understanding the physiologic events of normal pregnancy, the pathogenesis of preeclampsia, the abnormalities characteristic of various forms of heart disease, and various medical disorders. Studies have also been done to compare pulmonary artery catheterization and echocardiography assessments of hemodynamic parameters in critically ill patients with similar results.[80–83]

Pulmonary artery catheterization allows constant monitoring of the mixed venous oxygen saturation (SV_{O_2}), which reflects the balance between oxygen delivery and oxygen utilization. SV_{O_2} reflects tissue perfusion, the variation in oxygen requirements of different organs, and the affinity of hemoglobin for acceptance and subsequent release of oxygen. Noninvasive pulse oximetry uses spectrophotometry to detect arterial oxygen saturation by measuring the absorption of selected wavelengths of light in pulsatile blood flow, and calculates the percentage of oxyhemoglobin saturation. Pulse oximetry is useful as a continuous monitor of the adequacy of blood oxygenation. Thus, the noninvasive monitoring of echocardiography is definitely an alternative to the invasive technique of pulmonary artery catheterization. Especially in the patient where invasive monitoring is not feasible, as in thrombocytopenia, echocardiography is an alternative. However, in the unstable patient who requires minute-by-minute adjustments, definitely pulmonary artery catheterization is clearly more practical.

Obstetric intensive care

Maternal mortality rates have declined dramatically over the past 50 years, but there has been little change in the last decade.[84] Traditionally, hemorrhage, hypertensive disease of pregnancy, and obstetric infection have been the most frequent causes of maternal death in the USA.[85] However, recently thromboembolism is emerging as the leading cause of mortality in the USA.[86] Maternal-fetal intensive care units (MFICU) are being established in major centers nationwide in an attempt to reduce maternal mortality. There are some difficulties encountered in establishing such a unit.

The concept of the MFICU initially had a poor reception from obstetric nurses. Eventually, however, certain nurses took on ICU responsibilities, and, most importantly, recruitment of former medical ICU nurses into obstetrics ensued. As would be expected, territorial problems with the anesthesia service arose, and were resolved by appointing a staff member from each service for any patient with responsibility for pulmonary artery catheterization. Demonstrating to the medical intensivist our ability to manage critically ill patients is also a challenge. The MFICU is best utilized in managing acute-phase, critically ill patients. Patients with chronic medical conditions, such as prolonged adult respiratory distress, are best managed in the medical ICU, where personnel are more familiar with chronic respiratory care. Mabie and Sibai reported their experience with a three-bed, obstetric ICU.[87] The main indications for admission were hypertensive disorders (46%), massive hemorrhage (10%), and medical problems of pregnancy (44%). They concluded not only that the critically ill, pregnant patient can be managed in an obstetric ICU, but also that the obstetric ICU be a bona fide part of obstetric practice that has been incorporated into their training program.

The MFICU offers some distinct advantages to the critically ill, pregnant patient. It allows rapid access to central volume assessment and ventilatory support. Expertise in pharmacologic treatment, such as that required for septic shock, is necessary. Rapid access to intensive care facilities should be available in tertiary obstetrics centers. The obstetrician, either in the tertiary care center or community hospital, should recognize and prevent prolonged hypotension or hypoxia, and utilize invasive monitoring in an intensive care setting to improve survival for the obstetric patient.

References

1. Swan JHC, Ganz W, Forrester J et al. Catheterization of the heart in man with use of a follow-directed balloon-tipped catheter. N Engl J Med 1970; 283: 447–51.

2. Benedetti TJ, Cotton DB, Read JC et al. Hemodynamic observations in severe preeclampsia with a flow-directed pulmonary artery catheter. Am J Obstet Gynecol 1980; 136: 465–70.

3. Clark SL, Horenstein JM, Phelan JP. Experience with the pulmonary artery catheter in obstetrics and gynecology. Am J Obstet Gynecol 1985; 152: 374–8 .

4. Cotton DB, Bendetti TJ. Use of the Swan–Ganz catheter in obstetrics and gynecology. Obstet Gynecol 1980; 56: 641.

5. Clark SL, Greenspoon JS, Aldahl D, Phelan JP. Severe preeclampsia with persistent oliguria: management of hemodynamic subsets. Am J Obstet Gynecol 1986: 154: 490–4.

6. Clark SL, Montz FJ, Phelan JP. Hemodynamic alterations in the patient with amniotic fluid embolism: a reappraisal. Am J Obstet Gynecol 1985; 151: 617–21 .

7. Clark SL, Phelan JP, Montoro M, Mestman J. Transient ventricular dysfunction associated with cesarean section in a patient with hyperthyroidism. Am J Obstet Gynecol 1985; 151: 384–6.

8. Cotton DB, Gonik B, Dorman KF. Cardiovascular alterations in severe pregnancy-induced hypertension. Acute effects of intravenous magnesium sulfate. Am J Obstet Gynecol 1984; 148: 162.

9. Hankins GDV, Wendel GD, Cunningham FG, Leveno KJ. Longitudinal evaluation of hemodynamic changes in eclampsia. Am J Obstet Gynecol 1984; 150: 506–12.

10. Hauth JC, Hankins GD, Kuehl T et al. Ritodrine hydrochloride infusion in pregnant baboons. I. Biophysical effects. Am J Obstet Gynecol 1983; 146: 916–24.

11. Bowdle TA. Complications of invasive monitoring. Anesth Clin North Am 2002; 20: 571–88.

12. Lee W, Rokey R, Cotton DB. Noninvasive maternal stroke volume and cardiac output determinations by pulsed Doppler echocardiography. Am J Obstet Gynecol 1988; 158: 505–10.

13. Kaiser CW, Koornick AR, Smith N, Soroff HS. Choice of routine for central venous cannulation: subclavian or internal jugular vein? A prospective randomized study. J Surg Oncol 1981; 17: 345–54.

14. Mitchell SE, Clark RA. Complications of central venous catheterization. AJR 1979; 133: 467.

15. Patel C, Labby V, Venus B et al. Acute complications of pulmonary artery catheter insertion in critically ill patients. Crit Care Med 1986; 14: 195.

16. Clark SL. Pulmonary artery catheterization. In Clark SL, Cotton DB, Hankins GDV et al. (eds), Critical Care Obstetrics (3rd edition). Blackwell Scientific: Boston, MA, 1997, pp 111–17.

17. Lund-Johansen P. Newer thinking on the hemodynamics of hypertension. Curr Opin Cardiol 1994; 9: 505–11.

18. Visser W, Wallenburg HCS. Central hemodynamic observations in untreated preeclamptic patients. Hypertension 1991; 17: 1072–7.

19. Fisher ML, De Felice LE, Parisi AF. Assessing left ventricular filling pressure with directed (Swan–Ganz) catheters: detection of sudden changes in patients with left ventricular dysfunction. Chest 1975; 68: 542–7.

20. Lappas D, Lell W, Gabel JC et al. Indirect measurement of left atrial pressure in surgical patients: pulmonary capillary wedge and pulmonary diastolic pressure compared with left atrial pressures. Anesthesiology 1973; 38: 394–7.

21. Bader RA, Bader MG, Rose DJ, Braunwald E. Hemodynamics at rest and during exercise in normal pregnancy as studied by cardiac catheterization. J Clin Invest 1955; 34: 1524–36.

22. Groenendijk R, Trimbos MJ, Wallenburg HCS. Hemodynamic measurements in preeclampsia: preliminary observations. Am J Obstet Gynecol 1984; 150: 232–6.

23. Clark SL, Cotton DB, Lee W et al. Central hemodynamic assessment of normal term pregnancy. Am J Obstet Gynecol 1989; 161: 1439–42

24. Baek S, Makabali GG, Bryan-Brown CW et al. Plasma expansion in surgical patients with high central venous pressure (CVP): the relationship of blood volume to hematocrit, CVP, pulmonary wedge pressure, and cardiorespiratory changes. Surgery 1975; 78: 304–15.

25. Connors AF, McCaffree DR, Gray BA. Evaluation of right hearted catheterization in the critically ill patient without acute myocardial infarction. N Engl Med 1983; 308: 263–7.

26. Cotton DB, Gonik B, Dorman KF. Cardiovascular alterations in severe pregnancy-induced hypertension. Relationship of central venous pressure to pulmonary capillary wedge pressure. Am J Obstet Gynecol 1985; 151: 762.

27. Stetz CW, Miller RG, Kelly GE et al. Reliability of thermodilution method in determination of cardiac output in clinical practice. Am Rev Respir Dis 1982; 126: 1001.

28. Clark SL, Cotton DB, Lee W et al. Central hemodynamic assessment of normal term pregnancy. Am J Obstet Gynecol 1989; 161: 1439.

29. Gonik B. Septic shock in obstetrics. In Clark SL, Cotton DB, Hankins GDV et al (eds), Critical Care Obstetrics (3rd edition), Blackwell Scientific: Boston, MA, 1997, pp 423–45.

30. Parillo JE. Pathogenetic mechanisms of septic shock. N Engl J Med 1993; 328: 1471–7.

31. Shubin H, Weil MH, Carlson RW. Bacterial shock. Am Heart J 1997; 94: 112.

32. Easterling TR, Benedetti TJ, Schmucker BC. Antihypertensive therapy in pregnancy directed by noninvasive hemodynamic monitoring. Am J Perinat 1989; 6: 86–9.

33. Fukushima T. Hemodynamic patterns of women with chronic hypertension during pregnancy. Am J Obstet Gynecol 1999; 180: 1584–92.

34. Easterling TR, Benedetti TJ, Schmucker B et al. Maternal hemodynamics in normal and preeclamptic pregnancies: a longitudinal study. Obstet Gynecol 1990; 76: 1061–9.

35. Divertie MB, McMichan JC. Continuous monitoring of mixed venous saturation. Chest 1984; 85: 423–8.

36. Safar ME, London GM, Leveson JA, et al. Rapid dextran infusion in essential hypertension. Hypertension 1979; 1: 615–23.

37. Gibbs FA, Williams D, Gibbs EL. Modification of the cortical frequency spectrum by changes in CO_2 blood sugar, and O_2. J Neurophysiol 1940; 3: 49.

38. Trawbaugh RF, Lewis FR, Christensen JM et al. Lung water changes after thermal injury: the effects of crystalloid resuscitation and sepsis. Ann Surg 1980; 192: 479–90.

39. Kerr MG. Maternal cardiovascular adjustments in pregnancy and labor In: Goodwin JW, Goodden JO, Chance GW (eds), Perinatal Medicine: The Basic Science Underlying Clinical Practice, p. 395. Williams & Wilkins: Baltimore, MD, 1976.

40. Ueland K, Hansen JM. Maternal cardiovascular dynamics. II. Posture and uterine contractions. Am J Obstet Gynecol 1969; 103: 1.

41. Clark SL, Cotton DB. Clinical opinion: clinical indications for pulmonary artery catheterization in severe pregnancy induced hypertension. Am J Obstet Gynecol 1988; 158: 453.

42. Kleinerman J, Sancetta SM, Hackel DB. Effects of high spinal anesthesia on cerebral circulation and metabolism in man. J Clin Invest 1958; 37: 285–93.

43. Jansen RPS. Relative bradycardia. A sign of acute intraperitoneal bleeding. Aust N Z J Obstet Gynecol 1978; 18: 206–8.

44. Rackow EC, Weil MH. Recent trends in diagnosis and management of septic shock. Curr Surg 1983; 40: 181–5.

45. Harms BA, Kramer GC, Bodai BI et al. The effect of hypoproteinemia on pulmonary and soft tissue edema formation. Crit Care Med 1981; 9: 503–8.

46. Zarins CK, Rice CL, Peters RM, Virgilio RW. Lymph and pulmonary response to isobaric reductions in plasma oncotic pressure in baboons. Cir Res 1978; 43: 925–30.

47. Carey JS, Scharschmidt BF, Culliford AF et al. Hemodynamic effectiveness of colloid and electrolyte solutions for replacement of simulated operative blood loss. Surg Gynecol Obstet 1970; 131: 679–86.

48. Callender K, Levinson G, Shnider SM et al. Dopamine administration in the normotensive pregnant ewe. Obstet Gynecol 1978; 51: 586–9.

49. Counts RB, Haisch C, Simon TL et al. Hemostasis in massively transfused trauma patients. Ann Surg 1979; 190: 91–9.

50. American College of Physicians. Practice strategies for elective red blood cell transfusion. Ann Intern Med 1992; 116: 403–6.

51. Donaldson MDJ, Seaman MJ, Park GR. Massive blood transfusion. Br J Anaest 1992; 69: 621–30.

52. Roberts JM, Laros RK. Hemorrhagic and endotoxic shock: a pathophysiologic approach to diagnosis and management. Am J Obstet Gynecol 1971; 110: 1041–9.

53. Ledger WJ, Norman M, Gee C, Lewis W. Bacteremia in an obstetric-gynecologic service. Am J Obstet Gynecol 1975; 121: 205–12.

54. Blanco JD, Gibbs RS, Castaneda YS. Bacteremia in obstetrics: clinical course. Obstet Gynecol 1981; 58: 621–5.

55. Cavanagh D, Knuppel RA, Shepherd JH et al. Septic shock and the obstetrician/gynecologist. South Med J 1982; 75; 809–13.

56. Gibbs CE, Locke WE. Maternal deaths in Texas, 1969 to 1973. Am J Obstet Gynecol 1976: 126: 687–92.

57. Henderson DW, Vilos GA, Milne KJ, Nichol PM. The role of Swan–Ganz catheterization in severe pregnancy-induced hypertension. Am J Obstet Gynecol 1984; 148: 570–4.

58. Packman MI, Rackow EC. Optimum left heart filling pressure during fluid resuscitation of patients with hypovolemic and septic shock. Crit Care Med 1983; 11: 165–9.

59. Rolbin SH, Levinson G, Schider SM et al. Dopamine treatment of spinal hypotension decreases uterine blood flow in pregnant ewes. Anesthesiology 1979; 51: 37–40.

60. Schmidt CR, Frank LP, Estafanous FH. Utility of continuous pulmonary artery oximetry as an early warning monitor in cardiac surgery patients. Presented at the fifth annual meeting of the Society of Cardiovascular Anesthesiologists, San Diego, California, 1983.

61. Goldberg LI. Dopamine – clinical uses of and endogenous catecholamine. N Engl J Med 1974; 291: 707–10.

62. Rinaldo JE, Rogers RM. Adult respiratory distress syndrome: changing concepts of lung injury and repair. N Engl J Med 1982; 206: 900–9.

63. McHugh TJ, Forrester JS, Adler L et al. Pulmonary vascular congestion in acute myocardial infarction: hemodynamic and radiologic correlations. Ann Intern Med 1972; 76: 29–32.

64. Anderson RR, Holliday RL, Driedger AA et al. Documentation of pulmonary capillary permeability in the adult respiratory distress syndrome accompanying human sepsis. Am Rev Respir Dis 1997; 119; 869–77.

65. Thompson JS, Severson CD, Parmely MJ. Pulmonary 'hypersensitivity' reactions induced by transfusion of non-HLA leukoagglutinins. N Engl J Med 1971; 282: 1120–5.

66. Berkowitz RL. The Swan–Ganz catheter and colloid osmotic pressure determinations. In: Berkowitz RL (ed.), Critical Care of the Obstetric Patient, p. 1. Churchill Livingstone: New York, 1983.

67. Berkowitz RL. The management of hypertensive crisis during pregnancy. In: Berkowitz RL (ed.), Critical Care of the Obstetric Patient, p. 299. Churchill Livingstone: New York, 1983.

68. Strauss RG, Keefer R, Burke T et al. Hemodynamic monitoring of cardiogenic pulmonary edema complication toxemia of pregnancy. Obstet Gynecol 1980; 55: 170–4.

69. Cotton DB, Longmire S, Jones MM et al. Cardiovascular alterations in severe pregnancy-induced hypertension: effects of intravenous nitoglycerin couple with blood volume expansion. Am J Obstet Gynecol 1986; 154: 1053–9.

70. Schalekamp MDAH, Krauss XH, Schalekamp-Kuyken MPA et al. Studies on the mechanism of hypernaturiuresis in essential hypertension in relation to measurements of plasma renin concentration, body fluid compartments and renal function. Clin Sci 1971; 41: 219–31.

71. Sehgal NN, Hitt JR. Plasma volume expansion in the treatment of pre-eclampsia. Am J Obstet Gynecol 1980; 138: 165–8.

72. Ulrych M, Hofman J, Heil Z. Cardiac and renal hyperresponsiveness to acute plasma volume expansion in hypertension. Am Heart J 1964; 68: 193–203.

73. Gallery EDM, Delpado W, Gyory AZ. Antihypertensive effect of plasma volume expansion in pregnancy-associated hypertension. Aust N Z J Med 1981; 11: 20–4.

74. Cohn JD. Paroxysmal hypertension and hypovolemia. N Engl J Med 1966; 275: 643–6 .

75. Dangerous antihypertensive treatment. BMJ 1979; 2: 228.

76. Graham DI. Ischemic brain damage of cerebral perfusion failure type after treatment of severe hypertension. BMJ 1975; 4: 739.

77. Kirshon B, Lee W, Cotton DB et al. Effects of low dose dopamine therapy in the oliguric patient with preeclampsia. Am J Obstet Gynecol 1988; 159: 604.

78. Eisenhauer ED, Derveloy RJ, Hastings PR. Prospective evaluation of central venous pressure (CVP) catheters in a large city-county hospital. Ann Surg 1982; 196: 560–4.

79. Belfort MA, Mares A, Saade G et al. A re-evaluation of the indications for pulmonary artery catheters in obstetrics: the role of 2-D echocardiography and Doppler ultrasound. Am J Obstet Gynecol 1996; 174: 331.

80. Belfort MA, Rokey R, Saade GR et al. Rapid echocardiographic assessment of left and right heart hemodynamics in critically ill patients. Am J Obstet Gynecol 1991; 171: 884–92.

81. Belfort MA, Mares A, Saade G et al. Two-dimensional echocardiography and Doppler ultrasound in managing obstetrics patients. Obstet Gynecol 1997; 90: 326–30.

82. Nagueh SF. Noninvasive evaluation of hemodynamics by Doppler echocardiography. Curr Opin Cardiol 1999; 14: 217–24.

83. Penning S, Robinson KD, Major CA, Garite TJ. A comparison of echocardiography and pulmonary artery catheterization for evaluation of pulmonary artery pressures in pregnant patients with suspected pulmonary hypertension. Am J Obstet Gynecol 2001; 184: 1568–70.

84. Sachs BP, Brown DAJ, Driscoll SS et al. Maternal mortality in Massachusetts. N Engl J Med 1987; 316: 667.

85. Barno A, Freeman DW, Bellville TP. Minnesota maternal mortality study: five-year general summary 1950–1954. Obstet Gynecol 1957; 9: 336–44.

86. Keuritz AM, Hughes JM, Grimes DA et al. Causes of maternal mortality in the United States. Obstet Gynecol 1983; 145: 797.

87. Mabie WC, Sibai BM. Treatment in an obstetric intensive care unit. Am J Obstet Gynecol 1990; 162: 1–4.

34 Trauma in pregnancy

Jeffrey Hammond

In many respects, the history of surgery is the history of the development of trauma management. Today, trauma is a principal public health problem in every society, stretching across cultural and socioeconomic groups. Trauma remains the leading cause of death in all age categories from infancy to middle age (1–44 years) in the USA. With over 100 000 trauma deaths annually in the USA and three permanent disabilities for each death, trauma-related costs now exceed $400 billion annually.[1]

The ages in which women are most likely to become pregnant coincide with the time period when they are also most likely to sustain trauma. During the peak childbearing period of 20–29 years of age, at least 3% of all women involved in a police-reported motor vehicle crash were pregnant.[2] Trauma in some form complicates 6–7% of all pregnancies, and results in nearly twice as many deaths as annual maternal mortality.[3] Homicide is the most common form of trauma resulting in death, followed by motor vehicle crash, but falls, especially in the third trimester when gait and balance are impaired, are the most common cause of trauma. Motor vehicle crashes are the most common cause of fetal injury mortality.[4]

Severe trauma in a pregnant patient is a relatively uncommon event, however. One large multi-institutional study of over 27 000 female trauma admissions among 13 trauma centers identified 1.3% of the study cohort as pregnant.[5]

Important and predictable anatomic and physiologic changes occur with pregnancy. Domestic violence often increases during pregnancy. Significant fetal injury may be associated with apparently mild maternal trauma. Attention to these and other details is required to ensure optimal outcome for both patients: the mother and the fetus. A general maxim, however, is that to care best for the fetus, take care of the mother.

The pregnant trauma patient is best treated by a multidisciplinary team with an organized approach. The relatively low incidence of major trauma during pregnancy leaves emergency departments and trauma teams at risk of ignoring steps that may avoid adverse outcomes.

Trauma general principles: triage

The cornerstone of trauma care is the timely identification and transport to a trauma center of those patients most likely to benefit; that is, the principle of triage. Triage, adapted from a French military concept, is, at its simplest, the sorting of patients by need for treatment and an inventory of available resources to meet those needs. This may take place in the field or within the institution. Trauma triage is founded upon the recognition that the nearest emergency room may not be the most appropriate destination. On a more complex level, it involves the development of an algorithm that seeks to balance avoiding undertriage (and possible adverse outcome) while minimizing overtriage (and overloading the system).[6]

Various prehospital scoring mechanisms have been suggested to assist in the triage decision.[7] It has been hoped that some scoring technique would facilitate identification of the 5–10% of trauma patients estimated to require the sophisticated trauma center. Current triage schema tend to assess the potential for life- or limb-threatening injury, utilizing physiologic, anatomic, and/or mechanism of injury criteria.[1] In general, physiologic criteria offer the greatest yield, while anatomic criteria are intermediate and mechanism low yield. Highest yield criteria include prolonged prehospital time, pedestrian struck at greater than 20 mph, associated death of another vehicular occupant, and the physiologic criteria of systolic blood pressure less than 90 mmHg, respiratory rate less than 10 or greater than 29 breaths per minute, or Glasgow Coma Score (GCS) of less than 13.

The trauma survey

The basic tenets of trauma resuscitation focus on addressing the management decisions and treatment algorithms that present for the patient that survives to reach the emergency department. To focus on this, the revised Advanced Trauma Life Support Course (ATLS) retains the mnemonic: *ABC*, now expanded to ABCDE.[1] Efforts during the initial, *primary*, survey are directed at establishing a secure *airway*, using techniques of rapid-sequence intubation if necessary; identifying that the patient has adequate *breathing* by ruling out or treating immediately life-threatening chest injuries; and ensuring adequate *circulation* by control of obvious hemorrhage.

Expeditious hemorrhage control, through operative and nonoperative means, has received increased emphasis over volume normalization through fluid administration and blood pressure maintenance. Simply put, the best way to maintain or re-establish blood pressure is to stop the bleeding, rather than by use of pressors or large-volume administration. These treatment principles hold true in both the prehospital environment and the trauma center setting. In fact, effective trauma care is predicated on a seamless transition of care from emergency medical services (EMS) to the hospital team. This requires coordination, communication, and treatment plans that are integrated and follow a logical sequence.

The medical history obtained during the primary survey also focuses on the essential information. A more detailed history can be taken as time permits after the primary survey. The mnemonic *AMPLE* is useful and reminds the questioner to ask about the patient's *a*llergies, *m*edications, *p*ast medical history, *l*ast meal (or *l*ast menstrual period for women of child-bearing age) and *e*nvironment (i.e. circumstances of the injury). Prehospital personnel should be questioned about vital signs en route and other details that could enhance understanding of the patient's physiologic state.

The *primary* survey is brief, requiring no more than a few minutes. The cornerstone of the primary survey concept is the dictum to treat life-threatening injuries as they are identified. This deviates from the traditional conceptual approach to the patient taught in medical school, wherein treatment is delayed until a thorough history is obtained, a physical examination is performed, and all differential diagnoses are entertained. Management during the primary survey relies heavily on knowledge of the expected patterns of injury based upon the mechanism of transfer of kinetic energy. Laboratory tests and diagnostic radiology are not emphasized at this point. Radiography should be ordered judiciously and should not delay resuscitative efforts or patient transfer to definitive care. Appropriate basic monitoring includes pulse oximetry and cardiac rhythm monitoring.

Extending the alphabetical mnemonic, evaluation of *disability* directs the resuscitation team to assess neurologic function and assign a GCS.[8] The GCS was designed to translate a subjective impression of altered mental status (e.g., terms such as 'lethargy', 'stupor', or 'somnolence') into an objective scoring mechanism. The score derives from assessment of the patient's best motor, verbal, and eye-opening responses. The patient is always assigned the most favorable score (for example, if the patient is decorticate on one side and decerebrate on the other, the higher motor score is assigned), so the score is reported as a finite number and not a range. This is extremely important, since it allows early detection of progression of neurologic deficit. If, on the other hand, the GCS were reported as a range, such as 9–10, one could not determine whether a subsequent report of a GCS of 8–9 represented no change or a drop of 2 points. Often, the trauma patient arrives in the emergency

department intubated and/or therapeutically paralyzed. In these cases, the preintubation GCS should be elicited from the field personnel for use as the treatment baseline. Alternatively, the verbal component of the score can be predicted from the motor and eye-opening components by the following formula: derived verbal score = –0.3756 + (motor score × 0.5713) + (eye score × 0.4233).

Implicit in this neurologic assessment is the assumption that a spine injury is present until proven otherwise, dictating the need for vigilance in spine immobilization. This is especially true when concomitant head injury is present, and the head and neck axis should be considered as a single unit. Evidence of a significant intracranial edema or space-occupying lesion, such as a GCS less than 8 or focal findings on cranial nerve examination, dictate early diagnostic imaging and neurosurgical consultation. *Exposure* directs the examiner to remove all clothing and logroll the patient to evaluate fully for injuries.

The *secondary* survey naturally follows the primary survey, and it is here that a more thorough head-to-toe examination is performed. The secondary survey does not begin until the primary survey is completed and resuscitation is well underway. This stage can be thought of as 'tubes and fingers in every orifice'. Rectal and/or vaginal examination and both urinary catheterization and gastric tube placement occur during the secondary survey. In this survey, a complete neurologic examination is performed. Frequent reassessment of vital signs is emphasized.

In the pregnant patient, the secondary survey includes a fetal assessment, including an assessment of fundal height, an estimation of fetal age, and a bimanual examination. An obstetric ultrasound examination should be performed to determine the estimated fetal weight, viability, and biophysical profile and to rule out abruptio placentae. Fetal monitoring should be started early, and may show evidence of uterine irritability or preterm labor. A sterile speculum examination permits examination of the cervix. Evidence of ferning and blue discoloration of nitrazine paper facilitates differentiation of vaginal fluid between amniotic fluid and urine.

Radiologic investigation of the abdomen to identify intra-abdominal or pelvic injury and hemorrhage takes place in the secondary survey, and may take the form of diagnostic peritoneal lavage (DPL), ultrasound (focused abdominal ultrasound for trauma (FAST)), or computed tomography (CT) scanning (Table 34.1). The choice of the most appropriate method to evaluate the abdomen and pelvis will depend on the mechanism of injury, the index of suspicion for an intra-abdominal injury, the patient's physiologic status, associated and confounding injuries, the experience of the clinician, and the logistics of the emergency department.

DPL can be safely performed during any trimester with the open technique in the supraumbilical location. It is extremely accurate for solid organ injury, but its near 100% sensitivity may result in nontherapeutic laparotomy and it will have false negatives in the absence of free blood such as may be found in injuries confined to the retroperitoneum.

Table 34.1 Comparison of diagnostic methods to evaluate abdominal trauma

	DPL	Ultrasound	CT scan
Sensitivity/specificity	97–99% sensitive and specific for blunt trauma; poorer specificity (44–86%) for penetrating trauma	82–97% sensitivity; 95–100% specificity	85–100% sensitivity; 95–100% specificity
Accuracy	Poor. Only indicates presence of blood; does not indicate if bleeding ongoing	Same as DPL	Very accurate. Permits solid organ injury grading. Demonstrates retroperitoneum
Speed	Fast, but >10 minutes and training required	Fast, taking 5–6 minutes	>20 minutes. Requires time and patient transport
Risk	<=1% if done open/semi-open and proper technique	None	Risk related to contrast (allergy, renal insufficiency)
Pro	Very sensitive; objective. Guidelines for both blunt and penetrating trauma	Noninvasive, sensitive. Can be performed in resuscitation bay while other activities ongoing	Very specific with good sensitivity. Good for evaluating posterior injuries
Con	Not recommended if prior laparotomy; not useful for retroperitoneal injuries. High sensitivity may result in nontherapeutic laparotomy	Operator dependent; requires equipment. Not useful for penetrating trauma	May miss intestinal or diaphragmatic injuries. Suitable only for stable patients. Higher radiation exposure than other options

CT: computed tomography; DPL: diagnostic peritoneal lavage.

Similarly, ultrasound is designed to evaluate cases of hemoperitoneum; it may not be positive in the face of a contained solid organ hematoma. It has the advantage of being noninvasive and can also be valuable for fetal assessment. CT is most accurate, supplying anatomic detail of both intraperitoneal and retroperitoneal injury. The major disadvantage is lack of portability and immediacy, often requiring a move from the safety of the emergency department, and the radiation dose imparted to the fetus.

Trauma resuscitation

Definitive hemorrhage control rather than normalization of volume status is again emphasized as the target of shock management.[9] Blood loss may be estimated through assessment of blood pressure, heart rate, and skin color (Table 34.2). Invasive monitoring is not warranted. Hypovolemic hypotension requires 15–20% blood volume loss, but may be a late sign in young, pregnant patients with good compensatory mechanisms.

Failure to correct hypotension or tachycardia after rapid infusion of 2–3 l of crystalloid solution suggests a volume deficit of greater than 15% or ongoing losses. Blood transfusion, using type O if type-specific blood is not available, should be considered when blood loss exceeds 1 l or greater than 3 l of crystalloid are needed to maintain blood pressure. Type O-positive

Table 34.2 Estimated blood loss based on physical examination

	Class I	Class II	Class III	Class IV
Blood loss (ml)	Up to 750	750–1500	1500–2000	> 2000
Blood loss (% volume)	Up to 15%	15%–30%	30%–40%	> 40%
Pulse rate	< 100	> 100	> 120	> 140
Blood pressure	Normal	Normal	Decreased	Decreased
Respiratory rate	14–20	20–30	30–40	> 40
Urine output (ml/hr)	> 30	20–30	5–15	Negligible
Mental status	Slightly anxious	Mild anxiety	Anxious, confused	Lethargic

blood can be safely given to most patients, reserving the often difficult to inventory O-negative blood for women of childbearing age. Attention must be directed to avoiding the creation of a secondary injury or insult, primarily by avoiding hypotension or hypoxia. This is especially true in the management of closed head injury. Evidence from the Traumatic Coma Data Bank indicates that even a single episode of hypotension results in poorer outcomes after head injury.

Prophylactic antibiotics should be started for penetrating trauma or open fractures.[10] The tetanus immunization status of the patient must be ascertained. If the immunization status is uncertain, or the patient has a tetanus-prone wound, tetanus immunoglobulin should be administered with the tetanus toxoid booster. Tetanus-prone wounds include those greater than 6 hours old, crush injuries, burns and electrical injuries, frostbite, high-velocity-missile injuries, devitalized tissue, denervated or ischemic tissue, and direct contamination with dirt or feces.

Great care should be exercised during resuscitation efforts to protect against transmission of bloodborne diseases to the health-care staff. Epidemiologic studies have found that 1–16% of trauma patients are infected with the human immunodeficiency virus (HIV) at the time of presentation.[11] The incidence increases with the percentage of penetrating trauma within the case mix. The prevalence and risk of hepatitis B is even greater. Nevertheless, adherence to the principle of 'universal precautions,' that is, the practice of strict barrier techniques applied in all cases on the presumption that all patients are infected, is poor. Compliance with infection control standards cannot be achieved by passive informational techniques, but requires active and continuous in-service supervision.

During the secondary survey, injuries are cataloged and potentially life-threatening or disabling injuries are identified. A treatment plan and priorities are set. A basic principle of trauma resuscitation is the need for continual re-evaluation and reassessment. Some authors have published their experience with regard to a *tertiary* survey, which can identify up to a 5–10% missed injury rate.[12] While the majority of these delayed diagnoses are not life- or limb-threatening, some will in fact be significant. Finally, the leader of the resuscitation team must also be able to assess accurately his or her facility's ability to render definitive care, and arrange for transfer to a tertiary facility or trauma center if warranted. Transfer to a higher level of care must be accomplished through physician-to-physician communication in a timely fashion, and can be facilitated by pre-existing transfer agreements.

Trauma in pregnancy: physiologic considerations

The basic principles of trauma care for the pregnant patient remain essentially the same. The signs of shock may be masked, however, by the physiologic maternal hypervolemia. Blood volume increases during pregnancy from 20–25% during the first trimester to 30–50% above normal at term.[13] A relative increase in plasma volume compared to red cell mass results in a mild-to-moderate decrease in hematocrit, resulting in a dilutional 'physiologic' anemia of pregnancy, averaging 32–34% by week 34.

Cardiac output increases 30–40% by week 10, despite a small drop in central venous pressure. This is accomplished, in part, by an increase in heart rate. The pulse rate increases by 15–20 beats/minute by the third trimester. Additionally, systolic and diastolic blood pressure decrease by 15–20 mmHg in the first two trimesters. These physiologic changes, which help the pregnant patient meet the increased demands of the fetus and childbirth, may, in the trauma setting, mask or delay the recognition of shock. Changes in pulse and blood pressure may not become evident until 1.5–2 l of blood loss, 35% of blood volume, has occurred.

Fetal distress will predate maternal distress since the maternal circulation is preferentially maintained. The mother will attempt to maintain homeostasis at the expense of the fetus. The uterus is not a vital organ, so vasoconstriction in the face of hypovolemia in an effort to maintain maternal blood pressure will result in a 10–20% reduction in blood flow to the fetus even before maternal blood pressure is affected. It is therefore possible for the fetus to be in shock while the mother is not.

Crystalloid is the preferred agent for initial resuscitation; pressors should be avoided if possible since they may also decrease uterine blood flow due to vasoconstriction. Exceptions include cardiogenic shock from blunt cardiac injury (formerly called myocardial contusion) and neurogenic shock from an associated spinal cord injury. In both cases, blood pressure and cardiac output are often not maintained by volume infusion alone.

Beyond week 20 of pregnancy, the gravid uterus may mechanically compress the vena cava, resulting in reduced venous return and hypotension. This should be relieved by manual distraction of the uterus or logrolling the patient into the left lateral decubitus position.

The pregnant patient develops chronic compensated respiratory alkalosis. Placental progesterone stimulates the medullary respiratory center from the second trimester until term. The tidal volume and minute ventilation may increase by 40–50%. However, as the uterus enlarges, the diaphragms rise as much as 4 cm and functional residual capacity decreases by up to 20%.

The resultant decrease in serum bicarbonate coupled with a decreased hematocrit culminates in a reduced acid–base buffering capacity. This decreased oxygen reserve may become problematic, as the demands of the fetus and placenta result in a 15% increased maternal oxygen consumption. The end result is a diminished oxygen reserve and a greater intolerance for hypoxia than in the nonpregnant state. A P_{CO_2} of 40 mmHg in the last two trimesters may represent hypoventilation and a relative respiratory acidosis that could precipitate fetal distress.[14]

In addition to the cardiologic and pulmonary alterations of pregnancy, other organ systems may be altered. The pregnant patient is at greater risk of aspiration due to delayed gastric emptying and decreased gastric tone. The bladder, displaced anteriorly and superiorly by the uterus, becomes an intra-abdominal organ and is more susceptible to injury. Of importance to the trauma evaluation, the pregnant patient may exhibit a decreased response or absence of peritoneal signs in response to abdominal injury, as the growth and stretching of the abdominal wall leads to a desensitization to peritoneal irritation.[13]

Fetal considerations and outcome

The role of maternal shock and hypoxia in contributing to an adverse fetal outcome cannot be overemphasized. Fetal heart monitoring should be initiated on all patients beyond week 22 of gestation as soon as possible. This includes patients with no obvious signs of abdominal injury, as direct impact is not necessary for disorders to be present. Even minor trauma may cause adverse fetal outcomes in up to 7% of cases.[15] Patients should be monitored for at least 4 hours; presentation of disorder beyond 24 hours is unlikely. Reports of delayed placental abruption are probably delays in diagnosis rather than delays in presentation.[16]

The most common obstetric complication after trauma is premature uterine contractions leading to delivery. External fetal monitoring and ultrasound, especially if used together, will identify fetal or pregnancy-related complications within 4–6 hours.[16] The Kleihauer–Betke (K–B) test has poor sensitivity and marginal specificity, and therefore has limited usefulness in the setting of acute trauma. Although usually part of a routine maternal trauma workup, the K–B test has a wide range of variation, and false positives make interpretation difficult. No data suggest that a positive K–B test alters management except in those who are Rh-negative.[17]

The major causes of fetal mortality are abruptio placentae and maternal mortality. Maternal acidosis, reflecting an under-resuscitated state, is a predictor of fetal demise.[18] Routine serum bicarbonate assay in the emergency department is recommended.[19] Maternal traumatic brain injury is a predictor of fetal outcome, and even moderate brain injury, GCS 9–12, contributes to a higher negative outcome.[20]

The difference in elasticity between the uterus and the placenta may result in placental detachment during deceleration injuries. Vaginal bleeding is a grave sign and carries a prohibitive fetal mortality rate.[21] An Injury Severity Score (ISS) of 25 or greater is associated with a 50% fetal mortality rate.[5]

One should not assume that minimal maternal injury conveys minimal fetal risk. The risk of pregnancy loss may not correlate with the mother's abdominal AIS (abbreviated injury score), and pregnancy losses may occur in patients with abdominal AIS of zero.[22] Fetal death may occur with a very low or negligible ISS, especially in cases of domestic violence and assault.[23] In these cases, obstetric findings are present in virtually all cases. Complications are rare in the absence of uterine contractions, uterine tenderness, or bleeding.[24]

Little research has focused on the developmental outcomes to children involved in traumatic events while *in utero*.

Trauma radiology during pregnancy

One area of trauma management that clearly differentiates the pregnant from the nonpregnant patient is the approach to radiologic investigation. Appropriate radiographs should not be withheld, but, because of the risk to the fetus, radiographs should be individualized, shielding the uterus when possible. Every effort should be made to avoid duplicate or gratuitous radiography. Only those studies that will dictate a change in management should be performed.

The effects of radiation exposure are greatest from 2–7 weeks, during the period of major organogenesis. There is little risk of teratogenesis after 17–20 weeks, but there is an increased relative risk of growth retardation, CNS dysfunction, and childhood malignancies.

The amount of radiation that a fetus will receive during 9 months' gestation from natural sources is approximately 50–100 mrad.[25] A radiation dose of less than 1 rad is believed to carry minimal risk. Exposure to greater than 15 rad is associated with a 6% risk of mental retardation and 3% risk of childhood malignancy.[26] The current recommendation is to limit exposure to less than 5 rad, with most radiographic studies delivering mrad doses (Table 34.3). The clinician must be cognizant that fetal doses will depend upon the equipment and techniques used, the size of the fetus and mother, and the number of radiographs used.

Diagnostically, ultrasound can be considered a 'noninvasive DPL.'[27] Moreover, the use of abdominal ultrasound in patients with a positive serum beta-HCG can contribute to a statistically significant decrease in radiation exposure.[28] Ultrasound is not always an effective tool to diagnose placental abruption since there is considerable variation in expertise among sonographers. Abruptio placentae should be suspected

Table 34.3 Radiation exposure from common radiographic studies

Study	Dose to fetus in mrad
CXR (AP)	1
C-spine	1–10
Extremity	1–5
Pelvis	200–350
Hip and femur	125–400
IVP	500–880
Head CT	50
Abdomen CT	3000–9000

in the presence of one or more of the following ultrasound findings: retroplacental separation (it is a rare finding), preplacental hematoma (jelly-like movement of the chorionic plate with fetal movement), increased placental thickness and echogenicity, and subchorionic or marginal collection.

Perimortem cesarean section

Perimortem cesarean section is a procedure that is discussed far more often than it is performed. Approximately 150–200 successful cases had been reported in the literature by the mid-1990s.[29] Perimortem cesarean section may be indicated if the fetus is viable (at least 24–25 weeks' gestation), there is reasonable certainty of maternal death, and fetal life can be demonstrated by ultrasound, clinical examination, or heart activity. Survival is unexpected if there are no fetal heart tones at the time of c-section.[30]

The time interval without maternal circulation is critical in prognosis, as the incidence of neurologic sequelae increases with longer delivery times. No time should be wasted once the decision to proceed with cesarean section has been made. The overwhelming majority, 70%, of survivors of perimortem cesarean section were delivered in 5 minutes or less from the loss of maternal circulation.[31]

Cesarean section should be performed while open or closed cardiac massage is in progress, without aortic cross-clamping. As there have been reports of maternal revival after cesarean section and delivery of the fetus, this intervention should be viewed as perimortem rather than postmortem.[32]

Domestic violence

Overall, upward of one-third of all emergency room visits by women in the USA are the result of domestic violence.[33] Some 1–2 million US women suffer injuries due to domestic violence annually, and 30–50% of female homicides are committed by present or former partners.[34] The National Family Violence Study reported that 15% of pregnant women were assaulted by their partners in the first 4 months of pregnancy.[35]

Physicians and nurses in the emergency department and on trauma teams have a unique opportunity to intervene in the cycle of domestic violence. Health-care professionals are often sought out by victims of domestic violence for assistance in preference to police authorities. Research suggests that patients expect the treating physician to initiate a dialog about abuse.[36] Barriers to identification are well described. These include discomfort on the part of the physician to ask, lack of time, lack of an organized infrastructure of care once a patient is identified,

---

Table 34.4 Partner violence screen and SAFE screen

Partner violence screen

(1) Have you been kicked, hit, punched, or otherwise hurt by someone within the last year?
(2) Do you feel safe in your current relationship?
(3) Is there a partner from a previous relationship who is making you feel unsafe now?

SAFE screen
Stress/safety

　　What stress do you experience in your relationships?
　　Do you feel safe in your relationship?

Afraid/abused

　　What happens when you and your partner disagree?
　　Has your partner ever threatened or abused you or your children?

Friends/family

　　If you were hurt, did your family or friends know?
　　Could you tell them?
　　Would they be able to help you?

Emergency plan

　　Do you have a safe place to go in case of an emergency?
　　Would you like help in locating a shelter?
　　Would you like to talk with a social worker or counselor to develop an emergency plan?

and a sense of powerlessness when faced with this issue. This reluctance may be complicated by the physician's or nurse's personal exposure to child or spousal abuse.[37]

Women seen in the emergency room should be privately screened for domestic violence. The Partner Violence Screen[38] will uncover approximately 70% of abuse victims, and the questions incorporated into the SAFE mnemonic (Table 34.4) can be incorporated into the emergency department evaluation.[34] Comprehensive documentation, including photographic recording of injury, can assist the victim access social or legal services.

References

1. American College of Surgeons Committee on Trauma. Advanced Trauma Life Support. American College of Surgeons: Chicago, 1997.
2. Weiss HB, Strotmeyer S. Characteristics of pregnant women in motor vehicle crashes. Inj Prev 2002; 8: 207–10.
3. Fildes J, Reed L, Jones N et al. Trauma: the leading cause of maternal death. J Trauma 1992; 32: 643–5.
4. Weiss HB. The epidemiology of traumatic injury-related fetal mortality in Pennsylvania, 1995–1997: the role of motor vehicle crashes. Accid Anal Prev 2001; 33: 449–54.
5. Rogers FB, Rozycki G, Osler T et al. A multi-institutional study of factors associated with fetal death in injured pregnant patients. Arch Surg 1999; 134: 1274–7.
6. Eastman AB. Blood in our streets: status and evolution of trauma care systems. Arch Surg 1992; 127: 677–81.
7. Wisner DH. History and current status of trauma scoring systems. Arch Surg 1992; 127: 111–17.
8. Brain Trauma Foundation. Guidelines for the management of severe head injury. J Neurotrauma 1996; 13: 638–734.
9. Buchman TG, Menker JB, Lipsett P. Strategies for trauma resuscitation. Surg Gynecol Obstet 1991; 172: 8–12
10. Eastern Association for the Surgery of Trauma. Practice management guidelines for prophylactic antibiotics in penetrating abdominal injury and in open fractures. www.east.org, 1998.
11. Hammond JS, Eckes J, Gomez G et al. HIV, trauma, and infection control: universal precautions are universally ignored. J Trauma 1990; 30: 555–61.
12. Enderson BL, Reath DB, Meadors J et al. The tertiary trauma survey: a prospective study of missed injury. J Trauma 1990; 30: 666–9.
13. Shah AJ, Kilclined BA. Trauma in pregnancy. Emerg Med Clin North Am 2003; 21: 615–29.
14. Neufeld JD. Trauma in pregnancy, What if . . . ? Emerg Med Clin North Am 1993; 11: 207–24.
15. Pearlman MD, Tintinalli JE, Lorenz RP. A prospective study of outcome after trauma during pregnancy. Am J Obstet Gynecol 1990; 162: 1502–10.
16. Towery R, English TP, Wisner D. Evaluation of pregnant women after blunt injury. J Trauma 1993; 35: 731–5.
17. Dhanraj D, Lambers D. The incidences of postive Kleihauer-Betke test in low risk pregnancies and maternal trauma patients. Am J Obstet Gynecol 2004; 190: 1461–3.
18. Hoff WS, D'Amelio LD, Tinkoff, GH et al. Maternal predictors of fetal demise in trauma during pregnancy, Surg Gynecol Obstet 1991, 172: 175–80.
19. Scorpio RJ, Esposito TJ, Smith LG, Gens DR. Blunt trauma during pregnancy: factors affecting fetal outcome. J Trauma 1992; 32: 213–16.
20. Kissinger DP, Rozycki G, Morris JA et al. Trauma in pregnancy: predicting pregnancy outcome. Arch Surg 1991; 126: 1079–86.
21. Corsi PR, Rasslan S, de Oliveira LB et al. Trauma in pregnant women: analysis of maternal and fetal mortality. Injury 1999; 30: 239–43.
22. Baerga-Varela Y, Zietlow S, Bannon M et al. Trauma in pregnancy. Mayo Clin Proc 2000; 75: 1243–8.
23. Poole GV, Martin J, Perry KG et al. Trauma in pregnancy: the role of interpersonal violence. Am J Obstet Gynecol 1996; 174: 1873–7.
24. Goodwin TM, Breen MT. Pregnancy outcome and fetomaternal hemorrhage after noncatastrophic trauma. Am J Obstet Gynecol 1990; 162: 665–71
25. Benson JM. Radiation safety. J Fam Pract 1982; 15: 435–9.
26. Wagner LK, Lester RG, Saldana LR. Exposure of the Pregnant Patient to Diagnostic Radiations: a Guide to Medical Management. JB Lippincott: Philadelphia, 1985.
27. Rozycki G, Ochsner MG, Feliciano D et al. Early detection of hemoperitoneum by ultrasound examination of the right upper quadrant: a multicenter study. J Trauma 1998; 45: 878–83.
28. Bochicchio GV, Haan J, Scalea TM. Surgeon-performed focused assessment with sonography for trauma as an early screening tool for pregnancy after trauma. J Trauma 2002; 52: 1125–8.
29. Esposito TJ. Trauma during pregnancy. Emerg Med Clin North Am 1994; 12: 167–99.
30. Morris JA, Rosenbower TJ, Jurkovich GJ et al. Infant survival after Cesarean section for trauma. Ann Surg 1996; 223: 481–91.
31. Katz VL, Dotter DJ. Perimortem cesarian delivery. Obstet Gynecol 1986; 68: 571–6.
32. Pimental L. Mother and child. Emerg Med Clin North Am 1991; 9: 549–63.
33. Warner MW, Salfinger SG, Rao S et al. Management of trauma during pregnancy. Aust N Z J Surg 2004; 74: 125–8.
34. Guth AA, Pachter HL. Domestic violence and the trauma surgeon. Am J Surg 2000; 179: 134–40.
35. AMA Council on Scientific Affairs. Violence against women: relevance for medical practitioners. JAMA 1992; 267: 3184–9.
36. Caralis PV, Musiallowski R. Women's experiences with domestic violence and their attitude and expectations regarding medical care of abuse victims. South Med J 1997; 90: 1075–80.
37. Ernst AA, Houry D, Nick T, Weiss SJ. Domestic violence awareness and prevalence in a first-year medical school class. Acad Emerg Med 1998; 5: 64–8
38. Sisley A. Jacobs LM, Poole GV et al. Violence in America: a public health crisis. J Trauma 1999; 46: 1105–13.

35 Surgery during pregnancy

Asha G Bale, Steve H Kim, and Edwin A Deitch

The goal of this chapter is to provide an overview of a spectrum of common and/or important diseases that may require nongestational surgery in the pregnant patient. These surgical diseases range from processes causing abdominal pain to malignancies (Table 35.1). By necessity, this chapter cannot cover the entire field of surgery nor every aspect of each disease process. Thus, it will focus on providing the key information required to make an early and accurate diagnosis of the disease entities outlined in Table 35.1 as well as summarize the key principles of their therapy. Being familiar with this information is important, since up to 2.2% of pregnant women will require nonobstetric surgery during or immediately after the gestational period. Furthermore, making an early correct diagnosis and providing appropriate therapy is critical in limiting maternal and fetal morbidity and mortality. For example, as discussed in more detail in the specific sections of this chapter, making an early diagnosis of certain common surgical abdominal conditions, such as acute appendicitis and biliary tract disease,[1] can be difficult during pregnancy, since many of the normal physiologic changes of pregnancy (Table 35.2) are signs and symptoms of these surgical emergencies. In addition to making an early diagnosis and knowing the principles of treatment, it is also important to have a clear knowledge of the natural history of the disease as well as the effects of treatment on both the mother and the fetus. This knowledge of the natural history of disease and the consequences of immediate as well as delayed therapy is most important in the treatment of neoplastic and endocrine diseases diagnosed during pregnancy and will thus be covered in these sections of this chapter.

Table 35.1 Surgical diseases during pregnancy

Abdominal disease processes
  Pain (appendicitis, cholecystitis, pancreatitis, bowel obstruction)
  Bleeding (hepatic adenoma, splenic artery aneurysm)
  Inflammatory bowel disease
Deep venous thrombosis
Pregnancy-associated neoplasia and related endocrine issues

Table 35.2 Maternal physiologic changes during pregnancy

Clinical
  Dyspnea
  Peripheral edema
  Systolic ejection murmur
  Nausea
Cardiovascular
  Increased heart rate (to about 90)
  Decreased blood pressure (by about 5–10 mmHg)
  Increased cardiac output (by 30–50%)
  Decreased systemic vascular resistance (SVR)
  Increased blood volume and plasma volume (by 1–1.5 liters)
  Decreased venous return of blood to the heart
  Decreased iliac artery flow
Respiratory
  Elevated diaphragm
  Functional residual capacity (FRC) decrease by 15–20%
  Increased minute ventilation
  Pa_{O_2} increase (to approximately 105 mmHg)
  Pa_{CO_2} decrease (to approximately 30 mmHg)
  pH increase (to approximately 7.44)
Gastrointestinal
  Decreased gastric motility
  Mild elevation in alkaline phosphatase
Hematologic
  Hypercoagulability
  Decreased plasma total protein and albumin levels
Renal
  Dilation of collection systems
  Relaxation of bladder with increased capacity
  Increased glomerular filtration rate (GFR) by 30–50%

Abdominal diseases

Assessment of abdominal pain in the pregnant patient

Abdominal pain in the pregnant patient requires careful assessment, since movement of the abdominal viscera by the gravid uterus can make the diagnosis and treatment of otherwise routine problems quite challenging. Thus, a thorough history, physical examination, and appropriate laboratory and radiographic studies are required. In the small group of patients with obvious peritonitis on abdominal examination, limited studies are required prior to surgical exploration. However, in most gravidas, the abdominal examination is equivocal and further diagnostic evaluation is necessary. In this situation, the radiographic evaluation should begin with directed ultrasound and/or plain films (with pelvic shielding). Ultrasound can be useful in the diagnosis of appendicitis, adnexal masses, cholecystitis, or fluid in the peritoneal cavity. Bowel obstruction can be diagnosed by plain abdominal films. No further workup is needed if pneumoperitoneum is clearly seen on chest radiograph since laparotomy is the next step. Alternatively, the chest radiograph may demonstrate pneumonia, an occasional cause of abdominal pain.

If the diagnosis is still in doubt after these initial studies, judicious use of magnetic resonance imaging (MRI), computed tomography (CT) scan, and/or laparoscopy may be required. MRI is considered safe for the fetus, and may be a good alternative to a CT scan because of the absence of radiation exposure. CT scan is sensitive in detecting abdominal disorder, but fetal exposure to the ionizing radiation is not without its own risks. If possible, CT scan should be avoided during the first trimester when the risk of teratogenicity is the highest. Laparoscopy is a good option in the first and second trimesters and can be both diagnostic and therapeutic. It has been performed safely in patients with cholecystitis and appendicitis in all trimesters without undue risks to the fetus.[13,14] In general, a more thorough radiographic evaluation may be utilized in the third trimester, since the risk of fetal radiation exposure is low at this time and is outweighed by the risk of preterm labor from unnecessary surgery. Once the diagnosis is confirmed, operative or nonoperative management can proceed as appropriate. An algorithm summarizing the management of abdominal pain during pregnancy is illustrated in Figure 35.1.

Because of the potential need for radiographic testing in pregnant patients with abdominal pain, knowledge of the relative risks of radiation exposure to the fetus is critical. Basically, radiography of a pregnant patient necessitates balancing the fetal risk of radiation exposure to the potential maternal and fetal morbidity if a treatable diagnosis is missed. In general, fetal harm is more likely with higher radiation dose and earlier gestational age. During the first 2 weeks of pregnancy, at the time of implantation, radiation is associated with fetal loss. Fetal exposure to radiation during the time of organogenesis has been shown to be associated with congenital malformations, lower

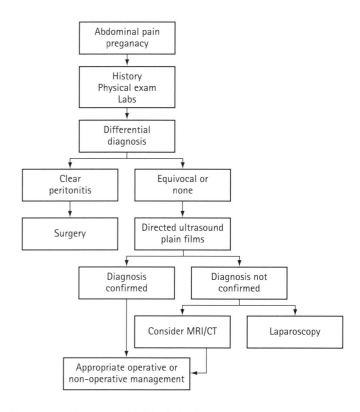

Figure 35.1 Management of abdominal pain during pregnancy.

IQ, and childhood cancer. The lowest threshold for these complications seems to be 100 mGy. Doses of 200–500 mGy (20–50 rad) may be associated with decrease in IQ and mental retardation. Doses greater than 500 mGy (50 rad) may cause growth restriction, CNS damage, and fetal death.[2] An additional, but rare, consequence of prenatal radiation exposure may be a slight increase in childhood cancer. The risk of induction of cancer can be estimated as 0.6% per mGy up to the age of 15 years.[3] All the above risks can be put into perspective by the knowledge that 15% of human embryos spontaneously abort, 2.7–3.0% of human embryos have major malformations, 4% have intrauterine growth restriction, and 8–10% have late-stage onset genetic disease.[4] Thus, the risk of radiation exposure to the fetus may be much smaller than the risk of spontaneous abortion in many cases.

Specific radiologic tests: indications and radiation risks

In choosing among the various radiographic tests available, one should initially attempt to use the test with the lowest radiation exposure to the fetus that has a reasonable chance of diagnosing the condition suspected. Ultrasound is frequently the initial test of choice, since it does not expose the fetus to radiation and has good sensitivity for diagnosing many of the entities associated with abdominal pain in the pregnant patient. Specifically, the appendix, pancreas, adnexae, and biliary tree are all assessable with this modality. Furthermore, rapid diagnosis of hemo-peritoneum is possible in situations of sudden cardiovascular collapse when intra-abdominal bleeding is suspected. Plain radiographs, CT scans, and fluoroscopy all expose the fetus to the risks of ionizing radiation (Table 35.3). The estimated fetal radiation dose is 2 mGy per plain film, 5 mGy per CT slice, and 10 mGy per minute of fluoroscopy when the fetus is in the field of radiation.[5] Films in which the fetus is not directly in the field (e.g., chest radiograph or skull film) expose the fetus to an absorbed dose of less than 0.01 mGy.[6] Shielding of the pelvis should be done routinely when studying the chest or upper abdomen to minimize fetal exposure to radiation.

Radiographic tests, such as a pelvic CT or a barium enema, in which the uterus is directly exposed to the x-ray beam, are associated with absorbed radiation doses to the embryo of about 20–80 mGy and 10–20 mGy, respectively,[6] while an abdominal CT, using the more modern scanners, has been estimated to expose the fetus to 29–42 mGy of radiation.[7] Nuclear medicine studies may be helpful in selected patients, since the radiation dose to the embryo/fetus is less than 10 mGy. Addition aids are adequate hydration of the mother and Foley catheterization for prompt removal of the isotope from the bladder to minimize fetal radiation exposure when nuclear medicine tests are utilized.[8]

Although limited information is available on the long-term effects of MRI on the fetus, one major advantage of MRI is that it does not require the use of ionizing radiation or the injection of contrast material. Thus, although the complete biologic effects of MRI are still unknown, it has been used successfully in all trimesters of pregnancy and appears to have minimal fetal risk. MRI has been used in several case reports to diagnose appendicitis during pregnancy and has been helpful in identifying patients with abdominal pain that do not require surgery.[9]

In summary, the judicious use of radiography in pregnant women can help the clinician to make a correct diagnosis and promptly treat surgical emergencies. In addition, judicious use of radiographic testing can reduce the number of negative surgical explorations, thereby reducing the risk of preterm labor. When using radiographic techniques associated with fetal radiation exposure, it is important to have a thorough discussion with the patient regarding the risks of radiologic examination of the fetus, so that an informed decision can be made. Another point to remember is that although a single radiographic study is usually not harmful, the increasing radiation dose of multiple examinations may be associated with an increased fetal risk. As a general rule, one should proceed with any necessary radiologic examination that is clinically indicated, since an early diagnosis and prompt therapy of operative abdominal disease processes is the best way to prevent maternal morbidity and premature labor.

Appendicitis

Appendicitis is the most common cause of a surgical abdomen in the pregnant patient, with an incidence of 1–2/1000 pregnancies. Pregnancy itself is not associated with an increase risk above that of the general population. The diagnosis of appendicitis in pregnancy may be difficult since the gravid uterus may displace the appendix and some of the symptoms of appendicitis, such as nausea and vomiting, can occur in a normal pregnancy. The usual presentation of appendicitis, which occurs in about 80% of patients, begins with periumbilical pain that moves to the right lower quadrant of the abdomen followed by anorexia, nausea, and vomiting. The evolution of this syndrome generally occurs over 12–24 hours. Fever and elevated white blood cell count are common, but they are later signs. As the pregnancy proceeds, the gravid uterus will push the appendix cephalad and rotate the appendiceal tip medially. The net result of this displacement of the appendix is the migration of pain from the right lower toward the right upper quadrant. However, even in this situation, the patient can usually pinpoint the exact site of tenderness, which at surgery will correspond to the anatomic location of the appendix. Ultrasound may be helpful in making the diagnosis of appendicitis if an inflamed appendix or periappendiceal fluid is visualized. An edematous appendix will be noncompressible on ultrasound. If the ultrasound is nondiagnostic, a CT scan can be used, since it has a high sensitivity (>90%) although it exposes the fetus to ionizing radiation. For this reason, some clinicians have begun using MRI as an alternative to the CT scan. A negative laparotomy rate of 20–50% has been reported in pregnant patients when they are operated on for clinical indications or when radiographic tests are not diagnostic.[8] In this situation, pyelonephritis has been found to be the most common postoperative diagnosis, highlighting the importance of a urine analysis in patients with possible appendicitis. Since a negative laparotomy is associated with minimal maternal morbidity, it is better to have a negative laparotomy than to miss the diagnosis. Thus, if appendicitis is suspected, operative management should not be delayed, since fetal risk increases from 2–8.5% in simple appendicitis to as high as 35% in cases of perforation.[10] Maternal mortality is less than 1–2%, with most deaths occurring when therapy is delayed.

Although the diagnosis in most patients with appendicitis is based on the clinical syndrome of pain migrating from the

---

Table 35.3 Estimated radiation exposure from radiography

Radiographic test	Estimated ionizing radiation exposure (mGy)
Chest radiograph	<0.01 mGy
Abdominal CT	29–42 mGy
Pelvic CT	20–80 mGy
Barium enema	10–20 mGy
Nuclear study	<10 mGy
Fluoroscopy	10 mGy per minute
Ultrasound	None
MRI	None

1 rad = 10 mGy.

epigastrium to the right side of the abdomen in association with nausea and vomiting, a significant subgroup of patients presents with atypical symptoms as well as advanced disease (that is, an abdominal phlegmon and/or periappendiceal abscess). If the patient has an atypical history or appears to have advanced disease on presentation, a CT scan can be very useful. For example, a CT scan is particularly helpful in distinguishing between patients with simple appendicitis and those with appendiceal phlegmon with or without accompanying periappendiceal abscess. If the patient with advanced appendiceal disease is hemodynamically stable without evidence of generalized peritonitis, then nonoperative management is preferred for several reasons. These include the difficulty of the operative procedure, the frequent need to do a right colectomy because of the inflamed nature of the cecum, and a much higher risk of operative complications. In fact, nonoperative therapy, consisting of broad-spectrum antibiotic therapy combined with percutaneous drainage of periappendiceal abscesses under ultrasound or CT guidance, has a high rate of success. In patients with advanced disease treated nonoperatively, consideration should be given to the performance of an interval appendectomy after delivery. The approach to the management of patients with appendicitis is summarized in Figure 35.2.

Biliary tract disease

The incidence of biliary disease in gravidas is reported to be 0.16%.[11] The pregnant patient with biliary colic usually presents with nausea, vomiting, and right upper quadrant abdominal pain, typically after ingestion of a fatty meal. These episodes usually start an hour after the meal and are self-limited, lasting about 2 hours. Unremitting pain in patients with biliary tract disease usually implies the development of acute cholecystitis. Ultrasound can confirm the presence of gallstones, and acute cholecystitis is suggested by the presence of pericholecystic fluid and gallbladder wall thickening over 3 mm. In general, treatment is symptomatic and hospitalization is not required in patients with biliary colic, unless there is persistent vomiting. In contrast, patients with acute cholecystitis require admission, intravenous fluids, and a course of antibiotics. Fortunately, more than 90% of pregnant patients with biliary tract disease resolve their acute episodes with conservative treatment alone.[12] Relapse rates prior to delivery have been reported to be as high as 69%, with medical management alone resulting in multiple hospitalizations during the pregnancy. Conservative treatment may be associated with premature contractions.[10,13] If repeated attacks of biliary colic or acute cholecystitis result in multiple admissions to the hospital, cholecystectomy should be considered during the first or second trimester. In the third trimester, attempts should be made to delay the cholecystectomy until after the delivery. If surgery is to be performed, laparoscopic cholecystectomy appears to be safe. Technical aspects to remember during laparoscopy include using lower-pressure pneumoperitoneum (9–12 mmHg) as well as an open technique to enter the peritoneum. In the third trimester, the gravid uterus may not allow sufficient pneumoperitoneum for laparoscopy; therefore, open cholecystectomy may be required. Open cholecystectomy is associated with a 12% risk of spontaneous abortion in the first trimester and a 40% risk of preterm labor in the third trimester.[14] The laparoscopic approach appears to result in lower risk of both complications. As with most operations, the second trimester is the most favorable time for elective or semielective surgery. Finally, in unstable patients, percutaneous cholecystostomy performed under ultrasound guidance followed by postpartum cholecystectomy is an option. The management approach to the patient with biliary tract disease is summarized in Figure 35.3. The management of patients with biliary pancreatitis will be covered in the next section.

Pancreatitis

First-trimester pancreatitis has an incidence of 1 out of every 10 000 live births. Gallstones are the most common etiology during pregnancy[15] followed by hyperlipidemia. The patient typically presents with nausea, vomiting, and epigastric pain radiating to the back. Laboratory values will show elevated amylase and lipase, with the latter being the more sensitive indicator. Electrolyte imbalances can occur with prolonged vomiting and should be expediently corrected. Although mild increases in alkaline phosphatase levels are normal during pregnancy, a disproportionate elevation associated with concomitant increases in bilirubin and transaminases suggests biliary obstruction and biliary pancreatitis. The severity of the pancreatitis can be estimated with Ranson's criteria or the APACHE II score. In patients with pancreatitis, an ultrasound should be done early in the clinical course to assess the gallbladder and common bile duct, focusing on whether the patient has gallstones with biliary obstruction. In severe cases, a CT scan of the abdomen with intravenous contrast should be done to deter-

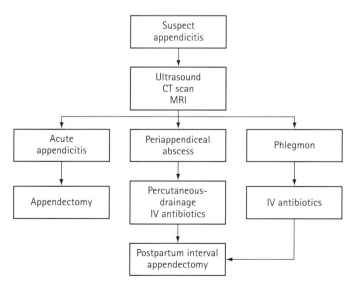

Figure 35.2 Management of appendicitis during pregnancy.

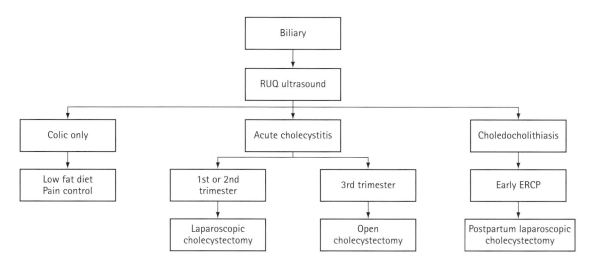

Figure 35.3 Management of biliary disease during pregnancy. RUQ, right upper quadrant.

mine the presence and extent of pancreatic necrosis, since the extent of pancreatic necrosis correlates with ultimate mortality. In most patients who develop pancreatitis, the disease process rapidly resolves over a few days and only symptomatic therapy is required. In fact, neonatal outcomes do not appear to be adversely affected if the mother has uncomplicated pancreatitis.[14] In the patient group with uncomplicated biliary pancreatitis, cholecystectomy during the pregnancy may be necessary, but an attempt should be made to defer this to the postpartum period.

In patients with severe gallstone pancreatitis, acute treatment involves aggressive hydration and, if there is obstruction of the common bile duct by gallstones, relieving this obstruction by endoscopic retrograde cholangiopancreatography (ERCP). The use of early ERCP, within the first 48 hours of a life-threatening attack of biliary pancreatitis, is based on several randomized, controlled trials in nonpregnant patients showing that this strategy decreases the mortality and morbidity by about threefold. Thus, ERCP should be strongly considered in pregnant patients, since several case reports indicate that ERCP is safe throughout pregnancy when combined with fetal monitoring and pelvic shielding to limit fetal radiation exposure. Obviously, fluoroscopy time should also be minimized. Because of the fetal risk of radiation, in the pregnant patient, ERCP should be restricted to therapeutic indications only, such as gallstone extraction, sphincterotomy, or biliary stent insertion.[16]

Patients with severe pancreatitis should be admitted to the intensive care unit where their cardiovascular, fluid, and oxygenation status can be monitored during the initial resuscitative phase of their illness, since they are at high risk of developing respiratory failure and/or hypovolemic shock. The prophylactic administration of broad-spectrum antibiotics is indicated if pancreatic necrosis involving more than 30% of the gland is present by CT scan. Imipenem is the antibiotics of choice, since it has good penetration into the pancreatic tissues and early pro-

phylactic use has been shown to reduce the mortality rate by over 50% in patients with necrotizing pancreatitis. Because gut bacterial translocation has been associated with the development of pancreatic sepsis and pulmonary injury, early enteral feeding is recommended to improve gut barrier function. In fact, early enteral feeding of liquid diets through a feeding tube, as opposed to total parenteral nutrition, has been shown to reduce morbidity in several series of patients with severe pancreatitis. In contrast to antibiotics and early enteral feeding, use of somatostatin does not appear to affect the course of pancreatitis. If there is CT scan evidence of pancreatic necrosis, and the patient does not improve or worsens in the first 10–14 days of admission, fine-needle aspiration of peripancreatic fluid is indicated to rule out bacterial infection. If the fluid is sterile, conservative treatment with antibiotics is continued for up to 3 weeks. However, if infection is diagnosed, surgical debridement of the pancreas should be performed. This will usually require serial visits to the operating room during the patient's hospital course. Figure 35.4 outlines the key elements of the care of patients with pancreatitis.

Intestinal obstruction

Small bowel obstruction is a rare event during pregnancy, occurring in about one in every 3000–6000 pregnant women. The most common cause of obstruction is adhesions from previous surgery. As the gravid uterus pushes the intestines cephalad, pre-existing adhesions may cause the bowel to twist on itself, causing obstruction. The second most common cause of obstruction during pregnancy is cecal volvulus, which is responsible for obstruction in about 25% of the patients. Pregnant patients are more prone to cecal volvulus than the general population, since the cecum is not completely fixed to the retroperitoneum and can twist on its mesentery as the uterus enlarges, displacing it from its normal location. Cecal volvulus may lead to cecal infarction if the blood supply is compromised.

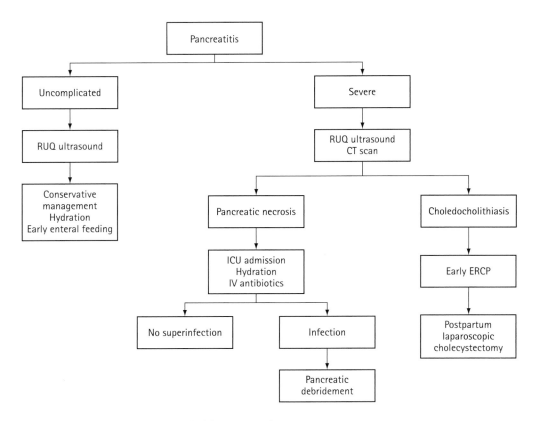

Figure 35.4 Management of pancreatitis during pregnancy. RUQ, right upper quadrant.

Patients with intestinal obstruction present with nausea, vomiting, abdominal distention, and pain. Usually, the pain is described as crampy and felt in the periumbilical region. Obstipation is generally the case, but stools can be passed from the colon distal to the obstruction. The patient may have symptoms and signs of dehydration along with electrolyte imbalances if prolonged vomiting is present. The physical examination should include inspecting the abdomen for scars, and a thorough search for incarcerated hernias, especially those in the inguinal and femoral regions. Abdominal distention may not be fully appreciated because of the gravid uterus. If the physical examination suggests peritonitis, or fever and leukocytosis are present, bowel ischemia should be suspected. Plain films will generally show a characteristic stepladder pattern of distended small intestine. Dilation of the small intestine, air fluid levels, and paucity of air in the colon are all findings suggestive of intestinal obstruction. If cecal volvulus is the cause of obstruction, a dilated cecum with an air-fluid level can be seen in the right lower quadrant on the plain film.

On presentation, patients should initially be treated with nasogastric tube decompression and intravenous fluids. Potassium and chloride replacement may be necessary. A Foley catheter should be placed to monitor urine output. It is important to try to determine whether the obstruction is partial or complete, since nonoperative resolution occurs in over 80% of patients with partial intestinal obstruction. In complete obstruction, plain films will show no air in the colon. Patients with findings of complete obstruction should undergo laparotomy early, since nonoperative therapy is not generally successful, and, if bowel ischemia develops, over half of the patients will go into preterm labor. Furthermore, for patients that develop shock or sepsis, fetal mortality approaches 50%.

Intra-abdominal bleeding

Liver adenoma

A ruptured hepatic adenoma is a cause of sudden hypotension and abdominal pain during pregnancy. Hepatic adenomas are benign, usually solitary liver lesions, whose growth is stimulated by estrogen. Thus, the high circulating estrogen levels during pregnancy can result in significant increases in adenoma size and a higher risk of spontaneous rupture, which can be lethal. This risk of rupture is higher in the postpartum period. Because of estrogen's effect on adenoma growth, nonpregnant women with known liver adenomas are advised to stop oral contraceptives and avoid pregnancy. This alone has led to regression of the tumor. If planning a pregnancy, a woman with a known liver adenoma should undergo prophylactic resection or ablation of the lesion beforehand. Emergent fluid resuscitation followed by hepatic artery embolization or surgical hepatic artery ligation is recommended for the pregnant patient with a known adenoma who presents in hemodynamic shock.

Splenic artery aneurysm

Rupture of a splenic artery aneurysm is a rare but documented cause of intra-abdominal hemorrhage during pregnancy. Increased circulating blood flow and portal hypertension during pregnancy are pathogenic factors leading to an increased risk of rupture. The patient presents with sudden cardiovascular collapse. Initially, ultrasound will show a hemoperitoneum. A CT scan can be done if the patient is hemodynamically stable. Once diagnosed, a ruptured splenic artery aneurysm can be treated with surgery or angioembolization. At the time of surgery, if the aneurysm is located in the proximal splenic artery, it is resected followed by reanastamosis of the splenic artery. If it is located distally near the spleen, splenectomy is usually also preformed with aneurysmectomy.[17] This condition can be fatal; therefore, a high index of suspicion is warranted.

Inflammatory bowel disease (IBD)

Women with active Crohn's disease are generally advised to avoid pregnancy because of the risk to the fetus. However, women with quiescent disease have safely carried their pregnancies to term with low maternal morbidity and mortality. Pregnancy in itself does not appear to influence the course of Crohn's disease, and women in remission do not appear to have complications during pregnancy. Neonatal birth weights are small for gestational age in about 25% of births with low birth weight being more common in women with ileal Crohn's disease and in those who have had previous bowel resection.[16] Acute exacerbations are seen in about 20–26% of pregnant women with Crohn's.[18,19] This rate is similar to the rate of acute exacerbation in nonpregnant women with Crohn's. Active Crohn's at the time of conception or acute exacerbations during the pregnancy predispose to preterm delivery, spontaneous abortion, fetal loss, and/or live-born babies with malformations.[17] In one cross-sectional study, while women with Crohn's disease were at increased risk of preterm delivery, low birth weight, and small for gestational age, births to women with ulcerative colitis had a significantly higher incidence of congenital malformations compared to healthy controls.[20]

Based on the above information, the goal of treatment in pregnant women with IBD is maintenance of remission throughout the pregnancy. It appears that active disease is more harmful to the fetus than the effects of the medications used to achieve remission; therefore, most medications taken for IBD should be continued before, during, and after the pregnancy. Sulfasalazine and 5-aminosalicylic acid have been used safely during pregnancy. Steroids can be used during pregnancy and do not have teratogenic effects. Women treated with steroids have higher rates of miscarriage and preterm births.[21] This observation may be a result of the severity of the disease itself. 6-Mercaptopurine and azathioprine should be used with caution, since both may cause impaired fetal immunity, growth retardation, or prematurity.[22,23] Cyclosporine should be used cautiously because it is associated with fetal growth restriction and prematurity. Methotrexate is associated with congenital malformations and should not be used during pregnancy. There are not enough data about the use of infliximab during pregnancy to assess its risks or safety. Although controversial, metronidazole and ciprofloxacin have been used for short periods during acute exacerbations without adverse effects, but the effects of longer periods of use, as is typical for Crohn's disease, are unknown.[20]

Deep venous thrombosis (DVT) during pregnancy

Pregnant women are 6–10 times more likely to develop DVT than nonpregnant women of the same age,[24] with DVT occurring in 0.05–0.1% of pregnant women. DVT is more common in the postpartum than the antepartum period. During pregnancy, the incidence is highest in the second trimester and is more common in the left lower extremity than the right. There are several etiologies proposed to explain the increased incidence of the development of a DVT during pregnancy. These include the mechanical effect of the gravid uterus compressing the veins of the lower extremities, creating venous stasis. Venous distensibility and capacity are also increased during pregnancy. In addition, pregnancy is a hypercoagulable state where the procoagulation factors II, III, and X are increased, and the levels of the anticoagulant factor protein S are decreased. The fibrinolytic system is inhibited in the third trimester and fibrin levels are increased. These are all favorable conditions for the development of DVT. The risk of developing DVT is higher with advanced maternal age, sepsis, hemorrhage, multiparity and cesarean section, or instrument-assisted delivery. Additional risk factors for the development of DVT include multiple pregnancy, high body-mass index, prolonged bed rest, and hypercoagulable disorder.[25]

The diagnosis of DVT and even pulmonary embolus is more difficult in the pregnant patient, since bilateral lower extremity edema and mild dyspnea are common during pregnancy. Thus, it is important to have a high index of suspicion and order an expedient duplex venous ultrasound if DVT is suspected. During performance of the ultrasound, the uterus should be displaced laterally after the second trimester to improve the accuracy of the test. Venography or serial noninvasive testing is recommended for high-risk patients whose venous duplex test is negative. The workup should include the search for an underlying hypercoagulable disorder, such as antithrombin III deficiency, protein C and protein S deficiency, activated protein C resistance, the presence of lupus anticoagulant factor, and hyperhomocystinemia. Once DVT is diagnosed, the treatment is anticoagulant therapy beginning with intravenous unfractionated heparin for 7–10 days (heparin does not cross the placenta), followed by low-molecular-weight heparin for the remainder of the pregnancy. It is unclear whether heparin should be held during labor. Thus, heparin can be given throughout labor, or it can be held once contractions start.

Warfarin should be prescribed postpartum for 6–12 weeks. Since pulmonary emboli occur more commonly during the postpartum than the antepartum period, if a pulmonary embolus is suspected during pregnancy, a ventilation perfusion scan should be rapidly obtained. In most patients, this scan will be diagnostic; however, if the reading is indeterminate, pulmonary angiography or a CT angiogram should be done to confirm the diagnosis. The initial treatment of pulmonary embolus is intravenous heparin, which is administered for 5–10 days, or low-molecular-weight heparin. Subsequently, subcutaneous heparin or low-molecular-weight heparin can be used for the remainder of the pregnancy. Warfarin should be used postpartum for 6 weeks or until 3 months of anticoagulation therapy has been completed. If there is a contraindication to anticoagulation in the patient with pulmonary embolus, a vena caval filter can be placed safely in pregnant females. Thrombolytic agents should not be used.

Pregnancy-associated neoplasia and related endocrine issues

Findings from a recent survey of the California State Cancer Registry revealed that the most common cancers associated with pregnancy were those of the breast, thyroid, and cervix followed by melanoma and Hodgkin's lymphoma (Table 35.4).[26] This section will focus on the most common nongynecologic neoplastic and related diseases of general surgical import in the pregnant patient as well as integrate important endocrine problems such as pheochromocytoma and hyperparathyroidism.

Diagnosis and management of puerperal breast masses

During pregnancy, alterations in breast texture, tenderness, and size make examination more difficult. Small masses are frequently missed as gestation progresses, thus mandating a careful baseline breast examination as soon as pregnancy is discovered.

Table 35.4 Incidence of neoplastic disease in the puerperium from the California Cancer Registry, 1991–1999

Cancer type	Incidence*
Breast	19.3
Thyroid	14.4
Cervix	12.0
Melanoma	8.7
Hodgkin's lymphoma	5.4
Ovary	5.2
Leukemia	4.3
Colorectal	2.8

*Per 100 000.

Mammography, ultrasound, and, more recently, MRI are the currently available imaging modalities for evaluating breast masses.[27] Due to the radiation dose, mammography is rarely used in women already pregnant. However, for women over age 40 who are considering pregnancy (especially those with a family history of breast cancer), it is prudent to obtain a mammogram prior to conception. The utility of screening mammography in women under the age of 40 has not been demonstrated.

Any suspicious findings on physical examination are initially evaluated with breast ultrasound. Common benign cystic lesions include galactoceles and abscesses. Needle aspiration is diagnostic and therapeutic for the former. Abscesses in the breast are treated with incision and drainage, with the caveat that a biopsy of the wall should also be done to rule out necrotic breast cancer. Benign solid masses include fibroadenomas, lactating adenomas, and hamartomas, all of which can grow to impressive size within the hormonal milieu of pregnancy. A typical history for these benign neoplasms is that of a long-standing mass that undergoes rapid growth as gestation progresses. Focal breast infarcts also may occur in pregnancy due to hypertrophy of normal breast tissue beyond its blood supply; the resulting area of fat necrosis may be indistinguishable from cancer on both physical examination and sonography, making biopsy mandatory.[28] Although it has shown promise, MRI of the breast is still in its infancy. Lack of ionizing radiation makes it theoretically advantageous for use during pregnancy. However, the increased vascular flow and permeability of gestational breast tissue may decrease the sensitivity of gadolinium-enhanced MRI to detect malignancy.[29] Other disadvantages include expense and lack of radiologic expertise required for its interpretation.

Any suspicious lesion should undergo biopsy by either fine-needle aspiration or core-needle biopsy. Although there have been anecdotal reports of milk fistulas with the latter technique,[30] this is an extremely rare complication. The large tissue samples resulting from core biopsies increase the sensitivity and specificity of the biopsy. Excisional biopsy is warranted only if the clinical and radiologic suspicion of breast cancer is high, and a diagnosis has not been achieved with needle biopsy. Benign lesions such as fibroadenoma, lactating adenoma, or hamartoma can be safely followed until the end of the pregnancy and excised postpartum if indicated. A suggested management algorithm for puerperal breast masses is shown in Figure 35.5.

Breast cancer and pregnancy

In the USA, about 25 000 women between the ages of 18 and 44 are diagnosed with breast cancer each year. Within this age group, the subset of *gestational* breast cancer (defined as during or within 1 year of pregnancy) numbers 500–1500 cases (about 1 in 3000 to 1 in 10 000 live births). Unfortunately, because of the relative rarity of these coincident diagnoses, few data are available beyond reviews of retrospective series and expert

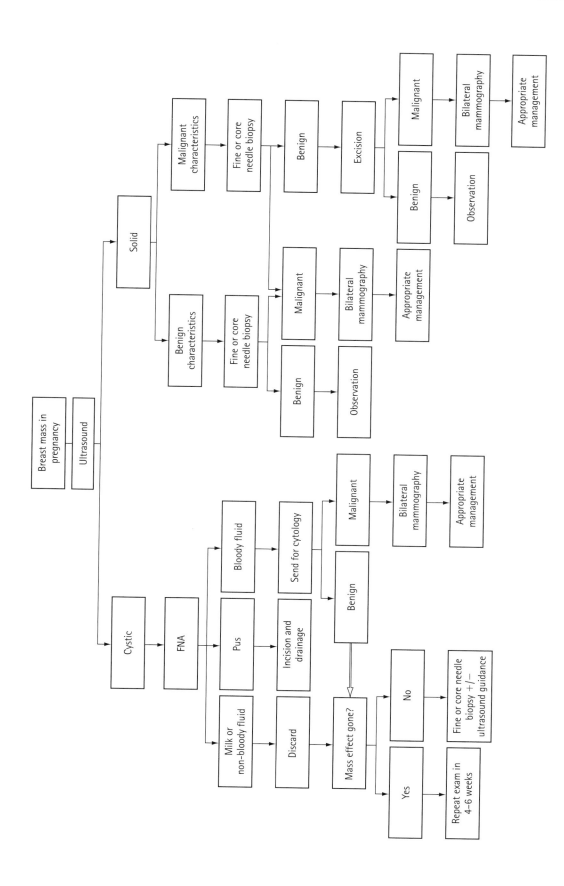

Figure 35.5 Management algorithm for breast masses in the puerperium. FNA, fine needle aspiration.

opinion. Prospective randomized data are absent. In addition to the complexity of the diagnostic and therapeutic issues, it is difficult to imagine a time during which the emotional consequences of a breast cancer diagnosis are more devastating.

Diagnosis

A high index of suspicion is required to make the diagnosis of gestational breast cancer. Ultrasound examination is often useful in differentiating solid lesions that are benign from those that are malignant. Cancers tend to be hypoechoic and spiculated, with heterogeneous internal echoes and acoustic shadowing (Figure 35.6). It is crucial to obtain this study *prior* to biopsy, since hematoma formation may hinder the interpretation of a subsequent ultrasound. After an ultrasound examination has been performed, a histopathologic diagnosis of palpable lesions may be attempted with a needle biopsy in the office. For lesions that are not clearly palpable, an ultrasound-directed needle biopsy is ideal. A nondiagnostic biopsy result from any mass that is clinically and/or sonographically suspicious mandates either repeat needle biopsy or a subsequent excisional biopsy.

Pretherapeutic staging

As always, preoperative staging begins with a thorough clinical examination. The size of the lesion and presence of skin or chest wall involvement should be documented. The axillary and supraclavicular lymph-node basins must also be carefully examined. A palpable supraclavicular node mandates fine-needle aspiration biopsy, as a positive result would preclude potentially curative surgery. Clinical staging (Tables 35.5 and 35.6) is important since it determines not only the initial treatment but also the extent of the pretreatment metastatic evaluation. Only liver chemistries and a chest radiograph with appropriate fetal shielding are required for clinical stage I or II

Table 35.5 Clinical TNM staging of breast cancer

Tis: carcinoma *in situ*
T1: tumor ≤2 cm
T2: tumor >2 cm but ≤5 cm
T3: tumor >5 cm
T4: tumor of any size with skin or chest wall involvement

N0: no palpable axillary lymph nodes
N1: palpable mobile axillary lymph nodes
N2: palpable fixed axillary lymph nodes
N3: palpable supraclavicular lymph nodes

M0: no metastasis
M1: metastatic disease present

T: tumor; N: nodes; M: metastasis.

disease, since the incidence of occult metastasis is less than 5%. For patients with more locally advanced cancers (clinical stage III), the significant incidence of metastasis (up to 25%) justifies bone scanning despite the radiation dose. MRI can be used to evaluate for visceral metastasis. Lastly, directed radiographic evaluation should be performed in patients of any clinical stage with symptoms (back or abdominal pain, weight loss) or significant laboratory abnormalities (e.g., elevated liver chemistries).

Treatment

The primary treatment of resectable breast cancer is surgery. The goals of surgery are as follows: (1) removal of the cancer with either mastectomy or lumpectomy; (2) staging of the axillary lymph nodes with sentinel lymph-node biopsy and/or axillary dissection. Modified radical mastectomy remains the standard local management of breast cancer in pregnancy, since

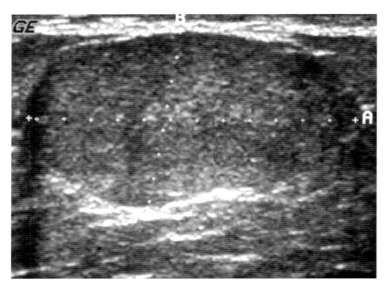
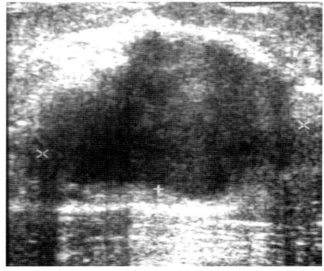

Figure 35.6 Ultrasound imaging of lactating adenoma (left) and gestational breast cancer (right). Note smooth regular border of the adenoma compared to irregularity, spiculation, and acoustic shadowing of the cancer.

Table 35.6 Clinical stage grouping of breast cancer

T	N	M	Stage
1	0	0	I
1	1	0	IIA
2	0	0	
2	1	0	IIB
3	0	0	
1	2	0	IIIA
2	2	0	
3	1	0	
3	2	0	
3	0–2	0	IIIB
Any	3	0	IIIC
Any	Any	1	IV

breast conservation therapy (lumpectomy followed by postoperative radiation) is essentially precluded by the fetal radiation risk. Furthermore, it has been hypothesized that the increased vascularity of the gestational breast may predispose to intramammary dissemination and an increased risk of local recurrence after lumpectomy. Small case series have described induction chemotherapy with subsequent breast conservation followed by postoperative, postpartum radiotherapy; however, long-term follow-up data on these patients is lacking.[31] Sentinel lymph-node biopsy is reserved for patients with breast cancer who do not have palpable lymphadenopathy. The radiation dose required for the procedure is negligible and therefore not contraindicated by fetal risk. There are no data on fetal toxicity or teratogenic effects of the isosulfan blue used in performing sentinel lymph node biopsy. There is about a 1% risk of severe maternal allergic reaction with the drug, leading some groups to avoid its use in pregnancy. Patients with sentinel lymph-node metastasis or palpable axillary nodes should undergo levels I and II axillary node dissection.

The role of therapeutic abortion in pregnant patients with breast cancer is frequently discussed. No data have ever definitively demonstrated that termination of pregnancy is of therapeutic benefit. Some old reports have even suggested that therapeutic abortion may have a *negative* impact on prognosis, but these studies are confounded by selection bias and staging discrepancies.[32,33] There is little question that abortion does make treatment decisions easier, since fetal risk is removed from consideration (e.g., radiation can be used with impunity). The decision for this step is therefore a highly personal one for the patient and family. Finally, it should be noted that fetal metastasis from maternal breast cancer has never been reported.

In addition to surgery, systemic chemotherapy and hormonal therapies are important components of the treatment of breast cancer. Chemotherapy can be given with relatively low fetal risk in the second and third trimesters. This point is illus-

trated by a retrospective French study in which 20 patients were given chemotherapy for breast cancer. Live healthy births were noted in 17 patients, spontaneous abortion occurred in both patients treated during the first trimester, and there was one intrauterine death in the second trimester.[34]. Although other groups have demonstrated similar results, it should be noted that long-term follow-up of infants born after this treatment is not available. The most commonly used agents are cyclophosphamide, doxo- or epirubicin, and 5-fluorouracil. The indications for chemotherapy are similar to those in nonpregnant women: (1) tumor size over 1 cm with poor prognostic characteristics (e.g., poorly differentiated or hormone receptor-negative) and/or (2) lymph-node metastasis. The timing of delivery should coincide with recovery from nadir white blood cell counts so that neonates are not born neutropenic. Chemotherapy is used more than hormonal therapy in pregnant women, since estrogen and/or progesterone receptor positivity of the tumors occurs less frequently in pregnant women than in age-matched controls (approximately 60% and 80%, respectively).[35] Consequently, in the absence of estrogen and/or progesterone positivity, hormonal treatment is often not useful. Tamoxifen has been associated with a significant risk of teratogenesis as well as spontaneous abortion and is not recommended antepartum.

Prognosis

Although the prognosis of gestational breast cancer stage for stage is similar to that of nonpregnant women, the overall prognosis is worse. Late diagnosis with resultant larger tumors and a higher rate of node positivity is thought to be primarily responsible for this unfortunate fact. However, one large study from France comparing 154 pregnant patients with 308 age-matched controls demonstrated that pregnancy was a significant and *independent* predictor of decreased survival.[35]

Future pregnancy in breast cancer survivors

Young breast cancer survivors contemplating pregnancy often receive conflicting advice. Unfortunately, for a small proportion of patients, the issue may be moot due to iatrogenic menopause from chemotherapy. This complication is related to type of drug, dose, and increasing patient age.[36] For example, in one study, 9% of women receiving doxorubicin were rendered permanently infertile.[37] In survivors capable of childbirth, there is no definitive evidence to suggest that future pregnancy worsens the ultimate prognosis.[38] Long-term overall survival tends to favor women who do experience post-treatment childbirth, a finding that most experts ascribe to the 'healthy mother effect'; that is, pregnancy is an indicator of good health and performance status.[39] The data on the interval from completion of treatment to the next childbirth are conflicting. Although two studies have shown a worse survival if this interval was less than 2 years, these studies are confounded by their retrospective nature and data collection mainly by physician investigator recall.[32,40] Other, similar studies have shown no difference in outcome with earlier pregnancy.[37] Given this uncertainty combined with the knowledge that breast cancer recurrence is most frequent in the first few years after treatment, most oncologists will advise prospective mothers to wait at least 1–2 years before getting pregnant. Certainly, this approach at least makes issues of further treatment less complicated in the event of recurrence.

General surgical endocrinology and the pregnant patient

Thyroid nodules and thyroid cancer

Although radionuclide scanning of the thyroid is contraindicated in pregnancy, evaluation of thyroid nodules is otherwise the same as that in nonpregnant individuals. Physical examination and fine-needle aspiration biopsy (with or without ultrasound guidance) are the primary diagnostic tools. As in the general population, well-differentiated thyroid cancers (papillary and follicular) are most common. Diagnosis during pregnancy has no negative prognostic import, and therapeutic abortion is not indicated. If discovered in the first half of pregnancy, these patients should undergo surgical resection during the second trimester. If thyroid cancer is found during the second half of pregnancy, it is usually prudent to delay the thyroidectomy until the postpartum period. Suppression therapy with exogenous thyroid hormone can be done during this period.

Medullary thyroid cancer (MTC) coincident with pregnancy is extremely rare. The diagnosis is suggested by the presence of a thyroid nodule associated with significant diarrhea; the latter is due to elevated serum levels of calcitonin. A thorough family history is important since approximately one-third of cases are hereditary, associated with either familial medullary thyroid cancer or type II multiple endocrine neoplasia. Genetic testing for germline mutations in the RET proto-oncogene should be performed in these patients. Due to its multifocality, total thyroidectomy with central neck lymph-node dissection is recommended. A careful evaluation for pheochromocytoma (see section below) should be done in suspected familial cases prior to delivery or any surgical intervention.

Hyperthyroidism

The diagnosis of hyperthyroidism is sometimes difficult in pregnancy because many of the hypermetabolic symptoms mimic that of gestation. Laboratory tests may also be equivocal, since pregnancy-related increases in thyroglobulin increase the protein-bound thyroid hormone (T_4) level (although not that of the free hormone). Hence, a high index of suspicion and measurement of both total and free T_4 is important for diagnosis. Graves' disease is the most frequent cause of puerperal hyperthyroidism and has an incidence of 0.2%.[41] Definitive treatment with radioactive iodine (RAI) is contraindicated in pregnant patients. Thus, the key goal is to achieve a euthyroid state with propylthiouracil (PTU) until RAI can be safely administered during the postpartum period. PTU is usually started at 100 mg t.i.d. and is adjusted according to the patient's clinical response with T_4 levels being monitored once a month. Neonatal hypothyroidism, as a consequence of PTU treatment,

has an incidence of 6–7% and is usually temporary.[41,42] Breast-feeding is not contraindicated with PTU treatment as the drug has limited transfer into breast milk. Thyroidectomy (ideally during the second trimester) is indicated only if there is a clear failure of medical management or in the rare instance of hyperthyroidism associated with a goiter large enough to cause airway compromise. Treatment of toxic multinodular goiters is similar to that for Graves' disease, while toxic uninodular goiters can be treated with either simple excision in the second trimester or percutaneous alcohol injection.[43]

Hyperparathyroidism

Although an uncommon problem, hypercalcemia during pregnancy can be associated with significant maternal and fetal morbidity. For the expectant mother, there is an increased risk above that of the general population of known hypercalcemia-related complications, such as nephrolithiasis (and associated urinary tract infection) and pancreatitis. Furthermore, hyperemesis gravidum seems to be significantly worsened by coexistent hypercalcemia. For the fetus, the risk of growth retardation, premature delivery, and miscarriage is significant and has been reported to be as high as 50% in untreated cases. Additionally, the fetal parathyroid glands are severely inhibited by the high maternal parathyroid hormone (PTH) level, resulting in neonatal hypocalcemia and tetany if maternal hyperparathyroidism is not recognized and treated.[44]

The most frequent presentation of hyperparathyroidism is an elevated calcium level on routine serum chemistries. The diagnosis of hyperparathyroidism is suggested by an elevation in the chloride/phosphate ratio greater than 33. Elevation in the serum PTH level is pathognomonic. A careful history can often elicit many of the above symptoms as well as more subtle changes often ascribed to pregnancy itself, such as fatigue, depression, and muscle weakness. Although coincidental hypertension is much more commonly due to preeclampsia (especially in the third trimester), it should also raise the possibility of pheochromocytoma and multiple endocrine neoplasia type IIA. A history of severe peptic ulcer disease may suggest the presence of a gastrinoma (a pancreatic islet cell tumor) and multiple endocrine neoplasia type I. These patients may also have pituitary neoplasms, most commonly prolactinomas; the latter often cause infertility.

In accord with the NIH Consensus Statement on treatment of hyperparathyroidism released in 1990, patients with serum calcium of $\geq$12 mg/dl and any evidence of not otherwise explainable renal dysfunction, nephrolithiasis, diminished bone density, or history of hypercalcemic crisis are considered surgical candidates. Surgery is also offered to young patients (under 50 years of age) and those unwilling or unable to continue medical follow-up. Those who are truly asymptomatic, have serum calcium under 12 mg/dl, and are willing to undergo careful surveillance need not have surgery.[45] Whether this latter guideline can be applied to pregnant women, given the previously described maternal and fetal risks, is controversial. If conservative management is elected on the basis of the above recommendations, careful maternal surveillance is mandatory, since early recognition and prompt treatment of neonatal hypocalcemia with oral or IV supplementation are crucial. Maternal acute hypercalcemic crisis mandates close monitoring of the mother and fetus. Management is initially with normal saline infusions. Once adequate volume repletion is achieved in accordance with urine output, IV furosemide can be administered to promote calcium excretion. Calcitonin is also given to lower serum calcium acutely. Bisphosphonates, such as etidronate, act to inhibit osteoclastic activity and should be used with trepidation in the pregnant patient, because they cross the placental barrier and their effects on fetal bone development are unknown. Once stabilized, semiurgent parathyroidectomy should be scheduled. Although best done during the second trimester, surgery should not be delayed in the third trimester if the mother has symptomatic hypercalcemia, as the risk of fetal morbidity and mortality with surgery appears to be outweighed by that from the disease itself.[44,46]

Pheochromocytoma

Although it is a rare disease, missing the diagnosis of pheochromocytoma in pregnancy can have lethal consequences for both mother and fetus.[47] The diagnosis should be suggested by hypertension (which can be sustained and/or episodic) that frequently predates the pregnancy and often requires more than one medication to be controlled. Preeclampsia is the most common cause of hypertension in pregnancy; however, it is relatively infrequent before the third trimester. Proteinuria is rarely associated with pheochromocytoma. As with hyperthyroidism, the symptoms of pheochromocytoma (headaches, palpitations, and anxiety) may be attributed to those of pregnancy, so a high index of suspicion is required. A careful family history is mandatory, since up to 25% of these tumors are genetic in origin; for example, they may be associated with multiple endocrine neoplasia type IIA (in association with hyperparathyroidism and medullary thyroid cancer) or von Hippel-Lindau disease among others.[48] As in the general population, the biochemical diagnosis of a pheochromocytoma is made by a 24-hour collection of urine for catecholamines and metanephrines. Rarely, patients with mainly episodic hypertension may require inpatient observation with plasma catecholamine levels sent at the time of the symptomatic and/or hypertensive event to establish the diagnosis. MRI can be used to image the adrenals and assess for bilateral or extra-adrenal disease. Not surprisingly, these two findings are more common in genetic syndromes. ^{131}I-MIBG scanning can localize extraadrenal pheochromocytomas; however, the utility of this nuclear medicine study in pregnancy is limited. Tumors larger than 6 cm or in an extra-adrenal location are more likely to be malignant (10% of pheochromocytomas); however, the only definitive criteria for malignancy is the presence of metastasis.[49] Percutaneous biopsy is contraindicated due to the possibility of precipitating a hypertensive crisis.

Treatment begins with medical control of the hypertension by alpha-adrenergic blockade. The typical first-line drugs are phenoxybenzamine (10 mg b.i.d.) or prazosin (1 mg b.i.d.). The dose is slowly escalated, usually over a period of a few weeks, until postural hypotension is achieved. It is important to avoid hypovolemia during this period. Persistent tachycardia and palpitations after adequate alpha blockade may suggest a tumor that predominantly secretes epinephrine, and is treated with beta-adrenergic blocking agents, such as atenolol or metoprolol. Patients presenting in hypertensive crisis require admission to the intensive care unit and treatment with hydralazine or nitroprusside. Potential fetal cyanide toxicity (which may partly be abrogated with sodium thiosulfate treatment) relegates nitroprusside to second-line drug status.[50] Adrenalectomy should be performed only after successful medical control of the hypertension. Due to the rarity of cases, evidence-based management strategies for timing and method of resection are lacking. In general, patients diagnosed in the first 26 weeks of pregnancy are advised to undergo adrenal resection in the second trimester once alpha- +/− beta-blockade has been achieved. Cases discovered in the third trimester can be resected under the same anesthetic immediately after elective cesarean section once fetal maturity is reached.[51,52] Alternatively, if the hypertension is well controlled, and it is felt that labor will not be prolonged (as shown by history of previous pregnancy), vaginal delivery with later elective adrenalectomy is feasible. Laparoscopic resection is quickly gaining acceptance as the standard of care in experienced hands due to its lower postoperative pain and recovery time.[53] There are no data to suggest carbon dioxide insufflation into the peritoneal cavity has any negative consequences to the fetus. In any event, whether done open or laparoscopically, it is critical that this rare and complex problem be managed in a multidisciplinary manner by an experienced team of surgeons, obstetricians, neonatologists, and anesthesiologists.

Melanoma

The incidence of melanoma is rising faster than that of any other malignancy, such that, in 2005, one in 50 Americans will be afflicted. The disease affects a much younger patient population than other cancers, with median age at diagnosis being in the mid-40s.[54] The diagnosis and treatment of melanoma in the puerperium is not appreciably different from that of any other patient. Suspicious cutaneous lesions are evaluated according to the 'ABCDE' rule. Asymmetry, border irregularity, color variegation, diameter greater than 10 mm and elevation, of a mole should all prompt expedient biopsy. A long-standing, benign-appearing mole that has undergone recent change in color, size, or ulceration also warrants further workup.[55] For small lesions, excisional biopsy with narrow margins (1–2 mm) should be done. Larger moles can be biopsied with a punch instrument, done in the part of the lesion that is thickest and/or most ulcerated.

The primary therapy of melanomas is surgical, with the extent of the surgery being related to the stage of the disease. Melanomas are staged according to thickness (mm), while the margin of a definitive surgical excision is determined by the depth of invasion. Tumors less than 1 mm thick are excised with 1-cm margins; tumors 1–2 mm in thickness, with 2-cm margins; and those over 2 mm in thickness, with at least 2-cm margins. Most of these procedures can be done under local anesthesia, thus negating the fetal risk of general anesthesia. Patients with palpable regional lymph nodes should undergo full lymphadenectomy. Patients without palpable regional nodes who have lesions over 1 mm in thickness are candidates for sentinel lymph-node biopsy to determine the extent of disease and plan the need for any further therapy. As discussed in the breast cancer section, the radiopharmaceutic dose has negligible fetal risk, but the isosulfan blue dye occasionally causes severe maternal allergic reactions, leading many surgical oncologists to perform the procedure only with the former in pregnant patients. A positive sentinel node usually leads to full lymphadenectomy.

Coincident pregnancy carries no negative prognostic implications in melanoma.[56] Therapeutic abortion is not indicated. Patients with stage IV disease who become pregnant should have the placenta carefully evaluated, since one study demonstrated a 22% risk of fetal metastasis if the placenta was also involved.[57]

References

1. Visser BC, Glasgow RE, Mulvihill KK et al. Safety and timing of nonobstetric abdominal surgery in pregnancy. Dig Surg 2001; 18: 409–17.
2. Timins JK. Radiation during pregnancy. N J Med 2001; 98: 29–33.
3. Kal HB, Struikmans H. [Pregnancy and medical irradiation; summary and conclusions from the International Commission on Radiological Protection. Publication 84]. Ned Tijdschr Geneeskd 2002; 146: 299–303.
4. Brent RL. The effect of embryonic and fetal exposure to x-ray, microwaves and ultrasound: counseling the pregnant and non-pregnant patient about these risks. Semin Oncol 1989; 16: 347–68.
5. Mann FA, Nathens A, Langer SG et al. Communicating with the family: the risks of medical irradiation to conceptuses in victims of major blunt-force torso trauma. J Trauma 2000; 48: 354–7.
6. Kusama T, Ota K. Radiological protection for diagnostic examination of pregnant women. Congenit Anom (Kyoto) 2002; 42: 10–14.
7. Damilakis J, Perisinakis K, Voloudaki A et al. Estimation of fetal radiation dose from computed tomography scanning in late pregnancy: depth-dose data from routine examinations. Invest Radiol 2000; 35: 527–37.
8. Steenvoorde P, Pauwels EK, Harding LK, et al. Diagnostic nuclear medicine and risk for the fetus. Eur J Nucl Med 1998; 25: 193–9.
9. Cobben LP, Groot I, Haans L et al. MRI for clinically suspected appendicitis during pregnancy. AJR Am J Roentgenol 2004; 183: 671–5.
10. Cameron J. Current Surgical Therapy, pp. 271–2. (7th edition). Mosby: St Louis, MO, 2001.
11. Swisher SG, Schmit PJ, Hunt KK et al. Biliary disease during pregnancy. Am J Surg 1994; 168: 576–9; discussion 580–1.
12. Ghuman E, Barry M, Grace PA. Management of gallstones in pregnancy. Br J Surg 1997; 84: 1646–50.
13. Muench J, Albrink M, Serafini F et al. Delay in treatment of biliary disease during pregnancy increases morbidity and can be avoided with safe laparoscopic cholecystectomy. Am Surg 2001; 67: 539–42; discussion 542–3.
14. Graham G, Baxi L, Tharakan T. Laparoscopic cholecystectomy during pregnancy: a case series and review of the literature. Obstet Gynecol Surg 1998; 5: 566–74.
15. Legro RS, Laifer SA. First-trimester pancreatitis. Maternal and neonatal outcome. J Reprod Med 1995; 40: 689–95.
16. Tham TC, Vandervoort J, Wong RC et al. Safety of ERCP during pregnancy. Am J Gastroenterol 2003; 98: 308–11.
17. Moser MA, Okun NB, Mayes DC et al. Crohn's disease, pregnancy, and birth weight. Am J Gastroenterol 2000; 95: 1021–6.
18. Morales M, Berney T, Jenny A et al. Crohn's disease as a risk factor for the outcome of pregnancy. Hepatogastroenterology 2000; 47: 1595–8.
19. Dominitz JA, Young JC, Boyko EJ. Outcomes of infants born to mothers with inflammatory bowel disease: a population based cohort study. Am J Gastroenterol 2002; 97: 641–8.
20. Gur C, Diav-Citrin O, Shechtman S et al. Pregnancy outcome after first trimester exposure to corticosteroids: a prospective controlled study. Reprod Toxicol 2004; 18: 93–101.
21. Connell W, Miller A. Treating inflammatory bowel disease during pregnancy: risks and safety of drug therapy. Drug Saf 1999; 21: 311–23.
22. Ferraro S, Ragni N. Inflammatory bowel disease: management issues during pregnancy. Arch Gynecol Obstet 2004; 270: 79–85. Epub 2003 Apr 30.
23. Kujovich JL. Hormones and pregnancy: thromboembolic risks for women. Br J Haematol 2004; 126: 443–54.
24. Toglia MR, Weg JG. Venous thromboembolism during pregnancy. N Engl J Med 1996; 335: 108–14.
25. D'Ambrosio R, Ricciardelli L, Lanni GL et al. [Intraperitoneal hemorrhage from rupture of an aneurysm of splenic artery: case report and literature review]. Ann Ital Cir 2003; 74: 97–101.
26. Smith LH, Danielsen B, Allen ME, Cress R. Cancer associated with obstetric delivery: results of linkage with the California cancer registry. Am J Obstet Gynecol 2003; 189: 1128–35.
27. Hogge JP, De Paredes ES, Magnant CM, Lage J. Imaging and management of breast masses during pregnancy and lactation. Breast J 1999; 5: 272–83.
28. Scott-Conner CE, Schorr SJ. The diagnosis and management of breast problems during pregnancy and lactation. Am J Surg 1995; 170: 401–5.
29. Talele AC, Slanetz PJ, Edmister WB et al. The lactating breast: MRI findings and literature review. Breast J 2003; 9: 237–40.
30. Schackmuth EM, Harlow CL, Norton LW. Milk fistula: a complication after core breast biopsy. AJR Am J Roentgenol 1993; 161: 961–2.

31. Kuerer HM, Gwyn K, Ames FC, Theriault RL. Conservative surgery and chemotherapy for breast carcinoma during pregnancy. Surgery 2002; 131: 108–10.

32. Clark RM, Chua T. Breast cancer and pregnancy: the ultimate challenge. Clin Oncol (R Coll Radiol) 1989; 1: 11–18.

33. King RM, Welch JS, Martin JK Jr, Coulam CB. Carcinoma of the breast associated with pregnancy. Surg Gynecol Obstet 1985; 160: 228–32.

34. Giacalone PL, Laffargue F, Benos P. Chemotherapy for breast carcinoma during pregnancy: a French national survey. Cancer 1999; 86: 2266–72.

35. Bonnier P, Romain S, Dilhuydy JM et al. Influence of pregnancy on the outcome of breast cancer: a case-control study. Société Française de sénologie et de pathologie mammaire Study Group. Int J Cancer 1997; 72: 720–7.

36. Surbone A, Petrek JA. Childbearing issues in breast carcinoma survivors. Cancer 1997; 79: 1271–8.

37. Sutton R, Buzdar AU, Hortobagyi GN. Pregnancy and offspring after adjuvant chemotherapy in breast cancer patients. Cancer 1990; 65: 847–50.

38. Velentgas P, Daling JR, Malone KE et al. Pregnancy after breast carcinoma: outcomes and influence on mortality. Cancer 1999; 85: 2424–32.

39. Sankila R, Heinavaara S, Hakulinen T. Survival of breast cancer patients after subsequent term pregnancy: 'healthy mother effect'. Am J Obstet Gynecol 1994; 170: 818–23.

40. Kroman N, Wohlfahrt J, Andersen KW et al. Time since childbirth and prognosis in primary breast cancer: population based study. BMJ 1997; 315: 851–5.

41. Lazarus JH, Kokandi A. Thyroid disease in relation to pregnancy: a decade of change. Clin Endocrinol (Oxf) 2000; 53: 265–78.

42. Kriplani A, Buckshee K, Bhargava VL et al. Maternal and perinatal outcome in thyrotoxicosis complicating pregnancy. Eur J Obstet Gynecol Reprod Biol 1994; 54: 159–63.

43. Wemeau JL, Do Cao C. [Thyroid nodule, cancer and pregnancy]. Ann Endocrinol (Paris) 2002; 63: 438–42.

44. Schnatz PF, Curry SL. Primary hyperparathyroidism in pregnancy: evidence-based management. Obstet Gynecol Surv 2002; 57: 365–76.

45. NIH Conference. Diagnosis and management of asymptomatic primary hyperparathyroidism: consensus development conference statement. Ann Intern Med 1991; 114: 593–7.

46. Kort KC, Schiller HJ, Numann PJ. Hyperparathyroidism and pregnancy. Am J Surg 1999; 177: 66–8.

47. Harper MA, Murnaghan GA, Kennedy L et al. Phaeochromocytoma in pregnancy. Five cases and a review of the literature. Br J Obstet Gynaecol 1989; 96: 594–606.

48. Neumann HP, Bausch B, McWhinney SR et al. Germ-line mutations in nonsyndromic pheochromocytoma. N Engl J Med 2002; 346: 1459–66.

49. Harrington JL, Farley DR, van Heerden JA, Ramin KD. Adrenal tumors and pregnancy. World J Surg 1999; 23: 182–6.

50. Shoemaker CT, Meyers M. Sodium nitroprusside for control of severe hypertensive disease of pregnancy: a case report and discussion of potential toxicity. Am J Obstet Gynecol 1984; 149: 171–3.

51. Botchan A, Hauser R, Kupfermine M et al. Pheochromocytoma in pregnancy: case report and review of the literature. Obstet Gynecol Surv 1995; 50: 321–7.

52. Freier DT, Thompson NW. Pheochromocytoma and pregnancy: the epitome of high risk. Surgery 1993; 114: 1148–52.

53. Brunt LM. Phaeochromocytoma in pregnancy. Br J Surg 2001; 88: 481–3.

54. Rigel DS, Carucci JA. Malignant melanoma: prevention, early detection, and treatment in the 21st century. CA Cancer J Clin 2000; 50: 215–36; quiz 237–40.

55. Whited JD, Grichnik JM. The rational clinical examination. Does this patient have a mole or a melanoma? JAMA 1998; 279: 696–701.

56. Driscoll MS, Grin-Jorgensen CM, Grant-Kels JM. Does pregnancy influence the prognosis of malignant melanoma? J Am Acad Dermatol 1993; 29: 619–30.

57. Alexander A, Samlowski WE, Grossman D, et al. Metastatic melanoma in pregnancy: risk of transplacental metastases in the infant. J Clin Oncol 2003; 21: 2179–86.

36 Urologic complications during pregnancy

Stuart S Kesler, Neel Shah, and Jonathan J Hwang

A wide range of urologic complications during pregnancy are possible, ranging from urinary tract infection to life-threatening trauma. The pregnant patient with urologic problems merits careful evaluation and requires special consideration due to potential risks to the developing fetus. Often, symptoms related to urinary tract abnormalities are misconstrued and dismissed as part of the normal physiologic response to pregnancy. This may lead to a delay in diagnosis and treatment. The evaluation and management of the pregnant patient may differ significantly from patients experiencing similar urologic complaints in a nonobstetric setting. Thus, a thorough understanding of potential urologic problems encountered during pregnancy is crucial in order to minimize morbidity to the mother and fetus through early recognition and intervention. This chapter will provide a comprehensive review of urologic complications and issues related to pregnancy.

Physiologic changes of pregnancy

The urinary tract undergoes dramatic physiologic alterations during pregnancy. Dilation of the renal pelvis and ureters, which begins in the first trimester and is present in about 90% of women by the third trimester, has been recognized as a physiologic response to mechanical and hormonal changes of pregnancy. This physiologic pyelouretectasis occurs only above the pelvic brim. The lower third of the ureters retain a normal caliber despite the fact that they must course around the rapidly enlarging gravid uterus. Lower ureteral dilation suggests ureterovesical junction obstruction, a condition which may have antedated the pregnancy. The right side is more often affected than the left. In a review of 220 excretory urograms during pregnancy, Schulman and Herlinger reported greater dilation of the right side in 86% of the cases.[1] This predilection is attributed to mechanical pressure at the pelvic brim by the dextrorotation of the pregnant uterus as it rises out of the pelvis, whereas the left ureter is protected by the sigmoid colon.[2] Hormonal changes leading to increased urinary tract compliance and reduced ureteral muscle tone are believed to be primarily responsible for dilation of the upper urinary system during the first trimester.[3,4]

Renal adaptations associated with pregnancy include a 30–50% increase in glomerular filtration rate and renal plasma flow.[5] These changes lead to a 25% reduction in serum creatinine and blood urea nitrogen levels. Serum levels of 1,25-dihydroxyvitamin D are found to be elevated during pregnancy, promoting a hypercalciuric state by increasing intestinal absorption of calcium and stimulating urinary calcium excretion.[6]

Urinary tract infection and pyelonephritis

Asymptomatic bacteriuria affects 2–7% of all pregnant women.[7,8] Although pregnancy itself is not believed to predispose women to urinary tract infections, approximately 25% of pregnant women with documented asymptomatic bacteriuria without treatment progress to pyelonephritis. Antimicrobial treatment of asymptomatic bacteriuria has been shown to reduce the incidence of pyelonephritis to 3–4%.[8] Prematurity, maternal hypertension, and maternal anemia have been associated with pyelonephritis during pregnancy.[9,10] Thus, routine screening early in pregnancy for asymptomatic bacteriuria is recommended.

An awareness of potential drug toxicities to the mother and fetus is important prior to antibiotic administration (Table 36.1). Continuous antibiotic suppression with nitrofurantoin has been advocated by some for frequent, recurrent urinary tract infections.[9] Recurrent or persistent bacteriuria episodes are associated with an increased risk of structural abnormalities of the urinary tract,[11] and these patients should undergo a complete, postpartum, urologic workup.

Table 36.1 Potential toxicity of antibiotics during pregnancy

Drug	Fetal	Maternal
Aminoglycosides	CNS toxicity, ototoxicity	Ototoxicity, nephrotoxicity
Cephalosporins	–	–
Chloramphenicol	Gray syndrome	Bone marrow toxicity
Clindamycin	–	Pseudomembranous colitis
Erythromycins	–	–
Isoniazide	Neuropathy, seizures	Hepatotoxicity
Metronidazole	–	Blood dyscrasia
Nitrofurantoin	G6PD hemolysis	Neuropathy, interstitial pneumonia
Penicillin	–	–
Quinolones	Bone growth malformation	–
Sulfonamides	G6PD hemolysis, kernicterus	–
Tetracycline	Tooth dysplasia, bone growth inhibition	Hepatotoxicity, renal failure
Trimethoprim/sulfamethoxazole	Folate depletion	Vasculitis

Hydroureteronephrosis and spontaneous renal rupture

Mechanical obstructive uropathy may cause acute pain, hypertension, or even acute renal failure.[12–14] In evaluating the pregnant patient with flank pain, it is important to differentiate upper tract dilation due to 'physiologic' hydronephrosis from clinically significant obstruction secondary to pre-existing congenital or acquired causes. Congenital ureteropelvic junction obstruction from intrinsic stenosis or extrinsic crossing vessels may be obscured or enhanced by hydronephrosis of pregnancy. Ureteral dilation below the pelvic brim strongly suggests pre-existing obstruction near or at the bladder. The detection of ureteral jets on bladder ultrasonography, either performed transvaginally or transabdominally, is an excellent screening method for confirming ureteral patency.[15,16]

Spontaneous rupture of the kidney or collecting system is a rare event, often presenting with flank pain, hematuria, hypotension, an expanding flank mass, or signs of an acute abdomen.[17] If unrecognized, rupture may lead to catastrophic consequences, including maternal shock and intrauterine fetal demise. Rupture associated with hydronephrosis of pregnancy is often preceded by abnormally massive dilation, repeated episodes of pyelonephritis, or a history of prior renal disease causing inelastic or scarred renal parenchyma. Oesterling et al described 16 cases of spontaneous rupture during pregnancy: 10 cases of collecting system rupture and six cases of renal parenchymal rupture.[18] Five cases occurred in the second trimester and 11 were diagnosed during the third trimester or immediately postpartum. Only three cases involved the left kidney, all of which had pre-existing renal disease. Of the six cases with parenchymal rupture, five were managed with a nephrectomy and one patient died prior to surgery. In contrast, only four of the 10 patients with renal pelvic rupture underwent nephrectomy. The remainder of patients were managed conservatively with successful renal salvage and appropriate internal (five) or external (one) drainage.

The greatest risk of renal rupture occurs between week 18 of gestation and the immediate postpartum period. A conservative approach with bed rest in the contralateral decubitus position should be attempted in cases recognized early. Symptomatic hydronephrosis can be managed with early urinary diversion, utilizing a percutaneous nephrostomy or internal ureteral stent. Since renal cell carcinoma is the most common renal neoplasm during pregnancy, and spontaneous rupture is possible, postpartum radiographic studies are important in those treated with successful renal salvage. Asymptomatic angiomyolipomas have the propensity to grow rapidly during pregnancy.[19] Therefore, to avoid the risk of spontaneous rupture, some have suggested that women who intend to conceive should undergo prophylactic angioembolization for tumors greater than 4 cm.[20]

Stone disease

Calculous disease in the pregnant patient often presents a major therapeutic and diagnostic challenge for physicians of various specialties. In addition to the welfare of the patient, the well-being of the fetus must be considered. Symptoms of ureteral colic often imitate those commonly seen in pyelonephritic patients, in pregnant females with other intra-abdominal disorder, and in the normal pregnancy state. In an attempt to avoid fetal radiation exposure, physicians often restrict imaging studies, thereby limiting their diagnostic accuracy. Thus, the diagnosis and management of urolithiasis in the pregnant woman can be quite complex and requires a thorough, systematic approach.

The overall incidence of urolithiasis during pregnancy is estimated to be one in 1500 pregnancies,[21] which approximates the incidence in nonpregnant women of childbearing age.[22]

Although 50–80% of stones in pregnant women pass spontaneously,[23] urinary calculi must be taken seriously, as they have been associated with premature labor.[21,24] Although right-sided hydronephrosis is more commonly identified during pregnancy, multiple investigators report equivalent stone rates bilaterally.[25] Approximately 90% of urinary stones occur during the second and third trimesters, making colic in the first trimester rare.

There is little difference in the presentation of urinary colic between the pregnant and nonpregnant female. Complaints of flank or abdominal pain, nausea, vomiting, dysuria, frequency, urgency, or any combination of the above are customary. In the setting of calculi, the incidence of hematuria is 50–75%. Mechanical and hormonal changes have both been found to cause vascular dilation of the ureter and renal pelvis, leading to bleeding. Therefore, hematuria alone is not enough to make the diagnosis. A thorough past medical history is vital to an accurate and timely diagnosis. Some 35–40% of patients were found to have prior urologic procedures or a history of stone disease.[25,26] Fever is not infrequent, but it is a more ominous sign and must be monitored closely. Physicians should maintain a high index of suspicion for obstructing urinary calculi, especially in patients diagnosed with pyelonephritis who fail to defervesce after at least 48 hours of intravenous antibiotic therapy. Peritoneal signs found on abdominal examination should raise suspicion of nonurologic etiology; differential diagnoses include appendicitis, pyelonephritis, cholecystitis, small and large bowel disease, and ovarian and uterine etiology.

As physicians may avoid studies utilizing ionizing radiation, the diagnosis of urinary calculi during pregnancy can often be challenging. Although a complete discussion about fetal radiation exposure is beyond the scope of this chapter, a brief discussion is as follows. Ionizing radiation induces cell death in mammalian cells through direct ionization, and also indirectly through involvement of free radical complexes with cellular structures. Fetal cells undergo accelerated proliferation and are thought to be more sensitive to radiation. Potential risk to the fetus is primarily dependent upon two factors, namely, gestational stage and radiation dose. Very early radiation exposure during preimplantation (0–2 weeks) can lead to either spontaneous abortion or no effect on the fetus (an all-or-none phenomenon). In early organogenesis (2–16 weeks), growth retardation and teratogenesis predominate. Later fetal stages seem to be more resistant to radiation, but functional disorders have been reported.[27] Embryos usually receive less than 100 mrad of radiation throughout an entire pregnancy due to background radiation, and the Radiation Safety Committee of the Centers for Disease Control and Prevention recommends that laboratory workers not exceed a cumulative dose of 500 mrad during pregnancy (1 Gy = 100 rad).[28] The carcinogenic effect of prenatal radiation exposure has been a highly controversial topic, with multiple studies reporting conflicting findings.[29,30] With the lack of overwhelming evidence to support or oppose an absolute radiation restriction, and due to the ever increasing reluctance of pregnant women to expose their fetus to radiation, the authors avoid this potential risk in the setting of urinary stones. Our approach is consistent with that of Loughlin, who states, 'It would therefore seem most prudent for the urologist to avoid any radiation to the fetus during gestation, unless the radiographic study is going to have a major impact on the management of the mother.'[31]

Numerous diagnostic tests, including standard radiography, ultrasound, computed tomography (CT), and magnetic resonance imaging (MRI), have been used to help identify stones during pregnancy. In the past, intravenous pyelography (IVP) and abdominal radiographs were commonplace during pregnancy, but an unwillingness to expose the fetus to radiation has limited their use in recent years. Still, some perform a limited IVP consisting of a scout film, a 30–60 minute film, and an optional delayed film.[32] The number of CT scans has also declined significantly, as they emit approximately 3000 mrad of radiation to the fetus. Estimated doses of radiation emitted from various radiographic procedures are listed in Table 36.2. Harmful fetal effects are not expected with exposures less than 5 rad.

Ultrasound appears particularly attractive as a first-line intervention because of the avoidance of radiation. Although this technology is most commonly utilized, it is also the most inefficient in diagnostic accuracy. With hydronephrosis of pregnancy extremely common, ultrasound is notoriously nonspecific for obstruction when calculi are not clearly identified.[25] Conversely, some describe satisfactory results with ultrasound confirmation alone.[33] Modern ultrasound has improved resolution and flow capabilities. Using color Doppler, some have associated the lack of ureteral jets,[34] or the presence of a dilated ureter below the iliac artery with obstruction.[32] Shokeir et al reported on 22 pregnant patients, using elevated renal resistive index to diagnose unilateral obstruction with sensitivity and specificity of 45% and 91%, respectively.[35] MRI has also been used to differentiate the physiologic hydronephrosis of pregnancy from pathologic obstruction with good results.[36] MRI has not been found to cause cellular mutagenesis and is believed to be safe during pregnancy.

The management of symptomatic urinary calculi in the pregnant female has been highly debated in the urologic literature. In the past, urinary diversion with ureteral stent or

Table 36.2 Estimated fetal radiation exposure from radiographic imaging

Radiographic examination	Fetal dose (mrad)
Upper gastrointestinal series	100
Pelvic film	200
Abdominal KUB	250
Lumbar spine film	400
Intravenous pyelogram	480
Retrograde pyelogram	600
Barium enema	1000
CT abdomen	3000

KUB, Kidney/ureter/bladder X-ray.

nephrostomy tube placement was the first intervention to treat the acute episode, with definitive stone removal performed postpartum. More recently, many have advocated therapeutic stone intervention during pregnancy. However, due to the high rates of spontaneous stone passage, the *initial* treatment modality should be conservative with hydration, antiemetics, and adequate pain control. Nonsteroidal anti-inflammatories (NSAIDs) may cause constriction of the fetal ductus arteriosus. Therefore, their use is strongly discouraged, especially after 32 weeks' gestation. *Immediate* surgical intervention is warranted in cases complicated by sepsis, intractable pain, renoureteral colic precipitating premature labor, a solitary kidney, or bilateral ureteral obstruction.

Endoscopic ureteral stenting is part of the urologist's routine stone management armamentarium. Local or intravenous sedation is usually sufficient. Ultrasound has replaced fluoroscopy in many institutions to confirm accurate stent placement.[37] Hyperuricosuria and absorptive hypercalciuria found during pregnancy may cause accelerated encrustation, requiring more frequent stent exchanges. These additional procedures may place the mother and fetus at increased risk.[38]

With the gravid uterus reaching maximum size during later stages of pregnancy, some believe that percutaneous nephrostomy tube placement may be more reasonable than internal ureteral stenting. Nephrostomy tube placement is routinely performed under ultrasound guidance and, like stent placement, does not require general anesthesia. We have not found ureteral stenting in the pregnant female to be significantly more challenging, and it is our preferred method of urinary diversion. Some studies have found significant degrees of discomfort and higher rates of infection with nephrostomy tubes compared with ureteral stents.[39] In select circumstances, percutaneous nephrostomy tube placement may achieve greater urinary diversion and prove to be the treatment of choice.

Percutaneous nephrolithotomy (PCNL) in the pregnant patient has been attempted by some, but is still highly controversial. Denstedt and Razvi reported a woman of 24 weeks' gestation who delivered prematurely 2 days after PCNL.[23] In concurrence with others,[39] we do not recommend PCNL in pregnant patients.

There are few studies evaluating extracorporeal shock wave lithotripsy (ESWL) during pregnancy. The general consensus has been that ESWL in the pregnant woman is contraindicated by both shock wave energy and radiographic imaging. Asgari et al reported on six women who were unknowingly pregnant at the time of their ESWL treatment.[40] No teratogenic malformations, chromosome abnormalities, or abortions were identified in those children. Ohmori et al reported on the effect of ESWL on pregnant mice fetuses.[41] The timing of ESWL treatment in relation to conception and the number of shock waves given were considered. A higher number of shocks given farther from the time of conception correlated with decreased fetal survival rates and histologic findings of brain, lung, and subcutaneous hemorrhages. More studies are required, but the present literature raises serious concerns about ESWL treatment during pregnancy. At our institution, it is mandated that all women of child-bearing age are required to have a preoperative beta-human chorionic gonadotropin (β-HCG) prior to ESWL and a positive test is considered an absolute contraindication.

Innovative techniques and technological advances have made an astounding impact on the field of endourology in recent years. Originally, some believed that the ureter of the pregnant female would be difficult to navigate secondary to distortion.[39] In reality, physiologic hydroureteronephrosis may make ureteroscopy easier. Over the past decade, a number of reports have supported the use of rigid and flexible ureteroscopy to treat pregnant women with calculi.[23,26,35,37,42,42–46] Modern ureteroscopes are less traumatic, and ureteroscopy may often be performed without fluoroscopy[47] or dilation of the ureteral orifice.[42] The majority of urologists maintain a temporary ureteral stent in place for 1–4 days after ureteroscopy. Some authorities prefer holmium:YAG laser lithotripsy to electrohydraulic lithotripsy for its low peak pressures.[48] Furthermore, some avoid using ultrasonic lithotripsy for fear of causing hearing injury to the fetus.[45] Continuous fetal monitoring must be maintained at all times throughout the operative procedure.

Ureteroscopy may also assist in differentiating ureteral colic from pain related to physiologic hydronephrosis. Ulvik et al detailed ureteroscopy in 24 pregnant patients.[45] In 48% of those cases, urinary calculi were *not* identified. Without undergoing ureteroscopy, these patients might have suffered from a stent or nephrostomy tube for the remainder of their pregnancy without justification.

To date, no major complications from ureteroscopy have been reported. Minor complications include fever in three patients (two had preoperative urinary tract infections) and one ureteral perforation managed with a ureteral stent.[45] Relative contraindications to ureteroscopy include an inexperienced ureteroscopist, inadequate endoscopic instruments, stone burden greater than 1 cm, multiple calculi, transplanted kidney, sepsis, and a solitary kidney.[49] Overall, ureteroscopy has been shown to be a safe and effective procedure for the diagnosis and treatment of urinary calculi in the pregnant patient.

Placenta percreta

Placenta percreta is defined as placental invasion through the uterine serosa into adjacent structures. Direct invasion into the bladder can lead to life-threatening hemorrhage at the time of delivery. Identified risk factors include multigravidity, previous cesarean section or prior uterine surgery, and endometrial curettage.[50] Patients with placenta percreta have a higher incidence of placenta previa than the general population.[51] Sonographic findings suggestive of placenta percreta include absent retroplacental space and vessels from the placenta penetrating into the bladder wall.[50] MRI may be indicated if ultrasound is inconclusive.[52] Cystoscopy may reveal posterior wall abnormalities and also offers the opportunity to 'protect' the ureters through ureteral stenting. Antepartum diagnosis may be the most important factor in management and in minimizing mortality and morbidity. Conservative management includes uterine and pelvic artery embolization with methotrexate therapy. Perioperative blood loss is decreased, but retained placental tissue may pose a serious risk of future hemorrhage.[53] Immediate surgical management includes hysterectomy with varying degrees of bladder repair. The intraoperative blood loss can be minimized with proper exposure, anterior wall cystotomy to define dissection planes, and prophylactic, bilateral, internal iliac artery ligation. Possible urologic complications include bladder laceration, ureteral injury, urinary fistula, and small bladder capacity.

Previous bladder augmentation or urinary diversion

There is limited experience regarding pregnancy in patients with urinary diversion or bladder augmentation. Chronic bacteriuria and recurring urinary tract infections are common in this patient population. Hill and Kramer found that urinary tract infections or pyelonephritis developed in 9 of out 15 pregnancies.[54] Therefore, some recommend antibiotic prophylaxis with routine urine cultures to decrease the risk of serious infectious episodes.[55–57] Close monitoring of renal function with routine blood work and monthly renal ultrasounds is important.

Obstetric indications should determine the preferred route of delivery. However, caesarean section should be considered in cases with artificial sphincter placement or bladder neck reconstruction.[31,54] During cesarean section, injury to the vascular pedicle of the cystoplasty is possible. To avoid this complication, a high uterine incision rather than a low transverse incision should be used. Urologic consultation may prove invaluable in complicated cases.

Urologic malignancy

Malignancy during pregnancy is an uncommon occurrence with an estimated incidence of approximately one per 1000 gestations.[58] Although the pregnant female undergoes immunologic changes that enable the fetus to survive, there is little evidence that pregnancy exacerbates the malignant course.[31]

Renal cell carcinoma, followed by angiomyolipoma, is the most common renal lesion discovered during pregnancy. Flank mass or hematuria is the presenting symptom in 88% and 47% of pregnant patients with renal tumors, respectively.[59] Attempts to avoid exposing the fetus to radiation restrict diagnostic evaluations of renal lesions to ultrasound or MRI. Management strategies for suspicious renal tumors are usually based upon the stage of pregnancy, but cases must be individualized according to the wishes of the mother and other family members. Most agree that a nephrectomy is warranted if renal malignancy is discovered in the first trimester, and that surgery should be post-poned until after delivery if the diagnosis is made in the third trimester.[60] Differences of opinion exist regarding second-trimester treatment. Some hold that one should postpone surgery until the third trimester,[61] while others advocate waiting until 28 weeks' gestation, testing for fetal lung maturity, and then proceeding with nephrectomy.[60] In this way, the morbidity of premature delivery is reduced.

Fewer than 30 cases of bladder cancer diagnosed during pregnancy have been reported in the literature. Rather than assume bleeding to be vaginal, physicians must be diligent to workup hematuria with cystoscopy and renal ultrasound. Cystoscopy may be performed throughout pregnancy. Some have even suggested that a well-performed bladder ultrasound can replace cystoscopy.[60] Bladder tumors should be resected transurethrally. Low-grade lesions may be followed, while high-grade lesions with muscle involvement may require cystectomy. Diagnosis in later stages of pregnancy requiring cystectomy may be postponed until after delivery, or may follow cesarean section.

Urinary tract injury

Obstetric injuries to the urinary tract, while much less common than gynecologic injuries, pose a serious risk to pregnant women. Urethral ischemia from prolonged labor may occur, but is infrequently seen in developed countries with modern obstetric practices. Cases of forceps-assisted delivery leading to bladder or ureteral damage have also been reported, but are exceedingly rare.[62] With nearly 25% of all deliveries in the USA performed by cesarean section,[63] the overwhelming majority of obstetric urinary tract injuries occur during this procedure. The most important concept pertaining to urinary tract injury is to maintain a high index of suspicion. Injuries discovered intraoperatively may be repaired immediately to minimize morbidity, while injuries identified in a delayed fashion may have devastating consequences, such as fistula formation.

The reported incidence of bladder injury during cesarean section ranges from 0.0016% to 0.94%.[63] Eisenkop et al reported a higher incidence of cystotomies during repeat than primary cesarean section: 0.6% and 0.19%, respectively. In that review of 52 bladder injuries, prior cesarean section with 'dense bladder adhesions' was cited as the most common factor associated with bladder injury.[64] In one large study, 75% (12/16) of cystotomies took place during emergent cesarean section.[62]

In performing a cesarean section, all of the aforementioned risk factors must be considered. The peritoneal cavity should be entered at the superiormost portion of the incision, especially in patients with prior surgery. Even in emergent conditions, a disciplined approach should be followed. Bladder drainage with an indwelling catheter is valuable. By preventing the gravid uterus from displacing the bladder superiorly, a urethral catheter may help avoid bladder injury upon entering the abdomen. In obtaining hemostasis, blind suturing or clamping should be strictly discouraged. Rather, the bleeding area should be compressed until identification of bleeding vessels and their anatomic relationship to the bladder and ureters is determined. If significant dissection occurs in the vicinity of the bladder, a thorough evaluation of bladder integrity must be performed. The instillation of methylene blue or indigo carmine into the bladder through a urethral catheter is the easiest method to detect bladder injuries. Once the diagnosis of a bladder injury is made, the limits of the defect should be clearly defined and all devitalized tissue debrided.

The incidence of ureteral injury during cesarean section ranges from 0.027% to 0.09%.[62,64] Both of these major studies reported equal injury rates in comparing the left and right ureters; however, others have found the left ureter to be more vulnerable.[65,66] Fortunately, the overall incidence of ureteral injuries is decreasing.[67] Intraoperative diagnosis of ureteral injury during cesarean section ranges from 25% to 71%. Injuries initially missed were usually diagnosed within 14 days. The predominant belief is that ureteral injuries result from hemostatic attempts at uterine incisions that extend into the broad ligament.[67] In a study evaluating 21 iatrogenic ureteral injuries from obstetric and gynecologic etiologies, Meirow et al associated enlarged uteri, adhesions in the pelvis, and significant hemorrhage with ureteral damage.[66] A complete understanding of pelvic anatomy and the course of the ureter is essential in the prevention of operative ureteral injury. As with bladder injuries, suspicion of a ureteral injury requires a thorough evaluation.

Several modalities have been described to assess ureteral integrity intraoperatively. Mattingly described a method of incising the ureter proximally and passing ureteral catheters distally to identify obstruction or injury.[68] Most authorities do not advocate this aggressive approach. Alternatively, diagnostic cystotomy or cystoscopy followed by intravenous injection of methylene blue or indigo carmine has been used to identify ureteral injuries. One should observe equal efflux of urine bilaterally. Urine flow asymmetry may suggest partial obstruction, and further evaluation by passing ureteral catheters in a retrograde fashion may be performed. Time should also be taken to look for blue dye in the retroperitoneal space.

Some signs and symptoms may alert the clinician to the possibility of a missed injury. Bladder injuries may present with oliguria, fever, suprapubic pain, abdominal distention, ileus, gross hematuria, or vaginal watery secretions. In addition to these findings, ureteral injuries may also present with flank tenderness and hydronephrosis. Numerous types of genitourinary fistulas are common with bladder and ureteral defects. Neuman et al reviewed 30 years of experience with ureteral injuries and found urinary leakage (44%), pain (33%), fever (5%), and urosepsis (12%) to be the most common presenting symptoms.[67]

The operative management of bladder injuries is determined by size, location, and, most importantly, timing of diagnosis. Depending upon the experience and comfort level of the obstetrician, urology involvement may not be mandatory for simple cystotomies. For more complicated repairs, intraoperative urology consultation is recommended. Fortunately, most cystotomies do not involve the ureteral orifices or trigone and a simple closure is satisfactory. If it is identified intraoper-

atively, our practice has been to perform a running closure of the mucosa with 3–0 chromic suture followed by a running, imbricating stitch of submucosa and muscularis with 2–0 or 3–0 chromic suture. A running third layer to reapproximate the serosa is placed if possible. Suturing the mucosa layer separately appears to minimize bleeding from mucosal edges. Use of silk or other nonabsorbable suture is contraindicated, as it may function as a nidus for calculi or infection. Filling the bladder with methylene blue allows the closure to be evaluated to determine whether additional sutures are needed. A suprapubic tube or abdominal drain is not routinely placed, but a urethral catheter remains for approximately 7–10 days. We do not traditionally perform a voiding cystourethrogram prior to catheter removal.

In Eisenkop et al's study of 52 cystotomies, patients without prolonged labor with ruptured membranes showed no benefit from antibiotic usage. Furthermore, only one patient had a documented urinary tract infection.[64] In Rajasekar and Hall's study, all 16 cystotomy patients were treated with prophylactic antibiotics. Six of these patients were documented to have urinary tract infections, resistant organisms requiring additional treatment.[62] Therefore, it is our practice to withhold prophylactic antibiotics, obtain intraoperative urine cultures, and treat expectantly.

Bladder injuries that involve the ureteral orifices or bladder trigone should be closely evaluated for ureteral injury as previously described. Like bladder injuries, management of ureteral injuries depends upon the time of diagnosis, location, and extent of injury. Intraoperative discovery and repair are almost always preferred to delayed correction to avert the cost and morbidity of subsequent procedures. Distal ureteral 'crush' injuries secondary to improperly placed sutures or clamps, where the tissue has not been devitalized, may be managed simply by removal of the offending agent and observation. If upon further inspection there is concern over tissue viability, an 8F double-J stent should be placed retrograde. The Foley catheter and stent are removed at 1 and 2 weeks, respectively.

Transection or severe 'crush' injuries of the ureter within 5 cm of the bladder are most definitively managed with neocystotomy. We usually perform a nonrefluxing reimplantation adhering to several important principles. First, a 5:1 ratio of submucosal tunnel length to ureteral caliber is utilized to prevent reflux. Next, anastamosis of bladder mucosa to ureteral mucosa and a tension-free anastamosis must be performed. Lastly, a temporary ureteral stent is placed.

Ureteral injuries 5–10 cm above the bladder can still be managed with neocystotomy; however, a psoas hitch is often required to allow the ureter sufficient length for a tension-free anastamosis.[69] This procedure mobilizes the bladder upward and secures it to the psoas fascia with absorbable suture. In some circumstances when additional length is needed, a Boari flap may be used. This technique, as shown in Figure 36.1, swings a flap of ipsilateral bladder cranially to meet the distal portion of ureter. Very rarely, when none of the above procedures are possible, transureteroureterostomy may be performed,

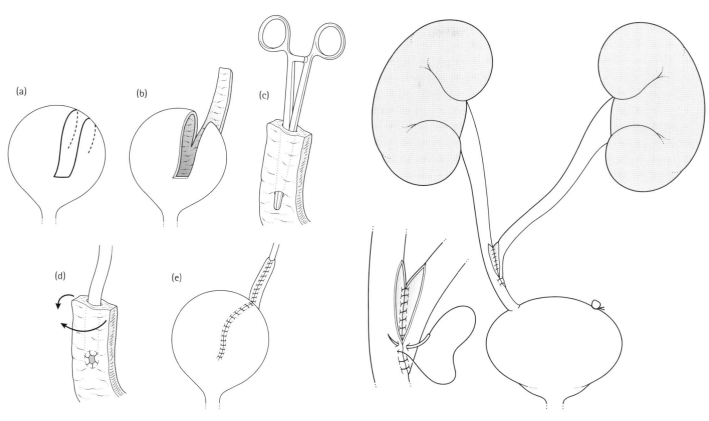

Figure 36.1 Boari flap used for lower ureteral replacement. (a) Selection of bladder flap; (b) rotation of flap; (c) development of antireflux submucosal tunnel in flap; (d) ureteral implantation completed (beginning tubularization of flap); (e) closure of flap and bladder.

Figure 36.2 Transureteroureterostomy.

as shown in Figure 36.2. In all cases of ureteral reimplantation, an abdominal drain, ureteral stent, and urethral catheter are left in place.

Proximal ureteral injuries are extremely rare during cesarean section. In such cases, ureteroureterostomy is often the procedure of choice. The ureteral edges are debrided, spatulated obliquely with Pott's scissors on opposite sides, and then reattached in an interrupted fashion, using 4-0 or 5-0 chromic suture (Figure 36.3). As in neocystotomy, an abdominal drain, stent, and catheter are left in place. Other options for managing proximal ureteral injuries include autotransplantation or interposition of a segment of ileum.

The management of ureteral injuries discovered postoperatively is more controversial. Some believe that a defect discovered within 10–14 days, in an otherwise uncomplicated patient, may still undergo immediate repair.[63] Others support urinary diversion with a percutaneous nephrostomy tube followed by future definitive repair. The literature lacks convincing statistical evidence to dictate the most appropriate time for repair, as most studies encompass only a handful of cases. In a review of over 300 genitourinary fistulas from 1970 to 1985, Lee et al stated that definitive repair should be delayed for 8–12 weeks.[70] This allows edema and inflammation to subside,

tissue to regain its blood supply, prior suture material to disintegrate, and tissue planes to be more easily dissected. Time may even prove to be therapeutic, as one study found that four out of 21 cases of ureteral obstruction spontaneously resolved after urinary diversion because of absorbed suture material.[66]

One of the most devastating consequences of urinary tract injury is genitourinary fistula formation. While a small percentage of fistulas resolve with urinary diversion alone, the vast majority require reoperation.[70] In addition to a thorough history

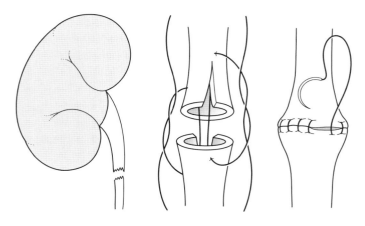

Figure 36.3 Repair of ureter by end-to-end anastomosis (ureteroureterostomy).

and physical examination, a complete diagnostic workup to define the fistula location and characteristics is necessary. This may consist of dye studies, cystography, CT scan, endoscopic evaluation, retrograde pyelogram, and/or intravenous pyelogram. A comprehensive review of genitourinary fistula repair is beyond the scope of this chapter; however, we strongly encourage a team approach with involvement of multiple specialties to confront these challenging issues.

References

1. Schulman A, Herlinger H. Urinary tract dilatation in pregnancy. Br J Radiol 1975; 48: 638–45.
2. Waltzer WC. The urinary tract in pregnancy. J Urol 1981; 125: 271–6.
3. Klarskov P, Gerstenberg T, Ramirez D et al. Prostaglandin type E activity dominates in urinary tract smooth muscle in vitro. J Urol 1983; 129: 1071–4
4. Hsia TY, Shortliffe LM. The effect of pregnancy on rat urinary tract dynamics. J Urol 1995; 154: 684–9.
5. Barron WM. Medical evaluation of the pregnant patient requiring nonobstetric surgery. Clin Perinatol 1985; 12: 481–96.
6. Gertner JM, Coustan DR, Kliger AS et al. Pregnancy as state of physiologic absorptive hypercalciuria. Am J Med 1986; 81: 451–6.
7. Lucas MJ, Cunningham FG. Urinary infection in pregnancy. Clin Obstet Gynecol 1993; 36: 855–68.
8. Whalley P. Bacteriuria of pregnancy. Am J Obstet Gynecol 1967; 97: 723–38.
9. Gilstrap LC, Leveno KJ, Cunningham FG et al. Renal infection and pregnancy outcome. Am J Obstet Gynecol 1981; 141: 709–16.
10. Schieve LA, Handler A, Hershow R et al. Urinary tract infection during pregnancy: its association with maternal morbidity and perinatal outcome. Am J Public Health 1994; 84: 405–10.
11. Zinner SH, Kass EH. Long-term (10 to 14 years) follow-up of bacteriuria of pregnancy. N Engl J Med 1971; 285: 820–4.
12. Quinn AD, Kusuda L, Amar AD, Das S. Percutaneous nephrostomy for treatment of hydronephrosis of pregnancy. J Urol 1988; 139: 1037–8.
13. Laverson PL, Hankins GD, Quirk JG Jr. Ureteral obstruction during pregnancy. J Urol 1984; 131: 327–9.
14. Homans DC, Blake GD, Harrington JT, Cetrulo CL. Acute renal failure caused by ureteral obstruction by a gravid uterus. JAMA 1981; 246: 1230–1.
15. Haratz-Rubinstein N, Murphy KE, Monteagudo A, Timor-Tritsch IE. Transvaginal gray-scale imaging of ureteral jets in the evaluation of ureteral patency. Ultrasound Obstet Gynecol 1997; 10: 342–5.
16. Matsuda T, Saitoh M. Detection of the urine jet phenomenon using Doppler color flow mapping. Int J Urol 1995; 2: 232–4.
17. Meyers SJ, Lee RV, Munschauer RW. Dilatation and nontraumatic rupture of the urinary tract during pregnancy: a review. Obstet Gynecol 1985; 66: 809–15.
18. Oesterling JE, Besinger RE, Brendler CB. Spontaneous rupture of the renal collecting system during pregnancy: successful management with a temporary ureteral catheter. J Urol 1988; 140: 588–90
19. Fernandez AM, Minguez R, Serrano P et al. [Rapidly-growing renal angiomyolipoma associated with pregnancy]. Actas Urol Esp 1994; 18: 755.
20. Yanai H, Sasagawa I, Kubota Y et al. Spontaneous hemorrhage during pregnancy secondary to renal angiomyolipoma. Urol Int 1996; 56: 188–91.
21. Drago JR, Rohner TJ, Jr, Chez RA. Management of urinary calculi in pregnancy. Urology 1982; 20: 578–81.
22. Coe FL, Parks JH, Lindheimer MD. Nephrolithiasis during pregnancy. N Engl J Med 1978; 298: 324–6.
23. Denstedt JD, Razvi H. Management of urinary calculi during pregnancy. J Urol 1992; 148: 1072–4.
24. Loughlin KR, Bailey RB, Jr. Internal ureteral stents for conservative management of ureteral calculi during pregnancy. N Engl J Med 1986; 315: 1647–9.
25. Horowitz E, Schmidt JD. Renal calculi in pregnancy. Clin Obstet Gynecol 1985; 28: 324–38.
26. Lifshitz DA, Lingeman JE. Ureteroscopy as a first-line intervention for ureteral calculi in pregnancy. J Endourol 2002; 16: 19–22.
27. Mayr NA, Wen BC, Saw CB. Radiation therapy during pregnancy. Obstet Gynecol Clin North Am 1998; 25: 301–21.
28. Ratnapalan S, Bona N, Koren G. Ionizing radiation during pregnancy. Can Fam Physician 2003; 49: 873–4.
29. Harvey EB, Boice JD Jr, Honeyman M, Flannery JT. Prenatal x-ray exposure and childhood cancer in twins. N Engl J Med 1985; 312: 541–5.
30. Brown RF. Radiation facts for public health officers. Calif Med 1960; 92: 16.
31. Loughlin KR. Management of urologic problems during pregnancy. Urology 1994; 44: 159–69.
32. Biyani CS, Joyce AD. Urolithiasis in pregnancy. I. Pathophysiology, fetal considerations and diagnosis. BJU Int 2002; 89: 811–18.
33. Hendricks SK, Ross SO, Krieger JN. An algorithm for diagnosis and therapy of management and complications of urolithiasis during pregnancy. Surg Gynecol Obstet 1991; 172: 49–54.
34. Deyoe LA, Cronan JJ, Breslaw BH, Ridlen MS. New techniques of ultrasound and color Doppler in the prospective evaluation of acute renal obstruction. Do they replace the intravenous urogram? Abdom Imaging 1995; 20: 58–63.
35. Shokeir AA, Mahran MR, Abdulmaaboud M. Renal colic in pregnant women: role of renal resistive index. Urology 2000; 55: 344–7.
36. Spencer JA, Tomlinson AJ, Weston MJ, Lloyd SN. Early report: comparison of breath-hold MR excretory urography, Doppler ultrasound and isotope renography in evaluation of symptomatic hydronephrosis in pregnancy. Clin Radiol 2000; 55: 446–53.
37. Scarpa RM, De Lisa A, Usai E. Diagnosis and treatment of ureteral calculi during pregnancy with rigid ureteroscopes. J Urol 1996; 155: 875–7.
38. Borboroglu PG, Kane CJ. Current management of severely encrusted ureteral stents with a large associated stone burden. J Urol 2000; 164: 648–50.

39. Kroovand RL. Stones in pregnancy and in children. J Urol 1992; 148: 1076–8.

40. Asgari MA, Safarinejad MR, Hosseini SY, Dadkhah F. Extracorporeal shock wave lithotripsy of renal calculi during early pregnancy. BJU Int 1999; 84: 615–17.

41. Ohmori K, Matsuda T, Horii Y, Yoshida O. Effects of shock waves on the mouse fetus. J Urol 1994; 151: 255–8.

42. Watterson JD, Girvan AR, Beiko DT et al. Ureteroscopy and holmium:YAG laser lithotripsy: an emerging definitive management strategy for symptomatic ureteral calculi in pregnancy. Urology 2002; 60: 383–7.

43. Rittenberg MH, Bagley DH. Ureteroscopic diagnosis and treatment of urinary calculi during pregnancy. Urology 1988; 32: 427.

44. Harmon WJ, Sershon PD, Blute ML et al. Ureteroscopy: current practice and long-term complications. J Urol 1997; 157: 28–32.

45. Ulvik NM, Bakke A, Hoisaeter PA. Ureteroscopy in pregnancy. J Urol 1995; 154: 1660–3.

46. Vest JM, Warden SS. Ureteroscopic stone manipulation during pregnancy. Urology 1990; 35: 250–2.

47. Shokeir AA, Mutabagani H. Rigid ureteroscopy in pregnant women. Br J Urol 1998; 81: 678–81.

48. Vorreuther R. New tip design and shock wave pattern of electrohydraulic probes for endoureteral lithotripsy. J Endourol 1993; 7: 35–43.

49. Biyani CS, Joyce AD. Urolithiasis in pregnancy. II. Management. BJU Int 2002; 89: 819–23.

50. Abbas F, Talati J, Wasti S et al. Placenta percreta with bladder invasion as a cause of life threatening hemorrhage. J Urol 2000; 164: 1270–4.

51. Hudon L, Belfort MA, Broome DR. Diagnosis and management of placenta percreta: a review. Obstet Gynecol Surv 1998; 53: 509–17.

52. Maldjian C, Adam R, Pelosi M et al. MRI appearance of placenta percreta and placenta accreta. Magn Reson Imaging 1999; 17: 965–71.

53. Butt K, Gagnon A, Delisle MF. Failure of methotrexate and internal iliac balloon catheterization to manage placenta percreta. Obstet Gynecol 2002; 99: 981–2.

54. Hill DE, Kramer SA. Management of pregnancy after augmentation cystoplasty. J Urol 1990; 144: 457–9.

55. Hensle TW, Bingham JB, Reiley EA et al. The urological care and outcome of pregnancy after urinary tract reconstruction. BJU Int 2004; 93: 588–90.

56. Volkmer BG, Seidl EM, Gschwend JE et al. Pregnancy in women with ureterosigmoidostomy. Urology 2002; 60: 979–82.

57. Creagh TA, McInerney PD, Thomas PJ, Mundy AR. Pregnancy after lower urinary tract reconstruction in women. J Urol 1995; 154: 1323–4.

58. Williams SF, Bitran JD. Cancer and pregnancy. Clin Perinatol 1985; 12: 609–23.

59. Walker JL, Knight EL. Renal cell carcinoma in pregnancy. Cancer 1986; 58: 2343–7.

60. Loughlin KR. The management of urological malignancies during pregnancy. Br J Urol 1995; 76: 639–44.

61. Hendry WF. Management of urological tumours in pregnancy. Br J Urol 1997; 80 (Suppl 1): 24.

62. Rajasekar D, Hall M. Urinary tract injuries during obstetric intervention. Br J Obstet Gynaecol 1997; 104: 731–4.

63. Davis JD. Management of injuries to the urinary and gastrointestinal tract during cesarean section. Obstet Gynecol Clin North Am 1999; 26: 469–80.

64. Eisenkop SM, Richman R, Platt LD, Paul RH. Urinary tract injury during cesarean section. Obstet Gynecol 1982; 60: 591–6.

65. Thomas DP, Burgess NA, Gower RL, Peeling WB. Ureteric injury at caesarean section. Br J Urol 1994; 74: 122–3.

66. Meirow D, Moriel EZ, Zilberman M, Farhas A. Evaluation and treatment of iatrogenic ureteral injuries during obstetric and gynecologic operations for nonmalignant conditions. J Am Coll Surg 1994; 178: 144–8.

67. Neuman M, Eidelman A, Langer R et al. Iatrogenic injuries to the ureter during gynecologic and obstetric operations. Surg Gynecol Obstet 1991; 173: 268–72.

68. Mattingly RF. Operative Gynecology, pp. 291–306. (5th edition). Lippincott: Philadelphia, 2004.

69. Ehrlich RM, Melman A, Skinner DG. The use of vesico-psoas hitch in urologic surgery. J Urol 1978; 119: 322–5.

70. Lee RA, Symmonds RE, Williams TJ. Current status of genitourinary fistula. Obstet Gynecol 1988; 72: 313–19.

37 Management of malignant and premalignant lesions of the female genital tract during pregnancy

Darlene G Gibbon, Wilberto Nieves-Neira, Allison Wagreich, and Lorna Rodriguez-Rodriguez

Complications in pregnancy due to cancer have been estimated at approximately 0.94–1 in 1000 pregnancies.[1–3] Cervical carcinoma is the most common cancer seen in pregnancy, occurring in approximately one in 2200 pregnancies.[4] Other malignancies encountered during pregnancy with decreasing frequency include breast cancer, melanoma, ovarian cancer, thyroid cancer, leukemia, lymphoma, and colorectal cancer.[5]

There is little prospective literature regarding the optimal management of gynecologic cancer in pregnancy. Because of the increasing trend of advanced maternal age at the time of first pregnancy, often associated with a history of assisted reproductive technologies, the treatment of gynecologic cancers during pregnancy challenges previously undisputed algorithms of pregnancy termination followed by cancer treatment. The major challenge for the medical team is the lack of prospective, randomized clinical trials to help create appropriate management guidelines.

This chapter will focus on the diagnosis and treatment of preinvasive and invasive gynecologic malignancies in the pregnant patient and will highlight some of the difficult management issues.

Preinvasive lesions of the cervix

Cervical cancer and dysplasia are associated with human papillomavirus (HPV) infection in 99.7% of cases worldwide.[6]

The HPV prevalence in pregnant patients has been reported as high as 42%.[7] Papillomaviruses are DNA-nonenveloped viruses and are members of the papovavirus family. There are over 100 subtypes of HPV. The subtypes infecting the genital tract are divided into those that are low and high risk by their oncogenic potential. The virus contains early and late genes. Two of the early genes, E6 and E7, encode proteins which interfere with cell-cycle control; E6 binds to p53 and E7 binds to pRB.[8]

Juvenile laryngeal papillomatosis is a rare condition caused by HPV. Because this condition is so uncommon, and HPV is very prevalent, the presence of HPV infection or genital warts is not an indication for cesarean delivery.

In a recent study, pregnant women were tested for HPV in the third trimester and again at the time of delivery.[9] Their newborns were tested after delivery for oral and genital HPV. Of the patients, 29% were HPV positive in the cervix during the third trimester and/or at the time of delivery, and 2% were HPV positive in the oral cavity. Of 68 male partners tested (oral only), 6% were positive. In the 571 newborns, less than 1% had genital infection and less than 1% had oral infection with HPV. Only one mother–infant pair was infected with the same HPV subtype. The authors concluded that type-specific vertical transmission of HPV is rare.

Cervical cytology in pregnancy

Cervical cytology is performed for the prevention and early detection of cervical cancer. Abnormal cytology can be further evaluated with colposcopy and cone biopsy. The rationale for cervical cytology in pregnancy is to screen at a time when the patient is more likely to seek medical care.

Cervical cytology is now reported with terminology from the 2001 Bethesda criteria.[10] Squamous abnormalities are atypical squamous cells of unknown significance (ASCUS), atypical squamous cells not excluding high-grade squamous intraepithelial lesion (ASC-H), low-grade squamous intraepithelial lesion (LSIL), and high-grade squamous intraepithelial lesion (HGSIL). Glandular abnormalities are atypical glandular cells of unknown significance (AGCUS) and adenocarcinoma in situ (AIS).

The American Society for Colposcopy and Cervical Pathology (ASCCP) has published consensus guidelines for the management of cytologic abnormalities, including guidelines for pregnancy, which are summarized below.[11]

ASCUS can be managed with repeat cytology and colposcopy, or triaged with HPV detection. HPV-positive patients are then evaluated by colposcopy. HPV-negative patients should be followed as in the nonpregnant patient with repeat cytology in 1 year. All patients with ASC-H need colposcopic evaluation.

Cervical dysplasia and colposcopy in pregnancy

During pregnancy, colposcopy is facilitated by easier visibility of the transformation zone, because there is eversion of the columnar epithelium and/or gaping of the external os.[8] However, colposcopy during pregnancy may be more difficult to interpret due to cervical edema, softening, cyanosis, and increased vascularity.[12] One nonneoplastic cervical change in pregnancy is deciduosis, in which edematous columnar epithelium is mixed with metaplastic epithelium and has a similar appearance to adenocarcinoma. Biopsy is used to distinguish deciduosis from adenocarcinoma.[8]

During colposcopic evaluation in the pregnant patient, endocervical curettage is not recommended because of the possibility of pregnancy disruption. Colposcopically guided biopsies may be performed for high-grade lesions and definitely should be done on lesions suspected of invasion. Because of increased vascularity, bleeding at biopsy sites can be brisk. Economos et al reported on 612 pregnant patients with abnormal cytology. They performed colposcopic biopsies in 449 patients and had no acute bleeding complications. Three patients experienced delayed bleeding, which was controlled with pressure.[13] In our institution, we use Surgicell to achieve hemostasis with great success.

Many authors have reported on the reliability of colposcopy in pregnant patients.[14–16] In a series of 265 pregnant patients with abnormal cytology, there were no missed cases of cancer.[16] Cytology was concordant (within one degree) with colposcopic biopsy in 84% of patients. Cervical conization was performed on 23 patients, and four patients were diagnosed with microinvasive cervical cancer. No patients with cytology of moderate dysplasia or less had microinvasive or invasive cancer. Therefore, the authors questioned the value of reassessment during pregnancy after the initial evaluation.

Conization during pregnancy

The goal of treatment of cervical dysplasia is to prevent the development of cervical cancer. Therefore, understanding the natural history of cervical intraepithelial neoplasia is important in any treatment decisions. The natural history includes regression, persistence, progression, and recurrence. In Ostor's meta-analysis of dysplasia in nonpregnant patients, CIN 1 (mild dysplasia) will regress 60% of the time, but it will progress to cervical cancer only less than 1%. CIN 3 (severe dysplasia) will regress 33% of the time while it may progress in 12% of the patients when left untreated.[17] The ASCCP guidelines recommend treatment of dysplasia in the nonpregnant patient, by conization or ablation, for CIN 2 or 3; treatment may also be offered for persistent CIN 1.[11] In the nonpregnant patient, cone biopsies can lead to perioperative complications, including hemorrhage and infection, as well as delayed complications, including cervical stenosis and preterm premature rupture of membranes in future pregnancies. Conization during pregnancy is associated with higher rates of hemorrhage and increased risk of preterm labor and delivery. Therefore, conization during pregnancy should be performed only when there is suspicion of microinvasion or invasion.[11]

Cold-knife conization is the standard procedure during pregnancy. Hannigan et al[18] reviewed their experience with 82 pregnant patients who had cervical conization. Two patients received blood transfusions. Ten patients (12.4%) had blood loss greater than 500 ml. Three patients required readmission for hemorrhage, and one of these patients was taken back to the operating room twice to obtain hemostasis. Seven patients terminated the pregnancy due to cervical cancer and four patients were lost to follow-up. Of the remaining 71 patients, three had spontaneous abortions after the conization. Of note, one of these patients had a combined cone-cerclage due to a history of a midtrimester loss.[18] Averette et al published their series of 180 conizations and found that 7% had blood loss in excess of 500 ml and 9% received blood products. Delayed bleeding occurred in 4% of the patients.[19] It is unknown whether combined cerclage-conization modifies the risk of preterm labor or of hemorrhage. We perform the procedure by the method of Goldberg et al in which McDonald cerclage is performed prior to cold-knife conization.[20]

Loop excision electrosurgical procedure (LEEP) has been studied in pregnancy. In one series by Robinson et al, 20 patients underwent LEEP.[21] Two patients required blood transfusion. One patient whose LEEP was performed at 27 weeks delivered at 28 weeks. Two additional patients delivered prior to 37 weeks. Three patients had specimens that were negative for dysplasia during pregnancy but had CIN 2–3 at postpartum evaluation. Margins were positive in eight patients (57%) out of the 14 with dysplasia in the specimen. Mitsuhashi and Sekiya reported on nine patients who underwent LEEP, with local anesthesia, prior to 14 weeks' gestation. No patients required transfusion. One patient did have cervical shortening at 21 weeks, had a cerclage placed, and delivered at term. Two patients had residual disease postpartum. The authors concluded that LEEP may be performed safely in the first trimester.[22] The utility of LEEP in pregnancy is limited by the high rate of positive margins.

Dunn et al reported on combined loop excision of the transformation zone (LLETZ)-cerclage. Thirteen patients were reported.[23] Bupivacaine (0.25% with 1:1000 epinephrine) was injected into the cervix, a McDonald cerclage was placed, and LLETZ was performed with top hat. The mean gestational age was 24 weeks. The final pathology was carcinoma *in situ* in nine patients, adenocarcinoma *in situ* in two patients, and microinvasion in two patients. Six (46%) patients had positive margins. There was no hemorrhage and one patient delivered prematurely at 36 weeks.

Follow-up in pregnancy

For the pregnant patient with an abnormal Pap smear, traditional recommendations have included repeat cytology in each trimester. The risk of cervical cancer in a patient with ASCUS or LSIL and a colposcopy with CIN 1 or less is less than 1%. Therefore, it would be reasonable to repeat the evaluation postpartum. Patients with HGSIL should be followed with repeat Pap smear and colposcopy early in the third trimester to rule out an invasive cancer prior to delivery. Education and counseling are an important part of the antepartum colposcopy, including visits to ensure postpartum follow-up.

Regression of cervical intraepithelial neoplasia in the postpartum period

HPV and cervical intraepithelial neoplasia can persist, progress, or regress when left untreated. As mentioned before, in the nonpregnant patient, the spontaneous regression rates are 60% for CIN 1 and 33% for CIN 3. In the pregnant patient, regression of HGSIL has been reported in 30–64%.[24–28] Siddiqui et al performed a retrospective analysis of 100 pregnant patients with abnormal cytology: 30 had HGSIL; 53, LSIL; and 17, ASCUS. The subjects had colposcopy at 12–24 weeks and postpartum cytology. The ASCUS, LSIL, and HSIL groups regressed in 76%, 64%, and 63% of the cases, respectively. Of six patients with carcinoma *in situ*, two regressed to LSIL and none progressed to invasion.[27]

In the pregnant patient, regression may be due to the natural history of the disease or to cervical remodeling after labor and delivery. Ahdoot et al performed a retrospective analysis of pregnant women with abnormal cytology and stratified the

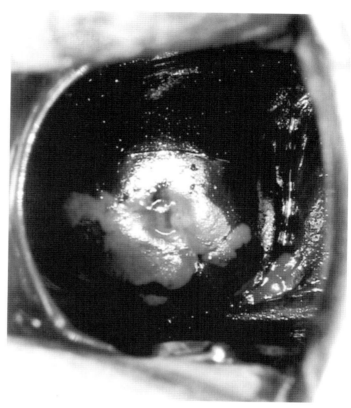

Figure 37.1 Lugol's solution on a cervix from a patient 6 weeks after delivery. Areas of nonstaining represent persistent HGSIL.

patients by route of delivery. The overall postpartum regression rate of the 59 patients with HGSIL was 48%. Of the 47 who delivered vaginally, 28 (60%) regressed postpartum, while none of the 12 patients delivered by cesarean section regressed.[26] It appears from retrospective data that the dysplasia regression rate is higher in the postpartum period than in the nonpregnant patient. A prospective study powered to detect an increase in regression from the baseline rate would provide useful information for both patients and physicians. Figure 37.1 shows a Lugol-stained cervix 6 weeks postpartum with persistent HGSIL.

Invasive cancer of the cervix

Diagnosis

Invasive cervical cancer is the most common gynecologic cancer during pregnancy (0.120 per 1000 deliveries).[29] Cervical cancer during pregnancy is usually diagnosed in an early stage.[29,30] The diagnosis of invasive cancer is frequently made by colposcopically guided biopsy or after a cone biopsy/cerclage procedure as described above. In some instances, it could also be made only by colposcopic examination if the patient refuses biopsy for fear of pregnancy loss.

Staging

Clinical staging is performed according to the International Federation of Gynecology and Obstetrics (FIGO) classification (Table 37.1). This provides the information necessary to determine prognosis and treatment plan. Pelvic examination is an integral part of cervical cancer staging. However, the pelvic examination to assess the parametrium and the cervix may be inaccurate, because the tissue around the cervix changes during pregnancy. Fortunately, new technologies, such as magnetic resonance imaging (MRI), are now available. The cervical anatomy can be adequately evaluated, as well as parametrial, rectal, or bladder involvement; pelvic and paraortic lymph-node enlargement; and hydronephrosis.[31,32] A chest MRI provides information regarding distant metastasis without exposing the fetus to ionizing radiation.

A recent prospective study of 35 children exposed *in utero* to MRI during the third trimester revealed no adverse effects.[33] Gadolinium-based contrast material that is routinely used for MRI crosses the placenta and appears in the fetal bladder, amniotic fluid, and gastrointestinal tract.[34] The safety of its use in pregnancy is not fully established, and therefore it is not rou-

tinely recommended at this time. Gadopentetate dimeglumine, a contrast imaging agent, is considered a pregnancy category C drug, as it has been shown to retard slightly development in rats when given in doses 2.5 times those administered to humans.[36]

Although the use of MRI in pregnancy has increased, there are no prospective data regarding fetal adverse effects in the first and second trimesters. Even in the third trimester, the longest prospective follow-up available for fetal MR exposure is 9 years. Therefore, the potential effects on reproductive function in this group of children, who are still prepubertal, has not been determined. This may be important because damage to Sertoli cells in fetal mice after MR exposure during the period of gonadal differentiation has been described.[36,37] At present, MRI appears to be relatively safe during pregnancy, and its use should not be discouraged if there is clinical indication.

Management

Once the diagnosis of cervical cancer has been made and the stage of the disease is known, the medical team needs to consider the prognosis and any theoretical effects of treatment delay versus the benefits of pregnancy prolongation. The plan should be presented to the parents with a full understanding of their religious and ethical concerns. The decision regarding immediate treatment versus delay is influenced by patient choice, gestational age, disease stage, and progression as well as tumor histology.

For early stage disease, such as stage IA1 or lower, with no lymphovascular space involvement, treatment delay until fetal maturity or delivery is acceptable. For stage IA2 or higher, treatment delay is acceptable if the disease is diagnosed in the third trimester. For cancer diagnosed prior to 24 weeks' gestation, the available data indicate similar outcomes for pregnant and nonpregnant patients if treatment is initiated in a timely fashion.[38,39] For patients who decide to delay treatment until delivery, the paucity of data regarding the effects of treatment delay in the first and second trimesters does not allow accurate counseling regarding prognosis.

Once the decision has been made by the mother or both parents regarding time of delivery or pregnancy termination, the treatment is either delayed until fetal maturity, or termination of pregnancy is induced and the cancer is treated as in the nonpregnant patient.

Immediate treatment

First and second trimesters

For stage IB1, surgery and radiation therapy are equally effective. The decision regarding surgery, including radical hysterectomy with lymphadenectomy and probably ovarian trans-position, is made as in the nonpregnant patient. Since these patients are usually young, ovarian preservation surgery is the treatment of choice. Although therapeutic outcomes are the same, there is a significantly higher amount of blood loss in the radical hysterectomy performed after hysterotomy or cesarean delivery.[40] This

Table 37.1 FIGO staging system for carcinoma of the cervix

Stage	Description
Stage I	*The carcinoma is strictly confined to the cervix*
IA	Invasive cancer identified only microscopically All gross lesions even with superficial invasion are stage IB cancers Invasion is limited to measured stromal invasion with maximum depth of 5 mm and no wider than 7 mm*
IA1	Invasion of stroma no greater than 3 mm in depth and no wider than 7 mm
IA2	Invasion of stroma greater than 3 mm and no greater than 5 mm and no wider than 7 mm
IB	Clinical lesions confined to the cervix or preclinical lesions greater than stage IA
IB1	Clinical lesions no greater than 4 cm in size
IB2	Clinical lesions greater than 4 cm in size
Stage II	*Vaginal or parametrial extension*
IIA	Extension to the upper two-thirds of vagina
IIB	Extension to parametria, but not to pelvic side wall
Stage III	*Pelvic side-wall extension, lower vaginal involvement, or hydronephrosis*
IIIA	Extension to the lower one-third of vagina
IIIB	Extension to pelvic side wall or hydronephrosis
Stage IV	*Mucosal involvement of bladder or rectum, or distant disease*
IVA	Mucosal involvement of bladder or rectum
IVB	Involvement of distant organs

*The depth of invasion should not be more than 5 mm taken from the base of the epithelium, either surface or glandular, from which it originates. Vascular space involvement, either venous or lymphatic, should not alter the staging.

is probably secondary to the increased vascularity of pregnancy, but also the uterine incision and the delivery of the placenta itself are major contributors to the blood loss. No other complications appear to be increased when compared to the nonpregnant state.[40,41]

For more advanced stages (with a few exceptions of very small vaginal involvement in a stage IIA), radiation therapy with concomitant cisplatin-based chemotherapy is the treatment of choice.[42,43] In this group of patients with a nonviable fetus, external pelvic radiation may be initiated immediately with the fetus *in utero*. This will most likely result in the death of the fetus and spontaneous abortion at about the time of completion of external radiation. However, the timing of abortion varies by gestational age. In the first trimester, the mean time to abortion is 33 days, with a range of 27–50 days.[44] In the second trimester, the mean time to abortion is 44 days, with a range of 33–66 days.[44] If spontaneous abortion has not occurred within 1 week of completion of external radiation, the uterus should be emptied by suction curettage or instrument evacuation for later gestations. There is a recent report of the use of misoprostol as an effective alternative to surgical evacuation once intrauterine demise is detected.[45] Once the fetus is evacuated, the first intracavitary implant can be placed without delay 2 weeks after completion of external radiation. There is no need for hysterotomy in these patients, since the tumor has already received a large dose of radiation and the risks of hemorrhage or tumor dissemination are minimal.

There has been some concern that if radiation is started late in the second trimester, the fetus may survive radiation. Some have advocated hysterotomy prior to initiation of radiation in order to avoid this possibility.[46,47] Stone et al reported the birth of a microcephalic infant with bilateral congenital hip deformity and aplastic anemia after radiation in the late second trimester.[48] Others have reported births of apparently normal infants in the same situation, although no follow-up data on the infants were provided to show that there were no late sequelae.[49] It appears that it would be reasonable to consider hysterotomy after 20 weeks' gestation to avoid the birth of a fully radiated, compromised infant.

Third trimester

After fetal maturity is achieved, cesarean section followed by radical hysterectomy or chemoradiation as indicated by stage should be performed. Exactly 214 radical hysterectomies have been reported in the literature.[50] Pregnancy results in a marked increase in blood supply to the uterus, cervix, and vagina. The interstitial edema of pregnancy makes development of surgical planes and identification of surgical anatomy considerably easier than in the nonpregnant state. The lymphatic tissue comes away from the pelvic vessels easily, the bladder and ureter are easily dissected from surrounding tissues, and the rectum is easily separated from the posterior vagina. The uterine vessels are markedly enlarged, and the veins are more fragile than in nonpregnant patients.

Treatment delay

An increasingly larger proportion of women are opting for treatment delay until after delivery. The effect of delaying therapy in women with stage IA2 or more is not known. Furthermore, there is no definition of what constitutes a safe treatment delay. Although prospective data are lacking, there are some facts to consider. First, therapy of cervical cancer is frequently delayed for about 6 weeks after diagnostic conization; therefore, a delay of 6 weeks should also be acceptable for the pregnant patient. Second, in the years 1993–2003, we found not a single report of a maternal death associated with treatment delay for early disease. However, cervical cancer diagnosed postpartum carries a worse prognosis than when diagnosed during pregnancy. Some interpret this observation as an outcome resulting from treatment delay. Alternatively, if the cancer was not clinically evident during pregnancy, it may be because it was small at the time, perhaps had fast growth rate, and therefore may carry a worse prognosis.

Treatment delay in advanced disease

For more advanced disease, treatment delays are not advisable. However, there are some anecdotal reports that neoadjuvant chemotherapy results in significant disease reduction and successful delivery with excellent infant outcomes.[51,52]

Mode of delivery

In advanced disease, it may be logical to deliver the fetus by cesarean section. In theory, vaginal delivery could result in dissemination of tumor in disrupted veins and lymphatics with an accompanying decrease in survival. Another concern is the possibility of life-threatening hemorrhage. There does not seem to be any adverse effect on the fetus from passing through a cervix involved with cancer. Moreover, vaginal delivery has not been found to affect maternal survival adversely. In a comprehensive review of the literature up to 1980, Hacker et al found that the overall survival of patients delivered vaginally to be 45.8% versus 32.7% for those delivered by cesarean section.[30] When analyzed by stage, survival after vaginal delivery was better in all categories. Since these data were retrospective, it was not possible to control for all confounding variables. However, it certainly appears that vaginal delivery does not result in decreased survival as compared to cesarean section. In Hacker et al's study there was an overall survival of 63.1% in patients undergoing a pretreatment abortion (spontaneous or induced). Lee et al noted a 90% survival in 20 patients with stage IB disease regardless of mode of delivery.[53] Ten patients were delivered by cesarean section and 10 were delivered vaginally. Despite these data, some advocate cesarean section to avoid uncontrollable hemorrhage in the presence of gross clinical lesions. The uterine incision during cesarean section should be classical and should begin above the vesicouterine reflection. This avoids the lower uterine segment, which may be involved with tumor. Figure 37.2 shows a radical hysterectomy specimen with a 14-week fetus *in utero*. If the patient delivers vaginally, a 4–6-week delay is often recommended to allow involution prior to radical hysterectomy. Patients in advanced labor can reasonably deliver vaginally if the cancer is small. A rare complication of vaginal delivery is recurrent disease in an episiotomy site. A total of 13 cases have been reported in the literature, and all were felt to occur as a result of tumor implantation during delivery rather than metastasis.[54]

Adnexal masses

Adnexal masses occur in from one in 81 to one in 2200 pregnancies, and of those surgically excised, 2.4–7.9 are malignant.[55–59] Recent publications have also found the rate of malignancy to be between 1–6%.[60–64] In the past, removal of an ovarian cyst during pregnancy was recommended due to the risk of malignancy as well as the danger of torsion (cysts greater than 5 cm), rupture, or hemorrhage leading to acute surgical

intervention and possible adverse pregnancy outcomes.[65] Several retrospective studies in the literature examine the risk of these complications in the presence of an adnexal mass found during pregnancy (Figure 37.3).

Historically, rates of ovarian torsion during pregnancy have been quoted to be 7–28%.[66–69] Hess et al reported that 28% (15/54) of patients with a persistent adnexal mass in pregnancy required emergency laparotomy.[57] In patients who underwent emergency laparotomy because of hemorrhage or torsion of an adnexal mass, spontaneous abortion or preterm delivery was more frequent than in patients who underwent elective laparotomy for removal of the adnexal mass. On this basis, they recommended that a pregnant woman with a persistent adnexal mass undergo elective removal of the mass in the second trimester of pregnancy.

Recent studies have shown a much lower incidence of ovarian torsion in pregnancy than previously described. Rates approaching 1% or less are recently reported.[60,71] The diagnosis of adnexal torsion in the third trimester of pregnancy appears to be an uncommon event. Two recent studies found a higher incidence of torsion in the first and early second trimesters of pregnancy, providing an argument against surgical intervention in the late second trimester to prevent ovarian torsion.[61,71] Zanetta et al detected 82 ovarian cysts in 79 of 6636 women screened from 1996 to 1999.[62] Three women were diagnosed with ovarian torsion in the first trimester and underwent surgical intervention. Of 72 women managed conservatively with the diagnosis of adnexal mass, one ovarian torsion diagnosed at 37 weeks required surgical intervention and cesarean delivery. Sherard et al followed nine patients with mature teratomas in

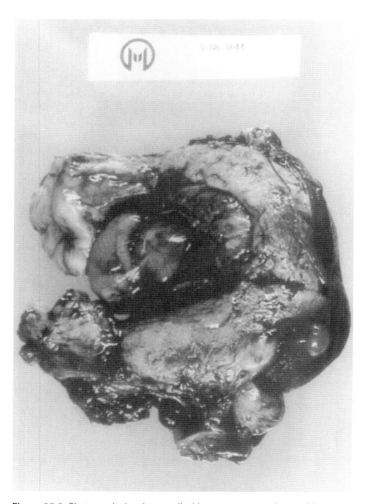

Figure 37.2 Photograph showing a radical hysterectomy specimen with a 14-week fetus *in utero*.

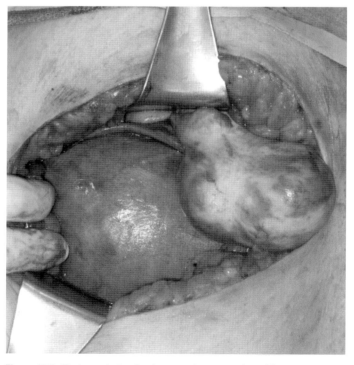

Figure 37.3 Photograph showing large ovarian cyst and gravid uterus.

his series of 56 patients. The average size was 6.3 cm and the follow-up period ranged from 7–26 weeks. There were no incidences of torsion in this group of patients.[63]

Rates of cyst rupture have previously been estimated to be 9–17%.[71,72] However, recent studies have found the rate of ovarian rupture and hemorrhage to be much lower at 0–0.8%.[64–67,75] The risk of an adnexal mass causing obstruction of labor is thought to be 17–21%.[69,76] However, the only recent review by Zanetta et al revealed that only two of 70 patients (2.6%) being conservatively managed underwent cesarean delivery to facilitate delivery.[75]

The recent literature suggests that the incidences of ovarian torsion, rupture, and hemorrhage of the adnexal mass in pregnancy are all much lower than previously reported. A possible explanation for this could be that recent technological advances have led to an increase in the number of asymptomatic adnexal masses being diagnosed by ultrasound, and not by symptoms or physical examination, when an adnexal mass would likely be larger to be clinically detected. The recently reported lower incidence of complications has led several authors to propose conservative management of *asymptomatic* adnexal masses in pregnancy that are not suspected of malignancy.[74,76]

As the number of adnexal masses diagnosed in pregnancy continues to increase, our ability to diagnose malignant adnexal masses needs to improve, so that unnecessary laparotomies can be avoided. Symptoms secondary to the adnexal mass or, in some cases, to a malignancy are often attributed to normal physiologic changes associated with pregnancy. Physical examination, radiographic imaging including ultrasonography and MRI, and serum tumor markers need to be utilized to improve the preoperative diagnosis of a possible malignancy and provide the information necessary to decide about surgical intervention.

Ultrasonography

The use of ultrasonography to make the preoperative diagnosis of an ovarian malignancy is well established in the nonpregnant patient, and it is based upon morphologic indices, as well as Doppler flow studies. Morphologic indices used in the characterization of an adnexal mass include size, solid or cystic components, internal or external excrescences, septations, and the presence of ascites. The clinical usefulness of Doppler flow in the evaluation of an ovarian mass in pregnancy is not well established; therefore, its routine use has not been established. Most importantly, the use of Doppler flow imaging in the diagnosis of borderline tumor of the ovary, the most common malignancy diagnosed during pregnancy, is difficult because there are no biologic, morphologic, or demographic parameters that are specifically predictive.[75]

There is uniform agreement that simple cysts detected by ultrasonography less than 5 cm in diameter are not associated with adverse outcomes and in the majority of cases resolve by the second trimester.[59,60,62,70] The corpus luteum of pregnancy, as well as other physiologic components of the ovary, including follicular cysts, is commonly transient during early pregnancy.

These cysts are generally small and asymptomatic, and resolve by the early second trimester. Bernhard et al found that 28% of women diagnosed with an adnexal mass in pregnancy had used ovulation-induction agents.[60] The majority of these masses (92%) resolved, and none required surgical intervention. No other study has noted the impact of ovulation induction on the presence or significance of adnexal masses in the pregnant patient.

Resolution of adnexal masses that are larger than 5 cm is also a common occurrence in the second trimester of pregnancy. Rates approaching 50–70% have been reported.[60,62] Traditionally, an adnexal mass 8 cm in diameter or greater was considered at risk of being malignant. However, Sherard et al found that the mean size for benign masses in their study was 7.6 cm (range 3–15 cm), and for malignant lesions 11.5 cm (range 6–17 cm).[63] Septations were found equally in benign and malignant lesions. However, internal excrescences were found in 50% of malignant adnexal masses and none in benign masses. Unfortunately, the use of only morphologic characteristics in cystic ovarian masses in pregnancy can be misleading. Low malignant potential tumors of the ovary have presented as simple cystic masses in several series.[59,61,63] In addition to malignant lesions such as dysgerminomas or immature teratomas, a solid adnexal masses can represent a fibroma, luteoma, cystic teratoma, or even fibroid.[61,63] In one series of 10 patients with fibroids who underwent surgical intervention for an adnexal mass, the preoperative ultrasound patterns were found to be solid (five patients), complex (three) and simple (two).[61] MRI can be beneficial in clarifying the origin of the adnexal mass, thus avoiding unnecessary surgical procedures.

While occasionally misleading, ultrasonography in general is very beneficial in the preoperative evaluation of adnexal masses during pregnancy. Attention needs to be given to the size of the mass, whether it is cystic or solid, and whether there are papillary excrescences. Factors that determine whether a mass will persist include the presence of symptoms, size, and complexity.[60] The use of MRI may further assist in the evaluation of adnexal masses in the pregnant patient.

Magnetic resonance imaging (MRI)

As reviewed in the cervical cancer section, MRI has not been shown to have adverse fetal effects, although it utilizes magnets to alter the energy state of hydrogen protons, thereby possibly inducing cell damage. The National Radiological Protection Board advises against its use in the first trimester, and this position is supported by the American College of Obstetrics and Gynecology.[77]

The use of MRI has been shown to be of value in the evaluation of adnexal masses during pregnancy. MRI signal features have been shown to improve characterization of the adnexal mass over ultrasonography and has improved accuracy in the diagnosis of the exact type of the adnexal mass.[78] The use of MRI has been especially beneficial in the diagnosis of uterine fibroids when solid adnexal masses are detected on ultrasonography.[79] MRI may be utilized in those situations in which ultrasonography alone is unable to determine the origin of an adnexal mass or its malignant potential, thereby avoiding an unnecessary surgical procedure in a pregnant patient.

Tumor markers

The use of serum tumor markers in the evaluation of an adnexal mass is complicated by the presence of pregnancy. Many of the germ cell tumor markers, including alpha fetoprotein (AFP), used in the diagnosis of endodermal sinus tumors, and human chorionic gonadotropin (HCG), used in the diagnosis of ovarian choriocarcinoma or embryonal carcinomas, are elevated in normal pregnancies. The use of an elevated maternal AFP screening has led to the diagnosis of an immature teratoma that was unsuspected in two asymptomatic patients.[80–85] Alternatively, lactate dehydrogenase (LDH) levels used in the diagnosis and monitoring of dysgerminomas undergo minimal change during pregnancy, except in women with preeclampsia or HELLP syndrome. Buller et al published a small series of two patients managed conservatively with the diagnosis of dysgerminoma and concomitant pregnancy through the monitoring of LDH.[86]

CA125 is a high-molecular-weight glycoprotein which is expressed in celomic epithelium during embryonic development and in more than 80% of nonmucinous, epithelial, ovarian carcinomas. It is often used in the preoperative evaluation of adnexal masses or in assessing treatment response in epithelial, ovarian carcinoma.[81,82] Measurements of CA125 in women with normal pregnancies reveal that the levels peak at 10 weeks' gestation and decrease to normal values during the second and third trimesters.[83,84] A transient increase in maternal serum CA125 is also seen after delivery.[84] Elevations in maternal serum CA125 are also observed in hydatidiform moles, threatened or spontaneous abortions, and pregnancies complicated by intrauterine fetal demise.[85,86] It has been hypothesized that CA125, which has been localized to the decidua vera, is released into maternal serum either when chorionic villi invades the decidua or disruption of decidua occurs, as during delivery or spontaneous abortions.[83,87,88]

Carcinoembryonic antigen (CEA) levels do not change during pregnancy and therefore may be useful in the evaluation of possible colon or breast carcinoma, or other malignancies.[87]

As in the nonpregnant patient, the use of tumor markers must be coupled with symptomatology, physical findings, and radiographic assessments in the evaluation of the potential malignancy of an adnexal mass in pregnancy.

Surgical management of the adnexal mass in pregnancy

A conservative approach should be taken to all asymptomatic adnexal masses detected during the first trimester unless there is concern of a possible ovarian malignancy. Surgical intervention during the first trimester is avoided due to the increased risk of spontaneous abortion.[89–91]

Asymptomatic adnexal masses detected during the second trimester need to be evaluated for their malignant potential, and possible risk of torsion, rupture, or labor dystocia. Recent studies suggest that the risk of torsion, rupture, or labor dystocia is small; therefore, management needs to be based on the risk of malignant potential. Several reports in the literature support the conservative approach to the management of benign-appearing ovarian masses, with surgical intervention in the postpartum period if indicated.[63,74,76]

For those women in whom surgical intervention is being considered, the clinician needs to keep in mind that there is increased morbidity, including preterm labor and fetal distress, with surgical intervention during the third trimester.[61,71] Whitecar et al found that patients undergoing laparotomy before 23 weeks had significantly fewer adverse pregnancy outcomes than those undergoing laparotomy after 23 weeks ($p = 0.005$; odds ratio, 0.15; 95% CI 0.03–0.69). Of the patients having surgery in the third trimester who delivered preterm, four delivered within 3 weeks of surgery, and one underwent emergency cesarean delivery for fetal distress 4 hours after laparotomy for removal of an adnexal mass.[61] Consequently, surgical intervention during the second trimester at approximately 16–18 weeks has been advocated as being the safest time to intervene.

Symptomatic adnexal masses in pregnancy need to be evaluated for malignant potential. The literature describes management utilizing surgical intervention with either laparotomy or laparoscopy, or the use of percutaneous cyst drainage. The use of cyst aspiration during pregnancy has been limited to unilocular simple cysts without solid or echogenic areas, septations, or papillary structures.[74,76] No adverse outcomes have been reported; all symptoms resolved and the patients were able to go on to deliver at term. The theoretical concern is that there could be development of peritonitis, either chemical, as is seen with the rupture of a mature teratoma, or infectious, spillage of mucinous material leading to the development of pseudomyxoma peritonei, or spillage of malignant cells into the abdominal cavity, leading to dissemination of disease. Cyst aspiration during pregnancy cannot be routinely recommended.

Laparotomy has been the approach most commonly used in the management of an adnexal mass in pregnancy and should still be the approach utilized when an ovarian malignancy is suspected. However, there is a growing body of evidence that laparoscopy may be a safe approach to the management of pregnant patients with benign-appearing, ovarian masses, based on the gynecologic and surgical experience of cholecystectomy and appendectomy. There have been acceptable outcomes, with the majority of studies noting no serious complications except for two fetal deaths, one due to unrelated obstetric causes and another due to intra-abdominal dissemination of a stage I immature teratoma after a solid ovarian mass was morcelated.[92–96] Open laparoscopy by the Hassan technique or placement of a 5-mm videolaparoscope in the left upper quadrant or 6 cm above the umbilicus should be utilized to introduce the

10-mm infraumbilical trocar, thereby decreasing the risk of injury to the gravid uterus. Secondary port site placement should be modified to a more caudal approach. Concerns regarding laparoscopic surgery in pregnancy include the possibility of hypercarbia and associated acid–base disturbances in the fetus secondary to insufflated carbon dioxide, and reduction in maternal diaphragmatic excursion and vena caval blood flow due to the increased maternal intraperitoneal pressure.

Regardless of which surgical approach is chosen, pelvic washings need to be performed at the beginning of the case, and the abdomen should be carefully explored to rule out disseminated cancer. Care must be taken to minimize uterine manipulation. A frozen-section analysis should be performed; if necessary, a gynecologic oncologist should perform the necessary staging procedure, including pelvic and periaortic lymph-node biopsies, omentectomy, and tumor debulking as far as is technically feasible. The contralateral ovary needs to be inspected prior to closure. In the presence of a viable fetus, fetal heart-rate monitoring should be performed before and immediately after surgery. After 20 weeks' gestation, uterine monitoring for contractions should be used to rule out uterine activity or preterm labor. There is no uniform consensus on the use of tocolytics after surgery. The majority of adnexal masses removed during pregnancy are mature cystic teratomas or benign cystadenomas (Table 37.2).

Ovarian cancer

Because of the younger age of patients, germ-cell tumors account for the larger proportion of ovarian malignancies found during pregnancy. Pregnancy does not appear to alter the prognosis of ovarian malignancy. There have been two reports of ovarian cancer metastasizing to the placenta.[97] In most instances, an ovarian malignancy is diagnosed at laparotomy for an adnexal mass and is generally confined to the ovary. A thorough staging laparotomy should be performed through a midline incision, including unilateral adnexectomy, peritoneal

Table 37.2 Histology of adnexal masses removed during pregnancy

Histologic type	Number	(%)	
Cystadenoma	450	(37.3)	
Dermoid	259	(21.5)	
Paraovarian/paratubal	192	(15.9)	(134/228 in one series)
Functional	149	(12.4)	
Endometrioma	35	(2.9)	
Benign stromal	17	(1.4)	
Leiomyoma	12	(1.0)	
Luteoma	7	(.6)	
Miscellaneous	49	(4.1)	
Malignant	36	(3.0)	
Total	1206		

washings, multiple peritoneal biopsies, partial omentectomy, and ipsilateral pelvic and para-aortic lymph node biopsies. Biopsy of the contralateral ovary is performed only if there is evidence of abnormality.

Germ-cell tumors of the ovary

Germ-cell tumors are the most common ovarian malignancies encountered during pregnancy, dysgerminomas being the most frequently seen. These tumors have a predilection for spread to the retroperitoneal lymph nodes, and unilateral pelvic and para-aortic lymph-node biopsies are considered especially important as part of the staging process. These tumors are prone to present acutely with severe abdominal pain, torsion, or incarceration in the cul-de-sac. In the pregnant patient found to have an ovarian dysgerminoma, a careful staging laparotomy with evaluation of the contralateral ovary should be performed. Although up to 24% of these patients may be expected to relapse, the overall survival for this group of patients can be expected to be greater than 90%. Approximately 65% of patients present with stage IA disease.[98]

Nondysgerminoma germ-cell malignancies are uncommon during pregnancy. Endodermal sinus tumors of the ovary are the next most commonly seen.[99,100] These tumors are rarely bilateral, and even patients with tumors apparently confined to the ovary have a significant recurrence rate. Therefore, postoperative adjuvant chemotherapy is recommended regardless of stage. Therapy should start within 1–2 weeks of surgery because of the potential for rapid growth of these tumors.

Epithelial cell tumors of the ovary

The diagnosis of invasive, epithelial ovarian carcinoma is uncommon during pregnancy. The majority of tumors diagnosed are of low malignant potential (LMP). Such tumors often present with early-stage disease, are managed surgically with unilateral adnexectomy and staging, and require only adjuvant therapy when metastatic implants have invasive features. MD Anderson published a series of 10 LMP tumors diagnosed during pregnancy and found that 8 of 10 tumors had evidence of microinvasion.[101] Three patients were found to have more aggressive tumors. One with metastasis to a superclavicular node, another with peritoneal implants, and a patient that required two surgical procedures, one at 24 weeks' gestation and the other at 2 months postpartum. All patients are alive without evidence of disease despite the aggressive behavior of their tumors during pregnancy. Various other reports in the literature support the more indolent behavior of these tumors during pregnancy, as would be expected.

Invasive, epithelial ovarian carcinomas are an unusual occurrence in pregnancy, as this is usually a diagnosis in older women. Many of the reported cases were in patients with early-stage disease.[102] There are also several case reports of epithelial ovarian cancer and synchronous, primary, endometrial cancer.[103,104] An unusual case has been reported in the literature of a patient who conceived spontaneously with bilateral, malignant ovarian masses *in situ* and disseminated disease.[105]

Sex cord-stromal tumors diagnosed during pregnancy

Malignant gonadal stromal tumors are extremely rare during pregnancy. The largest series was reported by Young et al, including 17 granulosa-cell, 13 Sertoli–Leydig-cell, and six unclassified sex-cord stromal tumors diagnosed during pregnancy or the puerperium.[106] All 36 patients presented with stage I disease and underwent unilateral adnexectomy, except for one patient with bilateral ovarian involvement. Ten of the tumors had ruptured preoperatively, two patients developing hemorrhagic shock, and in three patients, the tumor ruptured during removal. Four of the patients who had a ruptured tumor received postoperative radiation therapy or chemotherapy, and one of these patients had a small tumor implant on the contralateral ovary at second-look laparotomy. Twenty-six patients were followed for 1–3 years and remained alive without evidence of disease. Young et al noted that microscopic examination of many of the sex-cord stromal tumors in pregnancy differed from tumors in the same diagnostic categories occurring in the absence of pregnancy by having a disorderly arrangement of their cells, lacking recognizable differentiation in many areas, showing prominent edema, and containing unusually large numbers of lutein or Leydig's cells.[106]

Occasionally, benign ovarian lesions encountered in pregnancy can be confused with a sex cord-stromal tumor.[107,108] These lesions include the luteoma of pregnancy, hyperreactio luteinalis, solitary luteinized follicle cyst of pregnancy and puerperium, granulosa cell proliferation, hilus cell hyperplasia, and ectopic decidua. While they can simulate a neoplasm, all of these lesions will resolve spontaneously after termination of the pregnancy.

Chemotherapy for epithelial ovarian carcinoma

The concern regarding the administration of chemotherapy is the risk of teratogenesis in the first trimester and growth retardation, prematurity, developmental handicaps, and systemic toxicity in later pregnancy. There have been also reports of fetal myelosuppression.[109] The current recommendation for the management of primary, epithelial ovarian carcinoma is combination chemotherapy with paclitaxel and carboplatin. Traditionally, cyclophosphamide in combination with cisplatin has been used; therefore, much of the published literature refers to this combination.

The pharmacodynamics of cisplatin in pregnancy differ from those seen in the nonpregnant state. There is high protein binding of cisplatin; therefore, minimal changes in protein binding can result in large changes in the fraction of free drug that may cross the placenta and lead to fetal toxicity. The lower concentrations of protein and albumin levels seen in fetuses

and pregnant women than in nonpregnant women result in fetal and maternal exposure 50% higher in platinum levels at an equal total concentration.[110] This higher level of free drug may increase the risk of toxicity in both the mother and fetus. Studies using rat models show that cisplatin DNA adduct formation is increased in the fetal brain and liver mitochondria, suggesting that mitochondrial DNA in these organs may be a target of cisplatin genotoxicity.[111] Mitochondrial functional integrity has also been assessed with a pregnant rat model, and it was found that cisplatin exposure did not alter mitochondrial morphology or mtDNA quantity in fetal kidneys and livers; however, specific activities of oxidative phosphorylation enzymes for complexes II and IV were significantly decreased. These changes were assessed as being mild. There was no discernible mitochondrial toxicity in the fetal brain; however, severe toxicity was noted in the maternal rat kidney.

There have been two published cases of women who received chemotherapy for advanced-stage ovarian cancer in pregnancy using paclitaxel in combination with carboplatin or cisplatin.[113,114] Chemotherapy was administered in the early second trimester for the paclitaxel–carboplatin combination and the early third trimester for the paclitaxel–cisplatin combination. Chemotherapy was well tolerated, there was no evidence of fetal toxicity, and both infants were noted to have normal growth and development at 15 or 30 months.

Malfetano and Goldkrand reported on the use of cisplatin/cyclophosphamide chemotherapy in a pregnant woman with stage IIIC, epithelial ovarian cancer who underwent surgical debulking at 16 weeks' gestation.[115] The infant was delivered at term and at 19 weeks after delivery both mother and infant were healthy. Henderson et al also described the use of cisplatin and cytoxan followed by carboplatin and cytoxan after the patient developed ototoxicity.[116] Chemotherapy was administered from 19 weeks' gestation. Antenatal testing by serial ultrasound was normal, and no adverse fetal events were noted. The patient delivered a normal infant weighing 3600 g. Cisplatin-DNA adducts were detected in maternal blood, placenta, fetal amniotic cells, and cord blood. Other studies also report on the safe administration of cisplatin during pregnancy without adverse pregnancy outcome.[117]

Chemotherapy for germ-cell tumors of the ovary

Any patient diagnosed with a germ-cell tumor of the ovary, excluding patients with a stage IA, Grade I, immature teratoma or a stage I dysgerminoma, should receive adjuvant chemotherapy. The current recommendation is the use of bleomycin, etoposide, and cisplatin (BEP). Other active combinations include vincristine, actinomycin D, and cyclophosphamide (VAC); and vinblastine, bleomycin, and cisplatin (VBP).

Malone et al reported on a woman who received two courses of VBP during the early third trimester for an ovarian endodermal sinus tumor, after which she delivered a normal infant prematurely at 32 weeks, who did well.[118] Others have also reported on the administration of chemotherapy for the management of endodermal sinus tumors during pregnancy.[99,100] In both cases, chemotherapy was administered, and one fetus was noted to have ventriculomegaly after the patient developed lower abdominal pain 1 week after the administration of chemotherapy. Both patients were free of disease at the time of publication.

There are several reports of the administration of VAC during pregnancy.[80,120,121] All infants were developmentally normal and no adverse events were reported.

Vulvar dysplasia and condylomata

A significant increase in the incidence of HPV-associated disease of the vulva affecting young women has been noted over the last 20 years.[122] Manifestations include condylomata, vulvar intraepithelial neoplasia (VIN), and VIN-associated squamous cell carcinoma. Approximately 15% of vulvar cancers occur in women younger than 40 years.[123] As the age of childbearing is delayed in Western societies, the number of pregnant patients presenting with these problems is expected to increase. Increased awareness and early attention to vulvar symptoms during pregnancy are necessary. Yet, it remains a rare occurrence during pregnancy, and the literature on this topic consists of small series and case reports.

Pregnancy seems to stimulate the growth of condylomata acuminata, leading to significant discomfort. Larger lesions become symptomatic for pain and may compromise defecation and micturition, depending on the affected area. Bleeding and tissue trauma (from avulsion or erosion of the florid lesions) are of concern and may facilitate secondary bacterial infection. Extensive condylomata may obliterate the birth canal and require cesarean delivery due to either dystocia or the risk of hemorrhage.[124] Repair of lacerations or episiotomies may be difficult and wound healing may be poor.[125]

The use of topical agents during pregnancy is limited due to concerns over systemic absorption related to increased blood flow in the vulva during gestation. The only compound considered safe for use during pregnancy is trichloroacetic acid (TCA). TCA application (85% solution) has been used safely during pregnancy in combination with laser ablation.[126–128] Unlike podophyllin, TCA does not cause inflammation and therefore is better tolerated. However, it is an inconvenient therapy requiring repeated applications, since a single application is only 20–30% effective. Podophyllin use is contraindicated in pregnancy. It is a pregnancy category C product. There are no teratogenic effects of its topical applications in rabbits, but high-dose intraperitoneal administration is associated with embryotoxicity in rats. Podophyllin use has been associated with congenital malformations (simian crease), premature delivery, and intrauterine death. Severe systemic toxicity reactions, including coma and death, have been reported in nonpregnant individuals. Cytotoxic agents, including 5-fluorouracil cream and bleomycin, are also contraindicated due to concerns

related to systemic absorption. There are no reports on the use of imiquimod during pregnancy. It is a pregnancy category B product with no teratogenic effects noted on rats or rabbits.

Laser vaporization of vulvar condylomata during pregnancy is safe and effective. Arena et al reported on 115 pregnant patients undergoing laser ablation for genital condylomata.[127] Sixty (52.7%) of the patients had vulvovaginal disease. One ablation treatment was sufficient for 89 patients (92.2%) while eight (7%) required a second procedure. The failure rate, including persistent or recurrent lesions, was 7.8%. At 1 year postpartum, 83 patients (72.2%) remained free of HPV disease manifestations. Adelson et al reported no recurrences after laser ablation during pregnancy or at 6 weeks postpartum.[128]

The CO_2 laser is used to ablate lesions from the core outward to the level of surrounding epithelium. Low-power densities (400–500 W/cm^2) ensure elimination of surface epithelium to 1 mm in depth. The brushing technique described by Baggish to coagulate skin and mucosal surfaces superficially is used between confluent condylomas and the skin surrounding the lesion.[129] This treatment has been performed from early first trimester to 36 weeks of gestation without major complications. Adelson et al reporting on 16 patients undergoing laser ablation indicated an average length of procedure of 48 minutes, with 88% being completed in less than 1 hour.[128] Average blood loss was 25 ml. The average hospital stay was 3 days. Indwelling urethral catheters were used for patients with periurethral disease, and there was one patient with urinary retention due to edema. In the series of Arena et al, vulvar edema was the main surgical complication for three out of 115 patients (2.6%).[127] Laser treatment does not affect neonatal outcomes and mode of delivery. Cesarean delivery may be necessary if there are persistent clinical lesions. Premature uterine contractions occur in 6–37%, with spontaneous resolution or response to tocolysis.

There are no published studies of vulvar dysplasia during pregnancy. Close surveillance of patients with VIN I and VIN II, consisting of vulvoscopy throughout pregnancy and repeat biopsies for lesions manifesting changes, is recommended. Patients with VIN III can undergo wide local excision unless there are specific obstetric contraindications for surgery. If conservative management is undertaken, multiple biopsies of representative areas are advisable to document the absence of occult or microinvasive carcinoma. Lesions diagnosed in the late third trimester can be addressed at 6–8 weeks postpartum. Spontaneous regression of VIN II and III has been described and can occur during pregnancy.[130]

Vulvar carcinoma

Invasive vulvar carcinoma accounts for about 4% of gynecologic tumors. Approximately 15% of cases occur in women younger than 40 years of age.[123] It has been estimated that 5% of vulvar cancers are complicated by pregnancy, although no recent statistics have been published.[131] Overall, fewer than 50 cases of invasive squamous cell carcinoma of the vulva during pregnancy have been reported in the literature in English. DiSaia and Creasman estimated a frequency of one per 20 000 deliveries at his institution.[132] Most patients were 25–35 years of age, with the youngest patient 17 years old. As in the nonpregnant population, the most common histology is squamous cell carcinoma followed by melanoma, sarcoma, and adenoid cystic adenocarcinoma.

Treatment of vulvar carcinoma during pregnancy is essentially the same as for the nonpregnant patient. Recent trends for less radical surgery and individualization of surgical approach are applicable to the pregnant patient.[133] Microinvasive carcinoma (up to 1 mm in depth of invasion, no lymphovascular space involvement, and no confluent tongues of invasion) is treated with wide local excision, ensuring a 2-cm lateral clinical margin of resection. Unilateral stage I lesions (less than 2 cm in diameter) are treated with radical wide local excision or hemivulvectomy and ipsilateral, inguinofemoral lymph-node dissection. Lesions that cross the midline, clitoral lesions, and stage II or certain stage III lesions (lower vaginal involvement) are treated with radical vulvectomy and bilateral, inguinofemoral lymph-node dissection. The triple incision approach (separate incisions for the vulvectomy and lymphnode dissections) has significantly decreased postoperative wound morbidity by reducing the amount of tissues being resected. Surgery for invasive vulvar disease diagnosed in the first and second trimesters can be performed around week 18 of gestation. Acceptable outcomes have been obtained with surgery up to 36 weeks of gestation. After this gestational age, patients can be allowed to deliver vaginally and then be treated postpartum.[134] The increased vascularity of the vulva in the late third trimester is considered a risk factor for increased operative morbidity. This approach would also prevent disruption of an incompletely healed surgical wound by vaginal delivery. Radical vulvectomy may be performed as soon as 1 week postpartum.

There are no data to indicate the impact of mode of delivery on the course of the disease for untreated patients. The size and location of the lesion are factors to consider when deciding on cesarean delivery. It is conceivable that traumatic laceration of a large lesion at the time of vaginal delivery could result in tumor embolization. Vaginal delivery after radical vulvectomy is possible as long as the wound is well healed. Vulvar scarring or vestibular stenosis may require cesarean delivery. Patients that need adjuvant radiotherapy to the groin may be delivered by cesarean section once fetal lung maturity has been established.[135] There is no contraindication for future pregnancies after radical vulvectomy with or without lymphadenectomy.[134] Barclay reported 16 pregnancies after surgery for vulvar carcinoma.[136] The interval between surgery and pregnancy was between 6 months and 4½ years.

Endometrial carcinoma

Endometrial cancer is the most common gynecologic malignancy. Because it is a cancer of the menopausal years, it is rarely seen in pregnancy. The risk factors associated with endometrial cancer in premenopausal women, such as obesity and anovulation, are the same risk factors associated with infertility. Therefore, endometrial cancer in pregnancy is uncommon. The only cases reported were in association with a miscarriage or ectopic pregnancy, or were in the postpartum period. Therefore, the dilemma regarding the balance of fetal and maternal welfare is usually not a concern, and the management should follow standard care as for the nonpregnant patient. However, because this is a younger patient population interested in childbearing, conservative treatment with progestins can be considered with close surveillance to diagnose any possible recurrence. Jadoul and Donnez reviewed the literature from 1970 to 2001, and reported on 26 patients of less than 40 years of age who underwent conservative treatment of endometrial adenocarcinoma with subsequent pregnancy. A total of 31 pregnancies with good fetal outcomes were reported for these 26 patients.[137]

Conclusion

Optimal treatment of gynecologic cancers in pregnancy requires a multidisciplinary approach, including an obstetrician experienced in high-risk obstetrics, a gynecologic oncologist, a psychologist, a neonatologist, a radiation oncologist, and other specialists as indicated. With such an approach, in most cases, the management of cancers may be delayed without affecting the health of the mother, and therefore improving the health of the fetus.

References

1. Oduncu FS, Kimmig R, Hepp H, Emmerich B. Cancer in pregnancy: maternal-fetal conflict. J Cancer Res Clin Oncol 2003; 129: 133–46.
2. Smith LH, Danielsen B, Allen ME, Cress R. Cancer associated with obstetric delivery: results of linkage with the California cancer registry. Am J Obstet Gynecol 2003; 189: 1128–35.
3. Oehler MK, Wain GV, Brand A. Gynaecological malignancies in pregnancy: a review. Aust N Z J Obstet Gynaecol 2003; 43: 414–20.
4. Jolles CJ. Gynecologic cancer associated with pregnancy. Semin Oncol 1989; 16: 417–24.
5. Boulay R, Podczaski E. Ovarian cancer complicating pregnancy. Obstet Gynecol Clin North Am 1998; 25: 385–99.
6. Walboomers JM, Jacobs MV, Manos MM et al. Human papillomavirus is a necessary cause of invasive cervical cancer worldwide. J Pathol 1999; 189: 12–19.
7. Kemp EA, Hakenewerth AM, Laurent SL et al. Human papillomavirus prevalence in pregnancy. Obstet Gynecol 1992; 79: 649–56.
8. Singer A, Monaghan JM. Lower Genital Tract Precancer: Colposcopy, Pathology and Treatment, pp. 26–8. Blackwell Science: Oxford, 2000.

9. Smith EM, Richie JM Yankowitz J et al. Human papillomavirus prevalence and types in newborns and parents: concordance and modes of transmission. Sex Transm Dis 2004; 31: 57.

10. Solomon D, Davey D, Kurman R et al. The 2001 Bethesda System; terminology for reporting results of cervical cytology. JAMA 2002; 287: 2114–19.

11. Wright TC, Cox JT, Massad LS et al. 2001 Consensus guidelines for the management of woman with cervical cytological abnormalities. JAMA 2002; 287: 2120–9.

12. Baldauf JJ, Dreyfus M, Ritter J, Philippe E. Colposcopy and directed biopsy reliability during pregnancy: a cohort study. Eur J Obstet Gynecol Reprod Biol 1995; 62: 31–6.

13. Economos K, Veridiano NP, Delke I et al. Abnormal cervical cytology in pregnancy: a 17-year experience. Obstet Gynecol 1993; 81: 915–18.

14. Woodrow N, Permezel M, Butterfield L et al. Abnormal cervical cytology in pregnancy: experience of 811 cases. Aust N Z Obstet Gynaecol 1998; 38: 161–5.

15. Ueki M, Ueda M, Kumagai K et al. Cervical cytology and conservative management of cervical neoplasias during pregnancy. Int Gynecol Pathol 1995; 14: 63–9.

16. LaPolla JP, O'Neill C, Wetrich D. Colposcopic management of abnormal cervical cytology in pregnancy. J Reprod Med 1988; 33: 301–6.

17. Ostor AG. Natural history of cervical intraepithelial neoplsia: a critical review. Int J Gynecol Pathol 1993; 12: 186–92.

18. Hannigan EV, Whitehouse HH, Atkinson WD et al. Cone biopsy during pregnancy. Obstet Gynecol 1982; 60: 450–5.

19. Averette HE, Nasser N, Yankow SL, Little WA. Cervical conization in pregnancy: analysis of 180 operations. Am J Obstet Gynecol 1970; 106: 543–9.

20. Goldberg GL, Altaras MM, Block B. Cone cerclage in pregnancy. Obstet Gynecol 1991; 77: 315–17.

21. Robinson WR, Webb S, Tirpack J, et al. Management of cervical intraepithelial neoplasia during pregnancy with loop excision. Gynecol Oncol 1997; 64: 153–5.

22. Mitsuhashi A, Sekiya S. Loop electrosurgical excision procedure (LEEP) during first trimester of pregnancy. Int J Gynaecol Obstet 2000; 71: 237–9.

23. Dunn TS, Ginsburg V, Wolf D. Loop-cone cerclage in pregnancy: a 5-year review. Gynecol Oncol 2003; 90: 577–80.

24. Kiguchi K, Bibbo M, Hasegawa T, Kurihara S, Tsutsui F, Wied GL. Dysplasia during pregnancy: a cytologic follow-up study. J Reprod Med 1981; 26: 66–72.

25. Lundvall L. Comparison between abnormal cytology, colposcopy and histopathology during pregnancy. Acta Obstet Gynecol Scand 1989; 68: 447–52.

26. Ahdoot D, Nostrand V, Kristi M et al. The effect of route of delivery on regression of abnormal cervical cytologic findings in the postpartum period. Am J Obstet Gynecol 1998; 178: 1116–20.

27. Siddiqui G, Kurzel RB, Lampley EC, Kang HS, Blankstein J. Cervical dysplasia in pregnancy: progression versus regression post-partum. Int J Fertil 2001; 46: 278–80.

28. Strinic T, Bukovic D, Karelovic D, Bojic, Stipic I. The effect of delivery on regression of abnormal cervical cytologic findings. Coll Antropol 2002; 26: 577–82.

29. Barber HR, Brunschwig A. Gynecologic cancer complicating pregnancy. Am J Obstet Gynecol 1963; 85: 156–64.

30. Hacker NF, Berek J, Lagasse LD et al. Carcinoma of the cervix associated with pregnancy Obstet Gynecol 1982; 59: 735–46.

31. Okamoto Y, Tanaka YO, Nishida M et al,. MR imaging of the uterine cervix: imaging-pathologic correlation. Radiographics 2003; 23: 425–45.

32. Hannigan EV. Cervical cancer in pregnancy. Clin Obstet Gynecol 1990; 33: 837–45.

33. Kok RD, De Vries MM, Heerschap A et al. Absence of harmful effects of magnetic resonance exposure at 1.5 T in utero during the third trimester of pregnancy: a follow-up study. Magn Reson Imaging 2004; 22: 851–4.

34. Nagayama M, Watanabe Y, Okumura A et al. Fast MR imaging in obstetrics. Radiographics 2002; 22: 563–80.

35. Levine D, Barnes PD, Edelman RR. State of the art obstetric MR imaging. Radiology 1999; 211: 609–17.

36. Orth JM, Gunsalus GL, Lamperti AA. Evidence from Sertoli cell-depleted rats indicates that spermatid number in adults depends on numbers of Sertoli cells produced during perinatal development. Endocrinology 1988; 122: 787–94.

37. Carnes KI, Magin RL. Effects of in utero exposure to 4.7 T MR imaging conditions on fetal growth and testicular development in the mouse. Magn Reson Imaging 1996; 14: 263–74.

38. Hopkins MP, Morley GW. The prognosis and management of cervical cancer with pregnancy. Obstet Gynecol 1992; 80: 9–13.

39. van der Vange N, Weverling GJ, Ketting BW, et al. The prognosis of cervical cancer associated with pregnancy: a matched cohort study. Obstet Gynecol 1995; 85: 1022–6.

40. Monk BJ, Montz FJ. Invasive cervical cancer complicating intrauterine pregnancy; treatment with radical hysterectomy. Obstet Gynecol 1992; 80: 199–203.

41. Sivanesaratnam V, Jayalakshmi P, Loo C. Surgical management of early invasive cancer of the cervix associated with pregnancy. Gynecol Oncol 1993; 48: 68–75.

42. Rose PG, Bundy BN, Watkins EB et al. Concurrent cisplatin-based radiotherapy and chemotherapy for locally advanced cervical cancer. N Engl J Med 1999; 240: 1144.

43. Morris M, Eifel PJ, Lu J et al. Pelvic radiation with concurrent chemotherapy compared with pelvic and para-aortic radiation for high-risk cervical cancer. N Engl J Med 1999; 240: 1137–43.

44. Prem KA, Makowski EL, McKelvey JL Carcinoma of the cervix associated with pregnancy. Am J Obstet Gynecol 1966; 95: 99–108.

45. Ostrom K, Ben-Arie, Edwards C, et al. Uterine evacuation with misoprostol during radiotherapy for cervical cancer in pregnancy. Int J Gynecol Cancer 2003; 13: 340–3.

46. Peake JD. Carcinoma of the cervix complicated by pregnancy. South Med J 1960; 53: 34–9.

47. Stander RW, Lein JN. Carcinoma of the cervix and pregnancy. Am J Obstet Gynecol 1960; 79: 164–7.

48. Stone ML, Weingold AB, Sall S. Cervical carcinoma in pregnancy. Am J Obstet Gynecol 1965; 93: 479.

49. Danforth WC. Carcinoma of the cervix during pregnancy. Am J Obstet Gynecol 1937; 34: 365.

50. Nisker JA, Shubat M. Stage IB cervical carcinoma and pregnancy: report of 49 cases. Am J Obstet Gynecol 1983; 145: 203–6.

51. Tewari K, Cappuccini F, Gambino A et al. Neoadjuvant chemotherapy in the treatment of locally advanced cervical carcinoma in pregnancy. Cancer 1998; 82: 1529–34.

52. Marana HRC, de Andrade JM, da Silva Mathes AC et al. Chemotherapy in the treatment of locally advanced cervical cancer and pregnancy. Gynecol Oncol 2001; 80: 272–4.

53. Lee RB, Neglia W, Park RC. Cervical carcinoma in pregnancy. Obstet Gynecol 1981; 58: 584–9.

54. Goldman NA Goldberg GL. Late recurrence of squamous cell cervical cancer in an episiotomy site after vaginal delivery. Obstet Gynecol 2003; 101: 1127–9.

55. Beischer NA, Buttery BW, Fortune DW, Macafee CA. Growth and malignancy of ovarian tumors in pregnancy. Aust N Z Obstet Gynaecol 1971; 11: 208–20.

56. Chung A, Birnbaum SJ. Ovarian cancer associated with pregnancy. Obstet Gynecol 1973; 41: 211–14.

57. Hess WL, Peaceman A, O'Brien WF et al. Adnexal mass occurring with intrauterine pregnancy: report of fifty-four patients requiring laparotomy for definitive management. Am J Obstet Gynecol 1988; 158: 1029–34.

58. Koonings PP, Platt LD, Wallace R. Incidental adnexal neoplasms at cesarean section. Obstet Gynecol 1988; 72: 767–9.

59. Thornton JG, Wells M. Ovarian cysts in pregnancy: does ultrasound make traditional management inappropriate? Obstet Gynecol 1987; 69: 717–21.

60. Bernhard LM, Klebba PK, Gray DL, Mutch DG. Predictors of persistence of adnexal masses in pregnancy. Obstet Gynecol 1999; 93: 585–9.

61. Whitecar P, Turner S, Higby K. Adnexal masses in pregnancy: a review of 130 cases undergoing surgical management. Am J Obstet Gynecol 1999; 181: 19–24.

62. Zanetta G, Mariani E, Lissoni A et al. A prospective study of the role of ultrasound in the management of adnexal masses in pregnancy. Br J Obstet Gynecol 2003; 110: 578–83.

63. Sherard GB 3rd, Hodson CA, James WH et al. Adnexal masses and pregnancy: a 12-year experience. Am J Obstet Gynecol 2003; 189: 358–62.

64. Usui R, Minakami H, Kosuge S et al. A retrospective survey of clinical, pathologic, and prognostic features of adnexal masses operated on during pregnancy. J Obstet Gynecol Res 2000; 26: 89–93.

65. Mundell EW. Primary ovarian cancer associated with pregnancy. Clin Obstet Gynecol 1963; 6: 983.

66. Tawa K. Ovarian tumors in pregnancy. Am J Obstet Gynecol 1964; 90: 511–16.

67. Buttery BW, Beischer NA, Fortune DW, Macafee CA. Ovarian tumors in pregnancy. Med J Aust 1973; 1: 345–9.

68. Gray LA. Ovarian cysts and myomas of uterus during pregnancy. South Med J 1961; 54: 632–5.

69. Spencer CP. Pregnancy and ovarian cysts. BMJ 1920; 1: 79.

70. Hogston P, Lilford RJ. Ultrasound study of ovarian cysts in pregnancy: prevalence and significance. Br J Obstet Gynecol 1986; 93: 625–8.

71. Agarwal N, Parul, Krilani A et al. Management and outcome of pregnancies complicated with adnexal masses. Arch Gynecol Obstet 2003; 267: 148–52.

72. Struyk AP, Treffers PE. Ovarian tumors in pregnancy. Acta Obstet Gynecol Scand 1984; 63: 421–4.

73. Peterson WF, Prevost EC, Edmunds FT et al. Benign cystic teratomas of the ovary. Am J Obstet Gynecol 1955; 70: 368–82.

74. Caspi B, Levi R, Appleman Z et al. Conservative management of ovarian cystic teratoma during pregnancy and labor. Am J Obstet Gynecol 2000; 182: 503–5.

75. Zanetta G, Lissoni A, Cha S et al. Preoperative morphological and colour Doppler features of borderline ovarian tumors. Br J Obstet Gynaecol 1995; 102: 990–6.

76. Platek DN, Henderson CE, Goldberg GL. The management of a persistent adnexal mass in pregnancy. Am J Obstet Gynecol 1995; 173: 1236–40.

77. ACOG Committee on Obstetric Practice Committee Opinion. Guidelines for diagnostic imaging during pregnancy. 1995; 158.

78. Kier R, McCarthy SM, Scoutt LM et al. Pelvic masses in pregnancy: MR imaging. Radiology 1990; 176: 709–13.

79. Sherer DM, Maitland CY, Levine NF et al. Prenatal magnetic resonance imaging assisting in differentiating between large degenerating interamural leiomyoma and complex adnexal mass during pregnancy. J Matern Fetal Med 2000; 9: 186–9.

80. Montz FJ, Horenstein J, Platt LD et al. The diagnosis of immature teratoma by maternal serum alpha-fetoprotein screening. Obstet Gynecol 1989; 73: 522–5.

81. Kabawat SE, Bast RC, Bhan AK et al. Tissue distribution of a coelomic epithelium related antigen recognized by the monoclonal antibody OC125. Int J Gynecol Pathol 1983; 2: 275–85.

82. Kabawat SE, Bast RC, Welch WR et al. Immunopathologic characterization of a monoclonal antibody that recognizes common surface antigens of human ovarian tumors of serous endometrioid and clear cell types. Am J Clin Pathol 1983; 79: 98–104.

83. Kobayashi F, Sagawa N, Nakamura K et al. Mechanism and clinical significance of significance of elevated CA125 levels in the sera of pregnant woman. Am J Obstet Gynecol 1989; 160: 563–6.

84. Haga Y, Sakamoto K, Egami H et al. Evaluation of serum CA125 values in healthy individuals and pregnant woman. Am J Med Sci 1986; 292: 25–9.

85. Takahashi K, Yamane Y, Yoshino K et al. Studies on serum CA125 levels in pregnant woman. Acta Obstet Gynaecol Jpn 1985; 37: 1931–4.

86. Buller RE, Darrow V, Manetta A et al. Conservative management of dysgerminoma concomitant with pregnancy. Obstet Gynecol 1992; 79: 887–90.

87. Quirk JG, Bronson GL, Long CA et al. CA125 in tissues and amniotic fluid during pregnancy. Am J Obstet Gynecol 1989; 159: 644.

88. Cheli CD, Morris DL, Meaman IE et al. Measurement of four tumor marker antigens in the sera of pregnant woman. J Clin Lab Anal 1999; 13: 35–9.

89. Novak ER, Lambrou CD, Woodruff JD. Ovarian tumors in pregnancy: an ovarian tumor registry review. Obstet Gynecol 1975; 46: 401–6.

90. Booth RT. Ovarian tumors in pregnancy. Obstet Gynecol 1963; 21: 189–93.

91. White KC. Ovarian tumors in pregnancy: a private hospital ten year survey. Am J Obstet Gynecol 1973; 116: 544.

92. Stepp KJ, Tulikangas PK, Goldberg JM et al. Laparoscopy for adnexal masses in the second trimester of pregnancy. J Am Assoc Gynecol Laparosc 2003; 10: 55–9.

93. Canis M, Pouly L, Wattiez A et al. Laparoscopic management of adnexal masses suspicious at ultrasound. Eur J Obstet Gynecol Reprod Biol 1997; 89: 679–83.

94. Mathevet P, Nessah K, Dargent D, Mellier G. Laparoscopic management of adnexal masses in pregnancy: a case series. Eur J Obstet Gynecol Reprod Biol 2003; 108: 217–22.

95. Soriano D, Yefet Y, Seidman DS et al. Laparoscopy versus lapartotomy in the management of adnexal masses during pregnancy. Fert Steril 1999; 71: 955–60.

96. Moore RD, Smith WG. Laparoscopic management of adnexal masses in pregnant women. J Reprod Med 1999; 44: 97.

97. Patsner B, Mann WJ, Chumas J. Primary invasive ovarian adenocarcinoma with brain and placental metastases: a case report. Gynecol Oncol 1989; 33: 112–15.

98. Gershenson DM, Wharton JT, Kline RC et al. Chemotherapeutic complete remission in patients with metastatic ovarian dysgerminoma: potential for cure and preservation of reproductive capacity. Cancer 1986; 58: 2594–9.

99. Shimizu Y, Komiyama S, Kobayashi T et al. Successful management of endodermal sinus tumor of the ovary associated with pregnancy. Gynecol Oncol 2003; 88: 447–50.

100. Elit L, Bocking A, Kenyon C, Natale R. An endodermal sinus tumor diagnosed in pregnancy: case report and review of the literature. Gynecol Oncol 1999; 72: 123–7.

101. Mooney J, Silva E, Tornos C et al. Unusual features of serous neoplasms of low malignant potential during pregnancy. Gynecol Oncol 1997; 65: 30–5.

102. Rahman MS, Al-Sibai MH, Rahman J et al. Ovarian carcinoma associated with pregnancy: a review of 9 cases. Acta Obstet Gynecol Scand 2002; 81: 260–4.

103. Hoffman MS, Cavanagh D, Walter TS et al. Adenocarcinoma of the endometrium and endometrioid carcinoma of the ovary associated with pregnancy. Gynecol Oncol 1989; 32: 82–5.

104. Ojomo EO, Ezimokhai M, Reale FR et al. Recurrent postpartum haemorrhage caused by endometrial carcinoma co-existing with endometrioid carcinoma of the ovary in a full term pregnancy. Br J Obstet Gynecol 1993; 100: 489–91.

105. Bennett RA, Dodson WC, Olt GJ et al. Spontaneous conception in the presence of stage IIIC endometrioid ovarian cancer. Fert Steril 2001; 75: 623–4.

106. Young RH, Dudley AG, Scully RE. Granulosa cell, Sertoli-Leydig cell, and unclassified sex cord-stromal tumors associated with pregnancy: a clinicopathological analysis of thirty-six cases. Gynecol Oncol 1984; 18: 181–205.

107. Clement PB. Tumor-like lesions of the ovary associated with pregnancy. Int J Gynecol Pathol 1993; 12: 108–15.

108. Clement PB, Young RH, Scully RE. Ovarian granulosa cell proliferations of pregnancy: a report of nine cases. Hum Pathol 1988; 19: 657–62.

109. Garcia L, Valcacel M, Santiago-Borrero PJ. Chemotherapy during pregnancy and its effects on the fetus-neonatal myelosuppression. Two case reports. J Perinatol 1999; 19: 230–3.

110. Zemlickis D, Klein J, Moselhy G et al. Cisplatin protein binding in pregnancy and the neonatal period. Med Pediatr Oncol 1994; 23: 476–9.

111. Giurgiovich AJ, Diwan BA, Olivero OA et al. Elevated mitochondrial cisplatin–DNA adduct levels in rat tissues after transplacental cisplatin exposure. Carcinogenesis 1997; 18: 93–6.

112. Gerschenson M, Paik CY, Gaukler EL et al. Cisplatin exposure induces mitochondrial toxicity in pregnant rats and their fetuses. Reprod Toxicol 2001; 15: 525–31.

113. Mendez LE, Mueller A, Salom E, Gonzalez-Quintero VH. Paclitaxel and carboplatin chemotherapy administered during pregnancy for advanced epithelial ovarian cancer. Obstet Gynecol 2003; 102: 1200–2.

114. Sood AK, Shahin MS, Sorosky JI. Paclitaxel and platinum chemotherapy for ovarian carcinoma during pregnancy. Gynecol Oncol 2001; 83: 599–600.

115. Malfetano JH, Goldkrand JW. Cisplatinum combination chemotherapy during pregnancy for advanced epithelial ovarian cancer. Obstet Gynecol 1990; 75: 545.

116. Henderson CE, Elia G, Garfinkel D et al. Platinum chemotherapy during pregnancy for serous cystadenocarcinoma of the ovary. Gynecol Oncol 1993; 49: 92–4.

117. King LA, Nevin PC, William PP et al. Treatment of advanced epithelial ovarian carcinomas in pregnancy with cisplatin-based chemotherapy. Gynecol Oncol 1991; 41: 78.

118. Malone JM, Gershenson DM, Creasy RK et al. Endodermal sinus tumor of the ovary associated with pregnancy. Obstet Gynecol 1986; 68: 86S–89S.

119. Metz SA, Day TG, Pursell SH. Adjuvant chemotherapy in a pregnant patient with endodermal sinus tumor of the ovary. Gynecol Oncol 1989; 32: 371–4.

120. Frederiksen MC, Casanova L, Schink JC. An elevated maternal serum alpha-fetoprotein leading to the diagnosis of an immature teratoma. Int J Gynecol Obstet 1991; 35: 343–6.

121. Kim DS, Park MI. Maternal and fetal survival following surgery and chemotherapy of endodermal sinus tumor of the ovary during pregnancy: a case report. Obstet Gynecol 1989; 73: 503–7.

122. Joura EA, Losch A, Haider-Angeler MG et al. Trends in vulvar neoplasia. Increasing incidence of vulvar intraepithelial neoplasia and squamous cell carcinoma of the vulva in young women. J Reprod Med 2000; 45: 613–15.

123. Henson D, Tarone R. An epidemiologic study of cancer of the cervix, vagina, and vulva based on the Third National Cancer Survey in the United States. Am J Obstet Gynecol 1977; 129: 525–32.

124. Young RL, Acosta AA, Kaufman RH. The treatment of large condylomata acuminata complicating pregnancy. Obstet Gynecol 1973; 41: 65–73.

125. Snyder RR, Hammond TL, Hankins GDV. Human papillomavirus associated with poor healing of episiotomy repairs. Obstet Gynecol 1990; 76: 664–7.

126. Schwartz DB, Greenberg MD, Daoud Y, Reid R. Genital condylomas in pregnancy: use of trichloroacetic acid and laser therapy. Am J Obstet Gynecol 1988; 158: 1407.

127. Arena S, Marconi M, Frega A et al. Pregnancy and condyloma. Evaluation about therapeutic effectiveness of laser CO_2 on 115 pregnant women. Minerva Ginecol 2001; 53: 389–96.

128. Adelson MD, Semo R, Baggish MS, Osborne NG. Laser vaporization of genital condylomata in pregnancy. J Gynecol Surg 1990; 6: 257–62.

129. Baggish MS. Improved laser techniques for the elimination of genital and extragenital warts. Am J Obstet Gynecol 1985; 153: 545–50.

130. Jones RW, Rowan DM. Spontaneous regression of vulvar intraepithelial neoplasia 2–3. Obstet Gynecol 2000; 96: 470–2.

131. Collins CG, Barclay DL. Cancer of the vulva, and cancer of the vagina in pregnancy. Clin Obstet Gynecol 1963; 30: 927–42.

132. DiSaia PJ, Creasman WT. Clinical Gynecologic Oncology, pp. 439–40. (6th edition). CV Mosby: St Louis, MO, 2002.

133. Angioli R, Nieves-Neira W, Penalver MA. Treatment of malignancy of the vulva. In: Sciarra JJ, Dooley S, Depp R et al. (eds), Gynecology and Obstetrics Clinical Text, pp. Lippincott Williams and Wilkins, 2001.

134. Monaghan JM, Lindeque G. Vulvar carcinoma in pregnancy Br J Obstet Gynaecol 1986; 93: 785–6.

135. Gitsch G, van Eijkeren M, Hacker NF. Surgical therapy of vulvar cancer in pregnancy. Gynecol Oncol 1995; 56: 312–15.

136. Barclay DL. Surgery of the vulva, perineum and vagina in pregnancy. In: Barber HR, Graber EA (eds), Surgical Disease in Pregnancy, p. 320. Saunders: Philadelphia, 1974.

137. Jadoul P, Donnez J. Conservative treatment may be beneficial for young women with atypical endometrial hyperplasia or endometrial adenocarcinoma. Fertil Steril 2003; 80: 1315–24.

38 Gestational trophoblastic neoplasia

Jesús R Alvarez and Abdulla Al-Khan

The term 'gestational trophoblastic neoplasia' (GTN) is used to describe the spectrum of trophoblastic diseases, from hydatidiform mole to choriocarcinoma. The word 'hydatid' was first used by Aetius of Amida in the sixth century AD to describe the cystic and degenerative nature of the placental tissue. Although our knowledge of the etiology of these diseases is incomplete, they are the most curable type of gynecologic malignancy at the present time. Through the centuries, the disease has elicited the curiosity of historians, laymen, and physicians. The diagnosis, management, and follow-up of this disease is a multidisciplinary endeavor. The objective of this chapter is to provide an insight into the diagnosis and management of the disease and to discuss the future reproductive outcome of women affected by this disease.

Epidemiology

Hydatidiform mole is a rare complication of pregnancy. Its incidence varies among different ethnic groups and geographic areas. The incidence of molar pregnancies is generally expressed in relation to the total number of pregnancies in a given population. Most reports agree that the incidence of hydatidiform mole is greater in Southeast Asia than in the Western Hemisphere. The reported incidence of this disease in the Western countries is estimated to be 1/2000 pregnancies versus 1/77 for some countries in Asia such as Indonesia, China, and the Philippines. It is estimated that in the USA, one in 1500 pregnancies is complicated by trophoblastic disease. The reason for this difference in the rates of hydatidiform mole between The USA and Asian countries is uncertain. It may involve genetic, nutritional, immunologic, or environmental factors.[1–3]

Brinton, among others, has noticed an increased incidence of hydatidiform mole among women at the extremes of reproductive age.[3] The incidence seems to be higher among women over 40 years of age and those under 20. A recent case-control study from China confirmed these findings and also showed a protective effect associated with having a term live birth or stillbirth.[1] This study suggested an increased risk of hydatidi-

form mole among women with a history of two or more induced abortions. There also appears to be an increased risk in patients with a prior history of twins. Acacia et al found an increased incidence of hydatidiform mole among women with history of recurrent spontaneous abortion.[4]

Poor nutrition and low socioeconomic status may contribute to the high incidence of hydatidiform mole in Asia. High consumption of vitamin A has been associated with a higher incidence of molar pregnancy. However, a lower incidence has been found in women with high consumption of carotene and animal fat, but recent studies have not supported this concept. Brinton et al found no relationship between the risk of molar pregnancy and various dietary variables.[1] A higher incidence of hydatidiform mole has been found in chronic smokers (relative risk 4.2) and in patients with blood group B.

The incidence of choriocarcinoma differs from the incidence of molar pregnancy. There is a decline in incidence rate over the last 25 years, mainly due to early diagnosis and aggressive treatment of molar pregnancy (Table 38.1). In Europe and North America, the incidence of choriocarcinoma is in the range of 1/30 000–1/40 000 pregnancies. In Southeast Asia, the incidence seems to be about 1/3500–1/5000 pregnancies, and in Latin America at 0.2 cases per 10 000 pregnancies.

Patients with a history of hydatidiform mole have an increased risk of trophoblastic disease in a future pregnancy that is estimated to be as high as 1/50 for patients with two or more molar pregnancies. There are also reports of cases of familial trophoblastic disease. These observations suggest that there may be genetic susceptibility to this disease, but do not rule out a common environmental factor.

Pathogenesis and classification

Hydatidiform mole is an abnormal pregnancy that is characterized by abnormal fetal development and placental overgrowth. On a histopathologic basis, the abnormality can be classified as a complete hydatidiform mole (CHM) or as a partial hydatidiform mole (PHM). CHM and PHM can still be defined by specific characteristics that reflect their unusual genetic origin.[5–7]

Table 38.1 The Japanese trophoblastic disease classification

Hydatidiform mole

(1) Complete mole
   (a) Noninvasive complete mole
   (b) Invasive complete mole
(2) Partial mole
   (a) Noninvasive partial mole
   (b) Invasive partial mole

Choriocarcinoma

(1) Gestational choriocarcinoma
   (a) Uterine choriocarcinoma
   (b) Extrauterine choriocarcinoma
   (c) Intraplacental choriocarcinoma
(2) Nongestational choriocarcinoma
   (a) Choriocarcinoma of germ-cell origin
   (b) Choriocarcinoma derived from differentiation from other carcinomas

Placental site trophoblastic tumor

Persistent trophoblastic disease (histopathologic specimen not available)

(1) Postmolar persistent HCG
(2) Clinically invasive/metastatic mole
(3) Clinical choriocarcinoma

Hydatidiform mole is a neoplasm that originates from the fetal chorion. The microscopic characteristics required for diagnosis are: (1) an enlarged villi with hydropic or edematous stroma; (2) absence of vascularization in the villi; (3) excessive trophoblastic proliferation. In general, trophoblastic proliferation determines the benign or malignant character of the molar tissue. Trophoblastic proliferation involves both the cytotrophoblast cells and syncytiotrophoblast cells, as well as the intermediate elements.[1] Two different histologic classifications have been proposed in an attempt to correlate the clinical prognosis of hydatidiform mole with its histologic pattern.

Vassilakos and Kajii proposed a new classification scheme for molar pregnancy in 1976. Their work was later supported by investigators such as Szulman and Surti.[8] It is still the classification used. These investigators classified a molar pregnancy into a complete mole, or a partial mole, by morphologic and cytogenetic characteristics. Although the pathologic criteria used to define these two entities have changed with the advent of ultrasound and earlier termination of suspected molar pregnancies, CHM and PHM can still be defined by specific characteristics that reflect their unusual genetic origin.

A CHM is characterized by (1) the absence of normal chronic villi; (2) pronounced vesicular swelling of the villi; (3) the lack of an embryo, cord, or amniotic membranes, except in the rare case of a CHM with coexistent normal twin; (4) marked trophoblastic hyperplasia and anaplasia. Macroscopically, this provides the classical clinical description of molar tissue as a 'bunch of grapes'. Approximately 90% of the complete moles have a 46,XX chromosomal complement. The other 10% have a 46,XY complement. Chromosome-banding techniques, enzyme markers, and HLA antigen typing, can confirm the diploid chromosomal complement of paternal origin. A complete mole originates by the fertilization of an empty egg, or 'blighted ovum', by a haploid sperm, which later duplicates to give the 46,XX complement. The 46,XY mole originates by dispermy, or the fertilization of a 'blighted ovum' by two spermatozoa. The mechanisms involved in this abnormal fertilization pattern remain uncertain. The potential for malignancy is greater with a complete mole[8–10] than with its counterpart, the PHM.

A partial mole is defined as the coexistence of a hydatidiform mole with a fetus. Macroscopically, the hydatidiform changes are focal, with relatively small vesicles; therefore, its clinical diagnosis may be easily missed. The histopathologic assessment of a partial mole includes (1) focal hydropic swelling and cavitation of the villi; (2) focal mild to moderate hyperplasia, usually confined to the syncytiotrophoblast; (3) scalloping of the outline of the villi by trophoblastic inclusions; (4) identifiable fetal or embryonic structures. The embryo/fetus can survive to term, and in most cases demonstrates the stigmata of triploidy.[10] A chromosomally normal fetus may coexist with a PHM.[11–13] The cytogenetic evaluation of a partial mole reveals that most have a triploid karyotype. The additional set of haploid chromosomes can be supplied by either parent. Therefore, the origin of a partial mole may involve the phenomenon of dispermy with a normal egg, or the fertilization of an ovum that has not undergone the reduction division by a haploid sperm.[8] Although the malignant potential of a partial mole is less than that of a complete mole, these pregnancies should also be followed closely with human chorionic gonadotropin (HCG) titers after evacuation.[10] Sometimes the pathologic diagnosis of CHM is confounded by overlapping features with hydropic spontaneous abortion (HAS) and PHM, yet accurate classification of a given case is clinically important, since there are different consequences for the prognosis and management of each condition.[14,15] This scenario can be seen when (1) most of the products of conception is passed before presentation, (2) tissue is inadvertently discarded during the evacuation procedure or during its handling in the laboratory, and (3) when the need to re-evaluate a prior diagnosis calls for analysis of an archival specimen. In this case, it is possible to use flow cytometry for ploidy. The majority of PHMs are triploid,[16–18] while CHMs are usually diploid and occasionally tetraploid. Ploidy can also be determined by using paraffin-embedded tissue.[16,19] Cytogenetic analysis can detect the subset of HAS that is aneuploid[20] in addition to identifying triploid PHMs.[21] Fluorescence *in situ* hybridization using chromosome-specific probes on paraffin sections can serve as a substitute for karyotyping to evaluate the chromosomal status.[22] Immunohistochemistry for the imprinted gene product IPL/PHLDA2 has also been used to aid in the diagnosis.[23]

Clinical presentation

The clinical presentation of a gravida with molar pregnancy has changed over the last two decades due to early diagnosis by ultrasound and quantitative serum HCG estimation. The clinical symptoms may vary depending on whether the diagnosis is made early in the first trimester or in the second trimester. Although molar pregnancies are classified into the complete or partial types, they share some typical presenting features.

The titer of HCG is generally higher in a molar pregnancy than in a normal gestation. However, a single titer cannot be used as the only criterion for diagnosis.

The clinical examination of uterine size reveals a discrepancy between uterus size and dates in approximately 50% of the cases. The uterus can be enlarged by the presence of the proliferative tissue, and also by clotted blood. Uterine enlargement has been considered a risk factor for postmolar trophoblastic disease and for pulmonary embolization at the time of evacuation. Vaginal bleeding is a universal symptom of hydatidiform mole. A molar pregnancy may be erroneously diagnosed as a missed abortion until the products of conception are analyzed. Although many cases present with severe bleeding and anemia at the time of diagnosis, these problems can be minimized with early diagnosis and intervention.

Theca lutein cysts can be observed in 25–60% of molar pregnancies (Figure 38.1). These cysts are formed secondary to hyperstimulation of the ovaries by HCG secreted by the trophoblastic tissue. The diagnosis can be made clinically by palpation of an adnexal mass, or sonographically. The management is conservative, since these cysts regress after evacuation of the mole and normalization of the HCG titer unless there is acute torsion of an ovary secondary to the cysts. Approximately 20–26% of molar pregnancies present with hyperemesis gravidarum. This symptom is usually associated with enlarged uterus and/or elevated HCG titer. Other diagnoses such as multiple

gestation, central nervous system (CNS) tumors, and hyperthyroidism should be entertained. The occurrence of pregnancy-induced hypertension before 24 weeks' gestation has been regarded as a sine qua non of molar pregnancy. Subclinical or acute thyrotoxicosis can be seen in these patients due to high levels of serum HCG.

Postmolar trophoblastic disease can occur after either a partial or a complete mole. Therefore, it is imperative that such pregnancies undergo close surveillance of HCG titers after evacuation.[24] Reports from Berkowitz et al[2] and the review of Watson et al[10] summarized some interesting findings about the natural history of partial mole. Most of the patients had vaginal bleeding and absence of fetal heart activity as the presenting symptoms. The diagnosis was not suspected in most cases prior to the evacuation. In Berkowitz's series, the initial clinical diagnosis in 90% of the cases was missed or incomplete abortion. Only 7% of the patients in that series had HCG titers over 100 000 mIU/ml prior to evacuation, and none of their patients had theca lutein cysts. Only 10% of the patients developed nonmetastatic, persistent gestational trophoblastic disease. These authors therefore conclude that PHM usually does not present with the classical features of molar pregnancy, and meticulous pathologic review of the placental tissue must be done after a presumed missed or incomplete abortion.[25] Watson et al[10] noticed a significant difference in the maternal age of those patients with complete versus partial mole. Only 18% of the women with partial mole were younger than 20 years, compared to 27% with complete mole. As previously mentioned, the most common karyotype in a partial mole is triploidy. However, up to 30% of the reported cases have a normal 46,XX or XY karyotype.[10]

The management of those cases where a partial mole coexists with a chromosomally normal fetus is still controversial. In the past, most authors recommended termination of pregnancy after the diagnosis was made to avoid the risk of malignant sequelae. However, Thomas et al's[12] report of a preterm normal female delivered at 29 weeks' gestation contrasts with that traditional view. A conservative approach was also followed by Feinberg et al[11] in a case of a partial mole coexisting with a normal fetus. The neonatal outcome, in their case, was poor due to the extreme prematurity of the fetus at the time of delivery. Both authors conclude that the minimal obstetric workup required for cases identified by sonogram as a partial mole includes determination of the fetal karyotype, serial sonographic assessment of the pregnancy, serial determination of HCG levels and coagulation profile, thyroid workup and liver profile to assess common complications of molar pregnancies, and a chest radiograph to rule out metastasis. A progressive rise in HCG titers, development of obstetric complications, or evidence of metastasis is an indication for termination of the pregnancy. The long-term prognosis for these pregnancies is still uncertain.[11,12]

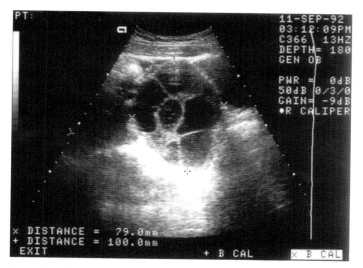

Figure 38.1 Theca lutein cysts.

Diagnosis

Several diagnostic modalities have been used to identify molar pregnancy, including HCG titers, amniography, sonography, computed tomography (CT) scan, and magnetic resonance imaging (MRI).

The most essential diagnostic modality remains histopathologic evaluation. Histologic examination is required for all cases of missed or incomplete abortions, and in elective terminations of pregnancy. Amniography is no longer used, since it requires the pregnancy to have been over for 14 weeks to allow the physician access into an abdominal uterus, and involves exposure to ionizing radiation.

Sonographic examination is the principal diagnostic tool for the diagnosis of molar pregnancy. Its advantages include the absence of ionizing radiation and the ability to identify a viable fetus and the presence of partial mole.[26] The introduction of vaginal sonography has facilitated the diagnosis of hydatidiform mole during the first trimester and in obese patients where the abdominal approach might be inconclusive.[27] Molar changes can be detected around 8 weeks of gestation by ultrasonography. The typical snowstorm pattern can be visualized with low-frequency ultrasound, but with high-frequency ultrasound, clearly defined cystic spaces representing hydropic villi can be seen (Figure 38.2). The use of MRI for hydatidiform mole has been advocated by Powell et al,[28] who stress that MRI can distinguish hemorrhage within the molar tissue from myometrial invasion.

Recently, the use of flow cytometry to distinguish between PHM and CHM has been advocated. Hemming et al[29] found that the hyperploid fraction is indicative of increased cell proliferation. The hyperploid fraction seen in complete moles is different from that found in normal placentas or partial moles. He also observed that specimens of tissue from persistent trophoblastic disease have the hyperploid fraction characteristics seen in the complete mole. Analysis of deoxyribonucleic acid (DNA) content by flow cytometry is easy and rapid. It can be performed both in fresh or formalin-fixed tissues even when the amount of tissue is insufficient for cytogenetic studies. This new technique is capable of identifying patients at high risk of persistent trophoblastic disease.[29] Flow-cytometry studies confirmed the cytogenetic analysis in all cases.[30]

All trophoblastic tissue produces HCG when viable tissue is present. This glycoprotein is composed of two dissimilar polypeptide subunits, the alpha and beta chains. The primary structure of the alpha subunits in all glycoprotein hormones is almost identical. The beta subunits have a unique amino-acid content and sequence, which confer the immunologic and biologic specificity on each hormone. The assay developed by Vaitukis in 1972 measures both intact HCG molecules and the subunits present in a given sample. The half-life of the complete HCG molecule is longer than that of its subunits, and is the predominant molecule measured with this assay. The development of monoclonal antibody technology led to radioimmunoassays that can distinguish between the intact HCG molecule and its free beta subunits of HCG. An increase of free beta subunits has been observed in patients who develop metastatic disease.[9]

Treatment and follow-up of nonmalignant gestational trophoblastic neoplasia

Prior to the termination of a molar pregnancy, a complete history, physical examination, chest radiography, and baseline laboratory studies are required. They serve to establish the patient's health status and to detect possible metastatic disease. In addition, these laboratory tests serve to disclose the presence of any complication of molar pregnancy (Table 38.2).

It is important to determine the patient's reproductive desires before a management plan is initiated. In patients who have completed their families, primary hysterectomy may be considered since it significantly decreases the risk of malignancy (3.5% vs 20%).[31] Approximately 25% of patients with molar pregnancy have prominent theca lutein cysts. Because these cysts regress spontaneously upon normalization of the HCG

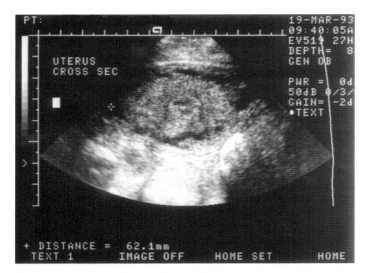

Figure 38.2 Sonogram of hydatidiform mole.

Table 38.2 Laboratory workup for molar pregnancies
Complete blood count with differential
Coagulation parameters – PT, PTT, fibrinogen, platelets
Liver function studies
Renal function studies
Thyroid function tests
Chest radiography
Serum and urine beta-HCG titers
Blood type and cross-match

PT = prothrombin time; PTT = partial thromboplastin time.

titers, the uterine adnexa need not be removed during the hysterectomy unless adnexal metastasis is seen.[31] These patients must be carefully followed after surgery with beta-HCG titers, since metastatic disease has also been described in 3% of cases of hydatidiform mole managed with hysterectomy.

The use of hysterotomy or uterotonics for evacuation of molar pregnancies is not recommended. The disadvantages of these methods include an increased incidence of hemorrhage, trophoblastic embolization, and the risk of retained molar tissue, as well as the common side effects produced by prostaglandins.[32]

The preferred method for evacuation of a molar pregnancy is suction curettage. The uterus can be completely evacuated by the vaginal route with this method with minimal danger of hemorrhage, even in cases of enlarged uterus. The patient must have typed and cross-matched blood prior to the procedure. Either general or conduction anesthesia can be used. In rare emergencies, paracervical block combined with intravenous narcotic analgesia can be used. The patient is placed in the lithotomy position, and the cervix is gently dilated to allow the introduction of a 9–12-mm plastic cannula into the uterine cavity. An oxytocin drip is initiated simultaneously with the activation of the suction pump. The curette is rotated in place until most of the molar tissue is evacuated. This should be associated with a decrease in the uterine size. The suction curette can then be removed and the remaining products removed by sharp curettage. This last specimen should be submitted for histologic investigation separately. The physician should exercise caution during the performance of the sharp curettage in order to avoid perforation or subsequent Asherman's syndrome.[32]

Controversy exists regarding the need for repeat curettage 7–10 days after the initial evacuation. The experience in Hong Kong of Lao et al[33] indicated that this procedure is not useful. Significant abnormality was found in less than 1% of the specimens, and the presence of trophoblastic tissue was not predictive of the subsequent blood HCG levels. Repeat curettage is indicated, however, for those patients with persistent vaginal bleeding.

Prophylactic chemotherapy has been suggested to decrease the incidence of persistent trophoblastic disease. A prospective, randomized study to assess the usefulness of prophylactic chemotherapy was performed at the Hanyang University Hospital of Seoul, South Korea, from 1978 to 1984.[34] The authors observed an increase in the cost of therapy, a higher degree of resistance to the chemotherapeutic agents, and a delay in diagnosis of persistent disease among these patients. However, they reported a decrease in the incidence of persistent disease among patients classified as high risk. There was no adverse effect on the reproductive performance of patients who received prophylactic chemotherapy. There is still concern about exposing all these patients to a potentially toxic treatment when approximately only 20% will be at risk of development of persistent GTN. Nevertheless, studies have shown that only 4% of patients with complete molar pregnancies develop local uterine invasion after being treated with a single dose of actinomycin D

prophylactically. None of these patient's had metastasis, and they all had complete remission after one additional course of chemotherapy.[35,36] Thus, the benefits of prophylactic chemotherapy are questionable, but may have a role in the management of high-risk patients especially when hormonal follow-up is unavailable.

After evacuation of a molar pregnancy, 80% of patients will need no further intervention.[37,38] However, it is prudent to follow these patients with serial beta-HCG titers to document the regression of blood titers. This should be done weekly until the beta-HCG levels are normal for 3 consecutive weeks, followed by monthly determinations until levels are normal for 6 months. There is cross-reactivity between HCG and luteinizing hormone (LH) because they share the same alpha chain. Therefore, the beta-subunit radioimmunoassay is the most reliable assay in the management of GTN.

The documentation of a rise or plateau in the beta-HCG titer on two or more occasions, and the demonstration of metastasis and/or histopathologic diagnosis of choriocarcinoma on a surgical specimen or in spontaneously passed tissue are considered diagnostic of persistent gestational trophoblastic disease. These patients require chemotherapy and consultation with a gynecologic oncologist.[39]

A patient may ovulate as early as 2–4 weeks after evacuation.[40] Therefore, an effective method of contraception should be started early to facilitate an adequate follow-up. All patients are advised to use contraception for 1 year after a normal beta-HCG titer is documented. The preferred method of contraception is debatable due to earlier reports suggesting an increased risk of persistent trophoblastic disease among patients using oral contraception. The studies of Yuen and Burch[41] and the report from the Gynecologic Oncology Group in the USA have shed new light on this controversy.[42] None of these studies showed evidence that women using oral contraception with 50 µg estrogen were at higher risk of postmolar trophoblastic disease than those using other modes of contraception. Women using barrier contraception have a relatively higher pregnancy rate at a time when contraception is a critical element for appropriate follow-up. Therefore, oral contraception is the preferred method for all patients with no specific contraindication to its use. The intrauterine device is an acceptable alternative for those patients for whom oral contraception is contraindicated.

The current management of molar pregnancy does not require hysterectomy; therefore, the fertility of these women can be preserved. In counseling these patients, the clinician should point out that a woman with one molar pregnancy can anticipate almost the same reproductive outcome as other women without that history. Their rate of term delivery is approximately 67%, and they are have a minimal increased risk of future obstetric complications. The risk of another episode of trophoblastic disease is 1/50–1/150 among women with a prior molar pregnancy. Recurrent molar pregnancy is usually characterized by worse histologic features and higher risk of gestational trophoblastic neoplasia. The physician and the patient should also be aware that even after an intervening normal pregnancy, these patients can develop choriocarcinoma. Therefore, a high degree of suspicion must be maintained in all future pregnancies of patients with a history of hydatidiform mole. The appropriate workup and diagnosis after an uneventful normal pregnancy must be followed. The physician should document the absence of molar changes in the placenta with the aid of sonography early in pregnancy. The placenta should be sent for histopathologic evaluation after delivery. An HCG titer should be obtained at the 6-week postpartum visit. Some patients might present during the postpartum period with abnormal uterine bleeding or an enlarged uterus. Any such abnormality during the puerperium should prompt a careful and detailed evaluation in these patients for recurrent GTN or metastatic disease.[25]

Medical complications of gestational trophoblastic disease

A relatively common complication is the development of trophoblastic hyperthyroidism. This entity includes a spectrum of clinical conditions involving a hypermetabolic state diagnosed clinically or by laboratory parameters. A hydatidiform-mole-induced thyrotoxicosis may present as a medical emergency. The HCG molecule has weak thyrotropin-stimulating effect on the thyroid gland when present in high concentrations. Accordingly, most cases of hyperthyroidism result from high levels of HCG. The clinical features can include palpable goiters, supraventricular tachycardia, weight loss, and fine tremors. The laboratory findings observed in these patients include normal or low thyroid-stimulating hormone levels (TSH), increased thyroxine (T_4) and triiodothyronine (T_3), and a suppressed response to thyroid-releasing hormone (TRH). The treatment of this entity is emergent evacuation of the molar pregnancy. A medical consultation may be necessary for patients with a hyperdynamic cardiac response in order to administer beta-blockers or sodium iodine prior to the procedure.

Another common complication of molar pregnancy is anemia resulting from excessive vaginal bleeding and loss of iron stores. A complication of having major blood loss is the development of disseminated intravascular coagulation (DIC). However, DIC could also be the presenting symptom of molar pregnancy. It is believed to be associated with the release of thromboplastic substances from the molar tissue into the maternal circulation. The treatment consists of evacuation of the molar tissue and correction of the fibrinogen and platelet depletion as needed. Infection associated with molar pregnancy is uncommon and can be appropriately controlled by broad-spectrum antibiotics.[26]

Respiratory complications can be the sequelae of metastatic disease, pulmonary edema, adult respiratory distress syndrome (ARDS), or trophoblastic embolization. All patients with pulmonary dysfunction require a thorough workup,

including physical examination with special attention to the respiratory system, chest radiography, arterial blood-gas determination, and possible placement of a pulmonary artery catheter. The finding of severe hypoxemia and/or pulmonary edema requires immediate intensive care and consultation with a pulmonary specialist. If respiratory compromise occurs prior to evacuation of the mole, the procedure should still be performed after supportive measurements have been established.[13,26]

The occurrence of subclinical trophoblastic embolization has been well documented by the finding of trophoblastic tissue in the lungs during autopsy[13] and by the recovery of multinucleated giant cells and large mononuclear cells from pulmonary artery blood specimens.[43] This phenomenon occurs in 2–3% of molar pregnancies and is more common in the presence of an enlarged uterus. The patient may be asymptomatic or have minimal symptoms at the time of the diagnosis. On the other hand, some patients may require oxygen support, sedation, steroids, and positive-pressure ventilation for their respiratory compromise.[26] Hankins et al studied the hemodynamic profile in six pregnancies with the diagnosis of mole prior to, during, and after evacuation, to assess the degree of thromboplastic embolization associated with pulmonary distress. They found that minimal thromboplastic embolization did not alter the hemodynamic parameters of the pulmonary or systemic circulations. They concluded that the pulmonary vascular reaction is not an anaphylactoid phenomenon, but is dose-related. Embolization sufficient to cause pulmonary compromise was rare. They postulated that the etiology of the pulmonary compromise in some patients could be overzealous fluid management for anemic patients with normal intravascular volume, or for those with altered hemodynamic parameters secondary to hypertensive disease. These authors suggest the use of a Swan–Ganz artery catheter in patients presenting with hydatidiform mole and hypertension and/or pulmonary dysfunction.[43]

Treatment and follow-up of malignant trophoblastic tumors

Malignant gestational trophoblastic tumors (GTT) can be categorized into metastatic and nonmetastatic disease. They are sensitive to chemotherapy, and complete remission can usually be achieved. Resistance to treatment is dependent on the patient's prognostic risk factors. A prognostic scoring system has been developed by the World Health Organization (Table 38.3). Multiagent chemotherapy should be administered if the prognostic scores are 8 or higher.[44]

Patients with locally invasive GTT will present clinically with persistently elevated serum beta-HCG levels, vaginal bleeding, uterine enlargement, or acute pelvic pain. Acute pelvic pain may occur secondary to myometrial invasion and erosion by the tumor causing intra-abdominal bleeding and necrosis. Histologically, nonmetastatic invasive GTT may have

Table 38.3 World Health Organization prognostic index for gestational trophoblastic disease

	Score (1, 2, or 4)			
Prognostic factor	0	1	2	4
Age (years)	<39	>39	–	–
Antecedent pregnancy	Mole	Abortion	Term	–
Interval (months)	<4	4–6	7–12	>12
HCG (mIU/ml)	$<10^3$	10^3–10^4	10^4–10^5	$>10^5$
ABO groups	–	0 or A	B or AB	–
Largest tumor	–	3–5 cm	>5 cm	–
Site of metastasis	Lung, pelvis, or vagina	Spleen or kidneys	Gastrointestinal tract or liver	Brain
Number of metastatic tumors	–	1–3	4–8	>8
Prior chemotherapy	–	–	Single	Multiple

Risk category for failing initial therapy given total score:
Low risk:	0–4
Intermediate risk	5–7
High risk:	>8

(Data from World Health Organization Scientific Group on Gestational Trophoblastic Disease, Technical Report Series No. 692. World Health Organization: Geneva, 1983)

features of choriocarcinoma or of hydatidiform mole. Locally invasive GTT occurs in 15–20% of patients after undergoing evacuation for molar gestation. Treatment should begin at once, regardless of their level and without waiting to see whether they decrease. Cure rate occurs in approximately 100% of the cases.

Placental-site trophoblastic tumor is another type of non-metastatic GTT. This rare condition can be found after a dilation and curettage for vaginal bleeding after any type of pregnancy. Placental-site trophoblastic tumors usually do not metastasize. They produce small amounts of HCG and placental lactogen, which may be used in the diagnosis and follow-up of the disease. These tumors fail to respond to chemotherapy, and their inconsistent production of HCG causes great concern. Therefore, if metastasis is not evident, hysterectomy is the treatment of choice.

Metastatic GTT occurs in approximately 4% of patients undergoing uterine evacuation for molar pregnancy. They tend to be hemorrhagic tumors. The symptoms are a result of bleeding at the metastatic site. Histologically, these metastases usually have features of choriocarcinoma. Metastatic GTT can be successfully treated with chemotherapy in over 70% of the cases. Metastasis usually occurs into the vagina, lungs, liver, and brain. This metastasis gives rise to the anatomic staging of GTT (Table 38.4).

Metastatic lesions to the vagina are friable, and appear to be red or purple. These lesions occur in 30% of patients with metastasis. A lesion to the vagina gives the patient stage II disease. Vaginal lesions can bleed profusely and may be managed by packing, hypogastric artery embolization, or wide local excision.

Pulmonary metastasis occurs in 80% of patients with metastatic GTT. Pulmonary involvement gives the patient stage III disease. Such metastasis can be seen in routine chest radiography as 'snowstorm' appearance, pleural effusions, densities, and wedge patterns similar to those seen with an embolism. Nevertheless, the most sensitive test for diagnosing pulmonary metastasis is a chest CT scan. A patient with pulmonary metastasis may have symptoms of hemoptysis, dyspnea, and shortness of breath, or be asymptomatic. Patients may also develop pulmonary hypertension. These lesions are usually responsive to chemotherapy, but, if they are resistant, thoracotomy and resection can be perform with great success.

Metastasis to brain, liver, kidneys, or the gastrointestinal tract categorizes the patient as having stage IV disease. At this stage, the disease is usually resistant to single-agent chemotherapy and should be treated with a combination regimen.

Liver metastasis can occur in 10% of patients with metastatic GTT. For diagnosis and follow-up, an abdominal CT scan can be used. Acute abdominal pain can be the presenting symptoms of hepatic lesions secondary to hemoperitoneum caused by hemorrhagic lesions. Exploratory laparotomy and hepatic resection may sometimes be needed for control of bleeding.

Brain metastasis can occur with metastatic GTT and patients can present with neurologic deficits secondary to spontaneous bleeding. If brain metastasis is diagnosed, emergent radiation with 2000–3000 cGy should be given along with a systemic multiagent chemotherapy regimen. A neurosurgical

Table 38.4 FIGO staging of gestational trophoblastic neoplasia

Stage I	Confined to uterine corpus
Stage II	Metastasis to vagina and pelvis
Stage III	Metastasis to lungs
Stage IV	Distant metastasis

team should be notified in case a craniotomy is needed for decompression and control of bleeding.

Chemotherapy

Chemotherapy is the treatment of choice for metastatic gestational trophoblastic tumors. This treatment should be given by a gynecologic oncologist or a medical oncologist.

For nonmetastatic GTT and low-risk metastatic GTT (stages II–III), single-agent chemotherapy with either methotrexate or actinomycin D has achieved excellent remission rates.[45] To determine the need of additional treatment, serum HCG is measured weekly, and the levels are curved to follow its regression. A second chemotherapy course can be given if the HCG level rises, or if the levels remain constant for 3 consecutive weeks.

A combination chemotherapy regimen is reserved for resistant tumors previously treated with a single chemotherapy course, high-risk patients with prognostic scores of 8 or greater, and patients with stage IV disease (Table 38.2). For chemorefractory GTT, 42% of patients undergoing surgery have achieved complete response.[46]

Methotrexate, actinomycin D, and cyclophosphamide (MAC) was the preferred combination chemotherapy regimen until recent years when effective protocols using etoposide were introduced. The new combination regimen of etoposide, methotrexate, actinomycin D, cyclophosphamide being (CTX), and vincristine (EMA-CO) has produced a 75–85% remission rate in patients with metastasis and high-risk scores.[47,48] New multiagent regimens have been developed. For brain metastasis, an 87% remission was reported with the use of EMA-CO in a small series of patients in 1996.[49] Recently, a regimen using platinum or taxol has been implemented for EMA-CO-resistant disease and metastatic placental-site trophoblastic tumors with great success.[50]

The major side effects of chemotherapy are neutropenia, hemorrhagic cystitis from the CTX, and severe renal toxicity (Table 38.5). The use of adequate hydration, and granulocyte colony-stimulating factor have reduced the incidence of this side effects. An observation has been made of an increased risk of secondary tumors since the addition of etoposide. An increased incidence of leukemia, colon cancer, melanoma, and breast cancer has been reported in patients treated with chemotherapy for GTN.[49] The use of chemotherapy agents on young women increases their risk of early menopause. Recent studies suggest that the combination of gonadotropin-releasing hormone agonists given concurrently with the chemotherapy regimen may prevent chemotherapy-induced ovarian failure.[51]

Patients successfully treated for GTN with chemotherapy can expect normal reproduction in the future.[52] Nevertheless, patients should be counseled to use a reliable form of hormonal contraception during the first year of remission, since there is a risk of 1–2% of having a second mole in a subsequent pregnancy.[53] It has also been reported that patients treated with chemotherapy are not at increased risk of having offspring with congenital anomalies.[54]

Table 38.5 Chemotherapy agents used in the treatment of GTN

Chemotherapy agent	Side effects
Methotrexate	Hepatotoxicity, myelosuppression, mucosal ulceration
Actinomycin D	Nausea and vomiting, myelosuppression, skin necrosis
Etoposide	Hypotension, myelosuppression, alopecia
Cyclophosphamide	Hemorrhagic cystitis, bladder fibrosis, myelosuppression, alopecia, amenorrhea, hepatitis
Vincristine	Cranial nerve palsies, neurotoxicity, alopecia
Cisplastin	Nephrotoxicity, tinnitus and hearing loss, nausea and vomiting, peripheral neuropathy, myelosuppression
Paclitaxel	Cardiac arrhythmia, myelosuppression, alopecia, allergic reactions
Bleomycin	Pulmonary fibrosis, dermatologic and anaphylactic reactions, fever

References

1. Brinton LA, Wu B, Wang W, Ershow AG. Gestational trophoblastic disease: case-control study from the People's Republic of China. Am J Obstet Gynecol 1989; 161: 121–7.
2. Berkowitz RS, Goldstein DP, Bernstein MR. Natural history of partial molar pregnancy. Obstet Gynecol 1983; 66: 677.
3. Pratola D, Wilkins P. The placenta, umbilical cord and amnio sac. In: Gompel C, Silvergery SG (eds), Pathology in Gynecology and Obstetrics, pp. 481–91. JB Lippincott: Philadelphia, 1985.
4. Acaia B, Parazzini F, LaVecchia C et al. Increased frequency of complete hydatidiform mole in women with repeated abortion. Gynecol Oncol 1988; 31: 310–14.
5. Szulman AE, Surti U. The syndromes of hydatiform mole. I. Cytogenetic and morphological correlations. Am J Obstet Gynecol 1978; 131: 665–71.
6. Szulman AE, Surti U. The syndromes of hydatiform mole. II. Morphologic evolution of the complete and partial mole. Am J Obstet Gynecol 1978; 132: 20–7.
7. Sebire NJ, Fisher RA, Ree HC. Histopathological diagnosis of partial and complete hydatiform mole in the first trimester of pregnancy. Pediatr Dev Pathol 2003; 6: 69–77.
8. Szulman AE, Surti U. The syndromes of partial and complete molar gestation. Clin Obstet Gynecol 1984; 27: 172–80.
9. Jones BW. Gestational trophoblastic disease. What have we learned in the past decade? Am J Obstet Gynecol 1990; 162: 1286–95.
10. Watson EJ, Hernandez E, Miyazawa K. Partial hydatidiform moles. A review. Obstet Gynecol Surv 1987; 42: 540–4.

11. Feinberg FR, Lockwood CJ, Salafia C, Hobbins JC. Sonographic diagnosis of a pregnancy with a diffuse hydatidiform mole and coexistent 46,XX fetus. A case report. Obstet Gynecol 1988; 72: 485–8.

12. Thomas EJ, Pryce WI, Maltby EL, Duncan SLB. The prospective management of a coexisting hydatidiform mole and fetus. Aust N Z J Obstet Gynaecol 1987; 27: 343–5.

13. Vejerslev L, Sunde L, Hansen B et al. Hydatidiform mole and fetus with normal karyotype: support of a separate entity. Obstet Gynecol 1991; 77: 868.

14. Berkowitz RS, Goldstein DP. Gestational trophoblastic disease. Cancer 1995; 76: 2079–85.

15. Sebire NJ, Fisher RA, Foskett M et al. Risk of recurrent hydatiform mole and subsequent pregnancy outcome following complete or partial hydatiform molar pregnancy. Br J Obstet Gynaecol 2003; 110: 22–6.

16. Fisher RA, Lawler SD, Ormerod MG et al. Flow cytometry used to distinguish between complete and partial hydatiform moles. Placenta 1987; 8: 249–56.

17. Lage JM, Driscoll SG, Yavner DL et al. Hydatiform moles: application of flow cytometry in diagnosis. Am J Clin Pathol 1988; 89: 596–600.

18. Lage JM, Popek EJ. The role of DNA flow cytometry in evaluation of partial and complete hydatiform moles and hydropic abortions. Semin Diagn Pathol 1993; 10: 267–74.

19. Hedley DW, Friedlander ML, Taylor IW et al. Method for analysis of cellular DNA content of paraffin-embedded pathological material using flow cytometry. J Histochem Cytochem 1983; 31: 1333–5.

20. Redline RW, Hassold T, Zaragoza M. Determinants of villous trophoblastic hyperplasia in spontaneous abortions. Mod Pathol 1988; 11: 762–8.

21. Szulman AE, Surti U. The syndromes of hydatiform mole. I. Cytogenetic and morphologic correlations. Am J Obstet Gynecol 1978; 131: 665–71.

22. Choi-Hong SR, Genest DR, Crum CP et al. Twin pregnancies with complete hydatiform mole and coexisting fetus: use of fluorescent in situ hybridization to evaluate placental X and Y chromosomal content. Hum Pathol 1995; 26: 1175–80.

23. Harashwardhan MT, David RG et al. Immunohistochemistry for the imprinted gene product IPL/PHLDA2 for facilitating the differential diagnosis of complete hydatiform mole. J Repro Med 2004; 49: 630–6.

24. Goldstein DP, Berkowitz RS, Bernstein MR. Reproductive performance after molar pregnancy and gestational trophoblastic tumors. Clin Obstet Gynecol 1984; 27: 221–7.

25. Caspi B, Elchalal U, Dgani R et al. Invasive mole and placental site trophoblastic tumor: two entities of gestational trophoblastic disease with a common ultrasonographic appearance. J Ultrasound Med 1991; 10: 517–19.

26. Kohorn EI. Molar pregnancy. Presentation and diagnosis. Clin Obstet Gynecol 1984; 27: 181–91.

27. Trimor-Tritsch IE, Rottem S, Blumenfeld Z. Pathology of the early intrauterine pregnancy. In: Timor-Tritsch IE, Rottem S (eds), pp. 109–24. Transvaginal Sonography. Elsevier: New York, 1988.

28. Powell MC, Buckely J, Worthington BS, Symonds EM. Magnetic resonance imaging and hydatidiform mole. Br J Radiol 1986; 59: 561–4.

29. Hemming JD, Quirke P, Womack C et al. Diagnosis of molar pregnancy and persistent trophoblastic disease by flow cytometry. J Clin Pathol 1987; 40: 615–20.

30. Fisher RA, Lawler SD, Ormerod MG et al. Flow cytometry used to distinguish between complete and partial hydatidiform moles. Placenta 1987; 8: 249–56.

31. Soper JT. Surgical therapy for gestational trophoblastic disease. J Reprod Med 1994; 39: 168–74.

32. Schlaerth JB. Methodology of molar pregnancy termination. Clin Obstet Gynecol 1984; 27: 192–8.

33. Lao TTH, Lee FHC, Yeung SSL. Repeat curettage after evacuation of hydatidiform mole. Acta Obstet Gynecol Scand 1987; 66: 305–7.

34. Kim DS, Moon H, Kim KT et al. Effects of prophylactic chemotherapy for persistent trophoblastic disease in patients with complete hydatidiform mole. Obstet Gynecol 1986; 67: 690–4.

35. Goldstein DP, Berkowitz RS, Bernstein MR. Management of molar pregnancy. J Reprod Med 1981; 26: 208–12.

36. Goldstein DP, Berkowitz RS. Prophylactic chemotherapy of complete molar pregnancy. Semin Oncol 1985; 22: 157–60.

37. A Ilancheran. Optimal treatment in gestational trophoblastic disease. Ann Acad Med Singapore 1998; 27: 698–704.

38. Soper JT, Lewis JL, Hammond CB. Gestational trophoblastic disease. In: Hoskins WJ, Perez CA, Young RC (eds), Principles and Practice of Gynecologic Oncology, pp. 1039–77. Lipincott-Raven: Philadelphia, 1997.

39. Lurain JR, Brewer JI, Torok EE, Halpern B. Natural history of hydatidiform mole after primary evacuation. Am J Obstet Gynecol 1983; 145: 591–5.

40. Pak-Chung H, Wong L, Ho-Kei M. Return of ovulation after evacuation of hydatidiform moles. Am J Obstet Gynecol 1985; 153: 638.

41. Yuen BH, Burch P. Relationship of oral contraceptives and the intrauterine contraceptive devices to the regression of concentrations of the beta subunit of human chorionic gonadotropin and invasive complications after molar pregnancy. Am J Obstet Gynecol 1983; 145: 214.

42. Curry SL, Schlaerth JB, Kohorn EL et al. Hormonal contraception and trophoblastic sequelae after hydatidiform mole (a Gynecology Oncology Group Study). Am J Obstet Gynecol 1989; 160: 805–9.

43. Hankins GD, Wendel GD, Snyder RR, Cunningham EG. Trophoblastic embolization during molar evacuation. Central hemodynamic observations. Obstet Gynecol 1987; 69: 368–72.

44. Gordon AN, Gerhenson DM, Copeland LJ, Stringer CA, Morris M, Wharton JT. High-risk metastatic gestational trophoblastic disease: further stratification into two clinical entities. Gynecol Oncol 1989; 34: 54–6.

45. Homesly HD. Single-agent therapy for nonmetastatic and low-risk gestational trophoblastic disease. J Reprod Med 1998; 43: 69–74.

46. Lehman E, Gerhenson DM, Burke TW et al. Salvage surgery for chemorefractory gestational trophoblastic disease. J Clin Oncol 1994; 12: 2737–42.

47. Bagshawe KD. Treatment of high-risk choriocarcinoma. J Reprod Med 1984; 29: 813–20.

48. Bolis G, Bonazzi C, Landoni F et al. EMA/CO regimen in high-risk gestational trophoblastic tumor (GTT). Gynecol Oncol 1988; 31: 439–44.

49. Rustin GJ, Newlands ES, Lutz JM et al. Combination but not single-agent methotrexate chemotherapy for gestational trophoblastic tumors increases the incidence of second tumors. J Clin Oncol 1996; 14: 2769–73.

50. Newlands ES, Mulholland PJ, Holden L et al. Etoposide and cisplastin/etoposide, methotrexate, and actinomycin D (EMA) chemotherapy for patients with high-risk gestational trophoblastic tumors refractory to EMA/cyclophosphamide and vincristine chemotherapy and patients' metastatic placental site trophoblastic tumors. J Clin Oncol 2000; 18: 854–9.

51. Blumenfeld Z, Avivi I, Linn S et al. Prevention of irreversible chemotherapy-induced ovarian damage in young women with lymphoma by a gonadotropin-releasing hormone agonist in parallel to chemotherapy. Human Reprod 1996; 11: 1620–6.

52. Berkowitz RS, IM SS, Bernstein MR, Goldstein DP. Gestational trophoblastic disease: subsequent pregnancy outcome, including repeat molar pregnancy. J Reprod Med 1998; 43: 81–6.

53. ACOG Practice Bulletin No. 53. Diagnosis and treatment of gestational trophoblastic disease. June 2004: 1365–77.

54. Green DM, Zevon MA, Lowrie G et al. Congenital anomalies in children of patients who received chemotherapy for cancer in childhood and adolescence. N Engl J Med 1991; 325: 141–6.

39 Quality of obstetric care: the medicolegal perspective

Marlene Schwebel and Curtis L. Cetrulo

With increasing professional liability settlements, many obstetric providers have faced new challenges in their practices.[1] Some physicians have gone as far as dropping obstetrics from their practice, while others have altered patient management by using defensive medical practices. A recent obstetrics and gynecology survey performed by a national physician search and consulting firm suggests that rising malpractice insurance premiums may result in a serious impact on the availability of obstetric services in the selected states surveyed.[2] Of the 268 responses, 95% of obstetricians and gynecologists reported experiencing rising malpractice insurance premiums. Thirty-nine percent reported discontinuing deliveries due to the malpractice premium crisis, while 83% stated that they would continue to perform deliveries in their state if malpractice insurance rates were reasonable.

While one solution to this problem would be tort reform, we must also consider the reality of professional liability litigation when injury occurs and the patient sues for professional liability. The purpose of this chapter is to introduce and familiarize the practitioner with the fundamental concepts of professional liability law as well as confidentiality, informed consent, and the medical record.

The law of torts

Professional liability claims in the USA are governed by the law of 'torts'. The word 'tort' is derived from the Latin 'tortus' meaning 'twisted'.[3] Generally, a tort has been defined as 'a private or civil wrong or injury, including action for bad faith breach of contract, for which the court will provide a remedy in the form of an action for damages'.[4]

As this definition suggests, tort law encompasses a multitude of wrongdoings, ranging from assault and battery to design, manufacture, and sale of defective products that cause injury.

Tort law is governed by 'common law', a body of rules and principles of actions that is derived from ancient usages and customs, or from the judgments and decrees of courts.[5] Therefore, tort law is distinguished from statutory law, the body of law which is created by legislative enactments, and from regulatory law, the body of law created by administrative bodies or regulatory agencies. The 'rules' of tort law will not be found in the statute books, code books, or published regulations; instead, they are defined primarily by the decisions, rulings, and opinions of courts of law as recorded over the centuries. Because tort law is defined by judicial decisions, it is continually evolving as new decisions are rendered. Each state has its own unique body of common law as defined by its own courts. Therefore, the law of torts is different in each state. Moreover, one state's court decision is not binding in another state, although decisions are often cited in other states for persuasive purposes.

Historically, the two generally recognized objectives of tort law have been to compensate the injured party at the expense of the wrongdoer and to discourage antisocial behavior.[6] Generally, tort law can be divided into three major categories: (1) the law of 'intentional torts'; (2) the law of 'strict liability'; (3) the law of 'negligence'.[7]

An 'intentional tort' is simply a tort in which the person committing the harm, or the 'tortfeasor', acts with the intention of harming another. For instance, the act of striking a person in anger and thereby causing injury is an intentional tort.

The law of strict liability determines liability without reference to the state of mind or degree of 'fault' of the tortfeasor. The law of strict liability is applied only to certain types of conduct. Historically, strict liability has been applied to activities that are deemed to be extremely dangerous such as the use of high explosives. More recently, strict liability has been more broadly applied to the manufacture of defective products.

'Negligence' is defined as the failure to use care as a reasonable, prudent person would use in similar circumstances.[8]

In the law of negligence, the standard of care is the degree of care, as a range of reasonableness, that a reasonable, prudent person should exercise in similar circumstances.[9] The majority of professional liability claims allege negligence on the part of the practitioner. The following sections of this chapter will discuss the necessary elements of the plaintiff's prima facie case in a professional liability case.

The prima facie case

In all civil litigations, the plaintiff bears the burden of proof in a professional liability action. Burden of proof is the obligation of a party to establish, by evidence, the necessary degree of belief concerning a fact or facts in dispute between the parties in the mind of the jury or the judge.[10] In civil litigation, the 'necessary degree of belief' is generally defined as 'more probable than not'. This is very different from a criminal case in which there is a much higher standard, namely, 'beyond a reasonable doubt'. In order to meet this burden of proof in a professional liability action, the plaintiff must prove all four of the following elements of his/her claim by a preponderance of the evidence which a jury finds to be credible:

(1) duty
(2) breach of the standard of care
(3) proximate causation
(4) injury (damages).

For instance, in order to establish liability in a professional liability case, the plaintiff must present evidence to establish that, more probable than not:

(1) The physician owed a duty of care to the patient.
(2) There was a breach of duty of the standard of care.
(3) The breach of the duty owed was the proximate cause of the injury.
(4) An injury, or damages, did occur.

Duty

When we refer to 'duty' as it relates to professional liability, it is generally the reference made to the obligation of the physician/health-care provider/hospital to the patient. Many cases have been argued on the issue of 'duty' and whether a duty existed between the physician and patient. The physician/patient relationship is a contractual agreement, and generally begins when the physician agrees to provide medical services to the patient that are commiserate with his abilities within acceptable standards of care. This is a consensual agreement between the physician and the patient and the duty exists whether or not a fee for the services was received. Unless this relationship is found to exist, a physician cannot be held liable for professional liability. In other words, without such a relationship, the physician owes no 'legal' duty to the would-be patient. It is important not to confuse the physician's 'legal'

duty with the physician's 'ethical' duty. The American Medical Association's Principles of Medical Ethics provide that a physician may serve, in the provision of appropriate patient care, except in emergencies, whomever the physician freely chooses to serve, without an obligation to accept any patient.[11] Duty to the patient by the physician may end when the treatment to the patient is complete or when the patient is referred to another health-care provider who has the medical ability to care for the patient and is willing to accept the patient. A standard of reasonableness is utilized when terminating the physician/patient relationship where the patient is referred to an alternative health-care provider. It is prudent to provide the patient with three alternative physicians/health-care providers within a reasonable specified period of time. The patient may also terminate the relationship by procuring care from another health-care provider.

Breach

Once duty has been established, the next requisite element is 'breach'. It must be proven that the physician breached the standard of care owed to the patient. The standard of care is the degree of care which a reasonable, prudent person would exercise given a particular set of circumstances. The legal definition of the standard of care in the medical profession is requiring the physician to possess and exercise the degree and skill of due care of the 'average qualified practitioner' in that medical specialty. Those practitioners who hold themselves out to be specialists will be held to a higher standard of care. The standards are derived in a large part from the publications of medical organizations in appropriate areas of specialization and from widely accepted medical authorities.

While physicians often refer to the standard of care in terms of 'negligence', the law interprets 'negligence' in a broader manner, including all four requisite elements of the prima facie case noted above, only one of which is the breach of the standard of care. The standard of care and a breach of that standard thereof is determined upon the unique facts of each case. Since the plaintiff has the burden of proof in a professional liability case, the plaintiff generally offers the assistance of expert opinion by expert witnesses.

Patients frequently confuse an unfortunate outcome with wrongdoing. The occurrence of an unfortunate result or the failure of improvement in a patient's condition does not, in and of itself, prove negligence. A breach of the standard of care must be proven in order to prove negligence. For example, a physician who fails to use ordinary skill and care in making a diagnosis and, as a result, undertakes an incorrect treatment, may be liable for the resulting harm to the patient. Additionally, if special knowledge of equipment is needed to treat a patient, a general practitioner may be under a duty to refer the patient to a specialist.

Where two acceptable 'schools of thought' exist, the fact that one physician adopts one method of treatment as opposed to the other does not constitute negligence. When either school of thought is acceptable, the plaintiff must prove that such treatment was not in accordance with accepted practice. In almost all cases, expert medical opinion will be necessary to determine whether the conduct of the physician breached the standard of care. Experts are generally necessary, as jurors cannot be expected to understand the medical concepts in a professional liability case and could not be expected to come to a decision purely based on speculation. However, a jury determines what is reasonable and is not bound to believe the testimony provided by experts. It is the plaintiff's obligation to show a causal relationship between the alleged negligence and the ensuing injury. In rare cases, expert opinion is not required. In these cases, the negligence is so apparent that it is within common knowledge. For instance, a sponge or instrument left in the operative site would speak for itself. This is known as the doctrine of *res ipsa loquitur* and is still utilized today in applicable cases.

Causation

The third requisite element in a professional liability case is causation. The plaintiff must prove in a standard of 'more likely than not' that 'but for' the physician's actions, the injury would not have occurred. Experts are enlisted to provide a medical opinion about the probability (more likely than not) that the medical treatment was the cause of the injury. The plaintiff must prove that a duty was breached and the breach of the duty was the 'proximate' (that is, primary, moving, or producing) cause of the injury in order to prevail in a claim of professional liability based on negligence theory. This is a significant burden for the plaintiff to prove. In professional liability cases, the causal connection between the negligence of the defendant and the injury must be established by expert testimony that the injury sustained, to a reasonable degree of medical certainty, was more probable than not a result of the physician's negligence.

The legal requirement for establishing cause is the 'probability' or 'greater that 50.1% rule', 'more probable than not', or 'within reasonable medical certainty'. Testimony provided that such a relationship is merely possible, conceivable, or reasonable, is insufficient to meet the burden of proximate causation. Therefore, the distinction between what is probable and what is merely possible is crucial.

The necessity of proving causation in order to recover on a professional liability claim is illustrated by the following example. Consider a case in which a patient had an abnormal labor with an arrest disorder and, at the same time, had hyperstimulation with oxytocin. In addition, there was prolonged second stage of labor without fetal heart-rate monitoring, and the baby was born with congenital anomalies incompatible with life. While it could be argued that the failure to manage properly the labor constituted malpractice, if there was no causal connection between the failure to manage the labor and the congenital anomalies, there will be no recovery against the physician.

The breach of the standard of care and causation must be established by expert testimony. Medical expert witnesses are professionals having the same medical degree and specialty who assist the court and jury by explaining, in lay terms, the medical facts of the case. Additionally, the medical expert is permitted to offer 'opinions' as to what he or she thinks, believes, or infers, regarding the medical evidence presented in the case as to the facts in dispute. However, in recent years, it has become increasingly necessary for experts to be prepared to back up their opinion with scientific proof.[12] This represents the change that occurred when the US Supreme Court ruled in *Daubert v. Merrell Dow Pharmaceuticals* that the trial judge must ensure that expert testimony is the result of a 'reliable foundation'.[13]

There are usually two different interpretations of the facts. The first is the facts as explained by the plaintiff's expert, and the second is often a very different set of facts as portrayed by the defendant's expert witness. It is then left to the jury or the judge to decide which set of facts is reasonable and most believable, and, thus, which opinion to find most credible. Ideally, the expert witness offers an unbiased opinion as to his or her interpretation of the facts. However, it has been suggested that often expert testimony is biased. Only a physician can offer expert opinion against another physician. There has been much debate about the competence of physicians offering opinion on standards of care in specialty areas Expert witnesses should have the same training, practices, and expertise as the defendant provider. Each discipline should provide expert opinion for that particular specialty. A pediatrician is qualified to offer expert opinion testimony against another pediatrician. One profession should not provide expert opinion on the standard of care for another profession. Recently, in a landmark court decision, the Illinois Supreme Court held that a physician is not qualified to offer expert opinion on standards of care for nursing, and that only a nurse is qualified to offer expert opinion regarding the standard of care for nurses.[14]

Injury (damages)

The fourth requisite element in a professional liability case is injury. The plaintiff must have sustained an injury in order to succeed in a professional liability suit. The injury must be causally related to the alleged negligence of the physician. Damages may be physical, emotional, or financial. Punitive damages may be recoverable in certain circumstances when there has been gross departure from the standard of care. Interestingly, in a recent decision by the New York Court of Appeals, it was held that a woman may recover for damages for emotional distress, despite the lack of physical injury, for medical malpractice that results in stillbirth or miscarriage.[15]

Confidentiality

Physician/patient confidentiality came about in the early 1900s in an effort for patients to be honest with their physicians when accessing medical care. The privilege of confidentiality belongs to the patient, not the physician. Additionally, physician/patient confidentiality does not cease to exist even after the patient dies.[16] One early case demonstrating confidentiality and the physician/patient relationship is *Humphers v. First Interstate Bank of Oregon*.[17] In this case, sealed adoption records were opened by the hospital on the basis of necessity after the defendant physician intentionally wrote a letter stating that it was imperative that the daughter given up for adoption (Dawn Kastning) contact her biologic mother because of a possible diethystilbestrol (DES) exposure. The suggestion of DES exposure was knowingly untrue. The plaintiff was unmarried at the time of the child's birth and had given her up for adoption. The plaintiff had since married, had a family of her own, and had never told anyone about the birth of this child. When Dawn Kastning contacted her biologic mother, Ramona Humphers, Mrs Humphers was outraged and sued the defendant physician for breach of confidentiality.

Another case involving breach of confidentiality is *Estate of Behringer v. Princeton Medical Center*.[18] In this case, the plaintiff, Dr Behringer, was hospitalized at the hospital where he practiced as an ear, nose, and throat specialist as well as a plastic surgeon. He was diagnosed with HIV/AIDS after being hospitalized with *Pneumocystis carinii* pneumonia. His chart was kept at the nurses' station without any protection. His diagnosis was soon known throughout the hospital. During his hospital stay and after he returned home, he received numerous calls from well-wishers, all of whom knew his diagnosis. He was subsequently banned from performing surgery at the hospital, and as word in the community grew, his office practice dwindled. One of the causes of action against the defendant hospital was for breach of confidentiality, as the hospital failed to take reasonable precautions regarding the patient's medical record.

What about when confidentiality comes into conflict with the duty to disclose? In a well-known case, *Tarasoff v. Regents of University of California*,[19] the psychiatrist treating a patient named Proddar knew that his patient presented a serious danger to Tatiana Tarasoff, as he had verbalized his intent to harm her. Proddar carried out his threat and killed Tatiana. The court held that the psychiatrist, Dr Moore, had a special relationship with Proddar (physician/patient relationship) but also had a duty to protect the identifiable victim from a foreseeable risk of harm and to warn her. This case dealt with the specialty of psychiatry and the special relationship between a psychiatrist and patient, but one can extrapolate the facts of this case to other medical disciplines, and consider whether the duty to warn identifiable third parties from foreseeable serious harm will follow the *Tarasoff* court holding. Of note is that *Tarasoff* is a California state court decision, and the court's decision is not binding in any other state. It has, however, been cited in court cases outside California for persuasive purposes.

In an effort to protect patient records from disclosure, the federal government became involved, and HIPAA (Health Insurance Portability and Accountability Act of 1996) was cre-ated. The privacy rule requirements of HIPAA became effective in 2003. This was intended to protect individual medical information while maintaining the communication of health information in order to provide and protect patient health information. Provisions of the privacy rule include but are not limited to patients' access to their medical records, notice of the provider's privacy practices, limits on how personal health information may be used, restriction of use of patient's health information for marketing, confidentiality protection utilizing state law, confidential patient communication, and complaints regarding privacy practices.[20]

In general, the HIPAA privacy rule requires the healthcare provider to establish privacy procedures for its practice. The provider must also implement a system for notifying patients about their privacy rights. The provider must give notice to every individual receiving care on the date of service. Additionally, the provider should also obtain the patient's written acknowledgment of receiving the notice and keep the acknowledgment copy. Providers must also provide training to their employees on privacy procedures and designate an individual to be responsible for overseeing the enforcement of privacy procedures. Although messages may be left at patients' homes, it is prudent to limit the amount and type of information. For instance, it is reasonable to leave the provider's name and number, requesting the patient to return the call. Additionally, patient requests that are reasonable, such as requesting that messages be left at an alternative telephone number or requesting that correspondence be mailed to an alternative address, should be accommodated. Sign-in sheets may be utilized as long as the information is limited. Medical information, such as the reason for the patient's visit, should not appear on the sign-in sheet.

Faxing of patient's health information records to another provider is allowed, but reasonable safeguards must be in place to protect the patient's confidentiality. An example would be to have the fax machine situated as a designated fax in a secure location away from unauthorized access, and confirming the fax number prior to sending the fax. Due to safeguard concerns, e-mail is not a good idea.

It is important to realize that the HIPAA privacy rule, although a federal regulation, does not pre-empt state law where state laws provide additional protection. For instance, when a state law requires reporting of a specific disease, the privacy rule does not supersede the state law.

Informed consent

Another area that can expose the physician to liability for professional liability is informed consent.

> 'Informed consent is the name for the general principle of law that a physician has a duty to disclose what a reasonably prudent physician in the medical community in the exercise of reasonable care would disclose to his patient as to whatever grave risks of injury might be incurred from a

proposed course of treatment, so that a patient, exercising ordinary care for his own welfare, and faced with the choice of undergoing the proposed treatment, or alternative treatment, or none at all, may intelligently exercise his judgment by reasonably balancing the probable risks against the probable benefits.'[21]

As demonstrated by this definition, informed consent does not merely necessitate the patient's signature on a consent form but also dictates a process in which the physician communicates with the patient, in detail, the proposed treatment or procedure. The American Medical Association states that the physician should discuss the following with the patient:[22]

(1) patient diagnosis, if it is known
(2) nature and purpose of the proposed treatment or procedure
(3) risks and benefits of the proposed treatment or procedure
(4) alternatives to the proposed treatment or procedure (regardless of cost or health insurance coverage)
(5) risks and benefits of alternative treatment
(6) risks and benefits of nontreatment or not undergoing the procedure.

The purpose of the doctrine of informed consent is that with communication of the above, a 'reasonable person' would be able to make an informed decision about consenting to or refusing the proposed treatment or procedure. Justice Cardozo, a leading jurist in the foundation of tort law, stated: 'Every human being of adult years and sound mind has a right to determine what shall be done with his own body.'[23] In a landmark case, *Canterbury v. Spence*, the doctrine of informed consent was applied.[24] In this case, the plaintiff suffered from back pain and consented to a laminectomy. The complaint cited several causes of action, including the failure to inform the patient, beforehand, of the risk of paralysis. The physician stated that the risk of the surgery was no more serious than that of any other operation. The day after surgery, the patient fell and became paralyzed. He sued the physician for lack of informed consent regarding the risk of paralysis. *Canterbury* established the 'reasonable person' standard – what a reasonable person in that situation would find 'material' in making the decision regarding the proposed treatment or procedure.

In *Truman v. Thomas*, the court held that the patient must be informed of the risks of nontreatment even if that patient refuses treatment.[25] In this case, a wrongful death action was brought against the decedent's physician for failure to provide information on the risk of refusal of treatment. Here, the plaintiff refused annual Pap smears, although this was recommended by her physician. The reason for refusal was cost and not wanting to have the screening test done. Interestingly, the medical record omitted any counseling or recommendation that the plaintiff have a Pap smear. This issue of documentation or lack thereof will be addressed in the next part of this chapter. The plaintiff brought a cause of action against the physician, stating that the risks of refusing a Pap smear, namely, the risk of not detecting cervical cancer,

was not discussed with the plaintiff and therefore the plaintiff was not afforded the opportunity to make an informed decision.[26]

From the doctrine of informed consent, we learn how important it is to document details of patient instruction, information, and detailed discussion in the patient's medical record. Since the medical record is scrutinized in a professional liability case for its information, it is prudent for the physician to take the time to document not only the examination but also the details pertaining to any proposed treatment or procedures and the patient's decision or lack thereof at that date of service. Documentation of informed refusal is as important as informed consent. Take, for instance, the case of an obstetric patient of advanced maternal age whom the physician counsels regarding advanced maternal age and the availability of genetic testing. The patient declines genetic amniocentesis and the chart does not reflect the physician's counseling or the patient's decision. The patient goes on to deliver a baby with Down's syndrome and sues the physician for not offering her this procedure. The medical record, if properly documented, would offer the necessary defense. Instead, it becomes the physician's nightmare. Another example is dealing with patients that may refuse blood transfusion, such as Jehovah's Witnesses. Alternatives and options must be discussed and clearly outlined.[27] This leads us to a discussion of one of the most important types of evidence in any professional liability case, the medical chart.

The importance of the medical chart

The importance of the medical chart in professional liability litigation cannot be overstated. Accurate and complete medical record keeping is the first principle of the practice of defensive medicine. The purpose of a hospital chart has always been to enable the physician to reconstruct the management of a patient as it occurred, and thus to make fully informed decisions about continuing management.[28] If this cannot be done, the chart is inadequate and the physician cannot credibly reconstruct his or her own management at a later date.

Recurrent themes in professional liability litigation include: 'It's what in the record that counts'; 'If it isn't charted, it didn't happen'; and 'If you didn't chart it, you didn't do it.' The medical chart is a witness that never dies.

Professional liability can be limited by assiduous attention to the medical record. Attention to risk factors and documentation of normal and abnormal findings, as well as appropriate assessment and explanation of any positive findings, need to be clearly elucidated in the medical record. Clear documentation of a logical plan based on a thorough clinical database is the cornerstone of better medical record keeping, and thus, the cornerstone of defensive medicine.

Communication is the key to effective risk management, and the medical record serves as a means of communication critical to the care of the patient. The medical record is the patient's health-care diary and reflects all significant medical events in the recent and remote past. To many, the accuracy and completeness of the medical record reflects the quality of the patient's care. A poor, incomplete, or sloppy record suggests that care was of a similar quality. It is often difficult to convince a judge or a jury that the care provided was any better than the record. As such, the medical record is crucial to the defense of a physician's professional performance. However, it is imperative not to alter records. This can lead to a disaster in litigation. A case that would have been defendable becomes a case that is impossible to win once altered records are discovered.[29] Moreover, there are penalties that can be imposed for altering records, such as cancellation of professional insurance, exclusion of coverage, criminal charges, and the possibility of the loss of professional license.[30] When the rationale behind medical judgment in patient care is absent from the record, or the medical record is silent as to crucial facts, the defensibility of professional performance suffers. The professional's judgment is less subject to second-guessing if the record is accurate, completely objective, and legible, and gives a plan of management that is rationale. The physician who tries to recall intention or rationale 5 or more years after the fact is no match for the expert with perfect hindsight who retrospectively reviews medical events. A documented prospective plan of management, therefore, is essential to successful defense of professional liability cases.

The obstetric record

At the first prenatal visit, an accurate and complete medical and surgical history should be obtained, documenting all events of the patient's pregnancy that might adversely influence the physiology of the mother, function of the placenta, or development of the fetus. Family medical history is also important. Risk factors for adverse perinatal outcome should be identified and documented. A detailed review of prior pregnancies should be documented, including outcomes. Additionally, it is important to obtain previous operative reports and records pertaining to past stillbirths, abortions, miscarriages, preterm deliveries, and infants born with congenital anomalies. Furthermore, it is prudent to request any pathology reports available, such as an autopsy report or a placental pathology report from a previous pregnancy loss. A referral to genetic counseling should be offered if applicable.

A comprehensive menstrual history must also be obtained to assist in determining gestational age. Previous menstrual periods, the last normal menstrual period, the interval between periods, the onset of menarche, and the usual amount and duration of bleeding should be documented. If birth-control pills were used prior to pregnancy, the date they were discontinued should be recorded. Any use of ovulation medication should also be recorded. If the date of conception is known, or the date of a positive pregnancy test is known, document it as well. Any history of vomiting and weight loss, fever, rashes, or bleeding prior to the first visit should be noted in the chart along with appropriate counseling and intervention.

Additional information that should be documented in the prenatal chart is a social history. This would include, but not be limited to, past and present use of tobacco, illicit drugs (marijuana, cocaine, heroin, Ecstasy, etc.), alcohol, prescription drugs and over-the-counter drugs. It is also important to document the tobacco, alcohol, and illicit drug use of the patient's partner. Other important social history includes information on the patient's home environment, especially any past or present domestic violence. Appropriate counseling with documentation should follow.

A complete physical examination should be performed and all findings documented. Special attention should be given to the patient's weight, vital signs, cardiovascular system, breasts, abdominal examination (including fundal height and location of the fetal heart rate), and pelvic examination (notably the size of the uterus and clinical pelvimetry). A urinalysis should be performed, and the results of glycosuria, ketonuria, and proteinuria should be documented. Other initial prenatal laboratory testing includes CBC, RPR (VDRL), blood type and Rh, antibody screen (indirect Coombs), hepatitis B surface antigen, rubella immunity screening, hemoglobin electrophoresis, urine culture, gonorrhea and chlamydia cultures and Pap smear. The patient should also receive instruction and counseling for HIV and cystic fibrosis and be offered testing. It is crucial that the instruction and counseling for HIV and cystic fibrosis and the patient's decision on whether or not to be tested be documented. First-trimester screening using nuchal lucency, maternal serum free beta-HCG, and pregnancy-associated plasma protein A (PAPP-A) should be offered if the patient presents within this gestational age.[31] QUAD screening information should be provided and the patient offered the screening test between 15 and 20 weeks' gestation.

Finally, at the first prenatal visit, the physician must assess and document the gestational age. To accomplish this accurately, the physician should utilize menstrual history, physical examination, and, if needed, ultrasound assessment.

As the course of prenatal care continues, additional information must be added at each subsequent visit, including maternal weight gain or loss, blood pressure, urine analysis, presence of edema, fetal heart rate, fundal height, gestational age, and any vaginal examination findings.

At later times during pregnancy, additional laboratory and diagnostic testing should be offered and performed, as well as accurately and timely documented in the prenatal chart. The patient should be provided with information and offered a QUAD screen between weeks 15 and 20, and genetic counseling/testing, if applicable, should be offered and documented. Diabetic screening, hemoglobin and hematocrit, and an antibody screen should be provided between 24 and 28 weeks. If the patient is Rh negative and not sensitized, Rhogam should be given and recorded at 28 weeks after appropriate patient instruction, counseling, and consent.

Routine prenatal visits should be scheduled and documented every 4 weeks until 28 weeks, then every 2 weeks until

36 weeks, and then weekly until delivery. Additional prenatal visits should be scheduled as necessary.

Among the most common allegations made in professional liability litigation is the charge that a physician failed to follow up abnormal findings. The abnormal findings which require intervention and which are most frequently overlooked are abnormal antenatal testing, hypertension, Rh sensitization, and lack of fetal growth. Therefore, every physician's office needs to have an organized system to record and notify patients about abnormal laboratory findings on a regular basis, and to initial and date abnormal findings as a record of review. Patient telephone contact should be documented, including, but not limited to, date, time, reason for telephone call, and advice provided to the patient. It is crucial that an updated prenatal record be available at the labor and delivery unit for review during the intrapartum admission.

Intrapartum events must be recorded with the same comprehensive attention to detail that characterized the documentation of the prenatal record. All contacts with the patient and all examinations must be dated and timed, and all details of the examination must be documented. With computerized records, it is prudent to check that all entries are complete and thorough. This includes, but is not limited to, date and time, vital signs, admission history, physical assessment of patient and fetus, and a detailed plan of care based upon the history and objective findings. If the plan of care or management changes during the inpatient admission, those changes must be documented as well as what was communicated to the patient. It is crucial to have fetal heart monitoring documentation besides an actual strip in case the actual strip is subsequently unavailable. There should be an adequate system in place to allow access and retrieval of the inpatient record, fetal monitoring strip, and other stored documentation for a minimum of 21 years. If the patient is admitted to labor and delivery but is discharged prior to delivery, it is imperative that there is detailed documentation of the assessment of both patient and fetus along with a discharge plan.

It is advisable to have a narrative report of all events and the delivery, as the narrative provides a detailed account of what has transpired. Checklists often are less than ideal and do not provide the full picture.

During the postpartum period, communication must exist between the pediatrician, neonatologists, and obstetrician to ensure accurate records of any events occurring during the neonatal course in the nursery. Any discrepancies between the obstetric record and neonatal record should be rectified. For instance, if the neonatal record refers to a forceps mark on the newborn's face and forceps were not utilized in the delivery, this discrepancy between the two records needs clarification.

While professional liability claims continue to burden the obstetric community and appear to be influencing how obstetricians and gynecologists practice, there are ways to reduce the risk of successful litigation through careful practices. Although there is no doubt than maintaining an accurate, legible, and carefully documented chart with a plan of care is time-consuming, it becomes crucial when that chart is subsequently scrutinized years later. A few extra moments spent documenting the medical record can be priceless years later when it serves to protect one's practice and credibility.

References

1. Rice B. Malpractice rates: how high now? Med Econ 2004; 81: 57–9.
2. Merritt Hawkins and Associates, Summary Report, 2003. Obstetric/Gynecology Malpractice Survey.
3. Black's Law Dictionary, (6th edition) p. 1489. 1990.
4. Ibid.
5. Black's Law Dictionary p. 276 6th edition, 1990.
6. Prosser W. Law of Torts (4th edition) p. 123. 1971.
7. Restatement (Second) of Tort – generally.
8. Black's Law Dictionary, p. 1032.
9. Black's Law Dictionary, p. 1404.
10. Black's Law Dictionary, p. 196.
11. American Medical Association, Principles of Medical Ethics, June 2001.
12. Peters JD. Evidence based medicine in courts. Trial 2002; 74–9.
13. *Daubert v. Merrell Dow Pharmaceuticals, Inc.*, 509 U.S. 579 (1993).
14. *Sullivan v. Edward Hospital*, No. 95409, 2004 WL 228956 (Ill. Feb 5, 2004).
15. *Broadnax v. Gonzalez* and *Fahey v. Canino*, 2 N.Y. 3d 148; 809 N.E. 2d 645; 777 N.Y.S 2d 416; 2004 N.Y.
16. *Prink v. Rockefeller Center*, 48 N.Y.2d 309, 398 N.E. 2d 517 (1979).
17. *Humphers v. First Interstate Bank* 684 P. 2d 581 (App. 1984).
18. *Estate of William Behringer M.D. v. the Medical Center at Princeton*, 249 N.J. Super. 597, 592 A. 2d 1251 (1991).
19. *Tarasoff v. Regents of University of California*, 17 Cal. 3d 425 (1976).
20. Summary of the HIPAA Privacy Rule, United States Department of Health and Human Services, OCR Privacy Brief, May 2003.
21. Black's Law Dictionary, p. 779.
22. American Medical Association, Office of the General Counsel, Division of Health Law, 1998 (updated 2003).
23. *Schloendorff v. Society of New York Hospital*, 211 N.Y. 125 (1914).
24. *Canterbury v. Spence*, 464 F.2d 722, 787 D.C. Cir. (1972).
25. *Truman v. Thomas*, 611 P. 2d 902 (Cal. 1980).
26. Ibid.
27. Gyamfi et al, Ethical and medicolegal considerations in the obstetric care of a Jehovah's Witness. Obstet Gynecol 2003; 102: 173–80.
28. Trial, May 1983.
29. Pennachio DL. Alter records, lose the case. Med Econ 2003; 80: 40, 43–4.
30. Ibid., p. 43.
31. First-Trimester Screening for Fetal Aneuploidy. ACOG Committee Opinion, No. 296. Obstet Gynecol 2004; 104: 215–17.

40 Patient safety

Richard M Weinberg

Emphasis on patient safety has increased in the past few years mostly in response to the Institute of Medicine report *To Err Is Human: Building a Safer Health System*. Obstetrician-gynecologists should incorporate elements of patient safety into their practices and also encourage others to use these practices.[1]

Current interest in patient safety began growing in the 1980s after the publication of Wennberg and Gittleson's study of practice patterns,[2] which demonstrated surprising variation in the distribution and use of medical resources in the USA. That publication, and many to follow, revealed unexplainable variation in practice patterns, and pervasive quality and safety problems throughout the USA. Despite the importance of this publication and many related papers, the topic of patient safety remained unexciting to most practicing physicians and health-care administrators.

Though clinicians and the public took little note of these studies, large health-care purchasers and politicians scrutinized them. The reports concluded that the problems of overuse, underuse, and misuse that contribute to variations in outcomes, unreliable quality, and inadequate patient safety were not simply the problems of a few incompetent practitioners; rather, they were the problems of the entire health-care system. Focusing much of their initial effort on physicians, the business professionals who made decisions about a substantial fraction of US health-care expenditures encouraged politicians and insurers to 'manage care' more directly. This resulted in review of plans of care,[3] contractual requirements for precertification and preauthorization, public reporting of physician errors and quality of care indicators,[4] and progressively more intrusive administrative supervision of documentation, billing, and clinical management decisions.[5]

Those administratively and contractually imposed processes did little to improve patient safety, largely because they were focused on identifying and punishing poor performers. Moreover, they increased physicians' overhead, diminished their autonomy, and made them angry, reducing their inclination to participate in projects designed to improve safety in a systematic manner. Finally, however, in 1999, physician interest in the topic of patient safety was galvanized by the report of the Institute of Medicine (IOM), entitled *To Err Is Human: Building a Safer Health System*.[6]

This famous IOM report (infamous to some) is often credited for establishing in the mind of the public a single concept: that 44 000–98 000 patients die annually from preventable accidents in US hospitals. The cost of these errors, alone, was at least $17 billion[7] in 1992 dollars, and the cost in human suffering is incalculable. Lost among the sensational headlines that often accompany media comments about *To Err Is Human* is the fact that this comprehensive report, compiled by a learned and respected group, reaffirmed the skills, dedication, and performance of health-care professionals but indicted the health-care system for the safety failures.

The report emphasized the complexity of health-care delivery – interactions of people and care processes, neither of which always respond in a predictable manner. Add to this mix of patients and processes the effects of allergies, idiosyncratic responses, patients' wishes, family members' needs, the selection and sequencing of tests, the availability of operating room time, administrative and contractual responsibilities, and regulatory constraints – and it becomes clear that managing the care of even a single patient is a complex affair, to say nothing of caring for hundreds of inpatients and hundreds of outpatients daily in hospitals.

The IOM report also emphasized the role of leadership in designing, implementing, and utilizing the systems necessary to prevent errors. Diagnostic and therapeutic options have been increasing rapidly. As the number of patients treated and the speed of patient throughput continue to increase, hospitals and clinicians need systems to manage routine processes and to provide decision support and fail-safe mechanisms that help to ensure patient safety. Leadership must provide the information management technology and the human resources necessary to ensure patient safety. Reason[8] has helped to explain the roles of clinicians and organizational leaders in patient safety by the concept of the 'sharp end and the blunt end' of health-care delivery.

Clinicians generally work at the 'sharp end' of health care, where each order written or surgical incision made affects a patient directly. Hospital board members, administrators, managers, and medical staff leaders are at the 'blunt end' of the system, where decisions are made that affect groups of patients or all patients. These decisions determine the constraints acting upon, and the resources available to, those working at the sharp end.

Errors do occur at the sharp end, but they are relatively infrequent. Today, physician sharp end errors are managed through the peer review process. Peer review has little effect on patient safety because it is focused on individuals, is retrospective, and infrequently addresses the real causes of errors. In management jargon, it is a quality-assurance process. Patient safety is a quality-improvement process: it is prospective, focused on processes and systems, and interdisciplinary in its approach. It is nonpunitive – seeking to 'fix the problem, not the blame'. The IOM report emphasized this and more, but much was lost because of the focus on the estimate of annual loss of life.

It is worth noting that physicians and a few other clinicians are the only members of the team who work regularly at both the sharp and the blunt end. This places physicians in a unique position to identify system and process problems and to work with administrators to find solutions. Physicians are increasingly participating in hospital and health system governance. Looking beyond self-interest and blame, these physician leaders have an opportunity to work with other members of the board to establish patient safety as an organizational strategic goal or competency. They can also work with their colleagues – in their leadership role – to educate them about patient safety and to help them understand the dual role of leader and participant physicians can play as members of the interdisciplinary teams needed to improve patient safety.

Achieving better patient safety, seen from the systems perspective, appears a daunting task. It seemed easier when we all thought that if each person did his or her job with diligence and care, everything would come out as intended. But it may not. Humans are fallible and have limitations. The processes of health care are becoming ever more complex, as diagnosis and treatment become more sophisticated. Budgets are tight and all members of the health-care team are being asked to work 'smarter and faster' even as occasional staffing shortages affect the daily chores of care delivery.

The initial step to improving safety is accepting health-care systems and processes, not individuals, as the cause of most errors. The next is to understand the five principles[9] identified in To Err Is Human as essential for improving patient safety. The first is to provide effective leadership to achieve greater safety. This includes the provision of the resources needed to achieve greater safety. Hospitals and health systems must invest more in technology and training to ensure safety. Physicians, too, must acknowledge their need for education and training in safety.

The second is to respect human limits in process design. Today, we rely far too much on memory and too little on the use of technology to provide reminders, forcing functions, and fail-safe mechanisms. Individual autonomy must be balanced differently against standardization to promote consistency and reduce errors.

Third, we must promote effective team functioning. This requires training as teams so we can function as teams. Anesthesiology is a specialty that has demonstrated the value of team training and the use of simulators,[10] that experience is being transferred to other venues of practice, and the operating room remains an excellent opportunity for simulations and team mock training. It also means eliminating the power or hierarchy gradients that inhibit the communication requisite for safety. Patients should also understand their care and be empowered to participate in the protection of their safety.

Fourth, we must anticipate the unanticipated. Just as we provide preventive maintenance for equipment, we must review our care processes regularly to identify the potential for error. Standardization and redundancy help identify unexpected events, while preparation and practice for mistakes in error-prone and high-risk processes improve outcomes when errors occur despite our vigilance.

Fifth, we must create a learning environment, one in which information about safety in our institutions flows freely. The information should include reliable data about errors and near misses in the organization. That, in turn, requires a blame-free, 'fair and just' culture that encourages and supports the reporting of all incidents. We will consider some practical steps for achieving patient safety in the section below on developing a patient safety program.

Mainstreaming patient safety

Patient safety moved from the shadows to the light of day with the publication of To Err Is Human. It galvanized not only physicians and others in health care to examine patient safety, but alerted the public and health-care purchasers to problems that appeared, in retrospect, to have been ignored or kept secret. One result has been a terrible blow to public confidence in our health-care system. A recent survey of 2012 US adults found that 40% believed that health-care quality had declined in the past 5 years, while only 17% noted improvement and 38% thought it remained unchanged.[11]

A survey of 400 practicing hospitalist physicians by Wachter revealed the opposite: 45% felt safety had improved, 17% felt it had declined, and 38% felt there had been no change. The impulse to assume that the difference in the opinions of patients and physicians is due to their perspectives, alone, should be tempered by a Leapfrog Group survey of more than 1000 hospitals, which showed wide variation in hospital conformance with the National Quality Forum safety practices.[12] With all this attention, it is clear that patient safety is no longer relegated to poorly attended quality improvement or risk management meetings – it has been thrust into the sight of senior managers, CEOs, and their boards – many of whom previously equated success – being busy and profitable – with quality and safety.

Now all of us – those at the sharp end and those at the blunt – are subject to scrutiny based on data and the research done by those of our colleagues who had the clarity of vision to understand the problem nearly two decades before their research was compiled to form the evidence basis for *To Err Is Human*. We are finally paying attention, but has it done any good? In 1999, the IOM report stated that we should set as our goal no less than a 50% reduction in preventable errors in the 5 years following the publication of the report. At the report's fifth anniversary in November 2004, there was no one with the temerity to suggest that we had even come close to that goal.

Comments by various authorities agreed that progress had occurred, but that 'the task is far from complete'.[13] The same group, including the coauthors of *To Err Is Human*, emphasized the need to establish a teamwork-oriented health-care culture, the continued development of information technology, and the need for federal support, in order that future patient safety efforts achieve meaningful progress.[14] Donald Berwick, MD, founder and CEO of the Institute for Healthcare Improvement (IHI) and coauthor of the IOM report, commented that the IOM report generated 'tremendous progress' in patient safety awareness (emphasis added), and Wachter noted that in a recent survey of 400 practicing hospitalists, nearly half attributed patient safety improvements to an 'overall increased sensitivity to the issue'.[14]

Many organizations are working, independently and in collaboration, to advance the patient safety agenda. Table 40.1 contains a list of national organizations that have invested all or part of their resources in efforts to improve patient safety. A few of these bear mention.

The Agency for Healthcare Research and Quality (AHRQ) is the USA's lead federal agency for research on health-care quality, costs, outcomes, and patient safety. AHRQ began operating in 1995 as the Agency for Healthcare Policy and Research (AHCPR), utilizing funds from the Congressional appropriations process. It was not fully authorized until the Healthcare Research and Policy Act of 1999, which changed the organization's name to AHRQ. AHRQ's mission includes both translating research findings into better patient care and providing policymakers and other health-care leaders with information needed to make critical health-care decisions. AHRQ's budget has grown over the past few years and in 2001–3, AHRQ distributed $69.6 million in research grants for projects in medical error reporting.[15] In comparison, federal medical information technology (IT) grants were $139 million; overall, the federal government invests 500 times as much in medical progress – through the NIH budget – as it invests in patient safety.[14]

The American Society for Healthcare Risk Management (ASHRM) is a personal membership group of the American Hospital Association (AHA). ASHRM provides educational tools and networking opportunities to health-care risk management professionals to help them with their goals of promoting quality care, maintaining a safe environment, and preserving human and financial resources in health-care organizations. Once a world apart from clinicians at the sharp end of health care, risk managers today are an integral part of the team working to manage the complexities of care delivery in a modern hospital.

The Foundation for Accountability (FACCT) is a nonprofit organization dedicated to helping US consumers make better health-care decisions. FACCT's agenda is based on the belief that the USA's ability to create a more responsive health-care system depends on informed, empowered consumers who help shape the system, hold it accountable for quality, and act as partners in improving health. As the US health-care enterprise increasingly responds to the consumer-driven[16] doctrines of the baby boomers, there can be little doubt that FACCT's perspective will contribute to the reshaping of the relationships between physicians, patients, and health-care organizations.

The Institute for Healthcare Improvement (IHI) is a Boston-based, independent nonprofit organization working to accelerate improvement in health-care systems by encouraging collaboration, rather than competition, among health-care organizations. Founded by CEO Donald Berwick, MD, MPP, a pediatrician and Harvard professor, IHI has gained worldwide acceptance as a resource for improving health-care safety. IHI has established as its measurable goals health care with no

Table 40.1 Patient safety organizations

Agency for Healthcare Research and Quality (AHRQ)	American Hospital Association (AHA)
American Society for Healthcare Risk Management (ASHRM)	Department of Veterans Affairs
Foundation for Accountability (FACCT)	Institute for Healthcare Improvement (IHI)
Institute for Safe Medication Practices (ISMP)	Leapfrog Group
National Business Coalition on Health (NBCH)	National Committee for Quality Assurance (NCQA)
National Forum for Healthcare Quality Measurement and Reporting (NQF)	National Patient Safety Foundation (NPSF)
Partnership for Patient Safety (P4PS)	Patient Safety Task Force
President's Advisory Commission on Consumer Protection and Quality in the Health Care Industry (1996–8)	Quality Interagency Coordination Task Force
Risk Management Foundation Center for Patient Safety	Society for Healthcare Consumer Advocacy
Society for Risk Analysis (SRA)	US Pharmacopoeia (USP)

Adapted from Association for Professionals in Infection Control and Epidemiology, with permission.

needless deaths, no needless pain or suffering, no helplessness in those served or serving, no unwanted waiting, and no waste. IHI works with individual health-care organizations and with small groups of organizations on process improvements demonstrated to improve safety, reduce waste, and favor evidence-based health-care delivery. Among American hospitals, IHI is the most recognized organization dedicated to improving safety.

The Leapfrog Group for Patient Safety was originally funded by the Business Roundtable, a group of large employers who felt they were unable to influence the quality and value of the health care they purchased. Leapfrog also receives funding through the Commonwealth Fund and the Robert Wood Johnson Foundation. Leapfrog works through its employer members and their health plans, encouraging them to provide incentives to hospitals that improve quality by implementing Leapfrog's quality and safety initiatives. Leapfrog became well known among hospitals because of its initiatives relating to intensivists, computerized provider order entry (CPOE), and selected surgical volumes; today many of its initiatives are aligned with those of JCAHO and the Center for Medicare and Medicaid Services (CMS).

The National Committee for Quality Assurance (NCQA) is a private, nonprofit organization that reports solely on the quality of managed health-care plans. It was formed in 1990 with the support of the managed care industry's main trade organization, the large employer community, and the Robert Wood Johnson Foundation. NCQA provides a certification program for managed care plans and information for purchasers through the Health Plan Employer Data and Information Set (HEDIS). Many NCQA indicators are related to quality and safety.

The National Quality Forum (NQF) is a nonprofit membership organization created to develop and implement a national strategy for health-care quality measurement and reporting. Headed by President and CEO Kenneth Kizer, MD, MPH, the NQF membership is a broad range of health-care providers, purchasers, professional and trade organizations, government organizations, and consumer organizations. Together, they are working to identify the principles and priorities that will guide a national measurement and reporting strategy to improve quality and safety.

The National Patient Safety Goals

The Joint Commission on Accreditation of Healthcare Organizations (JCAHO) occupies an important position in the patient safety movement in America. Because obstetric surgeons do much of their work in hospitals, understanding the JCAHO safety goals is worthwhile. JCAHO estimates that nearly 50% of its standards relate directly to patient safety.[17] Additionally, in 2001, JCAHO issued safety standards for hospitals and followed with standards for behavioral health care and long-term care in 2003 and standards for ambulatory care and home care

organizations in 2004. The JCAHO's National Patient Safety Goals (NPSGs) complement other elements of the organization's patient safety program, including the Sentinel Events Policy and Alerts; the implementation of the Universal Protocol for Preventing Wrong Site, Wrong Procedure, and Wrong Patient Surgery™; operation of the Office of Quality Monitoring; the Speak Up Initiatives; support for legislative initiatives and patient safety coalitions; and the Joint Commission Resources consulting subsidiary. In 2004, the JCAHO also began to develop program-specific NPSGs for its accreditation and certification programs.

The hospital requirements for 2003 comprised six NPSGs with 11 specific elements and the requirements for 2004 revised and expanded the list to seven NPSGs with 13 elements. All or some of the goals were applicable in eight health-care settings, including hospitals. The other settings included ambulatory services, behavioral health facilities, psychiatric hospitals, laboratories, home care organizations, and long-term care facilities (two subgroups). For 2005, there are 12 NPSGs, now applicable in 10 health-care settings, including hospitals, ambulatory care and office-based surgery, assisted living, behavioral health care, critical-access hospitals, disease-specific care, home care, laboratory, long-term care, and networks. In order to present a clear, relevant discussion of the NPSGs as they apply to obstetric surgeons, the comments that follow incorporate elements of the 2005 NPSGs and the older goals that have been revised, assimilated into the newer goals, or made part of the JCAHO hospital standards.

Patient identification

Various experts have estimated that as many as 85% of errors leading to serious patient harm are errors of patient identification. In a world where we increasingly must present multiple types of identification before using our credit cards, picking up theater tickets, or boarding a commercial airplane, it seems counterintuitive that a patient could be administered blood or even sent to the operating room without proper, reliable identification. Nonetheless, these are daily occurrences in many health-care institutions. The JCAHO goal of improving patient care identification is aimed at modifying traditional means of identification – memory, a cursory glance at an identification bracelet, a quick inquiry, 'Are you James?' – and ensuring more positive means.

JCAHO requires the use of two identifiers, neither of which may be the patient's room number, before administering medications or blood products, taking blood samples and other specimens for clinical testing, or providing any other treatments or procedures. The process further extends to any invasive procedure, before which the treating team must provide a final verification process to confirm the correct patient, procedure, site, and availability of appropriate documents. This verification must use active communication techniques. The nature of the information to be verified implies the active participation of the operating physician.

The Universal Protocol™

The Universal Protocol for Preventing Wrong Site, Wrong Procedure, and Wrong Person Surgery was adopted by JCAHO in 2003 and became a requirement in 2004. It was endorsed by nearly 50 professional health-care organizations and associations (Table 40.2). The Universal Protocol expanded and integrated a series of existing requirements in the 2003 and 2004 National Patient Safety Goals, and in 2005 the Universal Protocol became one of the JCAHO hospital standards. It remains linked to the 2005 NPSGs through the mention of the verification process in the goal of improving the accuracy of patient identification and in the goal requiring the elimination of wrong site, wrong procedure, and wrong patient surgery in the JCAHO's Disease-Specific Care programs. The Universal Protocol comprises several elements.

The first element is the preoperative verification process. This requires the development and use of a process – such as a checklist – to confirm that the appropriate documents, including radiographs, are available. The second is to implement a process for marking the operative site, with the patient's involvement. The third is to perform a 'timeout' immediately before starting the procedure.

Safety issues involving laterality or wrong-site surgery are relatively uncommon in obstetrics and gynecology, but errors do occur as in surgery performed on the wrong patient, or the wrong procedure on a correctly identified patient.[18] Among the issues that have been identified as possibly contributing to wrong-site surgeries are emergencies, morbid obesity or other unusual physical characteristics, time pressures, unfamiliarity of the team with the surgical or procedure suite setup, the presence of several surgeons during a procedure, and the performance of multiple procedures during a single encounter.

Obstetric surgeons may also be prone to other common surgical safety risks, including miscommunication among team members or with the patient's family, failure to verify the surgical site and procedure, and incomplete or missing preoperative checklists and patient assessments. The Universal Protocol seeks to reduce the risk of each of these problems, and the harm that may result from them, by establishing routine processes that eliminate the need to depend solely on the surgeon's memory to ensure that each element is carried out accurately and without fail.

JCAHO has provided detailed comments on the implementation of various aspects of the Universal Protocol[19] in its 'Frequently Asked Questions', available on the JCAHO website. The protocol requirements are quite specific and many of the items pertain directly to the physician. For instance, the site of the operation should be marked by the operating physicians with the participation of the patient (or the patient's legal surrogate, if the patient is unable to participate). The site is usually marked with a special surgical marker that will not wash off during the preparation of the site, and the marking should include the surgeon's initials. The use of an 'X' is not acceptable

---

Table 40.2 Organizations and associations endorsing the Universal Protocol

Accreditation Council for Graduate Medical Education	American Medical Group Association
Agency for Healthcare Research and Quality	American Nurses Association
American Academy of Ambulatory Care Nursing	American Organization of Nurse Executives
American Academy of Cosmetic Surgery	American Pediatric Surgical Association
American Academy of Facial Plastic and Reconstructive Surgery	American Radiological Nurses Association
American Academy of Family Physicians	American Society for Surgery of the Hand
American Academy of Ophthalmology	American Society of Anesthesiologists
American Academy of Orthopaedic Surgeons	American Society of General Surgeons
American Academy of Otolaryngology – Head and Neck Surgery	American Society of Ophthalmic Registered Nurses
American Academy of Pediatrics	American Society of PeriAnesthesia Nurses
American Association of Ambulatory Surgery Centers	American Society of Plastic Surgeons
American Association of Eye and Ear Hospitals	American Society of Plastic Surgical Nurses
American Association of Nurse Anesthetists	American Urological Association
American Association of Oral and Maxillofacial Surgeons	Association of American Medical Colleges
American College of Cardiology	Association of PeriOperative Registered Nurses
American College of Chest Physicians	Association of Surgical Technologists
American College of Emergency Physicians	Federated Ambulatory Surgery Association
American College of Foot and Ankle Surgeons	Federation of American Hospitals
American College of Obstetricians and Gynecologists	Medical Group Management Association
American College of Physicians	National Association of Medical Staff Services
American College of Radiology	National Patient Safety Foundation
American College of Surgeons	North American Spine Society
American Dental Association	Radiological Society of North America
American Hospital Association	Society of Thoracic Surgeons
American Medical Association	

because its meaning is ambiguous; similarly, contralateral marking is not acceptable. Nonoperative sites must not be marked, and adhesive markers should not be used.

Not all procedures or sites require marking. Table 40.3 includes a list of procedures and sites that do not require marking, subject to the understanding that a midline incision or endoscope insertion location that is the approach to a bilateral structure does require marking. The marking should be near the operative or insertion site and must be visible during the actual procedure. If this cannot be accomplished, the hospital should have a procedure for utilizing another method – for example, a temporary, special wristband for identifying the correct site.

The immediate preoperative 'timeout' must also be carried out according to a policy developed and implemented by the hospital or health-care organization – it should not be a department-specific policy. All timeout policies must include the following elements. The timeout must be an 'active' process involving the entire surgical team, by which the JCAHO means the surgeon, the anesthesia provider, and the circulating nurse. Other members of the team should be encouraged to participate. The timeout must be done immediately before the administration of anesthesia in the operating suite or procedure room. In addition to correct patient, procedure, and site, the timeout must verify the correct patient position and the availability of any unusual equipment necessary for the procedure. Finally, the timeout must be documented in the patient's record.

Some surgeons feel the Universal Protocol is an onerous, unnecessary burden and are reluctant to participate in its application. Hospital policies, however, must reflect the requirement for the Universal Protocol or an acceptable alternative, and patient safety experts all agree that the operating physician must participate as a member of the team, if not as its leader, in the active use of the hospital's version of the protocol, if patient safety is to be ensured. Professional and patient organizations, alike, have been encouraging patients and their surrogates to speak up and to ask questions that make the patient part of the process of ensuring the right procedure, in the right location, for each patient.

Effective communication

Improving the effectiveness of communication among caregivers is another important JCAHO patient safety goal that depends upon physician participation, in large part. The first element of this goal relates to the process for managing verbal and telephone orders and for receiving test results. It requires that the person receiving the order or result first write it down and then read it back to the person giving the order. While time-consuming, this process clearly has the potential to catch serious mistakes before they happen.

The next element requires each hospital to develop and adopt a standardized list of abbreviations, acronyms, and symbols that are not to be used throughout the organization. Among those suggested for inclusion by a variety of professional organizations are a number of the most commonly used abbreviations which, because of illegibility or ambiguity, may be misunderstood, resulting in serious harm. Table 40.4 gives a typical list.

Hospitals are now also required to measure, and improve, if needed, the time it takes to report critical test results to the patient's caregiver. For those laboratory results defined as 'critical' by the hospital, the result must be given directly to the licensed professional caring for the patient, rather than to a secretary or unit clerk. This approach reduces the potential for misunderstanding or for a report being lost.

Reducing risk of surgical fires

Obstetric surgeons and all others who perform office-based or ambulatory procedures should be aware of the NPSG requirements regarding the reduction of risk of surgical fires. All staff, including operating physicians and other licensed independent practitioners, must be trained specifically about how to control heat sources and manage fuels to reduce the risk of fire. The institution or practice must also establish guidelines to minimize oxygen concentrations beneath drapes.

Other JCAHO patient safety goals

While patient identification issues are responsible for most of the errors that result in patient harm, medication errors and near misses are, by far, the most frequent errors. JCAHO NPSGs require hospitals to remove concentrated electrolytes from all patient care units, standardize and limit the number of drug concentrations available in the organization, and identify a list of look-alike/sound-alike drugs used in the organization. They must also take action to prevent errors involving the interchange of the drugs.

A related goal will require all hospitals to perform medication reconciliation throughout the organization by 2006. For each patient entering care, the hospital will have to develop a list of medications the patient is receiving with the patient's participation and compare it to the hospital's formulary. Whenever the patient's setting is changed, within the institution or outside, the list will have to be communicated to the next provider of service. This requirement includes transfers between nursing units in hospitals. For organizations with electronic medical records (EMRs) and some with CPOE and/or pharmacy information systems with electronic medication administration records (MARs), this may not be too time-

Table 40.3 Sites and procedures not requiring marking

Single organ cases	Premature infants
Laparotomy/laparoscopy not for operation on a paired organ	Interventional cases without predetermined insertion site
Single-wound operative site	Midline sternotomy
Cesarean section	Teeth
Procedures on genitalia	True emergencies where delay might be harmful

Table 40.4 Typical 'do not use' list

Abbreviation	Intended meaning	Misinterpretation	Preferred practice
U or u	Unit	Read as a zero (0) or a four (4), causing a 10-fold overdose or greater (4U seen as '40' or 4u seen as '44').	Write 'units'
qd or QD qod or QOD	Once daily every other day	Misinterpreted as 'right eye' (OD – *oculus dexter* and administration of oral medications in the eye). QOD can be mistaken for 'I'	Write 'daily' Write 'every other day'
cc	Cubic centimeter	Misread as 'U' (units)	Write 'mL'
Trailing Zero (X.0mg); Lack of Leading Zero (.Xmg)		Decimal point is missed	Remember, 'Always lead, never follow)' Always write a leading zero before a decimal point and never write a zero by itself after a decimal point
MS, MSO$_4$ MgSO$_4$	Magnesium sulfate or morphine sulfate	Confused for one another – can mean morphine sulfate or magnesium sulfate	Write 'magnesium sulfate' or 'morphine sulfate'
IU	International unit	Misread as 'IV' (intravenous) or 10 (ten)	Write 'International Unit'
µg, mcg, mcgm	Microgram	Mistaken for 'mg' resulting in 1000-fold dosing overdose	Write 'microgram'
T.I.W.	Three times a week	Mistaken for three times a day or twice a week, resulting in an overdose	Write '3 times weekly' or 'three times weekly'
SC or sq	Subcutaneous	Mistaken for SL for sublingual, or '5 every'	Write 'subcut' or 'subcutaneous'
D/C	Discharge Discontinue	Premature discontinuation of medications when D/C (intended to mean 'discharge') has been misinterpreted as 'discontinued' when followed by a list of drugs.	Write 'discharge' or 'discontinue'
AS, AD, AU or OS, OD, OU	AS for OS AD for OD AU for OU	Mistaken for one another	Write: 'left ear', 'right ear', or 'both ears'; 'left eye', 'right eye', or 'both eyes'
Hs or qhs	Nightly at bedtime	Misread as every hour	Use 'nightly' or 'at bedtime'
< or >	Less than, more than	May be misinterpreted or confused with one another	Write 'less than' or 'more than'

consuming; for those dependent on manual records, the valuable goal of accurate medication reconciliation may require a significant alteration in work flow.

The NPSGs also focus on the safe use of infusion pumps, and require that all general-use and patient-controlled anesthesia (PCA) intravenous-infusion pumps be equipped with free-flow protection to prevent accidental overdosing.

The appropriate management of clinical alarm systems has been moved from the NPSGs for hospitals into the JCAHO hospital accreditation standards, but is worth mentioning. Reliable clinical alarm systems depend upon several elements to ensure safety and effectiveness. Alarms must be tested and given preventive maintenance regularly. When in use, the alarm audibility must be appropriate for the level of ambient noise, and the hospital should have a policy of identifying all who respond to alarms. Finally, the establishment of alarm parameters must be linked to the individual patient's physiologic requirements.

Nosocomial infections remain a significant and serious risk for hospitalized patients and continue to be a focus of safety efforts. The NPSGs require hospitals and their staff members, including physicians, to comply with the hand-hygiene guidelines promulgated by the Centers for Disease Control and Prevention (CDC). These guidelines address hand-washing and associated issues, such as the length of fingernails, the use of false fingernails and nail appliqués, and the appropriate use of alcohol-based hand cleaners in the clinical setting. Whenever a patient suffers a major permanent loss of function or unanticipated death due to nosocomial infection, the institution must perform a root cause analysis to determine the underlying cause of the occurrence and, if not already in place, establish policies and procedures to prevent recurrence of the event.

Finally, the NPSGs continue to focus on reducing the risk of patient harm from falls. Each patient's risk of falling must be assessed initially when the patient enters care and reassessed periodically. Particular attention must be paid to the patient's medication regimen, and action must be undertaken to reduce risks identified in the assessment/reassessment process.

The American College of Obstetricians and Gynecologists

After the publication of *To Err Is Human*, the American College of Obstetricians and Gynecologists (ACOG) reaffirmed its commitment to improving quality and patient safety in women's health care in a 2003 committee statement on patient safety in obstetrics and gynecology.[21] Citing the IOM report, as well as its own paper on ethics in obstetrics and gynecology and other references, this committee report codified ACOG's patient safety recommendations and identified seven objectives for obstetrician-gynecologists.

In urging its members to develop a commitment to a culture of patient safety, the ACOG opinion emphasized the need for teamwork and communication, including disclosure of errors, near misses, and adverse outcomes. The first ACOG objective also points out the importance of physicians assuming a leadership role at 'the blunt end' to ensure the availability of appropriate resources to achieve and maintain safety.

The second, third, and fourth ACOG objectives correspond to the JCAHO NPSGs. They are to: (1) implement recommended safe medication practices; (2) reduce the likelihood of surgical errors; (3) improve communication. ACOG's communication objective, however, focuses not on order and test result transcription but on another important aspect of communication – the creation of open, transparent communication between physicians and patients to enhance trust and patient satisfaction. It also addresses the need to communicate unanticipated outcomes and to use errors and near misses to develop programs to prevent their recurrence.

ACOG's fifth and sixth objectives are to identify and resolve system problems and to establish partnerships with patients. The former distinguishes between appropriate responses to errors that occur due to system problems and those due to willful violations of rules and regulations. In doing so, it re-emphasizes an earlier theme – namely, the need to disclose errors and near misses. The latter establishes the relationship between engaging patients in their health-care decision and their ultimate safety. This is an interesting alternative to the usual analysis that focuses on patient autonomy as the driving force behind making decision making a participatory activity.

The final ACOG objective is to make safety a priority in every aspect of practice. By restating this principle, the committee's opinion reaffirms both the importance of patient safety and the essential quality-improvement nature of the process of improving safety. For obstetrician-gynecologists interested in more information about patient safety and quality improvement, the ACOG website contains a Patient Safety Series of articles written for physicians, focusing on current concepts and their application in practice.[20]

Developing a patient safety program

Americans should be able to count on receiving health care that is safe. To achieve this, a new health care delivery system is needed – a system that both prevents errors and learns from them when they occur. The development of such a system requires, first, a commitment by all stakeholders to a culture of safety and, second, improved information systems.[21]

Adapting to a practice environment where safety is an issue of paramount importance is difficult for many physicians, not because they do not value safety – in fact, they value it highly – but because the new model requires physicians to confront and manage error in a new and difficult place. In the past, medicine required, above all, a strong sense of independent personal responsibility, expressed in the belief that if each professional is conscientious, errors will be prevented or minimized. Today, the notion that the responsibility to 'do no harm' is a personal responsibility is being replaced by the understanding that safety is a system property.

When this is coupled with another growing idea – that cooperation among professionals must supersede individual professional autonomy – it becomes clear that the stage is set for physician and hospital turmoil as both struggle to acknowledge, manage, and prevent errors. For many physicians who have been accustomed to a leadership role in their institutions, the path to future professional gratification and autonomy lies in leading the organization through the development and implementation of an effective patient safety program, rather than simply reacting to new rules, regulations, and care processes as others develop them.

Many authors and organizations have developed plans for developing patient safety programs. One that seems particularly adaptable to obstetricians and gynecologists is a practical approach advocated by Kenneth Kizer, MD, President and CEO of the National Quality Forum (Table 40.5). Kizer's 10 elements are helpful to physicians who wish to translate research and high-level recommendations into actionable items for their departments and institutions. With thought and deliberation, it will become clear which items need to be brought to realization through the medical staff's organizations, and which through the hospital. Working through the development of a patient safety program with professional colleagues is the best way to improve patient safety and to establish physician 'ownership' of the safety program. This, in turn, helps ensure physician satisfaction, rather than placing physicians in the awkward position of reacting to the sug-

Table 40.5 Practical approaches to developing a patient safety program

(1) Make patient safety a leadership priority – what is patient safety?

- A state of mind that recognizes the complexity and high-risk nature of modern health care
- A set of processes (reporting, investigating, analyzing, reducing hazards, improving)
- A set of outcomes (fewer efforts, less risk)

(2) Make a clear organizational commitment to patient safety (as reflected by infrastructure and dedicated resources) – what is an ideal infrastructure?

- Patient safety center
- Patient safety leader
- Patient safety event registry
- Patient safety oversight committee
- Lessons learned center
- Internal safety alert process

(3) Create a health-care culture of safety – what is a safety culture?

- Acknowledges high-risk, error-prone nature of modern health care
- Ensures widespread shared acceptance of responsibility for risk reduction
- Encourages open communication about safety concerns in a nonpunitive environment; freedom from fear in reporting problems
- Facilitates reporting of errors and safety concerns
- Learns from errors
- Embraces accountability for patient safety
- Ensures organizational structure, processes, goals, and rewards are aligned with improving patient safety

(4) Initiate routine safety assessments

- Implement the AHA–ISMP initiative to reduce medication errors
- Design and develop own audit instruments

(5) Implement known safety practices

- Educate patients and family members about their medications
- Implement mechanisms to ensure follow-up
- Implement a restraint-free policy
- Increase number of autopsies

(6) Incorporate patient safety into all health-care professional training

(7) Be accountable for patient safety

- Acknowledge error and resultant injury
- Apologize; say you are sorry
- Provide restorative or remedial care
- Conduct root-cause analyses
- Fix system or process problems

(8) Promptly and decisively deal with professional misconduct

(9) Support efforts to create a nonpunitive environment for health-care error reporting

(10) Make patient safety research a priority

Adapted from a presentation by Kenneth Kizer, MD, President and CEO, National Quality Forum, with permission.

gestions and policies created by other professionals and administrators.

One element that requires some further discussion is the creation of a 'nonpunitive' environment for health-care error reporting. This is a difficult but very important area, as it is easy to see that neither employees nor professional staff members are likely to report errors and near misses if the result will always be disciplinary action. Fortunately, much work has been done to help differentiate between blameless and blameworthy behavior.

Reason and Hobbs have suggested the use of the term 'just culture' to describe one in which the need to learn from mistakes is balanced against the need to take disciplinary action.[22,23] In general, those who have studied this problem have concluded that 'sharp end' workers should be protected from disciplinary action, with some exceptions, when reporting injuries, errors, or near misses, even if they were directly involved. This approach has been proved repeatedly in high-risk organizations, such as airlines, in nuclear power generation, and on aircraft carriers. The exceptions to the no-disciplinary-action policy are criminal behavior (for example, a physician, while inebriated, treating a patient), active malfeasance (purposeful violation of policies), and failure to report an injury in a timely manner.

Finally, obstetrician-gynecologists who choose leadership roles in developing and implementing patient safety programs must advocate, on behalf of their patients and themselves, investment in the information systems needed to ensure safe health care. These include systems that provide decision support (in the form of information, reminders, auto-stops, and other fail-safes) and systems to track near misses and minor injuries in order to identify care processes that are not fully satisfactory and track performance after process improvement.

Concluding remarks

I don't want to make the wrong mistake.

Yogi Berra

In a remarkable and incisive perspective paper of 2003, James Reinertsen, MD, pointed out that one of the most important reasons for the erosion of physician autonomy is the public perception that we have not consistently applied our scientific knowledge for the benefit of our patients.[24] Reinertsen was discussing the use of clinical guidelines and protocols, but his observation is equally true concerning patient safety.

In fact, the risk to physician autonomy may be even greater in this instance, given that it is easier for patients and their families to understand the issues surrounding the delivery of safe care and the results of errors than it is to understand the increasingly complex clinical issues that physicians treat, and the sophisticated clinical evidence that physicians utilize in decision making.

Working together and with other professionals and administrators, physicians can lead the transformation in medical care that is clearly in the wind. Physicians can demonstrate that their actions respect patient safety in all aspects, that the secrecy that characterized the guild mentality practice of medicine is giving way to transparency and information sharing, that the system anticipates each individual patient's needs, and that each of these characteristics helps to provide care that is effective and safe for each patient. When we have demonstrated these things, we will begin to restore the public trust in medicine.

References

1. Patient safety in obstetrics and gynecology. ACOG Committee Opinion No. 286, American College of Obstetricians and Gynecologists. Obstet Gynecol 2003; 102: 883–5.

2. Wennberg J, Gittleson A. Variations in medical care among small areas. Sci Am 1982; 246: 120–34.

3. Mechanic D. Managed care and the imperative for a new professional ethic. Health Aff (Millwood) 2000; 19: 100–11.

4. Eddy D. Performance measurement: problems and solutions. Health Aff (Millwood) 1998; 17: 7–25.

5. Gosfield A. Legal mandates for physician quality: beyond risk management. In: Gosfield A (ed.) Health Law Handbook. St. Paul, MN: West Group; 2001: pp. 285–321.

6. The Institute of Medicine. To Err Is Human: Building a Safer Health System. Washington, DC: National Academy Press; 2000.

7. King J, Pronovost P, Paine L, et al. Encourage a Culture of Safety: The Patient Safety Group Patient Safety Program. Boston, MA: The Patient Safety Group 2004.

8. Reason J. Human error. Cambridge, Cambridge University Press, 1992.

9. The Institute of Medicine. To Err Is Human: Building a Safer Healthcare System. Washington, DC: National Academy Press; 2000. Ch 8.

10. Gaba D. Patient Safety Via High Reliability Organization and Simulation. Presentation to the University HealthSystem Consortium 2004 Fall Quality Forum, Phoenix AZ.

11. PR Newswire, New York: PR Newswire Association LLC; 17 November 2004.

12. The Leapfrog Group Hospital Patient Safety Survey, April 2003–March 2004. Washington, DC: Leapfrog Group, 2004.

13. Altman DE, Clancy C, Blendon RJ. Improving Patient Safety – Five Years after the IOM Report. NEJM, 2004; 351: 20: 2041–3.

14. Wachter R. The End of the Beginning: Patient Safety Five Years After 'To Err Is Human.' Health Affairs, Web exclusive; 30 November 2004.

15. Morrissey J. Patient Safety Proves Elusive. Modern Healthcare, 1 November 2004.

16. Herzlinger R, Ed. Consumer-Driven Healthcare: Implications for Providers, Players and Policy-Makers. San Francisco, CA: Jossey-Bass, c2004.

17. www.JCAHO.org, Facts about patient safety. 2004.

18. Celestero R, Blute J. ACOG Clin Rev 2002; Vol 7, Issue 8.

19. www.JCAHO.org, Frequently Asked Questions about the Universal Protocol for Preventing Wrong Site, Wrong Procedure, Wrong Patient Surgery. 2004.

20. http://www.acog.org/

21. Patient Safety. Achieving a New Standard for Patient Care. Washington, DC: The National Academies Press, 2004: p. 1.

22. Reason J, Hobbs A. Managing Maintenance Error: A Practical Guide. Burlington, VT: Ashgate, 2003.

23. Marx D. Patient Safety and the 'Just Culture': A Primer for Healthcare Executives. New York, NY: Trustees of Columbia University, 2001.

24. Reinertsen J. Zen and the art of physician maintenance. Ann Intern Med 2003; 138: 992–5.

Index